FOOD, NUTRITION, AND DIET THERAPY

A TEXTBOOK OF NUTRITIONAL CARE

SEVENTH EDITION

Marie V. Krause, B.S., M.S., R.D.

*Formerly Dietitian in Charge of Nutrition Clinic
and Associate Director of Education,
Department of Nutrition, New York Hospital.
Therapeutic Dietitian and Instructor in Dietetics,
Mount Sinai Hospital, Philadelphia, Pa.
Therapeutic Dietitian and First Assistant to
Instructor in Nutrition, Department of Medicine,
University of Chicago Clinics.*

L. Kathleen Mahan, M.S., R.D.

*Lecturer, Nutritional Sciences;
Coordinator, Nutrition Services and Training,
Pediatric Pulmonary Disease Center,
University of Washington and
Children's Orthopedic Hospital;
Consulting Nutritionist, Private Practice,
Seattle, Washington
Formerly Assistant Professor and Director,
Program in Clinical Nutrition, College of Nursing
and Allied Health Sciences, Rush University,
Chicago, Illinois*

1984   **W. B. Saunders Company** Philadelphia/London/Toronto
Mexico City/Rio de Janeiro/Sydney/Tokyo

W. B. Saunders Company: West Washington Square
Philadelphia, PA 19105

1 St. Anne's Road
Eastbourne, East Sussex BN21 3UN, England

1 Goldthorne Avenue
Toronto, Ontario M8Z 5T9, Canada

Apartado 26370—Cedro 512
Mexico 4, D.F., Mexico

Rua Coronel Cabrita, 8
Sao Cristovao Caixa Postal 21176
Rio de Janeiro, Brazil

9 Waltham Street
Artarmon, N.S.W. 2064, Australia

Ichibancho, Central Bldg., 22-1 Ichibancho
Chiyoda-Ku, Tokyo 102, Japan

Listed here is the latest translated edition of this book together with the language of the translation and the publisher.

5th Edition (French) Les Editions HRW Ltee. Montreal, Quebec, Canada

Library of Congress Cataloging in Publication Data

Krause, Marie V.
    Food, nutrition, and diet therapy.

    Includes bibliographies and index.
    1. Diet therapy. 2. Nutrition. 3. Food.
I. Mahan, L. Kathleen. II. Title. [DNLM: 1. Diet
therapy. 2. Nutrition. WB 400 K91n]
RM216.K74   1984   615.8′54   83-20384
ISBN 0-7216-5514-9

Food, Nutrition and Diet Therapy: A Textbook of Nutritional Care   ISBN   0-7216-5514-9

Last digit is the print number: 9   8   7   6   5   4   3   2   1

Dedicated to my loving and supportive family—my parents Elsa and Richard, my husband Robert, and our daughter Carlin

L. KATHLEEN MAHAN

CONTRIBUTORS

ELIZABETH J. ADAMS, B.S.
Graduate student, Nutritional Sciences; Trainee, Pediatric Pulmonary Disease Center, University of Washington and Children's Orthopedic Hospital, Seattle, Washington

SAUNDRA N. AKER, R.D.
Clinical Instructor, Physiological Nursing; Affiliated Instructor, Nutritional Sciences, University of Washington; Director, Clinical Nutrition Unit, Fred Hutchinson Cancer Research Center, Seattle, Washington

ANDREA S. CARLSON, R.D., M.S.
Nutritionist and Coordinator for Women, Infants and Children Program, International District Community Health Center; Nutritionist, Central Seattle Community Health Centers, Seattle, Washington

CARRIE L. CHENEY, R.D., M.S.
Nutrition Research Analyst, Clinical Nutrition Unit, Fred Hutchinson Cancer Research Center, Seattle, Washington

DORICE M. CZAJKA-NARINS, Ph.D.
Dor-Art Associates, Downer's Grove, Illinois; Formerly Associate Professor, Clinical Nutrition, Rush University, Chicago, Illinois

HOLLY A. DIEKEN, R.D., M.S.
Doctoral Student, Department of Nutrition and Food Sciences, University of Tennessee, Knoxville, Tennessee; Formerly Lecturer, Nutritional Sciences, University of Washington, Seattle, Washington

NATALIE GONZÁLEZ, R.D., M.S.
Nutrition Consultant, Department of Social and Health Services, Division of Health, State of Washington, Olympia, Washington

BETTY LUCAS, R.D., M.P.H.
Lecturer, Nutritional Sciences; Nutritionist, Child Development and Mental Retardation Center, University of Washington, Seattle, Washington

MARY J. O'LEARY, R.D., M.S.
Coordinator, Neonatal Nutrition Services and Training; Teaching Associate, Department of Pediatrics, University of Washington, Seattle, Washington

PEGGY L. PIPES, R.D., M.P.H.
Lecturer, Nutritional Sciences; Assistant Chief Nutritionist, Child Development and Mental Retardation Center, University of Washington, Seattle, Washington

JANE M. REES, R.D., M.S.
Lecturer, Nutritional Sciences; Coordinator, Nutritional Services and Training, Division of Adolescent Medicine, Department of Pediatrics, University of Washington, Seattle, Washington

DEBORAH A. ROLAND, R.D., M.S.
Lecturer, Nutritional Sciences, University of Washington, Seattle, Washington

KARON J. SANDE, R.D., M.S.
Research Associate, Division of Endocrinology, Metabolism and Nutrition, Department of Medicine, School of Medicine, University of Washington, Seattle, Washington

CHEDWAH J. STEIN, R.D., M.S.
Nutrition and Diet Services, Portland, Oregon

CRISTINE M. TRAHMS, R.D., M.S.
Lecturer, Nutritional Sciences; Nutritionist, Biomedical Genetics, Child Development and Mental Retardation Center, University of Washington, Seattle, Washington

KATY G. WILKENS, R.D.
Nutrition Services Coordinator, Northwest Kidney Center, Seattle, Washington

JAYNE WILLIAMSON, R.D.
Clinical Dietitian, Regional Burn Center, Harborview Medical Center, Seattle, Washington

BONNIE S. WORTHINGTON-ROBERTS, Ph.D.
Professor, Nutritional Sciences; Chief Nutritionist, Child Development and Mental Retardation Center, University of Washington, Seattle, Washington

PREFACE
to the Seventh Edition

This seventh edition of Food, Nutrition and Diet Therapy continues to recognize the broad area nutrition occupies in the care of patients and the fact that nutritional care is provided by several different health professionals, the most prominent of whom are dietitians, nurses and physicians. Much nutrition education and training takes place in an interdisciplinary setting where nursing, dietetic and other health care students are receiving clinical experience, and this text is written for those students. Its purpose is to provide theoretical knowledge and clinical information that will be useful in the clinical learning situation.

Nutritional care of patients must include not only considerations of physiological requirements for nutrients but also the mental, emotional and social factors. For this reason discussions of the basis for diet therapy and nutritional care throughout this text include attention to the individual as a member of the community and his or her uniqueness in terms of nutritional needs, lifestyle, psychological status, the meaning of food and eating, and the stage of growth and development.

The first part of the book covers the basic science of nutrition and deals with normal nutrition and nutrition in the healthy individual. However, throughout this section are references to situations that the health student is likely to meet in clinical practice. This section can be used as the text for an undergraduate nutrition course. The second part, which covers nutritional care in various diseases, can be used as the text for a nutrition and diet therapy course, with the first part as a reference for more in-depth understanding of basic concepts.

An important enhancement to the first part is that guest authors have written chapters on nutrition throughout the life cycle. These authors are recognized authorities in each of these areas and have made the chapters current and practical. The old chapter on Nutrition in Childhood and Adolescence has been divided into two separate chapters dealing with each of these phases of human development and the pertinent nutrition information for working with each age group. We feel that this addition is of real benefit to the student because each topic is discussed in more detail. The new chapter on adolescence includes discussion of the nutritional issues in athletics, since these issues most frequently apply to this age group.

There are additional changes in Part 1. First is the omission of the chapter on Nutritional Deficiency Diseases and the incorporation of this material into the discussion of the appropriate deficiency syndrome in the chapters on Vitamins and Minerals. The discussion of protein-energy malnutrition has been incorporated into Chapter 38, Nutritional Care in Diseases of Infancy and Childhood. Second, we have moved the discussion of sodium, potassium and chloride into Chapter 8 on Water and Electrolytes so that they are discussed together, since we feel that they are now most likely to be taught that way. Third, Chapter 16 on Food Habits has been updated to include extensive discussion of the eating patterns of East Asians, so many of whom are refugees settling in North America. Added to Chapter 17, Food and Nutrition in the Community, is a succinct discussion of proposed dietary guidelines and the controversy that surrounds them.

Part 2, Diet Therapy and Nutritional Care in Disease, contains several chapters that are unique in nutrition textbooks. For example, Chapter 20 discusses The Computer in Nutritional Care. This chapter is meant to give the student an appreciation of the use of the computer to enhance nutritional care in both institutional and clinical settings and to provide a guide for further study and reading. Several of the chapters in Part 2, those on renal disease, burns and trauma, cancer, premature infants, and children with inborn errors of metabolism, are guest-authored by individuals working in each of these specialized areas. The material is still discussed with the same depth, but is made even more clinically relevant.

Other highlight changes in this section are the inclusion of a new exchange list for fat and cholesterol control in Chapter 28 and a clinically useful method for determining iron availability in Chapter 29. With the substantial interest in food allergies we felt compelled to greatly expand and update Chapter 31 on Food Allergy and Food Intolerance, which includes several clinically useful strategies and tools. Chapter 35 includes a comprehensive, current chart with the nutritional analysis of all the complete feedings and feeding modules used for patients with metabolic stress.

A major organizational change in this section is that celiac disease, previously covered in Chapter 38, Nutritional Care in Disease of Infancy and Childhood, is now covered in Chapter 23 in the discussion of malabsorption syndromes. This move was made after several recommendations that celiac sprue be discussed in the context of malabsorption syndromes because there are now many adults with celiac sprue.

Part 3 on Foods remains as a reference for the student faced with questions about food preparation and selection that may come up in the course of education of patients or discussion of the role of food in disease.

Finally, we have added several new appendices that we know will be useful to the teachers, students and clinicians using this book. The new Metropolitan Life Insurance Tables of average body weights, the HANES data on appropriate weights for adolescents and a table of the oxalate content of foods have been added with this edition. Also, the HANES data for determining percentiles for arm fat area and arm muscle area are included. We have brought these useful clinical tools together in one place so that they are convenient and easy to use for the student, teacher and clinician.

With the information presented here, we are confident that students will have the necessary information to understand the role of nutrition in health and disease and to make the most of their potential as health care professionals.

ACKNOWLEDGMENTS

With this edition we have several people to whom we would like to extend our most heartfelt appreciation. We would like to thank the following people for their help in critiquing various sections of the manuscript and giving their thoughtful and insightful comments:

Susan Adams, R.D.; Christopher Blagg, M.D.; John Brunzell, M.D.; Nancy Buergle, R.D.; Elizabeth Burrows, R.D., M.S.; Marion Childs, Ph.D.; Kenneth Crithman, M.D.; Beth Ann Cunningham, R.D., M.S.; Clifton Furukawa, M.D.; Elaine I. Hartsook, R.D., M.Ed.; Loretta Hoover, Ph.D.; Janet Jue-Mohney, R.D., M.S.; Joan Karkeck, R.D., M.S.; Polly Lenssen, R.D.; Donna Mueller, R.D., M.S.; Sue Olson, R.D.; Mary Podrabsky, R.D.; Nancy M. Robinson, Ph.D.; Ronald Scott, M.D.; David Simonowitz, M.D.; Susan Wagner, R.D.; Ann Weigle, R.D., M.S.; and Scott Weigle, M.D.

We would also like to thank those people who helped with the physical preparation and typing of the manuscript. Thank you to Sharon Feucht for research and editorial assistance, to Marie Haaneck for many of the new photographs, and to Ruth Boyd, B. J. Hayes, JoAnn Jarrett and Karen McMasters, who helped with some of the typing. We would also like to thank Janell Douglas, without whose tireless and relentless typing of the manuscript this edition would not have been possible. A tremendous thank you to Janell.

Lastly, a thank you to Katherine Pitcoff and Mark Coyle of W.B. Saunders Company, who were pleasant and professional to deal with and who made revising this text so gratifying.

CONTENTS

This section of the book deals with the information relative to normal nutrition and the foods that supply it. Special emphasis is given to the principles of optimum nutrition and their application to the life cycle; an appreciation of the importance of nutrition in providing and maintaining health; the background and knowledge for the application of nutrition to the student's personal needs; and the principles of learning and their application for teaching nutrition. Emphasis is placed on selection of foods required to meet the physiological and psychological needs of an individual and to conform to his or her socioeconomic background.

PART

1

SCIENCE OF NUTRITION

Introduction

Introduction—Nutrition in the Health of Individuals and Populations

The volume of scientific knowledge about nutrition is in the process of translation into action with a speed unparalleled in history. Much progress has been made to date in the understanding of foods and their relation to health. Most people concern themselves with food several times daily, and there is undoubtedly no practice or habit that can influence the health of an individual as much as the decisions that are made with regard to the kinds and amount of foods consumed. The body is made up of many materials, and these can be supplied by a wide variety of foods to insure good health. The body is, broadly speaking, the product of its nutrition. You are what you eat. Therefore, it is important that daily decision-making on this important aspect of health be properly guided and not conditioned by pseudoscientific or faddist influences.

Foods as Sources of Nutrients

Foods comprise all the solid and liquid materials taken into the digestive tract that are utilized to maintain and build body tissues, regulate body processes and supply heat, thereby sustaining life.

Foods are composed of various compounds, both organic and inorganic, so that any food is a chemical compound or mixture of chemical compounds. These compounds and elements of which foods are composed are proteins, lipids, carbohydrates, minerals, vitamins and water, and can be grouped as organic and inorganic compounds and elements.

ORGANIC COMPOUNDS. Proteins, lipids, carbohydrates, vitamins.

INORGANIC ELEMENTS. Water and minerals: calcium, phosphorus, sodium, potassium, chlorine, sulfur, iron, iodine, copper, magnesium, manganese, cobalt, zinc and others.

The constituents in food are known as *nutrients*. For all the nutrients essential to normal functioning, the body must depend on the wise selection of foods. If food is not properly chosen, there will be an inadequacy of one or more of the essential nutrients. An essential nutrient is one that must be provided to the body by food. It cannot be synthesized by the body. The nutrients that must be supplied in food and are essential for growth and normal functioning of the body are listed in the table below.

ESSENTIAL NUTRIENTS

Proteins as sources of the following amino acids:
  Histidine
  Isoleucine
  Leucine
  Lysine
  Methionine
  Phenylalanine
  Threonine
  Tryptophan
  Valine

Carbohydrate as a source of:
  Glucose

Fat as a source of:
  Linoleic acid

Minerals:
  Macro:
    Calcium
    Phosphorus
    Sodium
    Potassium
    Chloride
    Magnesium
    Sulfur
  Micro or trace minerals:
    Iron
    Iodide
    Zinc
    Copper
    Manganese
    Cobalt
    Fluoride
    Selenium
    Chromium
    Molybdenum

Fat-soluble vitamins:
  A
  D
  E
  K

Water-soluble vitamins:
  Thiamin (B_1)
  Riboflavin (B_2)
  Niacin (B_3)
  Pyridoxine (B_6)
  Cobalamin (B_{12})
  Ascorbic acid
  Folic acid
  Biotin
  Pantothenic acid
  Choline

Nutrition

Good nutrition is necessary for good health, and concern with food is important if certain illnesses are to be prevented. What is *nutrition*? It has different meanings. Many people identify it with that portion of nutrition that arouses their own interest. To some nutritionists, the subject is only biochemistry. To nurses, dietitians, nutritionists and physicians, nutrition may mean meals for the sick in terms of calories, protein, carbohydrate, fat, minerals and vitamins. To the layman, it represents food or it may mean a "special diet." By one definition, nutrition is "the combination of processes by which the living organism receives and utilizes the materials (food) necessary for the maintenance of its functions and for the growth and renewal of its components."[12]

Sir Harold Himsworth proposed that "nutrition is the analysis of the effect of food and its constituents on the living organism."[3] The science of nutrition is a young and dynamic biological science. It is based on the fundamental principles of chemistry and biology, biochemistry, microbiology, anatomy and physiology. The practice of nutrition is dependent upon the application of the principles of many sciences and the correlation of many disciplines, including among others agriculture, food technology, anthropology, psychology, sociology, economics, religion, communications and education.

Nutrition, in the concept of this book, is the relationship of food to the well-being of the human body. It includes (1) the metabolism of foods, (2) the nutritive value of foods, (3) the qualitative and quantitative requirements for food at different ages and developmental levels to meet physiological changes and activity needs, (4) the changes in nutrient and food requirements that accompany or prevent disease states, and (5) the economic, psychological, social and cultural factors that affect the selection and eating of foods. The science and practice of nutrition exist for and attempt to contribute to a more secure life, relatively free of disease and retarded mental and physical development.

Nutritional Status

Sometimes the term nutrition is used to refer to the nutritional status of an individual. "The condition of the body resulting from the utilization of the essential nutrients available to the body"[1] is termed the *nutritional status*. It may be good, fair or poor, depending on the intake of dietary essentials, on the relative need for them, and on the body's ability to utilize them.

Good nutritional status is essential for normal organ development and function; for normal reproduction, growth and maintenance; for optimum activity and working efficiency; for resistance to infection; and for the ability to repair bodily damage or injury. Poor nutritional status exists when a person is deprived of an adequate amount of the essential nutrients over an extended period of time. This is relative, because the body stores of some nutrients last longer than others. At times demands may go up, and intake, being constant, may become inadequate. The result is poor nutritional status.

Development of Knowledge and Research About Nutrition

During the eighteenth century, when scientific discoveries were changing concepts and causing intellectual ferment, the French chemist Antoine Laurent Lavoisier recognized the relationship of the process of respiration (intake of oxygen and output of carbon dioxide) to the metabolism of food. He had discovered the role of oxygen in combustion and investigated the relation of the burning flame to the metabolism of organic foods. Lavoisier is called the "father of nutrition." He, with the physicist Laplace, used guinea pigs for the first quantitative studies on respiration, and animals have continued to play a major role in nutritional studies. These early investigations were followed by intense interest in the energy value or calorie value of foods.

In 1896 W. O. Atwater, who has been called "the father of American nutrition," published the first extensive table of food values ever published in the United States. At that time, only proteins and calories were generally considered to be of nutritional importance. It was not until 20 years later that E. V. McCollum, one of the principal early workers in the field of accessory food factors, popularized the concept of "protective foods"—those primarily useful for their content of vitamins and minerals. Shortly after World War I, this resulted in a marked increase in the consumption of leafy vegetables, citrus fruit and milk.

At the same time Graham Lusk was exerting his far-reaching influence on dietary habits. An expert on calorie needs, it was he who first secured popular acceptance of the fact that adolescents required as much food as did adults. Space does not permit a comprehensive listing of all the other nutritionists who have contributed to our knowledge of the science of nutrition during the past century. Many men and women have contributed to the science of nutrition through their ideas, through equipment they have designed, and through the sciences of chemistry, physiology, biology, psychology and medicine. Some of the various pathways that have been used to accrue present knowledge in this field are summarized in the figure below.

An abundance of reading material on the history of nutrition is available for exploration by the interested student. Not only is it pleasant reading, but it is essential to present and future knowledge.[4, 5, 8–11]

National and International Nutritional Progress

In the history of nutrition science, one major trend is outstanding: the application has become ever broader. Prior to World War I, available knowledge was used mainly for the prevention and alleviation of dietary deficiency diseases in the individual or in small groups. The next step, an organized health approach, was planned distribution of preventive foods, such as butter (vitamin A), iodized salt and cod liver oil (vitamin D). Meanwhile, the isolation of vitamins progressed; and just before World War II, it became practical to improve staple foods with synthetic nutrients as a means of attacking deficiency diseases in large populations. Vitamin D was added to milk, and vitamin A to margarine. White flour and bread were enriched with thiamin, riboflavin, niacin and iron. Nationwide control of specific dietary diseases was now feasible, and a program was launched. Better nutrition education, a national school lunch program, improvements in agriculture practices, advances in food handling, preservation and distribution were included in the program.

In today's atmosphere of consumerism, nutrition has not escaped attention. People are becoming interested in nutrition and want to know more about their food and what is in it. Among the results of this interest have been nutritional labeling of foods, efforts by the food companies to provide nutritionally fortified foods, and methods of dating food that allow the consumer to know how long it has been on the shelf. These changes and more, all resulting

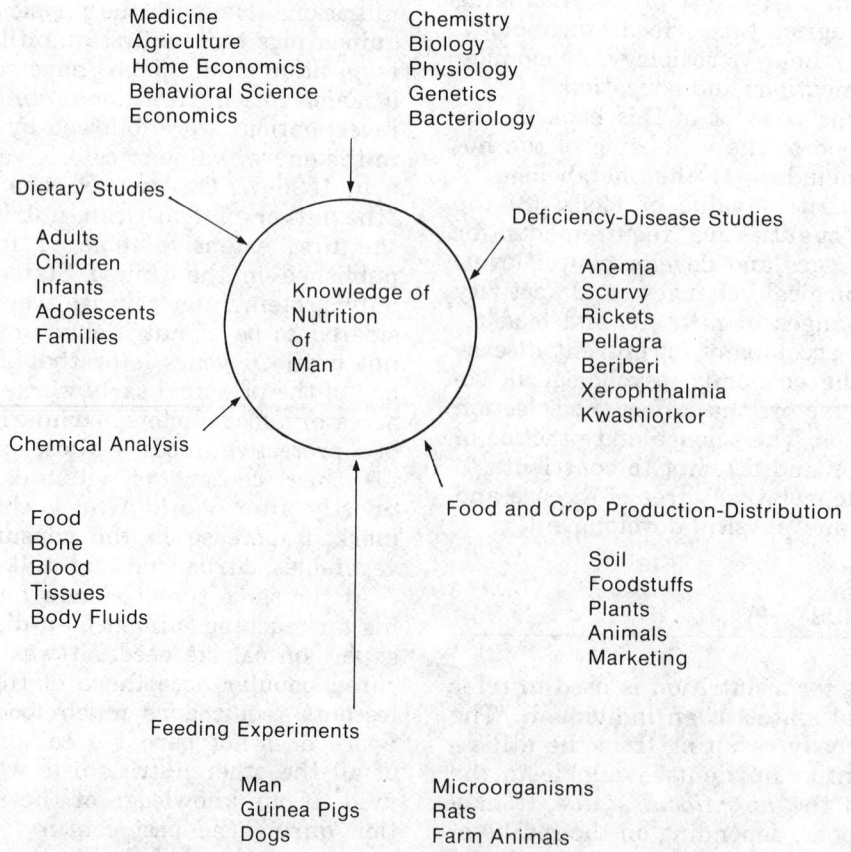

Contributing Fields:

Medicine
Agriculture
Home Economics
Behavioral Science
Economics

Chemistry
Biology
Physiology
Genetics
Bacteriology

Dietary Studies

Adults
Children
Infants
Adolescents
Families

Knowledge of Nutrition of Man

Deficiency-Disease Studies

Anemia
Scurvy
Rickets
Pellagra
Beriberi
Xerophthalmia
Kwashiorkor

Chemical Analysis

Food
Bone
Blood
Tissues
Body Fluids

Food and Crop Production-Distribution

Soil
Foodstuffs
Plants
Animals
Marketing

Feeding Experiments

Man
Guinea Pigs
Dogs

Microorganisms
Rats
Farm Animals

Methods and areas of investigations that led to the development of the science of nutrition. (After Lowenberg, M. E.: Food and Man. New York, John Wiley & Sons, Inc., 1967.)

from consumer interest, result in better food and nutrition for the American people.

EFFORTS TO IMPROVE NUTRITION IN THE UNITED STATES

The principal agencies of the federal government of the United States involved in public health nutrition programs are the Department of Health and Human Services and the Department of Agriculture. In the former department, the agencies dealing primarily with public health nutrition are the Public Health Service, the Children's Bureau and the Food and Drug Administration.

The Nutrition and Consumer Research Institute of the U.S. Department of Agriculture (USDA) coordinates nutrition services available to the public through federal, state and other agencies. This organization works through the research and education programs of the State Land Grant Universities. The Agricultural Research Service also conducts research in its laboratories in Beltsville, Maryland, and cooperates with State Experiment Stations' research programs. The standard food composition tables result largely from the food analysis data compiled and assembled by the USDA laboratories. Of great importance are the dietary surveys of the household consumption of foods in the United States performed by the USDA. The results of these studies have been published every 10 years since 1935, except in 1975. The sixth nationwide survey was started in 1977 and was completed in 1978. These surveys show trends in food and nutrient consumption in the United States.

In 1969 a White House Conference on Food, Nutrition and Health was held to explore what needed to be done in the United States (1) to improve the nutrition of the most vulnerable groups of people—the very poor, pregnant and nursing mothers, children and adolescents, and the aging; (2) to develop new technologies of food production, processing and packaging; (3) to improve nutrition teaching in the schools—from Head Start to nursing and medical schools; and (4) to improve Federal programs that affect nutrition such as food stamp, commodity distribution and school lunch programs. Surveys indicated considerable malnutrition (both undernutrition and overnutrition), anemia and degenerative disease in the United States (see Chapter 17).

In addition to these federal agencies, numerous private organizations devote some or all of their energies to nutrition—both basic and applied. Among these are professional organizations, members of which have carried on research and teaching in all aspects of nutrition.

In 1974 four private nutrition agencies formed the National Nutrition Consortium, Inc.* Concerned about the problems of the unusually low U.S. food production at the time and rising food costs and inflation, they formulated Guidelines for a National Nutrition Policy and presented them to the U.S. Senate Select Committee on Nutrition and Human Needs. This report identifies the considerations necessary for effective long-range governmental planning and implementation of food and nutrition programs in relation to the nation's health and other national responsibilities.[6] It is still speculation as to whether a national nutrition policy will be developed and implemented, but it certainly is needed.

INTERNATIONAL EFFORTS TO IMPROVE NUTRITION

The League of Nations planted the seeds for international cooperation in nutrition by publication of a document entitled "The Relation of Nutrition to Health, Agriculture, and Economic Policy." This famous report drew attention to the connections between food and health. Although World War II prevented the cooperative plans of the League of Nations from being put into full-scale use, a series of notable events insofar as nutrition was concerned took place in the United States during this period. In 1940, the Food and Nutrition Board of the National Research Council was established and accepted the responsibility of studying nutrition on a world-wide scale. This organization studied the substantial material on nutrition published by the League of Nations and published the first recommended daily dietary allowances in 1941. These allowances have been updated and revised approximately every five years, the most recent revision being published in 1980.[2] These recommended goals can be used in planning and in evaluating food supplies for healthy people from the nutritional point of view and are discussed in detail in Chapter 10.

After World War II, the Food and Agricultural Organization (FAO) and the World Health Organization (WHO) were created as divisions of the United Nations. FAO is dedicated to raising world-wide levels of nutrition and standards of living by securing improvement in the efficiency of production and distribution of food and agricultural products. To tackle this huge task, many sub-units of FAO were created, such as the Divisions of Nutrition, Economics, Forestry, Fisheries and Agriculture. As an example of

*American Institute of Nutrition, American Society for Clinical Nutrition, American Dietetic Association, and the Institute of Food Technology.

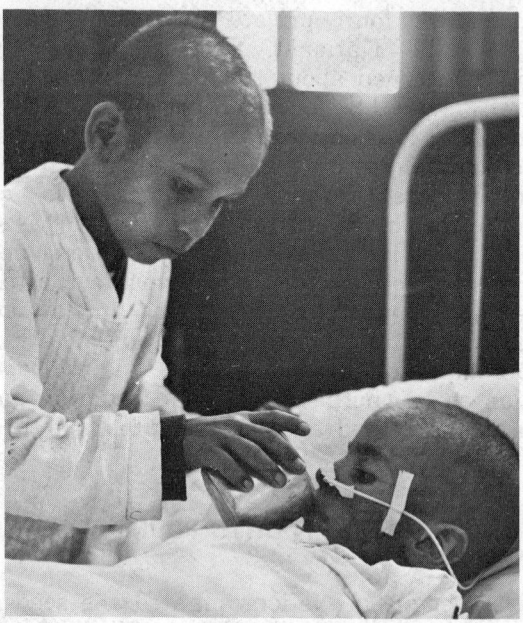

General Hospital, Guatemala City, Guatemala. Two victims of malnutrition—one recovering, the other one with a long way to go. There is almost a daily arrival of malnutrition cases at hospitals in Central America where, because of either ignorance or insufficiency, children's diets are often found to be extremely low in protein, vitamin A and riboflavin. Eggs, meat and citrus juices are not considered foods for children. The task of nutrition education undertaken by the Institute of Nutrition of Central America and Panama is a tremendous one when it is realized that these people have used the same low nutritive value foods for generations, have seen the ravages of resulting disease without determining the cause, and have made little change in their eating habits. (Photo by Maxine Rude. Courtesy of the World Health Organization.)

the work done by the FAO, one can point to the FAO-sponsored development of fish-farming. In this situation experts are asked to visit a country for a given period of time. There they establish centers for fish culture and train local personnel so that when they leave the country the work continues.

The World Health Organization (WHO) is the medically oriented unit of the United Nations. The Nutrition Division of WHO concerns itself primarily with the medical aspects of malnutrition as part of an overall effort to raise levels of nutrition throughout the world. As might be expected, much of the work of WHO and FAO overlaps. Indeed, it has become customary for these two organizations to convene joint committees to prepare authoritative reports on some pressing nutrition subjects, such as nutritional requirements.

Still another subdivision of the United Nations is the United Nations Children's Fund. This was originally called the United Nations International Children's Emergency Fund (UNICEF) and is still known by these initials. UNICEF is principally a supply agency and has

been active in bringing relief to children of the "have-not" nations through food distribution programs using surplus foods from the "have" nations. In recent years this agency has been primarily concerned with eradication of widespread malnutrition. UNICEF was awarded a Nobel Prize in 1965 for its great contributions to child health.

In the early seventies three agencies—FAO, WHO and UNICEF—began combining their efforts in the form of a new program—Applied Nutrition Program (APN). With a coordination of these agencies, there can be a multifaceted, interspecialty approach.

To this list of international agencies should be added the Agency for International Development, (AID) a U.S. government agency. Variously known in the past as the "Interdepartmental Committee for Nutrition in National Development (ICNND)" and the "Nutrition Section of the Office of International Research," this agency once had nutritional responsibilities principally at the international level. Its nutrition survey programs in more than 25 countries serve as models of excellence and its introduction of nutrition into long-range government planning will continue to bear fruit for years to come.

In 1960, FAO intensified its efforts to resolve the nutrition problems by launching a five-year Freedom from Hunger Campaign to dramatize the world's need for food. Attention was focused on information concerning research and national action programs. The United States, Canada and Australia, among other nations, contributed a great deal of financial and technical help and material toward providing food and other services to developing countries.

The widespread suffering from undernutrition, especially in the less developed countries, shows that a large segment of the world's population has not yet escaped the fear of malnutrition and hunger. The problem is not one of inadequate food production. Total food production during the past two decades has kept pace with population increases. For example, during the decade 1962 to 1972, world population increased 2.4 per cent and world food production increased 2.7 per cent.[7] The real problems are with the distribution and delivery of food, and the available income to buy food. In many nations food surpluses exist side by side with malnutrition and hunger; only the poor people go hungry. Governmental decisions also may prohibit ready access to available food.[13]

Another problem is the inability of governments to mount a continual, long-term effort against hunger. In a lecture in 1975, Adekke Boerma, Director-General of FAO of the United Nations, made the following statement in reference to the lack of progress against world hunger by the FAO since its inception over 30 years ago:

The fact is that, for most of the 30 years, the international community has been fighting the war against hunger in piecemeal fashion, without the over-all sense of commitment and integrated purpose which alone can win wars. Having failed to accept the necessary kind of general master strategy that John Boyd Orr (first Director-General) offered, it was unable or unwilling to replace it with anything comparable. And the reason for all this, as I indicated earlier, has quite simply been the lack of political will on the part of governments. So long as no major food crisis threatened, they felt no need for the kind of massive, concerted action that is required to overcome the world food problem once and for all. So the war drifted on, some advances being made here and there but with no frontal assault on the more difficult areas, with the result that the over-all shape of the struggle did not fundamentally change.[1]

What basically bothered the governments involved was the giving up of national sovereignty and control in order to come together and cooperate in feeding people who are hungry.

Another food crisis like a World War was needed to bring out the spirit of cooperation. Just such a crisis happened in the early 1970's after several years of bad weather and the realization that the North American grain reserves were dangerously low. In 1974 a United Nations World Food Conference met in Rome with the purpose of mounting a new attack against hunger. The achievements of the Conference were the following:

1. Adoption of a comprehensive series of resolutions for increasing agricultural production in developing countries.

2. Adoption of methods for increasing the flow of external financial resources to these countries to support their efforts.

3. Endorsement of an internationally coordinated system of nationally held grain reserves involving all countries who are in a position to participate.

4. Endorsement of a Global Information and Early Warning System on food and agriculture to be operated by FAO.

5. Recommendation of an improved policy of food aid with a minimum target of 10 million tons of grain per year.

6. Recommendation of the establishment of a World Food Council as an organ of the UN General Assembly, serviced within the framework of FAO, and headquartered in Rome with political authority for carrying out the other recommendations.

Although nothing new to FAO was presented at the conference, a very valuable outcome was the "concerted thrust of political will on the part of governments" against world hunger.[1] It remains to be seen what the long-term effects of this conference will be. The UN World Food Council, created as an outcome of this meeting to promote the implementation of the resolutions, has met yearly since the first Rome conference in 1974.

Nutrition in Preventive Health Care

In the last half century medical care, public health and scientific research have brought about dramatic progress in the betterment of health. Perhaps nothing is more indicative of this improvement than the increase in longevity. In 1900 the average span of life in the United States was about 49 years. Today the figure is over 70.

Much of this progress has been due to the control of preventable diseases, particularly those affecting the young, and nutrition has played a large part. Malnutrition adversely affects the life, development and health of more people in the world than any disease. It kills millions of infants and small children, especially in the technologically underdeveloped areas. More and more attention is being focused on preventive medicine or protective health than on curative measures. The World Health Organization defines health as "a state of complete physical, mental, and social well-being, and not merely the absence of disease infirmity."[14] Nutrition is one of the most important environmental factors affecting the state of an individual's or nation's health. Nutrition education programs in work, school and health settings can be successful in improving nutritional status and learning and working efficiency.

Nutritional Care in Disease

Nutritional care includes not only diet therapy, the use of food and nutrients to aid recovery from illness, but also other areas needed to apply the scientific principles of nutrition to benefit the health of an individual, such as food consumption information, nutritional status assessment, nutritional counseling and education, economic and social assistance to promote better dietary intake, and monitoring and evaluation of the individual's and community's health.

The nurse can play a large role in the nutritional care of patients. Together the dietitian and the nurse can devise ways of feeding those who have to be fed and to encourage those who need to consume an adequate amount of food.

The nurse knows whether the patient eats the food served, and how much is eaten. After consultation with the other members of the team concerning the nutritional welfare of the patients, the nurse can take the necessary steps to revise the dietary regimen or resolve the problems presented. Nutritional care should always be part of the total care plan for a patient (see Chapter 19).

A patient's eating habits are influenced largely be economic status, food idiosyncrasies, nationality or ethnic group, religion and social environment. During hospitalization, especially if it is prolonged, the nurse and dietitian/nutritionist have an opportunity to assist the person to improve the customary diet where indicated. Many patients utilize their hospitalization as a learning experience and are motivated to make changes in their food habits. Objectives for nutrition education in the care plans for these patients are especially useful.

Nutrition is considered one of the major health sciences and has an important place in health care today. Clinical nutrition research is expanding rapidly; it is a comparatively new science. Thus, many of the concepts and much of the knowledge gained so far must be considered as subject to modification when still more knowledge is obtained. The nutrition picture is constantly changing.

Problems and Suggested Topics for Discussion

1. What do the following terms mean: nutrition, nutritional status, health, and nutritional care? Explain the difference between food and nutrition.
2. How are nutrition and health related?
3. From the list of references select those pertaining to the history of nutrition and prepare a short report on some historical event in nutrition.
4. Analyze the community where you live and describe an example in which a community agency has fostered improved nutrition.
5. Explain how nutrition becomes an aspect of total nursing care.

Cited References

1. Boerma, A. H.: The 30 years' war against world hunger. Proc. Nutr. Soc., *34*:145, 1975.
2. Food and Nutrition Board, National Research Council: Recommended Dietary Allowances. 9th ed. Washington, D.C., National Academy of Sciences, 1980.
3. Himsworth, H.: What nutrition really means. Nutr. Today, *3*(3):18, 1968.
4. Lowenberg, M. E., et al.: Food and People. 3rd ed. New York, John Wiley & Sons, 1979.
5. McCollum, E. V.: A History of Nutrition—The Sequence of Ideas in Nutrition Investigations. Boston, Houghton Mifflin Company, 1957.
6. National Nutrition Consortium, Inc.: Guidelines for a National Nutrition Policy. U.S. Senate Select Committee on Nutrition and Human Needs, Washington, D.C., U.S. Government Printing Office, 1974. (Also in Nutr. Rev., *32*:153, 1974.)
7. Panel on Nutrition and the International Situation to the Senate Select Committee on Nutrition and Human Needs: National Nutrition Policy—Report and Recommendation VI. Washington, D.C., U.S. Government Printing Office, 1974.
8. Roe, D. A.: A Plague of Corn: The Social History of Pellagra. Ithaca, New York, Cornell University Press, 1973.
9. Todhunter, E. N.: Development of knowledge in nutrition, Part I: animal experiments and Part II: human experiments. J. Am. Diet. Assoc. *41*:328 and 335, 1962.
10. Todhunter, E. N.: Some classics of nutrition and dietetics. J. Am. Diet. Assoc., *44*:100, 1964.
11. Todhunter, E. N., Darby, W. J., and McNutt, K. W.: A Bedside Library for Nutrition Scholars in Present Knowledge in Nutrition. 4th ed. New York, The Nutrition Foundation, Inc., 1976, pp. 557–574.
12. Turner, D.: Handbook of Diet Therapy. 5th ed. Chicago, University of Chicago Press, 1970.
13. Wittwer, S. H.: Nutrition, agriculture and world health. Food Nutr. News, *55*(1):1, 1983.
14. World Health Organization—What It Is, What It Does. How It Works. Geneva, WHO, 1956.

Additional References

Bengoa, J. M.: Nutrition activities of the World Health Organization. J. Am. Diet. Assoc., *55*:228, 1969.

Briggs, G. M., and Calloway, D. H.: Bogert's Nutrition and Physical Fitness. 10th ed. Philadelphia, W. B. Saunders Company, 1979, Chapters 1 and 25.

Darby, W. J. (ed.): Food—The Gift of Osiris. 2 volumes. London: Academic Press, 1977.

Food and Agriculture Organization: Nutrition and Working Efficiency. Pamphlet. Rome, 1962.

Food and Nutrition. Science, *188*:501, 1975.

Hegsted, D. M.: Food and nutrition policy—now and in the future. J. Am. Diet. Assoc., *64*:367, 1974.

Joint FAO/WHO Ad Hoc Expert Committee: Energy and Protein Requirements. Technical Rep. No. 522, Geneva, WHO, 1973.

King, C. G.: Notes on history of nutrition in America. J. Am. Diet. Assoc., *56*:188, 1970.

Senate Select Committee on Nutrition and Human Needs: National Nutrition Policy Study—Report and Recommendation—IV. Washington, D.C., U.S. Government Printing Office, 1974.

NUTRIENTS IN FOOD—THEIR DIGESTION, ABSORPTION AND METABOLISM

Energy

Energy is defined as the capacity to do work or to produce a change in matter. When used in nutrition, the term energy deals with the chemical energy locked in foodstuffs because of the chemical bonding present in the nutrients. It also deals with the human body's requirement for energy to maintain life and work.

The ultimate source of all energy in living organisms is derived from the energy of the sun. Plants transform heat and light, through the action of chlorophyll with sunlight (photosynthesis), into energy which is stored as potential chemical bond energy within different foodstuffs, principally as carbohydrates, proteins and fats (see Chapter 2, Fig. 2–1). This chemical energy is used by animals, which are unable to use the energy of the sun directly.

The comparisons often drawn between a steam engine and the human body, while useful, may be misleading. The steam engine relies upon the combustion of fuel to yield heat to generate steam to perform work required. Although foods undergo combustion in the body and eventually yield heat, that heat is not productive. It is largely a byproduct of metabolism generated by the mechanical activity of muscles (mechanical energy). It is useful in that it does maintain body temperature. It is the chemical energy available from foods that is used for muscular work (kinetic energy), for brain and nerve activity (electrical energy) and in synthesis of body tissue (chemical energy). Energy is released by the metabolism of food and it must be supplied regularly to meet the energy needs for the body's survival.

Production of ATP for Storage of Energy

The foods from which energy is available (carbohydrate, alcohol, fat and protein) are converted in the body to glucose, fatty acids and amino acids before they reach the cell. Within the cell these nutrients react with oxygen to form carbon dioxide and water. This over-all reaction proceeds through a long series of steps, with the rates of reaction controlled by various enzymes. The energy produced is used to form *adenosine triphosphate (ATP)*. ATP is a nucleotide composed of adenine (nitrogen base), ribose (pentose sugar) and three phosphate radicals. The last two phosphate radicals in this compound are attached through an *energy-rich bond*, as shown in Figure 1–1. These bonds contain several times the energy of other chemical bonds and are very labile. ATP can release its energy instantly for mechanical work (muscle contraction), transport of material through cell walls and syntheses of chemical compounds. In the reaction ADP (adenosine diphosphate) or AMP (adenosine monophosphate) is formed. ADP and AMP can be rephosphorylated to ATP by the oxidative reactions. This process is continuous. ATP has been referred to as the energy currency of the cell, for it can be spent and remade again and again. *Creatine phosphate (CP)* is another energy-rich compound and is considered the "reser-

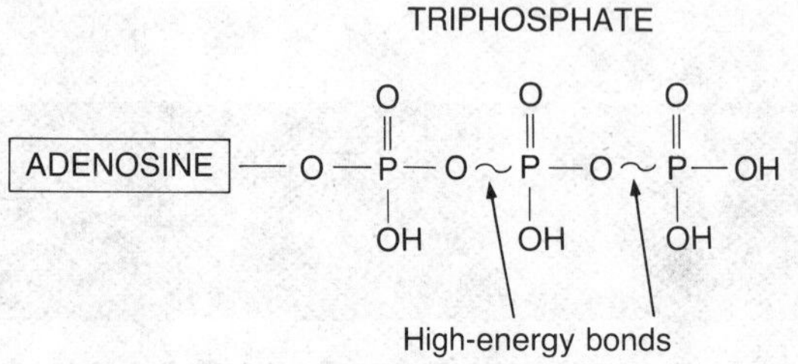

TRIPHOSPHATE

Figure 1–1. Simplified diagram of ATP.

voir" of high energy phosphate because it is stored in the body in larger quantities than is ATP.

Enzymes in Metabolism

The rapid chemical changes involved in ATP production and breakdown are brought about by the action of enzymes, coenzymes and hormones. They control biological oxidation of the cells. Every cell synthesizes the thousands of enzymes required for its metabolic processes.

Enzymes show a great deal of *specificity* in that each enzyme is so constructed that it will catalyze only one particular reaction. The compound being acted on by an enzyme is called the enzyme's *substrate*. It is thought that the enzyme and its substrate fit together like a lock and key during the catalytic process. The enzyme and substrate must fit together or the reaction will not take place. They first combine in a complex, then break apart, producing the new reaction products and the original enzyme, which is then ready to catalyze the reaction again.

Some enzymes (pepsin, for example) consist entirely of protein, while others may contain a non-protein portion. The protein part is called the *apoenzyme* and the non-protein part is called a *coenzyme*. Coenzymes are usually small, organic molecules (some of which are B vitamins) and almost always contain a phosphate group.

The reactions involved in cellular oxidation and formation of ATP require a series of enzymes with their coenzymes to effect the combination of hydrogen with oxygen to form water. These *oxidative phosphorylation enzymes* are believed to be arranged in an orderly fashion on the inner surface of the mitochondria (Fig. 1–2), thus facilitating rapid procession of the chemical reactions. For this reason the mitochondrion is called the "powerhouse" of the cell.

Hormones in Metabolism

Hormones, which are secretions of the endocrine glands, act as *chemical messengers* in energy production to *initiate or control* enzyme action. For example, the hormone thyroxine from the thyroid gland controls the body's metabolic rate; production of thyroxine, in turn, is controlled by thyrotropic hormone from the anterior pituitary gland. Another example is insulin, which is secreted by the pancreas and controls the rate of glucose utilization in the tissues.

The Calorie

The *calorie*, or small calorie, is a standard unit for measuring heat; it is the amount of heat energy required to raise the temperature of 1 gram of water by 1 degree Celsius (C. or centigrade). The *kilocalorie* is equal to 1000 small calories, or the amount of heat energy required to add 1 degree C. to the temperature of a kilogram of water. The term calorie is often used to mean either the small calorie or the kilocalorie. Since heat is one result of energy generated by the body, the calorie can serve as a measure of energy production. The kilocalorie, which may be abbreviated kcalorie, kcal. or Cal., is the unit of energy commonly used in studying human nutrition and is the unit that will be used most frequently in this book.

MEASUREMENT

The total caloric content (total energy) available from a food can be measured by means of a device called a bomb calorimeter, which is illustrated in Figure 1–3. This consists of a closed container in which the food is burned while the container is immersed in a known volume of water. The weighed food sample is burned in an oxygen atmosphere by igniting it with an electric spark. The rise in temperature of the water

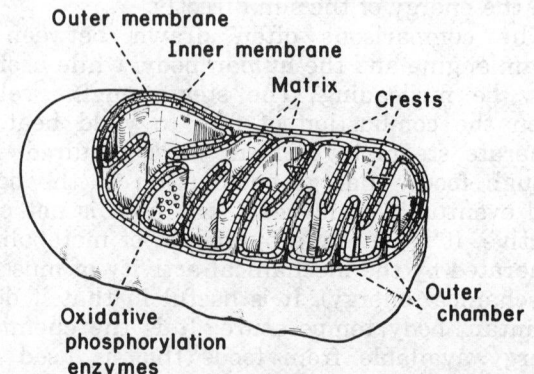

Figure 1–2. Structure of a mitochondrion. (Modified from De Robertis, E. D. P., Saez, F. A., and De Robertis, E. M. F., Jr.: Cell Biology. 6th ed. Philadelphia, W. B. Saunders Company, 1975. In Guyton, A. C.: Textbook of Medical Physiology. 6th ed. Philadelphia, W. B. Saunders Company, 1981.)

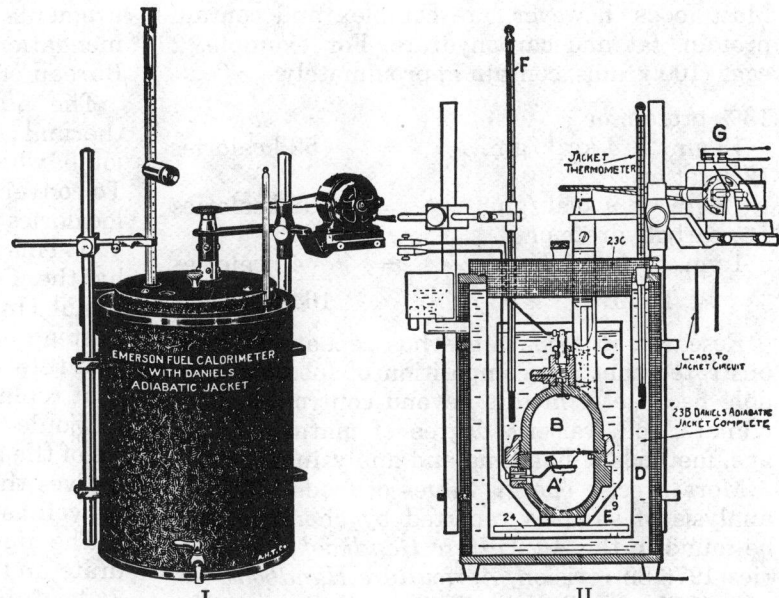

Figure 1–3. Bomb calorimeter as seen from the outside (I) and in longitudinal section (II). The water in the inner chamber (C) changes in temperature when the food in the food pan (A) is burned. The water in the outer chamber (D) acts as insulation, with the intervening air in the air space (E). The amount of heat produced is measured at F by the change in temperature of a measured amount of water. B is an oxygen chamber, and G is an electric motor for stirring the water.

after ignition of food can be used to calculate the heat energy or calories generated. Each food has a specific caloric value; that is, a given amount of food will yield a certain number of calories when it is burned or when it is metabolized in the body, and the caloric yield depends on the composition of the food in terms of protein, fat, carbohydrate and alcohol.

The amount of heat produced per gram of purified samples of protein, fat, carbohydrate and alcohol burned in the bomb calorimeter is as follows:

1 gm. of protein	5.65 kcalories
1 gm. of fat	9.45 kcalories
1 gm. of carbohydrate	4.10 kcalories
1 gm. of alcohol	7.10 kcalories

In the body some food is not completely digested and absorbed. Since the body is not completely efficient in this process, the extent to which the ingested nutrient is available to the cells, or its *digestibility*, is of importance. Normally about 98 per cent of the carbohydrate, 95 per cent of the fat and 92 percent of the protein is absorbed. However, there is a rather large variation in the digestibility of proteins.

As far as utilization by the cells is concerned, the calorie yield of carbohydrate and fat in the body is almost the same as in the bomb calorimeter because they are completely oxidized to carbon dioxide and water. This is not true of proteins. The amino (NH_2) group of the amino acids is not oxidized in the body as it is in the bomb calorimeter but is excreted in the urine, chiefly as urea, with smaller amounts of creatinine, uric acid and other compounds. The poten-

tial energy value of the energy-yielding nutrients in food is summarized in Figure 1–4.

The approximate kcaloric values 4, 9, 4 per gram of protein, fat and carbohydrate respectively can be used for all practical purposes to estimate the caloric values of foods in the average American mixed diet. Alcohol contains 7 kcal./gm.

CALCULATION OF FOOD ENERGY VALUE. The energy value of one tablespoon of oil (14 grams of fat) is approximately 126 kcalories (14 × 9).

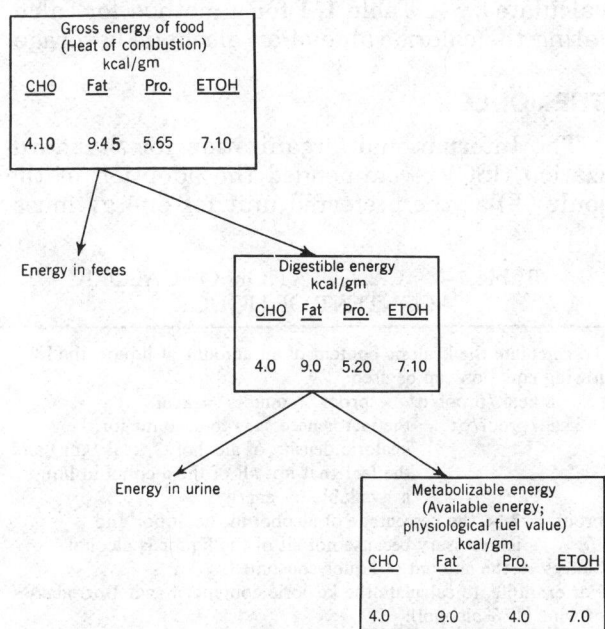

Figure 1–4. Energy value of food. (Adapted from Pike, R. L., and Brown, M. L.: Nutrition: An Integrated Approach, 2nd ed. New York, John Wiley and Sons, 1975.)

Most foods, however, are complex and contain protein, fat and carbohydrate. For example, 2 eggs (100 grams) contain approximately:

13% protein or
13 gm. × 4 kcal./gm. = 52 kcalories
12% fat or
12 gm. × 9 kcal./gm. = 108 kcalories
1% carbohydrate or
1 gm. × 4 kcal./gm. = 4 kcalories
Total 164 kcalories

Research in food values has repeatedly demonstrated that the composition of foods is variable because of factors beyond control, such as climate, soil, variety, degree of maturity, storage, methods of handling and analyzing.

More precise energy values of foods based on analysis of samples reported by chemists may be found in the *Agriculture Handbook*, No. 8 series 1976-82 revision, *Agriculture Handbook* No. 456, 1975, and *Bulletin (Home and Garden)*, No. 72, 1981, published by the United States Department of Agriculture (see Appendix Table 1). These tables are useful in calculating the specific nutritive value of each food. The values in Handbook No. 8 are given for 100-gram portions of food and household measures, whereas in Bulletin No. 72 and Handbook No. 456 values are listed for household measures only. Another source in which composition is given for common serving sizes of foods is *Bowes and Church's Food Values of Portions Commonly Used*, 13th edition, 1980. From tables of caloric values of foods (see Appendix Tables 1 and 2), the approximate caloric value of any diet can be calculated. See Table 1–1 for a method for calculating the caloric value of an alcoholic beverage.

THE JOULE

The International Organization for Standardization (ISO) recommended the adoption of the joule (J.) as the preferred unit for energy measurements in all branches of science. The recommendation was adopted by the U.S. National Bureau of Standards in 1964.

The nutritional kilocalorie is a measure of thermal energy and cannot be as precise as the joule, which is a measure of mechanical energy. To convert kilocalories to kilojoules, multiply kilocalories by 4.184 (or approximate by using 4.2). This is the conversion factor recommended by the Committee on Nomenclature, International Union of Nutritional Sciences. The Committee on Nomenclature of the American Institute of Nutrition in 1970 recommended that replacement of the kilocalorie (kcal.) by the kilojoule (kJ.) be effected as soon as the mechanics of the transition can be established. Table 10–3 gives the 1980 RDA for energy in MJ. (or kJ.) as well as in kilocalories.

The figures of 4 kcal. per gram of carbohydrate and of protein, 9 kcal. per gram of fat and 7 kcal. per gram of alcohol, converted to kilojoules and rounded off, would be 17 kJ. per gram for carbohydrate and protein, 38 kJ. per gram of fat and 29 kJ. per gram for alcohol.

Measurement of Energy Expenditure

The amount of energy generated by the body or the rate of metabolism can be measured by direct or indirect methods.

DIRECT CALORIMETRY. With the direct method the person is placed in a special calorimeter, and the amount of heat produced is measured. This method is very expensive, and there are few such large calorimeters available.

INDIRECT CALORIMETRY. The indirect method is a much simpler technique by which the rate of metabolism is measured by determining with a respiration apparatus the oxygen consumption and carbon dioxide production of the body in a given period of time. Using the *respiratory quotient*

$$RQ = \frac{\text{moles } CO_2 \text{ expired}}{\text{moles } O_2 \text{ consumed}},$$

these determinations are then converted into calories of heat produced per square meter of body surface per hour and expressed as caloric expenditure. This method is much more widely used and has the added advantages of mobility and low equipment cost.

This method may be applied when the body is lying at rest or engaged in various activities, as shown in Figure 1–5.

The respiratory quotient (RQ) depends on the fuel mixture (protein, fat and carbohydrate) being metabolized. For example, the RQ for carbohydrate is 1.00 because the same number of CO_2 molecules are produced as O_2 molecules con-

Table 1–1. CALCULATION OF CALORIC CONTENT OF LIQUOR

To calculate the kcaloric content of an amount of liquor, the following equation can be used:
.8 kcal./proof/oz. × proof × ounces = kcal.
.8 kcal./proof/oz. = the factor necessary to account for the kcaloric density of alcohol (7 kcal./gm.) and the fact that not all of the alcohol in liquor is available for energy.
proof = 2 × the percentage of alcohol in the liquor and is necessary because not all of the liquor is alcohol.
ounces = the amount of liquor consumed.
For example, to calculate the kcaloric content of two 4-oz. glasses of wine (12% alcohol):
.8 kcal./proof/oz. × 24 proof × 8 oz. = 154 kcal.

(From Gastineau, C. F.: Alcohol and Calories, Mayo Clin. Proc., *51*(2):88, 1976.)

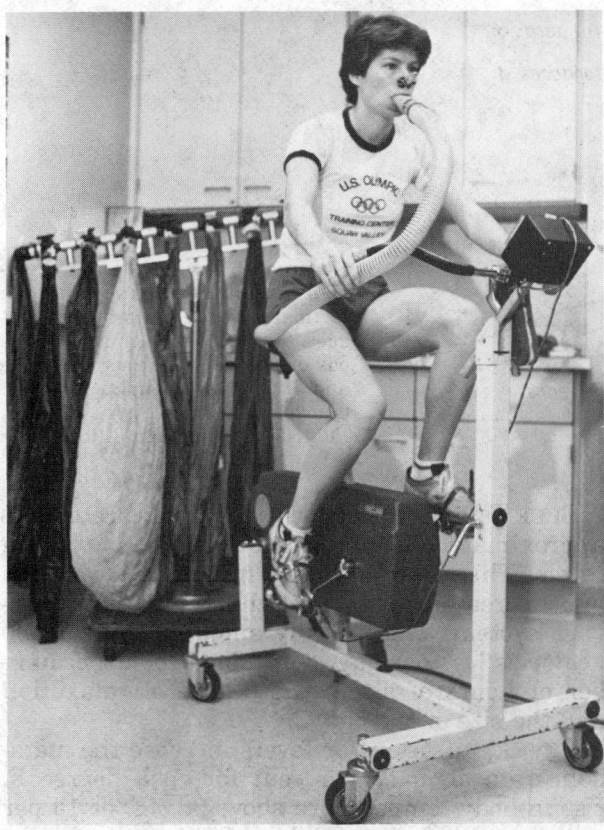

Figure 1–5. Indirect calorimetry using respirometer to determine energy expenditure of woman riding a bicycle.

sumed. The approximate RQ for fat is 0.7 and for protein 0.82. The RQ for a mixed diet is between 0.7 and 1.0 and generally is accepted as 0.82.[15] This means that the calorie equivalent of 4.825 kcal per liter of O_2 consumed (5.0 kcal./L O_2 for ease of calculation) can be used as an appropriate factor for estimating the body's energy expenditure.

Basal Metabolism

The *basal metabolic rate* (BMR) is the minimum amount of energy needed by the body at rest in the fasting state. It indicates the amount of energy needed to sustain the life processes: respiration, cellular metabolism, circulation, glandular activity and the maintenance of body temperature. It is usually measured by indirect calorimetry, with a tank type respiration apparatus, with the body at complete physical and mental rest, relaxed, but not asleep, at least 12 hours after the last meal and several hours after any strenuous exercise or activity and in a comfortable temperature and environment. Basal metabolic rate may range between 0.8 and 1.43 kcal./min. depending upon many factors.[15]

Resting metabolic rate (RMR) is the energy expenditure under similar conditions except after eating or exercise. Because the conditions for measurement are not as strict as with the BMR, the RMR is more frequently measured and used. A person's RMR is greater than the BMR and would include one or more of the many factors that raise the BMR.

PRIMARY FACTORS THAT AFFECT BASAL METABOLIC RATE

SURFACE AREA. The greater the body surface or skin area, the greater will be the amount of heat loss and, in turn, the greater the necessary heat produced by the body. For this reason estimation of the BMR takes into account the person's body surface area. It is interesting to note that a tall thin person has a larger surface area and, consequently, a higher basal metabolic rate than a short stout individual of the same weight.

SEX. Women, in general, have a metabolic rate about 5 to 10 per cent lower than men even when of the same weight and height (Fig. 1–6). This may be accounted for by a difference in body composition between the male and female. Generally speaking, women have more fat and less muscular development than men, and fat is less metabolically active than muscle. Cunningham proposes that based on lean body mass or active cell tissue, the BMR for males and females is similar.[5]

AGE. The metabolic rate is highest during the periods of rapid growth, chiefly during the first and second years, and reaches a lesser peak through the ages of puberty and adolescence in both sexes. The BMR declines about 2 per cent per decade during adult life, as shown in Figure 1–6, probably owing to reduced lean mass and a greater percentage of body fatness.[7, 20] The increased BMR in childhood results in greater heat production and accounts for the fact that a child will often refuse a jacket when his mother is chilly.

BODY COMPOSITION. A large proportion of adipose tissue lowers the basal metabolic rate since adipose tissue requires less oxygen and thus has a lower metabolic rate than muscle tissue. Athletes with greater muscular development show about a 5 per cent increase in basal metabolism over nonathletic individuals. In obese individuals it may be more accurate to determine the BMR using the lean body mass (LBM) rather than the surface area.[5]

ENDOCRINE GLANDS. The secretions of the endocrine glands, particularly those of the thyroid gland, are the principal regulators of the metabolic rate. When the supply of *thyroxine* is inadequate, the basal metabolism may fall by 30 to 50 per cent of the normal rate. If the thyroid gland is hyperactive, the basal metabolic rate

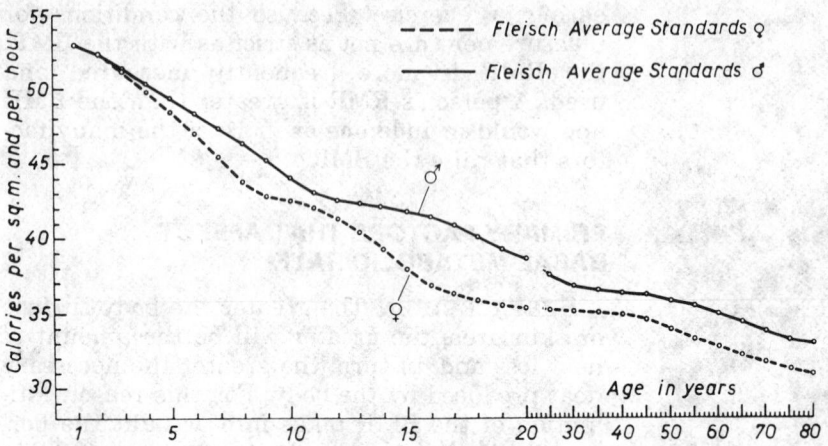

Figure 1–6. Average basal metabolic rates per m.² of surface area for males and females at different ages. (From Fleisch, A.: New Methods of Studying Gaseous Exchange and Pulmonary Function. 1960. Courtesy of Charles C Thomas, Publisher, Springfield, Illinois.)

may increase to almost twice the normal amount. In fact, an abnormal basal metabolic rate has been used as an indicator of thyroid function and malfunction. However, the BMR test is costly in both time and equipment and is therefore used infrequently.

The BMR in adult females fluctuates with the menstrual cycle. There is an average of 359 kcal./day difference in the BMR between its high point before menstruation and its lowest point about one week before ovulation.[17a]

The growth hormone can increase the BMR as much as 15 to 20 per cent, resulting from the stimulation of cellular metabolism.

Stimulation of the sympathetic nervous system, as during emotional excitement or stress, increases cellular activity by the release of the hormone *epinephrine* (adrenaline), which acts directly to cause glycogenolysis and increase basal metabolic rate. Other hormones, such as cortisol and insulin, may influence metabolic rate.

PREGNANCY. During pregnancy the adult female has an increased metabolic rate, which is thought to be due to increases in muscle development of the uterus, placenta and fetus and to respiration rate and cardiac work. The percentage of increase has been reported by Blackburn and Calloway to be 13 per cent when calculated on a per kg. basis. Because of increased weight, though, the total BMR increase was 28 per cent.[1]

SECONDARY FACTORS THAT AFFECT BASAL METABOLIC RATE

NUTRITIONAL STATUS. In conditions of marked undernourishment or prolonged starvation, an individual will demonstrate a lowered metabolism, often as much as 50 per cent below normal. This decrease in metabolism has been postulated to be due to an adaptive mechanism of the body that conserves energy and possibly to a decrease in mass of active tissue.

SLEEP. During sleep the metabolic rate falls approximately 10 per cent below that of waking levels. This drop is due to muscular relaxation and decreased activity of the sympathetic nervous system. This usually amounts to 40 to 80 kcalories less per day, depending upon the number of hours of sleep, the degree of relaxation and the size of the body.

FEVER. Infections or fevers increase the metabolic rate about 7 per cent for each degree F. rise in body temperature above 98.6°F. or 13 per cent for each degree C. above 37°C.

MUSCLE TONUS. The degree to which a person's muscles are relaxed affects the amount of energy used in the resting state and thus the metabolic rate. The less relaxed the muscles, the greater the metabolic rate. Emotional strain can cause increased tension in the muscles and thus increase the metabolic rate.

EXERCISE. BMR is measured with the individual in a state of rest. The effect of vigorous exercise is to increase the metabolic rate both during the exercise and for several hours after the exercise is completed.

Total Energy Requirement

The energy requirement of an individual takes precedence over all other needs. The minimum energy needs must be met first and other specific nutrients can be acquired later.

The three main factors that determine the total energy requirement of an adult are:
1. Basal metabolism
2. Physical activity
3. Specific dynamic action of food or diet-induced thermogenesis

In addition, other factors such as growth, pregnancy, lactation, recovery from illness and temperature regulation must also be considered.

BASAL ENERGY REQUIREMENT

Since it is usually inconvenient, expensive or impossible to actually measure an individual's BMR, it is usually calculated using one of many formulas that have been devised. Frequently the calculated BMR is referred to as the *basal energy expenditure* or *BEE*. To be most accurate these formulas should take into account age, sex and body surface area, the factors that most influence BMR. Harris and Benedict[11] devised a formula to give the standard BEE for an individual:

$$\text{BEE for a female} = 655.096 + 9.563(W) \\ + 1.85(H) - 4.676(A)$$
$$\text{BEE for a male} = 66.473 + 13.752(W) \\ + 5.003(H) - 6.755(A)$$

W = weight in kg., H = height in cm. and A = age in years. A nomogram for using the Harris-Benedict formula has also been developed.[17] Boothby and Sandiford have also devised a formula and the nomogram shown in Figure 1-7 to determine basal metabolic rate or expenditure. Using either one of these methods should produce a determination of BMR with an accuracy of ± 10 to 15 per cent.[2, 20]

The determination of the surface area has always been a frustration in BMR calculations. DuBois[6] has developed the most accurate formula for determination of body surface area:

$$\text{Surface area (m}^2\text{)} = .007184 \times W^{0.425} \times H^{0.725}$$

This formula is not valid in children under 6 years of age, however, and, Haycock[12] has described a method for determination of surface area in young children.

Fleisch[8] looked at all the formulas for calculating the BEE based on body surface area and came up with a weighted average that has been proposed to be the most accurate.[22] Figure 1-6 gives these average values in kcal./m.² for various ages and both sexes. It is possible to use the appropriate figure from this graph and the body surface area as determined by using the chart in Figure 1-7 to determine the BEE of an individual.

Another problem in calculating BEE is whether the increased surface area in an obese person does in fact increase the BEE as it would when BEE is determined by using body surface area. It is known that adipose tissue is not as metabolically active as fat-free mass. Thus, a determination based on surface area would result in an overestimation of BEE. Webb has shown that a more accurate determination for resting energy expenditure (REE) is made by using the lean body mass (LBM) as determined from underwater weighing (see Chapter 9) rather than the body surface area.[21] Cunningham proposes that a good prediction of BEE based on LBM is the following:

$$\text{BEE (kcal. per day)} = 501 + 21.6 \times \text{LBM.}[5]$$

It is also possible to partially correct the methods based on surface area by using the person's ideal body weight rather than the actual body weight if the person is obese or underweight. (See Appendix Table 27.)

Table 1-2 gives yet another method for determining BMR in persons of average height and weight. This method involves multiplying the weight in kg. × 1 kcal./kg. for males (.95 kcal./kg. for females) × 24 hours. This gives a good rough estimate of BEE.

For a young adult male whose ideal weight is 70 kilograms, the basal requirement would be 1680 kcalories (70 kg. × 1 kcal./kg. × 24 hr.) or 7030 kjoules. For a young adult female whose ideal weight is 55 kilograms, the basal requirement would be approximately 1254 kcalories (5246 kjoules).

No person could exist for very long receiving only sufficient energy to cover basal metabolic needs. The ordinary activities of life that require moving about and the various forms of muscular activity and the ingestion of food increase the energy needs of the body.

PHYSICAL ACTIVITY

Next to basal needs, physical activity is the greatest single factor influencing the energy needs of an individual. It may be as little as 10 per cent of the total energy requirement, as in the bedridden person, to as much as 50 per cent in the very active person or athlete.

A man doing heavy work (e.g., a miner) may need 4800 or more kcalories per day, while an individual of the same body build and age and height living in the same climate but doing sedentary work (e.g., an accountant) may require only 2500 kcalories. The inactive or sedentary person usually requires approximately 30 per cent additional calories above basal, whereas a lightly active person might need 50 per cent above basal, a moderately active person 75 per cent, and a very active person 100 per cent above basal. See Table 1-3 for descriptions of various levels of activity.

Levels of activity can be defined by stating the calorie expenditure per minute as shown in Table 1-3. The level of an activity can also be stated in *METs* or *metabolic equivalents*. A MET is a multiple of the resting metabolic rate (RMR) and is expressed in ml. of O_2 consumed

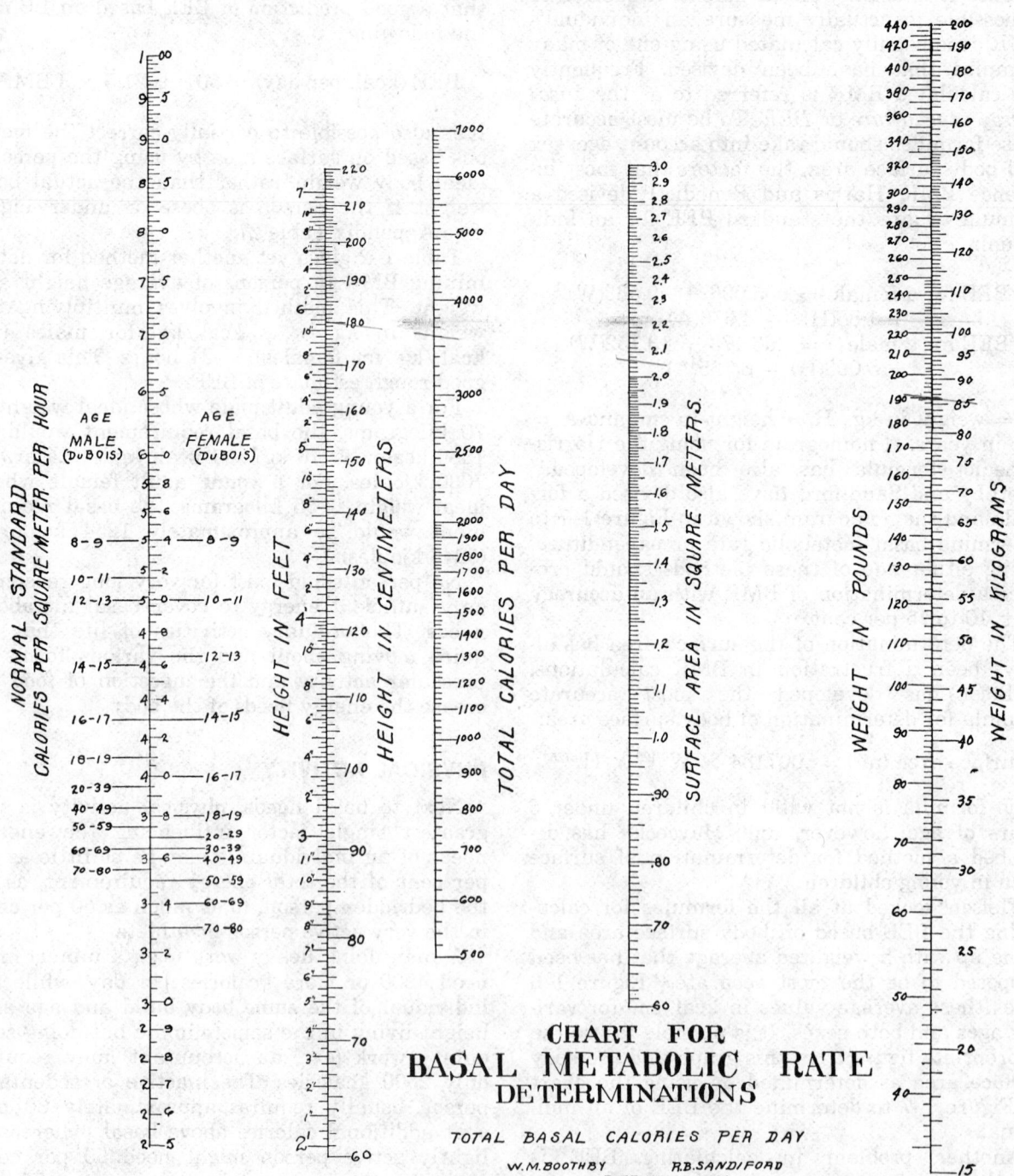

Figure 1–7. Place the chart on a flat, smooth table. Use only a ruler with a true straight edge. Do not draw lines on the chart but merely indicate their positions by the straight edge of the ruler. Locate the various points by means of needles (pin stuck through the eraser of a lead pencil). Locate the patient's normal weight on the scale on the right and his height on the scale second from the left. The ruler joining these two points intersects the scale second from the right at the patient's surface area. Locate the age and sex of the patient on the scale on the left. A ruler joining this point with the point already determined for the patient's surface area crosses the scale third from the left at the *basal* energy requirement. To convert kilocalories (kcal) to kJ., multiply by 4.184. (From Boothby, W. M., and Sandiford, R. B.: Nomographic charts for the calculation of the metabolic rate by the gasometer method. Boston Med. Surg. J., *185*:337, 1921.)

Table 1–2. CALCULATION OF BASAL ENERGY EXPENDITURE

Example: 20-year-old woman, 165 cm. in height, 55 kg. in weight (ideal body weight for this woman).

Method 1: .95 kcal./kg. IBW/hr. × IBW in kg. × 24 hr. = basal energy expenditure per day.

.95 kcal./kg. IBW/hr. × 55 kg. × 24 hr. = 1254 *kcal./day*

Method 2: Using the nomogram in Figure 1–7:
   a. place the end of a ruler at 55 kg. on the scale that measures weight in kg.
   b. place the other end of the ruler at 165 cm. on the scale that measures height in cm.
   c. the point 1.6 m.^{2} at which the ruler intersects the surface area scale gives the surface area of this woman.
   d. starting over again, place one end of a ruler at 1.6 m.^{2} on the surface area scale.
   e. place the other end of the ruler at 20–29 years on the right side of the scale on the left, which measures the age of females.
   f. the point at which the ruler now intersects the scale giving total calories is the basal energy expenditure per day for this woman.

1380 *kcal./day*

Method 3: Using the nomogram in Figure 1–7:
   a–c. same as in Method 2.
   d. now referring to Figure 1–6, determine the kcal./m.^{2} for a woman 20 years of age. It appears to be 35.5 kcal./m.^{2}.
   e. multiply 35.5 kcal./m.^{2} by 1.6 m.^{2} and then by 24 hours.

1363 *kcal./day*

The difference of 126 kcal. between the different methods of BMR determination is about 10 per cent, as would be expected.

per kg. of body weight per minute. An activity at 2 METs requires twice as much O_2 as resting metabolism and thus twice as many calories per minute as resting metabolism. See Table 1–4 for the energy expenditures of various activities. Individual energy expenditure varies considerably in a given activity. Most people have characteristic habits of motion. One person will sit quietly relaxed while another will unconsciously be making many habitual motions. The same is true in performing a task. One person will be very efficient and make few motions while another individual will expend much more energy making many unnecessary motions.

Body weight also affects energy expenditure. The greater the body weight, the greater the caloric expenditure for an activity. It takes more energy for an obese person to walk for 10 minutes than for a lighter weight person. For this reason activity can mean a large caloric reduction for an obese person in a weight reduction program.

Mental work does not appreciably affect the energy requirement. Fatigue after studying re-

Table 1–3. EXAMPLES OF DAILY ENERGY EXPENDITURES OF MATURE WOMEN AND MEN IN LIGHT OCCUPATIONS*

Activity Category	Time (hr.)	MAN, 70 KG. Rate (kcal./min.)	MAN, 70 KG. Total [kcal.(kJ.)]	WOMAN, 58 KG. Rate (kcal./min.)	WOMAN, 58 KG. Total [kcal.(kJ.)]
Sleeping, reclining	8	1.0–1.2	540(2270)	0.9–1.1	440(1850)
Very light	12	up to 2.5	1300(5460)	up to 2.0	900(3750)
Seated and standing activities, painting trades, auto and truck driving, laboratory work, typing, playing musical instruments, sewing, ironing					
Light	3	2.5–4.9	600(7520)	2.0–3.9	450(1890)
Walking on level, 2.5–3 mph, tailoring, pressing, garage work, electrical trades, carpentry, restaurant trades, cannery workers, washing clothes, shopping with light load, golf, sailing, table tennis, volleyball					
Moderate	1	5.0–7.4	300(1260)	4.0–5.9	240(1010)
Walking 3.5–4 mph, plastering, weeding and hoeing, loading and stacking bales, scrubbing floors, shopping with heavy load, cycling, skiing, tennis, dancing					
Heavy	0	7.5–12.0		6.0–10.0	
Walking with load uphill, tree felling, work with pick and shovel, basketball, swimming, climbing, football, jogging and other aerobic exercise.					
TOTAL	24		2740(11,500)		2030(8,530)

*Figures include BMR and SDA

Data from Durnin, J. V., and Passmore, R.: Energy, Work and Leisure, London, Heinemann Educational Books, 1967, p. 166. (Adapted from: Food and Nutrition Board, Recommended Dietary Allowances, 9th ed., Washington, D.C., National Research Council, NAS, 1980.)

Table 1-4. CALORIC EXPENDITURE DURING VARIOUS ACTIVITIES*

ACTIVITY	CAL./MIN.	ACTIVITY	CAL./MIN.	ACTIVITY	CAL./MIN.
Sleeping	1.2	Mopping floors	4.9	Handball and squash	10.0
Resting in bed	1.3	Repaving roads	5.0	Mountain climbing	10.0
Sitting, normally	1.3	Gardening, weeding	5.6	Skipping rope	10.0–15.0
Sitting, reading	1.3	Stacking lumber	5.8	Judo and karate	13.0
Lying, quietly	1.3	Chain saw	6.2	Football (while active)	13.3
Sitting, eating	1.5	Stone, masonry	6.3	Wrestling	14.4
Sitting, playing cards	1.5	Pick-and-shovel work	6.7	Skiing:	
Standing, normally	1.5	Farming, haying, plowing with horse	6.7	Moderate to Steep	8.0–12.0
Classwork, lecture (listen to)	1.7	Shoveling (miners)	6.8	Downhill Racing	16.5
Conversing	1.8	Walking downstairs	7.1	Cross-Country: 3–8 MPH	9.0–17.0
Personal toilet	2.0	Chopping wood	7.5	Swimming:	
Sitting, writing	2.6	Crosscut saw	7.5–10.5	Pleasure	6.0
Standing, light activity	2.6	Tree felling (ax)	8.4–12.7	Crawl: 25–50 yds/min	6.0–12.5
Washing and dressing	2.6	Gardening, digging	8.6	Butterfly: 50 yds/min	14.0
Washing and shaving	2.6	Walking upstairs	10.0–18.0	Backstroke: 25–50 yds/min	6.0–12.5
Driving a car	2.8	Pool or billiards	1.8	Breaststroke: 25–50 yds/min	6.0–12.5
Washing clothes	3.1	Canoeing: 2.5 MPH–4.0 MPH	3.0–7.0	Sidestroke: 40 yds/min	11.0
Walking indoors	3.1	Volleyball: Recreational–Competitive	3.5–8.0	Dancing:	
Shining shoes	3.2	Golf: Foursome–Twosome	3.7–5.0	Modern: moderate-vigorous	4.2–5.7
Making bed	3.4	Horseshoes	3.8	Ballroom: waltz-rhumba	5.7–7.0
Dressing	3.4	Baseball (except pitcher)	4.7	Square	7.7
Showering	3.4	Ping Pong–Table Tennis	4.9–7.0	Walking:	
Driving motorcycle	3.5	Calisthenics	5.0	Road–Field (3.5 MPH)	5.6–7.0
Metal working	3.5	Rowing: Pleasure–Vigorous	5.0–15.0	Snow: hard–soft (3.5–2.5 MPH)	10.0–20.0
House painting	3.7	Cycling: 5–15 MPH (10 speed)	5.0–12.0	Uphill: 5–10–15% (3.5 MPH)	8.0–11.0–15.0
Cleaning windows	3.8	Skating: Recreation–Vigorous	5.0–15.0	Downhill: 5–10% (2.5 MPH)	3.6–3.5
Carpentry	3.8	Archery	5.2	15–20% (2.5 MPH)	3.7–4.3
Farming chores	3.9	Badminton: Recreational–Competitive	5.2–10.0	Hiking: 40 lb. pack (3.0 MPH)	6.8
Sweeping floors	4.1	Basketball: Half–Full Court (more for fast break)	6.0–9.0	Running:	
Plastering walls	4.2	Bowling (while active)	7.0	12 min mile (5 MPH)	10.0
Truck and automobile repair	4.2	Tennis: Recreational–Competitive	7.0–11.0	8 min mile (7.5 MPH)	15.0
Ironing clothes	4.7	Water Skiing	8.0	6 min mile (10 MPH)	20.0
Farming, planting, hoeing, raking	4.7	Soccer	9.0	5 min mile (12 MPH)	25.0
Mixing cement		Snowshoeing (2.5 MPH)	9.0		

*Depends on efficiency and body size. Add 10% for each 15 lbs over 150, subtract 10% for each 15 lbs under 150.

(From: Sharkey, B. J.: Physiology of Fitness. Champaign, Ill., Human Kinetics Publishers, 1979.)

sults not from the mental work but from the physical activities or muscle tension that accompany the study habits.

The *state of health* may have a marked effect on physical activity. Such physiological and psychological stresses as fatigue, tension, depression and lack of sleep may influence the physical activity and total energy requirement.

A very low *environmental temperature* or a very high environmental temperature may increase slightly the energy needs. These additional calories are required to cover the work cost of maintaining body temperature at 37°C. The energy cost of work in cold weather is slightly greater than in warm weather. However, in extreme heat (greater than 86°F. or 30°C.) heavy activity or work requires greater energy expenditure owing to sweat gland activity. Nature, however, regulates heat loss very effectively in the various climates by enabling human beings to shiver or sweat as the temperature dictates.

SPECIFIC DYNAMIC ACTION OF FOOD OR DIET-INDUCED THERMOGENESIS

All foods give a stimulus to metabolism, but not all foods have the same effect on metabolism. This stimulus is called the *specific dynamic action* (SDA) or *calorigenic effect* of food. It is also called *diet-induced thermogenesis* because it may be related to brown adipose tissue[10] (see Chapter 27). Carbohydrate or fat increases the heat production by about 5 per cent of the total calories consumed. If the food intake is composed solely of protein, the increase may be as much as 30 per cent. If the food intake is very high in protein, about 15 per cent should be added.[14] This specific dynamic action effect of food is due to the energy needed not only for digestion of food but also for absorption and assimilation of nutrients. The mechanism of diet-induced thermogenesis is still not completely understood, but for a liberal mixed diet, about 10 per cent of total energy requirements for basal metabolism and muscular activity should be added to cover it. For some ill-understood reason, diet-induced thermogenesis may be enhanced by exercise.[4] The calorigenic effect of food after exercise was found to be nearly twice that when the body is at rest.[16]

The SDA is included in energy requirements determined for the resting state but not for the basal state. Therefore the RMR or REE includes the SDA. Energy requirements determined for the activities listed in Table 1–4 include the BMR, the SDA and the energy required for the activity.

GROWTH, PREGNANCY AND LACTATION

In the growing child, energy must be provided over and above that required for the basal met-abolic rate, physical activity and specific dynamic action. This additional energy is required to cover the cost of increasing body weight and height. Growing infants may store as much as 12 to 15 per cent of the energy value of their food intake in the form of new tissue. As a child becomes older, the rate of growth diminishes and the caloric requirement for growth is reduced. Although total energy requirements increase because of increased size, the energy requirement per unit of body size is smaller (see Fig. 1–6). The kcalorie allowances in Table 10–3 are proposed as average and approximate amounts for feeding groups of children. The needs of an individual child are governed by growth and physical activity (see Chapters 12 to 14).

Additional calories are required to meet the energy costs of pregnancy and lactation, which are also periods of growth (see Chapter 11).

ESTIMATION OF DAILY ENERGY REQUIREMENT OF AN ADULT

The total daily energy requirement is commonly estimated by adding together the requirement for basal metabolism, physical or muscular activity and the specific dynamic action (SDA) of food.

The method used depends on the degree of accuracy desired. For research purposes the individual has a basal metabolism determination. The energy cost of the daily activities is determined by the respirometer. The results of all activities added together would give the total energy requirement for physical activity. An additional 10 per cent would be added to account for the SDA and the total would be the energy requirement.

Another method involves estimating the amount of time during the day spent in various activities including sleeping, sitting, and so forth and then referring to Table 1–4 for the appropriate caloric expenditures. The sum of these would be the total energy expenditure for the day because BMR and SDA are included in the figures in Table 1–4. Table 1–3 shows how this was determined in a male and a female in light occupations.

A procedure that is less precise but accurate enough for many purposes is as follows:

1. *Determine the ideal body weight (IBW) of the individual in kilograms*. This can be determined from a record of the person's constant weight, from Appendix Tables 27, or from the rule of thumb presented in Table 1–5.

2. *Determine basal energy expenditure*:

male = 1.0 kcalorie (4.18 kJ.)/kg. of ideal body wt./hour × 24

female = 0.95 kcalorie (4.0 kJ.)/kg. of ideal body wt./hour × 24

Table 1–5. RULE OF THUMB DETERMINATION OF IDEAL BODY WEIGHT

Females:	100 lb. (45 kg.) for the first 5 ft. (152 cm.)
	plus
	5 lb. (2.2 kg.) for every inch (2.54 cm.) of height over 5 ft. (152 cm.)
Males:	110 lb. (45 kg.) for the first 5 ft. (152 cm.)
	plus
	5 lb. (2.2 kg.) for every 1 inch (2.54 cm.) of height over 5 ft. (152 cm.)
Example:	female, 165 cm. 45 kg. for 152 cm.
	plus
	2.2 kg. × 13 cm./2.54 cm. = 11.4 kg
	45 kg. + 11.4 kg. = 56.4 kg.

To adjust for frame size, 10 lb. (4.5 kg.) would be added in the case of a large frame or subtracted in the case of a small frame.

3. *Subtract* 0.1 kcalorie (0.42 kJ.)/kg. of ideal body wt./*hours of sleep.*

4. *Add activity increment.* (plus 30, 50, 75 or 100 per cent).

5. *Add specific dynamic action* (10 per cent of BEE plus activity increment).

6. *Sum* equals the *approximate daily calorie requirement.*

An even cruder method for estimating total energy requirements for the person at his or her ideal body weight is the following:

Multiply the IBW in kg. by one of these factors, which include basal, activity and SDA requirements:

sedentary: 30 kcal. (125 kJ.)/kg.
moderately active: 35–40 kcal.
(145–170 kJ.)/kg.
very active: 45 kcal. (190 kJ.)/kg.

The disadvantages of this method are that (1) no correction is made for sex or age, and (2) the estimation of activity is a rough one. See Table 1–6 for a summary of these two methods.

Even though several methods have been discussed for determining energy requirements it is necessary to remember that it is not exact. It

has been proposed that there is a regulatory mechanism in the human that allows adaptation to various energy intakes along with maintenance of stable weight and activity, and this may be within a range of ± 16 per cent of energy requirements.[19] This underscores the necessity of calculating individual energy requirements, monitoring weight and recognizing a possible variation of ± 16 per cent.

Energy Stores

A person who is exercising or fasting is relying on body energy stores. At first the energy comes from stored ATP and creatine phosphate. When this source is depleted after a few minutes, anaerobic glycolysis takes over, reconstituting ATP (see Chapter 5). The third and final source is oxidative phosphorylation of body nutrients—glycogen, fat and eventually protein. Then oxygen uptake is the limiting factor. Fat is carried as the primary energy store because it provides over twice as many calories per gram as glycogen or tissue protein. See Figure 1–8 for the difference between energy stores of a normal weight individual and an obese individual. The normal weight (69 kg.) individual has energy stores of 140,000 kcal., whereas the obese person (99 kg.) has stores of 320,000 kcal., over twice as much.

Recommended Energy Allowances

The recommendations for energy intake for adults, revised in 1980 by the Food and Nutrition Board, National Research Council, National Academy of Sciences, are given in Table 10–3. For the adult age categories, the recommenda-

Table 1–6. CALCULATION OF TOTAL ENERGY REQUIREMENT*

Example:		20-year-old female, 165 cm. tall and weighing 55 kg.
		Activity: light
Method 1:	a.	Determine IBW—55 kg. is IBW for this woman.
	b.	Basal needs = .95 kcal./kg. IBW/hr. × 55 kg. × 24 hr. = 1254 kcal. (5250 kJ.).
	c.	Sleep = .1 kcal./kg. IBW/hr. × 55 kg. × 8 hr. = 45 kcal.
		1254 kcal. − 45 kcal. = 1209 kcal.
	d.	Activity: light = 50% above basal = 625 kcal. (2600 kJ.)
		1209 kcal. + 625 kcal. = 1834 kcal. (7850 kJ.).
	e.	SDA = 10% above energy requirement = 184 kcal.
		1834 kcal. + 184 kcal. = *2022 kcal./day (8500 kJ/day)*
Method 2:		Factor for sedentary = 30 kcal./kg. IBW.
		Factor for moderately active = 35–40 kcal./kg. IBW.
		This woman has light activity, so use the factor of 33 kcal./kg. IBW/day.
		55 kg. × 33 kcal./kg. IBW/day = *1815 kcal./day (7600 kJ./day)*

*The difference of 207 kcal./day between these two calculations is a minor one (11 per cent). It is only a guideline and should be adjusted depending on whether the individual maintains her weight on this level of energy intake.

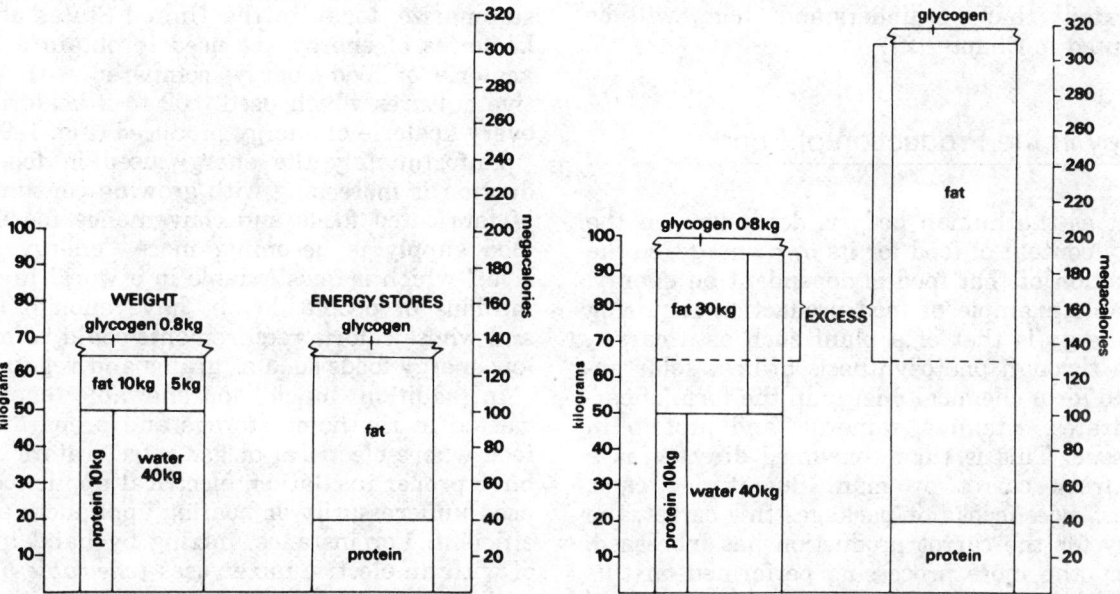

Figure 1–8. *A,* Body weight and energy stores of a normal adult weighing about 69 kg. *B,* Obese adult weighing 99 kg. Excess fat would supply total energy for three months. (From: Garrow, J. S.: The regulation of body weight. In Silverstone, T. (ed.): Obesity: Its Pathogenesis and Management. Publishing Sciences Group, 1975.)

tions are for adults living in a temperate climate and engaged in occupations requiring light activity. In this edition there is a separate table (Table 10–3) of recommended energy intakes with ranges for mean heights and weights. This focuses attention on maintenance of desirable body weight. In general, the trend is again for lower calorie allowances than were recommended in the previous editions (1958, 1963, 1968 and 1974) based on changes in the American way of life, new research information and concern for the large segment of the population which is now overweight. The average American male adult is 178 cm. (70 in.) tall, and the average female is 163 cm. (64 in.) tall. Accordingly, the average desirable weights are 70 kg. (154 lb.) and 55 kg. (120 lb.) throughout adult life. However, the body composition changes throughout adult life, because loss of lean body mass is compensated for by accumulation of body fat. A decrease in energy needed for each decade after age 22 is recommended. In order to better understand the use of the material, it is strongly advised that every student read and become familiar with the scientific basis for the allowances as revised in 1980.[9]

It is understood that energy allowances must be adjusted to meet the specific needs of an individual and to maintain body weight at the desired level. This is the final test of the adequacy of calculated or recommended energy allowances.

The energy allowances for pregnant and lactating women, infants, children and adolescents will be discussed in Chapters 11 through 14.

Excessive and Deficient Energy Intakes

Excessive energy intake is discussed in Chapter 27. Deficient energy intake is discussed with deficient protein intake as protein-energy malnutrition in Chapter 4.

Regulation of Energy Intake and Expenditure

The ability of the healthy, normal adult human being to control his energy intake in order to match his energy output is most remarkable. Body weight, the indicator of this balance, is quite stable. For instance, during a single year the average American adult male will ingest one million kcalories of which over 99 per cent will be expended. If only 1 per cent of these million kcalories (10,000 kcal.) was stored, this would result in a 3 lb. (1.4 kg.) weight gain for that year.[3] Thus the body's energy balance control is extremely sensitive. This balance between intake and expenditure depends on activity and the control of hunger, which depends on a multiplicity of factors.

Even more fascinating is the situation of obesity in which this controlling system has "failed." There has been too much hunger and either not enough activity to warrant the hunger or too little satiety. Why does this happen? A complete discussion of hunger and satiety, to the extent that we understand them, will be presented in Chapter 27.

Energy in the Production of Food

Just as the human body is dependent on the energy content of food for its own energy, so the production of that food is dependent on energy. A simple example of food production requiring low energy is that of a plant such as a carrot, which through photosynthesis utilizes solar energy to form chemical energy in the form of carbohydrates, vitamins, minerals and protein in its tissue. This is then consumed directly as a raw, fresh carrot by man. But if one cans, freezes, dices, cooks or packages this carrot, the energy for the carrot production has increased. In fact, the more processing performed on this carrot, the farther it is transported or the fancier its package, the more energy of production it represents.

About 13 per cent of the U.S. total energy consumption is used to bring food from the farm to the consumer, and meat processing makes up the largest segment of this energy cost. Animal protein is a very energy-expensive item because only 10 per cent of the plant protein fed to raise the animal is returned as animal protein.[13] To

summarize, today in the United States about 8 kcalories of energy are used to obtain a single kcalorie of food energy, compared with primitive cultures which used 0.02 to 2 kcalories for every kcalorie of energy produced (Fig. 1–9).

Unfortunately the energy used in food production is increasing with growing consumption of fabricated foods and convenience foods. The food supply is becoming more "energy intensive," which is questionable in a world in which millions of people do not have enough to eat and whose calorie requirements could be met by low-energy foods such as grains and vegetables.

In addition much nonrenewable energy is wasted in the home storage and preparation of food where electrical or gas refrigerators do not have proper insulation, electrical appliances are used unnecessarily or heating appliances are inefficient. For instance, mixing by hand instead of with an electric mixer uses *renewable* human energy instead of nonrenewable electrical energy. By using human energy one would expend additional kcalories and help avoid gaining that extra pound! People must become more conscious of personal use of nonrenewable energy in food preparation and make necessary changes to reduce that use if possible. To reduce the energy intensiveness of food production will require changes on the farm, in food processing and in the home.

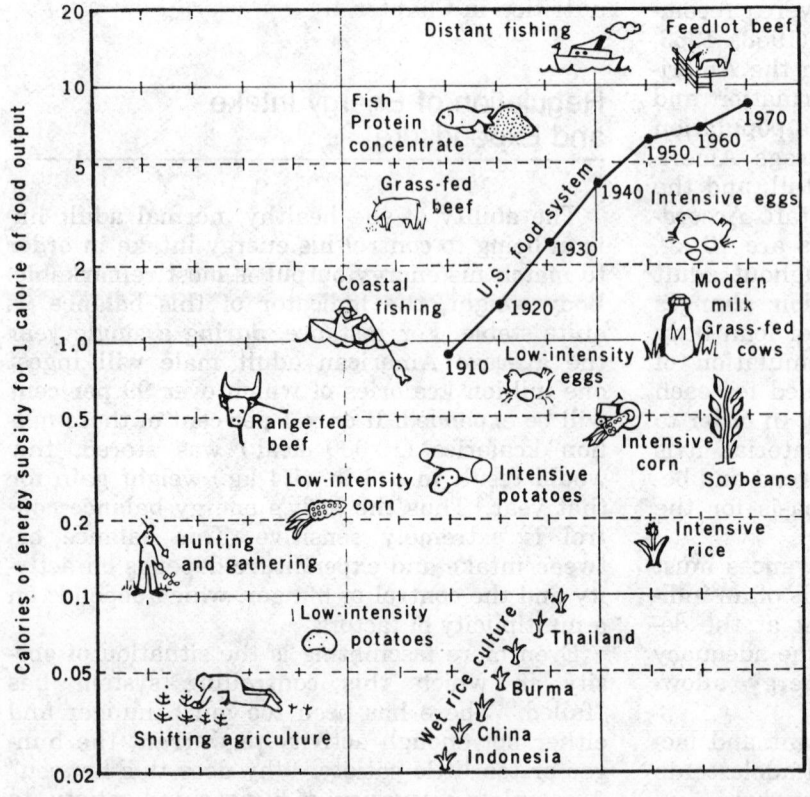

Figure 1–9. Energy subsidies for various food crops. The energy history of the U.S. food system is shown for comparison. (From: Steinhart, J. S., and Steinhart, C. E.: Energy use in the U.S. food system. Science, *184*: 307, 1974.)

Problems and Suggested Topics for Discussion

1. What does "calorie" mean? How is it used in nutrition?
2. (a) Consult food composition tables for the calorie values of food and list those which have 500 kcalories per serving, 200 kcalories per serving, 100 kcalories per serving and 50 kcalories per serving. (b) On the basis of the protein, fat and carbohydrate value, determine the energy value (kcalories) of:
   - 23 gm. whole wheat bread
   - 244 gm. whole milk
   - 190 gm. grapefruit sections
   - 150 gm. raw tomato
3. What is meant by basal energy expenditure and resting energy expenditure?
4. What is diet-induced thermogenesis? How is it determined?
5. Calculate your own basal energy expenditure and then your total energy requirement.
6. List the foods you have consumed during one 24-hour period and compute the total calorie value. Compare this total with the calorie allowance recommended by the Food and Nutrition Board of the National Research Council.

Cited References

1. Blackburn, M.W., and Calloway, D.H.: Basal metabolic rate and work energy expenditure of mature pregnant women. J. Am. Diet. Assoc., 69:24, 1976.
2. Boothby, W.M., Berkson, J., and Dunn, H.T.: Studies of the energy of metabolism of normal individuals: a standard for basal metabolism with a nomogram for clinical application. Am. J. Physiol., 116:468, 1936.
3. Bray, G.A., and Campfield, L.A.: Metabolic factors in the control of energy stores. Metabolism, 24:99, 1975.
4. Bray, G.A., Whipp, B.J., and Koyal, S.N.: The acute effects of food intake on energy expenditure during cycle ergometry. Am. J. Clin. Nutr., 27:254, 1974.
5. Cunningham, J.J.: An individualization of dietary requirements for energy in adults. J. Am. Diet. Assoc., 80:335, 1982.
6. Du Bois, E.F.: Basal Metabolism in Health and Disease. Philadelphia, Lea & Febiger, 1927, pp. 141–147.
7. Durnin, J.V., and Passmore, R.: Energy, Work and Leisure. New York, William Heinemann Educational Books, Ltd., 1967.
8. Fleisch, A.: New Methods of Studying Gaseous Exchange and Pulmonary Function. Springfield, Illinois, Charles C Thomas, Publisher, 1960.
9. Food and Nutrition Board, National Research Council: Recommended Dietary Allowances. 9th ed. Washington, D.C., National Academy of Sciences, 1980.
10. Glick, Z., Teague, R.J., and Bray, G.A.: Brown adipose tissue: thermic response increased by a single low protein, high carbohydrate meal. Science, 213:1125, 1981.
11. Harris, J.A., and Benedict, F.G.: A Biometric Study of Basal Metabolism in Man. Carnegie Institute of Washington, Publ. No. 279, 1919.
12. Haycock, G.B., Schwartz, G.J., and Wisotsky, D.H.: Geometric method for measuring body surface area: a height-weight formula validated in infants, children and adults. J. Pediatr., 93:62, 1978.
13. Hirst, E.: Living off the fuels of the land. Natural History, 82:21, 1973.
14. Latner, A.L.: Cantarow and Trumper Clinical Biochemistry. 7th ed. Philadelphia, W.B. Saunders Company, 1975, p. 451.
15. McArdle, W.D., Katch, F.I., and Katch, V.L.: Exercise Physiology: Energy, Nutrition and Human Performance. Philadelphia, Lea & Febiger, 1981, p. 105.
16. Miller, D.S., Mumford, P., and Stock, M.J.: Gluttony 2: thermogenesis in overeating man. Am. J. Clin. Nutr., 20:1223, 1967.
17. Rainey-MacDonald, C.G., Holliday, R.L., and Wells, G.A.: Nomograms for predicting resting energy expenditure in hospitalized patients. J. Parenteral Enteral Nutr., 6:59, 1982.
17a. Solomon, S.J., Kurzer, M.S., and Calloway, D.H.: Menstrual cycle and basal metabolic rate in women. Am. J. Clin. Nutr., 36:611, 1982.
18. Steinhart, J.S., and Steinhart, C.E.: Energy use in the U.S. food system. Science, 184:307, 1974.
19. Sukhatme, P.V., and Margen, S.: Autoregulatory homeostatic nature of energy balance, Am. J. Clin. Nutr., 35:355, 1982.
20. Tzankoff, S.P., and Norris, A.H.: Longitudinal changes in basal metabolism in man. J. Appl. Physiol., 45:536, 1978.
21. Webb, P.: Energy expenditure and fat-free mass in men and women. Am. J. Clin. Nutr., 34:1816, 1981.
22. Wilmore, D.W.: The Metabolic Management of the Critically Ill. New York, Plenum Medical Book Company, 1977, p. 818.

Additional References

Adams, C.F.: Nutritive Value of American Foods in Common Units. Agricultural Handbook No. 456. Washington, D.C., U.S. Department of Agriculture, 1975.
Briggs, G.M., and Calloway, D.H.: Bogert's Nutrition and Physical Fitness. 10th ed. Philadelphia, W.B. Saunders Company, 1979, Chapter 2.
Consumer and Food Economics Institute, Composition of Foods, Agricultural Handbook Vols. 8–1 to 8–9. Washington, D.C., U.S. Department of Agriculture, 1976–1982.
Cunningham, J.J.: Body composition and resting metabolic rate: the myth of feminine metabolism. Am. J. Clin. Nutr., 36:721, 1982.
Mahalko, J.R., and Johnson, L.K.: Accuracy of predictions of long-term energy needs. J. Am. Diet. Assoc., 77:557, 1980.
Miller, D.S.: Factors affecting energy expenditure. Proc. Nutr. Soc., 41:193, 1982.
Nutritive Value of Foods. Home and Garden Bulletin No. 72. Washington, D.C., U.S. Department of Agriculture, revised 1981.
Pennington, J.A.T., and Church, H.N.: Bowes and Church's Food Values of Portions Commonly Used. 13th ed. Philadelphia, J.B. Lippincott Company, 1980.
Pike, R.L., and Brown, M.L.: Nutrition: An Integrated Approach. New York, John Wiley & Sons, Inc., 1975, pp. 814–854.
Sharkey, B.J.: Physiology of Fitness. Champaign, Ill., Human Kinetics Publishers, 1979.
Sowers, M.F., et al.: Development and critical evaluation of the food nomogram. J. Am. Diet. Assoc., 79:536, 1981.

Carbohydrates

Carbohydrates furnish most of the energy that is needed to move, perform work and live; they are the starches and sugars. In the form of grains they furnish the major source of food for the people of the world and have the highest yield of energy per acre of land. However, the consumption of carbohydrates throughout the world is highly variable. In America about 45 per cent of the diet is composed of them, and an even higher proportion is used in other countries.[21] In the Orient, for example, where rice is a dietary staple, a higher proportion of calories is provided by carbohydrates. In the tropics carbohydrates may furnish as much as 90 per cent of the energy. Chapter 16 includes a discussion of grains used in the various countries. They are the cheapest, most easily obtainable, and most readily digested form of fuel. Since many of the foods that are high in carbohydrate content, such as bread, cereals, potatoes and other root vegetables are relatively inexpensive, the proportion of carbohydrates in the diet is greater at the lower economic levels. The chief sources of carbohydrates are grains, vegetables, fruits, syrups and sugars. That grains supply only carbohydrates is a popular misconception. Grains also supply a major portion of the protein for much of the world's population.

Definition and Composition

Carbohydrates are an important group of organic compounds that are composed of the three elements of carbon, hydrogen and oxygen. In their simplest form the general formula is $C_nH_{2n}O_n$. The hydrogen and oxygen are present in the same proportion as in water, H_2O, and there is one molecule of water for each carbon. From this comes the term carbohydrate, but this simple relationship gives no indication of the structure. More accurately the carbohydrates are defined as polyhydroxy aldehydes and ketones. They vary from simple sugars containing from three to seven carbon atoms to very complex polymers. Only the *hexoses* (six-carbon sugars) and *pentoses* (five-carbon sugars) and polymers built up from them play important roles in nutrition.

PHOTOSYNTHESIS. Plants store carbohydrates as their chief source of energy. Water, minerals and nitrogen in the soil are taken by the plant roots, trunk and branches to the leaves. The leaves absorb carbon dioxide (CO_2) from the air. The energy of sunlight acting on water (H_2O) and carbon dioxide in the presence of chlorophyll (the green coloring matter of leaves) enables the leaves to make sugar and release oxygen (O_2).

$$CO_2 + H_2O \xrightarrow[\text{plant enzymes}]{\overset{\text{sunlight}}{\text{chlorophyll}}} \text{Carbohydrate (CH}_2\text{O)} + O_2$$

This process of photosynthesis is illustrated in Figure 2–1. It involves the hydration of carbon dioxide to yield carbohydrate, and is nature's first step in the manufacture of all foods. The carbohydrate made in the leaves will be used in the growth of the plant (or tree) or will be stored energy in its leaves, stems, roots, seeds, pods and fruits. Thus, it can be said that the sun furnishes the energy for all living matter. To recover the locked-in energy of sunlight, the carbohydrate in plants is burned in the body and yields carbon dioxide and water. Not all the potential energy in sunlight is captured by photosynthesis; some is lost.

CLASSIFICATION

Carbohydrates are classified as monosaccharides, disaccharides, oligosaccharides and polysaccharides (Table 2–1). Monosaccharides (the simple sugars) cannot be hydrolyzed to a simpler form. Disaccharides may be hydrolyzed to give 2 molecules of the same or different monosaccharides. Oligosaccharides yield 3 to 10 monosaccharide units and polysaccharides more than 10 units—up to 10,000 or more.

Monosaccharides

The principal monosaccharides that occur free in foods are *glucose*, an aldohexose, and *fructose*, a ketohexose. They may exist in either an open-chain or a ring structure, as shown in Figure 2–2. When they are linked together as di- or polysaccharides they are held in the cyclic form. *Galactose* and *mannose*, two other aldohexoses

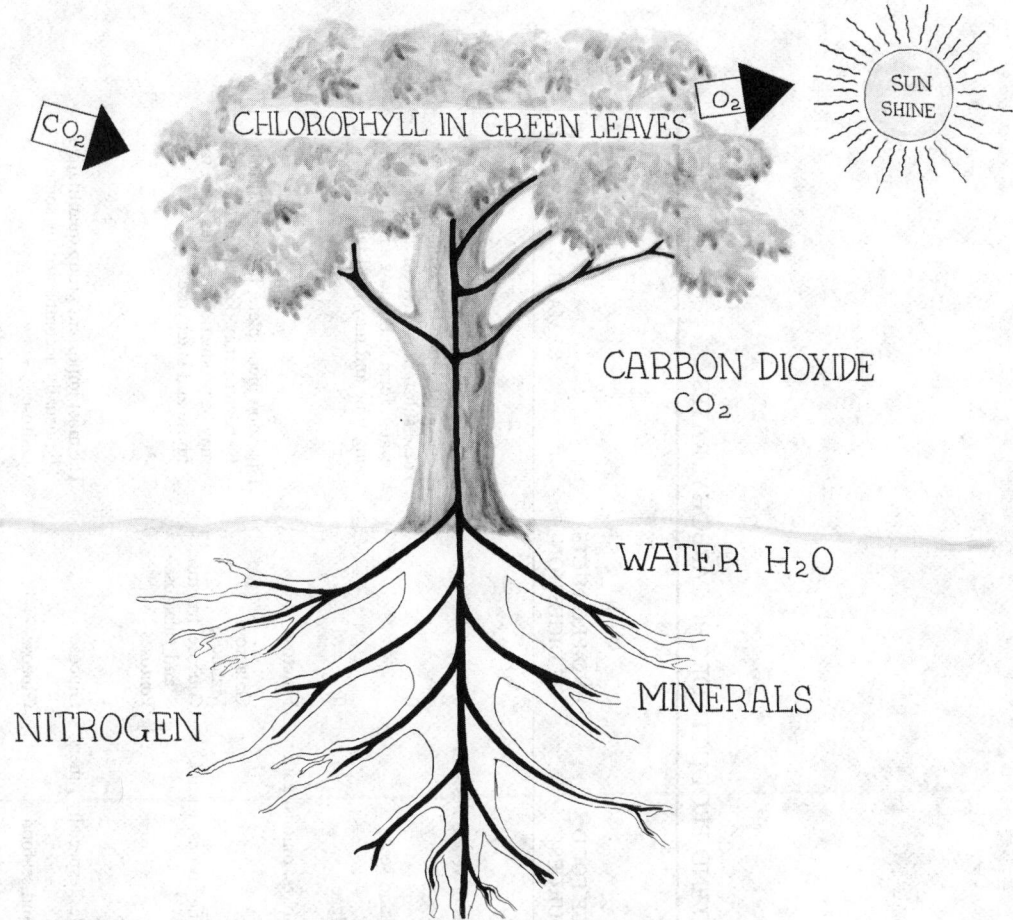

Figure 2–1. Synthesis of carbohydrates in plant life. Light from the sun is harnessed by the green chlorophyll of plant leaves. Cells in green leaves utilize this energy in synthesizing carbohydrates from the carbon dioxide in the air and the water in the soil. Carbohydrates are the chief form in which plants store potential energy.

which occur in bound form in food, have the same structure as glucose except for the orientation of the hydroxyl groups around the six carbon atoms.

Glucose (dextrose, grape sugar) is abundant in fruits, sweet corn, corn syrup, certain roots and honey. Glucose is the principal product formed by hydrolysis of more complex carbohydrates in the process of digestion. It is the form of sugar normally found in the blood stream. Glucose is oxidized in the cells to give energy and is stored in the liver and muscles as *glycogen*, a complex carbohydrate known as "animal starch." Under normal conditions the central nervous system can utilize only glucose as a major source of fuel. It is the best form of sugar to use when an immediate supply of sugar is needed, for it requires no changes in order to be utilized. It is relatively inexpensive and may be added to liquid foods to increase carbohydrate intake without seriously affecting the flavor of the food since it is only three fourths as sweet as cane sugar.

Sorbitol, a hexahydric alcohol derived from glucose, has a sweetening power similar to glucose (Table 2–2). Sorbitol is absorbed slowly and it serves to keep blood sugar levels high following a meal. It has been used in weight reduction as an aid to delay the onset of hunger sensations. It has the same energy value as glucose and is found in many fruits, vegetables and dietetic products.

Fructose (levulose, fruit sugar) is found together with glucose and sucrose in honey and fruit. It is the sweetest of the sugars. Technology has advanced to the point where levulose can be made from glucose. Now sweeteners containing glucose and levulose can be made from grains rather than only from the sugar beet and sugar cane. High-fructose corn syrup is an example.

Galactose is not found free in nature but is produced from lactose (milk sugar) by hydrolysis in the digestive process. It is found in nerve tissue.

Mannitol, a hexahydric alcohol derived from mannose, is found in foods. It is poorly digested

Table 2-1. TYPES, SOURCES AND END-PRODUCTS OF THE CARBOHYDRATES

CARBOHYDRATES	APPROXIMATE PERCENTAGE OF TOTAL CARBOHYDRATE INTAKE*	CHIEF FOOD SOURCES	END-PRODUCTS OF DIGESTION	REMARKS
POLYSACCHARIDES:				
a) Indigestible				
1. Cellulose	3	Stalks and leaves of vegetables; outer covering of seeds	0	May be partially split to glucose by bacterial action in large bowel
2. Hemicelluloses		Fruits	0	These substances have an affinity for water, form bulk, slow gastric emptying time and may bind bile acids
3. Pectins		Plant secretions and seeds		
4. Gums and mucilages				
5. Algal substances		Seaweeds and algae	0	
b) Partially digestible	2			
1. Inulin		Jerusalem artichokes, onions, garlic, mushrooms	Fructose	Digestion incomplete; further splitting by bacteria may occur in large bowel; may be production of flatus from raffinose and stachyose
2. Galactogens		Snails	Galactose	
3. Mannosans		Legumes	Mannose	
4. Raffinose		Sugar beets, kidney beans, lentils, navy beans	Glucose, fructose, and galactose	
5. Stachyose		Beans		
6. Pentosans		Fruits and gums	Pentoses	
c) Digestible				
1. Starch and dextrins	50	Grains; vegetables (especially tubers and legumes)	Glucose	The most important group quantitatively; usually accompanied by some maltose
2. Glycogen	Negligible	Meat products and seafood	Glucose	
DISACCHARIDES AND OLIGOSACCHARIDES:				
1. Sucrose	25	Cane and beet sugars, molasses, maple syrup	Glucose and fructose	
2. Lactose	10	Milk and milk products	Glucose and galactose	

		Synthetic products	Not metabolized	
3. Lactulose	Negligible†	Synthetic products	Not metabolized	Does not appear in foods; is synthetic, not digested, and is used as a laxative
4. Maltose and maltotriose		Malt products, some breakfast cereals	Glucose	
5. Trehalose		Mushrooms, insects, yeast	Glucose	
MONOSACCHARIDES:				
a) Hexoses:				
1. Glucose	5	Fruits; honey; corn syrup	Glucose	In fruits and vegetables the contents of glucose and fructose depend on species, ripeness, and state of preservation
–Sorbitol		Fruits, vegetables, dietetic products	Glucose	
2. Fructose	5	Fruits; honey	Fructose	
3. Galactose	0	0	Galactose	These monosaccharides do not occur in free form in foods; see under lactose and mannosans
4. Mannose	0	0	Mannose	
–Mannitol		Pineapples, olives, asparagus, sweet potatoes, carrots, dietetic products		
b) Pentoses:				
1. Ribose	0	0	Ribose	Ribose, xylose and arabinose do not occur in free form in foods. They are derived from pentosans of fruits and from the nucleic acids of meat products and seafood
2. Xylose	0	Fruits, vegetables, cereals, mushrooms, seaweed, dietetic chewing gum and other dietetic products	Xylose	
–Xylitol				
3. Arabinose	0	0	Arabinose	
CARBOHYDRATE DERIVATIVES:				
1. Ethyl alcohol	Variable	Fermented liquors	Absorbed as same	These substances are the products of natural or induced carbohydrate breakdown
2. Lactic acid	Negligible	Milk and milk products		
3. Malic acid	Negligible	Fruits		
4. Citric acid	Negligible	Fruits		

* Calculated from the average dietary of the middle-income group in the United States.

† Except in infant formulas.

(Adapted from Duncan, G. G. (ed.): Diseases of Metabolism. 5th ed. Philadelphia, W. B. Saunders Company, 1964, p. 106.)

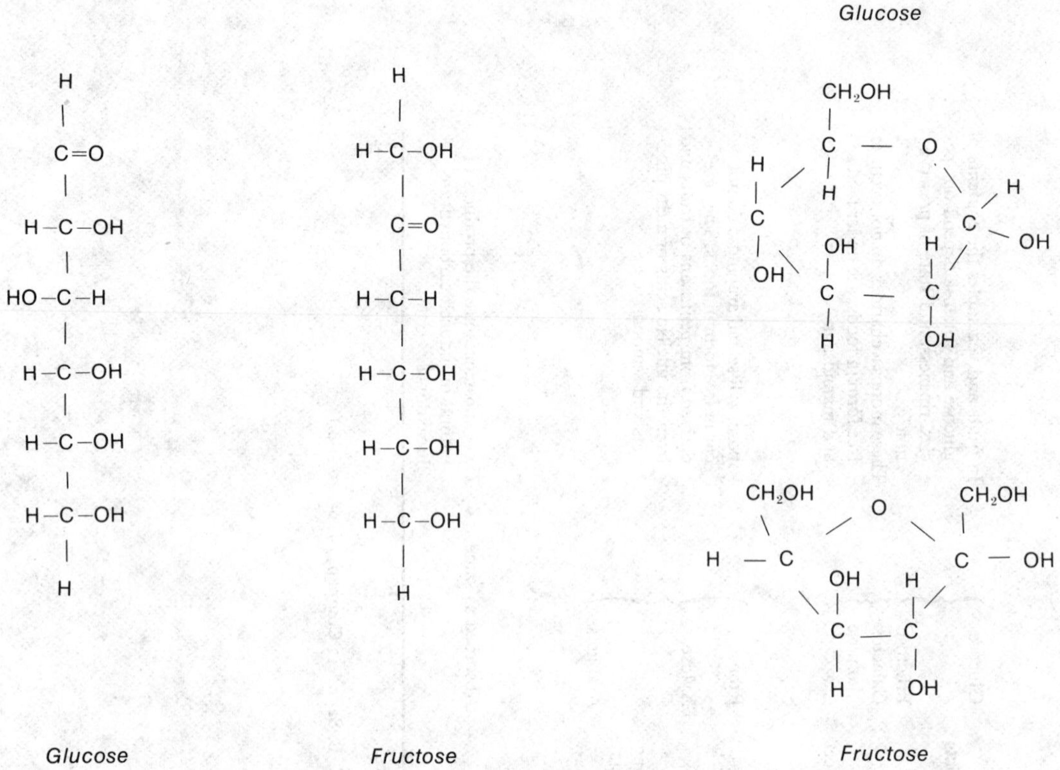

Glucose

Glucose   *Fructose*   *Fructose*

Figure 2–2. Structure of glucose and fructose.

and yields about one half as many calories per gram as glucose. It has been added to some foods for use as a drying agent. Pineapples, olives, asparagus, sweet potatoes and carrots, as well as sugarless gum and other dietetic products, contain some mannitol.

Mannose is not found free in foods but is derived from mannosans, which are found in manna and some legumes.

Several *pentoses* (five-carbon sugars) occur in bound form in food. *Ribose* and *deoxyribose* are derived from the nucleic acids of meat. They are essential components of nucleic acids and some coenzymes, but are not essential nutrients since they can be synthesized in the body. *Arabinose*

and *xylose* are constituents of the pentosans in fruits.

Xylitol, an alcohol of xylose with the sweetness of sucrose, is absorbed only one fifth as fast as glucose. For this reason it is used in sweetening foods for diabetics. It is also found in most fruits and vegetables. Because it is also less caries-promoting, it is also used in "sugar free" chewing gum.

Disaccharides

Disaccharides, or double sugars, are exemplified by sucrose (cane or beet sugar), maltose (malt sugar) and lactose (milk sugar). Each of the three double sugars is made up of two hexose molecules:

Sucrose = glucose and fructose
Maltose = glucose and glucose
Lactose = glucose and galactose

They are hydrolyzed by digestive enzymes to the constituent monosaccharides before absorption from the intestine.

Sucrose is ordinary table sugar. It is found mainly in sugar cane, sugar beets, molasses, maple syrup and maple sugar. When sucrose is hydrolyzed a 50:50 mixture of glucose and fructose forms. This mixture is called *invert sugar* and

Table 2–2. SWEETNESS OF SUGARS

SUGAR OR SUGAR PRODUCT	SWEETNESS VALUE
Levulose, fructose	173
Invert sugar	130
Sucrose	100
Glucose	74
Sorbitol	60
Mannitol	50
Galactose	32
Maltose	32
Lactose	16

From Freed, M.: Food Product Development, February–March, 1970.

frequently is seen on labels of foods. Sucrose is a very inexpensive and a common form of sugar in the diet.

Maltose or malt sugar does not occur free in nature. It is a so-called "derived" sugar, since it is a product of the digestion of starch by diastase, a plant enzyme obtained from sprouting grain. (This occurs in the manufacture of beer.) Maltose is formed from starch during digestion by the action of enzymes called *amylases*. The reaction begins with salivary amylase; other amylases are present in the intestine and pancreatic juice. Another enzyme, *maltase*, in the intestine hydrolyzes maltose to two molecules of glucose, in which form it is absorbed. Maltose is not readily fermented by bacteria in the colon.

Lactose is the principal sugar found in milk; 4 to 6 per cent in cow's milk and 5 to 8 per cent in human milk. It is not found in plants and is limited almost exclusively to the mammary glands of lactating animals. It is less soluble than the other common disaccharides and is only about one sixth as sweet as sucrose. It yields glucose and galactose upon hydrolysis and is digested more slowly than the other disaccharides. Some individuals have a deficiency of the enzyme *lactase*, which hydrolyzes lactose. Under such circumstances, some of this unhydrolyzed sugar passes into the large intestine, where it is fermented by intestinal bacteria and may have a laxative action. An excess amount may cause diarrhea, flatulence and abdominal cramping. Because lactose is less sweet than sucrose, it is often used to increase the calorie content of a liquid feeding without making it taste too sweet. However, it is difficult to dissolve and therefore not very practical. In the process of making cheese, some of the lactose in milk is converted to lactic and other acids, which contribute to the flavor. Lactose remains in the whey and is obtained commercially as a byproduct of the manufacture of cheese. As a consequence most cheese contains little or no lactose and thus can usually be tolerated in the lactase-deficient individual.

Lactulose, a new synthetic disaccharide, is composed of one molecule of galactose and one molecule of fructose. It is not metabolized by man and can therefore be used as a laxative.

Another synthetic sugar still in the experimental stage is *left-handed or L-sugar*. It has the same sweetening and textural properties as regular sugar, but it is not absorbed by the body or metabolized by bacteria. It is hoped that L-sugar can be used to sweeten dietetic foods.

Polysaccharides

The chief polysaccharides of interest in nutrition—starch, dextrin, cellulose, and glycogen—are assembled from glucose units. Other important plant and animal structures contain other monosaccharides. In some cases several different monosaccharides are combined in the polysaccharide molecule. As a group, polysaccharides are far less soluble and more stable than the monosaccharides. Starch and glycogen are completely digestible; other polysaccharides are partially or completely indigestible.

Starch occurs in two forms, *amylose* (long straight-chain glucose units) and *amylopectin* (branched arrangement of glucose units). It is found in grains, roots, vegetables and legumes. Starches are encased within the plant cells by cellulose walls in the form of granules of varying sizes and shapes and are typical for each starch. The composition of each starch differs, but all contain both amylose and amylopectin. Starches are insoluble in cold water and must be cooked. Cooking causes the granules to swell and the mixture to thicken or gel. Amylopectin in the starch granules participates in this process. Cooking softens and ruptures the cell to make the starch available for the enzymatic digestive processes in the intestine.

Modified food starch is very common in the food supply today. The natural starch structure is changed by a chemical process to make it a better thickening agent in foods such as salad dressing, pie filling, canned soup or gravy, canned pudding or baby food. Although structurally different, the energy value of the modified food starch is the same as for the natural starch—4 kcal./gram.

Dextrins are the intermediate products in the hydrolysis of starch to maltose and finally to glucose. This is accomplished by the action of dry heat (toasting of bread) or by enzymes during digestion. Dextrin is more soluble and sweeter than the original starch. Another commonly used product of the degradation of starch is *corn syrup*. Made from corn starch, corn syrup has the functions of giving sweetness or adding body or viscosity and is used in many food products from bakery products and confections to ice cream, beer and canned fruits.

Glycogen is a polysaccharide branched very much like amylopectin. Figure 2–3 illustrates the structure of glycogen. It is a very large molecule with a molecular weight from one million to four million. Glycogen is the storage form of carbohydrate in man and animals and is the primary and most readily available source of glucose and energy. Normally about three fourths of a pound or 340 grams of glycogen is stored in liver and muscle. Muscle glycogen is used directly for energy. Liver glycogen may be converted to glucose and carried by the blood to the tissues for their use. Very little glycogen is found in food. The small amounts in meat and seafood are largely converted to lactic acid at the time the animals are slaughtered.

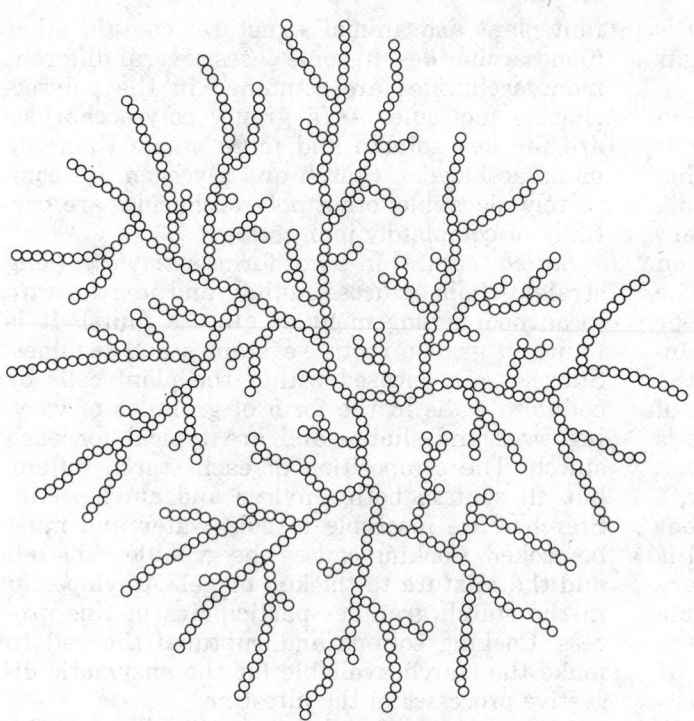

Figure 2–3. The structure of glycogen. (From: McGilvery, R. W.: Biochemistry: A Functional Approach. 2nd ed. Philadelphia, W. B. Saunders Company, 1979.)

Since the amount of glycogen stored at any time is very small, a constant supply of carbohydrate should be available to the body. Most of the carbohydrates consumed daily are in excess of the immediate energy needs and limited glycogen storage capacity. They are quickly converted into fats and stored in the adipose tissues. The dietary practice of "glycogen loading" is described in Table 14–7. The composition of carbohydrate in foods is given in Appendix Table 3.

POLYSACCHARIDES COMPRISING DIETARY FIBER. In the group of polysaccharides commonly referred to as *roughage* or *fiber* are the celluloses, the hemicelluloses, pectin, algal substances, gums and mucilages. These compounds in general are not energy sources because they are not hydrolyzed in the gut to yield simple sugars that can be absorbed.

Cellulose and hemicellulose are the cellular framework of plants. *Cellulose* resembles starch in that it is made up of many glucose molecules. The molecules are unbranched and resemble amylose, but they are not soluble in ordinary solvents. Whereas starch is readily digested by humans, cellulose is not. Humans do not have the enzyme needed to hydrolyze cellulose rapidly enough to make use of it. Ruminants can make use of cellulose, since it is digested by bacteria in the rumen.

The principal function of cellulose in human nutrition is to furnish indigestible "bulk," which promotes efficient intestinal function. Cellulose occurs in fruit, vegetable pulp and skin, stalks and leaves and the outer covering of grains, nuts, seeds and legumes.

Hemicelluloses or *non-cellulose polysaccharides* differ chemically from celluloses in that they may consist of hexoses, pentoses and acid forms of these compounds. Hemicelluloses hold water and produce bulk.

Pectin is made up of units of a derivative of galactose and is water soluble. It absorbs water, forms a gel, increases bulk, slows gastric emptying time and perhaps binds bile acids. Pectin, found in partially ripe fruit and fruit seeds and commercial preparations, is widely used for making jelly.

Gums and *mucilages* are similar to pectin except that the galactose units are combined with other different polysaccharides. They are found in plant secretions or seeds and perform functions similar to those of pectin in the human intestine.

Algal polysaccharides, another form of fiber, are found in seaweeds and algae. An example is carrageenan, which is used as a thickening agent and is listed on labels of many foods. Many other carbohydrate and noncarbohydrate gums are also used in food processing for the same functions of thickening and stabilizing.

The one non-carbohydrate occurring in the cell walls of plants that is considered part of dietary fiber is *lignin*. Lignin is a polymer of phenyl propyl alcohols and acids and is contained in the woody portions of fruit and vegetables and in wheat bran.

Synthetic fiber products, *methyl cellulose* and

carboxymethylcellulose, besides being used in laxatives, are used in the production of low-calorie foods because of their ability to produce bulk and a feeling of satiety. The use of synthetic celluloses is increasing rapidly in a society that demands satisfying but low-calorie foods.

Definition of Fiber in the Human Diet. The long-standing inattention to dietary fiber has resulted in a confusion about what actually is "dietary fiber." It is different from *crude fiber*, which is mainly lignin and cellulose and is the material in food remaining after a vigorous standardized treatment with acid and alkali. Most food composition tables give values for crude fiber.

Dietary fiber, the significant substance for man's digestive tract, contains two to five times more substances than just crude fiber.[18] In addition to lignin and cellulose, dietary fiber also includes hemicellulose, gums, pectin, and other carbohydrates not normally digested by man.[23] The best data on the dietary fiber content of foods are those of Southgate.[20]

OTHER POLYSACCHARIDES.[12, 17] The *mucopolysaccharides* occur in combination with protein in body secretions and structures and are responsible for the viscosity of body mucous secretions. They are not found in significant quantity in food. Some of the common mucopolysaccharides are *hyaluronic acids*, part of intercellular material; *chondroitin sulfate*, found in cornea, cartilage, skin, aorta and heart valves; *heparin*, present as a naturally occurring anticoagulant in blood; *keratosulfate*, related to blood group substances; and *dermatan sulfate*, present in the skin.

Function of Carbohydrates in the Body

The body tissues require a constant daily supply of carbohydrate in the form of glucose in all metabolic reactions. Comparatively little is stored. Approximately 110 gm. of glycogen is stored in the liver and approximately 225 gm. in the muscles, and there is about 10 gm. of glucose in the blood. For most individuals, the supply available from the storage depots would be insufficient for one day's need.

1. The principal function of carbohydrate is to serve as a major source of energy for the body. It must be supplied regularly and at frequent intervals in order to meet the energy needs of the body. Each gram of carbohydrate yields approximately 4 kcalories regardless of the source —monosaccharide, disaccharide or polysaccharide.

2. Carbohydrates exert a protein-sparing action. If insufficient carbohydrates are available in the diet, the body will convert protein to glucose in order to supply energy (*gluconeogenesis*). The energy needs of the body take precedence over all other needs. It has been found that for optimum utilization of amino acids for protein formation, carbohydrates must be supplied simultaneously with the essential amino acids. Protein utilization seems to be favorably affected by the presence of carbohydrates in the same meal, and nitrogen balance is improved.

3. The presence of carbohydrates is necessary for normal fat metabolism. If there is insufficient carbohydrate, larger amounts of fat are used for energy than the body is equipped to handle and oxidation is incomplete. There is an accumulation of acidic intermediate products (the ketone bodies), and acidosis results. Sodium combines with these acids so that they are excreted as sodium salts in the urine. This could lead to losses of fluid and sodium and cause dehydration and sodium imbalance.

4. In the liver, *glucuronic acid*, a metabolite of glucose, has an important function in combining with chemical and bacterial toxins, as well as some normal metabolites, and converting them into a form in which they may be excreted.

5. Glucose has a specific influence in that it is indispensable for the maintenance of the functional integrity of the nerve tissue and is the sole source of energy for the brain. Thus a constant supply of glucose from the blood is essential for the proper functioning of these tissues. Any lack of glucose or oxygen for its oxidation may cause irreversible damage to the brain.

6. Lactose remains in the intestines longer than the other disaccharides and thus encourages the growth of beneficial bacteria, resulting in a laxative action. One of the functions of these bacteria is believed to be the synthesis of certain vitamins (B-complex vitamins and vitamin K).

7. As previously described, cellulose and the closely related insoluble, indigestible carbohydrates aid in normal elimination. They stimulate the peristaltic movements of the gastrointestinal tract and absorb water to give bulk to the intestinal contents.

8. Carbohydrates or products derived from them serve as precursors to such compounds as nucleic acids, connective tissue matrix and galactosides of nerve tissue.

9. Foods that are usually considered for their carbohydrate content (e.g., cereals) also supply significant quantities of protein, minerals and B-vitamins.

METABOLISM OF CARBOHYDRATES

The digestion, absorption and metabolic breakdown of carbohydrates are discussed in Chapter 5. Figure 2–4 briefly summarizes and

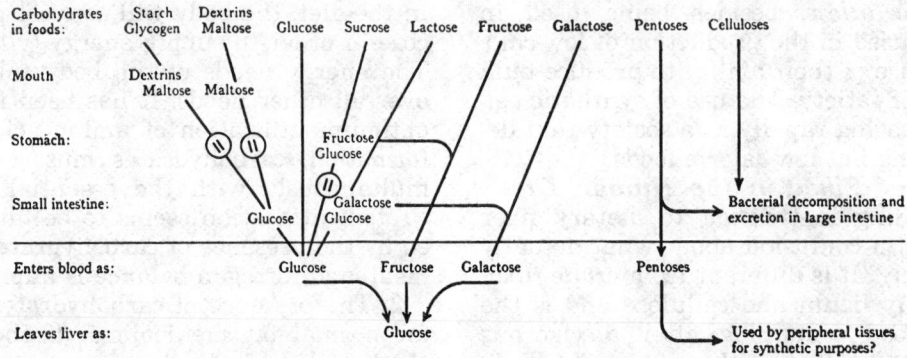

Figure 2–4. Products of carbohydrate digestion at various levels of the gastrointestinal tract and their subsequent fate. The ringed "ditto" signs indicate that the same products as at the preceding level continue to appear. (From Bondy, P. K., and Rosenberg, L. E.: Metabolic Control and Disease. 8th ed. Philadelphia, W. B. Saunders Company, 1980.)

reviews the digestion products of carbohydrates in the gastrointestinal tract and their subsequent fate, demonstrating the interrelations among carbohydrates.

Carbohydrates are absorbed through the intestinal mucosa as monosaccharides, primarily glucose with minor quantities of other sugars. All carbohydrate is then carried in the portal blood to the liver, after which it will be utilized in one of five ways. First, much of the glucose is used for immediate energy needs via oxidation (*tricarboxylic acid cycle*) to CO_2 and H_2O. This takes place in all tissues. Second, part is stored as glycogen in liver and muscle tissue. Third, some is converted to fatty acids and possibly stored as triglycerides in fat tissue (unfortunately an unlimited ability of the human body!). Fourth, a small amount is converted to other necessary carbohydrates, such as ribose, fructose (for spermatozoa), deoxyribose, glucosamine and galactosamine. Fifth, some becomes the carbon skeletons for the production by the body of the nonessential amino acids.

The utilization of glucose for energy involves a complex series of reactions, each one catalyzed by its specific enzyme and in many cases a B vitamin coenzyme. Energy is released, part of it as heat and part in the form of ATP (*adenosine triphosphate*), a special "high energy phosphate" or storage form of energy, which can be used as needed for muscular work, synthetic processes and other needs of the body. The first step in glucose metabolism is conversion of glucose to glucose-6-phosphate. From this point it may be broken down anaerobically to two three-carbon units, with release of a small amount of energy, and then via an active two-carbon unit, called *acetyl coenzyme A* or *acetyl-CoA*, to carbon dioxide and water, with liberation of a much larger amount of energy. These reactions occur in all tissues. Refer to the discussion on cell metabolism in Chapter 5.

Glycogen synthesis (*glycogenesis*) also starts by way of glucose-6-phosphate which can be envisioned as sitting astride the crossroads of carbohydrate metabolism. Figure 2–5 gives an abbreviated schematic outline of these reactions.

Fructose and galactose are converted to glucose in the liver and possibly to some extent in the intestinal mucosal cell. Some individuals lack the specific enzymes required for one or the other of these transformations. Mild to severe abnormalities in metabolism may result. Refer to the discussion on cell metabolism in Chapter 5.

Blood Sugar Regulation

The blood glucose is held at a remarkably constant level, 70 to 100 mg. per 100 ml. under fasting conditions. Some of the factors that influence the level of blood sugar are listed in Ta-

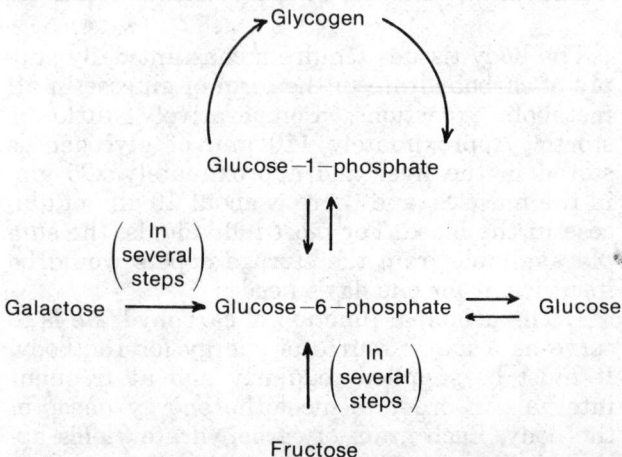

Figure 2–5. Summary of the overall process of glycogen formation and hydrolysis. Glycogen synthesis involves uridine diphosphate (UDP) and uridine triphosphate (UTP) as well as ADP and ATP.

Table 2–3. FACTORS INFLUENCING THE LEVEL OF BLOOD SUGAR

FACTORS THAT LOWER BLOOD SUGAR	FACTORS THAT INCREASE BLOOD SUGAR
Prolonged undernutrition	Excessive carbohydrate intake
Decreased absorption of glucose	Increased absorption of glucose
Increased exercise	Reduced exercise
Liver damage	Liver damage
Kidney abnormalities (renal glycosuria)	Hyperactivity of anterior pituitary
Anterior pituitary deficiency	Hyperactivity of adrenal cortex
Hypothyroidism	Diabetes mellitus
Adrenal insufficiency	Epinephrine
Insulin	Anesthesia
Sulfonylureas (stimulate insulin release)	Toxemias
Biguanides	Head injuries
	Fright and anger (stimulate epinephrine release)
	Glucagon
	Glucocorticoids
	Growth hormone
	Thyroxine

ble 2–3. The sugar level increases after a meal but returns to normal as the glucose is utilized and stored. As glucose in the blood is taken up by the tissues, liver glycogen is continually converted to glucose (*glycogenolysis*) and diffuses into the blood. Muscle glycogen is used only for energy and cannot be returned to the blood as glucose; however, lactic acid produced from muscle glycogen oxidation is carried to the liver, where it can be converted to glucose and glycogen (*Cori cycle*). If fasting is prolonged, gluconeogenesis occurs and amino acids and glycerol (from fat) are converted to glucose.

A battery of hormones is involved in the regulation of these reactions. *Insulin* is produced by the beta cells of the islets of Langerhans in the pancreas and affects carbohydrate metabolism by inducing the synthesis of certain enzymes. It has been called the "feasting hormone" because its liberation is enhanced by a high glucose level in the blood and to a lesser extent by the ingestion of protein or infusion of amino acids (particularly arginine) or ketone bodies. Hormones such as glucagon and the gastrointestinal hormones, stimulation of the vagus nerve, and certain drugs such as tolbutamide (an oral hypoglycemic agent) also stimulate its release. Insulin works to lower blood glucose by (1) increasing the facilitated diffusion of glucose into muscle and adipose cells, (2) promoting storage of glucose as glycogen in the liver and muscle cells and (3) enhancing the uptake of glucose by adipose and liver cells for conversion into fat. In summary then, insulin increases the rate of glucose utilization for all three purposes—oxidation, glycogenesis and lipogenesis.

Glucagon, produced by the alpha cells of the islets of Langerhans, has an effect exactly opposite to that of insulin. It causes a rise in the amount of sugar in the blood by increasing glycogenolysis and gluconeogenesis and stimulates the release of insulin from the pancreas. A similar form produced by the intestine (enteroglucagon) also stimulates the release of insulin but does not have glycogenolytic activity and appears to be under a different control than pancreatic glucagon. Thus, insulin and glucagon may be considered to be antagonists, and it is at least in part through their opposing effects that carbohydrate metabolism is maintained in a steady state.

Epinephrine, a hormone produced by the adrenal medulla gland, tends to favor the breakdown of liver and muscle glycogen to yield blood glucose (glycogenolysis) and decreases the release of insulin from the pancreas, thereby raising the blood sugar. The secretion of epinephrine is increased during anger or fear, and the increased formation of glucose that follows presumably serves as a source of extra energy to permit the body to respond more rapidly to the crisis.

Glucocorticoids, steroid hormones elaborated by the adrenal cortex, also influence blood glucose levels by stimulating gluconeogenesis. These hormones apparently reduce the utilization of glucose by the tissues and also increase the rate at which protein is converted into glucose. The net result of these two actions is to increase blood glucose; i.e., these steroid hormones counteract the action of insulin. Glucocorticoids also influence fat and protein metabolism, which will be discussed in Chapters 3 and 4.

When the blood glucose concentration is severely decreased, *thyroxine* secretion by the thyroid gland is increased. It stimulates hepatic glycogenolysis and gluconeogenesis, and the blood glucose concentration rises. Thyroxine also increases the rate of hexose absorption from the intestine.

Growth hormone, elaborated by the anterior pituitary gland, also raises the blood glucose. Growth hormone increases amino acid uptake and protein synthesis by all cells, diminishes cellular uptake of glucose and increases the mobilization of fat for energy. It spares both protein and carbohydrate.

In summary, the processes adding glucose to the blood and the processes removing glucose from the blood are in dynamic equilibrium depending upon the body's need for energy and the time since the last meal. Figure 2–6 summarizes this.

Metabolism of Ethyl Alcohol (Ethanol)

Ethyl alcohol is produced when yeast ferments carbohydrate. Every gram of alcohol yields approximately 7.0 kcal. when completely metabolized. It is rapidly absorbed from the stomach and small intestine, uniformly distributed throughout the body water, and rapidly oxidized with little or none stored. Small amounts are lost into the urine and into the respired air by diffusion. The "breath test" to determine whether a driver is intoxicated is a practical application of this physiological fact.

In the liver, ethyl alcohol is converted to acetaldehyde, and then to acetyl-CoA which, as has been discussed, may readily be utilized for energy. The rate of metabolism of alcohol is increased by fructose, but the effect varies with the individual. This is a possible reason for mixing alcohol with fruit juices or sugar-containing (fructose and glucose) mixers.

Experimental animals fed appreciable amounts of ethanol will grow about as efficiently as animals fed isocaloric quantities of carbohydrate or fat, if the protein, vitamin, essential amino acid and fatty acid requirements are met. Apparently, a high ethanol diet can provide the major portion of the energy needs of an individual; however, such a diet would be inadequate in all other respects.

This has been of necessity a very brief outline of carbohydrate metabolism. (The details of this very complex subject are presented in biochemistry texts listed at the end of this chapter.) Common abnormalities of carbohydrate metabolism are presented in Part 2. Diabetes mellitus is discussed in Chapter 25, carbohydrate malabsorption syndromes such as lactose intolerance in Chapter 23, and inborn errors of carbohydrate metabolism such as galactosemia in Chapter 39.

Daily Dietary Allowance

The body can utilize protein or fat for energy if carbohydrate is limited. However, if fat is serving as the main source of energy, intermedi-

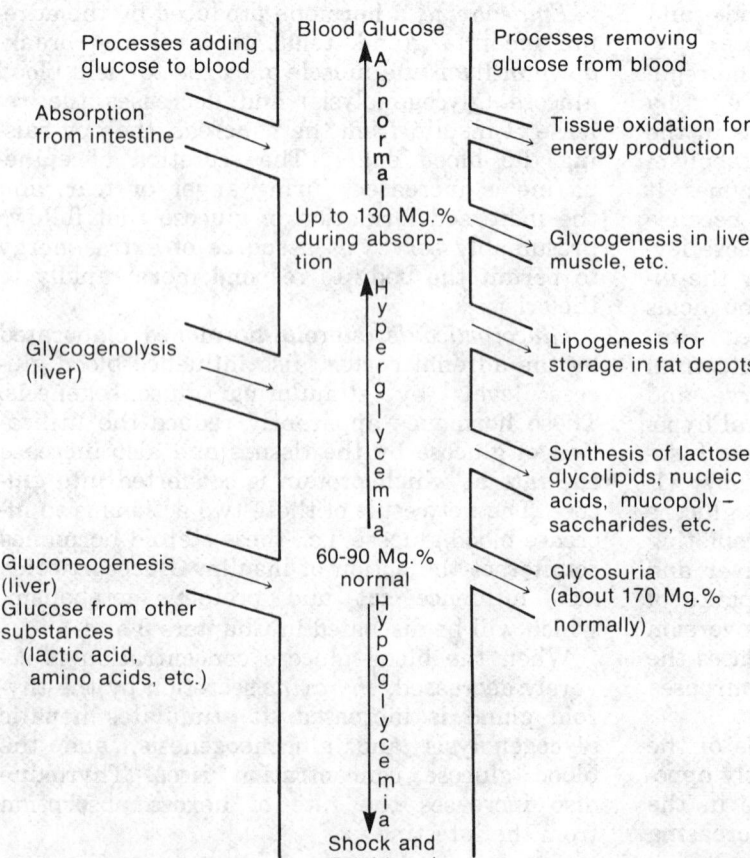

Figure 2–6. Blood glucose maintenance. (Adapted from West, E. S., et al.: Textbook of Biochemistry. 4th ed. New York, Macmillan Company, 1966.)

ates in the oxidative process are formed faster than they can be completely oxidized. Accumulation of these products causes acidosis. Utilization of protein for energy is wasteful because protein foods are expensive, the part burned for energy cannot be used for building body proteins, and the nitrogen is excreted in the urine and wasted.

There is no specific RDA for carbohydrate. According to the Food and Nutrition Board of the National Research Council in the 1980 revision,

Man, like most mammals, is capable of converting amino acids and the glycerol moiety of fats to glucose, and as a consequence there is no specific dietary requirement for carbohydrate. Nonetheless, it is generally agreed that a reasonable proportion of the calorie intake should be derived from carbohydrate. A diet devoid of carbohydrate is likely to lead to ketosis, excessive breakdown of tissue protein, loss of cations, especially sodium, and involuntary dehydration. These effects, produced by high-fat diets or fasting, can be prevented by the ingestion of 50–100 gm. of digestible carbohydrate per day. However, intakes considerably above this minimal level are desirable.[9]

Carbohydrate in the American Diet

TRENDS IN COMSUMPTION OF CARBOHYDRATES

Today's average American consumes a diet in which about 45 per cent of the calories come from carbohydrates, as shown in Table 2–4. Over the past 70 years carbohydrate consumption steadily declined until 1965, and since then there has been a slow increase in consumption. However, compared with the 1909–1913 intake of 492 gm. per person per day, the 1980 per capita consumption of 408 gm. per day is still much lower.

There has also been a decrease in per capita consumption of complex carbohydrate or starch. In 1909–1913, 68 per cent of the carbohydrate was complex; in 1980, 47 per cent was complex. The decrease in complex carbohydrate consumption is reflected in less consumption of grains, breads, cereals and potatoes, although this appears to be beginning to change.

Over half of the carbohydrates are consumed as sugars. Thus, about 17 per cent of the total energy in the diet comes from refined sugar, syrups, and other sweeteners. This is a per capita consumption of 143 pounds per year, up from 114 pounds in 1947–1949 and 91 pounds in 1909–1913.[24] The form of sugar has also changed over the past 50 years.[15] Whereas in 1949 the majority of sugar was eaten from the 5- or 10-pound bag of sugar in the home, today the majority is eaten in processed foods to which sugar or sweetener has been added in the processing.

The current trend appears to be one of continuing consumption of refined sugars, although this appears to be beginning to change with the increased consumption of sugar-free sodas and reduced-sugar products.

SUGAR AND HEALTH

Sugar, particularly sucrose, plays a role in the etiology of dental caries; however, it has been found that all forms of carbohydrate, including starch, can cause caries in the presence of the proper bacteria. Interestingly, the total amount of sugar consumed does not seem to be the deciding factor in the development of caries, but rather the physical form (sticky vs. liquid) and manner and frequency (a between-meal snack vs. part of a meal) with which it is eaten and the foods it is eaten with.[11] Bibby concludes that the increasing frequency of eating or

Table 2–4. CARBOHYDRATE AVAILABLE PER PERSON PER DAY AND PER CENT FURNISHED BY STARCH AND SUGARS

YEAR	GRAMS CARBO-HYDRATE	PER CENT STARCH*	PER CENT SUGARS†	PER CENT OF TOTAL K CALORIES
1909–1913	492	68.3	31.7	56.2
1925–1929	476	58.7	41.3	54.4
1935–1939	436	56.8	43.2	52.8
1947–1949	403	52.4	47.6	49.4
1957–1959	374	49.6	50.4	47.3
1965	374	48.8	51.2	47.0
1971	380	47.1	52.9	46.8
1974	385	46.5	53.5	45.9
1980	408	47.0	53.0	46.0

* Grains and starch vegetables.
† Fruits and sugar.
(Sources: Friend, B.: Nutrients in United States food supply. Am. J. Clin. Nutr., 20:911–912, 1967. Sugar: 1975. Washington, D.C., The Sugar Association, Inc., 1975. Friend, B., and Marston, R.: Nutritional Review. Consumer and Food Economics Institute, Agricultural Research Service, November, 1974. Welsh, S. O., and Marston, R. M.: Review of trends in food use in the United States, 1909–1980. J. Am. Diet. Assoc., 81:120, 1982.)

snacking and the popularity of mixtures of sugar and flour as snack items (e.g., pastries, cookies, cakes) may be the most important reasons for the increased incidence of dental caries in this country[1] (see Chapter 33).

The consumption of sugar (sucrose) has been postulated by several investigators to be a factor in the development of coronary heart disease.[10] A problem with making a definitive statement is that in the typical American diet it is difficult to separate the influence of dietary sucrose from dietary fat in the development of coronary heart disease. The evidence now is not strong enough to say that sugar consumption is a causative factor in the development of coronary heart disease[10] (see Chapter 28).

Sugar consumption has also been implicated in the increasing incidence of obesity. Again, there is no evidence to implicate sucrose any more than alcohol, fat or protein. Obesity results from an excess of calories regardless of the source. There can be the occasion, however, when similar to the alcoholic, the "carboholic" loses all control after the first bite of concentrated carbohydrate and goes on a binge with a resulting large intake of calories and eventual overweight[3] (see Chapter 27).

Within the past 10 years refined sugar has been implicated as a cause of disruptive and hyperactive behavior in children and youth. However, there are no scientific, well-controlled studies to document this suspicion (see Chapter 32).

DIETARY FIBER AND HEALTH

No longer can fiber avoid the attention of nutritionists. Its disappearance from the Western diet is being scrutinized as a factor in the etiology of diabetes, hyperlipoproteinemia, and common noninfective diseases of the colon such as constipation, hemorrhoids, diverticulosis and cancer.[5, 6] Several protective qualities have been attributed to dietary fiber. By affecting stool bulk, softness, and transit time, it is thought to be a factor in (1) lessening colonic pressure that may lead to diverticula[16] (see Chapter 23), (2) reducing the exposure of the gut mucosa to possible carcinogenic substances in the feces[4] (see Chapter 36), and (3) lowering blood cholesterol by binding with bile acids, thus leading to an increased cholesterol degradation and excretion via the bile acid pathways (see Chapter 28). However, the findings are not definitive enough yet to define an adequate or recommended level of fiber intake. Much of the evidence is epidemiological, comparing disease incidence in countries with high fiber intakes with the incidence in Western countries where the fiber intake is relatively low, but where a number of other factors are also different.

The dietary fiber content of a "typical" American diet has been estimated to be about 20 gm. per day.[19] This is much lower than the intake observed in some African tribes of as much as 150 gm. per day.[2]

The current guidelines for the proportions of complex carbohydrate and simple sugars in the diet recommended by various nutrition groups are discussed in Chapter 17.

COMMON SOURCES OF STARCHES AND SUGARS

The groups of food providing appreciable amounts of carbohydrate in the diet are (1) grains, (2) fruits, (3) vegetables, (4) milk, and (5) the refined sugars and concentrated sweets (Table 2–5).

Refined sugar, syrups and cornstarch are ex-

Table 2–5.   CARBOHYDRATE CONTENT OF SOME TYPICAL FOODS

SUGAR	CARBO-HYDRATE (Per cent)	STARCH	CARBO-HYDRATE (Per cent)
Concentrated Sweets		*Grain Products*	
Sugar: Cane, beet, powdered,	99.5	Starches: Corn, tapioca, arrowroot	86–88
brown, maple	90–96	Cereals (dry): Corn, wheat, oat, bran	68–85
Candies	70–95	Flour: Corn, wheat (sifted)	70–80
Honey (extracted)	82	Popcorn (popped)	77
Syrup: Table blends, molasses	55–75	Cookies: Plain, assorted	71
Jams, jellies, marmalades	70	Crackers, saltines	72
Carbonated, sweetened beverages	10–12	Cakes: Plain, without icing	56
Fruits		Bread: White, rye, whole wheat	48–52
Prunes, apricots, figs (cooked, unsweet)	12–31	Macaroni, spaghetti, noodles, rice (cooked)	23–30
Bananas, grapes, cherries, apples, pears	15–23	Cereals (cooked): Oat, wheat, grits	10–16
Fresh: Pineapples, grapefruits, oranges,		*Vegetables*	
apricots, strawberries	8–14	Boiled: Corn, white and sweet potatoes, lima,	
Milk		dried beans, peas	15–26
Skim	6	Beets, carrots, onions, tomatoes	5–7
Whole	5	Leafy: Lettuce asparagus, cabbage, greens,	
		spinach	4–3

a Kernel of Wheat

The kernel of wheat is a storehouse of nutrients needed and used by man since the dawn of civilization. Today's bread, flour and cereals—enriched, whole grain and restored—are one of four groups of food recommended for optimum nutrition by the U.S. Department of Agriculture. This popular, low-cost group includes such foods made from wheat as bread, rolls, biscuits, muffins, pancakes, breakfast cereals, macaroni, spaghetti and noodles. Nutrients listed below are considered esssential in human diet.

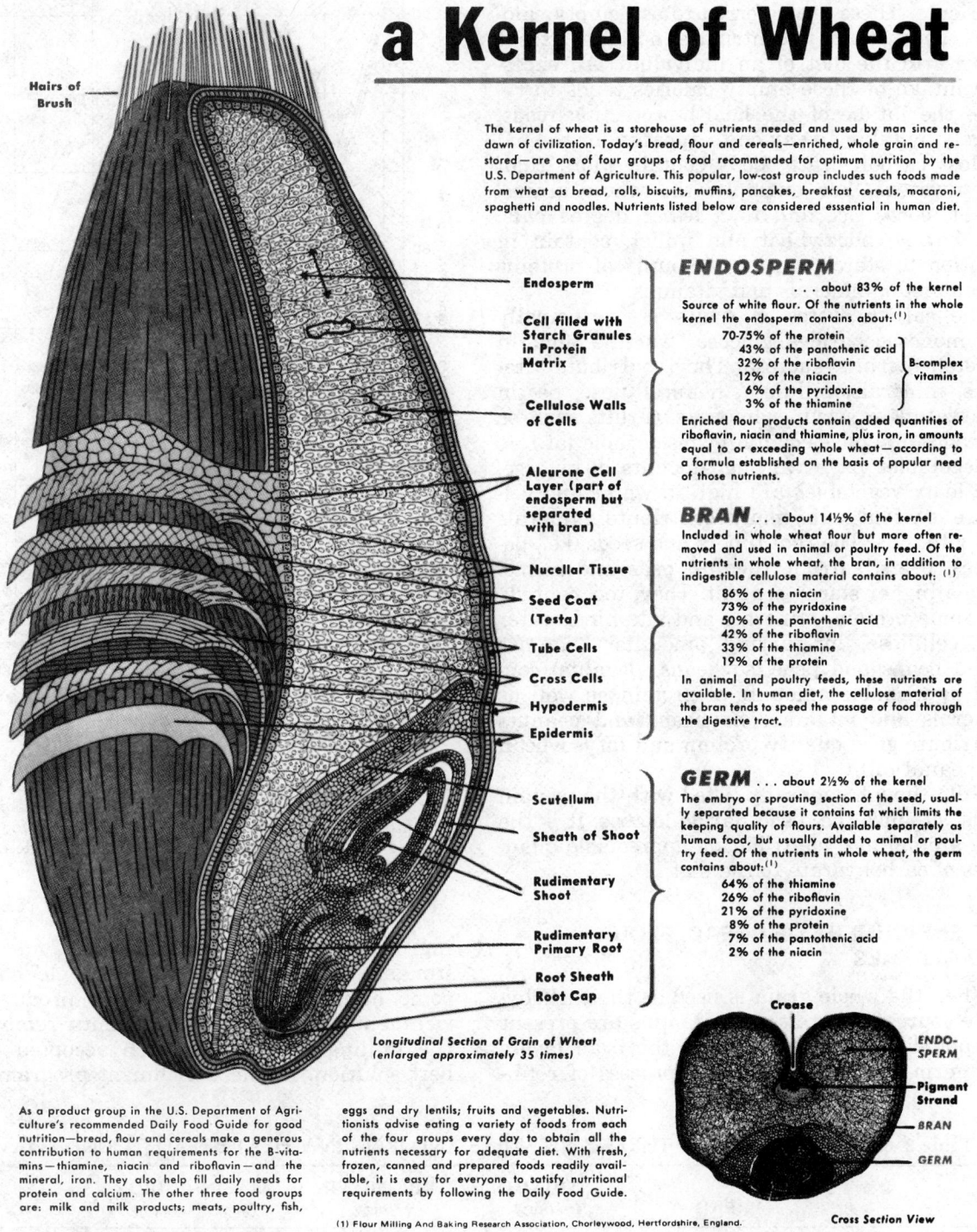

Hairs of Brush

Endosperm

Cell filled with Starch Granules in Protein Matrix

Cellulose Walls of Cells

Aleurone Cell Layer (part of endosperm but separated with bran)

Nucellar Tissue

Seed Coat (Testa)

Tube Cells

Cross Cells

Hypodermis

Epidermis

Scutellum

Sheath of Shoot

Rudimentary Shoot

Rudimentary Primary Root

Root Sheath

Root Cap

Longitudinal Section of Grain of Wheat (enlarged approximately 35 times)

ENDOSPERM
... about 83% of the kernel

Source of white flour. Of the nutrients in the whole kernel the endosperm contains about:[1]

70-75% of the protein
43% of the pantothenic acid
32% of the riboflavin
12% of the niacin
6% of the pyridoxine
3% of the thiamine

B-complex vitamins

Enriched flour products contain added quantities of riboflavin, niacin and thiamine, plus iron, in amounts equal to or exceeding whole wheat—according to a formula established on the basis of popular need of those nutrients.

BRAN ... about 14½% of the kernel

Included in whole wheat flour but more often removed and used in animal or poultry feed. Of the nutrients in whole wheat, the bran, in addition to indigestible cellulose material contains about: [1]

86% of the niacin
73% of the pyridoxine
50% of the pantothenic acid
42% of the riboflavin
33% of the thiamine
19% of the protein

In animal and poultry feeds, these nutrients are available. In human diet, the cellulose material of the bran tends to speed the passage of food through the digestive tract.

GERM ... about 2½% of the kernel

The embryo or sprouting section of the seed, usually separated because it contains fat which limits the keeping quality of flours. Available separately as human food, but usually added to animal or poultry feed. Of the nutrients in whole wheat, the germ contains about:[1]

64% of the thiamine
26% of the riboflavin
21% of the pyridoxine
8% of the protein
7% of the pantothenic acid
2% of the niacin

Crease

ENDO-SPERM

Pigment Strand

BRAN

GERM

Cross Section View

As a product group in the U.S. Department of Agriculture's recommended Daily Food Guide for good nutrition—bread, flour and cereals make a generous contribution to human requirements for the B-vitamins—thiamine, niacin and riboflavin—and the mineral, iron. They also help fill daily needs for protein and calcium. The other three food groups are: milk and milk products; meats, poultry, fish, eggs and dry lentils; fruits and vegetables. Nutritionists advise eating a variety of foods from each of the four groups every day to obtain all the nutrients necessary for adequate diet. With fresh, frozen, canned and prepared foods readily available, it is easy for everyone to satisfy nutritional requirements by following the Daily Food Guide.

(1) Flour Milling And Baking Research Association, Chorleywood, Hertfordshire, England.

Figure 2–7. Diagram shows the structure, composition and nutritive values of a kernel of wheat. © 1976, Wheat Flour Institute, Washington, D.C.

amples of pure carbohydrates, and many of the sweets such as candy, honey, jellies, molasses and soft drinks contain little, if any, of other nutrients. These are referred to as "empty calories" because they contribute nothing except calories to the diet of an individual. An excessive intake of these empty calories tends to reduce the intake of the health-protecting foods, largely by taking away one's appetite for them.

Most carbohydrate foods contain more than one nutrient. For example, the whole grains, wheat, corn, rice and to a lesser degree oats, rye, barley, buckwheat and millet, contain in addition to starch varying amounts of proteins (incomplete), minerals and vitamins.

The carbohydrates in fruits are principally the monosaccharides glucose, fructose and, in sweetened fruits, sucrose. They contribute vitamins, minerals, cellulose, hemicellulose, pectin and water, in varying amounts. (Fruits such as avocados and olives contain considerable fat.)

Vegetables have varying amounts of glucose. The leafy vegetables are high in water and cellulose content and many contribute minerals and vitamins. The root tubers and seeds (i.e., potatoes, beets, carrots, turnips, peas and beans) have a higher starch content. They, too, contribute some protein, minerals and vitamins, water and cellulose, in varying amounts. Legumes (dried beans and peas, soybeans, peanuts) contain appreciable amounts of protein as well as minerals and vitamins. Soybeans and peanuts contribute good quality protein and fat (soybean oil, peanut oil).

Milk, though generally listed with the protein foods, supplies the disaccharide lactose. It is the only animal food contributing appreciable quantities of carbohydrate to the diet.

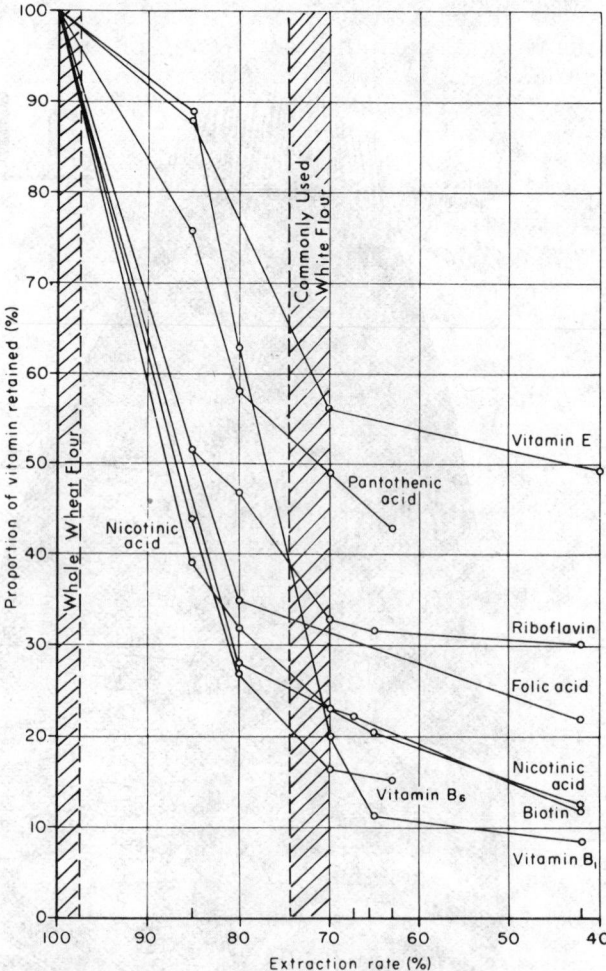

Figure 2–8. Relationship between extraction rate and proportion of total vitamins of the grain retained in flour. (Adapted from: Proposed Fortification Policy for Cereal-Grain Products. Washington, D.C., National Academy of Sciences, 1974.)

THE ENRICHMENT OF BREAD, FLOUR AND CEREALS

When the whole grain is used as the carbohydrate source, minerals and vitamins are present in appreciable amounts. When the bran layers and germ are removed by the process of refining, most of the thiamin, riboflavin, niacin and iron are lost (Fig. 2–7). Since people have become accustomed to the refined products, enrichment to replace the elements removed in the milling process has been accepted as the best solution. In the enrichment program these

Table 2–6. COMPARISON OF THREE B-VITAMINS AND IRON IN WHEAT BREAD (POUND LOAVES)

BREAD	THIAMIN (mg.)	RIBOFLAVIN (mg.)	NIACIN (mg.)	IRON (mg.)
Whole wheat made with 2% non-fat dry milk	1.17	0.56	12.9	10.4
White enriched* with 3 to 4% non-fat dry milk	1.8	1.1	15.0	11.3
White unenriched with 3 to 4% non-fat dry milk	0.31	0.39	5.0	3.2

*Enriched bread may also furnish, as an optional ingredient, added calcium salts in such quantity that each pound of the finished bread will contain 600 milligrams of calcium. (From Standards of Identity for Bakery Products, U.S. Dept. HEW, FDA, Federal Register 36:23074 (1971), 38:28558 (1973), 39:5188, (1974.)

three vitamins and mineral are added back to the level at which they are present in the whole grain flour. However, there are other vitamins, trace minerals and dietary fiber that are also removed but not replaced in the present enrichment program (Fig. 2–8).

The result of the enrichment of bread is seen in Table 2–6. Bread and flour enrichment is mandatory in most states and many other countries. It is widely practiced in those states without legal requirements. Almost 95 per cent of the white bread sold in the United States is enriched.[8] There also are federal standards for the enrichment of rice and corn grits. Nutrition scientists are in general agreement that this improvement in the nutritive quality of food has made a significant contribution to the improvement of nutrition and health.

Problems and Suggested Topics for Discussion

1. List the amounts of the various carbohydrate foods you consume during a period of 24 hours and a period of 3 days.
2. Evaluate the list of carbohydrate foods. Classify them into "sugars" and "starches." List the monosaccharides.
3. What percentage of calories in the daily diet should normally be consumed in the form of carbohydrate foods? When might this percentage be increased? Decreased?
4. Keep a record of your diet for one day. Calculate the carbohydrate and calorie content. What percentage of the calories were derived from carbohydrates? What percentage of the carbohydrate calories were derived from fruits, vegetables, breadstuffs and cereal foods? What percentage of the carbohydrate calories were derived from sugars, candy, soft drinks, cake and pie? List any changes you could make in carbohydrate content to improve your diet, and give reasons.
5. Why do you like to eat carbohydrate foods?
6. What factors tend to raise and to lower the blood sugar? What is the form of carbohydrate in the circulating blood? What is the normal concentration?
7. List the functions of carbohydrates in the body. What becomes of the carbohydrate eaten in excess of the body's daily need for energy?

Cited References

1. Bibby, B.G.: The cariogenicity of snack foods and confections. J. Am. Dent. Assoc., 90:121, 1975.
2. Bingham, S., and Cummings, J.H.: Sources and intakes of dietary fiber. In Spiller, G.A., and Kay, R.M. (eds.): Medical Aspects of Dietary Fiber. New York, Plenum Medical Book Company, 1980.
3. Bloom, W.L., and Clark, M.S.: Diagnosis and treatment of the obese carboholic. Obesity, 1:10, 1964.
4. Burkitt, D.P.: Epidemiology of cancer of the colon and rectum. Cancer, 28:3, 1971.
5. Burkitt, D.P.: Some diseases characteristic of modern western civilization. Br. Med. J., 1:274, 1973.
6. Burkitt, D.P., Walker, A.R., and Painter, N.S.: Dietary fiber and disease. JAMA, 229:1068, 1974.
7. Calloway, D.H.: Dietary components that yield energy. Environ. Bio. Med., 1:175, 1971.
8. Enriched Bread. Chicago, American Institute of Baking, 1976.
9. Food and Nutrition Board, Recommended Dietary Allowances. 9th ed. Washington, D.C., National Research Council, National Academy of Sciences, 1980.
10. Grande, F.: Sugar and cardiovascular disease. World Rev. Nutr. Diet., 22:248, 1975.
11. Gustafsson, B.E., et al.: The Vipeholm dental caries study: the effect of different levels of carbohydrates intake on caries activity in 436 individuals observed for 5 years. Acta. Odontol. Scand., 11:232, 1954.
12. Guthrie, H.A.: Introductory Nutrition. 3rd ed. St. Louis, C.V. Mosby Company, 1975.
13. Hardinge, M.G., Swarner, J.B., and Crooks, H.: Carbohydrates in foods. J. Am. Diet. Assoc., 46:197, 1965.
14. Nelson, R.A.: Role of unavailable carbohydrate (UC) in digestion. In White, P.L., Fletcher, D.C., and Ellis, M. (eds.): Nutrients in Processed Foods—Fats, Carbohydrates. Acton, Mass., Publishing Sciences Group, Inc., 1975.
15. Page, L., and Friend, B.: Level of use of sugars in the United States. In Sipple, H.L., and McNutt, K.W. (eds.): Sugars in Nutrition. New York, Nutrition Foundation Inc., Academic Press, 1974.
16. Painter, N.S., Almeida, A.Z., and Colebourne, K. W.: Unprocessed bran in treatment of diverticular disease of the colon. Br. Med. J., 2:137, 1972.
17. Pike, R.L., and Brown, M.L.: Nutrition: An Integrated Approach. 2nd ed. New York, John Wiley & Sons, Inc., 1975.
18. Scala, J.: Fiber. The forgotten nutrient. J. Food Technology, 28:34, 1974.
19. Southgate, D.A.T.: Chemical aspects. In Truelove, S.C., and Heyworth, M.F. (eds.): Topics in Gastroenterology. Oxford, Blackwell Scientific Publications, 1978, p. 13.
20. Southgate, D.A.T., et al: A guide to calculating intakes of dietary fiber, J. Human Nutr., 30:303, 1976.
21. Stare, F.J. (ed.): Sugar in the diet of man. World Rev. Nutr. Diet., 22:237, 1975.
22. Toscano, V.A.: Sugars and other carbohydrates. In White, P.L., Fletcher, D.C., and Ellis, M. (eds.): Nutrients in Processed Foods—Fats, Carbohydrates. Acton, Mass., Publishing Sciences Group, Inc., 1975.
23. Trowell, H.: Dietary fibre, coronary heart disease and diabetes mellitus. Plant Foods for Man, 1:11, 1973.
24. Welsh, S.O., and Marston, R.M.: Review of trends in food use in the United States, 1909 to 1980. J. Am. Diet. Assoc., 81:121, 1982.
25. White, P.L., Fletcher, D.C., and Ellis, M. (eds.): Nutrients in Processed Foods—Fats and Carbohydrates. Acton, Mass., Publishing Sciences Group, Inc., 1975.

Additional References

Anderson, T.A.: Recent trends in carbohydrate consumption. Ann. Rev. Nutr., 2:113, 1982.
Gray, G.M.: Carbohydrate digestion and absorption—role of small intestine. N. Engl. J. Med., 292:1225, 1975.
Guyton, A.C.: Textbook of Medical Physiology. 6th ed. Philadelphia, W. B. Saunders Company, 1981.
McGilvery, R.W.: Biochemistry: A Functional Approach. 2nd ed. Philadelphia, W.B. Saunders Company, 1979.
Martin, D.W.: Harper's Review of Biochemistry. 18th ed. Los Altos, California, Lange Medical Publications, 1981.
Mendeloff, A.I.: Dietary fiber and human health. N. Engl. J. Med., 297:811, 1977.
The role of fiber in the diet. Dairy Council Digest, 46:1, 1975.
Spiller, J.A., and Amen, R.J. (ed.): Fiber in Human Nutrition. New York, Plenum Press, 1976.
Sugar: 1975. Washington, D.C., The Sugar Association, Inc., 1975.
Worthington-Roberts, B.S.: Contemporary Developments in Nutrition. St. Louis, C.V. Mosby Company, 1981.

Lipids

The term lipid, often used interchangeably with the term fat, describes a heterogeneous group of compounds related to the fatty acids. They have the common properties of being (1) insoluble in water, (2) soluble in organic solvents such as ether and chloroform and (3) utilizable by living organisms. This group thus includes the ordinary fats and oils, waxes and related compounds. The principal foods contributing fat to the diet are butter, margarine, lard, vegetable oil, salad dressing, the visible fat of meat, the skin of chicken and the invisible fat found in cream, milk, milk products, egg yolk, meat, fish, poultry, nuts, seeds, olives, avocados and whole-grain cereals.

Classification and Composition

The principal groups of lipids important in nutrition are listed and classified in Table 3–1.

Most natural fats are composed of about 98 to 99 per cent triglycerides, and the vast majority of these are *long chain* triglycerides. The 1 or 2 per cent remaining include traces of mono- and diglycerides, free fatty acids, phospholipids and unsaponifiable matter containing sterols.

TRIGLYCERIDES

Like carbohydrates, *triglycerides* (the main component of ordinary fats and oils) are composed of carbon, hydrogen and oxygen. Structurally they are esters of a trihydric alcohol (glycerol) and fatty acids, as shown in Figure 3–1. Because of this structure triglycerides are also called *triacylglycerols*. The fatty acids can have from 4 to 30 carbon atoms and make up the bulk of the triglyceride. One hundred grams of fat will contain 95 grams of fatty acids.

FATTY ACIDS: SATURATED AND UNSATURATED. A fatty acid or hydrocarbon chain is described with regard to three characteristics: chain length, degree of saturation with hydrogen and location of the first double bond. The *length* is defined as the number of carbon atoms in the chain. For example, C_{16} denotes 16 carbons in the chain. Frequently, the terms "short"

(six or fewer carbons), "medium" and "long" (12 or more carbons) are used to describe the chains of fatty acids in triglycerides. The *degree of hydrogen saturation* is defined by the number of double bonds between the carbon atoms in the chains. A chain may contain all the hydrogen it can hold and have no double bonds, in which case it is called a *saturated fatty acid*. It may contain one double bond and be called a *monounsaturated fatty acid*, or it may be a *polyunsaturated fatty acid* and contain several double bonds, as shown in Figure 3–2. The *location of the first double bond*, as counted from the

Table 3–1. CLASSIFICATION OF LIPIDS IMPORTANT TO NUTRITION

I. *Simple Lipids*
  A. Fatty acids
  B. Neutral fats: Mono-, di-, triglycerides (esters of fatty acids and glycerol)
  C. Esters of fatty acids with high molecular weight alcohols
    1. Waxes
    2. Sterol esters
    3. Nonsterol esters
II. *Compound Lipids*
  A. Phospholipids: Compounds of fatty acids, phosphoric acid and nitrogenous base
    1. Lecithins
    2. Cephalins
    3. Sphingomyelins
  B. Glycolipids: Compounds of fatty acid combined with carbohydrate and a nitrogenous base
    1. Cerebrosides
    2. Gangliosides
  C. Sulfolipids: Sulfur-containing lipids
  D. Lipoproteins: Lipids in combination with protein
    1. Apolipoproteins
  E. Lipopolysaccharides: polysaccharide-containing lipids
III. *Derived Lipids*
  A. Fatty acids
  B. Glycerol: Water-soluble component of triglycerides and interconvertible with carbohydrate
  C. Mono- and diglycerides
  D. Sterols
    1. Cholesterol, ergosterol
    2. Steroid hormones
    3. Vitamin D
    4. Bile salts
  E. Fat-soluble vitamins
    1. Vitamin A
    2. Vitamin E
    3. Vitamin K
    4. Coenzyme Q (ubiquinone)

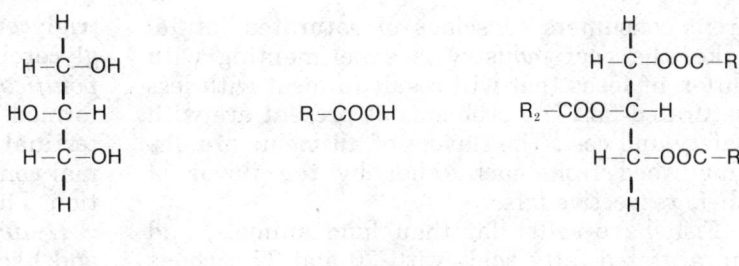

Figure 3–1. Structure of a triglyceride, which is an ester of glycerol and fatty acids.

Glycerol   Fatty Acid   Triglyceride

methyl end of the fatty acid, is the *omega (ω) number*, or "n" number. It is used only in reference to unsaturated fatty acids.

The whole series of saturated fatty acids has been found in natural fats. However, the only unsaturated fatty acids that naturally occur in large amounts contain 18 carbons, although there are small amounts of 16-, 20- and 22-carbon unsaturated fatty acids.

A convenient shorthand gives the number of carbon atoms, the number of double bonds and the ω number. For example, linoleic acid is designated as $C_{18:2\ \omega-6}$ because it has 18 carbons, 2 double bonds and the first double bond is at the sixth carbon. Besides this form of identification, fatty acids also have common names that usually indicate the fat from which they were isolated, e.g., linoleic from linseed oil and butyric from butter.

The diversity of natural fats is influenced by the properties of triglycerides in each fat, and the triglycerides are related to their fatty acids. The physical properties of the fatty acids are related to their chemical structure. The shorter and more unsaturated the fatty acids, the more liquid or soft the fat or oil is at room temperature. Solid fats such as mutton tallow contain large amounts of palmitic ($C_{16:0}$) and stearic ($C_{18:0}$) acids. Oils (fats that are liquid at room temperature) usually have a high proportion of oleic ($C_{18:1\ \omega-9}$) and linoleic ($C_{18:2\ \omega-6}$) acids.

The position of the fatty acids on the glycerol molecule also influences the properties, digestibility and absorption of the triglyceride. The ω number also affects the metabolism of the fatty acids.

Because of the large number of fatty acids in natural foods and the many possible combinations in the formation of triglycerides, there are a large number of different triglycerides in any fat.

SYNTHETIC FATS. *Medium chain triglycerides* are unnaturally occurring forms of fat that are absorbed and metabolized differently from long chain triglycerides. They are triglycerides composed of fatty acids with lengths of eight and ten carbon atoms and were formulated to provide a source of dietary fat for people with fat malabsorption problems. The principal fatty acid is octanoic acid ($C_{8:0}$).

Polyglycerol esters are synthetic hybrid fats made by the esterification of fatty acids. Although they look and taste like fat, they have fewer calories—6.5 to 8.5 kcal./gm. instead of 9 kcal./gm. for traditional fats. Food processors are using them to make low-calorie, palatable foods.

Another product, *sucrose-polyester (SPE)*, has been developed as a substitute for solid or liquid fat. It is made by combining fatty acids with sucrose, and looks and tastes like regular margarine or vegetable oil. It is being developed because it cannot be digested or absorbed by the body, and the food industry is also using it in the development of low-fat, low-calorie foods.

CHARACTERISTICS OF ANIMAL AND VEGETABLE FATS. There is considerable species variation in fats from animal sources. The major components of the fats of land animals are palmitic, stearic and oleic acids, with smaller amounts of linoleic acid and traces of arachidonic acid ($C_{20:4\ \omega-6}$). The fat of the herbivorous animals (beef and mutton tallow) is harder (more saturated) than pork and poultry fats. The degree of unsaturation of pork, beef and chicken fat may vary, depending on the diet of the animal. In fact, in response to pressure from associations concerned with heart disease and

$$CH_3(CH_2)_{16}COOH$$ Stearic Acid (Saturated)

$$CH_3(CH_2)_7CH=CH(CH_2)_7COOH$$ Oleic Acid (Mono-unsaturated)

$$CH_3(CH_2)_4CH=CHCH_2CH=CH(CH_2)_7COOH$$ Linoleic Acid (Polyunsaturated)

Figure 3–2. 18-Carbon fatty acids.

$$CH_3CH_2CH=CHCH_2CH=CH-CH_2-CH=CH(CH_2)_7COOH$$ Linolenic Acid (Polyunsaturated)

from consumers conscious of saturated fat intake, the beef industry is experimenting with different feeds that will result in meat with less saturated fat. The problems at present are with safety and cost. The flavors of all meats are distinguished from each other by the flavor of their respective fats.

Fish have softer fat than land animals, and unsaturated fatty acids with 20 and 22 carbons predominate in fish fat. In addition a majority of unsaturated fatty acids in fish are ω-3, as shown in Table 3–2. It appears that ω-3 unsaturated fatty acids have unique serum triglyceride lowering properties.[8] This is discussed further on page 565.

Vegetable oils are predominantly unsaturated, with a majority of the fatty acids being linoleic as shown in Table 3–2. An exception is coconut oil, which is almost completely saturated but has a low melting point because of a high content of medium chain fatty acids (8 to 12 carbons).

REACTIONS OF FATS. Enzymes of the digestive tract act as catalysts for the hydrolysis of triglycerides to their component fatty acids and glycerol. If the fat is hydrolyzed with alkali *(saponification)*, salts of the fatty acids or soaps are formed. Formation of insoluble soaps in the intestinal tract may be of concern in some abnormal conditions characterized by poor fat absorption. This is discussed further in Chapter 23.

Hydrogenation. Unsaturated fatty acids can add hydrogen to the double bonds, as shown in Figure 3–3. Thus, oleic acid, linoleic acid and linolenic acid when completely hydrogenated become stearic acid. Vegetable oils may be converted to solid fats by hydrogenation. Complete hydrogenation would produce a very hard and unpalatable fat. When the process is controlled, fat of any desired consistency can be prepared. Commercially hydrogenated vegetable oils can be manufactured that are solid cooking fats at room temperature.

Margarine is also made by hydrogenating oils but with additional processing to produce a product that will melt readily and simulate butter. It is emulsified with milk that has been cultured with a microorganism to add flavor. A

Table 3–2. FATTY ACID COMPOSITION OF COMMON DIETARY FATS AND OILS

SOURCE	18:2 ω-6 Linoleic	20:4 ω-6 Arachidonic	18:3 ω-3 Linolenic	20:5 ω-3 Eicosapentaenoic	22:6 ω-3 Docosahexaenoic	Saturated
Predominantly ω-6						
Safflower oil	73	—	0.5	—	—	9
Corn oil	57	—	1.0	—	—	13
Cottonseed oil	50	—	0.4	—	—	26
Sunflower seed oil	56	—	0.3	—	—	10
Peanut oil	29	—	1.0	—	—	19
Predominantly ω-3						
Linseed oil	15	—	55.0	—	—	13
Salmon oil	1	—	1.0	8	5	26
Cod liver oil	2	—	1.0	12	12	19
Channel catfish oil	6	2.0	0.7	4	9	26
Mackerel	2	2.0	1.0	10	16	35
Whale oil	1	4.0	—	3	7	19
Both ω-6 and ω-3						
Soybean oil	51	—	7.0	—	—	15
English walnut oil	55	—	11.0	—	—	11
Low in both ω-6 and ω-3						
Cow milk fat	2	—	1.0	—	—	62
Human milk fat	7	0.2	0.7	0.6	0.3	50
Lard	10	—	1.0	—	—	36
Chicken fat	17	—	1.0	—	—	33
Beef tallow	4	—	0.5	—	—	48
Egg yolk	11	6.0	0.2	—	—	53
Beef liver	10	6.0	0.5	—	—	39
Coconut oil	2	—	—	—	—	88
Olive oil	8	—	0.7	—	—	14
Cocoa butter	3	—	0.2	—	—	60
Palm oil	9	—	0.3	—	—	48

* Monounsaturated fatty acids constitute the remaining fatty acids. They are thought to have neutral effects upon plasma lipid levels.
Adapted from: Goodnight, S. H., et al: Polyunsaturated fatty acids, hyperlipidemia, and thrombosis. Arteriosclerosis, *2*:87, 1982.

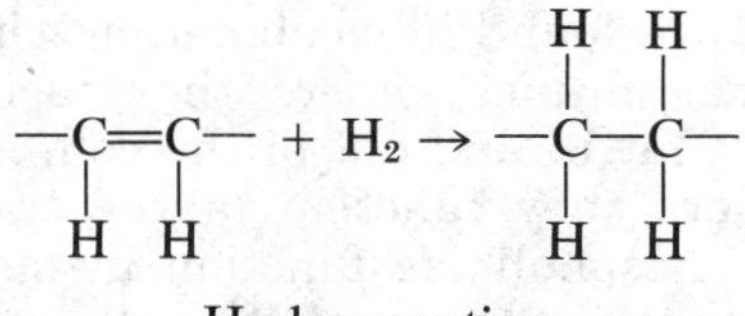

$$-\overset{\displaystyle H}{\underset{\displaystyle H}{C}}=\overset{\displaystyle H}{\underset{\displaystyle H}{C}}- \;+\; H_2 \;\rightarrow\; -\overset{\displaystyle H}{\underset{\displaystyle H}{C}}-\overset{\displaystyle H}{\underset{\displaystyle H}{C}}-$$

Hydrogenation

Figure 3–3. Hydrogenation.

yellow vegetable dye (beta carotene) and vitamins A and D are added to give the margarine the appearance and nutritive value of butter.

Two effects of hydrogenation are that it lowers the polyunsaturated fatty acid content of the fat and that *trans isomers* of the unsaturated acids are formed. Thus, the fatty acid composition of a partially hydrogenated vegetable oil retains little similarity to that of the natural oil. For example, trans polyunsaturated fatty acids have no essential fatty acid activity. These isomers are rare in nature, and their metabolism is unknown and requires further research. Unfortunately there is little information on these isomers, and they have generally been accepted as safe when in fact this may not be true.[1]

A spread of the same consistency but of higher linoleic acid content than butter may be prepared by mixing a portion of almost completely hydrogenated fat with some of the original oil. This procedure is used for some margarines, as some of the labels on "tub" or "soft" margarines show. Stick or "print" margarines contain an average of 31 per cent trans fatty acids, while tub margarines have an average of 17 per cent.[1]

Rancidity. When fats and oils are exposed to warm, moist air over a period of time, chemical changes occur that produce unpalatable flavors and disagreeable odors, commonly called rancidity. The oxygen of the air can attack the double bonds of the polyunsaturated fatty acids, forming peroxides which may be toxic in large amounts. Partial hydrogenation of oils decreases their tendency to oxidize and become rancid and thus increases their stability.

The oxidative process destroys vitamin A and vitamin E. Vitamin E is present in rather large amounts in vegetable fats. It is an antioxidant and protects against rancidity but in the process is, itself, inactivated. Fortification of fats or fatty foods with antioxidants such as butylated hydroxyanisole (BHA) and butylated hydroxytoluene (BHT) extends the storage time and protects essential nutrients. Precautions should be taken to lessen the danger of rancidity by storing fat-containing foods at low temperature and limiting the storage time.

Functions

FUNCTIONS OF TRIGLYCERIDES

ENERGY. Fats serve as a concentrated source of energy. Each gram of fat supplies 9 kcalories, which is more than twice the amount of energy supplied by each gram of carbohydrate. The main source of this energy is the fatty acids, which supply 40 to 50 carbon atoms for oxidation as compared with 3 from glycerol. Because of the high energy density and low solubility of fats, they are used as a storage form of energy. Not only ingested fat but carbohydrate and amino acids not immediately used by the tissues are converted to fat and stored in the adipose tissue. Up to two thirds of the total energy of the cells may be supplied by triglyceride rather than carbohydrate. Fat spares protein for tissue synthesis.

OTHER FUNCTIONS. Adipose tissue helps to hold the body organs and nerves in position and to protect them against traumatic injury and shock. The subcutaneous layer of fat insulates the body, which serves to preserve body heat and maintain body temperature. Fats aid in transport and absorption of the fat-soluble vitamins. Fats spare thiamin since they can be metabolized for energy, whereas the metabolism of carbohydrate requires thiamin. In the stomach fats depress gastric secretions and slow the emptying time of the stomach, thus providing a pleasant feeling of satiety after a meal. In addition, fats add to the palatability of the diet.

ESSENTIAL FATTY ACIDS (EFA). Three polyunsaturated fatty acids, namely, linoleic, linolenic and arachidonic acids, have essential fatty acid activity. However, only two—linoleic and linolenic—have been designated as essential fatty acids, and *linoleic acid* is the primary dietary EFA for humans.[8] *Arachidonic acid* can be synthesized from linoleic acid. The role of *linolenic acid,* which cannot be synthesized from linoleic acid, is still unclear, but it appears that it cannot be synthesized in the body.[3, 10] The essential fatty acids have important roles in fat transport and metabolism and in maintaining the function and integrity of cellular membranes. They also are a part of the fatty acids of cholesterol esters and phospholipids in plasma lipoproteins and mitochondrial lipoproteins. Serum cholesterol has been shown to be lowered by EFA, but the mechanism of this effect is not entirely clear.[3] Fatty acids with EFA activity are also precursors of a group of hormonelike compounds, *prostaglandins, thromboxanes* and *prostacyclins*, that participate in the regulation of blood pressure, heart rate, vascular dilation, blood clotting, lipolysis and the central nervous system.

DEFICIENCY. *Linoleic acid* was shown to be a dietary essential for infants by Hansen, Wiese and associates,[9] who found that linoleic acid would prevent or cure a characteristic dermatitis (eczema) observed in infants fed a fat-free diet as shown in Figure 3–4. The only reported instances of essential fatty acid deficiency in adults are associated with long-term fat-free intravenous feedings.

EFA deficiency in infants also causes a poor growth rate and lowered resistance to infections. It is now theorized that some of the manifestations of EFA deficiency may be due to resulting prostaglandin deficiency, since essential fatty acids are precursors of prostaglandins.[9]

LIPIDS WITH SPECIAL FUNCTIONS

PHOSPHOLIPIDS. Any lipid containing phosphorus is included in this classification. Phospholipids are the next largest lipid component of the body after the triglycerides. Phospholipids are formed in essentially all cells of the body, although a greater portion that enter the blood are formed in the liver cells and the intestinal mucosa. Because of their strong affinity for both water-soluble and fat-soluble substances in the molecule, large concentrations of phos-

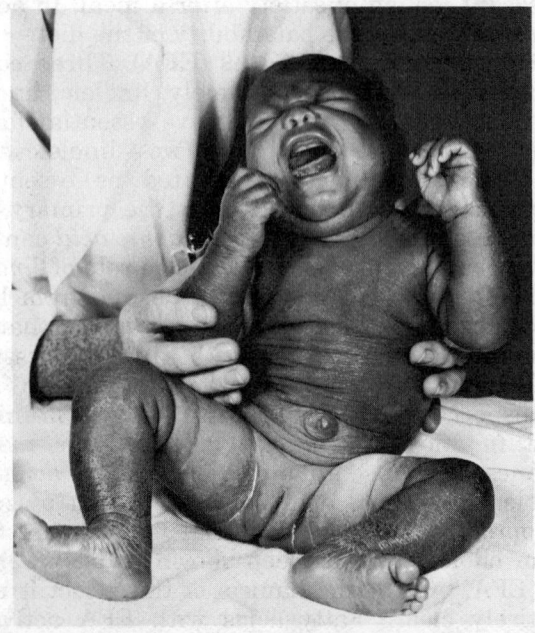

Figure 3–4. Thickening and dryness of the skin, oozing in the body folds and eruption in the diaper region caused by linoleic acid deficiency in infant having a low fat intake. (Photo courtesy of Dr. A. E. Hansen and The National Live Stock and Meat Board Food and Nutrition News, *29*, No. 5, 1958.)

pholipids are found in combination with protein in cell membranes, where they facilitate the passage of fat in and out of the cell, and in the blood where they function in the transport of fat. The phospholipids function in maintaining the structural integrity of the cells rather than as fat stores.

Lecithin (phosphatidylcholine) contains glycerol and fatty acids as well as phosphoric acid and the nitrogen-containing base choline. They are the most widely distributed of the phospholipids; liver, egg yolk and soybeans are especially rich in lecithin. Lecithin is added to food products such as cheese, margarine and confections to aid in emulsification. Lecithin functions in the transport and utilization of fatty acids through the enzyme *lecithin-cholesterol acyltransferase (LCAT)*. Lecithin is widely popularized as a remedy for hypercholesterolemia, but aside from its high linoleic acid content, lecithin has no effect upon lipid metabolism.[3] Lecithin in food or supplement is not absorbed as such from the gastrointestinal tract, but is mainly hydrolyzed into its constituent fatty acids and choline. The body can synthesize lecithin as it is needed.

Since it was shown that oral choline can affect the brain level of the neurotransmitter acetylcholine, choline has been given in the form of phosphatidylcholine or lecithin to treat various mental disorders (see page 666).

Phospholipids such as *cephalins* (which are similar in structure to lecithins), *lipontols* (which contain inositol, a compound with vitaminlike activity) and *sphingomyelins* (which contain no glycerol but a com plex amino alcohol) are found in rather high concentrations in nerve tissue. A *cephalin* is needed to form thromboplastin for the blood clotting process. *Sphingomyelin* is found in the brain and other nerve tissue as a component of the myelin sheath. This substance acts as an insulator around the nerve fibers. Egg yolk and liver are good sources of these phospholipids.

As a rule, the invisible and not the visible fat of both plant and animal tissue contains appreciable amounts of phospholipids. The amount in oils, lard and butter is small owing to the removal of most of the phospholipids in processing.

GLYCOLIPIDS. The glycolipids include the *cerebrosides* and *gangliosides*. They contain the base sphingosine and fatty acids with 22 and 24 carbons. The carbohydrate component of the cerebrosides is galactose; the gangliosides contain, in addition, glucose and a complex compound containing an amino sugar. Structurally both the cerebrosides and gangliosides are components of nerve tissue and certain cell membranes, where they play a role in fat transport.

LIPOPROTEINS. Lipoproteins are formed primarily in the liver and to a lesser degree in the intestine. They are found in cell and organelle membranes (mitochondria and lysosomes) and in the blood and function to transport insoluble lipids in an aqueous medium.

Lipoproteins are various combinations of triglycerides, phospholipids and cholesterol with protein (apoproteins). They are classified based on their electrophoretic mobility and density as (1) *chylomicrons* (formed in the chyle or lymph as lipids are absorbed), which consist of a core of triglyceride coated with phospholipid and protein; (2) *very low density lipoproteins (VLDL)*, which contain mostly triglycerides, little protein and some cholesterol; (3) *low density lipoproteins (LDL)*, which contain less triglyceride and more cholesterol and protein; and (4) *high density lipoproteins (HDL)*, which contain high concentrations of protein and low concentrations of triglycerides and cholesterol (see Fig. 28–4). *Non-esterified fatty acids* occur in combination with serum albumin. For further discussion of lipoproteins, see page 567.

HYDROCARBONS. Mention should be made here of the term "oil," a confusing word that may refer to fats in a liquid state or to other substances that have the same properties but have no relation to fats. An example is mineral oil, which is a hydrocarbon from petroleum. Motor oil is a hydrocarbon, and many hydrocarbon oils are physically like fats when cool (petroleum jelly, for example). Hydrocarbons have no nutritive value and are not metabolized or absorbed by the body. Some are used for specific purposes in medicine, such as mineral oil for its laxative and lubricating qualities in the bowel.

CHOLESTEROL

Cholesterol is a member of the large group of compounds called sterols. They all have the same complex ring structure, (as shown in Figure 3–5). The "-ol" ending indicates that cholesterol is an alcohol. *Cholesterol* is found only in animal tissues, but somewhat similar sterols are found in plants. *Ergosterol*, a yeast sterol, is converted to vitamin D_2 on exposure to ultraviolet light.

Beta-sitosterol, another plant sterol, is usually absorbed only slightly by the intestinal tract and largely passes out in the stool. In pharmacologic doses it has a hypercholesterolemic effect because it competes with cholesterol for absorption.[3]

Cholesterol is found not only as the free alcohol but also in combination with fatty acids as esters. It is an essential component of the structural membranes of all cells and is a major component of brain and nerve cells. It is found in

Figure 3–5. Cholesterol.

high concentrations in glandular tissues and in the liver, where it is synthesized and stored.

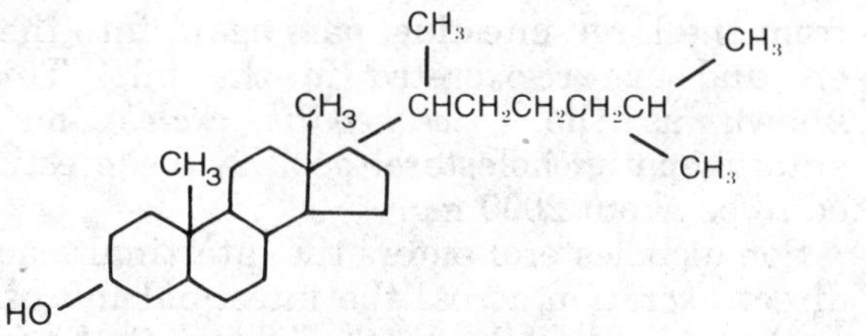

Not only is cholesterol present in foods consumed (exogenous cholesterol), but it also can be synthesized in the cell (endogenous cholesterol).

FUNCTION. The structural function of cholesterol is not entirely understood. It is, however, a key intermediate in the biosynthesis of a number of other important *steroids*. These include the bile acids, adrenocortical hormones, estrogens, androgens and progesterone. Cholesterol is a precursor of vitamin D (see Chapter 6). Cholesterol is coverted by the intestinal mucosa to 7-dehydrocholesterol, the provitamin of vitamin D_3, cholecalciferol. This transformation is also effected by skin and other tissues, upon exposure to ultraviolet light.

Cholesterol in the skin along with other lipids makes the skin resistant to the action of many chemical agents and to the absorption of water-soluble substances. Cholesterol and other lipids are highly inert to acids and certain solvents, which serve to prevent penetration into the body. Water evaporation from the skin is prevented by the presence of cholesterol and other lipids. Abnormal deposits of cholesterol in the tissues are associated with several conditions, including atherosclerosis (Chapter 28) and diabetes mellitus (Chapter 25).

ABSORPTION AND EXCRETION. Cholesterol esters are hydrolyzed in the intestinal tract, but the cholesterol is largely re-esterified during the process of absorption. It is incorporated into the chylomicrons formed in the intestinal wall and transported via the lymphatic circulation to the liver. The absorption of cholesterol is dependent upon the absorption of fat and is stimulated by the presence of fatty acids. In the blood, cholesterol is present free or esterified with fatty acids as part of the lipoprotein complex.

The principal products of cholesterol breakdown are the bile acids, which are formed in the liver and are delivered into the small intestine in the bile secretions. Thus the liver seems to control the rate of loss of cholesterol from the body. About 80 per cent of the cholesterol metabolized is converted to bile acids. Both bile acids and cholesterol are continually reabsorbed from the terminal ileum, and to a lesser extent from the large intestine, pass again into the liver, and are re-excreted in the bile. This is known as the *enterohepatic cycle*, and the enterohepatic cholesterol pool has been estimated to be about 2000 mg.

Some cholesterol enters the intestinal tract by direct excretion across the intestinal mucosa as well as via the bile. In the lumen of the intestine a portion is hydrogenated to *coprosterol* by intestinal organisms. Coprosterol cannot be absorbed and is excreted in the feces. Very little cholesterol is excreted in the urine; some is lost by way of the skin.

METABOLISM. The main sites of cholesterol synthesis are the liver cells and the intestinal cells, but it can also be synthesized in almost all other tissues. The liver enzyme *lecithin-cholesterol acyltransferase (LCAT)* esterifies cholesterol with fatty acyl residue from lecithin. These cholesteryl esters are rapidly transferred to other lipoproteins by apolipoprotein D; all of the cholesteryl esters found in VLDL, LDL and HDL are produced in this way. These cholesteryl esters in lipoproteins can then be hydrolyzed and excreted in the bile. Therefore this pathway of cholesterol transport helps to prevent accumulation of cholesterol in the body. The rate of endogenous cholesterol synthesis is variable and is dependent upon the amount already present in the body and somewhat upon the amount in the diet.

The physiological and metabolic relationships among dietary total fat, cholesterol, phospholipids, unsaturated fatty acids and atherosclerosis are complex and not completely understood, but are the object of much present-day medical research, as discussed in Chapter 28.

DIETARY SOURCES. Cholesterol occurs in largest amounts in egg yolk, liver, kidney, sweetbreads, brains and fish roe. Cholesterol is also present in smaller amounts in the fat of meat, whole milk, cream, ice cream, cheese and butter. Foods that are low in cholesterol or contain no cholesterol are fruits, vegetables, cereals, breadstuffs, sugars and syrups, egg white, low-fat fish, very lean meats, soup stock made without fat and skim milk. Table 3–3 and Appendix Table 5 give the cholesterol content of food. However, it must be pointed out that the amount synthesized and metabolized daily by the body itself is far greater than the amount usually consumed in the diet, of which only 40 per cent is absorbed.[4] Serum cholesterol is influenced by the amount present in the diet and also by the amount of fat, especially saturated fat, in the diet.

Regulation of Blood Lipid Levels Through Dietary Fat and Cholesterol Manipulation

The dietary fat intake has been shown to have an effect on the serum cholesterol level of individuals. Populations consuming diets high in fat usually have relatively high serum cholesterol levels. Populations with a low fat intake usually have relatively low serum cholesterol levels.

The total concentration of cholesterol in the blood plasma is highly variable and explained in detail in Chapter 28. The dietary factors that affect the plasma concentration of cholesterol may be summarized as follows:

1. A high intake of *dietary cholesterol* normally increases the blood cholesterol level a few milligrams per 100 ml. The liver normally com-

Table 3–3. CHOLESTEROL CONTENT OF SOME FOODS

	AMOUNT	MG. OF CHOLESTEROL
Kidneys	½ c. sliced pieces	562
Liver (beef, pork)	3 oz. slice (85 gm.)	372
Egg yolk	1 large yolk (17 gm.)	252
Custard, baked	½ c. (132 gm.)	139
Shrimp, canned	½ c. (64 gm.)	96
Crab, canned	½ c. (80 gm.)	80
Beef	3 oz. (85 gm.)	80
Halibut	1 fillet (125 gm.)	75
Pie, peach	⅛ of 9″ pie (114 gm.)	70
Chicken, breast	½ breast (80 gm.)	63
Lobster	½ c. of meat (72 gm.)	61
Oysters, canned	3 oz. (85 gm.)	38
Milk, whole	1 cup (244 gm.)	34
Cheese, cheddar	1 oz. (28 gm.)	28
Ice cream	½ c. (66 gm.)	26
Cheese, cottage, 1% fat	1 cup (267 gm.)	23

From Feeley, R. M., Criner, P. E., and Watt, B. K.: Cholesterol content of foods, J. Am. Diet. Assoc., *61*:134, 1972.

pensates for the high exogenous intake of cholesterol by synthesizing smaller quantities of endogenous cholesterol and converting more cholesterol into bile acids. However, these control mechanisms vary from one person to another and possibly from one race to another.

2. A diet containing only *saturated fat* (butter, coconut oil, fat of meat) increases the blood cholesterol level as much as 40 to 50 mg. per 100 ml.

3. Dietary intake of *monounsaturated fatty acids* has no effect on serum cholesterol.

4. A dietary intake of the *polyunsaturated fats* such as corn oil, cottonseed oil and safflower oil lowers serum cholesterol levels. This effect may vary depending upon the type of unsaturated fat and its ω number, as discussed earlier in this chapter.

5. Evidence suggests that *dietary fiber* may lower serum cholesterol by binding with bile acids and preventing their reabsorption, or by favoring the growth of intestinal flora, which produce secondary bile acids that are not as well absorbed as primary bile acids.[11]

Other factors such as an excess secretion of the *thyroid hormone* decrease the blood cholesterol levels. *Estrogens* decrease serum cholesterol and *androgens* increase serum cholesterol. In *diabetes mellitus* the blood cholesterol level rises, probably because of the increase in the mobilization of lipids. The blood cholesterol level rises along with blood triglyceride and phospholipid levels in *renal diseases*, resulting from a diminished removal of lipoproteins from the blood owing to an inhibition of lipoprotein lipase.

Cholesterol is further discussed under diseases of the gallbladder and in relation to atherosclerosis. Diets with modified cholesterol and fat content appear on page 581. Also, see Appendix Table 5 for fatty acid and cholesterol content of foods.

Metabolism and Storage of Fat

TRANSPORT OF FAT

Almost all the lipids of the diet are absorbed into the lymph from the intestinal mucosa. Only the medium chain fatty acids, absorbed directly into the portal blood, bypass the lymphatic system. The lipids are carried in the lymph as *chylomicrons*, droplets of fat with cholesterol and phospholipids with a small amount of protein (mainly *apolipoproteins* A and B) adsorbed to their outer surface. There are many different apoproteins, and they are important for the metabolism and storage of the lipoproteins in the liver and adipose tissue. Chylomicrons are large

enough that they can make the plasma appear milky after a meal containing fat if they are present in excessive amounts. They empty into the venous blood at the thoracic duct. In the lymph and blood, chylomicrons acquire additional apolipoproteins (mainly C and E). The chylomicrons are carried to the liver or are removed from the blood by the adipose tissue.

Within a few hours after eating, chylomicrons have been removed from the blood by the action of *lipoprotein lipase* on the endothelial cells lining the capillaries in the adipose tissue. Lipoprotein lipase hydrolyzes the triglycerides and phospholipids into fatty acids and glycerol, which can pass into the adipose cell. There they are re-esterified into triglycerides for storage.

In the liver lipids may be metabolized, stored or converted to lipoproteins, in which form they are carried in the blood to the tissues for immediate use for energy or special functions.

METABOLISM OF FAT

The first step in catabolism of triglyceride is hydrolysis to glycerol and fatty acid. The fatty acids are released as non-esterified fatty acids bound to serum albumin. Although a great deal of fatty acid is transported in this form, its level in the plasma remains low, since it is picked up by the tissues very rapidly. Normal plasma has a fatty acid concentration of about 15 mg. per 100 ml.

In the first stage of oxidation, fatty acids are broken down stepwise into two-carbon units complexed with coenzyme A (acetyl-CoA) as shown in Figure 3–6. This complex is also an intermediate metabolite in glucose metabolism and from this point fatty acids and glucose are oxidized by the same pathway. Glycerol also, after activation, may be converted to an intermediate of glucose oxidation. These steps are discussed in detail in Chapter 5.

Almost all tissues can utilize fatty acids for energy. They form a large portion of the energy for muscular tissue even when glucose is available. Glycerol can be oxidized in only a few tissues, so most of it is carried to the liver, where it can be oxidized for energy or used in the synthesis of new triglycerides.

The liver is a major center of lipid metabolism and is largely responsible for regulation of lipid levels in the body. Among its important functions are (1) synthesis of triglycerides from carbohydrate and, to a smaller extent, from protein; (2) synthesis of other lipids such as phospholipids and cholesterol from triglycerides; (3) desaturation of fatty acids (oleic acid is the predominant acid in human adipose tissue); and (4) degradation of triglycerides for use as energy. Even under normal conditions the liver produces

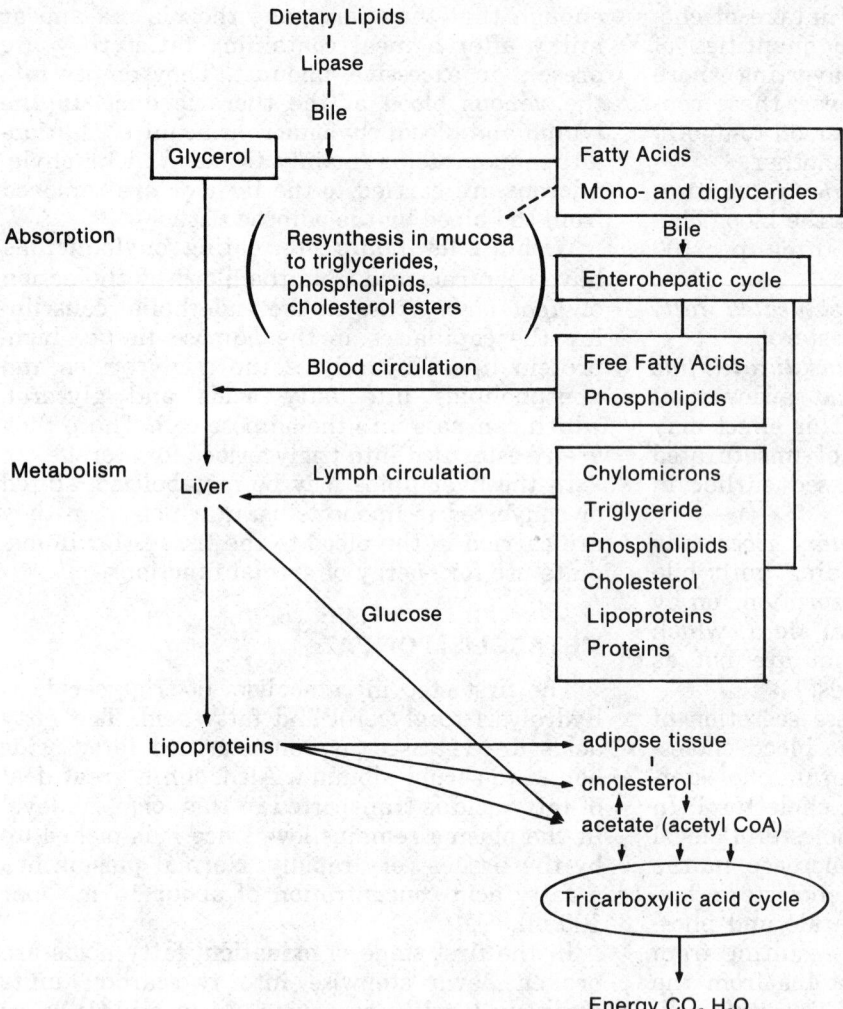

Figure 3–6. Brief summary of fat metabolism.

more acetyl-CoA than it can oxidize completely. Two molecules of acetyl-CoA condense to form acetoacetic acid, as shown in Figure 3–7.

The *acetoacetic acid* diffuses through the liver cell membranes and is carried to peripheral tissues, where it is converted again to acetyl-CoA and oxidized. When the body is relying almost entirely on stored fat for energy, as in uncontrolled diabetes mellitus or prolonged fasting or starvation, large quantities of triglyceride appear in the liver and the production of acetoace-

tic acid far outstrips the ability of the peripheral tissues to oxidize it, so that the level in the blood rises. Part of the acetoacetic acid is converted to beta-hydroxybutyric acid and acetone—the three compounds being known collectively as the *ketone bodies*. Acetoacidic acid and beta-hydroxybutyric acid are acids that must be carried in the blood and excreted in the urine in combination with base (sodium ion). This reduces the available base in the body and the condition, if unchecked, leads to a lowering of the pH of body fluids (*acidosis*) which may be fatal.

Hormonal Control of Fat Metabolism

The hormones that have marked effects on carbohydrate metabolism also affect fat metabolism.

1. *Insulin* inhibits fat utilization and increases fat synthesis. Insulin influences fat metabolism by activating lipoprotein lipase, which results in triglyceride hydrolysis and uptake of the result-

$$2\ CH_3CO\ CoA + H_2O \underset{\text{Other Cells}}{\overset{\text{Liver Cells}}{\rightleftharpoons}}$$

Acetyl-CoA

$$CH_3COCH_2COOH + 2\ H\ CoA$$

Acetoacetic Acid   Coenzyme A

Figure 3–7. Acetyl-CoA is converted to acetoacetic acid and coenzyme A in the liver, and these substances are converted back to acetyl-CoA in other tissues.

ing fatty acids by adipose tissue. Another enzyme, *hormone sensitive lipase (HSL)*, is also controlled by insulin; insulin decreases the activity of HSL. HSL causes the movement of fat out of the adipose tissue as free fatty acids.

2. *Thyroxine* increases mobilization of fats indirectly by increasing the rate of energy metabolism of each cell.

3. *Glucocorticoids* increase the rate of fat mobilization by increasing the fat cell membrane permeability.

4. *Adrenocorticoids* (especially adrenocorticotropic hormone (ACTH)) increase fat mobilization directly by increasing the activity of HSL.

5. *Epinephrine* and *norepinephrine* also increase the rate of fat mobilization by stimulating the activity of HSL and thus the release of free fatty acids from fat cells for metabolism.

STORAGE OF FAT

In the human body there are two kinds of body fat—white fat and brown fat. The vast majority of this fat is *white fat* composed of adipose cells that basically accumulate in three places; (1) subcutaneous tissue—50 per cent, (2) abdominal cavity, around the internal organs—45 per cent, and (3) intramuscular tissue—5 per cent. These fat cells store up to 95 per cent of their volume as triglycerides in liquid form. Fat storage is not static; there is a constant turnover of fat even though the amount remains the same.

Brown adipose tissue (BAT) is much less abundant and occurs only in certain areas of the body, particularly the interscapular region and the back of the neck. The amount of this fat is higher in the neonate and decreases with age, but it can be increased somewhat with extended exposure to cold since it functions in *thermo-genesis* a response to cold. Instead of releasing fatty acids into the blood, this fat cell has the ability to switch to oxidation of fatty acids for production of heat. The mitochondrial metabolism is changed so that oxidation and phosphorylation are uncoupled, and rather than the efficient entrapment of energy as ATP, the result is energy dissipated as heat, warming the body. As might be presumed, this *nonshivering thermogenesis* is especially active in the neonate, who must keep warm. Thermogenesis in relation to maintenance of body weight is discussed on page 524.

Changes in Fat Consumption

Fats supply roughly 43 per cent of the total calories available for consumption in the United States, and this reflects an upward trend from the years 1909–1913 when this proportion was 32 per cent. Total fat consumed from animal and vegetable sources has increased 35 per cent from 125 to 168 gm. per person per day from the period 1909–1913 to 1980.[15] The trend in fat consumption can be seen in Table 17–1. The consumption of vegetable fat during the same period has increased from 17 per cent of fat calories to 42 per cent, causing the animal fat component to fall from 83 to 58 per cent.[15] The most rapid increase in fat consumption, for the most part due to an increased consumption of salad and cooking oils, has occurred within the last 20 years.

The amount of fat in the diet has increased, but the percentage of total calories from *saturated* fatty acids has remained about the same at 13 to 15 per cent of total calories. As shown in Table 3–4, the ratio of polyunsaturated (lin-

Table 3–4. FATTY ACIDS AVAILABLE, PER PERSON PER DAY, AND PER CENT OF TOTAL CALORIES

YEAR	FATTY ACIDS			KCALORIES FURNISHED BY FATTY ACIDS			RATIO OF POLYUNSATURATED TO SATURATED FATTY ACIDS
	Total Saturated, gm.	Oleic Acid, gm.	Linoleic Acid, gm.	% Total Saturated	% Oleic Acid	% Linoleic Acid	
1909–1913	50.3	51.5	10.7	12.9	13.3	2.7	0.20
1925–1929	53.3	55.2	12.5	13.7	14.2	3.2	0.23
1935–1939	52.9	54.5	12.7	14.4	14.8	3.5	0.24
1947–1949	54.4	58.0	14.8	15.0	16.0	4.1	0.27
1957–1959	54.7	58.2	16.6	15.6	16.6	4.7	0.30
1965	53.9	58.8	19.1	15.2	16.6	5.4	0.35
1975	53.7	62.7	22.0	14.8	17.3	6.1	0.41
1980	58.0	66.8	25.1	14.8	17.1	6.4	0.43

(Adapted from Friend, B.: Nutrients in U.S. food supply. A review of trends 1909–1913 to 1965. Am. J. Clin. Nutr., *20*:911, 1967. Additional data from Marston, R., and Friend, B.: Nutrient Content of the National Food Supply, National Food Review, January 1978; and Brewster, L., and Jacobson, M. F.: The Changing American Diet. Center for Science in the Public Interest, Washington, D. C., 1982.)

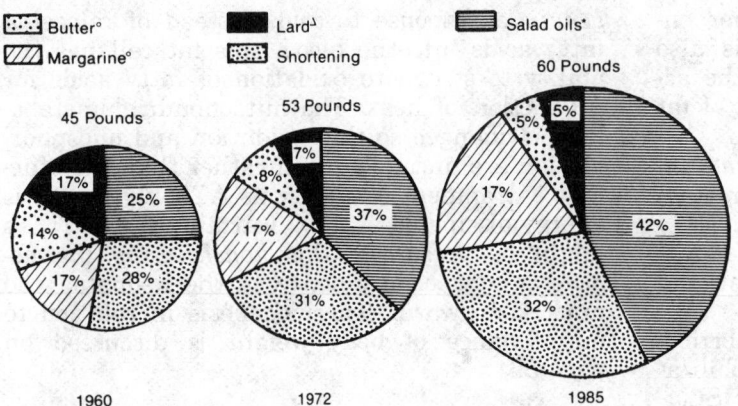

Figure 3–8. Average amounts and percentages of saturated and unsaturated fats in the U.S. diet. (From White, P. L., Fletcher, D. C., and Ellis, M.: Nutrients in Processed Foods—Fats and Carbohydrates. Acton, Mass., Publishing Sciences Group, 1975.)

oleic acid) to saturated fatty acids progressively increased from 0.21 in 1909 to 0.43 in 1980.[2] It should be pointed out that wastage, cooking and other losses are not considered in these statistics, so that the actual fat ingested is less than that available for consumption.

The trend toward a higher proportion of the energy intake in the form of vegetable fat is due to several factors: consumption of corn, cottonseed and soybean oils in salad and cooking; the trend toward the substitution of margarines for butter; the increase in poultry consumption; and processing technology, which permits the manufacture of shortening entirely from vegetable oils. Figure 3–8 shows this trend as well as a projection for 1985.

Current data on the actual *consumption* of nutrients by the U.S. population can be found in the Nationwide Food Consumption Survey of 1977–1978 (see page 344). This survey showed that the average fat intake of all of the individuals surveyed was 40.3 per cent of the total energy intake. Forty-one per cent of the fat in the diet came from meat, fish and poultry, 17 per cent from milk and milk products, 15 per cent from grain products and 10 per cent from fats and oils.

Recommended Allowance of Fat in the Diet

The requirement of the human for the essential fatty acids has been estimated to be approximately 1 to 2 per cent of the calorie intake (3 per cent for infants). For those with low fat intakes (25 per cent of total calories), the recommendation is 3 per cent of total calories as EFA. For those with higher fat intakes (35 per cent or more of total calories) no more than 8 to 10 per cent of total calories should be from linoleic acid.[7] Since fats are eaten for flavor and satiety, most diets contain much more than this level. There is disagreement among nutritionists regarding the optimum level of fat in the diet to

prevent heart disease, cancer and obesity. The Food and Nutrition Board in the Recommended Dietary Allowances makes this statement:[7]

Total fat intake, particularly in diets below 2000 kcal, should be reduced so fat is not more than 35 percent of dietary energy. There should be greater reduction in fats containing predominantly saturated fatty acids, such as those from animal sources, than in vegetable fats containing predominantly unsaturated fatty acids. These simultaneous changes in amount and type of dietary fat would increase the ratio of polyunsaturated to saturated fatty acids. The Committee on Dietary Allowances believes that, in view of the possible hazards of high intakes of polyunsaturated oils, an upper limit of 10 percent of dietary energy as polyunsaturated fatty acids is advisable.[7]

In the Report of the Inter-Society Commission for Heart Disease Resources the commission concluded that elevated serum cholesterol is a risk factor in the development of coronary heart disease and recommended dietary changes.[14] The American Heart Association recommends the following changes:

1. A caloric intake to achieve or maintain ideal body weight.

2. A reduction in total fat calories from 40–45 per cent to 35 per cent of total calories.

3. A reduction in dietary cholesterol to 300 mg. per day.

4. An increase in complex dietary carbohydrate to replace calories from fat.

Proposed recommendations for changes in dietary fat consumption are given in Table 17–7. See Chapter 28 for additional discussion of this topic.

Harm could result from severe reduction (less than 10 per cent of total calories) of dietary fat, both in quantity and in proportion to other nutrients. Prolonged low-fat regimens may lead to deficiencies of the essential fatty acids. Since dietary fat is the carrier of the four fat-soluble vitamins (A, D, E, and K) and carotene, deficiencies in these nutrients may develop during prolonged periods of fat restriction.

Cooking and Digestibility of Fats

Cooking by the usual methods has no appreciable effect on the fatty acids. However, heating fat at very high temperatures burns the fat, resulting in the decomposition of the fat and the production of the substance *acrolein*. Acrolein may be very irritating to the nasal passages and to the gastrointestinal mucosa. Properly fried foods should have no adverse effect on normal digestion, but digestion of improperly fried foods does involve more effort on the part of the digestive system.

Contrary to popular opinion, most fats are highly digestible; over 95 per cent of ingested fat is normally absorbed and utilized in the body. The absorption rate of fats varies, depending largely upon the melting point of the fat. Fats that are liquid at body temperature or more unsaturated are more rapidly absorbed than the solid fats. The rate of absorption is markedly enhanced by the presence of phospholipids and is also influenced by the quantity and type of mixture of fats eaten. In addition a *fatty acid binding protein (FABP)* in the mucosal cell may explain differences in rates of absorption of fatty acids. This protein exhibits an affinity for long chain unsaturated fatty acids.[12] The more rapidly absorbed fat is more quickly available to the tissues for energy. However, the more slowly absorbed fats remain in the intestines longer, thus extending the satiety period and producing much lower fluctuations in blood lipid levels following a meal.

Problems and Suggested Topics for Discussion

1. List the amount of various fat foods you consume during a period of 24 hours. Calculate the percentage of total calories that were derived from fat.
2. Classify the fats in your diet for 1 day into "invisible" and "visible" fat foods; saturated and unsaturated.
3. What percentage of the daily diet in the United States is consumed in the form of fat foods? What percentage is from saturated fat? From unsaturated fat?
4. Why do you like to eat fat foods?
5. How do you obtain essential fatty acid in your diet?
6. Explain what is meant by saturated fat, unsaturated fat and hydrogenation. Explain their importance in nutrition and health.
7. Explain the metabolism and storage of fats in the body after absorption.
8. What is ketosis? Under what conditions does it occur?
9. What are the functions of fats in the body?
10. Survey the literature and report on the most recent statements on fat intake in relation to heart disease and cancer.

Cited References

1. Brisson, G.J.: Lipids in Human Nutrition. Englewood, New Jersey, Jack K. Burgess, Inc., 1981.
2. Colburn, M., and Jacobsen, M.: The Changing American Diet, Update: 1982. Washington, D.C., Center for Science in the Public Interest, 1982.
3. Connor, W.E., and Connor, S.L.: The dietary treatment of hyperlipidemia: rationale, technique and efficacy, Med. Clin. N. Am., 66:485, 1982.
4. Connor, W.E., and Lin, D.S.: The intestinal absorption of dietary cholesterol by hypercholesterolemic (type II) and normocholesterolemic humans. J. Clin. Invest., 53:1062, 1974.
5. Fernstrom, J.D., and Wurtman, R.J.: Nutrition and the brain. Sci. Am., 230:80, 1974.
6. Food and Nutrient Intakes of Individuals in One Day in the United States, Spring, 1977. Nationwide Food Consumption Survey, 1977–1978, Preliminary Report No. 2. U.S. Department of Agriculture, Science and Education Administration, 1980.
7. Food and Nutrition Board, National Research Council: Recommended Dietary Allowances. 9th ed. Washington, D.C., National Academy of Sciences, 1980.
8. Goodnight, S.H., et al.: Polyunsaturated fatty acids, hyperlipidemia and thrombosis. Arteriosclerosis, 2:87, 1982.
9. Hansen, A.E., et al.: Role of linoleic acid in infant nutrition. Pediatrics, 31:171, 1963.
10. Holman, R.T., Johnson, S.B., and Hatch, T.F.: A case of human linolenic acid deficiency involving neurological abnormalities. Am. J. Clin. Nutr., 35:617, 1982.
11. Kritchevsky, D., and Story, J.A.: Binding of bile salts in vitro by nonnutritive fiber. J. Nutr., 104:458, 1974.
12. Ockner, R.K., et al.: A binding protein for fatty acids in cytosol of intestinal mucosa, liver, myocardium, and other tissues. Science, 177:56, 1972.
13. Privett, O.S., et al.: Studies of the effects of *trans* fatty acids in the diet on lipid metabolism in essential fatty acid deficient rats. Am. J. Clin. Nutr., 30:1009, 1977.
14. Report of Inter-Society Commission for Heart Disease Resources. Primary prevention of the atherosclerotic diseases. Circulation, 42:A55, 1970, revised April 1972.
15. Welsh, S.O., and Marston, R.M.: Review of trends in food use in the United States, 1909–1980. J. Am. Diet. Assoc., 81:121, 1982.

Additional References

Babayan, V.K.: Tailoring fats for technical and nutritional needs. In White, P.L., Fletcher, D.C., and Ellis, M. (eds.): Nutrients in Processed Foods—Fats, Carbohydrates. Acton, Mass., Publishing Sciences Group, Inc., 1975.

Danon, A.: Prostaglandins and fat metabolism. In White, P.L., Fletcher, D.C., and Ellis, M. (eds.): Nutrients in Processed Foods—Fats, Carbohydrates. Acton, Mass., Publishing Sciences Group, Inc., 1975.

Feeley, R.M., Criner, P.E., and Watt, B.K.: Cholesterol content of foods. J. Am. Diet. Assoc., 61:134, 1972.

Food Fats and Oils. 4th ed. Washington, D.C., Institute of Shortening and Edible Oils, Inc., 1974.

Goodhart, R.S. and Shils, M.E. (eds.): Modern Nutrition in Health and Disease. 6th ed. Philadelphia, Lea & Febiger, 1980, Chapter 5.

Guyton, A.C.: Textbook of Medical Physiology. 6th ed., Philadelphia, W.B. Saunders Company, 1981, Chapter 68.

Havel, R.J., Approach to the patient with hyperlipidemia. Med. Clin. N. Am., 66:319, 1982.

Latner, A.L.: Cantarow and Trumper Clinical Biochemistry. 7th ed. Philadelphia, W.B. Saunders Company, 1975, Chapter 2.

Rizek, R.L., Friend, B., and Page, L.: Fat in today's food supply—level of use and sources. J. Am. Oil Chemists' Soc., 51:244, 1974.

CHAPTER 4

Proteins

Definition and Importance

Protein derived its name more than a century ago from a Greek word meaning "of first importance." It was the first substance recognized as a vital part of living tissue. Proteins, the key components of all living organisms, are nitrogen-containing compounds that yield amino acids on hydrolysis. Proteins are the fundamental structural compounds of the cell; they are essential constituents of the nucleus and protoplasm of every cell. Proteins are the most abundant of the organic compounds in the body. Most of the protein is found in muscle tissue; the remainder is distributed in soft tissues, bones, teeth, blood and other body fluids. Hormones and enzymes are proteins. Since proteins serve such important and essential functions in the body, and since certain indispensable protein components can be obtained solely through dietary intake, it is obvious that the quality and amounts of protein in the daily diet and a knowledge of protein sources and of protein metabolism are matters of considerable importance to those interested in nutrition and health sciences.

The Composition and Nature of Proteins

Proteins, like fats and carbohydrates, contain carbon, hydrogen and oxygen but, in addition, they also contain about 16 per cent *nitrogen* along with sulfur and sometimes other elements such as phosphorus, iron and cobalt. The structural units of protein are the amino acids. They are united in long chains in various geometric structures and chemical combinations to form specific proteins, all of which are very large and complex molecules, each with its own physiological specificity. Despite their structural complexity, proteins can be broken down into their amino acid constituents by enzymes or by boiling with acids and alkalis under certain conditions. Pure dry proteins are fairly stable, but under the conditions in which they are found in foods they tend to decompose at room tempera-

tures, aided by bacterial action, and may form products that are toxic to the body; thus, the necessity for keeping protein foods such as eggs, fish, fowl, meat and milk refrigerated.

Plants obtain their nitrogen from the nitrates and ammonia in the soil, and from them synthesize their protein. Animals, in turn, obtain their required nitrogen from protein foods (plants and other animals). Animal metabolism, excretion and death finally return the nitrogen to the soil. This continuing process is known as the *nitrogen cycle.*

AMINO ACIDS

Twenty-two amino acids have been recognized as constituents of most protein. They are all alpha-amino carboxylic acids: that is, they have a basic amino group and an acid carboxylic group attached to the same carbon atom.

$$R-\overset{\overset{\displaystyle H}{|}}{\underset{\underset{\displaystyle NH_2}{|}}{C}}-COOH$$

They are differentiated by the remainder of the molecule (R), as illustrated above.

Amino acids, because they have both an acidic and basic group, have a buffer capacity. Depending on pH they can form salts with either acids or bases.

STRUCTURE OF PROTEINS

Amino acids join together to form proteins by means of the *peptide link:* the carboxylic carbon of one acid attaches to the nitrogen of another acid with a molecule of water being formed at the same time, as shown in Figure 4–1. The resulting compound has a free carboxyl group at one end and a free amino group at the other, so that the chain can continue to be built up from both ends.

Proteins vary in size from relatively small polypeptides such as ACTH with a molecular weight of 3200 (23 amino acid units) to very complex molecules with several hundred thousand amino acid units. The polypeptide chains take the form of a *helix.* Several chains may be

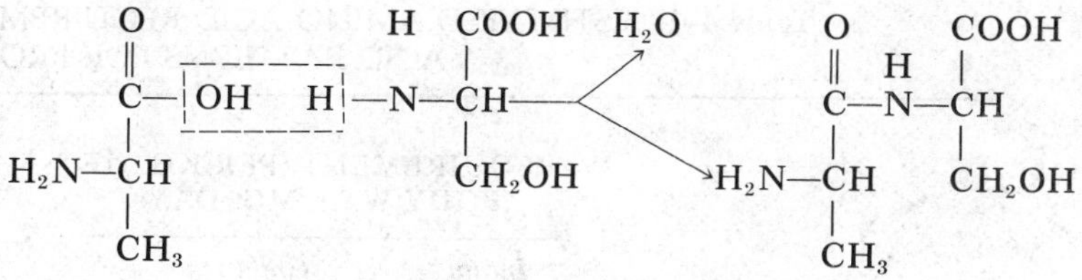

$$\underset{\text{Alanine}}{\overset{\displaystyle\overset{\text{O}}{\|}}{\underset{\underset{\text{CH}_3}{|}}{\underset{|}{\overset{\displaystyle\text{C}}{\underset{\displaystyle\text{H}_2\text{N}-\text{CH}}{}}}}\text{—OH}} \quad \underset{\text{Serine}}{\overset{\text{H COOH}}{\underset{\underset{\text{CH}_2\text{OH}}{|}}{\text{H}-\text{N}-\text{CH}}}} \quad \overset{\text{H}_2\text{O}}{\nearrow} \quad \underset{\text{Alanyl-serine}}{\overset{\displaystyle\overset{\text{O}}{\|}\ \ \text{COOH}}{\underset{\underset{\text{CH}_3}{|}}{\underset{\displaystyle\text{H}_2\text{N}-\text{CH}}{\overset{\text{H}\ |}{\text{C}-\text{N}-\text{CH}}}}}\text{CH}_2\text{OH}}$$

Figure 4–1. Formation of a dipeptide.

linked together (usually through the S-S link of cystine). In addition, the entire chain may be wound upon itself into a globular or other form —the whole being held rigid by interatomic forces such as hydrogen bonds. The structure of a protein may thus be considered at three levels: the *primary structure* is the number, kind, and order of the amino acids; the *secondary structure* is the helical form; and the *tertiary structure* is the spatial arrangement. It is because of the almost infinite possibilities of variation offered by these structures that there are millions of different proteins with specific properties and biological functions.

Studies on the shape of protein molecules indicate that there are two general types: globular proteins, with a length:width ratio less than 10, and fibrous proteins with a ratio greater than 10. The *fibrous proteins* are used in the formation of structural elements. They may have several helical peptide chains twisted together to form a stiff rod. They are characterized by low solubility and high mechanical strength. Collagen of connective tissue, keratin of hair and nails, and myosin of muscle tissue are examples of fibrous proteins.

Globular proteins are found in the extracellular fluid of plants and animals, and in conjugated form constitute most intracellular enzymes. They are very soluble and are easily denatured.* Some globular proteins of interest in nutrition are casein in milk, egg albumin, the albumins and globulins of blood plasma, and hemoglobin.

ESSENTIAL AMINO ACIDS

There are nine amino acids that are classified as essential, since they must be supplied to the body in the food. Body synthesis of these amino acids is lacking or so limited as to be insuffi-

cient to meet metabolic needs. These *essential amino acids* are:

valine	tryptophan
lysine	phenylalanine
threonine	methionine
leucine	histidine
isoleucine	

Histidine was first found to be required by infants, and work by Kopple and Swendseid suggests that it may also be essential for adults.[15] Without an adequate supply of the essential amino acids, protein cannot be synthesized or body tissue maintained.

The other amino acids that can be synthesized by the body in adequate amounts for normal function are termed *non-essential*:

glycine	proline
alanine	hydroxyproline
serine	citrulline
cystine	arginine
tyrosine	norleucine
aspartic acid	hydroxyglutamic acid
glutamic acid	

This is not to suggest that these amino acids are not essential constituents of the proteins, but rather that it is not essential to include them in the diet because the tissues can make their own supply from carbohydrate, fat and other amino acids. The estimated requirements for the essential amino acids for the infant and the adult are listed in Table 4–1.

Having stated the estimated requirements, the Food and Nutrition Board went on to define the "ideal" protein or the protein with the amino acid pattern that would best fulfill the requirements. In 1973 a committee of FAO/WHO also defined the amino acid pattern for the ideal protein, also shown in Table 4–1. They are somewhat different, which demonstrates that in this area of amino acid and protein requirements there are not clear-cut data and complete knowledge. Either of these patterns can be used to evaluate protein quality, and this will be discussed later in this chapter.

Because of growth, infants and children require more protein per kilogram of body weight, and a greater percentage of their protein must

---

*Conditions that do not hydrolyze peptide bonds may still destroy the biological nature and activity of the protein. These are heat, air, ultraviolet radiation, alcohol, strong acids or bases, detergents, salts of heavy metals, alkaloidal reagents such as tannic acid, and violent shaking. The protein usually coagulates after denaturation.

Table 4–1 ESTIMATED AMINO ACID REQUIREMENTS OF MAN AND AMINO ACID PATTERNS FOR PROTEINS

AMINO ACID	REQUIREMENT (PER KG. OF BODY WT.), MG./DAY*			AMINO ACID PATTERN FOR HIGH QUALITY PROTEINS, MG./G. OF PROTEIN	FAO/WHO†† PROVISIONAL AMINO ACID SCORING PATTERN MG./G. PROTEIN
	Infant† *(4–6 mo.)*	*Child* *(10–12 yr.)*	*Adult*		
Histidine	33	?	?	17	—
Isoleucine	83	28	12	42	40
Leucine	135	42	16	70	70
Lysine	99	44	12	51	55
Total *S*-containing amino acids (methionine and cystine)	49	22	10	26	35
Total aromatic amino acids (phenylalanine and tyrosine)	141	22	16	73	60
Threonine	68	28	8	35	40
Tryptophan	21	4	3	11	10
Valine	92	25	14	48	50

*FNB, Recommended Dietary Allowances, 9th ed., Washington, D.C., NRC, 1980.

†Two grams per kilogram of body weight per day of protein of the quality defined by the amino acid pattern would meet the amino acid needs of the infant.

††FAO/WHO, Energy and Protein Requirements, WHO Tech. Rep. No 522, 1973.

be composed of essential amino acids—approximately 43 per cent for the infant and 36 per cent for the child, compared with 19 per cent for the adult (Fig. 4–2).

SPECIAL FUNCTIONS OF AMINO ACIDS

Although virtually all the amino acids have certain unique functions in the body, a few are worth singling out. *Tryptophan* is a precursor of the vitamin niacin. Tryptophan is also a precur-

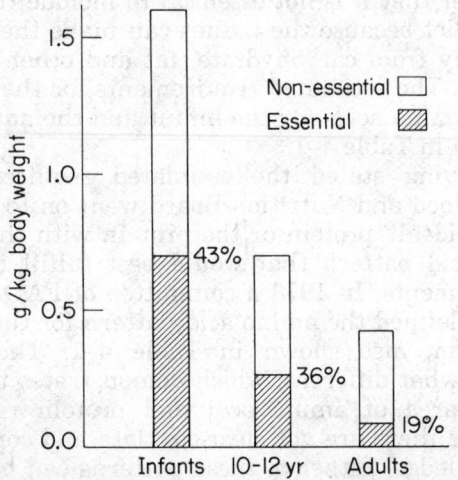

Figure 4–2. Proportion of total and essential amino acids required by various age groups as percentage of total nitrogen required. (From Scrimshaw, N. S.: Strengths and weaknesses of the committee approach: an analysis of past and present recommended dietary allowances for protein in health and disease. N. Engl. J. Med., *294*:136, 1976.)

sor of the neurotransmitter serotonin, which is discussed on page 666. *Methionine* is a principal donor of methyl groups for the synthesis of various compounds such as choline and creatine. Methionine is also a precursor of *cystine* and many other sulfur-containing compounds in the body. *Phenylalanine* is a precursor of *tyrosine* and together they lead to the formation of thyroxine and epinephrine. *Tyrosine* is the precursor from which the pigment of skin and hair is made. *Arginine* and *citrulline*, non-essential amino acids, are specifically involved in the synthesis of urea in the liver. *Glycine*, the simplest and perhaps most ubiquitous of the amino acids, combines with many toxic substances and converts them to harmless forms, which are then excreted. Glycine is also used in the synthesis of the porphyrin nucleus of hemoglobin and is a constituent of one of the bile acids (glycocholic acid). *Histidine* is essential for the synthesis of histamine which causes vasodilatation in the circulatory system. Creatine, synthesized from *arginine, glycine* and *methionine*, combines with phosphate to form creatine phosphate. Creatine phosphate is an important reservoir of high-energy phosphate in the cell. Glutamine, formed from *glutamic acid*, and asparagine, formed from *aspartic acid*, have important roles as reservoirs of amino groups throughout the body. In addition, glutamic acid is a precursor of the neurotransmitter gamma aminobutyric acid (GABA), which is discussed on page 666. Inborn errors of metabolism that involve amino acids are discussed in Chapter 39.

Classification of Proteins

It is difficult to devise a consistent system for classification of the multitude of proteins. The following system is based partly on solubility and characteristic physical properties and partly on chemical composition. They are grouped as simple proteins, conjugated proteins and derived proteins.

Simple proteins are those which yield only amino acids upon hydrolysis. They include the following, which exhibit various degrees of solubility: albumins, globulins, glutelins, prolamins and albuminoids. Those proteins which are soluble in water and dilute salt solution, such as albumins and globulins, are present in animal fluids, while less soluble ones such as myosin and muscle protein are present in tissues.

Conjugated proteins are combinations of simple proteins and some other non-protein substance, called a prosthetic group, attached to the molecule. They perform functions that neither constituent could properly perform by itself. These include:

1. Nucleoproteins—combinations of simple proteins and nucleic acid. Deoxyribose nucleoproteins are the principal constituents of the genes, and ribose nucleoproteins are necessary for the synthesis of proteins in cytoplasm.

2. Mucoproteins and Glycoproteins—combinations of proteins and large quantities of complex polysaccharides. Example: mucin found in secretions from gastric mucous membranes.

3. Lipoproteins—compounds of proteins and triglycerides or other lipids. Example: phospholipid or cholesterol found in cell and organelle membranes.

4. Phosphoproteins—phosphoric acid joined by ester linkages to proteins. Example: casein of milk.

5. Metalloproteins—compounds of metals (copper, magnesium, zinc, iron) attached to proteins. Example: ferritin, hemosiderin, transferrin.

Derived proteins are products formed in the various stages of hydrolysis of the protein molecule. For example, proteoses are formed early in the hydrolysis process, whereas peptones, polypeptides and peptides are products that form near the final stages of protein breakdown.

Nitrogen Balance

To determine the extent of protein utilization, the nitrogen balance is studied. The amount of nitrogen is an accurate index of the amount of protein involved. Most proteins contain about 16 per cent nitrogen, and this fact is utilized in determining the amount of protein in foods or body substances. The nitrogen content is determined chemically and this figure, multiplied by 6.25, gives the amount of protein present in the substance. Conversely, if the number of grams of protein present is known, dividing this figure by 6.25 gives the number of grams of nitrogen. Thus, if the amount of nitrogen that goes into the body in food and the amount that leaves the body in the excreta are determined, the portion used by the body can be calculated.

If the nitrogen intake and the nitrogen output are equal, the individual is in *nitrogen balance* or *equilibrium*. Should the intake of nitrogen be greater than the amount in urine, feces and integumental loss, the individual is in a state of *positive balance*; that is, the buildup (anabolism) or synthesis of tissue proteins is greater than the breakdown (catabolic) activities. This is seen in periods of growth, in pregnancy and when new tissue is being formed such as following injury, surgery or prolonged malnutrition. There is a net gain of protein in the body. Should the excretion of nitrogen be more than that consumed, a state of *negative balance* exists; that is, the rate of protein breakdown is exceeding the rate of protein synthesis as summarized in Table 4–2. Negative nitrogen balance will occur when the protein intake is below the amount required by the body, and when there is too little carbohydrate and fat in the diet to meet energy needs and the body is forced to burn protein to meet these needs.

Table 4–2 SUMMARY OF SIGNIFICANCE OF NITROGEN BALANCE DATA

CONDITION	MEASUREMENT	SIGNIFICANCE
Positive nitrogen balance	N intake > N excretion	Growth; anabolism
Nitrogen equilibrium	N intake = N excretion	Maintenance and repair of tissue
Negative nitrogen balance	N intake < N excretion	Wasting of body, loss of weight

(From Guthrie, H. A.: Introductory Nutrition, 4th ed. St. Louis, C.V. Mosby Co., 1979.)

An adult may be maintained in nitrogen and protein equilibrium at any level of nitrogen intake that is above the minimum requirement. The body adjusts the balance depending upon the amount of protein regularly consumed.

Evaluation of Protein Quality

COMPLETE AND INCOMPLETE PROTEINS

Proteins that contain all the essential amino acids in sufficient quantity and in the right ratio to maintain nitrogen equilibrium and permit growth of the young are known as *complete proteins*. Such proteins are ovalbumin, the main protein of egg, and casein, the principal protein in milk. Other complete proteins are those in meat, fish and poultry. Proteins that do not supply all the essential amino acids in appropriate amounts to maintain nitrogen equilibrium and growth are *incomplete proteins*. The proteins in vegetables and grains are classified as incomplete proteins. Proteins are also characterized by their *biological value*. The biological value is high or low depending upon the completeness with which a protein supplies the essential amino acids. Foods of high biological value are largely of animal origin. Grain and vegetable proteins, being incomplete proteins, are of only fair or low biological value.

The incompleteness of proteins may be partial or total. *Partially incomplete proteins* will sustain life but, lacking sufficient amounts of essential amino acids, will not support normal growth, as demonstrated in Figure 4–3. These are found in legumes (dried beans and peas, peanuts), nuts and grains. A food protein lacking an essential amino acid will not support life or growth. Zein, a protein in corn, and gelatin, an animal protein, are examples of *totally incomplete proteins*. Plant foods generally contain an insufficient quantity of lysine, methionine, threonine and tryptophan and so are incomplete proteins. The amino acids that plant foods do contribute, however, are important and should be utilized most effectively by being eaten simultaneously with small amounts of a complete protein food, by being served in a correct mixture of several plant foods that will give all the amino acids in appropriate amounts, or by being supplemented with synthetic amino acids to make a complete protein. This is discussed further on page 58.

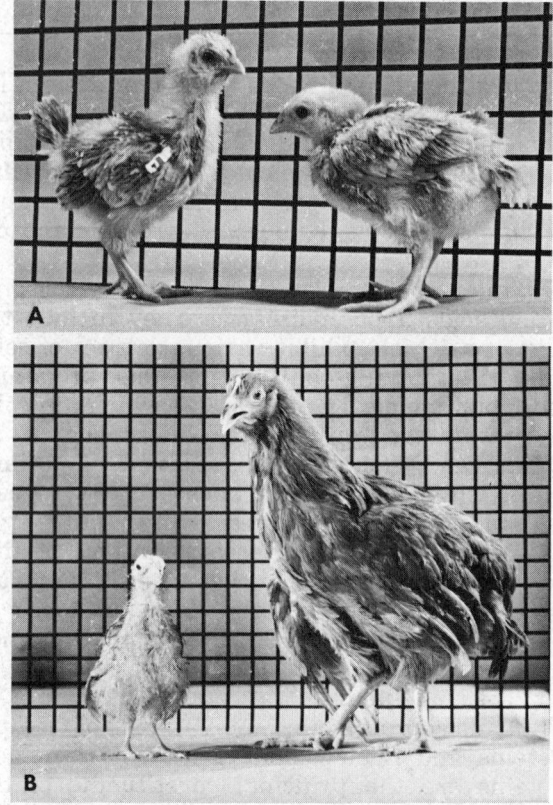

Figure 4–3. Effect of the amino acid tryptophan on growth and health. *A,* Week-old chicks. Chick at left to be fed a tryptophan-free diet. Chick at right will continue eating standard feed. *B,* Same chicks at nine weeks of age. The chick at left on tryptophan-free diet remains at approximately his week-old size. There are some changes in appearance, however, because most of the feathers, the beak and the eyes developed at normal rate. When tryptophan is restored to the diet, the chick will immediately begin to grow and mature, reaching maturation seemingly without ill effects. (Photos courtesy of Monsanto Chemical Company's Agricultural Experiment Farm, St. Louis, Missouri.)

AMINO ACID SCORE

The distribution of the essential amino acids in eggs and human milk has been recommended by the Joint Committee of FAO/WHO for use as the ideal reference pattern. However, in 1973 a new provisional amino acid scoring pattern was devised based on additional data on amino acid requirements.[5] Table 4–3 compares human milk protein, cow's milk protein and egg protein with the scoring pattern. A protein is compared with this amino acid reference pattern and receives an *amino acid or chemical score* by the calculation shown below.

$$\text{Amino acid score} = \frac{\text{mg. of an amino acid in 1 gm. test protein}}{\text{mg. of that amino acid in 1 gm. reference pattern}} \times 100$$

Table 4–3 COMPARISON OF HUMAN MILK, COW'S MILK AND EGG PROTEIN TO FAO/WHO STANDARD AMINO ACID PATTERN

AMINO ACID	FAO/WHO 1973 PROVISIONAL AMINO ACID SCORING PATTERN MG. PER G. OF PROTEIN	REPORTED COMPOSITION			
		HUMAN MILK		COW'S MILK	EGG
		RANGE	MEAN		
Histidine	*	18–36	26	27	22
Isoleucine	40	41–53	46	47	54
Leucine	70	83–107	93	95	86
Lysine	55	53–76	66	78	70
Methionine + cystine	35	29–60	42	33	57
Phenylalanine + tyrosine	60	68–118	72	102	93
Threonine	40	40–45	43	44	47
Tryptophan	10	16–17	17	14	17
Valine	50	44–77	55	64	66
Total	360	390–552	434	477	490
+ histidine		408–588	460	504	512

*Did not define for histidine
(From Joint FAO/WHO Ad Hoc Expert Committee, Energy and Protein Requirements, WHO Tech. Rep. No. 522, Geneva, Switzerland, 1973.)

The amino acid for which a protein has the lowest score is the *limiting amino acid* and becomes the chemical score for the protein. Proteins such as whole egg, human milk and cow's milk meet the reference pattern for all essential amino acids as shown in Table 4–3.

The amino acid score of a protein is a crude way to evaluate the quality of a protein because it does not take into account the digestibility of the protein, the availability of the amino acids, the utilization of those amino acids by the human body, or the ability of that protein to support cellular synthesis. Considering these biological factors, several measures of protein quality have been developed, but the most widely used is the net protein utilization.

NET PROTEIN UTILIZATION

Net protein utilization (NPU) measures the biological value (BV) or percentage of absorbed nitrogen utilized by the body and the digestibility of the protein under standard conditions of total dietary protein, total energy intake and nutritional status of the individual. NPU quantifies food nitrogen utilization and in simplistic terms is equal to the N retained/N intake, which is equal to

$$\frac{\text{N intake} - \text{N output}}{\text{N intake}}$$

The NPU will usually be less than the chemical score of a protein, as shown in Table 4–4.

An observation of interest is that as the amount of protein in the diet reaches the amount needed to maintain N equilibrium, a smaller percentage is retained, and thus the NPU for a protein seems to decrease. Why this happens is not clear, but on lower intakes of protein, the body seems to be more efficient in its protein retention and utilization. Possibly, the body has a survival mechanism providing for greater utilization of protein when protein intakes are low; however, even this ability is limited.

PROTEIN EFFICIENCY RATIO (PER)

This is the simplest test of protein quality. The PER is equal to the gain in weight of a growing animal divided by its protein intake during the study period. This gives an assessment of the nutritive value of a protein. A problem with this method is that some proteins are rated lower than their real value for human feeding because of the greater need for the sulfur-containing amino acid by the rat than by man.

Food Sources and Protein Complementation

Most people tend to ingest a mixture of foods in a meal, and the complete and incomplete proteins, in sufficient quantity, are apt to complement or supplement one another to provide all

Table 4–4 CHEMICAL SCORE AND NET PROTEIN UTILIZATION VALUES OF COMMON FOODS

PROTEIN	NEW PATTERN CHEMICAL SCORE	NPU MEASURED IN RATS
Whole egg	100	94
Human milk	100	87
Cow's milk	95	82
Soya bean	74	65
Sesame	50	54
Groundnut	65	47
Cottonseed	81	59
Maize	49	52
Millet	63	44
Rice, polished	67	59
Wheat, whole	53	48

(Adapted from Joint FAO/WHO Ad Hoc Expert Committee, Energy and Protein Requirements, WHO Tech. Rep. No. 522, Geneva, Switzerland, 1973, p. 67.)

the essential amino acids. The minimum daily protein requirement for the adult male, for example, is readily obtained in four slices of bread and one pint of milk as shown in Table 4–5.

When the use of a complete protein is restricted, mixtures of an incomplete protein with a small amount of a complete protein will supply the essential amino acids. Examples of this *complementation* are cereal with milk or macaroni and cheese. Small amounts of fish meal, meat sauce or skim milk may be added to vegetable or carbohydrate mixtures to provide the essential amino acids. Table 4–6 gives the amino acid contributions of vegetable proteins. Table 10–10 and Figure 10–2 show how foods can be eaten together to provide complete protein.

Products have been developed from incomplete proteins mixed together in proper proportions. One product, Incaparina, was developed by the Institute of Nutrition in Central America and Panama (INCAP). It consists of a mixture of ground maize, sorghum, cottonseed flour, torula yeast, calcium carbonate and vitamin A. Suitable products have been developed in other countries to meet the protein needs, especially of infants and children.

Enrichment of grains and legumes with amino acids that they lack (lysine to wheat, methionine to legumes) has also been done. However, if one amino acid is increased too greatly, the protein quality may be decreased, as evidenced by lower nitrogen retention.[12] Mutual complementation of proteins is most effective when two principles are kept in mind:

1. The lower the quality of protein, the more protein is required to meet the minimum requirements for amino acids and total protein. In a vegetable protein diet, more total protein is required than in a mixed vegetable and animal protein diet.

2. For maximal utilization of amino acids for protein synthesis, all amino acids should be present in the blood stream after absorption from the gastrointestinal tract. This means that complementary proteins should be eaten at the same time or after only a short interval.

Further discussion of protein complementation is found on page 227. The practical application of these principles with recipes is presented by Frances Moore Lappé in *Diet for a Small Planet.*

Metabolism of Proteins

The processes of digestion and absorption of proteins are discussed in Chapter 5. All proteins must be broken down into amino acids and di- or tripeptides by digestion before absorption and

Table 4–5 ESSENTIAL AMINO ACIDS SUPPLIED BY BREAD AND MILK (4 slices (100 gm.) of bread and 2 cups (480 gm.) of milk)

ESSENTIAL AMINO ACIDS	BREAD (White)–4 slices yield 8.5 gm. protein	MILK (Whole or skim)–2 cups yield 16.8 gm. protein	TOTAL	ADULT MINIMUM DAILY NEEDS (Male)
		Amounts in Grams		
Tryptophan	0.091	0.235	0.326	0.25
Threonine	0.282	0.773	1.055	0.50
Isoleucine	0.429	1.070	1.449	0.70
Leucine	0.668	1.651	2.319	1.10
Lysine	0.225	1.306	1.531	0.80
Methionine + cystine	0.342	0.562	0.904	1.10
Phenylalanine + tyrosine	0.708	1.670	2.378	1.10
Valine	0.435	1.152	1.587	0.80

The total amount of protein in bread and milk includes not only the essential amino acids listed but also the non-essential amino acids.

Table 4-6 AMINO ACID COMPOSITION OF SOME FOODS

ESSENTIAL AMINO ACIDS**	CHEESE EGGS MILK MEAT	CORN	CEREAL	LE-GUMES	WHOLE GRAINS (WITH GERM)	NUTS SEED OILS SOYBEANS	SESAME & SUN-FLOWER SEEDS	PEANUT PROTEIN	GREEN LEAFY VEG. LEAF PROT.	GELA-TIN*	YEAST
Cystine**			—	—			x				x
Methionine	x	x	x		x	—	x	—	—	—	x
Isoleucine	x										
Leucine	x		—		x					—	
Lysine	x	—		x	x	x	—	—		—	
Phenylalanine		—	—								
Threonine	x	—	—	x	—	x		—			x
Tryptophan				—	—		x	—		—	
Valine	x									—	

*Gelatin is not a good source of all essential amino acids.
**Not essential but added because hard to get in a vegetarian diet. Methionine and cystine can be compared as one.

Symbols: X = High amount of amino acid present in that food.
— = Low amount of amino acid present in that food.
Blank spaces indicate a general good balance of amino acids in the food.

(From Erhard, D.: Nutrition education for the "now" generation. J. Nutr. Educ., 3: 135, 1971.)

use by the body. In the lumen are large amounts of endogenous protein from cell sloughing and cell secretions, which combine with exogenous protein to present a fairly constant amino acid pattern. Absorption through the intestinal lumen is an active process, not simple diffusion, and it requires energy (ATP). There appear to be two systems, one for free amino acids and one for small peptides. The one for peptides appears to provide for intracellular hydrolysis of di- and tripeptides in the mucosal cell. As a group, the essential amino acids are better absorbed than non-essential amino acids. The amino acids are carried in the portal vein to the liver and then into the general circulation. Amino acids that are constantly being formed by breakdown of tissue proteins and non-essential amino acids synthesized in the body contribute to the circulating pool.

PROTEIN SYNTHESIS

The fundamental and most interesting use of the amino acid is as a building block for the body proteins, such as enzymes, hormones, vitamins and structural proteins. Each cell in the body has the capacity to synthesize an enormous number of specific proteins. For the synthesis of a protein all the essential amino acids must be available at the same time. Either the non-essential amino acids must be supplied as such or there must be suitable precursors, including amino groups from other amino acids, so that they can be synthesized. The synthesis of the characteristic proteins of each cell is controlled by the genetic material *deoxyribose nucleic acid (DNA)* in the nucleus. DNA is used as a template for *transcription* or the synthesis of *ribose nucleic acid* (RNA), of which there are several forms. One form, *messenger* or *mRNA*, carries the information to the cytoplasm where the proteins are synthesized. DNA and RNA are composed of nucleotide units consisting of ribose (or deoxyribose), phosphoric acid and one of the four cyclic nitrogenous bases (a purine or pyrimidine) as shown in Figure 4–4. They are strung together in long chains of pentose and phosphoric acid alternately with the purine and pyrimidine molecules as branches. DNA is a double-stranded molecule, the two chains in the form of a double helix held together by hydrogen bonds linking a purine and a pyrimidine. It may have a molecular weight of two billion, with a million or more bases arranged in a continuous line. RNA is a single strand. It is the sequence of the bases along the chain which specifies the arrangement of amino acids in the protein, each amino acid being defined by a set of three bases. In the cytoplasm are other RNA molecules, relatively small, one for each amino acid. These *t*

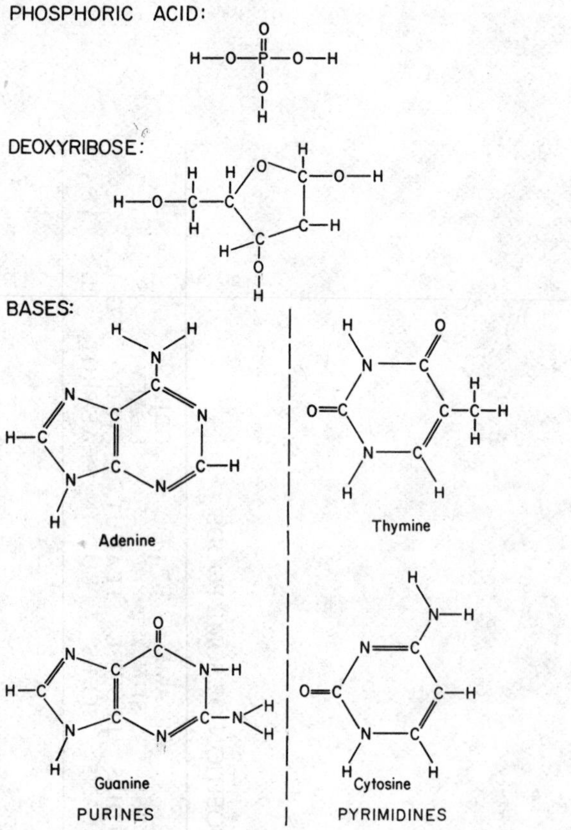

Figure 4–4. The basic building blocks of DNA. (From Guyton, A. C.: Textbook of Medical Physiology, 6th ed. Philadelphia, W. B. Saunders Company, 1981.)

(transfer) RNA's direct the amino acids to the appropriate position along the mRNA so that the peptide chain can be synthesized. In addition *r (ribosomal) RNA*, composed of a large and small RNA molecule, functions with the ribosome to bind tRNA to the ribosome and then provide enzymes that promote peptide linkage. This intricate process is summarized in Figure 4–5. Of course, among the proteins which must be synthesized are the enzymes needed to catalyze the synthesis. Energy for synthesis is supplied by ATP, itself a nucleotide.

PROTEIN CATABOLISM

There is no large reserve of free amino acids in the body, and any amount above that needed for synthesis of tissue protein and the varied non-protein nitrogen-containing compounds is metabolized. The amino group is detached from the amino acid before oxidation of the remaining portion of the molecule. Most of the amino nitrogen is converted to urea in the liver and excreted in the urine. The liver is the main location for deamination and other early steps in amino acid metabolism (including synthesis of non-essential amino acids). The carbon skeletons are converted into some of the same intermediates formed during glucose and fatty acid catabolism. These can be carried to the peripheral tissues, where they are used for oxidation to produce high-energy phosphate molecules (ATP). These fragments can also be used in synthetic processes to make glucose or fats. About 58 per cent of the protein consumed can be converted into glucose. The mechanisms of these reactions will be further discussed in Chapter 5.

Besides urea, the major excretory products are uric acid and creatinine. *Uric acid* is the end product of the metabolism of purines, important components of the nucleic acids. Disturbed metabolism of purines and uric acid is found in gout, which is discussed in Chapter 26. *Creatinine* is the excretion form of creatine, present in all muscle tissue and creatine phosphate, a store of high-energy phosphate. The amount of urea excreted is related to protein intake, while creatinine excretion is related to muscle mass and is relatively constant in any individual. In fact, it is so constant that it is often used to check the accuracy of 24-hour urine collections. Serum creatinine as a measure of protein nutriture is further discussed in Chapter 9.

METABOLIC POOL OF AMINO ACIDS

Metabolism of proteins is sometimes divided into two components: (1) *exogenous* metabolism, which includes the metabolism of all protein ingested in excess of essential body requirements and is obviously quite variable; and (2) *endogenous* metabolism, which includes all the necessary protein buildup and breakdown processes that are essential to life, growth and repair of the body. Creatinine excretion is regarded as a measure of the endogenous metabolism.

There is practically no storage of amino acids in the body. They are constantly being utilized to form other compounds and broken down to form new amino acids.

Any "storage" is in the form of cellular proteins themselves. There is an upper limit, however, after which excess amino acids are degraded and used for energy or stored as fat. As with fats and carbohydrates, there exists a state of dynamic equilibrium for amino acids, with constant buildup, breakdown, and interchange, and there exists a *metabolic pool* of amino acids in this state of dynamic equilibrium that at any given time may be called upon by the body for any appropriate need. The most active tissues for protein turnover are the plasma proteins, intestinal mucosa, pancreas, liver and kidney, while the muscle, skin and brain are much less active. Figure 4–6 summarizes the an-

abolic and catabolic reactions of amino acids. The direction taken depends on the supply of amino acids in the food and the needs of the body. Regulation is largely under hormonal control.

HORMONAL REGULATION

Hormones have anabolic and catabolic effects on protein metabolism. The *growth hormone* stimulates protein synthesis, thus increasing tissue concentration. *Insulin* also stimulates protein synthesis by accelerating amino acid transport across the cell membrane, and a lack of insulin reduces protein synthesis. *Testosterone* also stimulates protein synthesis during growth periods. The *glucocorticoids* stimulate gluconeogenesis and ketogenesis from proteins and decrease protein in most tissues except for plasma and hepatic protein, which are increased. *Thyroxine* indirectly affects protein metabolism by increasing the rate of metabolism in all cells. As a result it increases the rate of normal anabolic and catabolic reactions of protein. In physiological doses with adequate calories and amino acids present, it will produce protein synthesis. With inadequate calories or in large doses (unphysiological), thyroxine will have a catabolic effect.

Functions of Proteins in the Body

Dietary proteins furnish the amino acids for synthesis of tissue protein and other special metabolic functions. A concise summary of the numerous functions of proteins is as follows:

1. Proteins are used *to repair worn-out body tissue proteins* (anabolism) resulting from the continued "wear and tear" (catabolism) going on in the body. This is a function provided only by protein. No other nutrients can do it because the amino acid building blocks of tissue are available only from protein.

2. Proteins are used *to build new tissue* (anabolism) by supplying the necessary amino acid building blocks. This is the reason for an increased protein need during periods of growth, as in infancy, childhood, adolescence and pregnancy.

3. Proteins are a *source of heat and energy.* They supply 4 kcalories per gram, the same as does a carbohydrate, but in a more expensive fashion than a carbohydrate. Not only is protein a more expensive source of energy to buy and eat, but also it has a greater specific dynamic action than carbohydrate, which adds to the total energy expended by the body (5 per cent of calories for carbohydrate and fat versus as

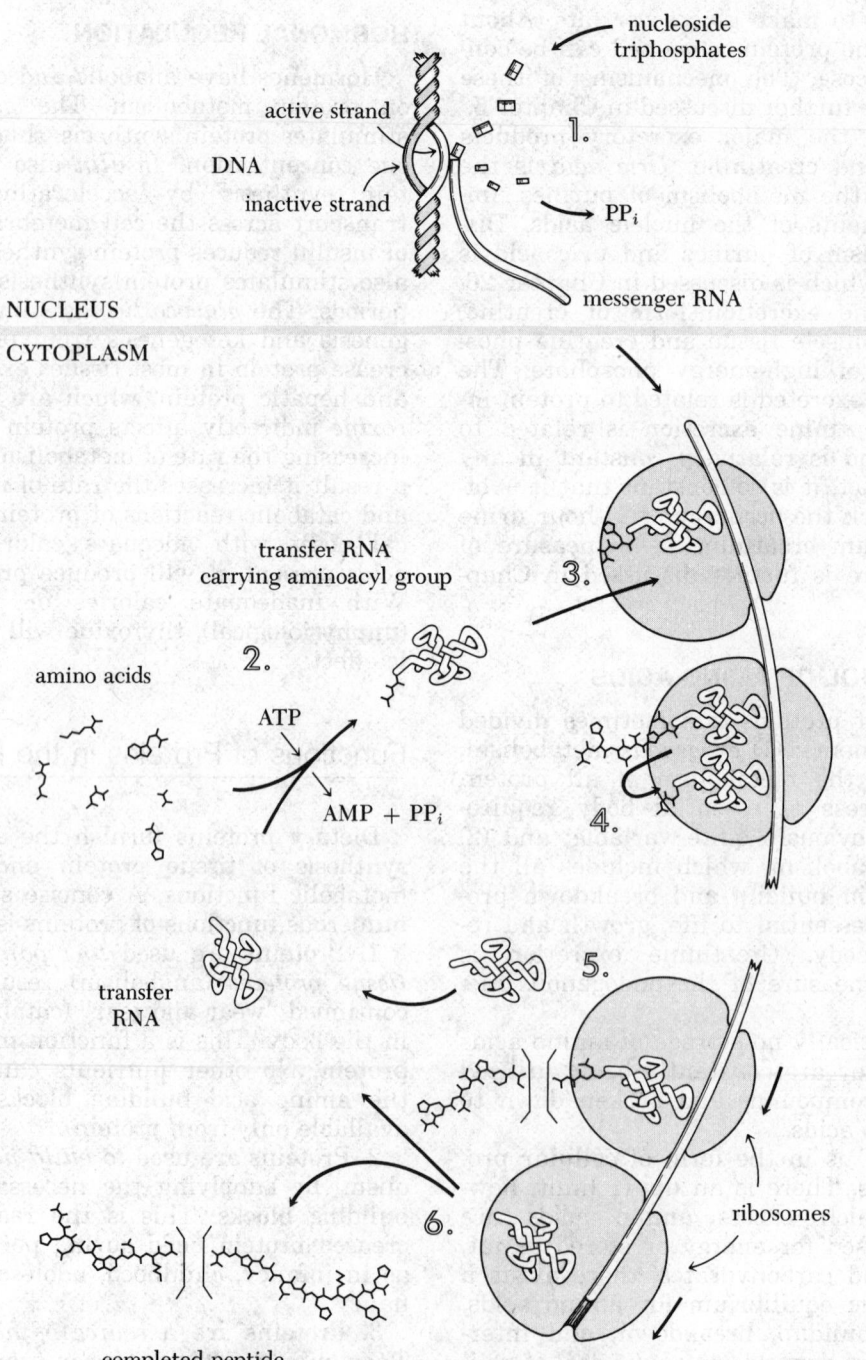

nucleoside triphosphates

active strand

DNA

inactive strand

1.

PPᵢ

messenger RNA

NUCLEUS

CYTOPLASM

transfer RNA carrying aminoacyl group

3.

amino acids

2.

ATP

AMP + PPᵢ

4.

transfer RNA

5.

ribosomes

6.

completed peptide

Figure 4–5. *See legend on opposite page*

much as 30 per cent for protein). However, in a mixed diet this difference is not significant. (See page 19 for definition of specific dynamic action.) Also, the excretion of nitrogen, the end product of protein metabolism, involves energy expenditure by the body. Carbohydrate, on the other hand, is cheap to obtain and burns completely to carbon dioxide and water.

4. Proteins *contribute to numerous essential body secretions and fluids.* Enzymes are proteins, and hormones have protein or amino acid components. Mucus, milk and sperm are largely protein, as is the fluid in which sperm are contained. About the only protein-free body fluids are bile and urine.

5. Plasma proteins of the blood, particularly albumin, are important in the *maintenance of normal osmotic relations* among the various body fluids. Indeed, one of the main signs of hypoproteinemia is the appearance of edema (excessive tissue fluid) as a result of a loss of osmotic balance.

6. Proteins *maintain the acid-base balance of blood and tissues.* Because of their unique structure proteins are able to combine with either acidic or basic substances and thus reduce their effect on fluid acidity.

7. Plasma proteins also function in the *transport of other substances.* Lipid-carrying proteins transport triglyceride, cholesterol, phospholipid and fat-soluble vitamins. Transferrin transports iron, and calcium is transported bound to a protein. Albumin carries free fatty acids and bilirubin. In addition many drugs are carried in the blood bound to albumin.

8. Proteins in the form of *immunoglobulins (or antibodies) play a role in the resistance of the body* to disease.

9. *Dietary proteins furnish the amino acids for a variety of metabolic functions.* Some of these have been discussed on page 54.

Recommended Protein and Amino Acid Allowances

The recommended daily allowance (RDA) for the 70-kg. man and 55-kg. woman is approximately 0.8 gm. of protein per kg. of ideal body weight per day.[9] This amounts to 56 and 44 gm. per day for the average man and woman, respectively (see Table 10–1), or approximately 8 to 9 per cent of the total daily calories.

The minimum requirement of protein needed to maintain nitrogen balance (see page 55) has been determined to be about 0.45 gm. per kg. ideal body weight daily, assuming adequate energy intake. An increase of 30 per cent is made to account for individual variation (0.45 × 1.30 = 0.585 gm./kg./day). This figure of 0.59 gm./kg./day is increased again to account for the fact that the mixed proteins in the U.S. diet have about 75 per cent efficiency of utilization. Thus the final recommended allowance for protein for the adult is 0.8 gm./kg./day based on ideal body weight.[9] For infants and children additional allowances are made for growth, and for the pregnant or lactating woman additional allowances are recommended for fetal development and milk production, as shown in Table 11–1).

The Joint Committee of FAO/WHO has also defined protein allowances by defining the "safe level" of protein intake in terms of the highest quality protein (egg or milk) as 0.52 to 0.57 gm./kg./day for the adult.[5] Table 4–7 gives

Figure 4–5. Schematic summary of protein synthesis. *Top, step 1.* A molecule of DNA in the nucleus unfolds, and one of its strands is used as a template to direct the formation of messenger RNA (mRNA) from nucleoside triphosphates, which lose inorganic-pyrophosphate (PP_1) as they attach to the growing RNA chain. The completed mRNA moves to the cytoplasm (*bottom*), where it binds ribosomes into a polysome, and acts as a template for protein synthesis.

The following steps are shown on separate ribosomes for clarity, but in fact they are repeated in sequence on each ribosome. The successive ribosomes group longer and longer peptide chains as they move down the molecule of mRNA.

Step 2. Meanwhile, amino acids are combined with specific molecules of transfer RNA (tRNA) in the cytoplasm by a reaction that also involves the cleavage of adenosine triphosphate (ATP) into adenosine monophosphate (AMP) and PP_1.

Step 3. The tRNA molecules, carrying the amino acids in the form of aminoacyl groups, diffuse to the polysome, where the growing peptide chain is on another molecule of tRNA already attached. The incoming tRNA, which bears the next group required for the growing peptide (in this case leucyl residue), has the proper configuration to complex with mRNA on the ribosome.

Step 4. When the proper tRNA is in place, the peptide chain is transferred onto the amino group of the new residue brought in by tRNA, so that the chain is now one residue longer.

Step 5. When the transfer of the previous step is completed, the previously bound tRNA no longer carries a peptide chain and is free to dissociate from the ribosome, returning to the mixed pool of tRNA in the soluble cytoplasm, where it is available for transport of another molecule of its specific amino acid. The ribosome now moves along the mRNA molecule to the position where the placement of the next amino acid will be directed.

Step 6. Steps 3, 4 and 5 are repeated. As each amino acid residue adds to the peptide chain, the ribosome moves down the mRNA molecule. When a ribosome has reached the end of the molecule, the peptide is completed and is detached into the soluble cytoplasm. The ribosome itself can then move free of the mRNA and be available for attachment to the beginning of yet another molecule of mRNA (not shown). (From McGilvery, R. W.: Biochemistry—A Functional Approach. 2nd ed. Philadelphia, W. B. Saunders Company, 1979.)

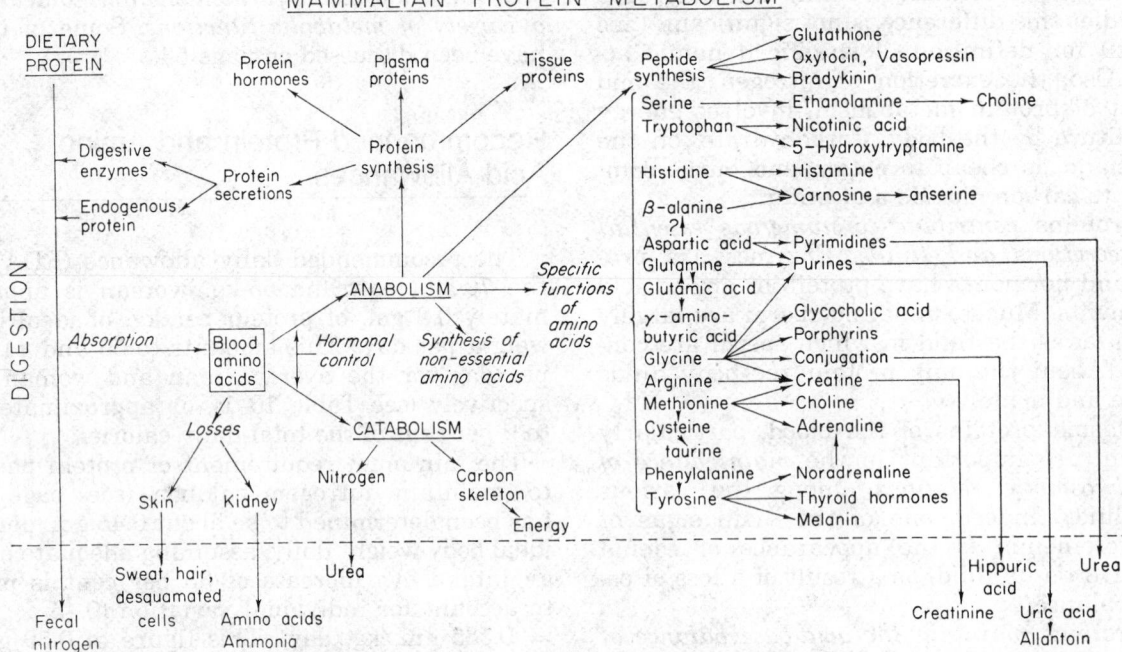

Figure 4–6. General features of protein metabolism. (From Munro, H. N.: An introduction to biochemical aspects of protein metabolism. In Munro, H. N., and Allison, J. B. (eds.): Mammalian Protein Metabolism. New York, Academic Press, 1964, p. 32.)

Table 4–7 SAFE LEVEL OF PROTEIN IN TERMS OF DIETS OF PROTEIN QUALITIES OF 60%, 70% AND 80% RELATIVE TO MILK OR EGGS

AGE GROUP	BODY WEIGHT (KG.)	SAFE LEVEL OF PROTEIN INTAKE		ADJUSTED LEVEL FOR PROTEINS OF DIFFERENT QUALITY (GM. PER PERSON PER DAY)		
		(gm. protein per kg. per day)	(gm. protein per person per day)	Score [a] 80	Score 70	Score 60
Infants						
6–11 months	9.0	1.53	14	17	20	23
Children						
1–3 years	13.4	1.19	16	20	23	27
4–6 years	20.2	1.01	20	26	29	34
7–9 years	28.1	0.88	25	31	35	41
Male adolescents						
10–12 years	36.9	0.81	30	37	43	50
13–15 years	51.3	0.72	37	46	53	62
16–19 years	62.9	0.60	38	47	54	63
Female adolescents						
10–12 years	38.0	0.76	29	36	41	48
13–15 years	49.9	0.63	31	39	45	52
16–19 years	54.4	0.55	30	37	43	50
Adult man	65.0	0.57	37	46 [b]	53 [b]	62 [b]
Adult woman	55.0	0.52	29	36 [b]	41 [b]	48 [b]
Pregnant woman, latter half of pregnancy			Add 9	Add 11	Add 13	Add 15
Lactating woman, first 6 months			Add 17	Add 21	Add 24	Add 28

[a] Scores are estimates of the quality of the protein usually consumed relative to that of egg or milk. The safe level of protein intake is adjusted by multiplying it by 100 divided by the score of the food protein. For example, 100/60 = 1.67, and for a child of 1–4 years the safe level of protein intake would be 16 × 1.67, or 27 gm. of protein having a relative quality of 60.

[b] The correction may overestimate adult protein requirements.

(From Joint FAO/WHO Ad Hoc Expert Committee, Energy and Protein Requirements, WHO Tech. Rep. No. 522, Geneva, Switzerland, 1973, p. 74.)

guidelines for increasing this amount depending on the quality of the protein in the diet. In addition, several argue that the estimated safe level of 0.57 gm./kg. for the adult male and 0.52 gm./kg. for the adult female are not adequate because the energy content of the diet can influence the nitrogen balance, and that adults at these levels did not maintain nitrogen balance.[10, 26] The magnitude of the change in nitrogen balance is 0.2 to 0.3 gm. of nitrogen for each 100 kcal. added to or subtracted from the diet.[9]

MEETING THE RDA FOR PROTEIN

The RDA of 0.8 gm. protein per kg. ideal body weight allows for intake of some proteins of low biological value. It is good nutritional practice to include at least one third of the protein intake from complete protein foods, although this is not absolutely necessary. Balanced and adequate protein intakes can be achieved by conscientious attention to the combination of incomplete proteins, but the protein requirement will be higher. Table 4–8 gives the protein content of various foods.

PROTEIN:CALORIE RATIO

If the fat and carbohydrate in a diet are supplied in adequate amounts to meet energy requirements, there can be nitrogen equilibrium even when the intake of protein is close to the minimum level. They will "spare" the proteins. Unless sufficient calories are available in the diet for energy needs, an increased amount of protein is metabolized to compensate for the dietary energy inadequacy. Carbohydrate seems to be more important than fat for "sparing protein." Although the mechanism is not understood, it is supposed that because carbohydrate provides a major source of oxaloacetate for the citric acid cycle and the carbon skeletons for non-essential amino acids, in the absence of adequate carbohydrate, protein must perform these functions, which fat cannot do. This is why inadequate carbohydrate intake can cause a negative nitrogen balance.

In 1975 the Protein-Calorie Advisory Group of the UN published a report stating a recommended protein:calorie ratio of 1:20, i.e., 5 to 5.5 per cent of the calories, should come from high quality protein.[21] This is the recommendation for a person with "moderate activity" who is consuming a high quality protein. "Light activity" with a lower calorie intake would require a higher concentration of protein in the diet and "heavy activity," usually with a greater energy intake, would require a lower percentage of calories from protein. The Department of Health and Social Security of the United Kingdom has also defined protein requirements based on energy intake and states that protein should be 10 to 15 per cent of total caloric intake, certainly high enough to allow a wide margin of safety.[24]

The 1973 FAO/WHO report states that populations of most countries, independent of income, select a diet containing approximately 11 to 13 per cent of the calories as protein.[5]

However, for much of the world's population income is a factor and the energy expenditure is high (and often not met by adequate energy intake) and the protein quality is low, meaning that the percentage of calories from protein may need to be higher.

Table 4–8 PROTEINS AVAILABLE IN COMMON FOODS

FOOD	CHIEF PROTEINS PRESENT	COMPLEMENT OF ESSENTIAL AMINO ACIDS	AVERAGE SERVING Grams of Proteins	AVERAGE SERVING Approximate Measure	WEIGHT GRAMS
Milk, whole	Casein and lact-albumin	Complete	9 gm.	1 glass (8 oz.)	244
Meat, lean	Albumin and myosin	Complete	22 gm.	3.0 oz.	85
Cheese, uncreamed cottage	Casein and lact-albumin	Complete	5 gm.	1 oz.	28
Egg	Ovalbumin and ovovitellin	Complete	6 gm.	1 egg	50
Navy beans	Phaesolin	Incomplete	7.5 gm.	½ cup	128
Peas, small, green	Legumin	Incomplete	4 gm.	½ cup	80
Corn, canned	Glutelin Zein	Incomplete Incomplete	2.5 gm.	½ cup	128
Wheat bread	Gliadin	Incomplete	2 gm.	1 slice	23
Soy beans	Glycinin Legumelin	Complete Incomplete	3 gm.	½ cup	54
Dry, nonfat milk	Casein and lact-albumin	Complete	6 + gm.	¼ cup	17.5 gm.

FACTORS AFFECTING PROTEIN REQUIREMENTS

EFFECT OF GROWTH. During growth the need for protein is greater than at any other time in a person's life. Thus, infants and children need relatively more than the adult allowance because they accumulate new tissue of high protein content. Recommended allowances for children are 2.2 gm. per kg. of body weight for the infant of 0 to 6 months of age, 2.0 gm. per kg. for the infant of 6 months to 1 year, 1.7 gm. per kg. for 1 to 3 years, 1.2 to 1.5 gm. per kg. for older children and 0.8 to 1.0 gm. per kg. for adolescents, as shown in Table 10–1 and discussed in Chapters 12 to 14.

EFFECT OF PREGNANCY AND LACTATION. Because pregnancy and lactation represent another form of growth, the mother has an additional need for protein. The RDA for pregnant women is 30 gm. above the normal allowance of 0.8 gm. per kg. of body weight. Lactation imposes an additional protein burden on the body inasmuch as 12 to 15 gm. of protein may be secreted daily in the breast milk. The RDA includes an intake of an additional 20 gm. of protein above the normal allowance during lactation (see Chapter 11). In all these periods of growth requiring additional amounts of protein, additional calories are also necessary.

EFFECT OF AGE. The protein allowance of 0.8 gm. per kg. of body weight is maintained throughout adult life. However, a higher proportion of protein in the diet is required to achieve this level when the total energy consumption is decreased with age. Protein requirements of the elderly are discussed in detail in Chapter 15.

EFFECT OF EXERCISE. The amount of physical work or exercise done is not of prime importance in determining protein allowance. Heavy work will require more expenditure of energy than light work will, but protein needs will not be increased, provided the energy requirement is satisfied. During the period when a person is getting into "top physical condition," additional protein may be helpful during the period of muscle growth and increased muscle mass, but this would be no more than 6 to 7 gm. per day.[4] The actual protein needs of the athlete are similar to those of the non-athlete, provided the calorie requirements are satisfied.

Profuse sweating from vigorous activity or exposure to a hot environment increases nitrogen loss from the skin; however, there is evidence that the skin loss of nitrogen is lessened as the body adapts to frequent profuse sweating.[3]

EFFECT OF ILLNESS, INFECTION AND SURGERY. Any physical illness increases protein breakdown in the body. Indeed, merely staying in bed and decreasing food intake for several days will put a person into negative nitrogen balance. It is important therefore that these factors be considered in diet planning for the ill and convalescent person. Surgery is frequently preceded by a poor or precarious protein balance that should, when time permits, be corrected before surgical procedures are undertaken. Surgery itself contributes to establishing or continuing a negative nitrogen balance, and such a balance retards wound healing and convalescence, as discussed in Chapter 34.

If the loss of protein is sudden, as occurs in hemorrhage following surgery or loss of plasma in burns, the patient will manifest shock. If the protein deficiency is gradual and prolonged, the following clinical signs of protein malnutrition may occur: loss of weight, skin changes (from soft, moist, pliable character to dry and scaly), reduced resistance to infection, impaired healing, hepatic insufficiency, nutritional edema, and changes in concentration of hemoglobin and plasma proteins.

Acute episodes of infection cause a negative nitrogen balance that depends on the severity and frequency of the infection and the response of the host, as discussed in Chapter 35. The negative nitrogen balance can be due to increased urinary nitrogen excretion caused by increased adrenocortical activity, decreased nitrogen absorption because of diarrhea, or anorexia. Protein supplementation during the infection does not prevent the negative balance, but it is important for replacing the nitrogen after the infection.

Protein Deficiency—Protein-Energy Malnutrition (PEM)

The adult or child apparently can, if necessary, get along on low protein intakes, depending upon the quality of protein ingested and the level of energy intake. The urinary nitrogen output of the person on a low protein intake falls drastically, which indicates an adaptation process going on within the body to compensate for the low protein intake. If the protein in the diet is suddenly decreased, a negative nitrogen balance will exist for four to five days. Then, equilibrium is re-established at a lower level. However, there is a critical point in protein requirement below which the body cannot adapt. Below this point protein deficiency is accompanied by edema, wasting of body tissues, weakness, and loss of vigor.

Protein deficiency is seen more often in children because of their higher requirements for protein and energy per kg. body weight, their greater susceptibility to factors preventing adequate intake, such as infections, and their inability to obtain food by their own means. Intrafamilial food distribution has been shown to lead to greater reduction of food intake by the young child than by the rest of the family during times of deprivation.[6] •

The term *kwashiorkor* was applied to severe protein deficiency in native children of the Gold Coast of Africa, in whose dialect it means "the disease of the deposed baby when the next one is born." It was first described in 1933 by C. D. Williams, a Jamaican pediatrician working in the region. The disease appears among infants and young children in the late breast feeding, weaning and post-weaning phases (usually between the ages of 1 and 4 years) wherever children are fed diets high in carbohydrate with low or poor quality protein. If untreated, it has a high mortality. Even among children receiving medical and hospital care, mortality still may be as high as 10 to 30 per cent.

ETIOLOGY

Kwashiorkor is caused by insufficient good quality protein and is often associated with a deficient energy intake. It is often aggravated by infectious processes and accompanied by other nutritional deficiencies such as severe vitamin A deficiency, which may result in permanent blindness. In most of the dietary patterns in areas where kwashiorkor is endemic, the intake of animal protein foods is extremely low. The concentration of protein in the diet may not be low, but the quality is low. Actual protein deficiency alone probably exists in only a very few places where the main staples are cassava, yams and sugar, which are low in protein concentration and quality.[13]

Besides existing in poor, destitute populations, protein-energy inadequacy problems can be secondary to other diseases. Serious caloric undernutrition occurs in association with chronic fevers such as tuberculosis, with malignancy, in diseases of the gastrointestinal tract that interfere with intake or absorption of food, and in patients with psychiatric problems. Protein deficiency is a complication of numerous pathologic states. Protein may be lost in malabsorption syndromes, or in the urine in certain diseases of the kidney. Iatrogenic protein-energy malnutrition can result from many modern medical treatments. Radiation therapy and chemotherapy for cancer can result in malabsorption, increased requirements and a consequent protein-energy deficiency.

Methods for assessing protein nutriture are given in Chapter 9 and in Appendix Table 36.

SYMPTOMS

Infants and children afflicted with the disease have a feverish, generally ill condition (Fig. 4–7) accompanied by the universal edema (Fig. 4–8), reddish pigmentation of the skin and hair, fatty liver and loss of enzymes from the pancreatic and intestinal secretions. Additional clinical symptoms are retardation of growth and maturation, weight loss (often masked by edema), diarrhea and a variety of dermatoses (Fig. 4–9). There is also a reduced number of T-cell lymphocytes and diminished cell-mediated immune response.[25] Consequently these children frequently suffer from secondary infections. The chronic form leads to retarded physical growth and development as illustrated in Figure 4–10, and increased susceptibility to acute and chronic infections.

More often protein deficiency accompanies inadequacy of energy intake and other nutritional problems and cannot be distinguished as a separate entity. The term *protein-energy malnutrition* (PEM) is used to describe a spectrum of clinical disorders caused by various degrees of deficiency and additional physiological insults and stresses. The term *marasmus* is also sometimes used to refer to a condition in which there is a deprivation of both energy and protein, a

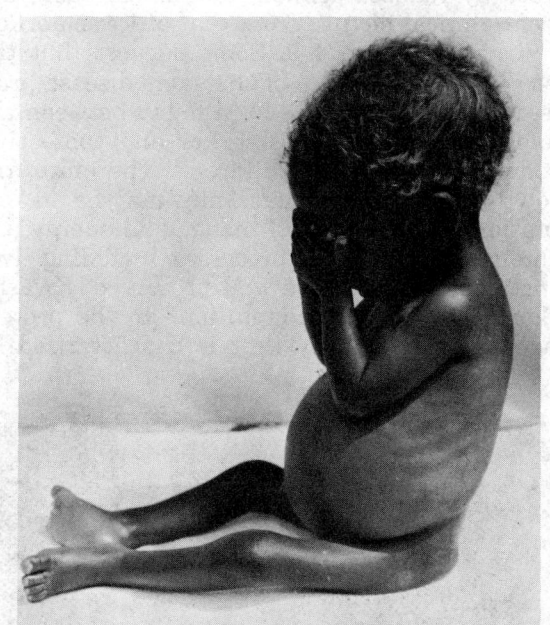

Figure 4–7. An African child suffering from kwashiorkor, the regional name for protein malnutrition. Note uncurled, graying hair, edema and skin lesions. The condition is common in areas where diets are high in starchy foods and low in protein and can be cured by protein-rich foods. (Courtesy Food and Agriculture Organization of the United Nations. Photo by M. Autret.)

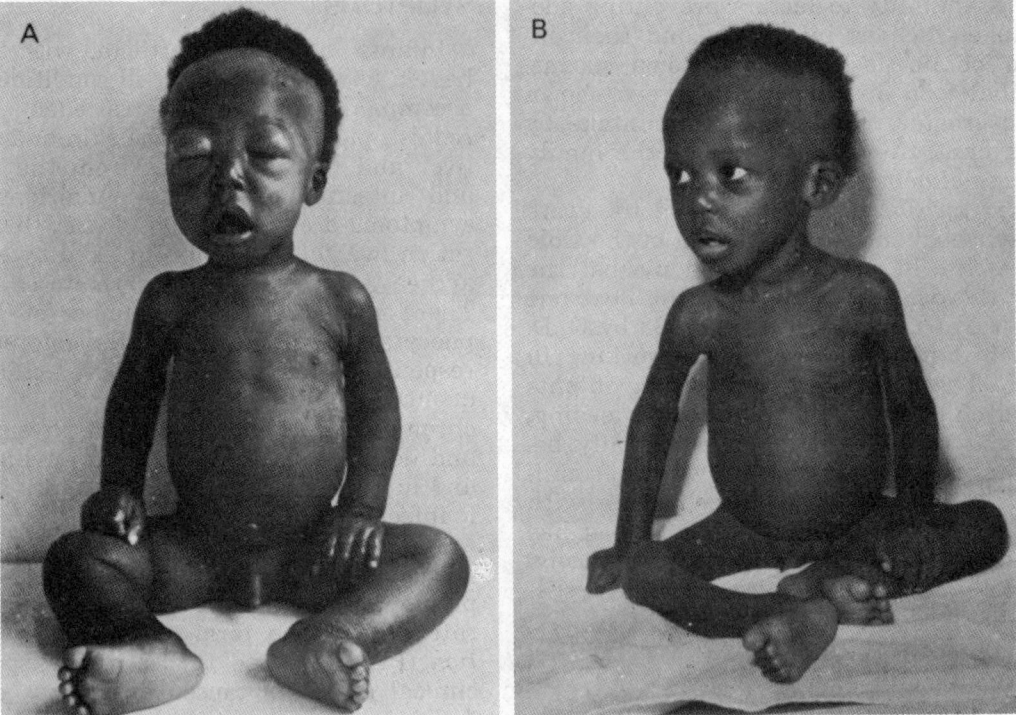

Figure 4–8. Child with kwashiorkor (*A*) on admission and (*B*) after the loss of his edema. (From: McLaren, D. S., and Burman, D.: Textbook of Paediatric Nutrition. 2nd ed. New York, Longman, 1982, p. 122, © 1982 by Longman Group Ltd.)

starvation condition, to which the child has adjusted by reduced growth. Marasmus has a different clinical picture from that of kwashiorkor, as shown in Table 4–9. Some suggest that the two diseases are facets of the same disease process. No differences have been found between the diets that produce kwashiorkor and those that produce marasmus in children.[11] Therefore, the growth retardation of marasmus may be an "adaptation" to the stress of inadequate energy and protein, and metabolic processes, including liver function, are able to be well preserved. Kwashiorkor may be a "dysadaptation" to the protein and energy deficiency that is characterized by

the edema and metabolic changes.[23] According to this view, such "dysadaptation" is frequently caused by an infection such as malaria, measles or gastroenteritis. The complex interrelationships between food intake, socioeconomic situation and infection in protein-energy malnutrition are shown in Figure 4–11.

Several clinicians have attempted to provide means of classifying the severity of protein-energy malnutrition. One system devised by the FAO/WHO Expert Committee on Nutrition is shown in Table 4–10. Other systems include the scoring system of McLaren, which is shown in Table 4–11.

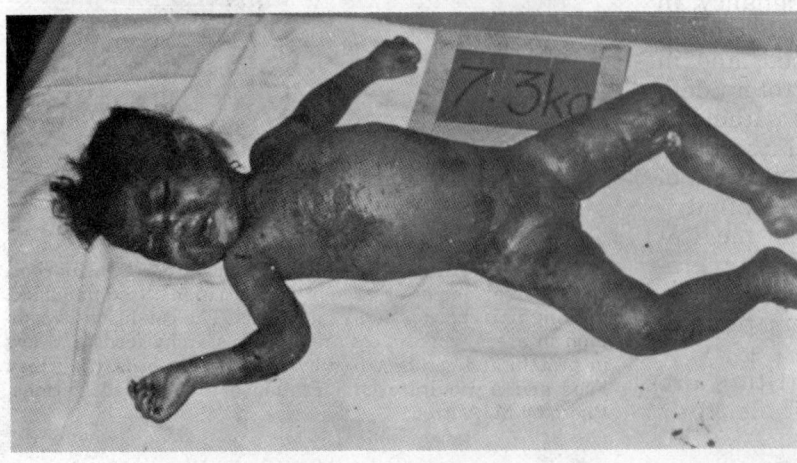

Figure 4–9. Dermatosis of kwashiorkor. (From: McLaren, D. S., and Burman, D.: Textbook of Paediatric Nutrition. 2nd ed. New York, Longman, 1982, p. 123. © 1982 by Longman Group Ltd.)

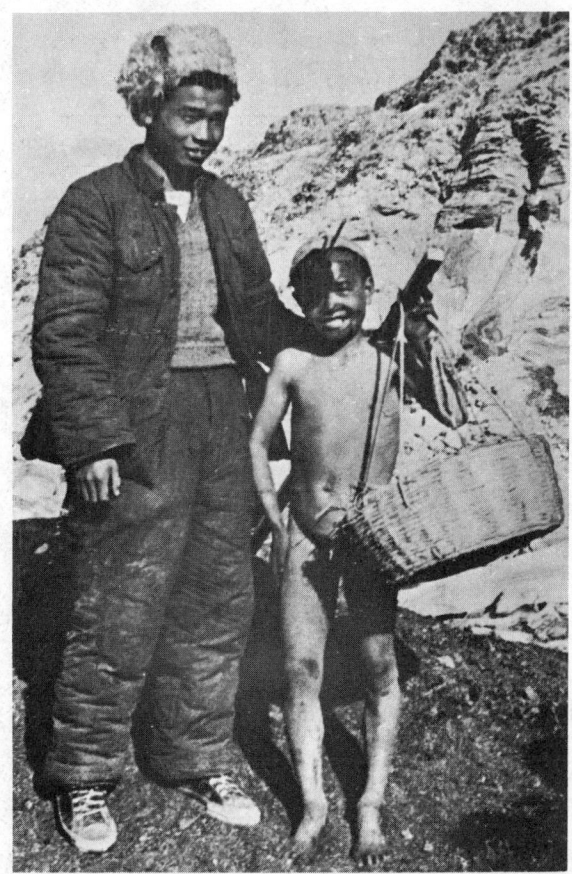

Figure 4–10. Two Asian boys of the same age. The boy on the right worked in a mine and received ordinary protein-poor local food. The other body spent four years in a boarding school were he was well fed. (Courtesy of Food and Agriculture Organization of the United Nations.)

TREATMENT AND PREVENTION

Clinical symptoms of kwashiorkor or PEM can usually be cured in four to six weeks with a diet adequate in energy, nutrients and high quality protein. However, the affected mental development in malnourished children may remain throughout life.

When rehabilitating the protein and energy malnourished adult or child it is important that all the other required nutrients be supplied also. For instance, protein rehabilitation without vitamin A can result in a vitamin A deficiency, as the protein vitamin A carrier, now available, depletes the liver of the small vitamin A stores that were present. Magnesium and potassium must also be given at the same time. Depletion of these electrolytes accompanies protein deficiency and may account for some of the neurological symptoms of the disease. Their repletion and balance are as important as the protein and energy intake.

The more difficult problem is the prevention of PEM. In areas of high prevalence, where eco-nomic factors and dietary customs limit the variability and availability of high-quality proteins or the total amount of food, prevention is difficult. Methods of preventing PEM lie in education, socioeconomic improvement, better food distribution, control of infectious disease and adoption of feeding patterns for infants and pre-school children that supply appropriate weaning foods containing higher-quality protein.

Excessive Intake of Protein

People on very high intakes of protein (up to 300 gm. per day) have been studied and found to have no apparent harm. The normal kidney can handle large amounts of nitrogenous waste without difficulty at least for a limited time, although this is being questioned with regard to the long-term health of the kidney.[1] Infants with normal immature kidneys do not tolerate excessive protein intakes (see Chapters 12 and 37). The consequences of excessive protein intake in chronic kidney disease are discussed in Chapter 30.

Meeting Protein and Energy Needs for the World Population

Intake of protein of inadequate quality is found in many parts of the world and frequently coincides with energy intakes below the recommended level. The situation of protein deficiency cannot be clearly separated from energy deficit, and in trying to remedy the problem a broader approach must be taken.[13, 17, 19]

In 1973 the FAO/WHO committee stated:

When intakes of both energy and protein are grossly inadequate, the provision of protein-rich food of animal origin may be a costly and inefficient way of improving diets, since energy can generally be provided more cheaply than protein of good quality.[5]

In 1974 McLaren stated:

Food consumption data and dietary surveys incriminate energy rather than protein deficit. Increasing the energy intake and not that of protein has produced catch-up growth in undernourished children. Lack of nutriment in general with an energy gap rather than a protein gap is the crux of the matter; but how to match the intake of the child with its requirements remains a problem of puzzling complexity.[17]

However, supplying nutritious food is not enough to prevent protein-energy malnutrition. The entire scope of the problem, including total food supply, housing, water, infections, digestibility of food and mother–child interactions,

Table 4–9 SOME CHARACTERISTICS OF MARASMUS AND KWASHIORKOR

	MARASMUS	KWASHIORKOR
General features		
Occurrence	World-wide	Limited
Usual age	Infancy	Second and third years
Adaptation to stress	Good	Poor
Response to treatment		
immediate	Poor	Good (occasional sudden death)
ultimate	Fair	Good
Long-term effects		
mental	Severe	Nil
physical	Severe	Mild
liver damage	Nil	Nil
Clinical signs		
Edema	Absent	Present
Dermatosis	Rare	Common
Hair changes	Common	Very common
Hepatomegaly	Common	Very common
Mental changes	Uncommon	Very common
Wasting of fat	Severe	Mild
of muscles	Severe	Mild
Anemia	Common and severe	Mild
Vitamin deficiencies	Uncommon	Common
Laboratory findings		
General		
Total body water	High	High
Extra-cellular water	Some increase	More increase
Body potassium	Some depletion	Much depletion
Malabsorption	Some	More
Fatty infiltration of liver	Absent	Severe
X-ray bone loss	Mild	Mild
Renal function	Impaired	Impaired
I.V. glucose tolerance	Normal	Impaired
Response to adrenaline	Exaggerated	Lowered
Serum		
Albumin	Slightly low	Very low
Enzymes (in general)	Normal	Low
Copper, zinc, sodium	Normal	Low
Non-essential/essential amino-acids	Normal	High
Triglycerides	Normal	Normal
Cholesterol	Normal	Low
Non-esterified fatty acids	Normal	High
β-Lipoprotein	High	Low
Insulin	Low	Low
Growth hormone	Low or normal	High
Glucose	Low	Very Low
Urine		
Urea/total N	Above 65 per cent	Below 50 per cent
Imidazole acrylic acid	Nil	Present
Hydroxyproline index	Low	Low
Liver		
Urea cycle enzymes	Low	Low
Amino-acid-synthesizing enzymes	High	High

(From McLaren, D. S.: Nutrition and Its Disorders. 3rd ed. Baltimore, Williams & Wilkins Co., 1981. © 1981 by The Williams & Wilkins Company.)

SOME CAUSES OF MALNUTRITION

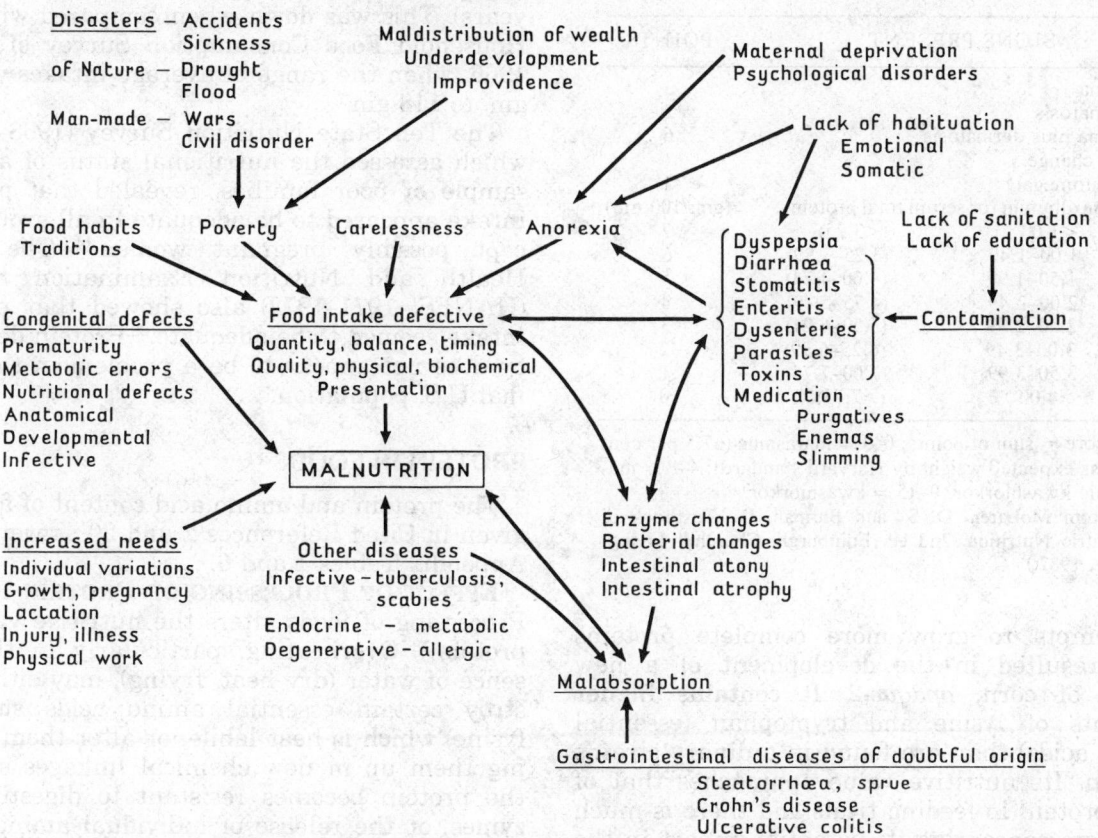

Figure 4–11. Some causes of malnutrition. (From: Williams, C. D.: Malnutrition. Lancet, 2:342, 1962.)

must be appreciated and changed or improved. "The malnourished child is deprived in many ways other than its nutrition and is a sick member of a sick community. The whole society is the patient."[16]

Correcting the problem will probably be better achieved through emphasis on better storage and distribution of the food that is produced in the country, so that the population can supply their food needs better. There must also be attention to controlling the growth of the popula-tion so that its growth does not outstrip the growth of the food supply.

SOURCES OF PROTEIN

In a number of the technically underdeveloped areas and countries, efforts to develop vegetable sources of protein have been, to a great extent, stimulated and aided by WHO, FAO, and UNICEF.

Table 4–10 "WELLCOME" CLASSIFICATION OF PEM

	BODY WEIGHT AS % OF STANDARD*	EDEMA	DEFICIT IN WEIGHT FOR HEIGHT†
Underweight child	80–60	0	Minimal
Nutritional dwarfing	<60	0	Minimal
Marasmus	<60	0	+ +
Kwashiorkor	80–60	+	+ +
Marasmic kwashiorkor	<60	+	+ +

*Standard taken as 50th percentile of the Harvard values.

†Weight for height $= \dfrac{\text{weight of patient}}{\text{weight of normal subject of same height}} \times 100$

(From FAO/WHO Expert Committee on Nutrition. Eighth Report. WHO Technical Report Series, No. 477, Geneva. WHO, 1971.)

Table 4–11 SCORING SYSTEM FOR SEVERE FORMS OF PEM

SIGNS PRESENT		POINTS
Edema		3
Dermatosis		2
Edema plus dermatosis		6
Hair change		1
Hepatomegaly		1
Serum albumin (or serum total protein)	(gm./100 ml.)	
<1.00	(<3.25)	7
1.00–1.49	(3.25–3.99)	6
1.50–1.99	(4.00–4.74)	5
2.00–2.49	(4.75–5.49)	4
2.50–2.99	(5.50–6.24)	3
3.00–3.49	(6.25–6.99)	2
3.50–3.99	(7.00–7.74)	1
≥4.00	(≥7.75)	0

Score = sum of points; 0–3 = marasmus (67.5 per cent or less expected weight by Harvard standard); 4–8 = marasmic kwashiorkor, 9–15 = kwashiorkor.

(From McLaren, D. S., and Burman, D.: Textbook of Pediatric Nutrition, 2nd ed. Edinburgh, Churchill Livingstone, 1982.)

Attempts to grow more complete proteins have resulted in the development of a new strain of corn, *opaque-2*. It contains higher amounts of lysine and tryptophan (essential amino acids) than are found in ordinary strains of corn. Its nutritive value approaches that of milk protein in feeding trials and there is much optimism concerning its potential impact in the corn-consuming countries of the world. Work is under way to develop soybean varieties containing larger amounts of methionine and wheat and sorghum containing more lysine.

However, the malnutrition problems of developing countries still exist. The energy gap is not resolved by additional protein and the problems of economics and getting the food to those who need it the most still exist.

Trends in Protein Content of the American Diet

Based on food disappearance data as listed in Table 17–1, the protein intake per capita for the U.S. is about the same as it was in 1909–1913. It dropped to a low of 90 gm. per day in 1935–1939 during the depression, but then it rose again.

The 1977–1978 Nationwide Food Consumption Survey, which surveyed the intake of 9620 individuals in one day in the spring of 1977 (see Chapter 17), showed that the average proportion of energy from protein was 16.6 per cent—more than adequate based on the RDA shown in Table 10–1. The average protein intake of all individuals was 165 per cent of the RDA and varied from 123 per cent for women 75 years and older to 210 per cent for 1 to 2 year olds.[8] The range of average intakes was 29 gm. (infants under 1 year) to 107 gm. (males age 15 to 18 years). This was down when compared with the Household Food Consumption Survey of 1965–1966, when the range of average intakes was 39 gm. to 118 gm.[7]

The Ten State Nutrition Survey (1968–1970), which assessed the nutritional status of a large sample of poor families, revealed that protein intake appeared to be adequate in all groups except possibly pregnant women.[14] The First Health and Nutrition Examination Survey (HANES, 1971–1972) also showed that protein intake seemed to be adequate.[22] Protein deficiency does not appear to be a problem in the normal U.S. population.

PROTEIN IN FOODS

The protein and amino acid content of foods is given in Cited References 2 and 20 as well as in Appendix Tables 1 and 6.

EFFECT OF PROCESSING OF PROTEIN FOODS. Processing of foods alters the nutritive value of protein.[18] Overheating, particularly in the absence of water (dry heat, frying), may either destroy certain essential amino acids such as lysine, which is heat labile, or alter them by tying them up in new chemical linkages so that the protein becomes resistant to digestive enzymes, or the release of individual amino acids in the intestinal tract is retarded. On the other hand, processing may have a favorable effect on protein foods by increasing the digestibility or increasing the liberation of individual amino acids.

Problems and Suggested Topics for Discussion

1. List the most popular protein foods. Classify them as to *complete* and *incomplete protein*.
2. What is meant by the term "essential amino acids"? Name them. What are the physiological functions of amino acids?
3. Give examples of specific functions of four of the amino acids.
4. List the amounts of various protein foods you consume during a period of 24 hours and a period of 3 days; calculate the protein content.
5. Evaluate the list of protein foods. Classify them into animal and vegetable-grain proteins. Which ones have high biological value? What percentage of your diet is protein? Was the total amount of protein consumed in 24 hours equally distributed throughout the day?
6. Design an adequate menu of complementary proteins for a vegetarian who does not eat eggs, milk products or animal flesh.
7. Plan a basic dietary pattern of protein foods you require daily. Divide into three meals, keeping in mind the quality and quantity of the protein.
8. What is the trend in protein consumption in the United States? What changes should be made?
9. What is meant by a negative nitrogen balance? When might this occur?

10. Using the ratio pattern for essential amino acids in Appendix Table 6, determine the balance of amino acids in your food intake for one day. Is your diet properly balanced in essential amino acids? If not, show how it can be corrected.
11. Why are proteins considered to be a wasteful source of energy?
12. Research the literature and discuss the controversy surrounding kwashiorkor, marasmus and PEM.

Cited References

1. Brenner, B.M., Meyer, T.W., and Hostetter, T.H.: Dietary protein intake and the progressive nature of kidney disease: the role of hemodynamically mediated glomerular injury in the pathogenesis of progressive glomerular sclerosis in aging, renal ablation and intrinsic renal disease. N. Engl. J. Med., 307:652, 1982.
2. Composition of Foods. Agricultural Handbooks, No. 8:1–9. Consumer and Food Economics Institute, U.S. Department of Agriculture, 1976–1982.
3. Consolazio, C.F., et al.: Comparison of nitrogen, calcium and iodine excretion in arm and total body sweat. Am. J. Clin. Nutr., 18:443, 1966.
4. Durnin, J.V.G.A.: Protein requirements and physical activity. In Pařízkova, J., and Rogozkin, V.A. (ed.): Nutrition, physical fitness and health. Baltimore, University Park Press, 1978.
5. Energy and Protein Requirements. Joint FAO/WHO Ad Hoc Expert Committee, World Health Organization, Tech. Report No. 522, Geneva, 1973.
6. Flores, M., et al.: Annual patterns of family and children's diets in 3 Guatemalan Indian communities, Br. J. Nutr., 18:281, 1964.
7. Food and Nutrient Intake of Individuals in the United States, Spring, 1965. Household Food Consumption Survey 1965–66, Report No. 11. Washington, D.C., U.S. Department of Agriculture, 1972.
8. Food and Nutrient Intakes of Individuals in 1 Day in the United States, Spring, 1977. Nationwide Food Consumption Survey, 1977–78, Preliminary Report No. 2. Washington, D.C., Science and Education Administration, U.S. Department of Agriculture, 1980.
9. Food and Nutrition Board, National Research Council: Recommended Dietary Allowances. 9th ed. Washington, D.C., National Academy of Sciences, 1980.
10. Garza, C., Scrimshaw, N.S., and Young, V.R.: Human protein requirements: a long-term metabolic nitrogen study in young men to evaluate the 1973 FAO/WHO safe level of egg protein intake. J. Nutr., 107:335, 1977.
11. Gopalan, C., and Narasinga Rao, B.S.: Nutritional constraints on growth and development in current Indian dietaries, Indian J. Med. Res. (Suppl.), 59:143, 1971.
12. Harper, A.E.: Amino acid excess. In White, P.L., and Fletcher, D.C. (eds.): Nutrients in Processed Foods—Proteins. Acton, Mass., Publishing Sciences Group, Inc., 1974.
13. Hegsted, D.M.: Protein needs and possible modification of the American diet. J. Am. Diet. Assoc., 68:317, 1976.
14. Highlights of the Ten-State Nutrition Survey, 1968–70. U.S. Department of Health, Education and Welfare, Pub. No. (HSM) 72–8134, 1972.
15. Kopple, J.D., and Swendseid, M.E.: Evidence that histidine is an essential amino acid in normal and chronically uremic men. J. Clin. Invest., 55:881, 1975.
16. McLaren, D.S.: Nutrition and Its Disorders, Baltimore, Williams and Wilkins Co., 1972.
17. McLaren, D.S.: The great protein fiasco. Lancet, 2:93, 1974.
18. Melnick, D.: The influence of heat processing on the functional and nutritive properties of protein food. Food Tech., 3:57, 1949.
19. Miller, D.S.: Protein-energy interrelationships. In Porter, J.W., and Rolls, B.A. (eds.): Proteins in Human Nutrition. New York, Academic Press, 1973.
20. Orr, M.L., and Watt, B.K.: Amino acid content of foods. Home Econ. Res. Rep. No. 4. Washington, D.C., U.S. Department of Agriculture, 1968.
21. PAG Bulletin, 5(3), September, 1975.
22. Preliminary Findings of the First Health and Nutrition Examination Survey, U.S., 1971–72, Dietary Intake and Biochemical Findings. U.S. DHEW Pub. No. (HRA) 74–1219–1, 1974.
23. Rao, K.S.: Evolution of kwashiorkor and marasmus, Lancet, 1:709, 1974.
24. Recommended Intakes of Nutrients for the United Kingdom, Report No. 120. Department of Health and Social Security, 1969.
25. Schopfer, K., and Douglas, D.S.: In vitro studies of lymphocytes of children with kwashiorkor. Clin. Immunol. Immunopathol., 5:21, 1976.
26. Scrimshaw, N.S.: Strengths and weaknesses of the committee approach—an analysis of past and present recommended dietary allowances for protein in health and disease. N. Engl. J. Med., 294:136, 294:194, 1976.

Additional References

Adibi, S.A.: Intestinal phase of protein assimilation in man. Am. J. Clin. Nutr., 29:205, 1976.
Allison, J.B., and Wannemacher, R.W.: The concept and significance of labile and over-all protein reserves of the body. Am. J. Clin. Nutr., 16:445, 1965.
Guggenheim, K.Y.: Nutrition and Nutritional Diseases. The Evolution of Concepts. Lexington, Mass., The Collamore Press, 1981.
Guyton, A.C.: Textbook of Medical Physiology. 6th ed. Philadelphia, W.B. Saunders Company, 1981.
Harpstead, D.D.: High-lysine corn. Sci. Am., 225(2):34, 1971.
Lappé, F.M.: Diet for a Small Planet. New York, Ballantine Books, 1971.
Leverton, R.M.: Amino acid requirements of young adults. In Albanese, A.A. (ed.): Protein and Amino Acid Nutrition. New York, Academic Press, 1959.
Munro, H.N., and Crim, M.C.: The proteins and amino acids. In Goodhart, R.S., and Shils, M.E.: Modern Nutrition in Health and Disease. 6th ed. Philadelphia, Lea & Febiger, 1980.
Nasset, E.S.: Amino acid homeostasis in the gut lumen and its nutritional significance. World Rev. Nutr. Diet., 14:134, Basel, Karger, 1972.
Rose, W.C., et al.: The amino acid requirements of man. J. Biol. Chem., 217:987, 1955.
Sanchez, A., et al.: Nutritive value of selected proteins and protein combinations. I. The biological value of proteins singly and in meal patterns with varying fat composition. II. Biological value predictability. Am. J. Clin. Nutr., 13:243, 1963.
The uses of energy and protein requirement estimates: Report of a workshop. Food and Nutrition Bulletin, 3:45, Jan. 1981.
Viteri, F.E.: Primary Protein-Energy Malnutrition: Clinical, Biochemical and Metabolic Changes. In Suskind, R.M. (ed.): Textbook of Pediatric Nutrition. New York, Raven Press, 1981.
Watson, I.D.: The Double Helix: A Personal Account of the Structure of DNA. New York, Academic Press, 1968.
Worthington-Roberts, B.S.: Proteins and Amino Acids. Contemporary Developments in Nutrition. St. Louis, C.V. Mosby Company, 1981.

Digestion, Absorption and Cell Metabolism

Most of the major nutrients in foods are bound in large molecules that cannot be absorbed from the intestine because of size or because they are not water-soluble. The reduction of these large molecules into smaller, readily absorbed units and conversion of the insoluble molecules into soluble forms is the work of the digestive tract.

The Digestive System

The digestive system extends from the mouth to the anus, as illustrated in Figure 5–1. It consists of the alimentary canal and the exocrine and endocrine functions of its appendage organs, e.g., the liver and biliary tree and the pancreas.

The functions of the digestive system include: (1) receipt, maceration and transport of ingested substances and waste products; (2) secretion of acid, mucus, digestive enzymes, bile and other materials; (3) digestion of ingested foodstuffs; (4) absorption; (5) storage of waste products; (6) excretion; and (7) certain ancillary functions.

MOUTH. The mouth receives food into the alimentary canal, reduces it in size by chewing and mixes it with saliva, mucus and the digestive enzyme ptyalin (salivary amylase).

ESOPHAGUS. The esophagus transports food and liquids from the oral cavity and pharynx to the stomach.

STOMACH. The stomach and first portion of duodenum participate in the storage, digestion and transport of ingested materials. The stomach secretes hydrochloric acid, intrinsic factor, the inactive protease pepsinogen, gastric lipase, mucus and the gastrointestinal hormone gastrin. Only very lipid-soluble substances and weak acids such as alcohol and aspirin (acetylsalicylic acid) are absorbed from the stomach.

SMALL INTESTINE. The small intestine functions to secrete and to participate in digestion, absorption and transport of ingested materials. It consists of the duodenum, jejunum and ileum. Just past the pyloric sphincter are Brunner's glands, which secrete the much needed mucus to protect the duodenal mucosa from chyme acidity. The duodenum receives the secretions of the large accessory glands of digestion—the pancreas and the liver. The small intestine functions to continue digestion and to absorb the end products of digestion of carbohydrates, proteins and fats. It secretes the enzyme enterokinase, and its epithelial cells contain several peptidases, sucrase, lactase, alpha-dextrinase, maltase, amylase and small quantities of enteric lipase. The gastrointestinal hormones secretin and enterogastrone are formed in the wall of the duodenum.

LARGE INTESTINE AND RECTUM. The large intestine and rectum absorb water, electrolytes and, in reduced amounts, some of the final products of digestion. They also provide temporary storage for waste products, which serve as a medium for bacterial synthesis of some vitamins.

ANUS. The anus controls defecation. Power for this function is provided by the propulsive contractions of the colon and rectum, which are normally coordinated with the involuntary and voluntary portions of the anal sphincter.

PANCREAS. The pancreas produces secretions required for the digestion and absorption of food. Enzymes excreted include pancreatic lipase, cholesterol esterase, pancreatic amylase, ribonuclease, deoxyribonuclease, carboxypolypeptidase, trypsin and chymotrypsin (in their respective inactive forms, e.g., procarboxypolypeptidase, trypsinogen and chymotrypsinogen). These are activated by trypsin only after they are in the intestinal lumen. Under the influence of secretin, the pancreas secretes fluid containing large amounts of the bicarbonate ion. Important endocrine secretions of the pancreas are insulin and glucagon.

LIVER AND BILIARY TRACT. The major functions of the liver include the metabolism of protein, carbohydrate and lipid; the conjugation and detoxification of hormones, toxins and drugs; and the synthesis of proteins. In addition, the metabolism of bile pigments and bile salts takes place within the liver, and these products, important in the digestion and absorption of fats, are secreted into the duodenum through the biliary tract.

Each of these functions will be discussed in more detail.

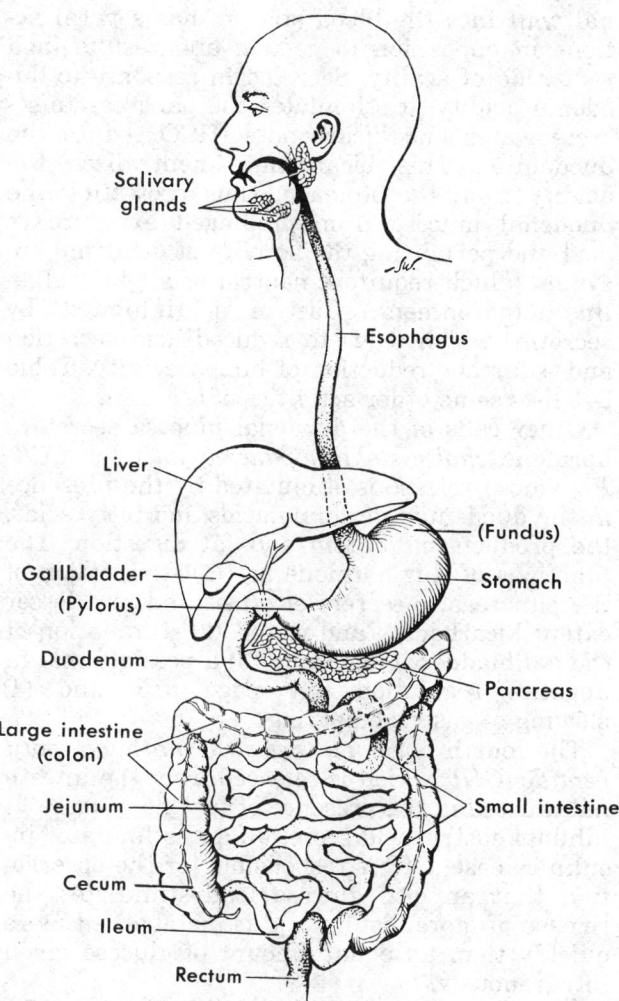

Figure 5–1. The digestive system.

Digestion and Absorption

Digestion and absorption do not take place one step at a time as isolated functions. They are continuous processes with many mechanical and chemical reactions taking place simultaneously; a defect in one phase hampers the other.

Normally, 92 to 97 per cent of the mixed American diet is digested and absorbed. Foods are prepared for ingestion in a variety of ways and combinations; processing methods and cooking may begin a slight breakdown of complex compounds such as starch and collagen before they are eaten. Water, monosaccharides, alcohol and inorganic ions are usually absorbed in their original form. The di- and polysaccharides, lipids and proteins must be converted to their simple constituents before they are absorbed.

A brief review of this subject is included for the purpose of integration. For additional details, consult a textbook on physiology or biochemistry.

DIGESTION

Digestion is a series of physical and chemical changes by which food taken into the body undergoes hydrolysis (addition of water) and is broken down in preparation for absorption from the intestinal tract into the blood stream.

The physical changes in food are brought about by grinding, crushing and mixing of the food with the digestive juices and propulsion of the mass through the digestive tract. The propulsive force of the gastrointestinal tract resides in the circular and longitudinal smooth muscles contained in its walls. These muscles churn and push the food mass (chyme) along the digestive tract in rhythmic waves (peristalsis) toward the anus. During the propulsion of the chyme through the gut, it is mixed at appropriate times with the digestive juices, which begin their chemical changes of food. The active materials in the digestive juices that cause this chemical breakdown are enzymes, both endoenzymes and exoenzymes. The whole process is regulated through neural and hormonal mechanisms.

REGULATION OF GASTROINTESTINAL ACTIVITY

NEURAL MECHANISMS. The neural control of gastrointestinal contractile and secretory activity is composed of two parts—a local system of internal plexuses and an external system of nerve fibers from the autonomic nervous system. The most common chemical messenger of this system is the neurotransmitter *acetylcholine*.

The local system consists of the *myenteric* plexus and the *submucosal plexus*. Located in the gut wall or mucosa are receptors sensitive to the composition of the chyme (acidity, for instance) and lumen stretch (fullness, for example). These receptors send impulses to the internal plexuses. From the plexuses impulses then go out on efferent fibers to muscle cells and secretory cells of the intestinal tract.

The autonomic innervation comes from the sympathetic postganglionic fibers, which run along blood vessels, and the parasympathetic preganglionic fibers in the vagus nerve. The *vagus nerve* has branches to the stomach, small intestine and upper portion of the large intestine and carries impulses, either excitatory or inhibitory. This activity does not control but rather influences the local activity in the plexuses. An example of vagal activity is the stimulation of acid secretion from parietal cells which accompanies the sight or smell of food (the cephalic phase of digestion). Because of its ability to stimulate gastric acid secretion, the vagus nerve is frequently cut as a treatment for peptic ulcer disease when constant hyperacidity is present.

HORMONAL MECHANISMS. Our knowledge of the hormonal control of the gastrointestinal tract is mushrooming, as evidenced by the continual discovery of "candidate hormones" (a term coined by Grossman[2]). These candidate hormones are identified substances that could have definite physiological functions and thus be termed hormones after additional study. Present knowledge indicates that hormonal regulation of the gastrointestinal system is controlled by many hormones, of which only four are fairly well defined: gastrin, secretin, cholecystokinin and gastric inhibitory polypeptide.

Gastrin is released from G cells in the antral mucosa of the stomach, the duodenum and jejunum. Like all of the gastrointestinal hormones, gastrin is released into the blood stream, is carried in the venous system to the heart, and does not have its particular effect on gastrointestinal cells until it returns via the arterial blood flow. Thus a gastrointestinal hormone can affect any portion of the gastrointestinal (GI) system regardless of where it was produced. The release of gastrin from the antral mucosa of the stomach is initiated by (1) distention of the antrum (as after a meal), (2) impulses from the vagus nerve (as at the thought of food), and (3) the presence in the antrum of secretagogues, such as partially digested proteins, food extracts (e.g., bouillon), alcohol and caffeine. Unfortunately the intestinal release of gastrin is not as well understood as the gastric release.

The functions of gastrin are many, but the most important one is to increase gastric secretion through stimulation of parietal cell acid secretion, chief cell enzyme secretion and gastric antral motility. Some other effects are listed in Table 5–1. Through a feedback mechanism, gastrin release is inhibited when the lumen pH gets too low, and thus acid secretion is reduced.

Secretin, a hormone released from the duodenal wall into the blood stream, has several actions in opposition to gastrin and results in a reduction of acidity. Secreted in response to duodenal acidity, it stimulates the pancreas to secrete water and bicarbonate (HCO_3^-) into the duodenum. This bicarbonate neutralizes the acidity from the stomach, thus protecting the duodenal mucosa from prolonged exposure to acid and permitting the activity of duodenal enzymes, which require a neutral or slightly alkaline environment. Gastrin is inhibited by secretin, which leads to reduced acid secretion and a further reduction of lumen acidity. Table 5–1 lists some other activities of secretin.

Other cells of the duodenal mucosa secrete a hormone *cholecystokinin-pancreozymin*, or *CCK-PZ*, whose release is stimulated by the presence in the duodenum of amino acids and fatty acids, the products of protein and fat digestion. The functions of this hormone are (1) stimulation of the pancreas to secrete enzymes and to a lesser extent bicarbonate and water, (2) stimulation of the gallbladder to contract, (3) a possible role in appetite regulation (see page 515) and (4) slowing of gastric emptying.

The fourth hormone is *gastric inhibitory polypeptide (GIP)*, which is released from the intestinal mucosa in the presence of fat and glucose. It inhibits gastric acid secretion and stimulates insulin release. GIP is responsible for the observation that an oral glucose load stimulates the release of more insulin and is metabolized more quickly than an equal amount of glucose given intravenously.

Candidate Hormones. Several other peptides have been isolated from the gastrointestinal tract that do not qualify as hormones. Some of these candidate hormones are *enteroglucagon, vasoactive intestinal peptide, motilin, somatostatin,* and *pancreatic polypeptide.* Their actions are summarized in Table 5–1.

Paracrine and Neurocrine Mechanisms. Many of these substances described in the gastrointestinal endocrinology literature may be

Table 5–1. IMPORTANT FUNCTIONS OF GASTROINTESTINAL HORMONES AND CANDIDATE HORMONES

CANDIDATE HORMONE	SITE OF RELEASE	STIMULANT OF RELEASE	ORGAN AFFECTED	EFFECT ON ORGAN
Gastrin	Antral mucosa of stomach	Polypeptides Amino acids	Esophagus	Increases resting pressure of lower esophageal sphincter
	Duodenum	Caffeine	Stomach	Stimulates secretion of HCl and pepsinogen by parietal and chief cells, respectively
	Jejunum	Alcohol		
		Food extracts		Increases gastric antral motility
		Distention of stomach antrum	Gallbladder	Weakly stimulates contraction of gallbladder
		Vagal nerve	Pancreas	Weakly stimulates pancreatic secretion of bicarbonate

Table 5–1. IMPORTANT FUNCTIONS OF GASTROINTESTINAL HORMONES AND CANDIDATE HORMONES *(Continued)*

CANDIDATE HORMONE	SITE OF RELEASE	STIMULANT OF RELEASE	ORGAN AFFECTED	EFFECT ON ORGAN
Secretin	Duodenal mucosa	Gut acidity (pH < 4–5)	Esophagus	Reduces resting pressure of lower esophageal sphincter
			Stomach	Reduces gastric and duodenal motility
				Stimulates pepsinogen secretion
				Inhibits gastrin-stimulated gastric acid secretion
			Duodenum	Decreases motility
				Increases mucous output of Brunner's glands
			Pancreas	Increases output of H_2O and bicarbonate
				Increases some enzyme secretion from the pancreas as well as insulin release
			Liver	Increases volume and electrolyte output of bile
Cholecystokinin-pancreozymin (CCK-PZ)	Duodenal mucosa	Amino acids (esp. tryptophan) HCl Fatty acids (<9c.) Food	Small bowel	Increases motility
			Gallbladder	Causes contraction of gallbladder
			Pancreas	Stimulates enzyme secretion of pancreas
				Potentiates effect of secretin on pancreas
				Slows gastric emptying
				May mediate feeding behavior
Gastric inhibitory polypeptide (GIP)	Small intestine	Glucose Fat	Stomach	Inhibits gastrin-stimulated gastric acid secretion
			Pancreas	Stimulates insulin secretion

CANDIDATE HORMONE				
Enteroglucagon and glucagon	Duodenum Jejunum	Carbohydrate Long chain triglycerides	Liver	Stimulates glycogenolysis
			Pancreas	Inhibits pancreatic enzyme secretion
			Small intestine	Inhibits motility
Vasoactive intestinal polypeptide (VIP)	Neurons in small intestine	Fat Ethanol Increased gut acidity (?)	Liver	Increases glycogenolysis
			Pancreas	Increases output of H_2O and bicarbonate
				Releases insulin and glucagon
			Small intestine	Increases intestinal secretions
			Stomach	Inhibits gastric acid output
			Other	Vasodilates with hypotensive effect
Motilin	Duodenum Jejunum	Alkalinity in the duodenum	Stomach	Decreases gastric emptying
				Regulates gut motility (?)
Somatostatin	Antrum of stomach Upper small intestine Hypothalamus primarily	Gastric and duodenal acidity Amino acids Fat (?)	Pancreas	Inhibits release of insulin and glucagon
				Decreases pancreatic enzyme production
			Stomach	Inhibits gastrin release
			Gallbladder	Inhibits contraction
			Other	Suppresses secretion of growth hormone
				Suppresses secretion of thyroid-stimulating hormone
Pancreatic polypeptide	Pancreas	Ingestion of a meal— vagal stimulation	Pancreas	Decreases secretion of trypsin
Others Chymodenin Bulbogastrone Urogastrone Gastrone Enterooxyntin Enterocrinin Villikinin Incretin		Little is known about the role and physiological importance of these substances		

active in the *paracrine* system. Like the hormonal mechanisms, the paracrine mechanisms employ messengers, in this case called gastrointestinal peptides. Their action is restricted to target cells within the reach of the messenger by diffusion through the intercellular space. They are not released into the general circulation. Enterogastrone, gastric inhibitory polypeptide, vasoactive intestinal peptide, motilin, pancreatic polypeptide, enteroglucagon, somatostatin and possibly others are gastrointestinal peptides thought to be part of the paracrine system (see Table 5–1).

The *neurocrine* system includes those peptides which have been found in both the brain and the digestive tract mucosa. Physiological mechanisms involving neurocrines are just beginning to be defined, but the concept of neurocrine release is important to understanding of the mechanisms regulating digestive function. Cited references 4 and 5 provide excellent reviews of the paracrine and neurocrine systems.

In the healthy person these neural, endocrine and paracrine mechanisms, of which we understand so little, beautifully regulate and orchestrate the complex, interrelated and simultaneously occurring processes of digestion and absorption.

DIGESTION IN THE MOUTH. In the mouth the teeth function to grind and crush the food into small particles. Simultaneously, the food mass is moistened and lubricated by saliva secreted by three pairs of glands: the parotid, submaxillary and sublingual glands.

These three pairs of glands produce about 1.5 liters of saliva daily. There are two types of saliva. One type is a serous secretion and contains *alpha-amylase (ptyalin)*, which begins the digestion of starch; the other contains mucus, a protein that makes particles of food stick together and lubricates the mass for easier swallowing. The masticated food mass, called a bolus, passes back to the pharynx under voluntary control, but from there on and through the esophagus the process of swallowing is involuntary. Peristalsis then moves the food rapidly into the stomach.

DIGESTION IN THE STOMACH. There is a mixing and propulsion of the food particles with gastric secretions in wavelike contractions. The churning and mixing waves are usually described as going from the fundus to the antrum and pylorus. In the process of gastric digestion the food becomes semiliquid (chyme) and contains approximately 50 per cent water.

Active chemical digestion begins in the middle portion of the stomach. An average of 2000 to 2500 ml. of gastric juice is secreted daily and contains the enzymes, mucus and hydrochloric acid necessary for digestion. Foodstuffs, when taken alone, leave the stomach in the following order: carbohydrate first, protein next, and then fat. But when carbohydrate, protein and fat are mixed, they all take longer. The stomach normally is emptied in one to four hours, depending upon the amount and kinds of foods eaten.

DIGESTION IN THE SMALL INTESTINE. The small intestine, which has a total length of about 22 feet, is divided into three sections: the duodenum, the jejunum and the ileum, as shown in Figure 5–1. The acidic chyme slowly moves in spurts of a few milliliters through the exit valve (pylorus) at the junction of the stomach and duodenum into the duodenum, where it mixes with duodenal juices, bile (produced by the liver and stored in the gallbladder until needed), and the secretions from the pancreas.

The valves (sphincters) guarding the entrance to and the exit from the stomach prevent backflow of the mixture from the stomach into the pharynx and from the duodenum into the stomach. These structures open and close at the proper time; but because the nervous system influences their behavior, they often become too energetic during emotional upsets. When the exit pyloric valve tightens or goes into spasms, the pain is excruciating. Irritation from nearby ulcers also may alter the performance of this structure. The chyme moves down the small intestine at a rate of 1 cm. per minute and takes from three to ten hours to travel the entire length to the ileocecal valve. Most of the digestion process is completed in the duodenum, and the remainder of the small intestine (jejunum and ileum) functions principally in the absorption of nutrients.

ABSORPTION

ABSORPTION FROM THE SMALL INTESTINE. The remarkable structural feature of the small intestine is its tremendous absorptive area. The inner lining of the intestine, the mucosa, is in immediate contact with the products of digestion. The mucosa is folded to form *valvulae conniventes*. Covering these folds are fingerlike projections called *villi*. The absorptive surface is further increased by the existence on each villus of *microvilli*, which make up the so-called *brush border*. The convolutions, villi and their microvilli give the small intestine an enormous absorptive surface of about 250 square meters, which rests on a supporting structure called the lamina propria. The lamina propria is composed of connective tissue in which are suspended the blood and lymph vessels. These vessels receive the absorbed nutrients from the mucosal cells. Figure 5–2 schematically represents the intestinal mucosa, and Figure 5–3 illustrates a villous absorptive or epithelial cell.

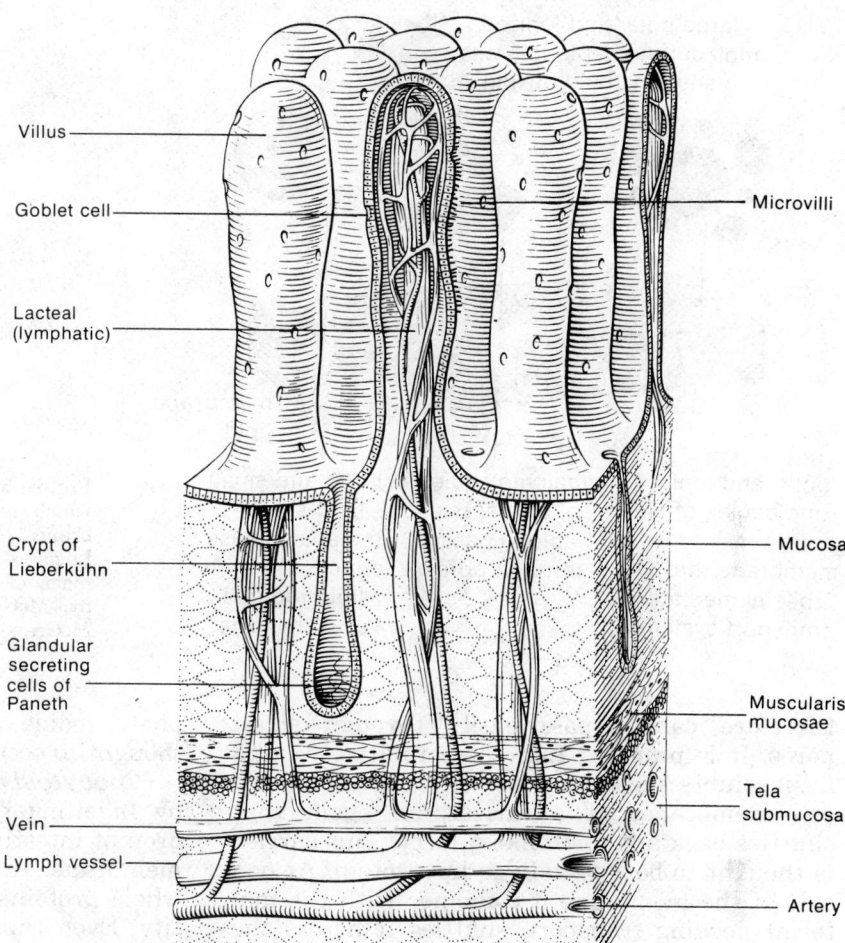

Villus

Goblet cell

Lacteal
(lymphatic)

Microvilli

Crypt of
Lieberkühn

Glandular
secreting
cells of
Paneth

Mucosa

Muscularis
mucosae

Tela
submucosa

Vein

Lymph vessel

Artery

Figure 5–2. Diagram of villi of human intestine showing their structure and blood and lymph vessels. (From Villee, C. A., and Dethier, V. G.: Biological Principles and Processes. 2nd ed. Philadelphia, W. B. Saunders Company, 1976.)

THE MECHANISM OF ABSORPTION. Absorption is an extremely complex process and not all its ramifications are completely understood. It is not simply a matter of diffusion of the nutrients through the mucosal cells into the blood stream for transport to other parts of the body. Diffusion does occur in certain instances; however, other more intricate processes are also involved and explain how large amounts of nutrients constantly enter and leave the cell. Physiologists and biochemists discuss current absorption theory in terms of pores, carriers, pumps and pinocytosis, as shown in Figure 5–4. These mechanisms, though not proven fact, may also apply to other tissues, such as liver, muscle and kidney.

Pores. The presence of a layer of lipoprotein in the wall of the microvilli makes the cell relatively impervious to water and water-soluble substances. It is postulated that these lipoprotein cell membranes are perforated by thousands of tiny pores that permit water, certain electrolytes and very small water-soluble molecules to enter the cell.

Carriers. Amino acids, simple sugars and fats have molecules larger than water molecules and

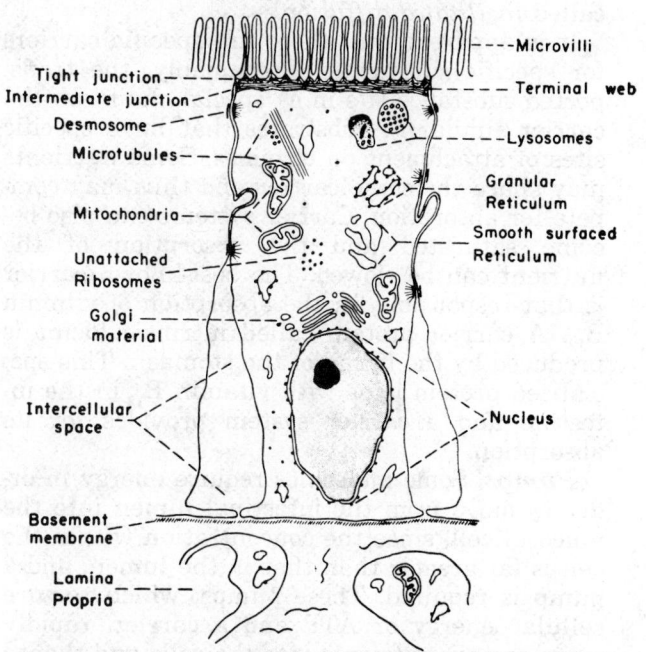

Microvilli

Tight junction

Terminal web

Intermediate junction

Desmosome

Lysosomes

Microtubules

Granular
Reticulum

Mitochondria

Smooth surfaced
Reticulum

Unattached
Ribosomes

Golgi
material

Intercellular
space

Nucleus

Basement
membrane

Lamina
Propria

Figure 5–3. Schematic diagram of a villous absorptive cell. (From Trier, J. S.: Structure of the mucosa of the small intestine as it relates to intestinal function. Fed. Proc., *26*: 1392, 1967.)

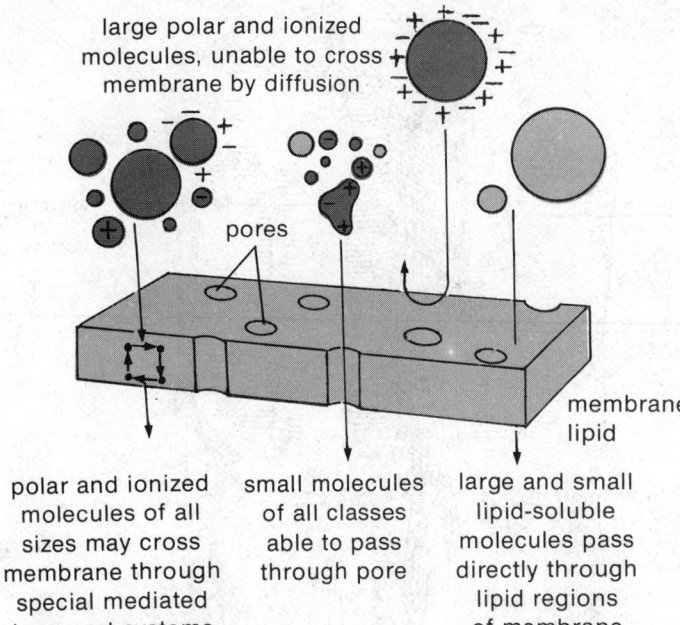

large polar and ionized molecules, unable to cross membrane by diffusion

pores

polar and ionized molecules of all sizes may cross membrane through special mediated transport systems

small molecules of all classes able to pass through pore

large and small lipid-soluble molecules pass directly through lipid regions of membrane

membrane lipid

Figure 5–4. Summary of the various pathways by which molecules can cross intestinal cell membranes. (From Vander, A. J., Sherman, J. H., and Luciano, D. S.: Human Physiology: The Mechanisms of Body Function, 3rd ed. Copyright © 1980 by McGraw-Hill, Inc. Used by permission of McGraw-Hill Book Company.)

therefore cannot pass easily through small pores. It is proposed that these relatively large fat-insoluble substances are escorted across the cell membranes by a carrier, an agent that shuttles back and forth like a ferry. This carrier is thought to be a protein or lipoprotein. At one side of the membrane it combines with the material needing transport, shuttles it across the cell membrane and then releases it into the interior of the cell. In so doing, it is then free to return for another load. This system is also called *facilitated diffusion.*

It is apparent that there are specific carriers for specific substances. Presumably, the transported substance sits in a "special chair" on the carrier similar to substrates that have specific sites of attachment on enzymes. Some nutrients may share the same carrier and thus may compete for absorption. Carrier systems can also become saturated and the absorption of the nutrient can be slowed. The best-known carrier is that responsible for the absorption of vitamin B_{12}. A carrier protein called intrinsic factor is produced by the lining of the stomach. This specialized protein joins with vitamin B_{12} in the intestine and a carrier system provides for its absorption.

Pumps. Some molecules require energy in order to move from the intestinal lumen into the mucosal cell, since the concentration within the cell is far greater than that in the lumen, and a pump is required. These pumps, which require cellular energy or ATP and a carrier, rapidly move certain nutrients into the cells and thence into the blood supply. The absorption of glucose, sodium, galactose, potassium, magnesium, phosphate, iodide, calcium, iron and amino acids is thought to occur in this manner.

Pinocytosis. Pinocytosis has been described by Ingelfinger[3] as a "drinking in" of a small drop of intestinal contents by the epithelial cell membrane. In this way, large particles such as whole proteins may be absorbed in small quantity. Even though it is doubtful that many nutrients are normally absorbed via pinocytosis, the movement of foreign proteins, which somehow find their way across the gastrointestinal tract into the blood stream and cause allergic reactions, may be a result of pinocytosis.

ABSORPTION FROM THE LARGE INTESTINE. The large intestine is approximately 5 feet long and consists of the cecum, colon and rectum, as shown in Figure 5–1. It is the site of the absorption of water, salts and some of the vitamins. The residue in the intestine is now in a semisolid state. Most of the water in the 500 to 1000 ml. of chyme that enters the colon each day is absorbed, leaving 100 to 200 ml. of fluid to be excreted in the feces. In the large intestine the sodium ion is actively absorbed by the mucosa, and because of the electrical potential thus created across the membrane, chloride and other negative ions as well as water move out of the colon into the intestinal mucosa. In addition, the large intestine serves to permit bacteria to reduce materials resistant to the previous digestive processes. Normally, as the contents of the colon move forward at 5 cm. per hour, almost everything of nutritional value is utilized. The waste is composed mostly of cellulose, a number of other polysaccharides and related substances such as pectins and pentosans and other indigestible fibers. The feces contain some water, dead mucosal cells, bacteria and some fat (2.5 to 5 per cent), which comes from the unabsorbed fatty acids from the diet, fat formed by bacterial action and fat found in the sloughed epithelial cells. Passing of feces through the anus, or defecation, occurs with varying frequency, ranging from after every meal to once every 3 or more days.

Digestion and absorption do not always proceed in an orderly fashion. An irritant such as an infection may increase the rate of peristalsis, causing the intestinal contents to pass through the intestinal tract rapidly (diarrhea). If the condition becomes chronic, a considerable loss of body water and electrolytes may result, causing dehydration and electrolyte imbalance. When the contents pass through too slowly, so that a large amount of water is removed, the feces become excessively hard (constipation). Some of the diseases and disturbances are discussed in Chapters 22, 23 and 24.

The Digestive Enzymes—Their Relation to Digestion and Absorption

The digestive enzymes are both exoenzymes and endoenzymes. Those enzymes concerned with metabolism of the cell are usually retained within the cell and are called *endoenzymes*. Those enzymes which are released by the cell and catalyze reactions in the environment of the cell are called *exoenzymes*. The latter are synthesized within specialized cells in the liver and pancreas, extruded and then delivered into the lumen of the intestine where they exert their catalytic action. The endoenzymes are localized in the lipoprotein membranes of the mucosal cells and attach their substrates as they enter the cell. Thus these cells have both a digestive and an absorptive function. Table 5–2 summarizes the enzymatic digestion and absorption of food. A discussion of the digestive enzymes is best considered in terms of the nutrient being digested and absorbed.

CARBOHYDRATE DIGESTION AND ABSORPTION. In the mouth, the enzyme *salivary amylase (ptyalin)*, which is neutral or slightly alkaline, starts the digestive action on starch, hydrolyzing it to dextrins (or isomaltose) and maltose. Approximately 1500 ml. (3 pints) of saliva is secreted daily. The activity of amylase continues in the stomach until the hydrochloric acid destroys it. If the digestible carbohydrate remained in the stomach long enough, the acid hydrolysis could reduce much of it to the monosaccharide stage. However, the stomach usually empties itself before this can take place, and carbohydrate digestion takes place almost en-

tirely in the small intestine, with the greatest activity in the duodenum. *Amylase* from the pancreas breaks the starches into dextrins and maltose, and maltase from the mucosal cells changes maltose to glucose, as illustrated in Figure 5–5. This breakdown occurs on the surfaces of the epithelial cells lining the intestines, the so-called *brush border* composed of microvilli. These outer cell membranes contain the endoenzymes *sucrase, lactase, maltase* and *isomaltase* (or *alpha-dextrinase*), which act on sucrose, lactose, maltose and isomaltose, respectively.

The resulting monosaccharides—glucose, galactose and fructose—pass through the mucosal cell and are actively absorbed using carriers, as depicted in Figure 5–6. They pass into the blood stream and travel via the portal vein to the liver. In the case of glucose and galactose, there is one carrier system that is dependent upon the presence of sodium. Because it is the same active transport mechanism, glucose and galactose compete for absorption. Fructose is absorbed by a not fully understood facilitated diffusion mechanism that is less than half as rapid as the active absorption. Other sugars, such as mannose, xylose and arabinose, are absorbed even more slowly, as Table 5–3 indicates.

From the mucosal cell the glucose and galactose travel to the liver, and from the liver, glucose is transported to the tissues, although some glucose is stored in the liver and muscles as glycogen until needed. A small amount of fructose may be converted to glucose before it passes from the intestinal cell into the blood stream, but most is transported as fructose to the liver where, like galactose, it is converted to glucose.

Glucose is the principal carbohydrate used by the body and is the sugar normally found in the blood. Within 30 minutes to 1 hour after a meal, the blood glucose reaches its highest level of 130 to 150 mg. per 100 ml. Fructose and galactose are found in the systemic circulation only after very large ingestion of these sugars by normal people, and in persons with liver damage. Lactose can be found in the blood of some normal lactating women, and fructose is commonly seen in seminal fluid. In some gastrointestinal disease conditions, disaccharides can be found in the urine, showing that they were absorbed from the GI tract. It is not understood how this happens.

Some forms of carbohydrate cannot be digested by man. Cellulose, hemicellulose, and lignin are among these and are excreted in the feces unchanged. Further discussion of fiber can be found on page 36. Neither salivary amylase nor pancreatic amylase has the ability to split the cellulose bond. The termite, cow and other lower animals, however, can digest cellulose with ease.

Table 5–2. SUMMARY OF ENZYMATIC DIGESTION AND ABSORPTION

SECRETION AND SOURCE OF SECRETION	ENZYME	SUBSTRATE	ACTION AND PRODUCTS OF ACTION	ABSORPTION
Saliva from salivary glands in mouth	Ptyalin (salivary amylase)	Starch	Hydrolysis to form disaccharides (dextrins and maltose) and branched oligosaccharides	
Gastric juice from gastric glands in stomach mucosa	Rennin	Casein (milk protein)	Curdles casein to prepare it for pepsin action (? presence in human infant)	
	Pepsin	Protein (presence of HCl)	Hydrolysis of peptide bonds to form polypeptides and amino acids	
	Lipase (tributyrinase)	Fat (tri-butyrin)	Hydrolysis to form free fatty acids	
Exocrine secretion from pancreas	Trypsin (activated trypsinogen)	Protein and polypeptides	Hydrolysis of interior peptide bonds to form polypeptides	
	Chymotrypsin (activated chymotryp-sinogen)	Proteins and peptides	Hydrolysis of interior peptide bonds to form polypeptides	Pinocytosis of small peptides
	Carboxy-polypeptidase	Polypeptides	Hydrolysis of terminal peptide bonds (carboxyl end) to form amino acids	Amino acids absorbed into blood
	Ribonuclease	Ribonucleic acids	Hydrolysis to form mononucleotides	
	Deoxyribo-nuclease	Deoxyribo-nucleic acids		
	Elastase	Fibrous protein	Hydrolyis to form peptides and amino acids	
	Lipase	Fat (presence of bile salts)	Hydrolysis to form simple glycerides, fatty acids and glycerol	
	Cholesterol esterase	Cholesterol	Hydrolysis to form esters of cholesterol and fatty acids	Micelles → mucosal cells → chylo-microns → lymph
	α-Amylase	Starch and dextrins	Hydrolysis to form dextrins and maltose	
Small intestine enzymes, most of which located in the "brush border"	Carboxypepti-dase Aminopeptidase Dipeptidase	Polypeptides	Hydrolysis of peptide bonds to form amino acids	Amino acids absorbed into blood
	Nucleosidase	Nucleotides	Hydrolysis to form nucleosides and H_3PO_4	
	Nucleosidase	Nucleosides	Hydrolysis to form purines, pyrimidines and pentose	
	Enterokinase	Trypsinogen	Activates to trypsin	
	Lipase (enteric)	Monoglycerides	Hydrolysis to fatty acids and glycerol	Micelles → mucosal cell → chylo-microns → lymph
	Sucrase	Sucrose	Hydrolysis to glucose and fructose	Glucose, galactose and fructose absorbed into blood
	α-Dextrinase (isomaltase)	Dextrin (isomaltose)	Hydrolysis to glucose	
	Maltase	Maltose		
	Lactase	Lactose	Hydrolysis to glucose and galactose	

There are no digestive enzymes in the large intestine. Digestion and absorption are completed by the time the colon is reached. Only water, salt, vitamins and minerals are absorbed thereafter.

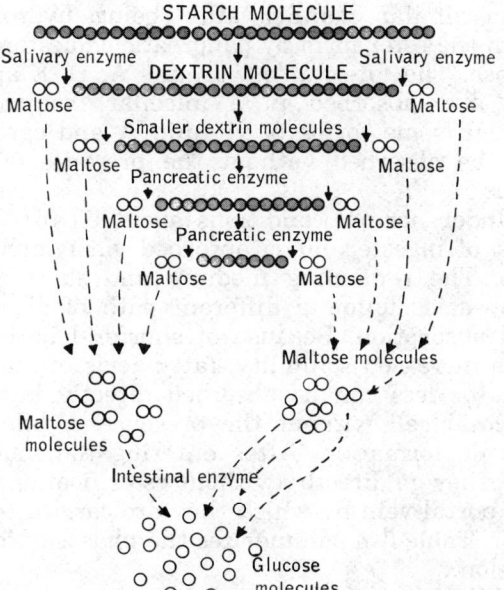

Figure 5–5. Breakdown of starch molecule to glucose. Gradual breaking down of large starch molecules by enzymes in digestion. The disaccharide maltose is split off by enzymes in the saliva and pancreatic juice, with smaller and smaller dextrin molecules formed as intermediate products, until the starch has been completely reduced to maltose. An intestinal enzyme then acts on the maltose molecules, splitting them into molecules of the monosaccharide, or simple sugar, glucose. (From Briggs, G. M. and Calloway, D. H.: Bogert's Nutrition and Physical Fitness. 10th ed. Philadelphia, W. B. Saunders Company, 1979.)

FAT DIGESTION AND ABSORPTION. Fat digestion starts in the stomach with the action of *gastric lipase* (tributyrinase), but it is only able to break naturally occurring short chain triglycerides (found in butter) into fatty acids and glycerol. It is unable to attack the larger molecules of unemulsified fat; therefore, its digestive activity is minimal. The presence of fat in the diet causes food to be retained in the stomach for a longer time. As mentioned, fat eaten with a meal enters the small intestine and stimulates the release of enterogastrone, which inhibits gastric secretion and motility. Food may remain in the stomach as much as four hours or longer before being discharged into the small intestines, which gives a prolonged feeling of satiety. In the small intestine bile acts on the larger fat molecules to break them into smaller fat particles (emulsification).

Bile is a secretion of the liver composed of bile acids (glycocholic and taurocholic acids), bile pigments (which color the feces), inorganic salts, some protein, cholesterol, lecithin, and many compounds metabolized and secreted by the liver, such as detoxified drugs. There are no enzymes in bile. From its storage place in the gallbladder, about 2 pints (1 liter) daily are secreted when it is called into the duodenum by the stimulus of food in the duodenum and stomach.

The emulsification by bile acids makes the fat globules more accessible to digestion by pancreatic lipase and, to a lesser extent, by enteric lipase, which usually splits off two of the three fatty acids from triglycerides. These resulting free fatty acids and monoglycerides along with bile salts form complexes called *micelles* that attach themselves to the surface of the microvilli, and the lipid part of the complex enters the cell presumably by simple diffusion. The bile salts are then released from their lipid components and re-enter the lumen of the gut. Most of the bile salts are actively reabsorbed in the terminal ileum and are recycled back to the liver to enter the gut via the liver and gallbladder. This efficient recycling is known as the *enterohepatic* circulation of bile acids. The pool of bile acids may circulate anywhere from 3 to 15 times per day, depending on the amount of food ingested.

The fatty acids and monoglycerides, now in the mucosal cell, are further digested into free fatty acids and glycerol. They are then

Figure 5–6. Digestion and absorption of carbohydrates. Sodium and either glucose or galactose combine with carrier. The sugar–carrier–sodium ion complex is transported across the cell membrane into the interior of the cell. Once inside the cell, the glucose diffuses passively across the serosal membrane, and the sodium is actively pumped back out of the cell. The driving force for glucose transport against a concentration gradient is the gradient of sodium ion across the membrane that contains the glucose carrier. (Modified from Greene, H. L.: Developmental Nutrition: Carbohydrate Absorption. No. 12. Ross Laboratories, 1976.)

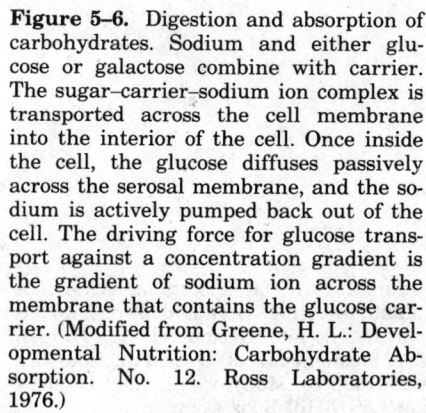

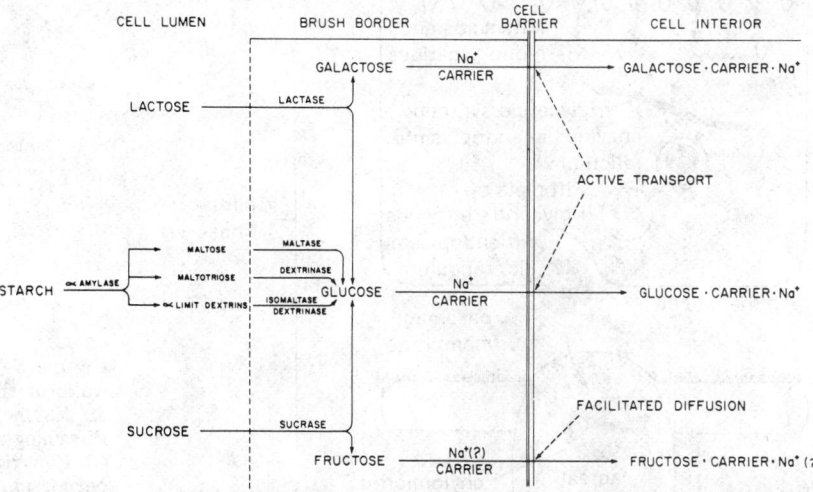

Table 5–3 RELATIVE RATES OF TRANSPORT OF SUGARS COMPARED WITH GLUCOSE

Galactose	1.1
Glucose	1.0
Fructose	0.4
Mannose	0.2
Xylose	0.15
Arabinose	0.1

From Guyton, A. C.: Textbook of Medical Physiology. 6th ed. Philadelphia, W. B. Saunders Company, 1981.

reassembled to form triglycerides, which along with cholesterol and phospholipids are surrounded by a protein coat, betalipoprotein, forming *chylomicrons*, as shown in Figure 5–7. The chylomicrons pass into the lacteals of the villi and are transported by the lymph vessels to the thoracic duct, which empties into the blood stream at the junction of the left internal jugular and left subclavian veins. The triglycerides in the form of chylomicrons are then carried to the liver and adipose tissue for metabolism and storage. Cholesterol is absorbed

in a similar manner after being hydrolyzed from the ester form by pancreatic cholesterol esterase. The fat-soluble vitamins A, D, E and K are also absorbed in a micellar fashion, although some forms of vitamin A and carotene can be absorbed without the presence of bile acids.

Under normal conditions about 60 to 70 per cent of ingested fat is absorbed via lymph vessels. The remaining medium and short chain fatty acids follow a different path of digestion and absorption. Because of shorter length and thus increased solubility, fatty acids of ten carbons or less can be absorbed directly into the mucosal cell without the presence of bile and micelle formation. After entering the mucosal cell, they go directly (without esterification) into the portal vein by which they are carried to the liver. Table 5–4 summarizes the phases of fat digestion.

The finding that shorter chain fatty acids (ten carbons or less) are absorbed quite differently than long chain fatty acids is of clinical usefulness. There are individuals who cannot efficiently absorb the usual types of dietary fat (long

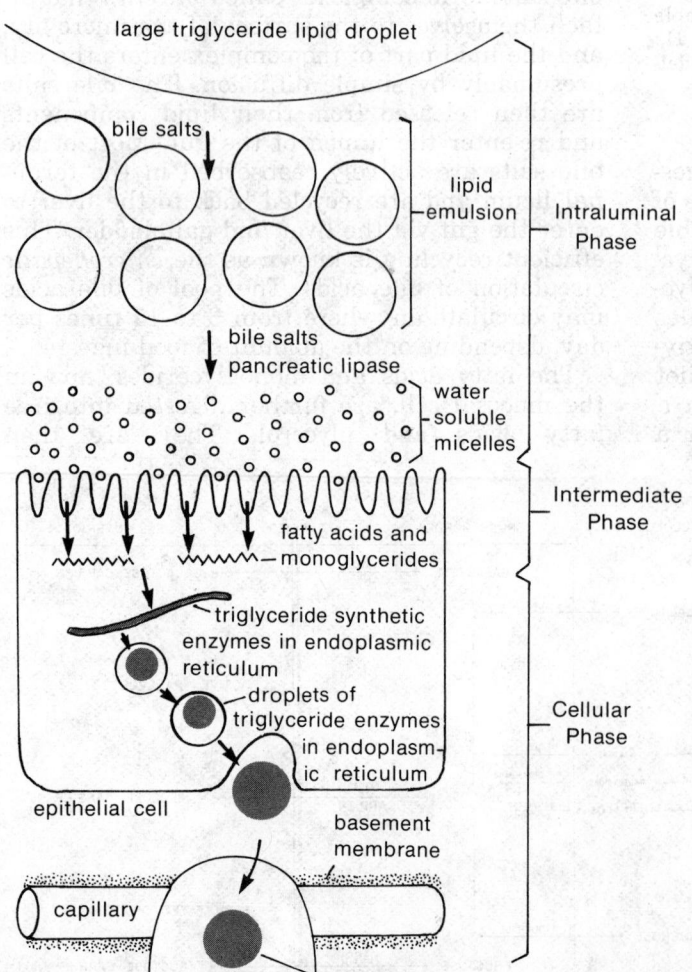

Figure 5–7. Summary of fat absorption across the walls of the small intestine. (Adapted from Vander, A. J., Sherman, J. H., and Luciano, D. S.: Human Physiology: The Mechanisms of Body Function, 3rd ed. Copyright © 1980 by McGraw-Hill, Inc. Used by permission of McGraw-Hill Book Company.)

Table 5–4.   THREE PHASES OF FAT DIGESTION AND ABSORPTION (LONG CHAIN TRIGLYCERIDES, CHOLESTEROL AND PHOSPHOLIPIDS)

1. Intraluminal:	Emulsification—formation of smaller fat droplets to increase surface area of fat. Action of bile acids helps.	
	Lipolysis—hydrolysis of triglycerides to glycerol, fatty acids and monoglycerides by lipases.	
	*Micelle formation—grouping of fatty acids, monoglycerides, phospholipids, cholesterol and bile acids into lipid soluble molecules.	
2. Intermediate:	Mucosal Uptake—release of fatty acids, monoglycerides and/or phospholipids and cholesterol into mucosal cells and return of bile acids to lumen.	
3. Cellular:	*Esterification—resynthesis of triglycerides from glycerol and fatty acids.	
	*Chylomicron formation—coating of cholesterol, triglyceride and phospholipid with single protein coat so that it is water soluble.	
	*Lymphatic delivery—release of chylomicrons into lacteal of villus with subsequent travel through lymphatic system to be emptied into blood stream via left internal jugular or left subclavian vein for transport to liver.	

*Denotes steps unnecessary in the digestion of medium and short chain triglycerides. Their transport is via the portal system, not the lymphatic system.

chain triglycerides) because they lack necessary bile salts for micellar formation or the means for transporting triglycerides out of the intestinal epithelial cells into the lymphatics (abetalipoproteinemia). In these cases *medium chain triglycerides,* C_8 and C_{10}, which bypass micellar formation and chylomicron formation, are used for the fat in the diet.

Increased motility, intestinal mucosa changes, and the absence of bile decrease absorption of fat, and undigested fat will appear in the feces —a condition known as *steatorrhea.* In the healthy adult only about 5 gm. of fat daily should remain in the feces.

PROTEIN DIGESTION AND ABSORPTION. Protein must be broken down into its constituents, the amino acids, to leave the cells in the lining of the intestine and pass through the capillary wall into the intracellular spaces and through the cell membrane into the cell. This involves breaking the peptide linkages that join the amino acids. Protein digestion begins in the stomach where the acid medium changes the preenzyme *pepsinogen* to *pepsin,* which hydrolyzes the protein into simpler molecules—polypeptides, proteoses and peptones. Unlike any of the other proteolytic enzymes, pepsin is able to digest collagen, the connective tissue of meat. However, in the total process of protein digestion the contribution of the stomach is small.

Intraluminal Phase. Movement of partially digested protein into the duodenum signals the beginning of the intraluminal phase of protein digestion. When the chyme reaches the intestinal mucosa, it causes the mucosa to release *enterokinase,* an enzyme that transforms inactive pancreatic *trypsinogen* into active trypsin. Trypsin in turn activates the other pancreatic proteolytic enzymes. Pancreatic *trypsin, chymo-*

trypsin and *carboxypolypeptidase* break down intact protein and continue the breakdown started in the stomach until simple peptides and amino acids are formed.

Surface Membrane Phase. Proteolytic peptidases located on the brush border also act on polypeptides, changing them to amino acids, dipeptides and tripeptides.

There is a distinct mechanism that involves the transport of some dipeptides and tripeptides across the membrane. It has a higher maximal rate of uptake than the amino acid carrier system.[1] It appears that whether the intestinal brush border membrane hydrolyzes dipeptides and tripeptides down to single amino acids or transports them across the membrane as peptides is dependent upon the luminal concentration of oligopeptides and the presence of certain inhibiting peptides.

Whole proteins may also be absorbed, presumably by pinocytosis. Fortunately this is very active in the newborn infant and accounts for the fact that the newborn breast-fed infant can absorb the protein antibodies in human colostrum and thus gain some of the immunity of the mother.

There are at least two distinct active transport systems for amino acids, one for neutral amino acids and the other for basic amino acids.[1] Via these systems, amino acids are absorbed from the lumen of the small intestine into the mucosal ells, enter the blood stream and are then sent to the liver via the portal vein. There they are released into general circulation and carried to the various tissues and cells or built into new protein, as demanded by the body.

Cytoplasmic Phase. There is a third phase of protein digestion that can take place within the mucosal cell cytoplasm. This is hydrolysis of dipeptides and tripeptides to their constituent amino acids by the peptide hydrolases located within the mucosal cells. This completes protein digestion. However, after a protein meal, probably small amounts of peptides still escape hydrolysis and enter the portal circulation as dipeptides.[1]

Some amino acids may remain in the epithelial cell to be used in the synthesis of intestinal enzymes and new cells. Almost all of the protein has been absorbed by the time it reaches the end of the jejunum, and only 1 per cent of ingested protein will be found in the feces. Throughout the intestinal length not only is ingested protein absorbed, but also most of the endogenous protein from intestinal secretions and desquamated epithelial cells.

Most amino acids, especially alanine, stimulate the release of insulin, particularly in the presence of an elevated blood glucose concentration.

OTHER NUTRIENTS. The vitamins, minerals and fluids are being absorbed simultaneously through the intestinal mucosa. Discussion of the absorption of individual vitamins can be found in Chapter 6 and of individual minerals in Chapter 7. Each day about 8 liters of fluid from the body pass back and forth across the membrane of the gut to keep the nutrients in solution. Figure 5–8 illustrates the present

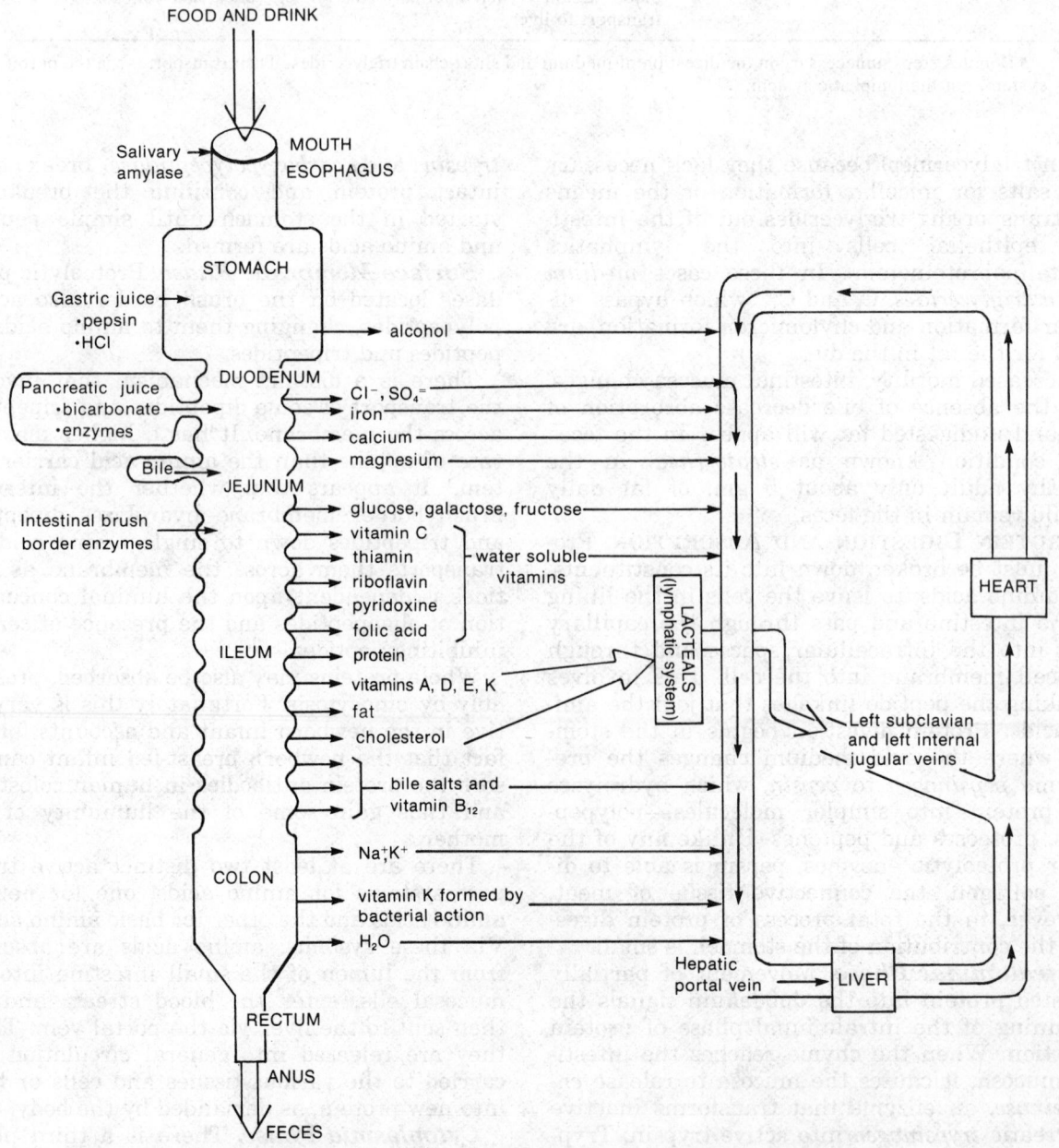

Figure 5–8. Sites of secretion and absorption in the gastrointestinal tract.

understanding of the sites and routes of absorption of nutrients.

Factors Affecting Digestion

The term *digestibility* has several meanings. Atwater used the term to mean the proportion of food material actually digested. From his studies Atwater found that over 90 per cent of the food in a mixed diet is utilized. The average coefficients of apparent digestibility (availability as Atwater used the term) for the nutrients in different food groups and for nutrients in a mixed diet are shown in Table 5–5.

PSYCHOLOGICAL FACTORS. Sight, smell, taste and even the thought of food increase secretions of saliva and the stomach juices and increase muscular activity of the gastrointestinal tract. The phrase "the sight of food makes my mouth water" applies to the psychic factor of digestion. Attractive food presentation in happy surroundings enhances digestion; unattractive food and unfamiliar tastes of food can retard digestion. Anger, fear, fright and worry have a depressing effect on the secretions and may delay digestion. Anger and fear produce an immediate effect in slowing down the process of digestion, and worry tends to produce a delayed effect. Emotions stimulate the hypothalamus, which activates the autonomic nervous system to depress secretions, inhibit peristalsis and increase the tone of the sphincters. The propulsion of food through the gastrointestinal tract is slowed considerably. However, emotional stimuli may increase gastric secretion during the interdigestive period. The presence of this highly potent secretion when there is no food upon which to act is irritating to the intestinal mucosa and accounts for the play of emotional factors in the etiology of peptic ulcers. These are important points to remember when assisting individuals with dietary problems. The appearance of the food served, the combinations and the tastes of food along with the existing emotional stresses have an impact on the digestion of food.

MECHANICAL FACTORS. These are the physical changes brought about by the grinding, crushing and mixing of the food that occurs in the gastrointestinal tract. They facilitate the mixing of the food with the digestive juices and propel the mass through the digestive tract. Movements in the stomach are weak and shallow in the fundic wall and are strong and vigorous in the pyloric region. In the intestines the chyme is propelled caudally by waves of rhythmic contractions (peristalsis), mixed, and brought into contact with the intestinal mucosa. Layers of circular and longitudinal muscles produce segmentation movements.

In general, properly cooked foods are more di-

Table 5–5 PER CENT DIGESTIBILITY OF NUTRIENTS

FOOD GROUP	PROTEIN	FAT	CARBO-HYDRATE
	Per Cent	*Per Cent*	*Per Cent*
Animal Foods	97	95	98
Cereals	85	90	98
Legumes, dried	78	90	97
Sugars and starches			98
Vegetables	83	90	95
Fruits	85	90	90
Vegetable foods	84	90	97
Total food*	92	95	97

*Weighted by consumption statistics based on a survey of 185 dietaries.

From Merrill, A. L., and Watts, B. K.: Energy Value of Foods—Basis and Derivation. Washington, D.C., U.S. Department of Agriculture, Handbook No. 74, 1955.

gestible than raw foods. Proper cooking of meat, for example, loosens the connective tissue, aids chewing and makes the meat more accessible to the digestive juices. Bolting of food has the result of introducing large chunks into the stomach, bypassing the benefit of mastication to break it down. It is an added tax on the digestive system. Small, frequent meals may be more easily digested than three large meals, an important factor to remember when feeding the sick.

CHEMICAL FACTORS. These apply to the chemical reactions between food and the secretions of the digestive system. Fatty and improperly fried foods in which *acrolein* is produced will retard the flow of digestive juices, while meat extracts, for example, will stimulate digestion.

Some foods agree with many people and disagree with others. Personal idiosyncrasy or an allergy may account for this. It has been suggested that there are people who are peculiarly sensitive to some chemical substances or to their physical states. For example, why do some people have distress from drinking orange juice? Although orange juice is considered a very easily digested food, there are those in good physical condition who claim it causes genuine distress, especially if ice cold and ingested when the stomach is empty.

There is evidence showing that digestive enzymes in the jejunum change in response to dietary substances. The change seems to take two to five days, the estimated turnover time of a human intestinal epithelial cell.[6] As these mechanisms of change become defined, some of the mystery surrounding individual intolerances of foods and indigestion will probably be dispelled.

BACTERIAL ACTION. The gut microflora make up a complex community in which about 100 species have been identified in the normal intestinal tract. At birth the gastrointestinal tract is essentially sterile, but implantation of various microorganisms soon takes place. *Lactobacillus* is the first organism to appear and is the chief component of the flora until the infant begins to eat solid foods. *Escherichia coli* become predominant in the distal ileum and the primary colonic flora appear to be *anaerobic* (that is, they grow in an environment without molecular oxygen), with species of the genus *Bacteroides* most frequent. Lactobacilli are also present in the stools of most persons on an ordinary mixed diet.

Normally, there is very little bacterial action in the stomach, as the hydrochloric acid acts as a germicidal agent. However, in conditions in which there is decreased secretion of hydrochloric acid, resistance to bacterial action is lowered. Occasionally gastritis, an inflammation of the gastric mucosa, may be due to bacterial inflammation.

Bacterial action is most intense in the large intestine, with 10^{11} organisms per gm. feces, compared with 10^5 for the stomach, duodenum, jejunum and upper ileum and 10^8 per gm. for the distal ileum. Colonic bacteria contribute to the formation of (1) gases (hydrogen, carbon dioxide, oxygen, ammonia, methane), (2) acids (lactic, acetic, etc.), and (3) various toxic substances (indole, phenol, etc.). Many of these products account for the odor of feces.

Although dietary intake alters the fecal flora, the response varies markedly from time to time and from individual to individual. The ingestion of carbohydrate, in general, leads to increased fermentation in the large intestine; protein yields increased putrefaction. If large amounts of carbohydrate or protein reach the large intestine as a result of faulty absorption in the small intestine, bacterial action may give rise to the formation of excessive gas and also of certain toxic substances. Some of these toxic substances have been suspected in the etiology of colonic cancer. An example is cyclohexylamine, a potentially carcinogenic agent that is formed by intestinal bacterial action on cyclamate, a nonabsorbed artificial sweetener.

Intestinal flora plays a much more important role in nutrition than was previously considered. Some of the intestinal organisms have the ability to synthesize a number of the vitamins of the B complex (especially biotin and folic acid) and vitamin K. In addition, they contribute toward maintaining the intestines in a healthy condition. The organic acids produced help to check the growth of some of the less desirable bacteria.

Metabolism

Absorbed nutrients, including water and electrolytes, are carried in the blood stream and enter the body's metabolism.

Metabolism comes from a Greek word, "metaballein," meaning to change or alter. Broadly speaking, metabolism may be defined as tissue change. It is the chemical process of transforming nutrients into complex tissue elements and of transforming complex body substances into simple ones, along with the production of heat and energy.

The two main phases of metabolism are anabolism and catabolism. *Anabolism* includes the chemical changes whereby simple substances are combined to form more complex substances with the net result that new cellular materials are produced and energy is stored. This is necessary for growth and for maintenance and repair of body tissues. *Catabolism* includes those processes concerned with the breaking down of the complex substances into simpler constituents for energy production or excretion. These processes occur constantly and simultaneously in the body. When anabolism exceeds catabolism, growth occurs. If catabolism exceeds anabolism, the breakdown is faster than the building up processes, making the body lose substance and weight. In health, a balance is maintained between these two constantly operating opposing processes so that body weight and tissue substance are maintained, or added to if desired.

The amount of food consumed can have a profound effect on whether anabolism or catabolism will predominate in a given situation. The person who consumes less food than he requires loses weight because the catabolic state predominates. The person who consumes more food than required gains adipose tissue and is in an anabolic state.

Other factors that increase anabolism are rest and certain endocrine secretions such as insulin and some adrenal and sex hormones (for example, during adolescence increased secretions of sex hormones stimulate growth).

Some factors that increase catabolism are fever, bacterial toxins, fractures, burns and certain endocrine secretions such as thyroxine and cortisone.

The metabolism of glucose, triglycerides, fatty acids and amino acids is regulated and controlled by cellular enzymes, their coenzymes (many of which are the B vitamins), other cofactors (many of which are trace minerals) and hormones. The end products of catabolism of glucose, fatty acids and amino acids are the same, namely, carbon dioxide and water. In addition to carbon dioxide and water, the end products of amino acid metabolism are the nitrogenous wastes in the urine.

In earlier chapters the general metabolism of the carbohydrates, fats and proteins has been described. The present discussion will consider the nutrition of the individual cells, the intricate biochemical pathway by which the chemical energy of the foods is made available to the cells as needed, and the mainly catabolic steps by which the three major nutrients enter this pathway. The same preliminary steps are needed whether the nutrients are used immediately for energy or are transformed for other use or storage. Figure 5–9 shows the location within the cells of the processes to be described.

ADENINE NUCLEOTIDES. The source of energy for the body is the oxidation of food. This energy must be in a utilizable form and for many processes, notably muscle contraction, it must be immediately available. The energy is trapped in certain organic phosphates and is released

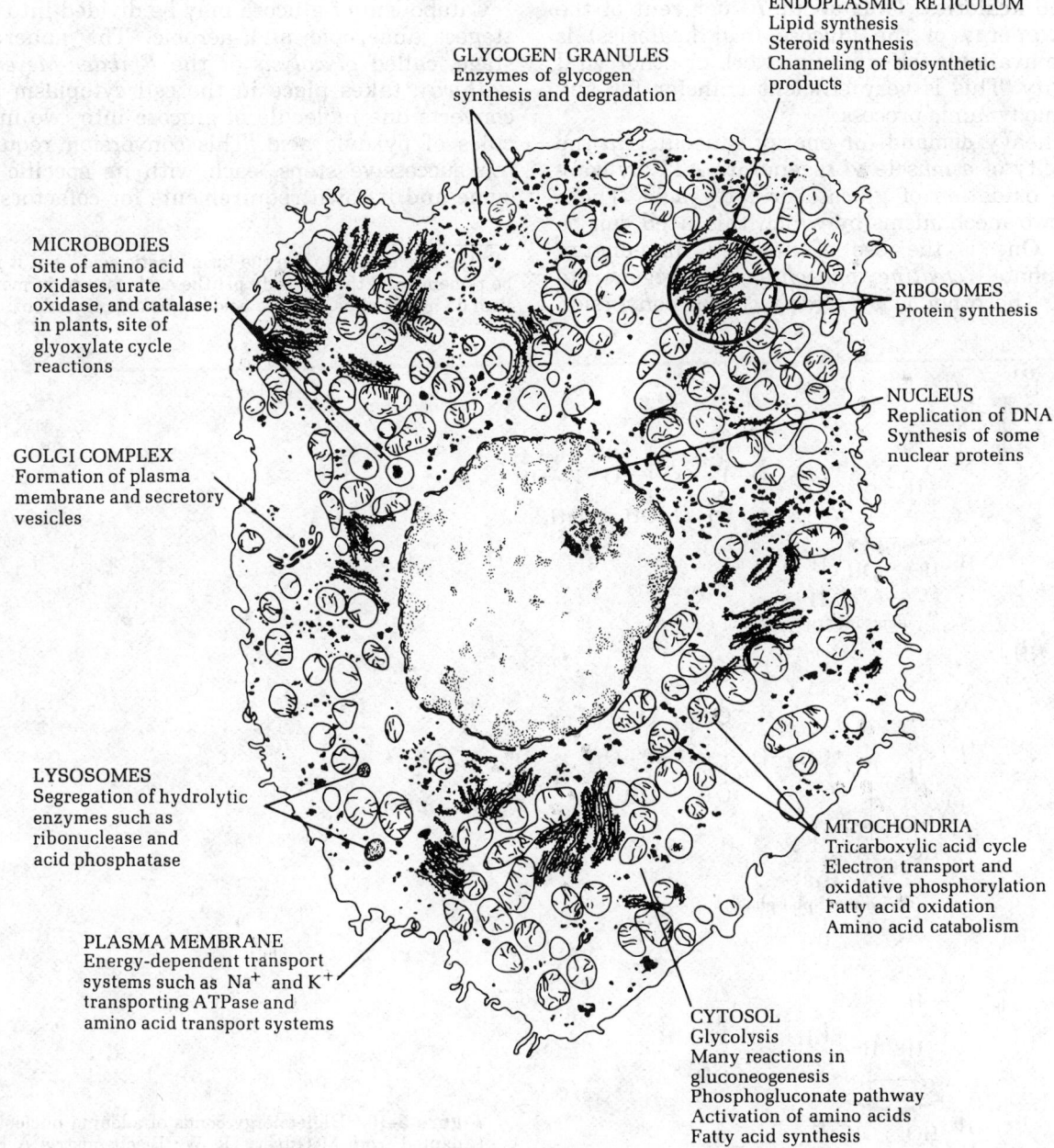

Figure 5–9. Compartmentation of some important enzymes and metabolic sequences in the liver cell of the rat. Traced from an electron micrograph. (From Lehninger, A. L.: Biochemistry, 2nd ed. Worth Publishers, 1976.)

very rapidly when the compounds are hydrolyzed. The most important of these are the adenine nucleotides *adenosine triphosphate (ATP)* and *adenosine diphosphate (ADP)*, as shown in Figure 5–10. *Adenosine monophosphate* (AMP) does not have a high-energy bond. ATP is rightly called the "energy currency" of the cell (see page 9). Hydrolysis of the terminal phosphate group of ATP or ADP releases a large amount of energy and the linkage is called a "high-energy phosphate bond" ($\sim$). When ATP is hydrolyzed, 12 kcalories are released per molecule. In the full oxidation of one molecule of glucose 38 high-energy phosphate bonds are formed, a total of 456 kcalories. Thus about 70 per cent of the total energy of the glucose (646 kcalories) is made available for muscular work or other vital activity. This is very efficient transfer for any thermodynamic process.

A heavy demand for energy can outstrip the capacity of a muscle to regenerate ATP by complete oxidation of glucose or fatty acid. There are two mechanisms by which this need can be met. One is the use of another high-energy phosphate, *creatine phosphate*, to regenerate ATP. The other is by *glycolysis*, the conversion

of glucose to lactic acid,* which will be discussed in the next section.

GLUCOSE. Every cell in the body is able to utilize glucose for production of energy. However, it must first be phosphorylated to *glucose-6-phosphate (G-6-P)* by hexokinases before it can enter the metabolic pathways in the cell. In most tissues this reaction is irreversible and the G-6-P must continue down the metabolic pathway. The two exceptions are liver and kidney tissue, which have the enzyme glucose-6-phosphatase necessary to release free glucose. Glucose-6-phosphate serves as a link between the major pathways of glucose metabolism.

Catabolism of glucose may be divided into two stages: anaerobic and aerobic. The anaerobic stage, called *glycolysis* or the *Embden-Meyerhof pathway*, takes place in the cell cytoplasm and converts one molecule of glucose into two molecules of pyruvic acid. This conversion requires ten successive steps, each with its specific enzyme and its own requirements for cofactors. In

---

*It is convenient to use the term "lactic acid," but it must be remembered that at body pH the acids formed in metabolism do not exist as the free acid but as organic anions.

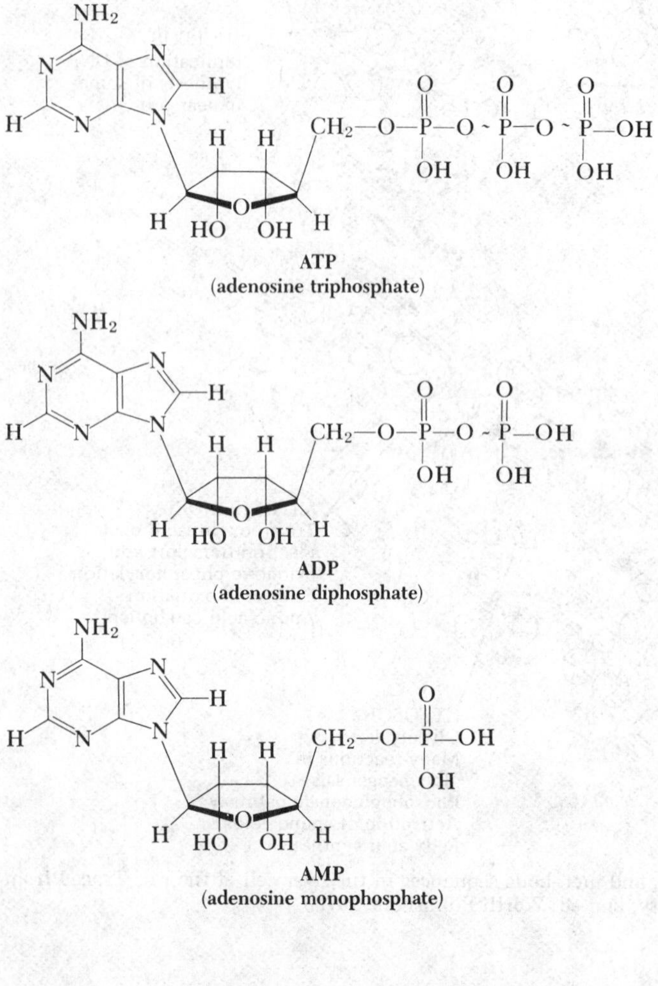

ATP
(adenosine triphosphate)

ADP
(adenosine diphosphate)

AMP
(adenosine monophosphate)

Figure 5–10. High-energy bonds of adenine nucleotides. (Adapted from McGilvery, R. W.: Biochemistry: A Functional Approach. 2nd ed. Philadelphia, W. B. Saunders Company, 1979.)

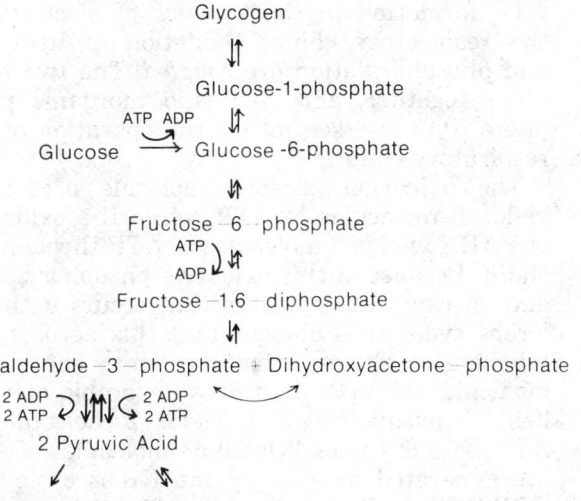

Glycogen

⇅

Glucose-1-phosphate

⇅

ATP ADP

Glucose ⟶ Glucose-6-phosphate

⇅

Fructose-6-phosphate

ATP

⇅

ADP

Fructose-1.6-diphosphate

⇅

Glyceraldehyde-3-phosphate + Dihydroxyacetone-phosphate

2 ADP
2 ATP   2 ADP
             2 ATP

2 Pyruvic Acid

Aerobic Pathway   2 Lactic Acid
(Krebs Cycle)

Figure 5–11. Simplification of Embden-Meyerhof anaerobic pathway.

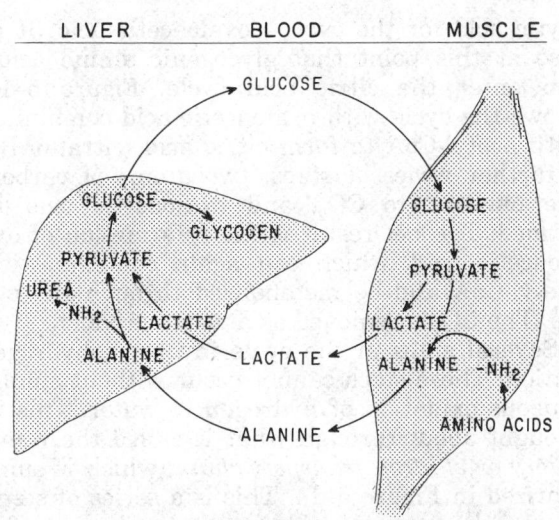

Figure 5–12. The relationship between the metabolism of muscle and liver during gluconeogensis. Note the parallelism of the lactic acid (Cori) cycle and the alanine cycle. The latter represents the major pathway by which the amino groups from muscle amino acids are conveyed to the liver to conversion to urea. (From Felig, P.: Disorders of carbohydrate metabolism. In Bondy, P. K., and Rosenberg, L. E. (eds.): Metabolic Control and Disease. 8th ed. Philadelphia, W. B. Saunders Company, 1980.)

the process two molecules of ATP are used and four are produced; thus, there is a net gain of two molecules of ATP available for immediate energy needs. Figure 5–11 gives an abbreviated outline of this pathway. There is no involvement of oxygen in this series of reactions. If there is heavy demand for muscular work and there is insufficient oxygen to continue with the aerobic pathway, the anaerobic reaction may go one step further with reduction of pyruvic acid to lactic acid (lactate). The lactic acid will diffuse out of the cells and its level in the blood stream will rise. This allows the concentration of pyruvic acid and H^+ in the cell to remain low, and thus the anaerobic glycolysis can continue longer and provide energy to the cell.

When O_2 is again present (as after completion of an exercise when "catching one's breath") the lactic acid can either be converted to glucose in the liver and be used directly for energy, or be converted into glycogen. This system in the muscle and liver whereby the following occurs— blood glucose → muscle glycogen → lactic acid → liver → glucose-6-phosphate → blood glucose— is called the Cori cycle and is outlined in Figure 5–12. Some pyruvate is also converted to alanine in the muscle and recycled in the same manner as lactate, and this is known as the alanine cycle. The steps indicated in the diagram can all occur in the reverse direction, but in a few steps the reverse reaction is catalyzed by a different enzyme.

Anaerobic glycolysis production of energy is inefficient, producing only two moles of ATP. However, it is necessary and life-saving during muscular activity and periods of oxygen shortage. The heart muscle has the unique ability to

utilize lactic acid and convert it to pyruvic acid, which is oxidized for energy production via the Krebs cycle.

The second stage of carbohydrate metabolism, which cannot take place without the presence of molecular oxygen, is the oxidative decarboxylation of pyruvate followed by entry into the cycle that is variously referred to as the aerobic cycle, Krebs cycle, tricarboxylic acid cycle or citric acid cycle. Pyruvic acid or pyruvate may be regarded as the starting point of the cycle, and it moves into the mitochondria for this oxidation.

It was early recognized that the first step involved oxidative decarboxylation of pyruvic acid with formation of CO_2 and acetic acid. The acetic acid was in some active form; the nature of this acid form was elusive but was finally identified as a combination of acetic acid with a derivative of pantothenic acid. The coenzyme was called coenzyme A and the active molecule acetyl-CoA. The reaction also involves lipoic acid and three other vitamins—thiamin, riboflavin and niacin. It is not surprising that thiamin deficiency may be associated with elevated blood pyruvate due to an impairment in its conversion to acetyl-CoA.

In another reaction, an adjunct to the Krebs cycle, pyruvic acid may combine with a molecule of CO_2 to form oxaloacetic acid. The significance of this reaction is that the body has the ability to assimilate CO_2 and synthesize the catalytic acid for the cycle—oxaloacetic acid. It is also at this point that glycogenic amino acids can enter the citric acid cycle. Figure 5–13 shows the cycle with oxaloacetic acid combining with acetyl-CoA to form citric acid (citrate). By a further series of steps, two atoms of carbon are oxidized to CO_2, and oxaloacetic acid is formed. The net result is the reformation of oxaloacetic acid, which can again combine with acetyl-CoA and be metabolized through the cycle. The CO_2 is removed as a waste product.

Several steps in the cycle involve dehydrogenation. These steps cannot occur without simultaneous oxidation of hydrogen to water. This is brought about through what is called the *respiratory or electron transport chain*, which is summarized in Figure 5–14. This is a series of steps involving alternate oxidation and reduction of a sequence of coenzymes, culminating in the combination of hydrogen with oxygen to form water. The whole process is called *oxidative phosphorylation*. If the hydrogen were combined with oxygen directly, much energy would be wasted as heat. Instead, the respiratory chain allows the capture of this energy by the formation of ATP. Figure 5–14 shows the sites of the

ATP formation in the transfer of electrons in the respiratory chain. Oxidation of hydrogen and phosphorylation are *coupled*. The two must occur together, and ADP and inorganic phosphate (P_i) are essential for the operation of the respiratory chain.

The oxidation of each molecule of NADH yields 3 molecules of ATP, while the oxidation of $FADH_2$ yields 2 molecules of ATP through the chain. Because of this oxidative phosphorylation and entrapment of energy that occurs with the Krebs cycle, it is obvious that this aerobic metabolism of glucose yields far more energy, 36 molecules of ATP, than does anaerobic metabolism to pyruvate, which yields 2 molecules of ATP. Two of the additional 34 molecules of ATP are generated directly by the Krebs cycle (the GDP-GTP), and the remaining 32 are generated by the respiratory chain shown in Figure 5–14.

Studies of cell structure at the molecular level have shown that these enzyme systems are not randomly dispersed in the cell, but are arranged in an orderly fashion on the matrix and inside wall of the *mitochondria* of the cell (see Fig. 1–2). Because this is the site of ATP generation, the mitochondrion has been called the cel-

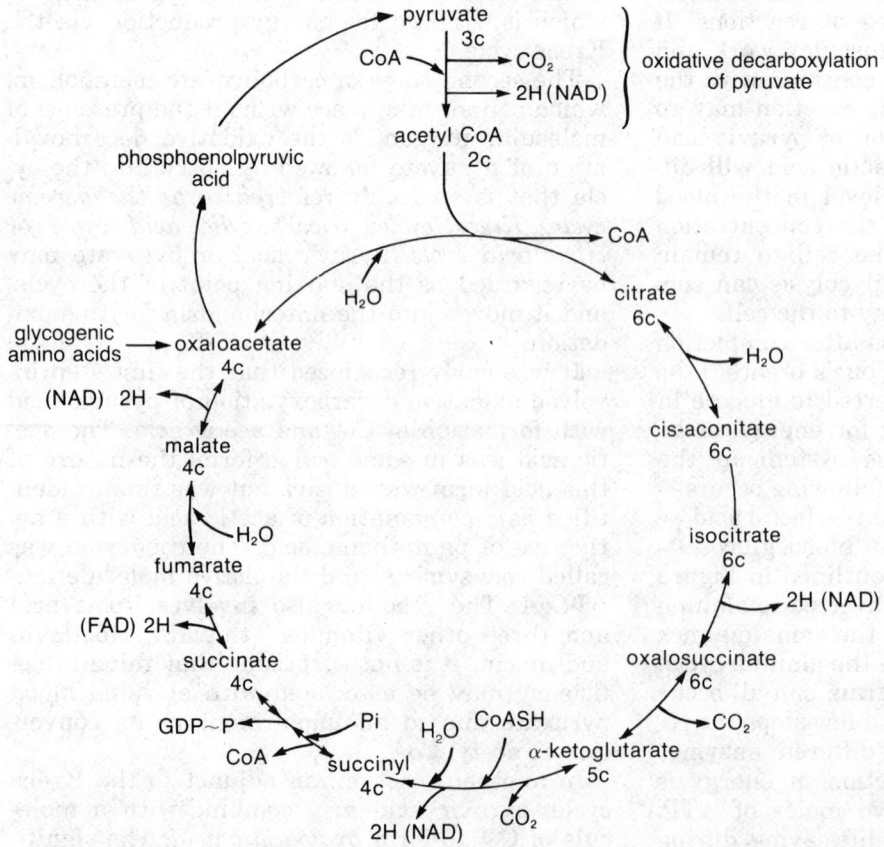

Net reaction per mole pyruvate: 1 Acetyl CoA + 3 H_2O + 1 Pi → 2 CO_2 + 8 H + 1 CoA + 1 GDP~P

Figure 5–13. The Krebs or citric acid cycle.

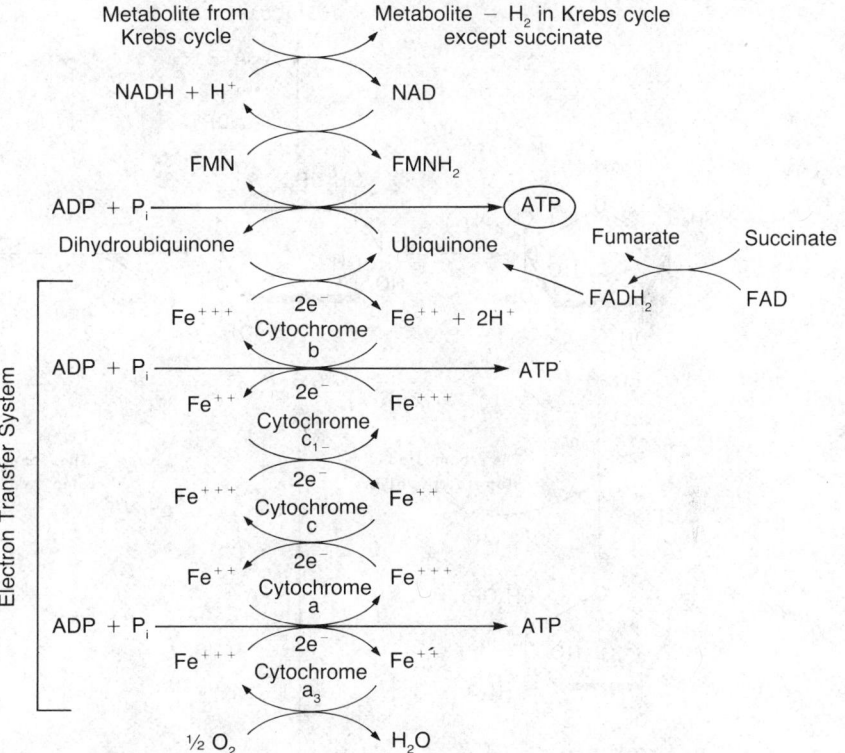

Figure 5–14. Oxidative phosphorylation at the respiratory chain level. Nicotinamide adenine dinucleotide (NAD), flavin adenine dinucleotide (FAD) and flavin mononucleotide (FMN) are coenzymes that are reduced as a result of oxidation of substrates in the Krebs cycle. They are reoxidized by the enzymes of the respiratory chain with entrapment of energy as ATP and the formation of water. P_i = inorganic phosphate; ATP = adenosine triphosphate; ubiquinone = coenzyme Q.

lular "powerhouse." Other activities such as fatty acid and amino acid synthesis are carried out by the mitochondria, but the entrapment of energy is the most important.

An additional anaerobic pathway of glycolysis that is important to mention is the *pentose phosphate shunt* or *hexose monophosphate shunt.* This pathway is useful in at least three ways: (1) it does not require ATP like the Embden-Meyerhof pathway; (2) it is one of the few reactions that produce reduced nicotinamide adenine dinucleotide phosphate (NADP), a coenzyme involved in the transfer of hydrogens (or electrons) and which is required in some cellular reactions such as the synthesis of fatty acids; and (3) it provides a means for synthesis of ribose and deoxyribose necessary for synthesis of nucleotide and nucleic acid. This pathway is very active in mammary gland, testis, adipose, leukocyte, adrenal cortex and liver tissue, but almost nonexistent in muscle tissue (striated muscle). Figure 5–15 is an abbreviated diagram of the hexose monophosphate shunt.

GALACTOSE AND FRUCTOSE. Galactose is easily converted in the liver to uridine diphosphoglucose (UDP-glu), which can be incorporated into glycogen or converted to glucose-1-phosphate, which can then be metabolized in the glucose pathways.

After absorption, fructose is converted to fructose-1-phosphate by fructokinase. Fructose-1-phosphate is then split to two 3-carbon fragments:

$$\text{Fructose} + \text{ATP} \rightarrow \text{fructose-1-phosphate} + \text{ADP} \rightarrow \text{glyceraldehyde} + \text{dihydroxyacetonephosphate}$$

The cellular entry of fructose does not appear to be insulin-dependent. However, as can be seen in Figure 5–16, fructose can be converted to glucose eventually, causing a rise in blood glucose if present in a large amount.

Sugars can be reduced to form alcohols such as sorbitol and myoinositol or oxidized to form acids such as ascorbic acid (vitamin C). The reduction pathway or *polyol pathway* is important in galactosemia or diabetes mellitus, where the level of blood glucose or galactose is high. In these situations the reduction of these sugars in the cell is increased and there is a buildup of the alcohol sorbitol that is thought to account for many of the complications of diabetes, particularly cataracts.

It is of interest to note here some of the roles of the vitamins in tissue metabolism. All the B-complex vitamins are known to function as coenzymes in metabolic reactions. Thiamin pyrophosphate is the coenzyme for decarboxylation of alpha-ketoglutarate. Transamination requires vitamin B_6 coenzyme. Coenzyme A is a derivative of pantothenic acid, and riboflavin and nic-

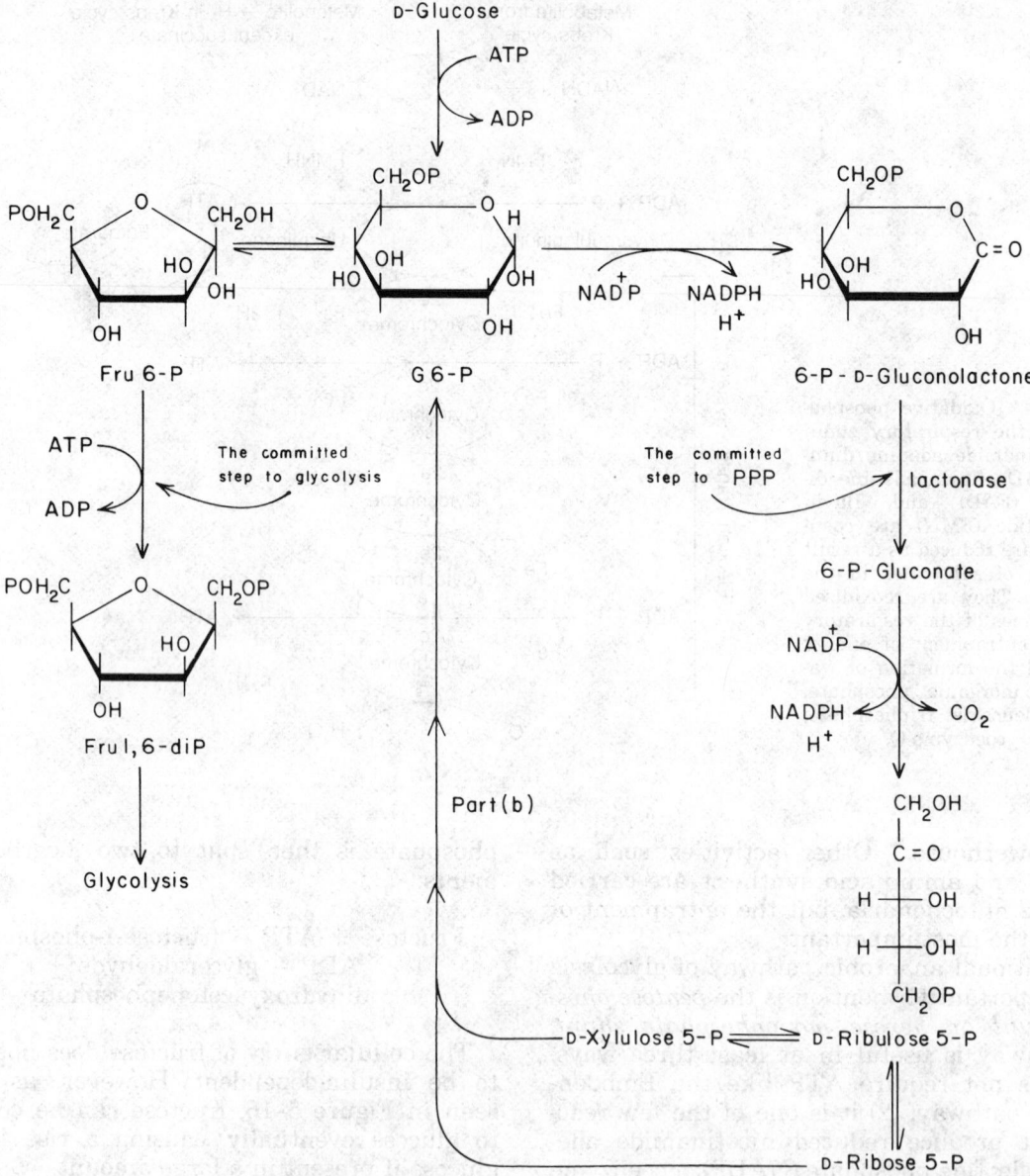

Figure 5–15. Pentose phosphate pathway or hexose monophosphate shunt. G 6-P = glucose-6-phosphate; Fru 6-P = fructose-6-phosphate. (From Montgomery, R., et al.: Biochemistry: A Case-Oriented Approach. 4th ed. St. Louis, C. V. Mosby, 1983.)

otinic acid are constituents of coenzymes of the respiratory chain. The role of vitamin E is less clear, but it also appears to be involved in electron transport in conjunction with the cytochromes.

FATS. The first step in utilization of fat in the body is hydrolysis to fatty acids and glycerol. This takes place largely in the adipose tissue by the enzyme *lipoprotein lipase*. This enzyme is located on the lumen surface of the capillary endothelial cell and is activated by insulin. Once activated, it hydrolyzes triglycerides and phospholipids into glycerol and fatty acids, which can diffuse into the fat cell. Glycerol diffuses back into the plasma since it can only be oxi-

dized for energy in the liver and kidney cell. There it is converted to glycerophosphate and is either reincorporated into triglycerides or (more likely) converted to glucose.

Fatty acids in the adipose tissue cells are resynthesized into triglycerides for storage, and the glycerol for this resynthesis comes from glucose, which also enters the adipose cell when insulin is present.

The activity of *lipoprotein lipase* varies with the state of the individual. In times of energy excess such as after a meal, the lipoprotein lipase is active in adipose tissue when triglycerides are being taken out of the blood for storage. In energy-deficient situations such as fasting,

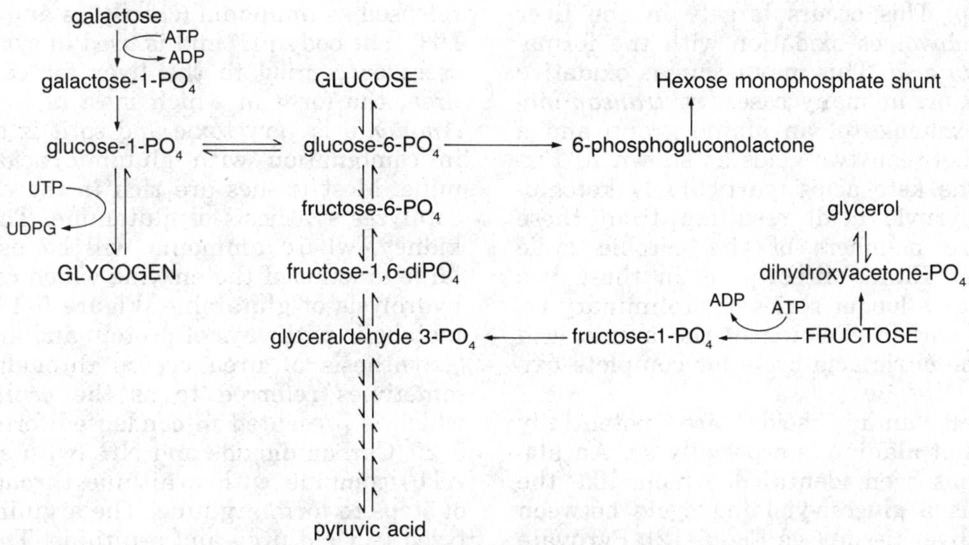

Figure 5–16. Metabolism of fructose and galactose and major pathways of carbohydrate metabolism. UTP = uridine triphosphate, UDPG = uridine diphosphoglucose.

the activity is high in muscle tissue when fatty acids need to be taken up for oxidation for energy.

Fatty acids are released from the adipose cells by the action of a *cellular lipase* in the adipose cell. They are carried in the blood bound to albumin as *free fatty acids* or *nonesterified fatty acids* (FFA or NEFA.) They travel to the liver, which can convert them to acetoacetic acid, beta-hydroxybutyric acid, and acetone *(ketone bodies)*, which can be utilized by muscle tissue for energy. As early as 1905 Knoop proposed that fatty acids are metabolized by beta oxidation (the beta carbon is the second from the carboxyl carbon). The chain is shortened by two carbons at a time, forming in each step acetic acid and a shorter fatty acid chain. This is still recognized as the major pathway of fatty acid oxidation and is directly associated with oxygen uptake. Oxygen must be available for beta oxidation; in an anaerobic situation, as in very strenuous exercise, fat catabolism is halted. The mechanisms have been worked out as illustrated in Figure 5–17. The fatty acid forms an active complex with coenzyme A, this initial step being supplied with energy by ATP. Note that the final product of the reaction is acetyl-CoA, which is then oxidized via the citric acid cycle to achieve energy as the end result.

It is interesting to note that the breakdown of fatty acids depends upon an adequate supply of oxaloacetic acid, which is mainly generated from carbohydrate metabolism. The acetyl-CoA from beta oxidation must combine with oxaloacetic acid to form citric acid in the Krebs cycle. Thus, complete fatty acid catabolism requires a continual background of glucose catabolism in

order to provide the pyruvic acid to make the necessary oxaloacetic acid. In situations of severe carbohydrate limitation, the acetate fragments produced from beta oxidation cannot be accommodated in the Krebs cycle and build up in extracellular fluids. They are readily converted to ketones and excreted in the urine and expired air.

AMINO ACIDS. It is impossible in a brief summary to show the catabolic pathways for all the amino acids. Important common steps may be illustrated. One of these steps is removal of the

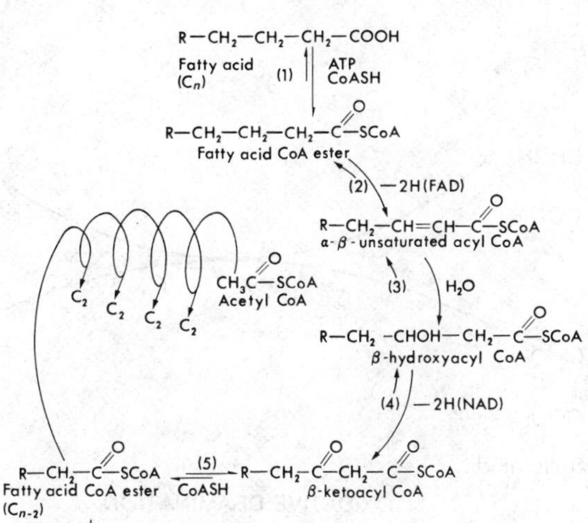

Figure 5–17. Fatty acid oxidation. Enzymes are: (1) acyl CoA synthetase, (2) acyl CoA dehydrogenase, (3) enoyl CoA hydrase, (4) Beta-hydroxyacyl CoA dehydrogenase and (5) Beta-ketoacyl thiolase. (From Pike, R. L., and Brown, M. L.: Nutrition: An Integrated Approach, 2nd ed. New York, John Wiley & Sons, 1975, p. 510.)

amino group. This occurs largely in the liver and usually involves oxidation with the formation of a *keto acid*. This may occur as oxidative *deamination* or, in many cases, as *transamination*, with exchange of an amino group and a keto group between two acids as shown in Figure 5–18. The keto acids (particularly ketoglutaric and pyruvic acid) resulting from these reactions are members of the aerobic cycle (Krebs cycle). Either directly, as in these two cases, or after a longer series of preliminary reactions, the carbon skeleton of the amino acid can enter the citric acid cycle for complete oxidation.

Almost all amino acids are potentially glucogenic, but alanine is especially so. An alanine cycle has been identified, which, like the Cori cycle, is a glucose-yielding cycle between muscle and liver tissue (see Fig. 5–12). Pyruvate from glucose oxidation in muscle is transaminated to form alanine, which is transported to the liver where it is deaminated and the carbon skeleton is reconverted to glucose. This alanine cycle is significant as a source of glucose during periods of low exogenous glucose supply. It is also a way to move nitrogen from the muscle to the liver without the formation of ammonia.

The amino group of the amino acids is usually released as ammonia (chiefly as ammonium ion, NH_4^+, at body pH) and is used in synthetic processes or carried to the liver for conversion to urea, the form in which most of it is excreted. *Ammonia* is very toxic and so it is transported, in combination with glutamic acid, as glutamine. Most tissues are rich in the enzyme that catalyzes synthesis of glutamine. The liver and kidney, where ammonia will be used, have a large amount of the enzyme which catalyzes the hydrolysis of glutamine. Figure 5–19 shows the metabolic pathways of protein and amino acids.

Synthesis of urea occurs through a process sometimes referred to as the *ornithine cycle*, which is presented in condensed form in Figure 5–20. Carbon dioxide and NH_3 (with energy from ATP) combine with ornithine through a series of steps to form arginine. The arginine is hydrolyzed to yield urea and ornithine. Thus an ornithine molecule is used over and over in the formation of arginine and urea.

COMMON METABOLIC PATHWAY. Figure 5–21 is an integration of the metabolic pathways that have been described. It shows how carbohydrate, fat and protein may be utilized for energy by a common pathway; how carbohydrate may be converted to fat for storage or to cholesterol via acetyl-CoA; how some amino acids may be converted to glucose and some to fat; and how

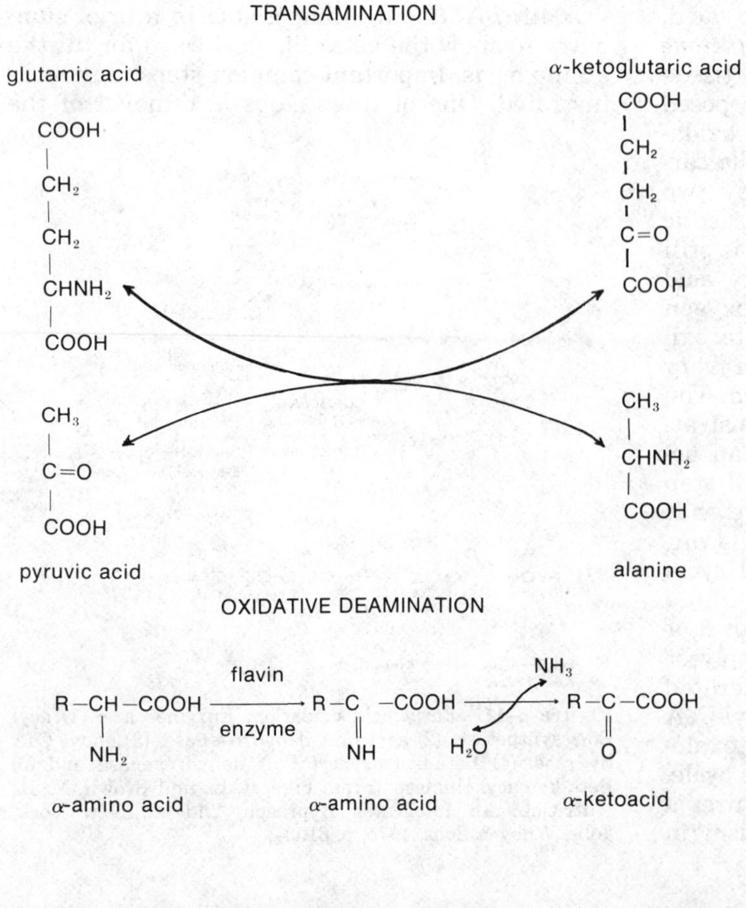

Figure 5–18. Transamination and deamination.

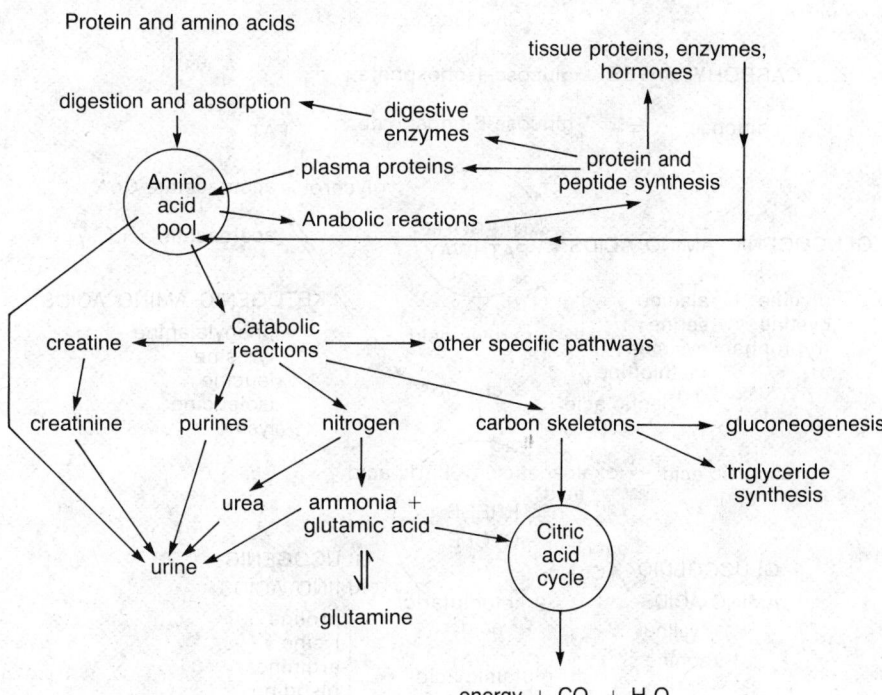

Figure 5–19. Protein and amino acid metabolism.

some of the non-essential amino acids are synthesized. It should be noted that the step from pyruvic acid to acetyl-CoA is not reversible, so fatty acids cannot be used for net gain of carbohydrate. It is by these interrelationships, and only a few of many have been shown, that the body can function smoothly under a variety of dietary and metabolic conditions.

HORMONAL CONTROL OF METABOLISM

In the presence of appropriate hormonal action, an enzyme in the plasma membrane, *adenyl cyclase*, forms *cyclic 3′:5′-AMP*, cAMP, from ATP. cAMP activates protein kinase, which can then activate other necessary enzymes within the cell, resulting in a biochemical amplification. Cellular reactions are terminated by the conversion of cyclic AMP to 5′-AMP. Thus, synthesis and catabolism of substances within the cell are controlled by enyzmes activated by intracellular cAMP concentrations, and cAMP concentrations are controlled by adenyl cyclase, which is controlled hormonally. A second method for hormonal control of enzymatic activity is enzyme induction by direct effect of hormone on transcription of enzyme synthesis.

Adenyl cyclase in particular cells is only activated by certain hormones for which that cell has hormone-binding receptors. Receptors for both adrenalin and insulin have been identified

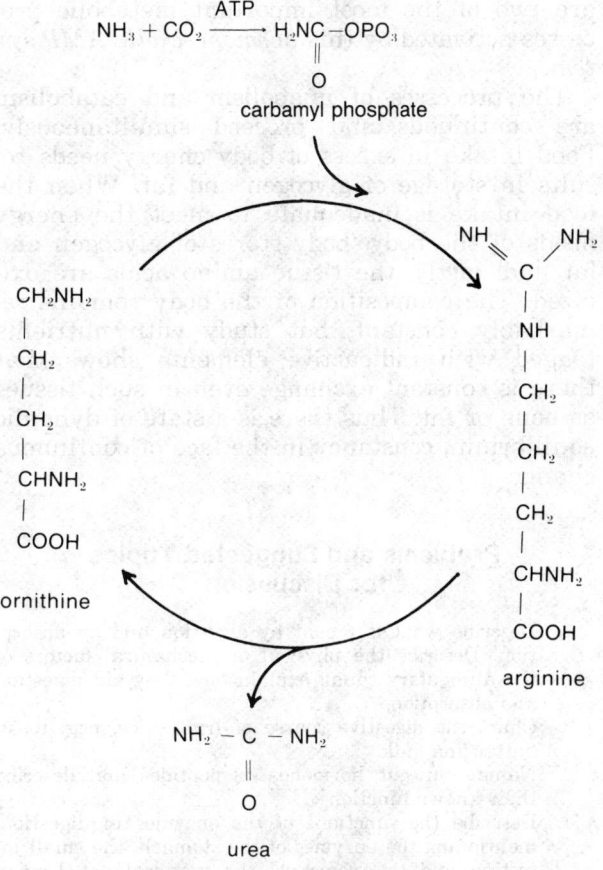

Figure 5–20. Urea formation.

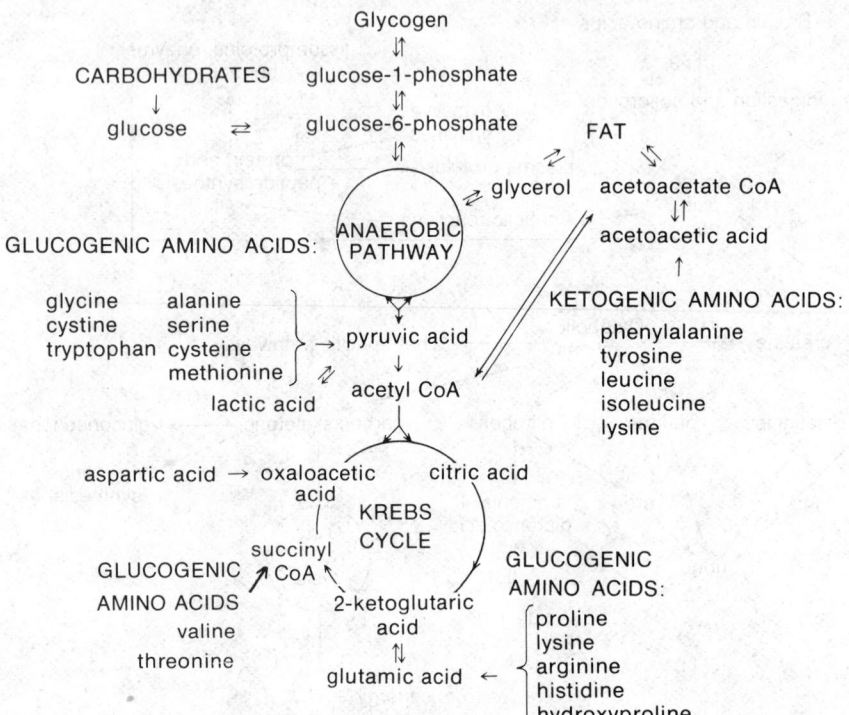

Figure 5–21. Metabolic integration of carbohydrate, fat and protein.

on adipose cells. Lipolysis and glycogenolysis are two of the most important metabolic processes activated by this *hormone–cyclic AMP system.*

The processes of anabolism and catabolism are continuous and proceed simultaneously. Food intake in excess of body energy needs results in storage of glycogen and fat. When the food intake is inadequate to meet the energy needs of the body, body stores of glycogen and fat and, lastly, the tissue amino acids are oxidized. The composition of the body remains remarkably constant, but study with nutrients tagged with radioactive elements shows that there is constant exchange even in such tissues as bone or fat. Thus there is a state of dynamic equilibrium, constancy in the face of continuous change.

Problems and Suggested Topics for Discussion

1. Describe what is meant by digestion and by absorption. Describe the physical or mechanical factors of the alimentary canal; explain how they aid digestion and absorption.
2. Chart the digestive course of fruit juice, egg, toast, butter and milk.
3. Name four gut hormones or peptides and describe their known functions.
4. Describe the functions of the enzymes in digestion, mentioning the enzymes of the stomach, the small intestine and the pancreas; the material acted upon (substrate); and the products of the action.
5. Describe the function of bile.
6. Compare the rate of digestion and absorption of carbohydrate, protein and fat. Explain.
7. Trace the catabolism of glucose through its various pathways.
8. Which substance is common to fat, carbohydrate and protein metabolism?
9. Explain where individual B vitamins function in the metabolism of carbohydrate, of protein and of fat.

Cited References

1. Adibi, S.A.: Role of small intestine in digestion of protein to amino acids and peptides for transport to portal circulation. In Winick, M. (ed.): Nutrition and Gastroenterology. Current Concepts In Nutrition, Vol. 9. New York, John Wiley & Sons, 1980.
2. Grossman, M.I.: Candidate hormones of the gut. I. Introduction. Gastroenterology, *67*:730, 1974.
3. Ingelfinger, F.J.: Gastrointestinal absorption. Nutr. Today, *2*:2, 1967.
4. Johnson, L.R.: Gastrointestinal Physiology. 2nd ed. St. Louis, C. V. Mosby, 1981.
5. Rayford, P.L., Miller, T.A., and Thompson, J.C.: Secretin, cholecystokinin and newer gastrointestinal hormones. N. Engl. J. Med. Part 1, *294*:1093, 1976; Part 2, *294*:1157, 1976.
6. Rosenweig, N.S., and Herman, R.H.: Time response of jejunal sucrase and maltase activity to a high sucrose diet in normal man. Gastroenterology, *56*:500, 1969.

Additional References

Bondy, P.K., and Rosenberg, L.E.: Metabolic Control and Disease. 8th ed. Philadelphia, W. B. Saunders Company, 1980.
Briggs, G.M., and Calloway, D.H.: Bogert's Nutrition and Physical Fitness. 10th ed. Philadelphia, Saunders College Publishing, 1979.

Davenport, H.W.: Physiology of the Digestive Tract. 5th ed. Chicago, Year Book Medical Publishers, 1982.

Drasar, B.S., and Hill, M.T.: Human Intestinal Flora. New York, Academic Press, 1975.

Floch, M.H.: Nutrition and Diet Therapy in Gastrointestinal Disease. Topics in Gastroenterology. New York, Plenum Medical Book Company, 1981.

Gangl, A., and Ockner, R.K.: Intestinal metabolism of lipids and lipoproteins. Gastroenterology, 68:167, 1975.

Grossman, M.D.: Physiologic effects of gastrointestinal hormones. Fed. Proc., 36:1930, 1977.

Guyton, A.C.: Textbook of Medical Physiology. 6th ed. Philadelphia, W. B. Saunders Company, 1981. Part XI, pp. 783–835.

Latner, A.L.: Cantarow and Trumper Clinical Biochemistry. 7th ed. Philadelphia, W. B. Saunders Company, 1975.

Lehninger, A.L.: Biochemistry. 2nd ed. New York, Worth Publishers, Inc., 1975.

Levitt, M.D.: Intestinal Gas. Warren-Teed G.I. Tract, 4(2):15, 1974.

Levitt, M.D., and Bond, J.H.: Volume, composition and source of intestinal gas. Gastroenterology, 59:921, 1970.

Liebow, C.: Enteropancreatic circulation of digestive enzymes. Science, 189:472, 1975.

Luckey, T.D.: Introduction: the villus in chemostat man. Am. J. Clin. Nutr., 27:1266, 1974.

McArdle, W.D., Katch, F.I., and Katch, V.L.: Exercise Physiology. Energy, Nutrition and Human Performance. Philadelphia, Lea & Febiger, 1981.

McGilvery, R.W.: Biochemistry—A Functional Approach. 2nd ed. Philadelphia, W. B. Saunders Company, 1979.

Pearse, A.G.E., Polak, J.M., and Bloom, S.R.: The newer gut hormones. Gastroenterology, 72:746, 1977.

Phillips, S.F.: The structure and function of the large intestine. Nutr. Today, 16(6):4, 1981.

Pike, R.L., and Brown, M.L.: Nutrition: An Integrated Approach. 2nd ed. New York, John Wiley & Sons, Inc., 1975.

Rosensweig, N.S.: Adaptive effects of dietary sugars on intestinal disaccharidase activity in man. In Sipple, H.L., and McNutt, K.W. (eds.): Sugars in Nutrition. New York, Nutrition Foundation, Inc., Academic Press, 1974.

Vander, A.J., Sherman, J.H., and Luciano, D.S.: Human Physiology: The Mechanisms of Body Function. 3rd ed. New York, McGraw-Hill Book Company, 1980.

Winick, M. (ed.): Nutrition and Gastroenterology. Current Concepts in Nutrition, Vol. 9. New York, John Wiley & Sons, 1980.

CHAPTER 6

Vitamins

DEFINITION. *Vitamins* are a group of unrelated organic compounds needed only in minute quantities in the diet but essential for specific metabolic reactions within the cell and necessary for normal growth and maintenance of health. Many act as coenzymes or a prosthetic group of enzymes responsible for promoting essential chemical reactions. They are often called "accessory food factors" in view of the fact that they do not supply calories nor contribute appreciably to body mass. Animals fed on pure mixtures of carbohydrate, fat, protein, water, and minerals fail to grow properly and thrive because, as is now known, they lack vitamins. Vitamins vary widely in chemical structure and in their body functions. Some are relatively simple, while others are quite complex. With a few exceptions the body cannot synthesize vitamins; they must be supplied in the diet or in addition to the diet. Certain vitamins (K, thiamin, folacin and B_{12}) to some extent may be formed by microorganisms in the intestinal tract, and it is known that vitamins A, choline and niacin can be formed if their precursors are supplied. Vitamin D can be synthesized in the skin upon exposure to sunlight. Considering new evidence it is becoming increasingly difficult to differentiate between hormones and those vitamins that can be partially synthesized by the body. They are somewhat similar in their organic structure and modes of action.

FUNCTION. Vitamins have different functions in various animal species. For the most part, this discussion will be restricted to the functions known for man and to the effects of deficiencies in man. Vitamins regulate metabolism, help convert fat and carbohydrate into energy, and assist in forming bones and tissues. Although a great deal is known about the vitamins, investigations continue to determine their biochemical structures and functions.

HISTORY. Vitamin investigation began with the search for the unknown accessory dietary factors that would prevent or cure the classic deficiency diseases. People have died or have lived miserable existences in poor health because of vitamin deficiencies, and the solutions to such medical riddles as pellagra, scurvy, rickets, night blindness and hemorrhagic disease of the newborn, to name a few, through the elucidation of the etiological role of vitamin deficiences in these diseases, are among the brightest chapters in medical and nutritional history.

With the possible exception of scurvy, the classic vitamin deficiency diseases have largely disappeared in the United States. They do, however, exist in a number of developing countries, through either a scarcity of food or ignorance of the basic food principles. The reader is urged to consult treatises on the development of vitamin knowledge for stimulating and interesting reading on vitamin history.[22, 46, 50]

Although history cites evidence as far back as the ancient Egyptians that indicates a knowledge of vitamins, the modern story dates back only to the close of the nineteenth century. Christiaan Eijkman in 1897 described a disease in chickens and pigeons resembling beriberi in man. He induced this disease by feeding milled rice exclusively. The symptoms could be cured by feeding the rice polishings. This recognition of the importance of other factors, besides carbohydrate, fat and protein, in promoting healthy nutrition stimulated investigations by many workers and led to the modern concept of vitamins. Today approximately 14 vitamins are known or believed to be important to human well-being, and the existence of several more has been postulated.

NOMENCLATURE. The term "vitamine," meaning a vital amine, was introduced by Casimir Funk (a Polish chemist working at the Lister Institute in London) in 1912 to designate the accessory food factors necessary to life. The final "e" has been dropped, since the chemical nature of these various substances has been proved and most of them are not amines.

The vitamins were originally named by letter or by their function. For example, vitamin B was commonly called the antineuritic or antiberiberi vitamin because it was found to be definitely useful in preventing the onset of these conditions. When it was found that the semipurified materials contained several active substances, additional letters or numerical subscripts were used to identify the newly discovered vitamins. This led to some confusion. As each vitamin was isolated in pure form and its chemical structure determined, specific names were assigned. At present the names are generally related to the chemical structure. The original names of some of the vitamins are still in use. See Table 6–1 for the current nomenclature of the original vitamins.

CLASSIFICATION. It is convenient to divide the vitamins into two groups on the basis of solubility: (1) the fat-soluble vitamins A, D, E and K, which are found in foods in association with lipids, and (2) the water-soluble vitamins, which are vitamins of the B complex and vitamin C. As more is being learned about the vitamins it is becoming apparent that the differences between these two groups concern more than just solubility. Although the modes of action of the fat-soluble vitamins are not nearly as clear as those for the water-soluble vitamins, it is evident that their activities are different from the coenzyme activities of water-soluble vitamins.

RECOMMENDED DIETARY ALLOWANCES (RDA). Much work has been done to determine requirements of vitamins for the various age groups and in circumstances of additional needs such as pregnancy and lactation. The National Research Council's Food and Nutrition Board has established desirable levels, as revised in 1980, for those vitamins whose requirements are known to be essential for health. These allowances, which are listed in Table 10–1, are intended to apply to persons whose physical activity is considered "normal" (neither sedentary nor heavy physical activity) and who are living in a temperate climate, and to provide a safety margin for each vitamin over the minimal level that will normally maintain health.

THE U.S. RDA (U.S. RECOMMENDED DAILY ALLOWANCE). There is a difference between the RDA established by the Food and Nutrition

Table 6–1. NOMENCLATURE OF THE VITAMINS*

ORIGINAL NAME	CURRENT NAME
Vitamin A (anti-infective)	Vitamin A (retinol)
Vitamin B₁ (antiberiberi, antineuritic)	Thiamin (vitamin B₁)
Vitamin G (B₂)	Riboflavin
Pellagra preventative factor	Niacin (nicotinic acid, niacinamide)
Vitamin B-complex	Vitamin B₆ (pyridoxine)
	Vitamin B₁₂ (cyanocobalamin)
	Folacin (folic acid, pteroylglutamic acid)
	Pantothenic acid
	Biotin
Vitamin C	Vitamin C (Ascorbic acid)
Vitamin D	Vitamin D (calciferol)
Vitamin E	Vitamin E (α-tocopherol)
Vitamin K	Vitamin K (menaquinone and phylloquinones)

*Only those vitamins proved to be essential to human nutrition are listed here.

Board[24] and the U.S. RDA established in 1973 by the Food and Drug Administration for the purpose of nutrition labeling of foods. In essence, the U.S. RDA represents the highest allowance of each nutrient for persons from 4 years of age through adult life, with the exception of pregnant or lactating women. For a complete explanation of the U.S. RDA and its use see page 229.

The possibility of *biochemical individuality* is being studied at present, and there is some evidence to indicate that it might exist. Applied to human nutrition and particularly to vitamin requirements, it may mean that individuals have different requirements for various nutrients.[84] However, much more research is needed on this subject before it can be put to clinical use.

With every innovation enthusiasm usually runs high, and since the early part of the twentieth century virtually all ailments have been blamed at some time on a shortage of vitamins. Under these circumstances it is not surprising that the vitamins should become imbued in the minds of many lay and professional people with far-reaching therapeutic qualities that they do not possess. However, it is also important that the nature of these substances and their highly specific role in human nutrition be appreciated.

Vitamins taken in excess of the finite amount utilized in the metabolic processes are valueless, since they will have no substrate upon which to act. Excessive water-soluble vitamins are excreted, mainly in the urine, and an excessive intake of fat-soluble vitamins will result in increased storage, having little or no beneficial effect, but rather, taken to extreme, producing actual toxicity.

VITAMIN SUPPLEMENTATION. There is no reliable evidence that vitamin supplementation increases immunity in the otherwise well-nourished individual, nor will there be that extra surge of energy so confidently expected by some when taking a multivitamin capsule. Although certain vitamin requirements may be increased by prolonged muscular exertion, the extra vitamins will be automatically provided if the exertion is counterbalanced calorically by the consumption of a reasonably mixed diet. Routine vitamin supplementation of the diet, as a prophylactic measure, is not justified, except in the case where the diet is known to be chronically poor, unbalanced or composed in large part of processed and unenriched and unfortified foods. Individuals likely to require vitamin supplementation include pregnant women, the elderly who are not eating well, and chronically ill people who take many medications or who are not able to maintain their weight by oral intake.

A vast amount of money is expended annually on vitamin concentrates that might better be used for providing health-building foods. Healthy persons who eat well-balanced meals rarely require vitamins as medication. Clinically manifested vitamin deficiencies are uncommon in this country except in alcoholics, the very poor or persons with gastrointestinal or psychological diseases. However, there possibly could be more subclinical vitamin deficiency than we realize because tests for blood and tissue levels of nutrients are not yet as sensitive as necessary.

Synthetic vs. Natural. There is no evidence for the claim of the superiority of natural vitamins over synthetic vitamins. The structure of the vitamin is the same regardless of whether it was made in a laboratory or by a plant or animal, and it performs the same functions. Although the body cannot tell the difference, the consumer can tell the difference by the price of natural vitamins, which often is twice that of the synthetic vitamins.

STANDARDIZATION. The early method of determining the vitamin potency of a food was of necessity based upon the direct measurement of its biological activity in preventing or curing certain specific pathological conditions in a predetermined experimental animal. This is known as the *bioassay* method and expresses measurement in terms of units. At present, however, amounts of all vitamins are expressed in terms of actual weight of material as determined by chemical or microbiological assay.

STABILITY. In general, the fat-soluble vitamins are fairly stable to ordinary cooking methods and are not lost in the cooking water. On the other hand, the water-soluble vitamins may be destroyed by overcooking and are easily dissolved in cooking water. A good rule to follow is to avoid long cooking at high temperature in the presence of air or under alkaline conditions, and to use as little water as is feasible. Steaming or pressure cooking of vegetables is a good method for retaining vitamins. Washing, dicing and failure to store under refrigeration are among other factors that cause loss of vitamins.

The potency of vitamins is directly related to their length of storage time.

TERMINOLOGY. *Avitaminosis* means "without vitamins" and is a term applied to severe vitamin deficiency. For example, in cases of severe or complete deficiency of B complex, the term "avitaminosis B" is used. Less severe grades of deficiency would be "deficiency of B complex." On the other hand, it is now known that excessive intake of certain vitamins can cause clinical abnormalities, characteristic of *"hypervitaminosis."*

Fat-Soluble Vitamins

Although vitamins A, D, E and K have the similar properties of being soluble in lipids and insoluble in water, they are dissimilar in many more ways. Each has a distinct physiological role.

These vitamins are absorbed along with dietary fats, and conditions interfering with fat absorption will also interfere with absorption of fat-soluble vitamins. They can be stored in the body to some extent and are not normally excreted in the urine. *Mineral oil* interferes with absorption, and if used it should be taken on rising or long enough after a meal to prevent interference with the utilization of the fat-soluble vitamins. Antibiotics and certain other drugs interfere with absorption, and these are discussed further in Chapter 21. Various disease states such as malabsorption syndromes also decrease the absorption of vitamins or increase their requirements. There are RDAs for vitamins A, D and E, but vitamin K has only a range of estimated safe and adequate daily intake.

VITAMIN A (Retinol)

HISTORY. Vitamin A was the first fat-soluble vitamin to be recognized. Two groups of research workers, McCollum and Davis at the University of Wisconsin and Osborne and Mendel at Yale University, made the discovery almost simultaneously in 1913. They found that young animals became unhealthy and failed to grow on diets lacking natural fats. They also observed that, following a lack of growth, the eyes became inflamed and infected but could be quickly relieved by the addition to the diet of a natural fat, such as butterfat or cod liver oil. These changes are illustrated in Figure 6–1. In 1924, Bloch, working in Denmark, demonstrated that *xerophthalmia* in children could be prevented by feeding them butterfat or cod liver oil.

Vegetable foods also had vitamin A activity which was found to be related to their content of carotenoids—*carotene, cryptoxanthin* and other yellow pigments frequently found in association with chlorophyll and largely responsible for the color of red and yellow vegetables. By 1932 it was found that the carotenes were precursors of vitamin A. *Beta carotene* is the most active, one molecule yielding two molecules of vitamin A, but the body is only 50 per cent efficient at this conversion. *Alpha and gamma carotenes* yield only one molecule of vitamin A, the other half of the carotene molecule being inactive. Carotene is referred to as a *provitamin*. Animals cannot synthesize it but can convert it to vitamin A. The human diet includes not only the provitamin in vegetable foods but the vitamin itself preformed, from animal foods and fish oils.

CHEMISTRY AND UTILIZATION. Vitamin A has been isolated in pure form as pale yellow crystals that are fat-soluble and has been synthesized chemically. The condensed formula, $C_{20}H_{29}OH$, indicates that it is an alcohol. It has been named *retinol* because it has a specific function in the retina of the eye. Natural vitamin A usually is found as long-chain *retinyl esters*. Metabolically active forms of the vitamin include the corresponding aldehyde and acid (*retinoic acid*). Vitamin A is rather stable to heat and light, so

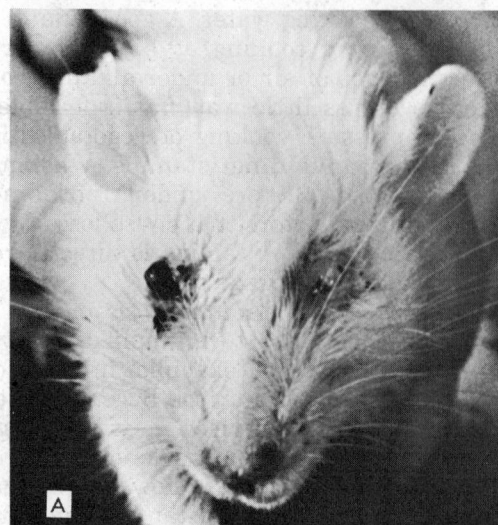
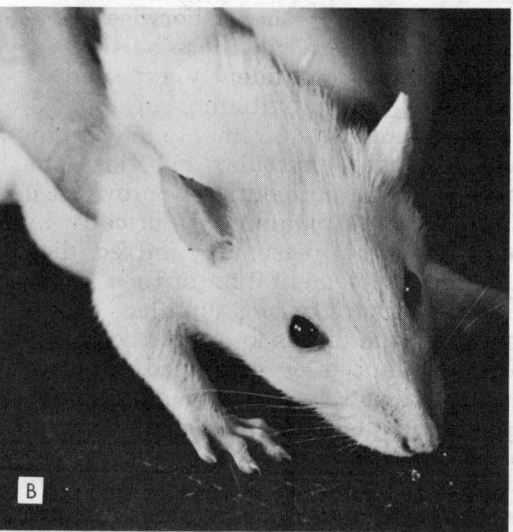

Figure 6–1. *A,* Typical eye condition produced by lack of vitamin A in the diet. *B,* Eyes restored to normal by feeding vitamin A. About 0.001 mg. of vitamin A daily will cause resumption of growth and cure symptoms of vitamin deficiency in the white rat. (Courtesy of E. R. Squibb and Sons.)

most processing and cooking cause little loss of vitamin A.

ABSORPTION, TRANSPORT, STORAGE AND EXCRETION. The dietary vitamin A esters are hydrolyzed in the lumen of the small intestine to form retinol. Retinol passes across the mucosal cell wall, where it is again esterified, and is carried as retinyl ester to the liver, where it is stored. Carotenoids are only partially absorbed as such from the intestine. Sixty to 70 per cent of the beta carotene that is absorbed is converted to retinyl esters after absorption. Twenty to 30 per cent enters the circulation as beta carotene. Both liver and intestinal mucosa have enzymes that catalyze reduction of the aldehyde to the alcohol. Since vitamin A and the carotenoids are fat-soluble, the factors that affect the absorption of fat (such as bile salts and lipases) affect their absorption. The absorption of retinoic acid is different from that of retinol or retinyl esters in that it enters the circulation via the portal system rather than through the lymphatic system.

In the blood stream vitamin A is transported with the lipids in the form of chylomicrons and lipoproteins in the lymph. It then enters the blood stream and is carried to the liver. Retinol is mobilized from the liver bound to *retinol-binding protein (RBP)*. RBP complexes with serum prealbumin. Adequate dietary protein and zinc appear to be necessary for retinal mobilization.[70] RBP transports vitamin A in the circulation and then may be removed from circulation by the kidney. Figure 6–2 gives the pathway by which dietary vitamin A reaches the target cells.

Retinoic acid is likely transported bound to serum albumin. It is rapidly metabolized and excreted in the urine and bile. The liver and kidney have the necessary enzymes to form retinoic acid from retinol.[64] The liver is considered the storage site of vitamin A, with small amounts in the fat depots, lungs, and kidneys. Through the years the liver accumulates a reserve supply which reaches its peak in adult life. Approximately 90 per cent of the vitamin A in the body is stored in the liver. This storage capacity allows for a temporarily reduced daily intake of vitamin A.

FUNCTIONS

Vision. Vitamin A is essential to the integrity of photoreception in the rod and cone cells in the retina because it is a chromophore of the visual pigments. The elucidation of the biochemical role of vitamin A in the visual system is a result largely of the investigations of Nobel Prize–winning Wald and coworkers.[81] The 11-cis isomer of vitamin A aldehyde (retinal) is combined with the protein *opsin* (rhodopsin in the rods and iodopsin in the cones). Light changes

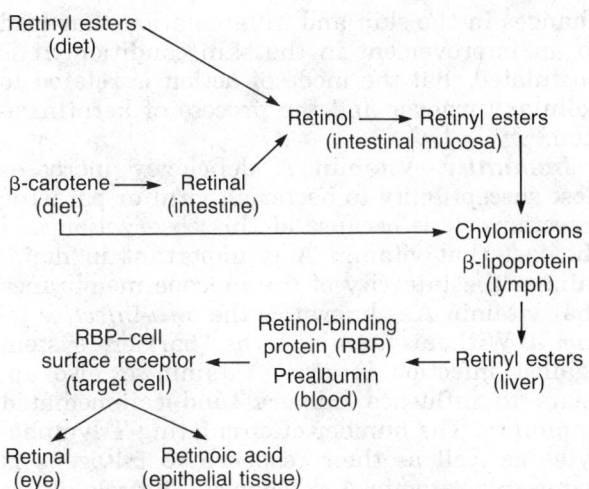

Figure 6–2. The pathway by which dietary vitamin A reaches target cells of an organ.

the 11-cis configuration to the all-trans form of the retinaldehyde. This causes visual excitation. When there is a deficiency of vitamin A the rods and cones cannot adjust to light changes. The rod cells are particularly sensitive to vitamin A deficiency, and for that reason night blindness is an early consequence when these cells are deprived of vitamin A. Night blindness or poor dark adaptation correlates with the blood retinol level. An injection of vitamin A corrects this condition within a matter of minutes.

Growth and Bone Development. Vitamin A is necessary for growth and development of skeletal and soft tissues through its effect upon protein synthesis and differentiation of the bone cells. It appears that the active metabolite in this capacity is retinoic acid and not retinol. A normal intake of vitamin A helps to provide for normal bone development. It also is necessary for enamel-forming epithelial cells in the development of teeth.

Epithelial Tissue Development and Maintenance. Retinoic acid also plays a role in the maintenance of normal epithelial structures. It is necessary in the differentiation of basal cells into mucous epithelial cells. A deficiency of this vitamin is accompanied by keratinization of the mucous membranes that line the respiratory tract, the alimentary canal and the urinary tract, and by keratinization of the body skin and epithelium of the eye, which lowers the protective barrier role played by these membranes in protection of the body against infection.

Retinoic acid applied topically is being used on a trial basis in the treatment of acne vulgaris, ichthyosis, psoriasis, keratosis and other skin disorders. It does not produce systemic effects of toxicity, but it does cause cytologic changes in the skin and inflammation that lead to an improvement in the skin condition. It is postulated that the mode of action is related to cellular turnover and the process of keratinization.[27, 44]

Immunity. Vitamin A deficiency increases host susceptibility to bacterial, viral or parasitic infections. It is because of this observation and the fact that vitamin A is important in maintaining the integrity of the mucous membranes that vitamin A is known as the *anti-infective vitamin.* Without vitamin A the "barrier" system against infection is gone. Vitamin A also appears to influence humoral and cell-mediated immunity. The number of circulating T lymphocytes as well as their response to mitogens is reduced in vitamin A deficiency. The role of nutrition in the immune response is further discussed on page 707.

Reproduction. Animal studies have shown that vitamin A intake must be increased above that required for good growth in order to assure normal reproduction and lactation. Retinol seems to be the form of the vitamin active in maintaining reproductive function. Although the role of vitamin A in reproduction is not clear, it may be an involvement in steroid hormone synthesis or a more basic role in cellular differentiation.

Anti-Cancer Function. Several studies indicate that retinoid (retinol, retinyl esters and ethers, retinoic acid and retinoic acid esters) deficiency enhances susceptibility to carcinogenesis both in experimental animals and in humans. Retinoids seem to have a role in promoting normal differentiation of epithelial cells and maintaining the controls which prevent the development of malignancy in these cells. In carcinogenesis there is a "dedifferentiation" of epithelial cells. For this reason, analogues of vitamin A or retinoids such as 13-cis retinoic acid are being used in humans to treat cancers (particularly of the skin, lungs, bladder or breast) that involve epithelial tissues. It appears that the inhibitory effects of retinoids are not the result of inhibition of the initiation of carcinogenesis, but rather the prevention of progression of premalignant disease to malignant disease. Chapter 36 further discusses the role of vitamin A in the etiology of cancer.

MEASUREMENT. The *international unit* (I.U.) of vitamin A activity was originally defined as the amount required per day to promote growth in a white rat receiving an otherwise vitamin A–free diet. This may now be expressed in chemical terms as 0.300 μg. of crystalline vitamin A alcohol. The unit for beta carotene is 0.6 μg. Thus dietary carotene has only about one half the activity of preformed vitamin A (retinol). However, because of the poorer absorption of

Table 6–2. RETINOL EQUIVALENTS

1 retinol equivalent = 1 μg. retinol
= 6 μg. β-carotene
= 12 μg. other provitamin A carotenoids
= 3.33 I.U. vitamin A activity from retinol
= 10 I.U. vitamin A activity from β-carotene

the provitamins as compared with retinol, the measurement of vitamin A activity in the diet as I.U. constantly had to be qualified as being from provitamins or retinol itself. In 1967 an FAO/WHO Expert Committee recommended that vitamin A activity be stated as an equivalent weight of retinol, *retinol equivalents* (*R.E.*), and not as I.U., which is a measure of vitamin A activity regardless of its absorption. For example, 1 retinol equivalent is equal to 1 μg. of retinol, 6 μg. of beta carotene or 12 μg. of other provitamin carotenoids, as shown in Table 6–2. The Food and Nutrition Board of the NRC/NAS adopted this recommendation and the 1980 RDA for vitamin A is stated in μg. and R.E.

RECOMMENDED DIETARY ALLOWANCE. The requirement appears to be proportional to body weight. The 1980 RDA for the adult male is 1000 R.E. (750 as retinol and 250 as beta carotene) or 5000 I.U. (half from retinol and half from beta carotene). The RDA for women is lower, 800 R.E. (4000 I.U.), to allow for smaller body size. Both are about twice that required to meet the minimal needs. During pregnancy 1000 R.E. (5000 I.U.) are recommended, and during lactation 1200 R.E. (6000 I.U.). Children need 400 to 1000 R.E. (2000 to 5000 I.U.) daily, the amount increasing from infancy to 14 years. The RDA are interpolations based on a few studies in infants, children and adults, since requirements for vitamin A have not been exactly determined for any age group.

In the United States, according to the Food and Nutrition Board, approximately 50 per cent of the vitamin A intake is in the form of the provitamin (carotene).

Data on vitamin A status from the U.S. Ten-State Nutrition Survey, 1968–70, revealed that in the low-income populations studied, there was a relatively high prevalence of low plasma vitamin A levels in children. This was most marked in the Spanish-American population.[76] Serum levels of vitamin A for healthy adults are about 30 to 65 μg. per 100 ml. (100 to 200 I.U. per 100 ml.), levels of 20 μg. per 100 ml. or less being indicative of marginal vitamin A status. Because vitamin A is stored, serum vitamin levels do not reflect recent vitamin A intake. Serum carotenoid level would more accurately

Table 6–3. VITAMIN A CONTENT OF SOME FOODS*

FOOD	I.U.
Liver, beef, 100 gm.	43,900
Carrots, raw, 1	11,000
Sweet potato, baked, 1 sm.	8,100
Spinach, cooked, ½ cup	7,300
Apricots, dried, 8 lg. halves	5,500
Squash, winter, ½ cup	4,200
Cantaloupe, ¼ melon	3,400
Broccoli, 1 stalk	2,500
Crab, 100 gm.	2,170
Peach, 1 med.	1,330
Halibut, 125 gm.	850
Egg yolk, 1	580
Milk, whole, 1 cup	370
Cheese, cheddar, 1 oz.	370
Orange, 1 med.	300
Butter, 1 tsp.	165
Margarine, fortified, 1 tsp.	165
Apple, 1 med.	140
Peanuts, raw, 100 gm.	16

*Preformed vitamin A and carotene forms.

reflect this. Since vitamin A is efficiently stored in the liver, well-nourished persons have at least a several months' supply that the body can utilize.

SOURCES. The leading dietary sources of vitamin A are listed in Table 6–3. The dietary sources of *preformed vitamin A* are chiefly liver, kidney, butter and fortified margarine, egg yolk, whole milk and cream, cheese made with whole milk or cream and fortified skim milk. The *carotene* forms are found in dark green, leafy and yellow vegetables (collards, spinach, carrots, sweet potatoes, squash) and yellow fruit (apricots, peaches, cantaloupe). The deeper the green or the yellow of a vegetable, the more carotene (provitamin A) it contains. Cod and halibut fish oils are usually sources for therapeutic doses of vitamin A.

DEFICIENCY. If the diet is inadequate in vitamin A, a primary deficiency may occur. "Secondary" or "conditioned" deficiencies occur when a bodily dysfunction interferes with the absorption, storage or transport of vitamin A, as in malabsorption due to bile acid insufficiency, protein-energy malnutrition, liver disease or abetalipoproteinemia. Studies in animals indicate that the rate of vitamin A metabolism is determined by supply; as a deficit develops, the animal slows the rate of vitamin A metabolism in an attempt to conserve the available supply.

Prolonged deficiency of vitamin A may produce skin changes, night blindness and corneal ulcerations. In extreme deficiency states, the mucous membranes of the respiratory, gastrointestinal, and genitourinary tracts may be affected.

Night Blindness (Nyctalopia). Night blindness is attributed to functional failure of the retina in the proper regeneration of rhodopsin. The ability to perceive details at low levels of illumination is related to tiny nerve endings called rods, which are found along with cones in the retina. Cones are concerned primarily with day sight and the perception of color, and the rods control night vision. Individuals afflicted with night blindness (nyctalopia) cannot see in a dim light or at twilight. Impairment of dark adaptation, the ability to adapt from a bright light or glare to darkness (encountered in night driving or on entering a dark room from a brightly lighted one), is symptomatic of vitamin A deficiency. Special photometric instruments are used in the dark adaptation test to measure vitamin A deficiency.

Xerophthalmia or Xerosis Conjunctivae. Xerophthalmia, one of the serious eye conditions caused by vitamin A deficiency, occurs rarely in the United States and is usually associated with malabsorption, chronic cachexia and weight loss from a debilitating disease such as cancer. It is more commonly found in developing countries throughout much of the world. It is associated with atrophy of the periocular glands, hyperkeratosis of the conjunctiva and, finally, involvement of the cornea, leading to softening or *keratomalacia* and blindness. Table 6–4 describes the progression of eye disease caused by vitamin A deficiency. Unfortunately it proceeds more rapidly and is most severe in very young children. It also may progress quickly to keratomalacia without the presence of *Bitot's spots* (Fig. 6–3). Avitaminosis A is reported to be the leading cause of preventable blindness in India and in Southeast Asia today. It appeared in epidemic form in Denmark during World War I, when dairy products were replaced in the diets by fats lacking vitamin A. Although most common in infants and young children, it may appear at any age.

Table 6–4. XEROPHTHALMIA OF VITAMIN A DEFICIENCY

Stage I   *Xerosis of conjunctiva* — dryness with "lack luster" appearance, thickening, wrinkling, and diffuse pigmentation of conjunctiva.

Stage II *Bitot's Spots* — usually triangular-shaped collections of desquamated keratinized epithelial cells and mucous.

Stage III *Xerosis of cornea* — dryness of cornea leading to keratinization and a hazy or milky appearance.

Stage IV *Keratomalacia* — ulceration, distortion and softening of the cornea with eventual perforation and iris prolapse and infection.

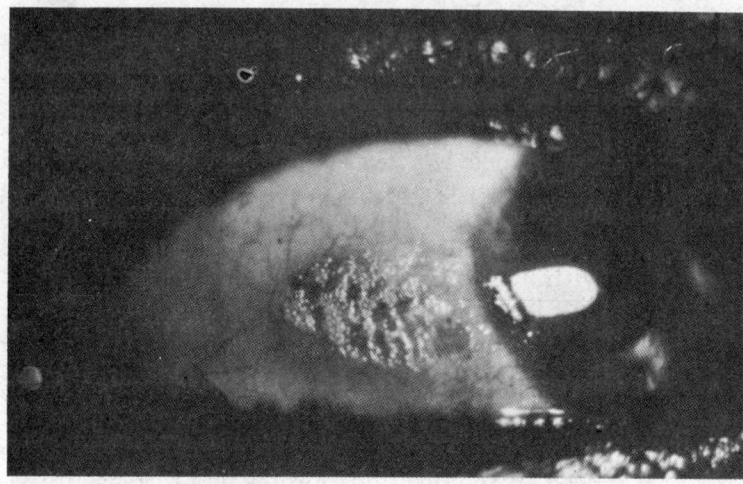

Figure 6–3. Bitot's spot. (From McLaren, D. S., and Burman, D. (eds.): Textbooks of Paediatric Nutrition. New York, Longman, © 1976 by Longman Group Ltd.)

Cutaneous Changes. Characteristic changes in the skin texture as a result of vitamin A deficiency are the "goose flesh" or "toad skin" (*follicular hyperkeratosis*) appearance as shown in Figure 6–4, or the "fish skin" or "alligator skin," known as *xeroderma*, shown in Figure 6–5. In follicular hyperkeratosis, the hair follicles are blocked with plugs of keratin from their epithelial lining. Not only is it seen with vitamin A deficiency, but also it may be caused by essential fatty acid deficiency, a vitamin B deficiency, exposure to sunlight or lack of cleanliness. The skin becomes dry, scaly and rough. At first the forearms and thighs are affected, but in advanced stages, the entire body may be involved. "Xeroderma" means dryness of the skin, and often a layer of fine, dry dandruff is seen over the skin, particularly the legs.

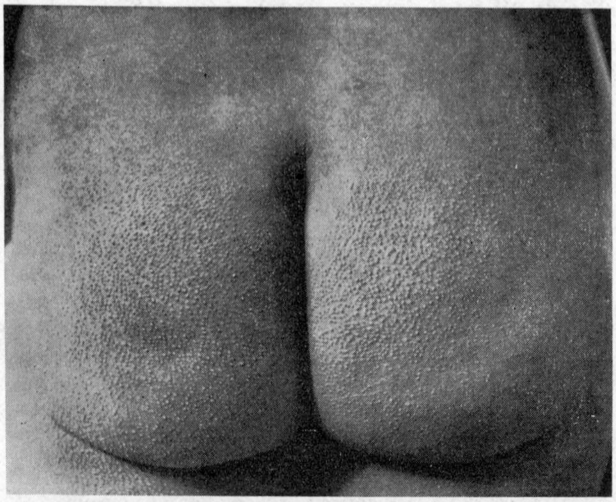

Other symptoms of vitamin A deficiency are loss of appetite, inhibited growth, skeletal abnormalities and decreased resistance to infections. Vitamin A deficiency causes keratinization of taste buds and loss of the sense of taste. This may be cause for the loss of appetite which is characteristic of deficiency.

Prevention and Treatment of Avitaminosis A. There is evidence that mild avitaminosis A, manifested by low serum vitamin A levels, does exist among the poor in this country. However, the Ten-State Nutrition Survey, which reported these findings, did not include clinical examination for night blindness. No xerosis, Bitot's spots or keratomalacia was noted.[76] Acute vitamin A deficiency is treated with large doses of vitamin A orally and correction of the usual concomitant protein-energy malnutrition. The various symptoms of vitamin A deficiency respond to diet and supplementation in about the same order as they appear. For example, night blindness, an early manifestation of vita-

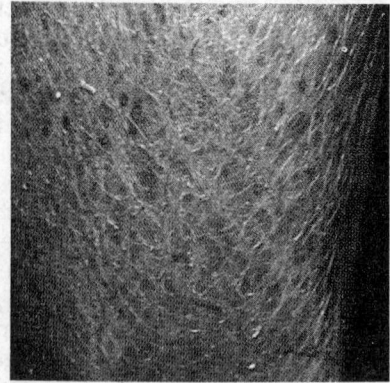

Figure 6–4. Vitamin A deficiency showing early follicular hyperkeratosis resembling "goose flesh." (Reproduced by courtesy of Section of Dermatology and Syphilology, Mayo Clinic, Rochester, Minn.)

Figure 6–5. Vitamin A deficiency showing advanced xerosis, usually called ichthyosis, resembling "fish skin." (From Jolliffe, N. (ed.): Clinical Nutrition. 2nd ed. New York, Harper & Bros., 1962.)

min A deficiency, responds very quickly. On the other hand, the skin abnormalities may take several weeks to disappear.

To prevent avitaminosis, the production and consumption of food sources of carotene and retinol must be increased in the developing countries of the world through agricultural and educational guidance. Whenever economically feasible, enrichment with vitamin A of popular foods might be considered.

India and Guatemala are considering fortifying tea and sugar, respectively, with a water-miscible form of vitamin A. In India and Bangladesh large prophylactic doses (200,000 I.U.) of retinol are given to children every six months in an attempt to avoid vitamin A deficiency and blindness. This therapy has proved to be effective because it can be incorporated into routine child health care. Since the most severe forms affect the infant and young child, special attention should be focused on infant and child feeding that provides adequate vitamin A.

TOXICITY. In individuals consuming normal doses no toxic effects are observed. *Hypervitaminosis A* has been observed in adults taking in excess of 50,000 I.U. per day for several years, or in the case of the synthetic water-soluble form, 18,500 to 60,000 I.U. for a period of months. Children taking in excess of 25,000 I.U. daily of the fat-soluble form for periods of time can develop toxic reactions.[82] Table 6–5 lists the signs of vitamin A toxicity. Drowsiness, vomiting and bulging of the fontanelle are the prominent symptoms in children receiving overdoses of vitamin A. Loss of appetite, coarsening and loss of hair, scaly skin eruptions, cracks at the corners of the mouth, irritability, double vision and skin rashes are among the symptoms of prolonged excessive intake.

Enlargement of the liver and spleen are advanced symptoms of hypervitaminosis. Portal hypertension and ascites with cirrhosis-like changes have also been reported in two adults taking over 100,000 I.U. per day for eight years.[66] Hepatotoxicity from 40,000 to 50,000 I.U. of vitamin A daily for seven years without the other signs of vitamin A toxicity has been reported in a man who also had protein malnutrition.[83] There was massive accumulation of vitamin A in the liver, but serum vitamin A and RBP were below normal, probably because of the lack of RBP synthesis.

Prolonged, severe hypervitaminosis A will result in bone fragility, thickening of the long bones, deep bone pain, and inability to walk.

If vitamin A toxicity is detected and stopped in time, the symptoms disappear in a few days after the vitamin is withdrawn, although this may take longer depending on the amount of vitamin A that has been ingested and the extent

Table 6–5. SIGNS OF VITAMIN A TOXICITY

Serum vitamin A of 250–6600 I.U./100 ml.
Bone pain and fragility
Hydrocephalus and vomiting (infants and children)
Dry, fissured skin
Brittle nails
Hair loss (alopecia)
Gingivitis
Cheilosis
Anorexia
Irritability
Fatigue
Hepatomegaly and abnormal liver function
Ascites and portal hypertension

of the liver stores of vitamin A. It is obvious that the "tolerance" to massive oral doses of vitamin A varies widely.

Hypercarotenemia, also called *hypercarotenosis*, from the ingestion of large amounts of foods containing carotene results merely in deposition of carotene in tissues, particularly the skin and eyes, and gives the person a disturbing yet harmless orange appearance. It can occur secondarily in diabetes mellitus, hypothyroidism or anorexia nervosa.

VITAMIN D (Calciferol)

HISTORY. The isolation of vitamin D was delayed because of its confusion for a time with vitamin A. Both of these vitamins are fat-soluble; hence, they occur together in nature.

Since the Middle Ages cod liver oil has been used as a remedy for rickets, but not until the period of World War I was the cause of rickets and the scientific basis for its cure established. It was next found that rickets could be counteracted by a fat-soluble factor that McCollum separated from vitamin A in 1922. In 1924 Steenbock and Hess independently and simultaneously discovered that ultraviolet irradiation gave antirachitic properties to certain foods. In 1930 vitamin D was isolated in crystalline form and named *calciferol*. In 1936 Windaus demonstrated that the natural prehormone found in the skin which becomes calciferol on ultraviolet irradiation was *7-dehydrocholesterol*. In 1968 Blunt, De Luca and Schnoes discovered that the metabolically active form of vitamin D was not calciferol but 25-hydroxycholecalciferol, which was synthesized in the body from calciferol. Since this time, more metabolites have been found and the metabolism of vitamin D has been clarified further.

ABSORPTION, TRANSPORT AND STORAGE. Vitamin D can be acquired either as *preformed vitamin D* by ingestion or by exposure to sunlight. Ingested vitamin D is absorbed with the fats from the intestine with the aid of bile. Vitamin

D from the skin is absorbed into the blood stream. Both are carried in the blood stream, bound to *vitamin D plasma binding protein* (DBP), to the liver and transformed into the active form. Storage sites of vitamin D and its active forms are liver, skin, brain, bones and probably other tissues.

METABOLISM. Vitamin D_3 is formed in the body by the *action of sunlight* (ultraviolet rays) on 7-dehydrocholesterol in the skin. Since the provitamin can be synthesized in the body and needs only sunlight as an activator, classification of the active compound as a vitamin is not strictly accurate. In fact, it might more appropriately be called a prohormone; its active metabolite is a hormone. Tracer studies indicate that vitamin D_3 (cholecalciferol) is converted in the liver by a hydroxylase to the biologically active metabolite *25-hydroxycholecalciferol* (25-OHD_3 or 25-HCC), which is five times as potent as vitamin D_3. 25-OHD_3 is also the dominant vitamin D sterol in the blood. It appears that the blood level of 25-OHD_3 is dependent on vitamin D intake or exposure to sunlight. The most active form of vitamin D_3, though, is *1,25-(OH)$_2$D$_3$ (calcitriol).* It is produced by the kidneys, which convert 25-OHD_3 to 1,25-dihydroxycholecalciferol (1,25-(OH)$_2$D$_3$). It is ten times as potent as vitamin D_3 and is the form that is presently thought to act on the intestine to increase calcium and phosphate absorption and on the bone to increase calcium and phosphate mobilization. Unlike other steroid hormones, it has a short plasma half-life (two to five hours). Figure 6–6 summarizes the metabolism of vitamin D. Several other naturally occurring vitamin D metabolites have been identified, but their roles are not defined at present.

Since calcitriol is produced by the kidney and functions elsewhere, it is considered a hormone, with the intestine and bone as its target organs. In keeping with its hormonal status, its synthesis is *feedback regulated* by the level of serum calcium and phosphorus. A low serum calcium results in increased production of 1,25-(OH)$_2$D$_3$, and a resulting hypercalcemic effect and less synthesis of 24,25-(OH)$_2$D$_3$, another metabolite found in the blood. (The function of this metabolite is not clear at present but it appears to be important in mineralization.) When the serum calcium approaches normal, the synthesis of 1,25-(OH)$_2$D$_3$ is stopped and that of 24,25-(OH)$_2$D$_3$ stimulated. It appears that parathyroid hormone, which is released in response to low serum calcium, is the mediator that stimulates the production of 1,25-OH$_2$D$_3$ by the kidney in response to a low serum calcium level. Thus it is proposed that the level of calcium in the diet affects serum calcium, which in turn affects PTH secretion, and PTH controls kidney syn-

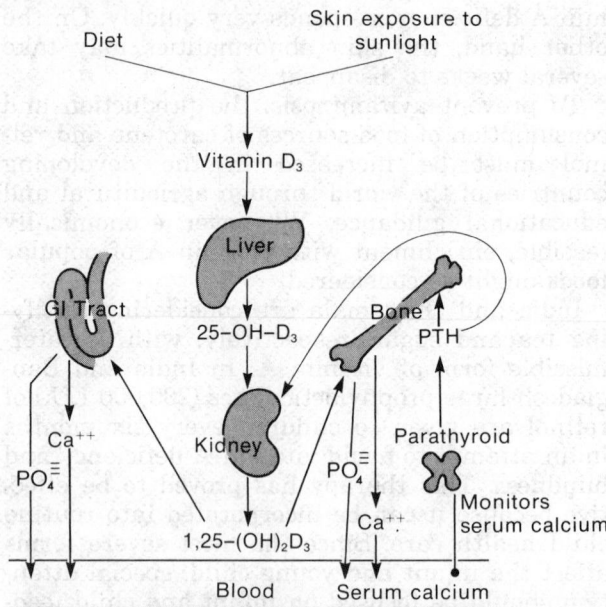

Figure 6–6. The metabolism and functions of vitamin D. Vitamin D_3 (cholecalciferol) is changed to its biologically active forms, 25-OHD_3 and 1,25-(OH)$_2$D$_3$. 1,25-(OH)$_2$D$_3$ acts on the intestine to increase calcium and phosphate absorption and on the bones to increase calcium and phosphate resorption.

thesis of 1,25-(OH)$_2$D$_3$. The intestine is then acted upon by 1,25-(OH)$_2$D$_3$, which increases absorption of calcium and acts on the bone to increase calcium mobilization. Dietary phosphate has a similar effect on 1,25-(OH)$_2$D$_3$ production, but does not require the intermediate action of parathyroid hormone. When serum phosphate is low, 1,25-(OH)$_2$D$_3$ production is stimulated and acts to stimulate the intestinal phosphate-transport system to be more efficient in absorption. It also acts to mobilize phosphate from bone.

During phases of rapid growth, pregnancy or lactation, plasma levels of 1,25-(OH)$_2$D$_3$ are elevated, presumably because of the need for large amounts of calcium for mineralization of bone.

In summary, proper calcium and phosphorus homeostasis requires functioning kidneys, liver and intestine, parathyroid hormone, calcitonin, and adequate dietary calcium, phosphorus, and vitamin D.

FUNCTIONS. The active form of vitamin D_3, 1,25-(OH)$_2$D$_3$, is essential for normal growth and development and is important for the formation of normal bones and teeth. Like other steroid hormones, 1,25-(OH)$_2$D$_3$ is localized in the nuclei of target organs through a receptor mechanism. It is thought to induce the formation of proteins that transport calcium or phosphorus. Along with parathyroid hormone and thyrocalcitonin, vitamin D has an important role in the maintenance of the appropriate serum levels of calcium and phosphorus to support normal mineralization of bone. The appropriate level of serum calcium is also important in the function of the neuromuscular system. In accordance with this overall purpose, 1,25-$(OH)_2D_3$ has the following functions:

1. It stimulates the active, energy-requiring intestinal absorption of calcium. This is through stimulation of the synthesis of *calcium-binding protein (CaBP)* in the brush border of the intestinal mucosa. Alkaline phosphatase, whose synthesis is also induced by 1,25-$(OH)_2D_3$, may also be involved.

2. It stimulates the active phosphate-transport system in the intestine.

3. In conjunction with parathyroid hormone, it acts to mobilize calcium from bone in order to maintain proper serum calcium levels.

4. It mobilizes phosphate from the bone in order to maintain serum phosphate levels.

5. In a minor way, it acts to increase the reabsorption of calcium by the kidney.

6. It increases renal tubular reabsorption of phosphate.

Other functions for vitamin D_3 are being discovered. Receptors for 1,25-$(OH)_2D_3$ have been found not only in intestinal, renal, parathyroid and skeletal tissues, but also in skin, breast, pancreas and connective tissue.[75] For example, 1,25-$(OH)_2D_3$, which is present in the beta cells of the pancreas, may have a role in insulin secretion, possibly through maintenance of serum calcium, which is important for adequate insulin secretion.[80]

MEASUREMENT. One International Unit of vitamin D is the equivalent of 0.025 μg. of cholecalciferol (D_3). For all practical purposes, the U.S.P. unit and I.U. are identical. The 1980 RDA are expressed as micrograms of cholecalciferol. One microgram of cholecalciferol equivalent is equal to 40 I.U. of vitamin D activity and 0.714 μg. of 25-$(OH)D_3$.

RECOMMENDED DIETARY ALLOWANCE. There is no established requirement for vitamin D. The 1980 RDA inclusion of an allowance for vitamin D for adults draws attention to the fact that vitamin D is required throughout life, and that dietary vitamin D is required if exposure to sunlight is inadequate. The normal adult is presumed to obtain sufficient vitamin D from exposure to sunlight and from the incidental ingestion of small amounts with food, such as fish and vitamin D fortified milk.

The need for supplemental vitamin D by vigorous adults is believed unnecessary unless they are shielded from sunlight, as in the case of persons living in smoggy sunless areas; wearing clothes that cover the body; working at night and staying indoors during the day, or being house-bound as elderly persons may be. This may be even more of a problem in people with dark skins in these situations because the heavy pigment can prevent up to 95 per cent of ultraviolet radiation from reaching the deeper layers of the skin where vitamin D is synthesized.[45] In these special cases a small daily supplement of vitamin D is believed desirable.

The Food and Nutrition Board set the daily allowance of vitamin D at 10 μg. (400 I.U.) for infants, children and adolescents who have no exposure to ultraviolet light. With cessation of bone growth, calcium needs decrease, so the RDA for the adult is set at 5 μg. or 200 I.U. of vitamin D. For women during pregnancy and lactation, adequate vitamin D is needed to promote efficient use of the increased calcium and phosphorus in the diet. An additional 5 μg. of cholecalciferol is recommended. There will be no benefit from the provision of adequate vitamin D unless the calcium and phosphorus requirements are met also.

DIETARY SOURCES. Vitamin D is found in only small and highly variable amounts in butter, cream, egg yolk and liver. The best food sources are the fish liver oils. In recent years approximately 98 per cent of all fluid milk has been fortified with vitamin D, usually 400 I.U. per quart. Most dried whole milk and evaporated milk are fortified as well as some margarines, butter, certain cereals and infant formula products. The milk used to make cheese usually is not vitamin D–fortified. Table 6–6 gives the

Table 6–6. VITAMIN D CONTENT OF UNFORTIFIED FOODS (INTERNATIONAL UNITS/100 GM. UNLESS OTHERWISE STATED)

Butter	35
Cheese	12–15
Cream	50
Egg yolk	25 I.U./average yolk
Halibut	44
Herring	
Fresh, raw	315
Canned	330
Liver	
Beef, raw	9–42
Calves, raw	0–15
Lamb, raw	17–20
Pork, raw	44–45
Chicken, raw	50–67
Mackerel	
Fresh, raw	1100
Milk	
Cow's	0.3–4 I.U./100 ml.
Human	0–10 I.U./100 ml.
Oysters	5 I.U./3–4 medium-sized
Salmon	
Fresh, raw	154–550
Canned	220–440
Sardines	
Canned	1150–1570
Shrimp	150

(From Avioli, L. V. In Improved vitamin D bone therapy. *Med. World News,* October 19, 1973, p. 34.)

vitamin D content of several foods. Vitamin D is remarkably stable, and preparations or foods containing it can be warmed or kept for long periods without its deterioration.

There are at least 11 sterols with vitamin D activity but only those called D_2 and D_3 are of practical importance. *Ergosterol*, a plant sterol, becomes ergocalciferol (D_2) when irradiated with ultraviolet light. 7-Dehydrocholesterol, found in the skin, becomes *cholecalciferol* (D_3) upon irradiation. Ergocalciferol is prepared commercially for use as a vitamin supplement. Cholecalciferol is the form synthesized in animal tissues and is the chief form in the fish oils.

Traditionally both human and unfortified cow's milk were considered to be poor sources of vitamin D, providing only 15 to 40 I.U. per liter as analyzed using the lipid fraction of milk. However, reports in the early 1970's suggested that both types of milk contained quantities of vitamin D sulfate adequate to meet the infant's need of 400 I.U. per day.[42, 77] As a consequence many clinicians recommended that nursing infants no longer needed a vitamin D supplement. However, more recent reports have not confirmed the finding of adequate quantities of vitamin D sulfate in human or bovine milk, and moreover suggest that the vitamin D sulfate has low biological activity.[30, 61] It has also been found that the main antirachitic sterol in milk is 25-OHD$_3$, which is bound to whey protein in fresh milk. Upon standing, however, it dissociates and migrates into the fat portion. This may explain the discrepancy. Although the vitamin D activity is only 25 I.U. per liter it may be as 25-OH-D$_3$, which is better utilized than vitamin D.[31] It is still recommended that nursing infants be given a vitamin D supplement, especially if the mother is expressing and storing milk before it is fed to her infant.

DEFICIENCY

Rickets. Vitamin D is needed to prevent and to cure *rickets*, a disease associated with malformation of bones due to deficient deposition of calcium phosphate (*hydroxyapatite*). In rickets the bones are not strong and rigid and cannot stand the ordinary stresses and strains expected of them, so that knock-knees, bowlegs, pigeon breast, and frontal bossing of the skull appear. If the disease is not treated, death eventually results from internal organ impairment from structural collapse.

When a deficiency of vitamin D occurs, and calcium is not well absorbed, the renal threshold for phosphate excretion is lowered and more phosphate than normal is excreted in order to maintain a balance between calcium and phosphorus in the blood. Parathyroid hormone activity increases, and this may account for skeletal and biochemical abnormalities seen in the disease.

The existence of rickets has been noted throughout the world, its frequency and severity varying in different localities. Supplementation of foods with vitamin D has almost eliminated the disease as a pediatric problem in North America. However, children with rickets still appear. Prolonged breast feeding without vitamin D supplementation or omission of fortified formula or milk from the diet of a young child can lead to rickets. It can occur in children who have a malabsorptive disease that deters the absorption of vitamin D and calcium. It also can occur in children receiving long-term anticonvulsant therapy for epilepsy. This drug–nutrient interaction is discussed further in Chapter 21.

In general, the disease has been reported to be more prevalent in the north temperate zone and less frequent in the tropical and subtropical areas, where infants and children have more opportunity to be exposed to the sun. However, rickets can occur even in sun-rich areas if the custom is total body covering that eliminates skin exposure to the sun.

Particularly vulnerable are dark-skinned children whose families are living in northern countries such as England or Scotland.[12, 72] In addition to the lack of exposure to sun, their diet often contains little natural vitamin D, since their mothers often do not use typical vitamin D–fortified products such as margarine or milk in cooking. These children respond well to vitamin D supplementation.[26] In the U.S., black children are at greater risk for vitamin D deficiency than are white children.[6, 65] The reason for this is that increased skin pigment (melanin) in black children reduces the amount of vitamin D made after an exposure to sunlight.[12]

Moderate vitamin D deficiency can easily occur in the elderly and may account for the fragility of their bones. Many elderly are housebound and do not get out of their homes and into the sunshine often enough. This is especially likely in an inner-city community in a temperate climate.

On the other hand, there are a group of cases that occur in a heterogeneous class of people in whom active rickets persists despite the administration of conventional doses of vitamin D. *Hypophosphatemic vitamin D refractory rickets* of the simple type, resulting from renal tubular dysfunction, is the most common. It may be classified as an inborn error of metabolism and is genetically determined. However, not all examples of vitamin D refractory rickets have an inherited background established. This form of rickets may develop in infancy but not infrequently appears in late childhood, or it may not appear until adult life. Currently, oral administration of massive doses of vitamin D_2 (50,000 to 500,000 I.U. per day) are used, but the treatment of choice is use of one of the active metab-

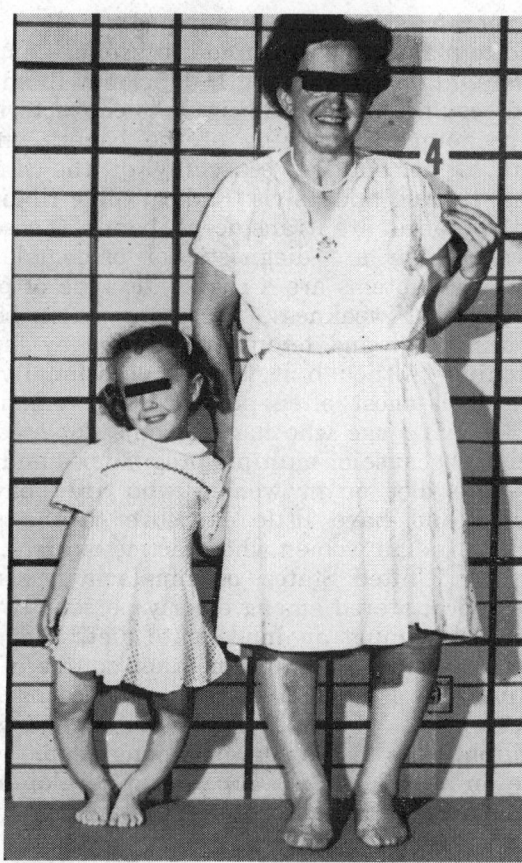

Figure 6–7. Illustration of hypophosphatemic vitamin D–refractory rickets of simple type. Mother and four-year-old daughter show typical deformities. (Courtesy of Fraser, D., and JAMA, *176*:281, 1961.)

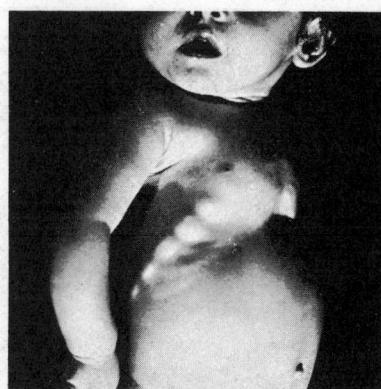

Figure 6-8. Child suffering from rickets. Note rachitic rosary and pot belly. (From Jolliffe, N. (ed.): Clincal Nutrition. 2nd ed. New York, Harper & Bros., 1962.)

olites of vitamin D_3—25-OHD_3 or 1,25 $(OH)_2D_3$ or a synthetic analogue. Use of these forms will bypass the metabolic defect that is causing the vitamin D–deficient state and rickets. Rickets is rarely completely cured and the stature remains short, as shown in Figure 6–7.

Synthetic analogues and available active metabolites of vitamin D_3 are discussed further on 622. Osteomalacia in renal disease is discussed on page 614.

SYMPTOMS. The first visible symptoms of rickets are profuse sweating and restlessness; in addition, the sleeping infant with rickets often moves his head from side to side and rubs off his hair. Contrary to the usual deficiency disease symptoms, the patient does not become thin or emaciated. Often parents will not recognize the symptoms of rickets until the child starts to walk. The legs will bow because the bones are soft and not strong enough to support the child's weight. A pot belly and beading of the ribs (the rachitic rosary), as illustrated in Figure 6–8, may pass unobserved in a plump, yet malnourished baby. If the deficiency appears during the third or fourth month of life, when the skull is growing rapidly, the structure

of the head will be larger than normal. The shape is inclined to be square, with bulging on the sides and front. Lesser defects sometimes ensue when the ailment is mild.

The softened and deformed bones cause other deformities such as pigeon chest, enlarged wrists and ankles (Figs. 6–9 and 6–10), and bowed legs or knock-knees (Fig. 6–11). The severity of the condition may be determined chemically through studies of the calcium, 25-OHD_3 and phosphorus content of the blood and clinically with roentgenograms of the bones. There may be an increase in the serum concentration of alkaline phosphatase, an enzyme released by the osteoblasts, because it cannot be used in growth owing to deficiency of calcium. Radiological evidence is a loss of metaphyseal definition.

Because teeth are made up of material similar to bone, it is believed by many authorities that vitamin D has a related effect on the development of teeth. Delayed tooth development may be a sign of subclinical rickets.

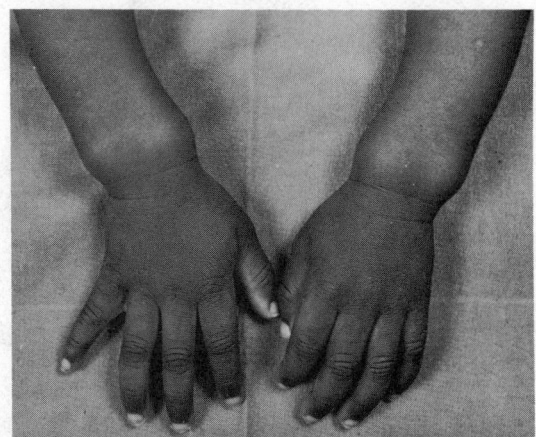

Figure 6–9. Rickets. Note the marked enlargement of wrists. (Courtesy of University of Rochester, Rochester, New York.)

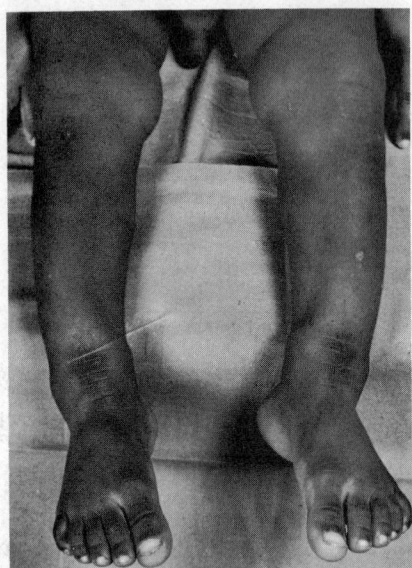

Figure 6–10. Rickets. Note the bowing and increase in width at epiphyses. (Courtesy of University of Rochester, Rochester, New York.)

PREVENTION AND DIETARY TREATMENT. To prevent rickets in the newborn baby, the importance of starting the administration of vitamin D in appropriate amounts early and continuing throughout the growth period cannot be emphasized too much. If rickets is present, massive doses of vitamin D are given. Vitamin D concentrates of the fish liver oils, such as cod liver oil, are often prescribed. One teaspoon (4 ml.) of cod liver oil contains 360 I.U. of vitamin D. Irradiated ergosterol is also an excellent source. However, mothers should be warned against the simultaneous use of several preparations, since it is possible to give too much.

The therapeutic dose of vitamin D is 25 to 125 μg (1000 to 5000 I.U.) per day, depending on the severity of the rickets. Calcium supplements should also be given in severe cases. In addition,

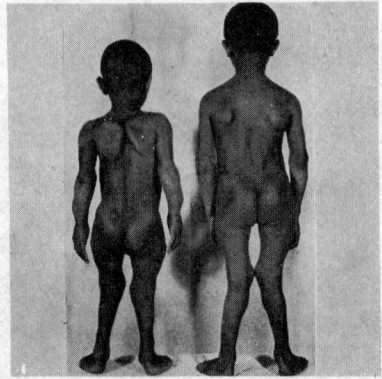

Figure 6–11. Rachitic deformities. Note knock-knees and enlarged joints. (From Jolliffe, N. (ed.): Clinical Nutrition. 2nd ed. New York, Harper & Bros., 1962.)

the mother should be encouraged to allow the child to play in the sunshine if possible.

Osteomalacia. Vitamin D deficiency in adulthood results in osteomalacia. It is characterized by pronounced softening of the bones, which leads to deformities, especially of the limbs, spine, thorax, and pelvis. Radiographic findings in the bones are translucent bands (Looser's zones), which are diagnostic of osteomalacia. Typical symptoms are a rheumatic type of pain and general weakness. There may also be a waddling gait and tetany manifested by facial twitching. Although it is seen occasionally in men, it is most often observed in women of child-bearing age who have become depleted of calcium because of multiple pregnancies and inadequate diet or in women who are heavily clothed and have little exposure to the sun (such as Indian women who practice purdah).

In the United States, osteomalacia is sometimes encountered among elderly persons living alone, consuming an inadequate diet, and getting inadequate sunshine or other source of vitamin D. It is seldom encountered among the lower classes who wear less clothing and who work outdoors in the sun, or among people who have an abundant diet. It can also develop as a consequence of malabsorption of vitamin D from chronic digestive disease.

Secondary hyperparathyroidism may accompany cases of osteomalacia. This is due to the constant hypocalcemia that induces parathyroid activity. If hyperparathyroidism is also present, the bones will also exhibit lesions of osteitis fibrosa cystica,[62] which is discussed in Chapter 33.

Osteomalacia is frequently confused with a disease having similar symptoms, osteoporosis, which is discussed on page 673. They frequently occur together.

PREVENTION AND TREATMENT. Prevention of rickets and osteomalacia is possible through the supply of adequate vitamin D, calcium and phosphorus in the diet. Vitamin D must be assured from either sunshine, ultraviolet lamp, natural food source, fortified food source, or a concentrated supplement. If osteomalacia is already present, doses of vitamin D are usually 1000 to 5000 I.U. per day unless there is evidence of malabsorption, in which case the dose should be 50,000 I.U. daily. Calcium supplements may also be necessary. The pain and weakness will usually disappear within 1 to 2 months after treatment is started.

TOXICITY. It is known that hypervitaminosis D can occur and cause pathological changes in the body when vitamin D is taken in excess. These changes, consequences of hypercalcemia, are excessive calcification of bone, and calcification of soft tissues such as the kidney (including

Table 6–7. SIGNS OF VITAMIN D TOXICITY

Excessive calcification of bone
Kidney stones
Metastatic calcification of soft tissues
  (kidney and lung)
Hypercalcemia
  Headache
  Weakness
  Nausea and vomiting
  Constipation
  Polyuria
  Polydipsia

kidney stones), lungs and even the tympanic membrane of the ear, which can result in deafness. Headache and nausea are often among the subjective findings, which are listed in Table 6–7. Infants given excessive amounts of vitamin D may suffer gastrointestinal upsets, bone fragility, retarded growth and mental retardation.

Vitamin D toxicity develops over time and there is individual variation in susceptibility to vitamin D toxicity. Toxicity should always be monitored in an individual receiving large doses of vitamin D (25 μg. or more) for an extended period of time.

Because present intake of vitamin D seems to be more than adequate for the U.S. population, it has been suggested that perhaps fortification of foods other than those already standardly fortified (milk and margarine) should be reduced or discontinued. This would apply mainly to cereal products.

VITAMIN E (Tocopherol)

HISTORY. Vitamin E was first discovered by Evans and Bishop in 1922 when they found that rats reared on a basic diet failed to reproduce until they were given a substance isolated from vegetable oils, after which they produced robust offspring. It was given the name of vitamin E or antisterility vitamin. Evans, Emerson and Emerson isolated a pure fraction from the unsaponifiable fraction of wheat germ oil in 1936, and it was chemically identified in 1938 and named tocopherol (after the Greek word *tokos*, which means offspring).

CHEMISTRY. Vitamin E activity in foods comes from four different *tocopherols* (alpha, beta, gamma, delta) and the *tocotrienols*. They are oily yellow liquids, insoluble in water but soluble in fat solvents.

They are fairly stable to heat and acids and unstable to alkalies, ultraviolet light, and oxygen. They are destroyed when in contact with rancid fats, lead, and iron. Since they are insoluble in water, there is no loss by extraction in cooking. Freezing and deep-fat frying destroy most of the tocopherol present. Esters of tocoph-

erol such as tocopherol acetate are not appreciably destroyed. The tocopherols protect vitamin A, carotene and vitamin C in foods from oxidative destruction. Their most important chemical characteristic is their antioxidant property.

ABSORPTION, TRANSPORT AND STORAGE. Vitamin E is thought to be absorbed in the same way as the other fat-soluble vitamins in the presence of bile salts and fat. An increase in linoleic acid and polyunsaturated fatty acids depresses the absorption of vitamin E by reducing micelle formation, which is necessary for vitamin E absorption.[52] Vitamin E should be ingested in larger amounts when the diet is high in polyunsaturated fat.

Plasma vitamin E is carried by the lipoproteins, so conditions that alter blood lipoprotein concentration will alter plasma tocopherol levels.

Vitamin E is stored primarily in the fatty tissues and not in the liver, unlike the other fat-soluble vitamins. The pituitary and adrenal glands have high concentrations of vitamin E.

FUNCTIONS. The function of vitamin E at the molecular level in the biological processes of the body is not fully determined.

Antioxidant Functions. Vitamin E acts *in vitro* as a lipid antioxidant. It serves to prevent the formation of peroxides from polyunsaturated fatty acids, thus preventing the oxidation of the unsaturated fats. Vitamin E also helps to enhance the activity of vitamin A by preventing its oxidation and loss of activity in the intestinal tract.

Vitamin E appears to protect cellular and subcellular membranes from deterioration caused by lipid peroxidation. It is a scavenger of free radicals that contain oxygen. When insufficient vitamin E is present, free radicals are able to catalyze lipid peroxidation of membranes and their destruction. This causes abnormal structure and function of the cell membrane, mitochondria and the lysosomes.

This ability of vitamin E to protect the membrane lipid has been related to aging, which is also characterized by cell membrane deterioration from lipid peroxidation. Vitamin E appears to control some of these processes.

A theory relating vitamin E, selenium, glutathione peroxidase, cystine and polyunsaturated fats in the cell membrane has been proposed. Selenium, which activates glutathione peroxidase, destroys peroxides after they are formed and before they can cause membrane damage. Sulfur-containing amino acids such as cystine maintain tissue glutathione levels. While adequate levels of vitamin E appear to protect the organism from excessive oxidative damage, there is no evidence that increased amounts will prevent or delay the aging process.

It has also been postulated that the antioxidant properties of vitamin E may have a protective effect for lung tissue exposed to ozone, an oxidant in smog. At present, this has only been demonstrated in rats, and more information is needed regarding its applicability to human populations.

While some authorities feel that the functions of vitamin E are only those of an antioxidant, there are others who feel that vitamin E has additional non-oxidant functions. Some of these specific functions will be discussed.

Specific Functions. Vitamin E modulates prostanoid biosynthesis. *Prostanoids* are compounds derived from polyunsaturated fatty acids and include thromboxanes, prostacyclins, leukotrienes and three series of primary prostaglandins. These compounds have profound and diverse physiological functions. For example, thromboxane A_2 (TXA$_2$) and prostacyclin (PGI$_2$) are involved in platelet aggregation and homeostasis; primary prostaglandins affect blood pressure, the reproductive process and other functions long associated with essential fatty acids. Arachidonic acid is the most common prostanoid precursor—PGI$_2$ and the thromboxanes arise from arachidonic acid.

It is not clear whether the mechanism by which vitamin E modulates prostanoid synthesis is an antioxidant mechanism. The effect of vitamin E appears to be different depending upon the tissue involved. For example, low vitamin E status decreases the production of prostaglandins by microsomes from muscle, testes, bursa and spleen, while it enhances their production by platelets during blood coagulation.

Findings from animal research suggest possibilities for the role of tocopherols in human nutrition. However, the many previous enthusiastic claims for vitamin E in relieving or preventing ischemic heart disease, thrombophlebitis, fibrocystic breast disease, rheumatic fever, muscular dystrophy, menstrual disorders, toxemias of pregnancy, spontaneous abortion, and sterility have not been substantiated. The reader is cautioned against acceptance of claims for usefulness of this vitamin (and for so many other vitamins and drugs) until long-term, controlled, and careful studies are completed.

MEASUREMENT. One milligram of d,l-alpha-tocopheryl acetate is the standard. One milligram of d,l-alpha-tocopherol, the naturally occurring form, is equal to 1.49 I.U. of vitamin E activity or 1.49 mg. d,l-alpha-tocopheryl acetate. However, this international unit for vitamin E is no longer used. Instead, the 1980 RDA is expressed as milligrams of alpha-tocopherol equivalents. One milligram of d,l-alpha-tocopherol equals one alpha-tocopherol equivalent (α-T.E.).

To calculate the total vitamin E activity of mixed diets the number of milligrams of tocopherols other than alpha-tocopherol should be multiplied by various factors given in Table 6–8. When these are added to the number of milligrams of alpha-tocopherol, the sum is the total milligrams of α-T.E. If only alpha-tocopherol in a mixed diet is reported, the value in milligrams should be multiplied by 1.2 to account for these other tocopherols present. This will give an approximation of the total vitamin E activity as milligrams of α-T.E.

RECOMMENDED DIETARY ALLOWANCE. The allowance for infants is 3 to 4 mg. α-T.E.; for children and adolescents the range is 5 to 10 mg. α-T.E.; for the adult male and female, 10 and 8 mg. α-T.E., respectively; and in pregnancy and lactation, 10 and 11 mg. α-T.E., respectively. The RDA for infants with low birth weight includes 0.5 mg. α-T.E. (0.7 I.U.) per 100 kcal. provided in formulas and at least 0.75 mg. α-T.E. (1.0 I.U.)/gm. linoleic acid plus an oral supplement of 3.3 mg. α-T.E. (5 I.U.) of water-soluble alpha-tocopherol. The requirement for vitamin E increases as the intake of polyunsaturated fatty acids (PUFA) in the diet is increased. The average daily intakes of Americans have been estimated at between 7.4 and 9.0 mg. α-T.E. and 21 gm. PUFA.[8, 10] This is equivalent to an alpha-tocopherol:PUFA ratio of approximately 0.4, which appears to be adequate.[8] A great deal more information is needed about the dietary factors that influence vitamin E requirements. As already alluded to, oxidizing agents, ozone and polyunsaturated fatty acids increase the requirement for vitamin E, whereas sulfur-containing amino acids and selenium reduce the need for this vitamin.

SOURCES. Vitamin E is the most widely available of any of the vitamins in common foodstuffs. Wheat germ oil is the richest source of the vitamin, but other cereal germs, green plants, egg yolk, milk fat, butter, meat (especially liver), nuts, and vegetable oils (soybean, corn, cottonseed) also contain it. Table 6–8 gives the alpha-tocopherol content as well as the total alpha-tocopherol equivalents of selected foods. Appendix Table 8 contains vitamin E content of additional foods.

In the customary United States diet about 64 per cent of the vitamin E intake is supplied by salad oils, margarine and shortening; about 11 per cent by fruits and vegetables; and about 7 per cent by grains and grain products. It is produced synthetically, also.

DEFICIENCY. Newborn infants have low tissue concentrations of vitamin E because there is little transfer across the placenta. A hemolytic anemia has been noted in infants, especially premature infants who have serum alpha-to-

Table 6–8. COMPARISON OF SOME REPRESENTATIVE FOODS AS SOURCES OF VITAMIN E

FOOD	TOTAL VITAMIN E*	ALPHA TOCOPHEROL	ALPHA-TOCOPHEROL EQUIVALENTS†
	mg./100 gm. Food		
Oils			
Coconut	3.58	0.35	0.78
Cod liver, commercial	21.96	21.96	21.96
Corn, refined	83.17	14.26	21.10
Cottonseed, refined	65.24	35.26	38.26
Olive	12.64	11.92	11.99
Palm, refined	35.53	18.32	21.82
Peanut, refined	25.00	11.62	12.92
Rapeseed, refined	44.81	17.65	20.35
Safflower seed, refined	38.10	34.05	34.40
Sesame seed, refined	29.07	1.38	4.07
Soybean, refined	93.74	10.99	17.43
Sunflower seed, refined	63.62	59.50	59.85
Wheat germ	254.58	149.44	183.00
Wrasse liver, non-commercial	250.67	250.67	250.67
Other Foods			
Almond, raw	24.48	23.96	24.01
Bean			
kidney, dry	2.08	tr.	0.21
soy, dry	20.43	0.85	2.03
Beef, skeletal muscle, raw	0.43	0.41	0.41
Bread, white, U.S.	1.19	0.12	0.20
Butter, U.S.	1.58	1.58	1.58
Carrot, raw	0.51	0.44	0.46
Corn, fresh	7.78	1.20	1.86
Eggs, whole large, raw	1.06	0.70	0.74
Herring, light muscle, frozen	2.00	2.00	2.00
Infant formulas			
milk-fat based, unfortified	0.04	0.03	0.03
soybean-oil based, unfortified	1.94	0.46	0.59
Margarine, soybean and cottonseed oils—stick	45.49	11.15	13.87
Milk			
cow, commercial	0.09	0.06	0.06
human	0.99	0.88	0.90
Peanut, raw	16.37	8.33	9.13
Pecan, raw	19.86	1.24	3.10
Spinach, raw	3.00	1.88	1.90
Tomato, raw	0.49	0.34	0.35
Walnut, English, raw	19.62	0.84	2.63
Wheat germ	27.56	14.07	17.38

*Total of measured tocopherols and tocotrienols, not based on activity.

†Expressed as alpha-tocopherol equivalents using the following biologic activity factors: beta-tocopherol, 0.4; gamma-tocopherol, 0.1; delta-tocopherol, 0.01; alpha-tocotrienol, 0.3, beta-tocotrienol, 0.05, gamma-tocotrienol, 0.01.

(From McLaughlin, P. J., and Weihrauch, J. L.: Vitamin E Content of Foods. J. Am. Diet. Assoc., 75:647, 1979.)

copherol levels of less than 0.5 mg./dl. It appears to be due to a relative vitamin E deficiency caused by the feeding of formulas high in polyunsaturated fatty acids and iron. Because of formula changes, it now is only rarely seen. The amount of vitamin E in human milk is apparently sufficient to meet the infant's requirement. Chapter 37 discusses this further.

A common instance of what appears to be a vitamin E deficiency is the muscle weakness, ceroid deposition in smooth muscle, creatinuria (resembling that in muscular dystrophy) and he-

molysis in patients with severe fat malabsorption syndromes caused by celiac disease, cystic fibrosis, sprue and other diseases. These patients also have low levels of vitamin E in their serum. This suggests a neurological role for vitamin E.[34] Alpha-tocopherol is also used to treat intermittent claudication (tension and pain in the legs when walking).[28]

It is well established that a deficiency of vitamin E causes a variety of symptoms in many species of animals. Some of these symptoms are fetal reabsorption, testicular atrophy, embryonic abnormalities, muscular dystrophy, anemia, myocardial degeneration, encephalomalacia and liver necrosis.

TOXICITY. Most individuals studied while taking large doses of vitamin E have not shown toxic effects.[23] This is fortunate considering the large amounts with which many people medicate themselves. However, recent evidence suggests that high levels of vitamin E may interfere with vitamin K activity in particular individuals,[18, 35] leading to an anticoagulant effect and prolonged blood clotting time. This may be particularly likely in patients receiving anticoagulants for a coronary condition,[19] or in those with vitamin K inadequacy due to liver disease. Large doses may be more toxic than known. Some of the isolated and inconsistent adverse effects from doses of 400 I.U. or greater for a period of time are hypertension, thrombophlebitis, pulmonary embolism and fatigue. Many more have been suspected.[63] In addition, doses of 600 I.U. per day have caused significant reduction of thyroid hormone and elevation of serum triglyceride levels in females.[78]

VITAMIN K

HISTORY. In 1935 Dam in Copenhagen discovered a severe hemorrhagic disease in newly hatched chickens on a ration adequate in all known vitamins and dietary essentials. When the chickens were given hog liver fat or alfalfa, normal clotting time was restored. It was suggested that the hemorrhage in chicks was due to a fall in prothrombin, a compound required for normal clotting of blood. Dam named the antihemmorrhage factor vitamin K, or "Koagulationsvitamin." In 1939 vitamin K was isolated and only a few months later it was synthesized.

CHEMICAL AND PHYSICAL PROPERTIES. There are at least three forms of vitamin K all belonging to a group of chemical compounds known as *quinones*. The naturally occurring vitamins are K_1 (*phylloquinone*), which occurs in green plants, and K_2 (*menaquinone*), which is formed as the result of bacterial action in the intestinal tract. Vitamin K_1 was isolated from alfalfa and K_2 from putrefied fish meal. Water-soluble forms of K_1 and K_2 are also available. The fat-soluble synthetic compound, *menadione* (K_3), is about twice as potent biologically as the naturally occurring vitamins K_1 and K_2 on a weight basis because it lacks the long side chain of the natural vitamin. The body must add the side chain to the menadione before it can function as vitamin K. None of the forms of vitamin K are stored in appreciable amounts.

STABILITY. Vitamin K is fairly resistant to heat, but sunlight destroys the K_1. There is no destruction in ordinary cooking methods and, since vitamin K is fat-soluble, there is no loss in cooking water. All vitamin K compounds tend to be unstable to alkali.

ABSORPTION AND TRANSPORT. The absorption of vitamin K requires bile and pancreatic juice. After absorption in the upper intestine, vitamin K is incorporated into chylomicrons and lipoproteins. From the upper intestinal tract it is carried to the liver. People with hyperlipidemia, especially hypertriglyceridemia, also have raised plasma levels of vitamin K.[69]

FUNCTION. In the liver vitamin K functions as an essential cofactor for an enzyme (carboxylase) that converts specific glutamic acid residues of precursor proteins to a new amino acid, *alpha-carboxyglutamic acid* (Gla) in the completed proteins. These proteins include the vitamin K–dependent blood clotting factors *prothrombin* (*factor II*) and *factors VII, IX and X*. Several other Gla-containing proteins are found in tissues as well. This fact leads to the speculation that vitamin K may have functions in addition to its role in blood clotting. For example a vitamin K–dependent Gla-containing protein called "osteocalcin" has been found in the bone and kidney. Since Gla is a calcium-binding amino acid, it may be that as part of "osteocalcin" it modulates calcium deposition in bone matrix.[29, 55] It is the calcium-binding action of Gla that gives prothrombin its unique place in coagulation.

The coumarin anticoagulant drugs (warfarin and dicumarol) act to prevent coagulation by antagonizing the action of vitamin K, but it is not completely clear how this is done.

The clotting mechanism, of which the final step is the conversion of *fibrinogen*, which is soluble, to *fibrin*, which is insoluble and forms the clot, is complex, as shown in Figure 6–12. The extrinsic clotting system is activated by injury and the intrinsic system is activated by platelets.

MEASUREMENT. At present there is no standard unit to measure vitamin K activity. One of the most commonly used measurements, however, is the Thayer-Doisy unit, which is equal to 1 µg. of pure vitamin K_1.

RECOMMENDED DIETARY ALLOWANCE. No specific estimate of vitamin K requirement has been made for human beings, but it is known that materials containing vitamin K activity in doses of 1 to 2 mg. will correct vitamin K deficiency in most cases. The estimated safe and adequate intake for young infants is based on 2 µg./kg. assuming no intestinal synthesis. The suggested intake for an adult is 70 to 140 µg. per day, an amount easily supplied by the diet. See Table 10–2 for an estimated safe and adequate intake for all ages.

SOURCES. Vitamin K is found in large amounts in green leafy vegetables, especially cabbage, broccoli, turnip greens and lettuce. Wheat bran, cheese, egg yolk and liver contain

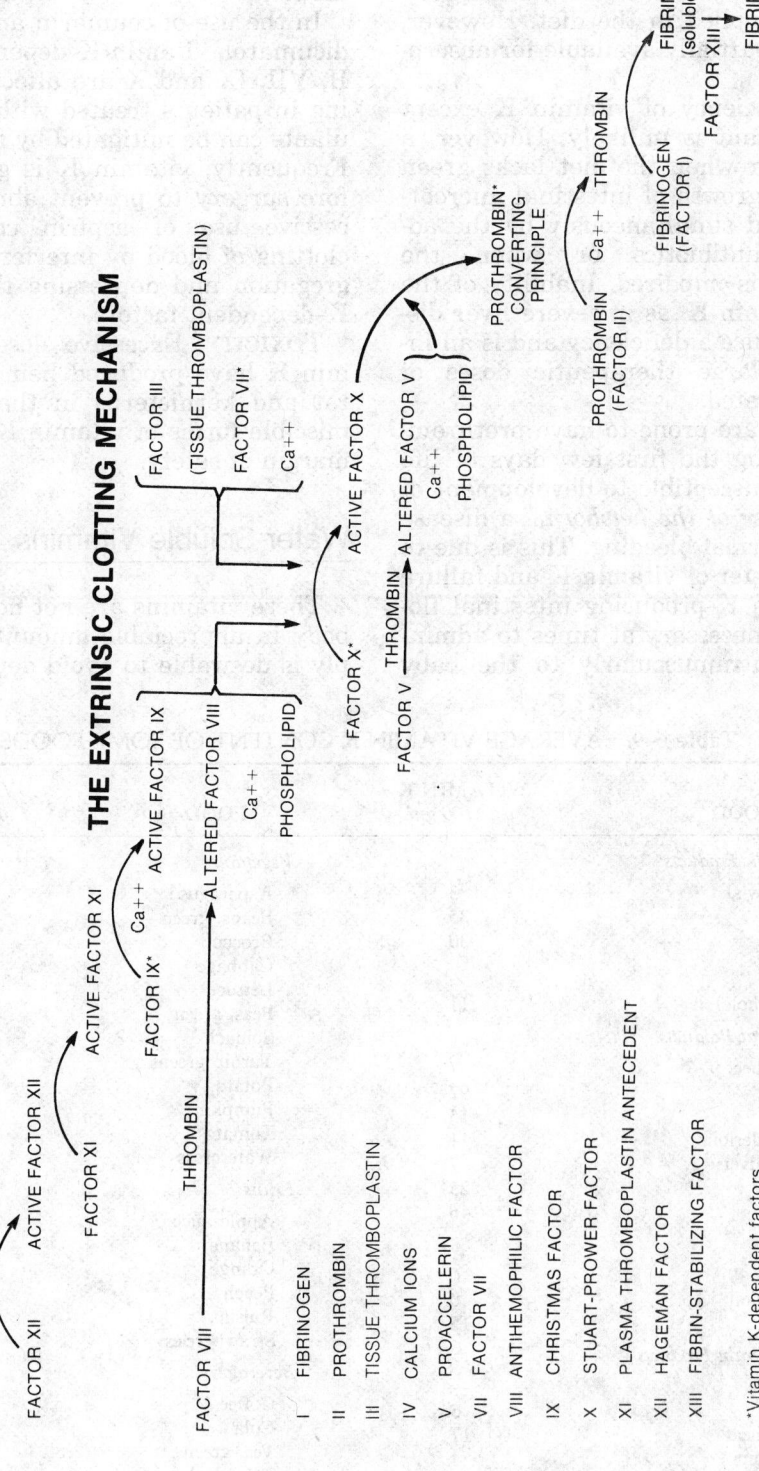

Figure 6-12. Cascade theory of blood coagulation. (Adapted from Sauberlich, H. E., Skala, J. H., and Dowdy, R. P.: Laboratory Tests for the Assessment of Nutritional Status. Cleveland, Ohio, CRC Press, 1974, p. 85.)

THE INTRINSIC CLOTTING MECHANISM

FACTOR XII → ACTIVE FACTOR XII

FACTOR XI → ACTIVE FACTOR XI

FACTOR IX* → ACTIVE FACTOR IX* Ca++

THROMBIN

FACTOR VIII → ALTERED FACTOR VIII Ca++ PHOSPHOLIPID

THE EXTRINSIC CLOTTING MECHANISM

FACTOR III (TISSUE THROMBOPLASTIN)

FACTOR VII* Ca++

→ ACTIVE FACTOR X

FACTOR X*

FACTOR V THROMBIN → ALTERED FACTOR V Ca++ PHOSPHOLIPID

→ PROTHROMBIN CONVERTING PRINCIPLE

PROTHROMBIN (FACTOR II) Ca++ THROMBIN

FIBRINOGEN (FACTOR I) → FIBRIN (soluble) FACTOR XIII → FIBRIN (insoluble)

I   FIBRINOGEN
II   PROTHROMBIN
III TISSUE THROMBOPLASTIN
IV   CALCIUM IONS
V   PROACCELERIN
VII FACTOR VII
VIII ANTIHEMOPHILIC FACTOR
IX   CHRISTMAS FACTOR
X   STUART-PROWER FACTOR
XI   PLASMA THROMBOPLASTIN ANTECEDENT
XII HAGEMAN FACTOR
XIII FIBRIN-STABILIZING FACTOR

*Vitamin K-dependent factors

117

smaller amounts. Table 6–9 lists the vitamin K content of a variety of foods. An average mixed diet provides about 300 to 500 μg. of vitamin K daily.[54] Vitamin K_2 has been shown to be formed by bacterial action of the flora of the human lower intestinal tract, so that an important supply of this vitamin may be available to the body even if it is not supplied in the diet. However, this source is only partially available for absorption.

DEFICIENCY. Deficiency of vitamin K except in the newborn infant is unlikely. However, a deficiency can occur when the diet lacks green vegetables and the growth of intestinal microorganisms is inhibited simultaneously by the administration of antibiotics or when the absorption of lipid is impaired. Inability of the liver to utilize vitamin K, as in severe liver disease, may also produce a deficiency and is an instance in which large therapeutic doses of vitamin K are indicated.

Newborn infants are prone to have prothrombin deficiency during the first few days of life and are therefore susceptible to development of *"hemorrhagic disease of the newborn,"* a disease manifested by abnormal bleeding. This is due to poor placental transfer of vitamin K and failure to establish vitamin K–producing intestinal flora. Therefore, it is necessary at times to administer vitamin K intramuscularly to the baby

upon delivery as a preventive measure against this disease. Shearer recommends vitamin K supplementation to the mother before delivery,[69] but this is controversial. Shearer substantiates this recommendation because of the low vitamin K content of breast milk of unsupplemented mothers.

In the use of coumarin anticoagulants such as dicumarol, vitamin K–dependent clotting factors II, VII, IX and X are affected. Excessive bleeding in patients treated with coumarin anticoagulants can be mitigated by the use of vitamin K. Frequently, vitamin K is given to patients before surgery to prevent abnormal bleeding. Excessive use of aspirin can prevent normal clotting of blood by interfering with platelet aggregation and depressing the levels of vitamin K–dependent factors.

TOXICITY. Excessive doses of synthetic vitamin K have produced hemolytic anemia in the rat and kernicterus in the infant. The water-miscible forms of vitamin K have a much wider margin of safety.

Water-Soluble Vitamins

These vitamins are not normally stored in the body in appreciable amounts; thus, a daily supply is desirable to avoid depletion and interrup-

Table 6–9. AVERAGE VITAMIN K CONTENT OF SOME FOODS

FOOD	VITAMIN K μg./100 gm.	FOOD	VITAMIN K μg./100 gm.
Milk & Milk Products		*Vegetables*	
Milk (cow's)	3	Asparagus	57
Cheese	35	Beans, green	14
Butter	30	Broccoli	200
Eggs		Cabbage	125
Hen's (whole)	11	Lettuce	129
		Peas, green	19
Meat & Meat Products		Spinach	89
Ground beef	7	Turnip greens	650
Beef liver	92	Potato	3
Ham	15	Pumpkin	2
Pork tenderloin	11	Tomato	5
Chicken liver	7	Watercress	57
Pork liver	25	*Fruits*	
Bacon	46	Applesauce	2
Fats		Banana	2
Corn oil	0	Orange	1
Safflower oil	0	Peach	8
Beef fat	15	Raisins	6
Cereals & Grain Products		Strawberries	—
Rice	—	*Beverages*	
Maize	5	Coffee	38
Whole wheat	17	Cola	2
Wheat flour	4	Tea, green	712
Bread	4	Tea, black	—
Oats	20		

(From Olson, R. E.: Vitamin K. In Goodhart, R. S., and Shils, M. E. (eds.): Modern Nutrition in Health and Disease. 6th ed. Philadelphia, Lea & Febiger, 1980, p. 172.)

tion of normal physiologic functions. Most of them are components of essential enzyme systems and are normally excreted in small quantities in the urine.

VITAMIN B COMPLEX

HISTORY. Originally vitamin B was recognized as the preventive factor in the disease beriberi. Today at least ten separate B vitamins have been identified and found to play important roles in nutrition.

In 1897 Eijkman, a Dutch physician in Java, observed that chickens in the prison yard showed symptoms similar to those of his beriberi patients. The chickens ate the polished-rice table scraps discarded from the prisoners' meals, developed the malady and died. Eijkman found that addition of rice bran to the rice cured and prevented the beriberi in fowls. Although the findings were wrongly interpreted and shelved for years, the work of Eijkman laid the foundation for the conduct of future experiments. It was not until about 1911 that Funk and others described vitamin B.

Since later work showed that the original vitamin B actually consisted of several necessary accessory food factors, the anti-beriberi portion was christened B_1, or thiamin, and the other parts were labeled B_2 and so forth as they were discovered. Today the members of the B complex are commonly referred to by their chemical names. Thiamin is B_1, riboflavin is B_2, pyridoxine is B_6, and there are also niacin (nicotinic acid), pantothenic acid, folacin, biotin, inositol, choline and cyanocobalamin (B_{12}).

The grouping of all these water-soluble compounds under the term "B-complex" is based upon their common source distribution, their close relationship in vegetable and animal tissues, and their intimate functional *interrelationships*.

FUNCTION. The B group, in general, plays an essential role in the metabolic processes of all living cells by serving as cofactors in the various enzyme systems involved in the oxidation of food and production of energy. They function as *coenzymes* or as a prosthetic group bound to an apoenzyme, an enzyme protein. Coenzymes and prosthetic groups function similarly, since both contain one of the active sites of the enzyme complex to which the substrate molecule is attached. There exists such a close interrelationship among the B vitamins that an inadequate intake of one may impair the utilization of others. Therefore, single discrete deficiencies of the B group are seldom seen clinically, although the signs and symptoms of deficiency of a particular member of the group may predominate. Furthermore, the use of a single member of the group therapeutically may create a vitamin imbalance and precipitate deficiency of other members of the group. Thus, therapy with vitamin B should generally consist of therapy with all vitamin B complex members rather than with any single substance of the group. Dry yeast is the richest natural source of the B complex.

Thiamin (Vitamin B₁)

HISTORY. Thiamin has been known as the antineuritic vitamin because it is needed for normal functioning of the nervous system. Its deficiency in animals causes hindquarter paralysis. The symptom recognized by Eijkman in chickens and pigeons, and the beriberi described by workers in the Orient, was found to be concerned with the B_1 or thiamin fraction of the original B vitamin. In 1926 Jansen and Donath isolated thiamin in crystalline form, and in 1936 R. R. Williams accomplished the synthesis and determined the chemical formula. The vitamin was named thiamin to designate the presence of sulfur and an amino group in the complex molecule.

CHEMICAL CHARACTERISTICS AND STABILITY. Pure thiamin hydrochloride has been isolated and is a crystalline yellowish white powder with a salty, nutlike taste, and is water-soluble. The dry vitamin is fairly stable, but solutions of it are unstable in the presence of heat or alkali. It is heat stable in acid solution. Loss of the vitamin in cooking is extremely variable, depending on the pH of the food, time, temperature, quantity of water used and discarded, and whether the water is chlorinated.[86] Freezing has little or no effect on the thiamin content of foods. *Thiaminase* present in uncooked freshwater fish and shellfish destroys approximately 50 per cent of the thiamin. Tea also contains an antithiamin factor (ATF).

ABSORPTION, SYNTHESIS AND STORAGE. Thiamin is absorbed readily in the acid medium of the proximal duodenum and to some extent in the lower duodenum. The maximum amount that can be absorbed is 5 mg. per day and any taken in excess of this will be excreted in the feces. When lumen concentration of the vitamin is low, an active, possibly sodium-dependent process of absorption operates, and when lumen concentrations are high, a passive diffusion takes place. Thiamin is phosphorylated in the mucosal cell to *thiamin phosphate*, and in this form is carried to the liver by the portal circulation. It is not stored in any great quantity in the body and must, therefore, be supplied daily. The vitamin can be synthesized by microorganisms in the intestinal tract of animals and man, but the amount available to the human body to supplement the dietary supply seems to be small. Thiamin is excreted in the urine in amounts that reflect the intake and the amount stored.

FUNCTIONS. Thiamin is necessary throughout life for tissue respiration. It combines with phosphorus to form the coenzyme *thiamin pyrophosphate* (TPP), which functions as a cocarboxylase. TPP is required for the oxidative decarboxylation of pyruvate to form active acetate and then acetyl coenzyme A, the central compound of the Krebs cycle. TPP is required for the oxidative decarboxylation of other alpha-keto acids such as alpha-ketoglutaric acid and the 2-keto-carboxylates derived from amino acids methionine, threonine, leucine, isoleucine and valine. TPP is also the coenzyme for the transketolase reaction, which functions in the pentose phosphate shunt, an alternate pathway for glucose oxidation. This cycle provides pentose phosphate for nucleotide synthesis and reduced NADP for various synthetic pathways such as fatty acid synthesis.

TPP has a specific role in neurophysiology separate from its coenzyme function. It appears to function at the nerve cell membrane to allow displacement so that sodium ions can freely cross the membrane.[59]

Thiamin is needed for the metabolism of carbohydrates, fats and proteins. However, all the evidence from the effects of thiamin deficiency link it with disturbance of carbohydrate metabolism, especially in the brain. The thiamin requirement is linked to carbohydrate intake. This indicates that the decarboxylation of pyruvate, which is concerned only with carbohydrate metabolism, is the one which suffers first during thiamin inadequacy.

RECOMMENDED DIETARY ALLOWANCE. Many factors influence the thiamin needs of an individual. Among these are body weight, energy intake, and the small amount synthesized in the intestinal tract. The amount of thiamin required is related to the amount of carbohydrate in the diet. Liberal amounts of fat in the diet exert a thiamin "sparing" effect, and such a diet will require less thiamin than will a high carbohydrate diet of the same caloric value. The Food and Nutrition Board recommends 0.5 mg. per 1000 kcal. for all ages (see Table 10–1). This allows for a margin of safety. A thiamin intake of 1.0 mg. per day is recommended for older adults even though they consume less than 2000 kcal. daily because it is believed that older persons use thiamin less efficiently. A minimum of 1 mg. per day is also recommended when energy intakes are restricted. This will maintain body stores. The allowance for pregnancy is 0.6 mg. per 1000 kcal., or about an additional 0.4 mg. per day. Recommended intake during lactation is 0.6 mg. per 1000 kcal., amounting to an additional 0.5 mg. per day. The allowance should be increased under certain conditions, such as hyperthyroidism, infections, and excessive exercise.

Findings from the Ten-State Nutrition Survey, 1968–70, revealed adequate thiamin nutriture among the population studied.[76]

SOURCES. Thiamin is found in a large variety of animal and vegetable materials but in abundance in only a few foods. Lean pork, fresh and cured, and wheat germ are outstanding sources. Liver and all organ meats, liver sausage, lean meats, poultry, egg yolk, fish, dry beans and peas, soybeans, peanuts and whole grain and enriched breads and cereals are excellent sources. Milk and milk products, fruit and vegetables are not rich in thiamin, but when consumed in sufficient quantities they contribute significantly to the day's total intake of thiamin. Appendix Table 1 gives the thiamin content of foods.

DEFICIENCY. Clinical signs of thiamin deficiency in adults primarily involve the nervous and cardiovascular systems. Animals and humans with mild deficiencies may show mental confusion, muscular weakness, peripheral paralysis, calf muscle tenderness, muscle fatigue, emotional instability, depression, irritability, loss of appetite, loss of interest in daily tasks, and general lethargy. Thiamin status of an individual is assessed by measuring the urinary excretion of thiamin or the erythrocyte transketolase–TPP effect (ratio).

Beriberi. Prolonged severe thiamin deficiency causes beriberi, a disease formerly quite common in the Orient owing to the high consumption of *milled* rice and foods with antithiamin factors (ATF) (see page 119).

CLASSIFICATION. Beriberi is classified into several types. The *acute, mixed type* of beriberi is characterized by nervous and cardiac symptoms producing neuritis and heart failure. There are two other types, namely, the "dry" and the "wet" beriberi. In the *"dry" type* of the disease the nervous manifestations, with loss of function or paralysis of the lower extremities, as shown in Figure 6–13, are predominant; hence the term *polyneuritis* is synonymous. In the *"wet" type* the edema of heart failure is the most striking sign. The edema is due to biventricular heart failure with pulmonary congestion. Pyruvate, which is an important fuel for oxidation in cardiac muscle, cannot be decarboxylated and oxidized in the citric acid cycle because of thiamin deficiency, so heart failure results. Indefinite digestive disorders and emaciation are additional symptoms. Table 6–10 lists the clinical features of beriberi.

A large number of diseases may have symptoms resembling those of beriberi, so the diagno-

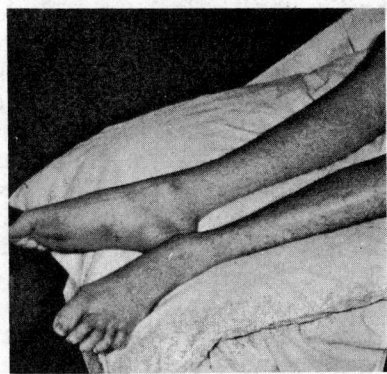

Figure 6–13. Advanced polyneuropathy with muscle atrophy and foot and toe drop in a patient with dry beriberi. (From Jolliffe, N. (ed.): Clinical Nutrition. 2nd ed. New York, Harper & Bros., 1962.)

Table 6–10. CLINICAL FEATURES OF THIAMIN DEFICIENCY

Early stage of deficiency:	Anorexia Indigestion Constipation Malaise Heaviness and weakness of legs Calf muscle tenderness "Pins and needles" and numbness in legs Anesthesia of skin, particularly at the tibia Increased pulse rate and palpitations
Wet beriberi:	Edema of legs, face, trunk and serous cavities Tense calf muscles Fast pulse Distended neck veins High blood pressure Decreased urine volume
Dry beriberi:	Worsening of polyneuritis of early stage Difficulty walking Wernicke-Korsakoff syndrome: encephalopathy may occur —loss of immediate memory —disorientation —nystagmus (jerky movements of eyes) —ataxia (staggering gait)
Infantile beriberi (2–5 months of age):	Acute —decreased urine output —excessive crying; thin and plaintive whining —cardiac failure Chronic —constipation and vomiting —fretfulness —soft, toneless muscles —pallor of skin with cyanosis

sis of beriberi should be confirmed by the erythrocyte transketolase activity test.

INCIDENCE. Beriberi occurs primarily among population groups that subsist on a diet of highly polished rice. In the United States it occurs most commonly in alcoholics because of poor intakes, decreased absorption, and phosphorylation defects. It is related to the *Wernicke-Korsakoff syndrome*, which is described in Table 6–10. Infantile beriberi occurs in breast-fed infants of mothers who have the disease. Since foods, especially rice, have been enriched with thiamin, and milling practices have been used that remove less of the bran, the incidence of beriberi has fallen dramatically. Although beriberi is rare in the United States, mild and borderline cases of thiamin deficiency are not uncommon.

TREATMENT AND PREVENTION. Thiamin as either thiamin hydrochloride or a derivative such as thiamin propyl disulfide (TPD) is used to treat beriberi. The effect of treatment in wet beriberi is rapid, with easier breathing, slower pulse rate and diuresis within a few hours of thiamin administration. A daily oral dose of 10 mg. should be continued until return to complete health. The recovery in dry beriberi is not as rapid. Infantile beriberi is treated by giving thiamin to the lactating mother and the infant.

Since most patients suffer from multiple deficiencies, frequently the B-complex concentrate is prescribed. If the damage to the nervous system is not too great, the response to treatment is usually good. In cases where acute heart failure has developed, the outlook is grave.

Education to prevent deficiencies is of primary importance. In Burma, Thailand and Vietnam, beriberi became prevalent after gasoline-driven mills began to be used in processing rice. This removed much more of the thiamin-containing rice bran than had been lost with the traditional method of manually pounding the grain. Rice is still being highly polished by the machines, but more thiamin is being consumed in other foods as these countries become more developed. In addition, manufacturers of cereals and millers of flour are restoring vitamins to their products, thereby enriching cereals and flours to normal potency. In Japan and the Philippines beriberi has practically disappeared as a result of the prophylactic use of thiamin and the enrichment of rice.

TOXICITY. There are no known toxic effects from thiamin.

Riboflavin (Vitamin B₂)

HISTORY. The existence of a yellow-green fluorescent pigment in milk whey was recognized in 1879. The biological significance of this pigment was not understood until 1932 when a group of German workers isolated "Warburg's yellow enzyme" from yeast and demonstrated that the material was necessary for activity of an intracellular respiratory enzyme. Almost simultaneously other investigators were studying a food factor that aided growth of laboratory animals. In 1933 Kuhn and coworkers isolated the pigment from milk. They noted, however, that it did not have all the activities ascribed to vitamin B_2. The compound was synthesized in 1935 by Kuhn and coworkers and given the name *riboflavin*. Later investigations differentiated it from the pellagra-preventive factor with which it had first been confused.

CHEMICAL CHARACTERISTICS AND STABILITY. Riboflavin belongs to a group of yellow fluorescent pigments called flavins. The flavin ring is attached to an alcohol related to ribose. It has been synthesized and in pure state appears as yellow crystals. It is stable to heat, oxidation, and acid; it is sparingly soluble in water but disintegrates in the presence of alkali or light, especially ultraviolet. Owing to its heat stability and limited water solubility, very little is lost in the cooking and processing of foods. However, because it is sensitive to alkali, the addition of baking soda to soften dried peas or beans for faster cooking destroys much of their riboflavin content.

It has been demonstrated that bottled milk left outside in sunlight will lose a significant amount of riboflavin. Milk in paper containers is protected against such losses. Sun drying of fruits and vegetables as practiced in some countries can also cause considerable destruction of the riboflavin content.

ABSORPTION, TRANSPORT AND EXCRETION. Riboflavin is easily absorbed through the walls of the proximal small intestine, where there is a specialized riboflavin transport process. The absorption of riboflavin is increased by the presence of food in the gastrointestinal tract. Only 15 per cent of the vitamin is absorbed when taken alone, and 60 per cent of a 30 mg. dose is absorbed when taken with food.[38] A decreased gastrointestinal transit time when food is present allows for greater absorption. It is phosphorylated to *flavin mononucleotide* (FMN), and then carried by the blood to the tissues of the body and excreted in the urine. The amount excreted depends upon the intake and relative need of the tissues. Loss of riboflavin accompanies a loss of protein from the body. Although small amounts of riboflavin are found in the liver and kidney, it is not stored to any great degree in the body and must therefore be supplied in the diet regularly.

FUNCTIONS. Riboflavin combines in the tissues with phosphoric acid to become part of the structure of two flavin coenzymes, FMN and *flavin adenine dinucleotide* (*FAD*). These coenzymes are the prosthetic group of the *flavoprotein* enzymes, which catalyze oxidation–reduction reactions in the cells and function as hydrogen carriers in the mitochondrial electron transport system. They are coenzymes of the dehydrogenases, which catalyze the first step in oxidation of several intermediates in glucose metabolism and of fatty acids. They are also active in oxidation deamination of amino acids. Riboflavin also is involved in the activation of vitamin B_6 and the conversion of folic acid to its coenzymes.

Riboflavin is present in free form in the retina in large amounts, but its function there is still not clear. Riboflavin is essential for growth and is thought to have multiple functions in production of corticosteroids, formation of red blood cells, gluconeogenesis and thyroid enzyme regulating activity.

RECOMMENDED DIETARY ALLOWANCE. The riboflavin requirements of the human, according to the 1980 RDA, are related to energy intake. The recommended amount for people of all ages is 0.6 mg./1000 kcal. See Table 10–1 for exact amounts. During pregnancy an increase of 0.3 mg. per day and for lactation an additional daily intake of 0.5 mg. are recommended. Possibly there is an increased requirement for riboflavin during use of oral contraceptives.[1, 60]

Adequacy of riboflavin is determined by urinary excretion of riboflavin. According to the Ten-State Nutrition Survey, 21.9 per cent of all blacks tested had riboflavin excretion levels suggestive of deficient or low riboflavin intake. Deficient or low intake was much less prevalent in other groups.[76] Perhaps these findings will direct more attention to possible riboflavin deficiency, which is usually ignored because it is rarely incapacitating.

SOURCES. Riboflavin is widely distributed in foods but in small amounts. The best daily sources in average servings are milk (fresh, canned or dried), cheddar cheese and cottage cheese. Organ meats (liver, heart, kidney, liverwurst) contain appreciable amounts of riboflavin, and other lean meats, eggs and green leafy vegetables are important sources in the amounts usually consumed. Breads and cereals enriched with riboflavin provide lesser amounts of riboflavin but contribute appreciably to the total daily intake. Appendix Table 1 gives the riboflavin content of foods. There is some synthesis of riboflavin by gut microorganisms but not in appreciable amounts.

DEFICIENCY. Early symptoms of riboflavin deficiency are soreness and burning of lips, mouth and tongue; photophobia; lacrimation; burning and itching of eyes; and loss of visual acuity. Severe riboflavin deficiency or ariboflavinosis is usually found in individuals who consume a marginal diet devoid of animal protein sources

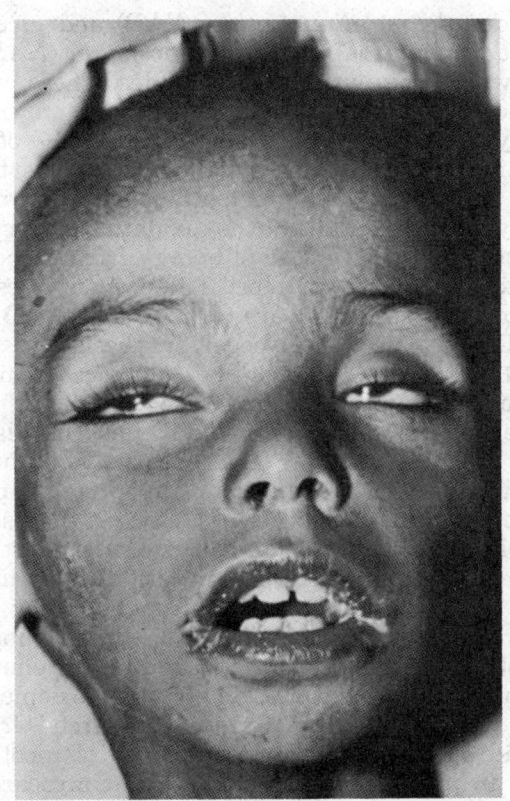

Figure 6–14. Angular stomatitis and cheiloses. (From McLaren, D.S., et al.: Vitamin deficiency. In McLaren, D.S., and Burman, D.: Textbook of Paediatric Nutrition. New York, Longman. ©1976 by Longman Group Ltd.)

and leafy vegetables. The intake of riboflavin must be low for several months for signs of deficiency to develop. It is characterized by the development of *cheilosis* (fissuring of the lips), *angular stomatitis* (Fig. 6–14) (cracks in the skin at the corners of the mouth), a greasy eruption of the skin in the nasolabial folds, scrotum or vulva (Fig. 6–15), a purplish swollen tongue and capillary overgrowth around the cornea of the eye. Table 6–11 summarizes signs of possible riboflavin deficiency.

The angular stomatitis of ariboflavinosis can easily be mistaken for the effects of ill-fitting dentures, and poor hygiene may cause dyssebacea of the nasolabial folds similar to that seen in riboflavin deficiency. Since riboflavin deficiency rarely appears alone, but is usually in the presence of multiple nutritional deficiencies, and because its symptoms are not specific for riboflavin deficiency alone, its diagnosis is difficult. Similar symptoms are characteristic of niacin, iron and pyridoxine deficiencies. A history of a dietary intake of less than 0.6 mg. of riboflavin per day for several months also helps to confirm the diagnosis of ariboflavinosis. Urinary excretion of riboflavin metabolites as well as measurement of *erythrocyte glutathione reductase activity* before and after addition of

FAD is used to assess riboflavin status, as explained in Chapter 9. A urinary excretion of less than 27 μg. of riboflavin per gm. of creatinine is also suggestive of deficiency.

Supplements of the crystalline riboflavin in oral doses of 5 mg. two or three times per day, as well as other B-complex factors, are often prescribed, especially if the underlying cause of the deficiency is faulty utilization or poor absorption of the vitamin. The lesions respond rapidly and heal within a few days or weeks.

PREVENTION. In many developing countries, conditions do not permit use of dairy products and meat. For such areas, an effective remedial step for increasing the riboflavin intake is the enrichment of the basic grain of the country—rice, wheat or corn.

TOXICITY. There is no known toxicity for riboflavin.

Niacin (Nicotinic Acid)

HISTORY. It has been known for several centuries that pellagra occurred mainly where people used corn as a staple of the diet. It was described by Casál of Spain early in the 18th century and the disease was common in Italy at about the same time. Pellagra was described first in United States in the early 1900's. The United States Bureau of Public Health selected

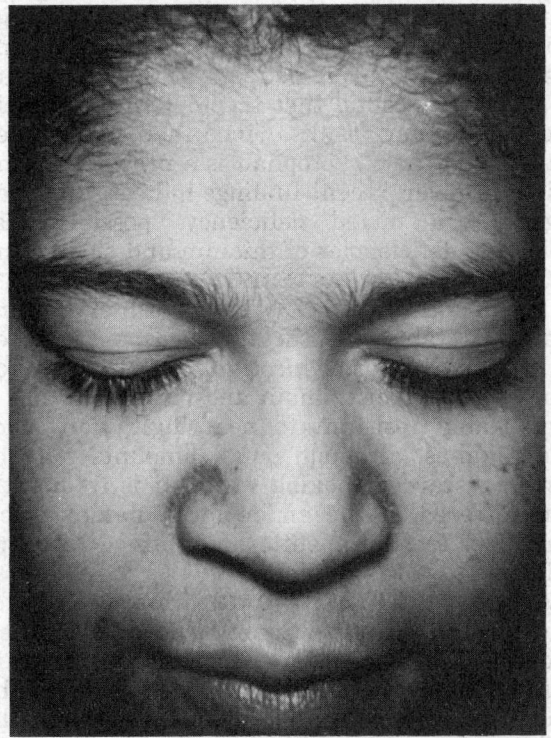

Figure 6–15. Riboflavin deficiency. Seborrheic dermatitis of nasolabial folds. (From Rivlin, R. S. (ed.): Riboflavin. New York, Plenum Press, 1975.)

Table 6–11. SIGNS OF POSSIBLE RIBOFLAVIN
DEFICIENCY

Soreness and burning of lips, mouth and tongue*
Cheilosis*
Angular stomatitis*
Glossitis*
Seborrheic dermatitis of nasolabial folds, vestibule
    of nose, and sometimes the ears and eyelids,
    scrotum and vulva
Ocular pathology (sometimes)
    —inflammation of conjunctiva
    —superficial vascularization of cornea
    —ulcerations of cornea
    —photophobia
Anemia—normocytic and normochromic
Neuropathy
Purplish or magenta tongue*
Hypertrophy or atrophy of tongue papillae*

*Tongue and mouth changes are difficult to differentiate
from those in niacin, folic acid, thiamin, vitamin B_6 or
vitamin B_{12} deficiency.
(Adapted from Goldsmith, G. A.: Riboflavin deficiency.
In Rivlin, R. S. (ed.): Riboflavin. New York, Plenum
Press, 1975.)

Joseph Goldberger to investigate the problem of
pellagra that was rampant in the southern
states. The condition based on evidence was related to a poor diet (high in cornmeal) as the
cause. A diet of good quality protein foods prevented pellagra. Following the discovery in 1937
by Elvehjem that the disease blacktongue in
dogs is due to a niacin deficiency, human pellagra was recognized by Spies and others as a niacin deficiency condition. In 1945 Krehl and
associates, in treating pellagra at the University
of Wisconsin, found that tryptophan and niacin
produce similar results. Since then it has been
established that tryptophan is a precursor of niacin. However, recent findings indicate that pellagra is a mixed deficiency, possibly also
involving deficiencies of thiamin and riboflavin.

CHEMICAL CHARACTERISTICS AND STABILITY.
Niacin, or *nicotinic acid*, is a whitish crystalline
material, stable when dry. It is easily converted
to the active form *nicotinamide*. It is much
more stable than thiamin and riboflavin, and is
remarkably resistant to heat, light, air, acids
and alkalies, although small amounts may be
lost in discarded cooking water. It is frequently
administered in the amide form, namely nicotinamide, for therapeutic doses, since nicotinic
acid acts as a vasodilator.

ABSORPTION AND STORAGE. Absorption takes
place in the intestine. Some forms of niacin, especially that in cereals, are bound and unavailable for absorption. Little storage occurs in the
body, and any excess is eliminated through the
urine.

FUNCTIONS. Nicotinamide functions in the
body as a component of the coenzymes *nicotin-*

amide adenine dinucleotide (*NAD*) and *nicotinamide adenine dinucleotide phosphate* (*NADP*),
known as the pyridine nucleotides. These coenzymes are involved with respiratory enzymes.
They serve as hydrogen acceptors capable of accepting and releasing hydrogen atoms as they
are removed by the dehydrogenase enzymes.
They are essential in the oxidation–reduction
reactions in the release of energy from carbohydrates, fats and proteins. These coenzymes in
their reduced forms are NADH and NADPH.
NAD is also used in glycogen synthesis.

CLINICAL USES. Niacin, but not nicotinamide,
in massive doses of 3 gm. or more per day will
lower serum cholesterol. The effect of niacin
may be due to an interference of lipoprotein
production or a stimulation of lipoprotein lipase
which degrades lipoprotein. However, the use of
niacin in reducing serum cholesterol is questionable because of evidence showing that it inhibits
the use of free fatty acids for energy by the
heart muscle. Consequently, the heart muscle
must rely on glycogen and stored fat for energy,
with the result that muscle glycogen is depleted.
The Coronary Drug Project Research Group
found only slight benefit from use of nicotinic
acid in protecting against recurrent myocardial
infarction.[17]

Massive doses of niacin have also been used
in the treatment of schizophrenia, but this is
questionable therapy.[3] See Chapter 32 for more
discussion of this topic.

RECOMMENDED DIETARY ALLOWANCE. The
Food and Nutrition Board recommended allowances for niacin are expressed as niacin
equivalents (N.E.), with 60 mg. of tryptophan
being regarded as equivalent to 1 mg. of niacin.
This is based on the average ability to convert
tryptophan to niacin, although the amount of
tryptophan required by different individuals to
make 1 mg. of niacin varies from 34 to 86 mg.
The RDA is based on energy intake and is set at
6.6 N.E. per 1000 kcal., but not less than 13
N.E. with intakes below 2000 kcal. Thus, the
RDA falls between 13 and 14 N.E. for women
and between 14 and 18 N.E. for men, varying
with the energy requirement. The RDA is increased by 2 N.E. during pregnancy and by 5
N.E. during lactation. For children over six
months of age and adolescents, the RDA is 6.6
N.E. per 1000 kcal., but not less than 8 N.E. For
infants less than six months old the RDA is 8
N.E. per 1000 kcal. See Table 10–1 for the niacin RDA, which includes dietary sources of niacin plus 1 N.E. for each 60 mg. of dietary
tryptophan. Excessive dietary leucine increases
the requirement for niacin.

SOURCES. Both niacin and its precursor, tryptophan, are included in determining the niacin
content of foods. Most diets consumed in the

United States average 500 to 1000 mg. or more of tryptophan daily and 8 to 17 mg. of preformed niacin, for a total of 16 to 34 N.E. Lean meats, poultry, fish and peanuts are rich daily sources of both. Organ meats, brewer's yeast, peanuts and peanut butter are the richest sources of niacin. Vegetables and fruits are poor sources. Milk and eggs contain small amounts of niacin but are excellent sources of tryptophan. To a lesser extent, beans, peas, other legumes, most nuts, and whole grains or enriched cereals also contain niacin and tryptophan.

Most foods rich in animal protein are also rich in tryptophan. A dietary intake of 60 gm. predominantly complete protein provides 0.6 gm. tryptophan. A simple approximation of tryptophan intake can be made by assuming that dietary protein contains 1 per cent tryptophan. If more precision is required the following approximations can be used: corn products 0.6 per cent, other grains, fruits and vegetables 1.0 per cent, meats 1.1 per cent, and eggs 1.5 per cent.

Since nutrient composition tables give only the milligrams of preformed niacin in food, the total nicotinamide equivalent of the diet is underestimated.[33] To determine intake accurately it is necessary also to consider the tryptophan in foods. Table 6–12 shows the niacin equivalents of selected foods. Some niacin may be synthesized by intestinal bacteria.

DEFICIENCY. The symptoms of niacin deficiency are many. In the early stages muscular weakness, anorexia, indigestion and skin eruptions occur. Severe deficiency of niacin leads to pellagra, which is characterized by dermatitis, dementia, diarrhea (the "3 D's" of pellagra), tremors, and sore tongue ("beef tongue"). The skin develops a cracked pigmented scaly dermatitis in the parts exposed to sunlight, as shown in Figure 6–16. Lesions appear in many parts of the central nervous system resulting in confusion, disorientation and neuritis. Many digestive abnormalities develop in niacin deficiency causing irritation and inflammation of the mucous membranes of the mouth and the gastrointestinal tract. Clinical symptoms of severe riboflavin deficiency appear. In fact, many of the niacin deficiencies are similar, owing to the close interrelationships of riboflavin and niacin in cell metabolism.

In addition, the role of corn in the production of this disease has been recognized. Frequently those people who suffer from pellagra are on very inadequate diets in which corn is a mainstay. There is very little niacin in the diet and the tryptophan in the corn is unavailable and

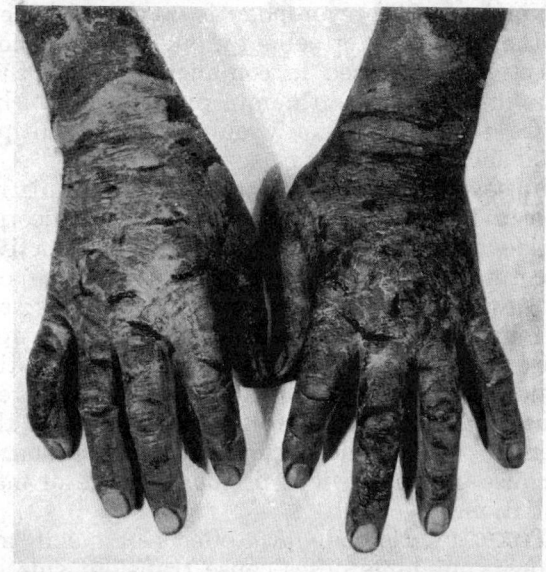

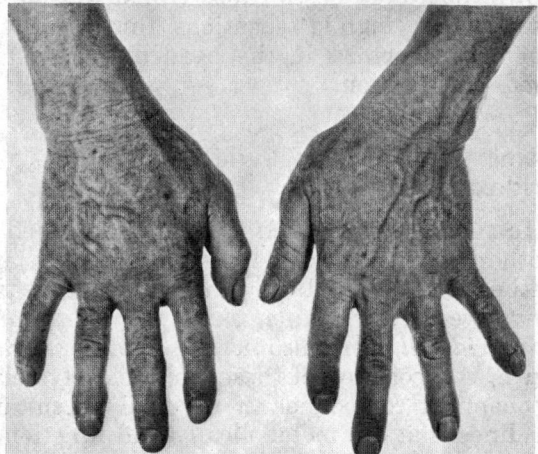

Figure 6–16. *Top,* Lesions on the backs of the hands are typical of pellagra. *Bottom,* The same patient after two weeks of nicotinamide therapy. (From Spies: Rehabilitation through Better Nutrition.)

Table 6–12. NIACIN EQUIVALENTS IN REPRESENTATIVE FOODS

FOOD	NIACIN	TRYPTOPHAN	NIACIN EQUIVALENTS
	mg./1000 cal.		*per 1000 cal.*
Cow's milk	1.2	673	12.4
Human milk	2.5	443	9.9
Beef, round	24.7	1,280	46.0
Whole eggs	0.6	1,150	19.8
Salt pork	1.2	61	2.2
Wheat flour, white	2.5	297	7.4
Corn grits	1.8	70	3.0
Corn	5.0	106	6.7

(From Horwitt, M. K., Harper, A. E., and Henderson, L. M.: Niacin-tryptophan relationships for evaluating niacin equivalents. Am. J. Clin. Nutr., *34*:423, 1981. Originally printed in Horwitt, M. K., et al.: Tryptophan-niacin relationships in man. Studies with diets deficient in riboflavin and niacin, together with observations on excretion of nitrogen and niacin metabolites. J. Nutr., *60* [Suppl. 1]:1, 1956.)

cannot be absorbed from the intestine. Subsequently, there is no tryptophan to be metabolized to niacin and a niacin deficiency state results. In corn-based diets, such as that of Mexicans in which the corn is soaked in lye before use, the alkali makes the tryptophan available for absorption, and niacin deficiency is infrequent.

Leucine and Vitamin B₆ Relationship. An excess of leucine in the diet, as in the case of the sorghum or millet eaters in central India, also seems to be associated with the occurrence of pellagra. It appears that excess leucine in the diet results in increased requirements for vitamin B_6. Since B_6 in the diet may already be low, this precipitates a B_6 deficiency. Several of the enzymes in the tryptophan–niacin pathway are B_6–dependent. In the presence of a deficiency of this vitamin, there are disturbances in this pathway and deficient niacin production, which can eventually result in pellagra.

Niacin and/or tryptophan is now used widely in the treatment of pellagra, but they are most effective when used in conjunction with other vitamins, especially thiamin and riboflavin, because pellagrins usually suffer from multiple deficiencies.

In severe cases of pellagra, oral administration of 150 to 600 mg. nicotinic acid or nicotinamide per day in several doses is effective. Nicotinamide is preferred because it does not cause the unpleasant flushing and burning sensations that accompany nicotinic acid therapy. Within 24 hours there is a response to nicotinamide, with cessation of diarrhea and less redness of the tongue. Unfortunately, some of the mental problems do not ever respond, probably because of the previous prolonged state of malnutrition.

TOXICITY. No real *toxic* effects of niacin are known, but large doses cause transient side effects such as tingling sensations, flushing of the skin and throbbing in the head because of its vasodilating action.

Vitamin B₆ (Pyridoxine, Pyridoxal and Pyridoxamine)

HISTORY. In 1938 *pyridoxine* was identified as another fraction of the vitamin B complex, and synthesized in 1939. Later it was found that two derivatives of pyridoxine, namely, *pyridoxamine* and *pyridoxal*, were also active. Therefore, vitamin B_6 is a complex of these three closely related chemical compounds of naturally occurring pyridines that are metabolically and functionally interrelated. Pyridoxine or B_6 is the term used to designate this group of vitamins.

CHEMICAL PROPERTIES. Pyridoxine, a white, crystalline, odorless compound, is soluble in water and alcohol. It is stable to heat in an acid medium and relatively unstable in alkaline solutions, but very unstable to light. Freezing of vegetables leads to a 20 per cent loss of pyridoxine.

ABSORPTION AND EXCRETION. Pyridoxine is absorbed in the upper small intestine, probably by simple diffusion. The lower the intestinal pH, the greater the B_6 absorption. Pyridoxine is excreted from the body primarily as pyridoxic acid.

FUNCTIONS. Pyridoxine is found in cells in the active form as *pyridoxal phosphate* (*PLP*) or as *pyridoxamine phosphate*, coenzymes that function in protein, fat and carbohydrate metabolism. Their primary function as coenzymes for many chemical reactions, however, is related to protein metabolism. PLP functions in the reactions involved in the non-oxidative degradation of amino acids, namely:

1. Transamination, the transfer of the amino group (NH_2) from one amino acid to form a different amino acid and the keto-analogue of the original amino acid. Transaminase activity in tissues is low in pyridoxine deficiency.

2. Deamination, the removal of amino groups from some amino acids not needed for growth, thus rendering the carbon residues available for energy.

3. Desulfuration, transfer of the sulfhydryl group (HS) from one amino acid (methionine) to another (serine) to form cysteine.

4. Decarboxylation, the removal of the carboxyl group (COOH) from certain amino acids to form another compound. This decarboxylation is required for the synthesis of the *neurotransmitters* serotonin, norepinephrine and histamine from tryptophan, tyrosine and histidine.

In addition, pyridoxal phosphate is necessary for the formation of alpha-aminolevulinic acid, a precursor of heme in hemoglobin.

As already mentioned, vitamin B_6 is essential for the formation and metabolism of tryptophan and for the conversion of tryptophan to nicotinic acid (niacin). In this reaction PLP plays a role in niacin supply. An individual with pyridoxine deficiency when given the tryptophan load test will accumulate *xanthurenic acid* (an intermediary product in the conversion of tryptophan to niacin). The amount can be measured in the urine and is used as an indication of the extent of available pyridoxine.

Pyridoxine as a part of the enzyme phosphorylase facilitates the release of glycogen from the liver and muscle as glucose-1-phosphate. It is also involved in the conversion of the essential unsaturated fatty acid linoleic acid to the biologically important arachidonic acid. The formation of sphingolipids involved in the development of the myelin sheath surrounding nerve cells is also vitamin B_6–dependent.

Pyridoxine is involved in the maintenance of

cellular immunity. In rats even a prenatal deficiency of vitamin B₆ adversely affects immunological competence in later life. It is not known whether this applies to humans.

Gamma-aminobutyric acid (GABA) has a neurotransmitter inhibitory role in the brain and PLP regulates its synthesis. Chapter 32 further discusses neurotransmitters. Pyridoxine is transported to the brain and CSF by a saturable transport process. This mechanism can maintain high brain pyridoxine levels even at low plasma concentrations, but it also maintains a homeostasis preventing the brain levels from getting too high. It has been theorized that certain brain conditions such as dementia exist because of inadequate cerebral uptake of certain vitamins, particularly B_6.[71]

RECOMMENDED DIETARY ALLOWANCE. Results from a study by Baker and coworkers[7] with young adult male subjects indicate that the requirement is directly related to protein intake. They conclude that the optimal daily vitamin B_6 requirement (as pyridoxine hydrochloride) for subjects on a high protein intake (100 gm.) appears to be 1.75 to 2.0 mg. per day; on a low protein intake (30 gm.) the requirement appears to be 1.25 to 1.5 mg. per day. In the 1980 revision, the Food and Nutrition Board provides for a margin of safety in recommending a level of 2.2 mg. per day for adult males and 2.0 mg. for adult females, as listed in Table 10–1. The need increases in pregnancy to an additional allowance of 0.6 mg. per day for a total allowance of 2.6 mg. per day. During lactation the RDA is 2.5 mg. per day. Vitamin B_6 requirements are possibly increased with aging and in special situations such as radiation exposure, cardiac failure,

isoniazid therapy and use of oral contraceptives containing estrogen.

The 1980 RDA for young children has been increased by 35 to 50 per cent and for older children by about 10 per cent on the basis that vitamin B_6 requirement should be related to the protein intake. A recommended dietary allowance of 0.3 mg is considered adequate for the young infant. For older infants (six months to one year of age) consuming a mixed diet, a daily allowance of 0.6 mg. of vitamin B_6 is recommended.

SOURCES. The best sources of pyridoxine are yeast, wheat germ, pork, glandular meats (especially liver), whole grain cereals, legumes, potatoes, bananas, and oatmeal. Milk, eggs, vegetables and fruit contain small amounts. See Table 6–13 for the pyridoxine content of selected foods. It is in most common foodstuffs and probably some can be synthesized by the intestinal flora.

DEFICIENCY. Adults who were given a B_6 antagonist (deoxypyridoxine) developed depression, nausea, vomiting, seborrheic dermatitis, mucous membrane lesions and peripheral neuritis.[79] Ataxia, hyperacusis, hyperirritability, altered mobility and alertness, abnormal head movements and convulsions are characteristic of vitamin B_6 deficiency.

Isoniazid (INH; isonicotinic acid hydrazide), used as a chemotherapeutic agent for tubercular patients, is a potent antagonist of B_6. Patients develop peripheral neuritis and many of the symptoms of pyridoxine deficiency. The enzyme involved in decarboxylation of amino acids apparently is inactivated when isoniazid combines with PLP. Urinary excretion of vitamin B_6

Table 6–13. PYRIDOXINE (B₆) CONTENT OF SELECTED FOODS (MG./100 GM.)

Egg, white	.002	Prunes, dried	.24
Milk, human	.01	Egg, yolk	.30
Orange juice	.028	Chicken, dark meat	.325
Apple	.03	Peanut butter	.33
Bread, white	.04	Avocado	.42
Milk, whole	.04	Tuna, canned	.425
Yogurt	.046	Halibut	.43
Cornflakes	.065	Beef	.435
Apricots	.07	Pork	.45
Cheese, cheddar	.08	Banana, raw	.51
Potatoes, mashed	.091	Rice, brown	.55
Tomato, raw	.10	Chicken, light meat	.683
Frankfurter	.14	Salmon, fresh	.70
Oatmeal	.14	Walnuts	.73
Rice, white	.17	Soybeans, dry	.81
Brussels sprouts	.175	Liver, beef	.84
Bread, whole wheat	.18	Wheat germ, toasted	1.15
Corn, canned	.2	Sunflower seeds, kernels	1.25
Cauliflower	.21	Yeast, dry active	2.0

(From Orr, M. L.: Pantothenic Acid, Vitamin B₆ and Vitamin B₁₂ in Foods. Home Econ. Res. Rep., No. 36, Agricultural Research Service, USDA, Washington, D.C., 1969.)

is greatly increased. The same is true with the medication penicillamine.

Vitamin B_6 deficiency has been shown to increase urinary oxalate excretion and has been implicated in renal calculus formation. This has been attributed to an inability to convert glyoxalate to glycine and reflects the importance of this vitamin in metabolism of glycine and serine. Renal calculi are discussed in Chapter 30.

Pregnant women on "normal" diets have manifested pyridoxine deficiency when given the tryptophan load test and the abnormality was corrected by the administration of the vitamin. The placenta actively transports pyridoxine to attain a fivefold increase in fetal blood as compared with the mother. The vitamin has been used in the treatment of nausea and vomiting of pregnancy and following radiation treatment with apparently good results. However, its efficiency in this use has not been proved. This is discussed further on page 254.

Fifteen to 20 per cent of women taking oral steroid contraceptives have been shown to have increased urinary excretion of tryptophan metabolites, suggestive of B_6 deficiency. This and accompanying states of malaise, depression, and glucose intolerance are relieved by 10 to 15 mg. of vitamin B_6 daily. Whether these effects of oral contraceptives represent a true vitamin B_6 deficiency is debatable (see Chapter 21).

Vitamin B_6 deficiency may accompany alcoholism, since alcohol and alcoholic liver disease can interfere with normal B_6 metabolism.

Central nervous system abnormalities appear in extreme pyridoxine deficiency. Infants fed a liquid milk formula in which much of the vitamin was unknowingly destroyed in processing (autoclaving, high temperatures) developed irritability and convulsions. Infants recovered rapidly after an injection of the vitamin. It is apparent that enzyme systems of the central nervous system have a low order of binding capacity with coenzyme pyridoxal phosphate, making them susceptible to deficiency with resultant derangement of cellular metabolism and clinical abnormalities.

A deficiency syndrome has been identified in mentally retarded children with uncontrollable convulsions from birth due to inborn error of B_6 metabolism. It is thought that these children are unable to synthesize GABA. Correction of the convulsions requires daily ingestion of large amounts of the vitamin and must be started in the neonatal period in order to prevent the development of irreversible mental retardation. Another form in children with cryptogenic epilepsy, which occurs at several years of age, requires large doses of pyridoxine in order to correct the tryptophan load test and improve the EEG and seizure manifestations.

TOXICITY. Side effects, such as sleepiness, may follow injection of large doses (100 mg.) of pyridoxine.

Folacin (Folic Acid or Pteroylmonoglutamate)

Folacin has been known under several names in the study of unidentified growth factors in bacteria and experimental animals and in the study and treatment of anemias. It was synthesized in 1946 and established as a dietary essential for man, many animals and microorganisms.

CHEMICAL AND PHYSICAL PROPERTIES. Folacin is a water-soluble, yellow, crystalline compound that belongs to a group of compounds known as "pterins" (Greek, "wing"; they were found in pigment of butterfly wings), and is also known chemically as pteroylglutamic acid, folate and *Lactobacillus casei* factor. *Pteroylglutamic acid* is formed by the linkage of three compounds: pteridine and para-aminobenzoic acid (PABA) conjugated with one, three or seven molecules of glutamic acid. Some of the glutamic acid molecules must be split off to form an unconjugated folic acid molecule, pteroyl*mono*glutamic acid (PGA), which is the active form and is referred to as *folic acid*. This is done with the aid of specific enzymes and vitamin B_{12}.

Some forms of folacin are heat stable, whereas others are rapidly destroyed by heat. Some are destroyed by acid, whereas other forms are stable at low pH. There is considerable loss of folic acid in vegetables during storage at room temperature, and additional loss can occur during processing at high temperatures. In dried milk, for example, folic acid activity is destroyed.

ABSORPTION, METABOLISM AND STORAGE. Folacin, usually present in the polyglutamate form in food, is broken down to the monoglutamate form by folyl conjugase from the pancreas and mucosal conjugase from the intestinal wall.[37, 39] It is then absorbed possibly by active transport and diffusion. It appears that folic acid absorption is decreased in an alkaline gastrointestinal tract.[47] During absorption or after entrance into the liver or both, monoglutamic acid is changed to *methyltetrahydrofolic acid* and stored. The exact amount of food folate that is absorbed is not clear, but it is assumed that all of the free folic acid (PGA) and a good portion of the polyglutamates are absorbed. Folic acid in the presence of NAD is reduced to *tetrahydrofolic acid* (THFA). THFA unites with a single carbon unit to form formyltetrahydrofolic acid or *citrovorum* factor, which is much more stable. Folic acid is an indispensable component of tissues, without which there is serious interference with cellular metabolism.

FUNCTIONS. *Tetrahydrofolic acid* is a carrier for the single carbon groups (formyl, hydroxymethyl, or methyl groups) from one substance to another. It plays an important role in the synthesis of the purines guanine and adenine and of the pyrimidine thymine, compounds which are utilized for the formation of nucleoproteins DNA (deoxyribonucleic acid) and RNA (ribonucleic acid), which are essential to cell division and the transmission of inherited traits.

Tetrahydrofolic acid participates in the interconversion of serine and glycine, the oxidation of glycine, methylation of homocysteine to methionine with B_{12} as cofactor, and the methylation of the precursor ethanolamine to the vitamin choline. The conversion of nicotinamide to *N*-methyl nicotinamide by addition of a single carbon (methyl group) and the oxidation of phenylalanine to tyrosine require folacin.

Folacin is required for one step in the conversion of histidine to glutamic acid. An impaired metabolism of histidine results in accumulation of the intermediary product, formiminoglutamic acid (FIGLU), which is excreted in the urine.

Folacin is essential for the formation of both red and white blood cells in the bone marrow and for their maturation. It serves as a single carbon carrier in the formation of heme.

RECOMMENDED DIETARY ALLOWANCE. It has been estimated that daily intakes of folacin by healthy individuals vary over a wide range.[24] The daily recommendations are 0.4 mg. for adults, 0.8 mg. during pregnancy and 0.5 mg. during lactation. Other stressful situations, including disease states and the consumption of alcohol, increase the requirement for folacin. The 1980 RDA for folacin for all age groups are listed in Table 10–1.

SOURCES. Folacin occurs widely in foods, and an adequate supply is easily obtained. It usually appears in the polyglutamate form. The best sources are liver, kidney beans, lima beans and fresh dark-green leafy vegetables, especially spinach, asparagus and broccoli. Good sources are lean beef, potatoes, whole wheat bread and dried beans. Poor sources include most meats, milk, eggs, most fruits and root vegetables. The folacin contents of various foods are listed in Table 6–14 and Appendix Table 7. The availability of folacin measurable in foods varies depending upon the presence of conjugase inhibitors, binders or other unknown factors. Probably 25 to 50 per cent of dietary folacin is nutritionally available. Intestinal bacteria synthesize large amounts of folacin, which add to the daily balance.

DEFICIENCY. Folacin deficiency may be the most common hypovitaminosis of humans, af-

Table 6–14. FOLACIN CONTENT OF SOME FOODS

	FOLACIN μg./100 gm.	
	Free	*Total*
Wheat germ	257	328
Yeast		
brewer's	175	3909
active, dry	140	4090
Wheat bran	134	258
Egg yolk	121	152
Liver, beef, raw	80	219
Spinach (cooked)	60	91
Romaine lettuce	60	179
Whole wheat flour	40	54
Fresh orange juice	34	55
Cabbage, raw	33	66
Almonds, raw	33	96
Fresh orange	32	46
Whole wheat bread	27	58
Broccoli (cooked)	27	56
Banana	22	28
White flour, all purpose	18	21
White bread	13	39
Beans, white, baked in tomato sauce	8	24
Milk, whole	5	5

(From Perloff, B. P., and Butrum, R. R.: Folacin in selected foods. J. Am. Diet. Assoc., *70*:161, 1977.)

fecting mainly the indigent of the world. Deficiency of folacin results in poor growth, megaloblastic anemia and other blood disorders, glossitis, and gastrointestinal tract disturbances arising from inadequate dietary intake, impaired absorption, excessive demands by tissues of the body or metabolic derangements. Protein malnutrition may impair the utilization and function of folacin, and conditions in which the demands for folacin are unusually great, such as pregnancy, hemolytic anemia, leukemia and Hodgkin's disease, and the use of certain drugs, can cause a deficiency. Untreated gluten-sensitive enteropathy and tropical sprue lead to folate malabsorption, as does alcohol. It is also suspected that folate absorption is less effective in the elderly.[39]

The main metabolic consequence of folic acid deficiency is altering of DNA metabolism. This results in changes in cellular nuclear morphology, especially in those cells with the most rapid rates of multiplication—red blood cells, leukocytes and epithelial cells of the stomach, intestine, vagina and uterine cervix.

In pernicious anemia, folic acid will produce marked alleviation of the anemia, but the gastrointestinal symptoms and neurologic lesions progress. This is referred to as the "masking effect" of folacin in pernicious anemia, which is described in Chapter 29.

TOXICITY. No toxicity from folic acid has been reported with daily doses as high as 15 mg.

However, excessive folate may interfere with the pharmacological action of anticonvulsant drugs, as discussed in Chapter 21.

Vitamin B$_{12}$ (Cobalamin)

In 1948 this compound was isolated from liver extract and shown to have high potency against pernicious anemia. It contains the heavy metal cobalt, chelated in a large tetrapyrrole ring very similar to the porphyrin ring of heme. The form of the vitamin originally isolated contained cyanide, which is ordinarily considered to be very toxic. Cobalamin is the generic name of vitamin B$_{12}$ because of the presence of cobalt. Several of the different cobalamin compounds exhibit vitamin B$_{12}$ activity. Of these compounds cyanocobalamin and hydroxycobalamin are the most active forms. The functional forms of the vitamin are called cobamide coenzymes.

Vitamin B$_{12}$ is the extrinsic factor of food necessary for treatment and prevention of pernicious anemia. It is considered to be identical with the anti–pernicious anemia factor and the erythrocyte maturation factor of Castle, as well as with the so-called animal protein factor.

CHEMICAL CHARACTERISTICS AND STABILITY. Vitamin B$_{12}$ is a red crystalline substance that is water-soluble. The red color is due to the presence of cobalt in the molecule. Vitamin B$_{12}$ is slowly destroyed by dilute acid, alkali, light and oxidizing or reducing agents. Approximately 70 per cent of the vitamin activity is retained during cooking.

Cyanocobalamin is the most stable form and therefore the form in which the vitamin is produced commercially from bacterial fermentation.

ABSORPTION, TRANSPORT AND STORAGE. Cobalamin is poorly absorbed from the intestinal tract unless the *intrinsic factor* (a mucoprotein enzyme called Castle's intrinsic factor) in the gastric secretion is present. The presence of hydrochloric acid is necessary to split vitamin B$_{12}$ from its peptide bonds. The intrinsic factor combines with vitamin B$_{12}$ in the food and in the bound form becomes adsorbed to a receptor in the membranes of the ileum, through which it is transported into the cells in pinocytic vesicles. Calcium is necessary for the transfer. There is an enterohepatic circulation of B$_{12}$ that recycles it from bile and other intestinal secretions. This is a reason why B$_{12}$ deficiency takes so long to develop in the human.

Absorption may also occur by simple diffusion, accounting for absorption of about 1 to 3 per cent of the vitamin consumed in ordinary diets. Absorption of B$_{12}$ appears to decrease with aging and with deficiency of iron and B$_6$ and increases during pregnancy. Normal people absorb about 30 per cent of a test dose of cyanocobalamin. However, in individuals with low intakes, absorption may increase up to 70 per cent.[24]

After absorption, cobalamin is transported in the blood stream again bound to serum proteins, *transcobalamin I and II* (II being more important), and circulates to the various tissues. The tissues of normal persons contain vitamin B$_{12}$ in varying amounts, with the highest concentration found in the liver and to some extent in the kidney. It is released as needed to the bone marrow and other tissues of the body. The body store of the vitamin (approximately 2000 µg.) is substantial. It may take five or six years for deficiency symptoms to appear after the body's supply from the natural sources has been restricted. An excess intake of the vitamin is excreted in the urine.

FUNCTIONS. Cobalamin has various physiological roles at the cellular level. It is essential for normal function in the metabolism of all cells, especially for those of the gastrointestinal tract, bone marrow, and nervous tissue, and for growth. It participates with folic acid, choline and methionine in the transfer of methyl groups in the synthesis of nucleic acids, purines and pyrimidine intermediates. Cobalamin coenzymes are necessary for reducing RNA to DNA, which functions in the promotion of growth and in red blood cell maturation. Vitamin B$_{12}$ affects myelin formation. It is involved in protein, fat and carbohydrate metabolism. It is related to folate metabolism in that B$_{12}$ is necessary for removal of a methyl group from methylfolate and for generation of tetrahydrofolate necessary for DNA synthesis. This is further discussed on page 596.

RECOMMENDED DIETARY ALLOWANCE. Human requirements for this factor are minute but essential. Doses of 0.5 to 1.0 µg., injected parenterally, have relieved pernicious anemia, and large doses have relieved or prevented progression of the neurologic complications of pernicious anemia. The 1980 revision of the Recommended Dietary Allowances suggests 3 µg. daily for adults, and 4 µg. during pregnancy and lactation. Allowances for older infants have been increased fivefold and for young children between 50 and 100 per cent in the 1980 recommendations, which are listed in Table 10–1. These changes resulted from relating the RDA for vitamin B$_{12}$ to growth rates. A diet containing 15 µg. daily will gradually replenish depleted stores. The "average" diet contains 5 to 15 µg. of vitamin B$_{12}$ per day.[24]

SOURCES. Vitamin B$_{12}$ is present in animal protein foods, including those listed in Table 6–15. Liver and kidney are richest sources; fresh milk, eggs, fish, cheese and muscle meats are

Table 6–15. VITAMIN B$_{12}$ CONTENT OF
SELECTED FOODS
(μG./100 GM.)

Milk, whole	.4
Chicken, fried	.42
Frankfurters, cooked	1.3
Egg	2.0
Beef, round	2.65
Oysters	18.0
Clams, canned	19.1
Liver, beef	80.0

(From Pennington, J. A.: Dietary Nutrient Guide. Westport, Connecticut, AVI Publishing Co., 1976.)

good sources. Pasteurized and evaporated milk have lost 40 to 90 per cent of the vitamin. Limited bacterial synthesis in man occurs in the colon, past the terminal ileum, so it is not absorbed.

DEFICIENCY. Failure to absorb vitamin B$_{12}$ because of the absence of intrinsic factor in the gastric secretion results in a deficiency state. This failure can result from surgical resection of the intrinsic factor–secreting portions of the stomach (fundus and cardia) or of the absorbing surfaces of the ileum. Small bowel diverticula, intestinal infestations, sprue and other malabsorption syndromes may induce a vitamin B$_{12}$ deficiency state.

Vegans (persons living exclusively on vegetables) have a low dietary intake of vitamin B$_{12}$. They usually have low serum levels of this vitamin and are likely to become deficient. With deficiency a megaloblastic anemia develops; this disease is discussed on page 595.

In the nervous system, B$_{12}$ deficiency causes demyelination of the large nerve fibers of the spinal cord. The result is a progressive neuropathy beginning in the peripheral nerves.

TOXICITY. No toxic effects are known.

Pantothenic Acid

HISTORY. The synthesis of pantothenic acid was completed in 1940. It is a part of coenzyme A, which functions in two-carbon unit metabolism.

CHEMICAL CHARACTERISTICS AND STABILITY. Pantothenic acid is a white, crystalline compound (calcium pantothenate), bitter to the taste, more stable in solution than in dry form and easily decomposed by acid, alkali and dry heat. It is water-soluble and stable in moist heat in neutral solution.

FUNCTIONS. Pantothenic acid is known to be essential in the intermediary metabolism of carbohydrate, fat and protein. As part of coenzyme A it has many metabolic roles in the cells. Because pantothenic acid is incorporated into CoA

on which acetylation and other acylation reactions depend, it is involved in the release of energy from carbohydrate and in the degradation and metabolism of fatty acids. Besides functioning in the transfer of acetate groups to the citric acid cycle, CoA is involved as an acceptor acetate group for amino acids, vitamins and sulfonamides. It is involved in the synthesis of cholesterol, steroid hormones, porphyrin for hemoglobin and phospholipids. It is known to be essential in the metabolism of man, chicks, dogs and rats, and prevents graying of the hair in certain animals.

RECOMMENDED DIETARY ALLOWANCE. According to the Food and Nutrition Board's 1980 revision a daily intake of 4 to 7 mg. is probably adequate for adults and there is evidence that a higher intake may be needed during pregnancy and lactation. However, there is not enough evidence to define a recommended allowance. Usual intake of pantothenic acid in the American diet is about 7 mg. per day with a range of 5 to 20 mg. Estimated safe and adequate intakes for other age groups based on proportional energy needs are in Table 10–2.

SOURCES. Pantothenic acid is present in all plant and animal tissue, hence its name meaning "widespread." Egg, kidney, liver, salmon, whole-grain cereals, legumes and yeast are the best sources. Cauliflower, broccoli, beef (lean), potatoes (white and sweet), tomatoes, and molasses are good sources. Table 6–16 presents the pantothenate content of some foods. It is also possibly synthesized by the intestinal flora.

Much of the pantothenate in meat is lost during thawing and approximately 33 per cent is lost in cooking. About 50 per cent is lost in the milling of flour.

DEFICIENCY. Pantothenic acid is so widely distributed in foods that a deficiency disease due to lack of the vitamin has not been observed in

Table 6–16. PANTOTHENIC ACID CONTENT OF
SELECTED FOODS
(MG./100 GM.)

Liverwurst	2.24
Cheerios	1.34
Wheat germ	1.22
Chicken, baked with skin	1.20
Salami	.99
Beef, chuck steak, pan broiled	.85
Tomato paste, canned	.77
Potato chips	.71
Sweet potatoes, canned	.40
Oatmeal, regular	.27
Potatoes, baked	.31
Orange juice, frozen, reconstituted	.19
Applesauce, canned, unsweetened	.08

(From Walsh, J. H., Wyse, B. W., and Hansen, R. G.: Pantothenic acid content of 75 processed and cooked foods. J. Am. Diet. Assoc., 78:140, 1981.)

man. Deficiency induced by administering an antagonist to volunteer subjects produced numerous physical and biochemical disturbances. Some of the subjects experienced dermatitis, burning sensations, especially of the feet, and pain in the arms and legs. Others noted loss of appetite, nausea and indigestion. Most became quarrelsome, sullen and depressed. Fainting attacks were common; the pulse tended to be rapid. An increase in susceptibility to infection seemed to follow. Pantothenic acid deficiency in both animals and man results in loss of antibody production. Pantothenic acid has been reported to improve the stress reactions of well-nourished subjects and to relieve the burning feet syndrome.

TOXICITY. No serious toxic effects of this substance are known; however, ingestion of large amounts may cause diarrhea.

Biotin

HISTORY. Biotin was first isolated in 1936 and synthesized in 1943. Previously it had been observed that chicks and rats developed a syndrome manifested by eczema, accompanied by alopecia around the eyes of the rats, when fed large amounts of raw egg whites. The syndrome was cured by adding egg yolks to the diet of the affected animals, and the corrective factor in the yolk was named vitamin H. This proved to be the same as a potent growth factor in yeast called coenzyme R, and the factor was renamed biotin.

CHEMISTRY AND STABILITY. Biotin is a monocarboxylic acid, stable to heat, soluble in water and alcohol, and susceptible to oxidation.

FUNCTION. Biotin is essential for the activity of many enzyme systems. It functions as the coenzyme for the process of carbon dioxide fixation (enzymatic reactions involving the addition or removal of carbon dioxide to or from active compounds). The synthesis and oxidation of fatty acids require biotin as a coenzyme. Biotin has a role in deamination as a coenzyme in the removal of NH_2 from certain amino acids (notably aspartic acid, threonine and serine). It is closely related metabolically to folic acid, pantothenic acid and vitamin B_{12}.

RECOMMENDED DIETARY ALLOWANCE. In 1980 the Food and Nutrition Board, National Research Council, stated that 100 to 300 μg. of biotin per day is the probable daily intake by Americans, and will meet the needs of most healthy adults. Although an RDA cannot at present be established, estimated safe and adequate intakes for adults are 100 to 200 μg. and the amounts recommended for others are listed in Table 10–2.

SOURCES. Biotin is found in a great many foods, and a considerable amount is synthesized by intestinal bacteria and absorbed by the body. Good sources are kidney, liver, egg yolk, some vegetables (mushrooms), a number of fruits (bananas, grapefruit, watermelon, strawberries), peanuts and yeast. Poor sources are meat, some fruits, and cereal grains. Biotin is frequently added to multiple vitamin preparations even though its need has not been definitely established.

DEFICIENCY. In animals deficiency of biotin is associated with the characteristic dermatitis and can be produced only by adding egg white to a biotin-deficient diet. Thus, it has been known in animal research as the "egg-white-injury" factor. *Avidin*, a material in raw egg white, combines with biotin in the intestine, making it unavailable to the body. Biotin deficiency symptoms have also been induced in human beings by feeding raw egg whites, and the symptoms have been alleviated by giving a biotin concentrate. The experimental diet for man of 200 mg. of dried egg white daily[74] induced the deficiency. This amount or its equivalent in raw egg white ingested daily in the American diet is unusual, since it would be about 24 egg whites. The occasional raw egg white would not precipitate a deficiency state. Avidin in raw egg whites is denatured upon cooking.

Possible biotin deficiency has also been described in patients receiving total parenteral nutrition (TPN) for several years.[36, 49] Neither the TPN solution nor vitamin supplements given to these patients contained biotin. Symptoms were skin lesions over the nose and mouth, depression, hyperesthesia and paresthesia (especially over the extremities), muscle pain, depression, conjunctivitis, blepharitis and progressive loss of hair and hair color. Sixty micrograms of biotin added daily to the TPN cleared most symptoms within two to three weeks, and by three months all signs of biotin deficiency had resolved.

TOXICITY. There are no known toxic effects from biotin.

VITAMIN C (Ascorbic Acid)

HISTORY. Vitamin C is the antiscorbutic vitamin, the preventive of and cure for scurvy. Many dramatic stories are in the scientific literature relating the use of citrus fruits for the cure of scurvy, the dreaded disease of explorers and voyagers. This disease was first described during the Crusades, and remained common among soldiers and sailors until the Dutch authorities discovered that the feeding of oranges, lemons or limes prevented it. English sailors are called by the nickname "limey," actually a misnomer, since early rations included not limes but lemons as a scurvy preventive. The specific relationship between scurvy, citrus foods and ascorbic acid was not established until the twentieth century.

Although vitamin C was isolated in 1928 by Albert Szent-Györgyi, who found it in adrenal tissue and in orange and cabbage and identified it as *hexuronic acid*, it was not until 1932 that C. Glenn King at the University of Pittsburgh reisolated the compound from lemons and identified it as vitamin C, having the properties of preventing and curing scurvy in guinea pigs. Shortly thereafter its correct structural formula was established and synthesis was accomplished. It is known as L-*ascorbic acid* in the reduced form and as L-*dehydroascorbic acid* in the oxidized form. Ascorbic acid is the accepted name of the vitamin.

CHEMICAL CHARACTERISTICS AND STABILITY. Chemically, ascorbic acid is a white, water-soluble crystalline material that is stable in dry form. In solution it is easily oxidized, especially on exposure to heat. Oxidation can be accelerated by the presence of copper or iron and by alkaline pH. Consequently, much ascorbic acid is lost in cooking or thrown out in the cooking water. Bruising, cutting, and allowing fruit and vegetables to be kept exposed to the air cause much loss of ascorbic acid. Less destruction and more retention of the vitamin occurs when the food is cooked quickly in small amounts of boiling water or steamed, and covered tightly. Quick freezing of foods preserves the vitamin. Refrigeration aids retention. Use of sodium bicarbonate in cooking vegetables to preserve and improve the color is very destructive of the vitamin. The ascorbic acid content of fruits and vegetables varies with the conditions under which they are grown and the degree of ripeness when harvested.

Ascorbic acid is a hexose derivative and classified as a carbohydrate closely related to the monosaccharides. The reduced ($C_6H_8O_6$) form is the most active form and is readily oxidized to form dehydroascorbic acid ($C_6H_6O_6$). Dehydroascorbic acid may be reduced back to the original form (reversible oxidation–reduction). Both forms are antiscorbutic. Further oxidation of dehydroascorbic acid produces diketogulonic acid, which has no antiscorbutic acid properties and cannot be reduced to form dehydroascorbic acid again. Fruits and fruit juices vary in their content of active ascorbic acid. For example, fresh orange juice has the greatest proportion of active ascorbic acid, followed by frozen orange juice concentrate and then pasteurized orange juice.[32]

In plants several simple sugars are converted to ascorbic acid, but in animals that can synthesize vitamin C, glucose and to some extent galactose are the precursors for the vitamin.

ABSORPTION AND STORAGE. Ascorbic acid is easily absorbed from the small intestine by an active mechanism and probably by diffusion and carried to the tissues by the blood. It readily passes into tissues of the adrenals, kidney, liver and spleen, most of which appear to be in equilibrium with serum level. It is stored in these tissues to some extent (1.5 gm.) through tissue saturation but should be supplied daily. Excess amounts ingested over the saturation level of various tissues are excreted in the urine as oxalic, threonic and dehydroascorbic acids and some is oxidized and exhaled as carbon dioxide. A very small amount is lost in the feces. It requires approximately 3 months for scurvy to develop in a person on a vitamin C–deficient diet.

FUNCTIONS. Ascorbic acid has multiple functions in the body, either as a coenzyme or cofactor. Its function at the cellular level has not been resolved. It appears to be present and essential to the normal functioning of all cellular units including subcellular structures such as ribosomes and mitochondria. The ability of ascorbic acid to lose and take on hydrogen gives it an essential role in metabolism.

Ascorbic acid is required for production and maintenance of *collagen*, a protein substance bound in all fibrous tissue (connective tissue, cartilage, bone matrix, tooth dentin, skin and tendon). The integrity of cellular structure depends on it. Ascorbic acid is involved in the hydroxylation of proline to form *hydroxyproline* in the synthesis of collagen. Ascorbic acid maintains this intercellular cement substance with preservation of capillary integrity. This promotes healing of wounds, fractures, bruises, pinpoint hemorrhages and bleeding gums; and reduces liability to infections. A high level of ascorbic acid is present during healing and in scar tissue.

Vitamin C is essential for the oxidation of phenylalanine and tyrosine and for the conversion of folacin to tetrahydrofolic acid (THFA). It is also helpful in the reduction of ferric iron to ferrous iron in the intestinal tract to facilitate absorption, and in the transfer of iron from plasma transferrin to liver ferritin. This function of vitamin C is discussed further in Chapter 29.

It is also necessary for the conversion of tryptophan to 5-hydroxytryptophan and the neurotransmitter serotonin, and in the formation of the neurotransmitter norepinephrine from dopamine.

Ascorbic acid also participates in the hydroxylation of certain steroids synthesized in adrenal tissue. Under stress, when adrenal cortical hormone activity is high, ascorbic acid concentration in the tissue is decreased. Injection of ACTH causes considerable loss of ascorbic acid from the adrenal cortex. During periods of emotional, psychological or physiological stress, the urinary excretion of ascorbic acid is increased.

The relationships of vitamin C to heart disease and cancer are discussed in Chapters 28 and 36, respectively.

Adequate tissue concentration of ascorbic acid may help the body to maintain resistance to infection. Whether this is actually true, and the mechanisms by which it might happen, have not been proved. It could be through influence on the immunological activity of leukocytes, the production of interferon, the process of inflammatory reaction or the integrity of the mucous membranes. The value of large amounts of ascorbic acid to prevent and cure the common cold has been reported, but these findings are still controversial.

Vitamin C and the Common Cold. Interest in the use of vitamin C for treatment of the common cold dates from the 1940's, but it was not really popularized until Linus Pauling, a Nobel laureate, wrote his book that made claims for vitamin C as a protective agent against the common cold.[56] There have been subsequent books also making claims for vitamin C.[57, 73] Sales of the vitamin skyrocketed in the presence of a great deal of controversy among nutrition authorities regarding this new information. In subsequent years several studies have been performed that tend to modify the original hypothesis:

1. Anderson and colleagues conducted a double-blind, large-scale trial on 818 individuals. One group consumed a placebo, and a second group took 1 gm. of vitamin C daily and 4 gm. daily during the first 3 days of a cold. Anderson found that those taking vitamin C did experience less illness, but the differences were smaller than those claimed and statistically were not significant. However, when those taking vitamin C did contract a cold, it was less severe and resulted in 30 per cent fewer days of disability.[4, 5]

2. In a study involving 641 children taking a placebo or 1 to 2 gm. of vitamin C, Coulehan and colleagues found a decrease of 28 to 34 per cent in the number of days of sickness in those children contracting a cold who were also taking vitamin C. Coulehan did not find that vitamin C prevented getting a cold.[21] However, a more recent study by the same investigator could not confirm the effectiveness of 1 gm. daily doses in reducing the severity of cold symptoms.[20]

3. Wilson and colleagues have found that prophylactic doses of 200 to 500 mg. daily resulted in reduced cold symptoms in girls, but had no effect in boys.[85]

4. Miller and coworkers conducted a double-blind study on co-twins ranging in age from 6 to 15 years receiving a placebo or 500 to 1000 mg. per day depending on their size. They showed that the observed effects on cold symptoms of vitamin C were a 28 per cent reduction in incidence, a 17 per cent reduction in total severity, and a 21 per cent variation in total duration. The effect of vitamin C seems to be more pronounced in younger females. The authors concluded that even though large doses of vitamin C may have a detectable prophylactic effect in some age and sex groups, the genetic, environmental or subjective factors would appear to account for a substantially greater fraction of the total morbidity.[51]

5. Carr and colleagues studied a series of pairs of monozygotic twins aged 14 to 64 years who received either 1 gm. of vitamin C daily or placebo for 100 days. They concluded that vitamin C perhaps reduces the incidence, severity and duration of a cold by at best 20 per cent. The perception of treatment was important, as those who thought they were on a "high dose" reported markedly fewer, shorter and less severe colds than their co-twins who thought they were on a "low dose." In addition, there were significant correlations between cold symptoms reported and the personality trait of neuroticism.[11]

In summary, one can conclude that large doses of vitamin C may have small effects on the severity and duration of the symptoms of a cold and the effect seems to be greater in females, especially young females.

One investigator concluded that ascorbic acid had an antihistaminic effect.[9] Other work has shown that persons with low plasma ascorbic acid levels have elevated blood histamine levels and that supplementation with ascorbic acid lowers blood histamine.[15]

RECOMMENDED DIETARY ALLOWANCE. According to the Food and Nutrition Board, the minimal daily intake of ascorbic acid needed to prevent scurvy is approximately 10 mg.; however, this does not provide acceptable reserves of the vitamin. At the onset of scurvy, plasma ascorbic acid levels range from 0.13 to 0.24 mg./dl. With vitamin C intakes of 60 to 75 mg. per day, serum ascorbic acid levels are 0.75 mg./dl. Even higher serum levels are maintained with higher vitamin C intakes, but the maximal serum level appears to be 1.4 mg./dl. To saturate the leukocytes of adults and maintain a desirable body pool of the vitamin, intakes of 60 mg. of vitamin C or more are necessary.[24] Whether there is value in larger daily doses of vitamin C is still debatable.

The revised recommended allowances (1980) are 60 mg. daily for adult females and males, an increase of one third over the 1974 recommendations. The basis for this was information suggesting that the efficiency of absorption of ascorbic acid is only 85 per cent and that iron absorption is improved by ascorbic acid. Infants need 35 mg. daily the first year. For children up to age 11 years, an allowance of 45 mg. per day is recommended, and for older children up to 60 mg. per day. Thus, the recommended intake of vitamin C per kg. of body weight is greater for children than for adults. A daily allowance of 80 mg. is recommended in pregnancy and 110 mg. during lactation, as listed in Table 10–1. Except for infants, these allowances are all higher than the 1974 RDA.

Several factors may alter the need for vitamin C. Under acute emotional or environmental stress, such as trauma, fever, infection or elevated environmental temperatures, increased intakes of vitamin C are required to maintain normal plasma levels. Cigarette smoking and the use of oral contraceptive agents lower plasma vitamin C levels, but the significance of these effects in terms of vitamin C requirements is not known. There appears to be a physiological difference in the metabolism of vitamin C in males and females.[24]

SOURCES. Ascorbic acid is widely found in citrus fruits, raw leafy vegetables, and tomatoes. Canned or frozen citrus fruit and tomatoes are good and inexpensive sources of ascorbic acid where fresh fruits are not abundant or not obtainable. Strawberries, cantaloupe, cabbage and green peppers are good sources. Potatoes are considered a good source when properly prepared because of the quantity eaten. Table 6–17 lists the vitamin C content of selected fruits and vegetables. *Isoascorbic acid*, which possesses little if any vitamin C biological value for humans, is often used as a preservative in food. Unfortunately, present methods of analysis do not distinguish between this compound and ascorbic acid. Milk, eggs, meat and poultry contain little or no ascorbic acid.

DEFICIENCY. Although not common, deficiency of ascorbic acid is likely to occur in people who consume a diet devoid of fruits and vegetables, alcoholics, aged people on very limited diets, severely ill people under chronic stress, and infants fed diets of exclusively cow's milk. The earliest signs of ascorbic acid deficiency may begin during the first month of deprivation, depending on the rate of catabolism. Deficiency appears after the serum level has fallen below 0.2 mg./dl. Severe deficiency of ascorbic acid causes scurvy. It is characterized by decreased urinary excretion, plasma concentration, and tissue and leukocyte concentration of ascorbic acid. Other symptoms include weakness, poor appetite and growth, anemia, tenderness to touch, swollen and inflamed gums, loosened teeth, swollen wrist and ankle joints, shortness of breath, petechial hemorrhages from the venules, beading or fracture of ribs at costochondral junctions, fracture of epiphyses, and multiple subcutaneous and subperiosteal hemorrhages with pain on motion of the body. Wounds may fail to heal and scars of previous wounds may break down. Secondary infections develop easily in the bleeding areas. All these characteristics have been attributed primarily to collagen defects. However, vitamin C may be involved in some way in the clotting mechanism, and this may be the mechanism by which its deficiency leads to these bleeding abnormalities.

Neurotic disturbances consisting of hypochondriasis, hysteria and depression followed by decreased psychomotor performance have been reported in ascorbic acid deficiency.[40] Although scurvy is rare today, dietary surveys indicate that many Americans receive insufficient amounts of this vitamin for optimal health.

Apparently cigarette smoking adversely affects the body's ability to utilize ascorbic acid. Less ascorbic acid is available in smokers for utilization and storage, indicating the lower amount absorbed. Smokers appear to oxidize more ascorbic acid to dehydroascorbic acid, which isomerizes to diketogulonic acid in the gastrointestinal tract due to the secretion of an oxidative enzyme, ceruloplasmin. Ceruloplasmin is involved in the oxidation of serotonin and serotonin is known to be released by nicotine. The average smoker probably needs twice as much ascorbic acid as the non-smoker to have a comparable blood level.[58]

TOXICITY. Excess ascorbic acid excreted in the urine gives a false-positive test for sugar. It has been implicated in the formation of urate and oxalate stones,[43] but recent evidence shows that massive vitamin C ingestion (9 gm. daily) produces only a small increase in urinary oxalate concentration and no change in urate or inorganic phosphate.[68]

It has also been reported that those on massive intakes of vitamin C have a "rebound" scurvy when they stop taking the massive doses. This is possibly due to a high rate of vitamin C catabolism as an adaptation to hypersaturation. This catabolism does not return to a normal level immediately upon reducing vitamin C intake, and a vitamin C deficiency state results.[48]

A summary of the information on vitamins can be found in Table 6–18.

Other Vitamin-like Factors

This chapter might be summarized by stating that, to date, the metabolic function in man of the following vitamins has been clearly demonstrated: vitamins A, D, E, K, ascorbic acid, thia-

Table 6–17. VITAMIN C CONTENT OF SELECTED FOODS

FOOD	AMOUNT	VITAMIN C (mg.)
Kiwi	1	265
Broccoli		
fresh	1 whole stalk	162
frozen, chopped	½ cup	52
Brussels sprouts	8	146
Peppers, sweet green	1	94
Cantaloupe	½ melon (5-in. diameter)	90
Collards (cooked)	½ cup	72
Peppers		
sweet	1	70
immature, green chili sauce (canned)	½ cup	83
mature, red chili sauce (canned)	½ cup	37
Orange	1 (2½-in. diameter)	66
Orange juice		
fresh	½ cup	62
frozen, diluted	½ cup	60
canned	½ cup	50
Kale, cooked	½ cup	51
Turnip greens	½ cup	50
Strawberries	½ cup	44
Grapefruit juice		
canned, unsweetened	½ cup	42
Tomatoes		
fresh	1 (3-in. diameter)	42*
canned	½ cup	21
juice	½ cup	20
Mango	½ cup	40
Papaya	½ cup (½-in. cubes)	39
Lemon	1 (2½-in. diameter)	39
Grapefruit	½	37
Honeydew melon	¹/₁₀ melon (6¼-in. diameter)	35
Cauliflower, cooked	½ cup	35
Mustard greens, cooked	½ cup	34
Potato		
baked, then peeled	1 medium	31
boiled, then peeled	1 medium	22
peeled, then boiled	1 medium	18
mashed	½ cup	11
French fries	10	7
chips	10	3
Watermelon	1 slice (6-in. diameter × 1 in.)	30
Sweet potato		
baked or boiled	1 medium	25
Spinach		
fresh	½ cup	25
frozen	½ cup	25
canned	½ cup	16
Cabbage, cooked	½ cup	24
Tangerine	1 (2¼-in. diameter)	22
Cabbage, shredded	½ cup	21
Okra, cooked	10 3-in. pods	21
Cranberry juice cocktail (Vitamin C added)	½ cup	20

*Vitamin C content depends on type of cultivation and harvest and time of year.

min, riboflavin, niacin, folic acid, B_{12}, B_6, pantothenic acid and biotin.

There are many other food factors, some of which have no known specific functions, and others that have functions known for certain animal species. A brief presentation of a few with vitamin-like properties follows.

BIOFLAVONOIDS

Flavonoids were used clinically for the first time in 1936 by Szent-Györgyi to treat patients with pathological conditions characterized by increased permeability and fragility of the capillary wall. However, subsequent work did not

Table 6-18. SUMMARY OF INFORMATION ON VITAMINS

FAT-SOLUBLE VITAMINS

Name	Daily Recommended Allowances for Adults	Sources	Stability	Biological Role
Vitamin A (retinol; provitamin A; α, β, γ carotene)	800 R.E. females; 1000 R.E. males	Liver, kidney, milk fat, fortified margarine, egg yolk, yellow and dark green leafy vegetables, apricots, cantaloupe, peaches.	Stable to light, heat and usual cooking methods. Destroyed by oxidation, drying, very high temperature, ultraviolet light.	Essential for normal growth, development and maintenance of epithelial tissue. Essential to the integrity of night vision. Essential for health of the eyes. Helps provide for normal bone development and influences normal tooth formation. Toxic in large quantities.
Vitamin D (calciferol)	Sunlight and normal diet are usually adequate. 7.5 μg. (300 I.U.) ages 19–22; 5 μg. (200 I.U.) after 22; 10 μg. (400 I.U.) in children, pregnancy and lactation.	Vitamin D milk, irradiated foods, some in milk fat, liver, egg yolk, salmon, tuna fish, sardines. Sunlight converts 7-dehydrocholesterol to cholecalciferol.	Stable to heat and oxidation.	Really a prohormone. Essential for normal growth and development; important for formation of normal bones and teeth. Influences absorption and metabolism of phosphorus and calcium. Prevents and cures rickets and osteomalacia. Toxic in large quantities.
Vitamin E (tocopherols and tocotrienols)	8 α-T.E. females; 10 α-T.E. males	Wheat germ, vegetable oils, green leafy vegetables, milk fat, egg yolk, nuts.	Stable to heat and acids. Destroyed by rancid fats, alkali, oxygen, lead, and iron salts, and ultraviolet irradiation.	Is a strong antioxidant. As such may help prevent oxidation of unsaturated fatty acids and vitamin A in intestinal tract and body tissues. Protects red blood cells from hemolysis. Role in reproduction (in animals). Role in epithelial tissue maintenance and prostaglandin synthesis.
Vitamin K (phylloquinone and menaquinone)	Not established. 70–140 μg. considered safe and adequate for healthy persons.	Liver, soybean oil, other vegetable oils, green leafy vegetables, wheat bran. Synthesized in intestinal tract.	Resistant to heat, oxygen, and moisture. Destroyed by alkali and ultraviolet light.	Aids in production of prothrombin, a compound required for normal clotting of blood. Toxic in large amounts.

WATER-SOLUBLE VITAMINS

Name	Daily Recommended Allowances for Adults	Sources	Stability	Biological Role
Thiamin (vitamin B_1)	0.5 mg. per 1000 kcalories; older person 1.0 mg. per day.	Pork, liver, organ meats, legumes, whole grain and enriched cereals and breads, wheat germ, potatoes. Synthesized in intestinal tract.	Unstable in presence of heat or alkali or oxygen. Heat stable in acid solution.	Prevents beriberi. As part of cocarboxylase, aids in removal of CO_2 from alphaketo acids during oxidation of carbohydrates. Essential for growth, normal appetite, digestion and healthy nerves.
Riboflavin (vitamin B_2)	0.6 mg. per 1000 kcalories. Older persons and when intake less than 2000 kcal, 1–2 mg. per day.	Milk and dairy foods, organ meats, green leafy vegetables, enriched cereals and breads, eggs.	Stable to heat, oxygen, and acid. Unstable to light (especially ultraviolet) or alkali.	Essential for growth. Essential for health of the eyes. Plays enzymatic role in tissue respiration and acts as a transporter of hydrogen ions. Coenzyme forms FMN and FAD. Prevents fissures at corners of mouth, around nose and ears, eye irritation, photophobia.

Table continued on the following page

Table 6–18. SUMMARY OF INFORMATION ON VITAMINS (*Continued*)

WATER-SOLUBLE VITAMINS

Name	Daily Recommended Allowances for Adults	Sources	Stability	Biological Role
Niacin (nicotinic acid and nicotinamide)	13–18 N.E. or 6.6 N.E. per 1000 kcal.	Fish, liver, meat, poultry, many grains, eggs, peanuts, milk, legumes, enriched grains. Synthesized by intestinal bacteria.	Stable to heat, light, oxidation, acid and alkali.	As part of enzyme system, aids in transfer of hydrogen, acts in metabolism of carbohydrates and amino acids. Prevents pellagra, nervous depression, neuritis. Involved in glycolysis, fat synthesis and tissue respiration. Requirement related to tryptophan.
Vitamin B_6 (pyridoxine, pyridoxal and pyridoxamine)	2.2 mg. males; 2.0 mg. females	Pork, glandular meats, cereal bran and germ, milk, egg yolk, oatmeal, and legumes. Synthesized by intestinal bacteria.	Stable to heat, light and oxidation.	As a coenzyme, aids in the synthesis and breakdown of amino acids and in the synthesis of unsaturated fatty acids from essential fatty acids. Essential for conversion of tryptophan to niacin. Prevents hypochromic anemia, seborrheic dermatitis, mucous membrane lesions and peripheral neuritis. Essential for normal growth. Leucine increases the requirement for B_6.
Folacin (folic acid)	400 μg.	Green leafy vegetables, organ meats (liver), lean beef, wheat, eggs, fish, dry beans, lentils, cowpeas, asparagus, broccoli, collards, yeast. Synthesized in intestinal tract.	Stable to sunlight when in solution; unstable to heat in acid media.	Appears essential for biosynthesis of nucleic acids. Essential for normal maturation of red blood cells. Functions as a coenzyme: tetrahydrofolic acid.
Vitamin B_{12} (cyanocobalamin)	3 μg.	Liver, kidney, milk and dairy foods, meat, eggs. Vegans require supplement.	Slowly destroyed by acid, alkali, light and oxidation.	Involved in the metabolism of single-carbon fragments. Essential for biosynthesis of nucleic acids and nucleoproteins, and thereby in normal red blood cell formation; role in metabolism of nervous tissue. Involved with folate metabolism. Related to certain anemias, especially pernicious anemia. Related to growth.
Pantothenic acid	Level not yet determined but 4–7 mg. believed safe and adequate. Supplied in normal diet.	Present in all plant and animal foods. Eggs, kidney, liver, salmon and yeast are best sources. Possibly synthesized by intestinal bacteria.	Unstable to acid, alkali, heat and certain salts.	As part of coenzyme A, functions in the synthesis and breakdown of many vital body compounds. Essential in the intermediary metabolism of carbohydrate, fat, and protein.

show them to be a vitamin, so the name vitamin P, which they had been called, was replaced in 1950 by the term bioflavonoids. They do have biological activity, but there is no evidence that they are essential or that they serve any unique role in nutrition or in the prevention or treatment of disease in humans. Despite claims of usefulness, there is no accepted role for bioflavo-noids in vascular purpura, degenerative vascular disease, hypertension, rheumatic fever, arthritis or cancer.

SOURCES. Flavonoids are the pigments in fruits and vegetables and are concentrated in the skin, peel and outer layers—those areas most susceptible to light. Citrus fruits contain 50 to 100 mg. of bioflavonoids per 100 gm. of

Table 6–18. SUMMARY OF INFORMATION ON VITAMINS (*Continued*)

WATER-SOLUBLE VITAMINS

Name	Daily Recommended Allowances for Adults	Sources	Stability	Biological Role
Biotin	Not known but believed 100 to 200 μg. will provide safe and adequate intake.	Liver, mushrooms, peanuts, yeast, milk, meat, egg yolk, most vegetables, banana, grapefruit, tomato, watermelon, and strawberries. Synthesized in intestinal tract.	Stable.	Probably as essential component of a coenzyme. Appears to be involved in synthesis and breakdown of fatty acids and amino acids through aiding the addition and removal of CO_2 to or from active compounds, and the removal of NH_3 from amino acids. It is closely related metabolically to folic acid and pantothenic acid.
Vitamin C (ascorbic acid)	60 mg.	Puerto Rican cherry, citrus fruit, tomato, melon, peppers, greens, raw cabbage, guava, strawberries, pineapple, potato.	Unstable to heat, alkali, and oxidation, except in acids. Destroyed by storage.	Essential for growth. Possibly functions as coenzyme in the metabolism of amino acids, particularly phenylalanine and tyrosine; facilitates conversion of folic acid to folinic acid and is essential for many hydroxylation reactions. Role in tooth and bone formation. Maintains intracellular cement substance with preservation of capillary integrity. Promotes healing of wounds and fractures; and reduces liability to infections. Enhances absorption of iron. Essential for production of collagen, the basic substance of connective tissue. Related in some way to biosynthesis of steroid hormones. Prevents scurvy.

fresh material. Leafy vegetables are good sources, but most root vegetables, with the exception of red onions, are not. Tea, coffee, wine and beer also contain appreciable amounts of bioflavonoids. The typical American mixed diet contains about 1000 mg. of flavonoids daily.

CHOLINE

Choline has been known for over a century as an essential component of animal tissues and it is classified as having vitamin-like activity in experimental animals. Man, however, can synthesize choline from methionine or from serine, provided that enough methionine is present to supply methyl groups and with vitamin B_{12} and folacin to act as coenzymes. However, the rate at which it is synthesized is insufficient to meet the need of most higher animals. For this reason choline is considered an essential nutrient.

However, there have been no experimental efforts to develop choline deficiency in humans, so proof of its need in the diet is lacking. Choline cannot be considered a vitamin for humans. Choline is widely distributed in animal and plant tissues, and in an average diet no inadequacy of it will occur.

FUNCTIONS. The function of choline in man is in the metabolism of and in the transport of fat from the liver, preventing the development of fatty liver. As a component of several phospholipids, it functions in triglyceride transport and cell membrane structure. In the liver choline forms *lecithin* (phosphatidylcholine). During the process fatty acids are removed from the glycerides of the liver, resulting in the decrease of triglyceride content in that organ. Because of this effect, choline is said to be lipotropic.

Choline is also a component of another phospholipid, *sphingomyelin*, in the brain and nerve tissue. As a precursor for *acetylcholine,* choline plays a role in the transmission of nerve impulses, as discussed on page 666. As a dietary source of labile methyl groups, it is involved in transmethylation.

RECOMMENDED DIETARY ALLOWANCE. Daily requirements are not known and no toxic effects have been observed. The amount required is influenced by the amount and type of fat, total energy, type of carbohydrate, amount of protein and amount of cholesterol in the diet. The average diet has been estimated to contain 400 to 900 mg. per day of choline, according to the 1980 revision of the Recommended Dietary Allowances. This amount is apparently adequate for health but should not be equated with dietary requirement.

SOURCES. The richest known dietary source is egg yolk. Other food sources are liver, brain, kidney, heart, lean meat, yeast, soy beans, peanuts, peas, other legumes, and wheat germ. Fruit, fruit juices, milk and vegetables generally are not sources of choline. Neutral fats are essentially devoid of choline.

DEFICIENCY. Deficiency in animals is associated with fatty deposition in the liver and hemorrhagic kidney disease. Choline deficiency in man has not been demonstrated.

Administration of pharmacologic doses of choline seems to alleviate symptoms of tardive dyskinesia and Huntington's disease in human beings, but the dosage required to achieve this effect, up to 20 gm. daily, appears to be beyond the specific dietary needs for choline.

INOSITOL

Inositol has long been known as a chemical compound, but only since 1940 has it been considered a vitamin. It is found in fruits, grains, vegetables, nuts, legumes and organ meats (liver, heart). It occurs abundantly in the average diet usually as inositol phopholipids and as *phytic acid* (inositol hexaphosphate). Phytic acid interferes with the absorption of calcium, iron and zinc, as discussed in Chapter 7. Inositol content of various foods can be found in cited Reference 2. It is estimated that a mixed North American diet provides the adult with 300 to 1000 mg. daily.[2, 13]

FUNCTIONS. Myoinositol, known as "muscle sugar," is the only one of the nine isomers of inositol that has metabolic importance. It is a cyclic six-carbon compound with six hydroxyl groups and a structure resembling glucose. It occurs in animal tissues as a component of phospholipids. It is concentrated in the brain and cerebrospinal fluid but occurs in skeletal and heart muscles and other tissues. The level of free inositol is especially high in all of the organs of the male reproductive tract, particularly in semen.

It is possible that the importance of inositol in human nutrition has been underestimated. Inositol's physiological role is related to its presence in phosphatidylinositol and thus to the function of phospholipids in cell membranes. Its functions include the mediation of cellular responses to external stimuli, nerve transmissions, and regulation of enzyme activity. It is considered to have lipotrophic activity by having a role in phospholipid synthesis and thus affecting the function of the lipid transporting molecules, lipoproteins. There is still a question as to whether inositol is a vitamin for humans. It is an essential growth factor for human cells in vitro. It also is synthesized by normal intestinal bacteria, making the confirmation of its essentiality more difficult.

Inositol metabolism is affected by dietary choline content, the amount and degree of saturation of dietary fat and the specific fatty acid composition.

DEFICIENCY. Because diabetic patients show high myoinositol metabolism levels in urine, and lowered levels in nerve membranes, there have been attempts to explain diabetic peripheral neuropathies on the basis of change in myoinositol metabolism. However, findings have not been consistent. Diabetic rats showed an impaired ability to maintain normal concentrations of inositol in the peripheral nerve, which was related to decreased motor nerve conduction velocity. This was reversed with inositol supplements.[25] The inositoluria that is seen in human diabetes may arise from an inhibitory effect of glucose on renal tubular reabsorption of inositol. Hyperglycemia may also impair inositol transport, resulting in a relative intracellar deficiency in man. Inositol given orally increased the neurophysiological measurements in diabetic patients.[67] Inositol may have a therapeutic role in diabetic neuropathy.[14]

Inositol deficiency in animals produces an accumulation of triglyceride in liver, intestinal lipodystrophy and other abnormalities. Signs of inositol deficiency have not been found in humans and a deficiency is not likely, considering the widespread occurrence of inositol in food. However, it possibly could occur in infants on non–cow's milk formulas, so the American Academy of Pediatrics has recommended its addition to non–cow's milk protein formulas as a preventive measure.[16]

TOXICITY. No toxic effects have been reported. Patients with chronic renal failure show elevated serum inositol levels. These levels may be neurotoxic, but there is no evidence that a reduction in plasma inositol levels by dietary modification will be beneficial.

LIPOIC ACID

Lipoic acid, a fat-soluble, sulfur-containing fatty acid, is not a true vitamin, since it can be synthesized in the body. It functions as a coenzyme and is essential, together with the thiamin-containing enzyme TPP, for reactions in carbohydrate metabolism that convert pyruvic acid to acetylcoenzyme A. Lipoic acid with two sulfur bonds combines with the TPP to reduce pyruvate to active acetate. It joins the intermediary products of protein and fat metabolism in the Krebs cycle in the reactions involved in producing energy from these nutrients. A metal ion (magnesium or calcium) is involved in this oxidative decarboxylation along with the vitamins thiamin, pantothenic acid, niacin, riboflavin and lipoic acid.

No dietary requirement for lipoic acid for humans is known. The amounts needed to participate in the reactions in the tissues may be synthesized in the body. It is found in liver and yeast.

UBIQUINONE (Coenzyme Q)

A lipid-like substance similar to vitamin K, ubiquinone belongs to a group of compounds known as ubiquinones, which are a group of coenzymes. Attached to the basic quinone ring structure are 30 or more carbon atoms in a side chain. Coenzyme Q is present in all cell nuclei and microsomes. It is concentrated in the mitochondria and functions in the respiratory chain in which energy is released from energy-yielding nutrients as ATP. The ubiquinones appear to be synthesized in the body and cannot be classified as vitamins.

Antivitamins (Vitamin Antagonists or Antimetabolites)

There are a growing number of instances of antivitamin activity of special interest in nutrition. An antivitamin or antagonist may be defined as a substance or condition that interferes with the synthesis or metabolism of vitamins. Many vitamin antagonists are compounds similar in structure to the active vitamin molecule. They can prevent incorporation of the vitamin units in the coenzyme structure by attaching themselves to the enzyme. They block the action of the coenzyme, which results in a true vitamin deficiency. Experimental vitamin deficiencies have been produced by using vitamin antagonists. An established example of another type of antivitamin is avidin, found in raw egg white, which combines with biotin and forms a compound which cannot be absorbed from the intestinal tract. Isonicotinic acid hydrazide (INH), which is used as a chemotherapeutic agent in the treatment of tuberculosis, is an antagonist for pyridoxine. Aminopterin, a drug used in the treatment of leukemia, is an antagonist of folacin. Dicumarol, which is an anticoagulant, acts as an antagonist to vitamin K.

Problems and Suggested Topics For Discussion

1. Evaluate your dietary pattern for the foods high in vitamins A, D, thiamin, riboflavin, niacin, and ascorbic acid. Make suggestions for improvement.
2. Select references from the suggested reading list pertaining to vitamins and vision, thiamin and nerve function, folic acid and anemia, vitamin B_6 and depression, and the relationship of hormones and vitamins, for either an oral or written report.
3. What are the functions of vitamins A, D, E and K?
4. List the fractions of the vitamin B complex that are recognized as necessary for humans. What is the function of each?
5. What effects may handling, storage, and cooking of foods have on vitamins A, thiamin, riboflavin, niacin, folic acid, B_{12} and ascorbic acid?
6. Does the normal healthy person on an adequate well-rounded diet need vitamin supplements? Explain.
7. Search the literature and make a list of drugs with antivitamin activity that are of special interest in nutrition.
8. List the vitamins that should be supplied daily. List the vitamins stored in the body. List the vitamins that are known to be synthesized in the body.

Cited References

1. Admed, F., Bamji, M.S., and Iyengar, L.: Effect of oral contraceptive agents on vitamin nutrition status. Am. J. Clin. Nutr., 28:606, 1975.
2. Alam, S.Q.: Inositols, IX. Biochemical systems. In Sebrell, W.H., and Harris, R.S. (eds.): The Vitamins. Vol. III, New York, Academic Press, 1971, pp. 380–394.
3. American Psychiatric Association Task Force on Vitamin Therapy in Psychiatry: Megavitamin and Orthomolecular Therapy in Psychiatry. Washington, D.C., Publications Services Division, Am. Psychiatric Assoc., 1973.
4. Anderson, T.W.: Large scale trials of vitamin C. Ann. N.Y. Acad. Sci., 258:498, 1975.
5. Anderson, T.W., Reid, D.B., and Beaton, G.H.: Vitamin C and the common cold: a double-blind trial. Can. Med. Assoc. J., 107:503, 1972.
6. Bachrach, S., Fisher, J., and Parks, J.S.: An outbreak of vitamin D deficiency rickets in a susceptible population. Pediatrics, 64:871, 1979.
7. Baker, E.M., et al.: Vitamin B_6 requirement for adult men. Am. J. Clin. Nutr., 15:59, 1964.
8. Bieri, J.G., and Evarts, R.P.: Tocopherols and fatty acids in American diets. J. Am. Diet. Assoc., 62:147, 1973.
9. Bouhuys, A.: Colds and antihistamine effects of vitamin C. N. Engl. J. Med., 290:633, 1974.
10. Bunnell, R.H., et al.: Alpha-tocopherol content of foods. Am. J. Clin. Nutr., 17:1, 1965.
11. Carr, A.B., et al.: Vitamin C and the common cold: a second MZ Cotwin control study. Acta. Genet. Med. Gemellol., 30:249, 1981.

12. Clemens, T.L., et al.: Increased skin pigment reduces the capacity of skin to synthesize vitamin D₂. Lancet, 1:74, 1982.

13. Clements, R.S., Jr., DeJesus, P.V., Jr., and Winegrad, A.I.: Raised plasma-myoinositol level in uraemic and experimental neuropathy. Lancet, 1:1137, 1973.

14. Clements, R.S., Jr., and Reynertson, R.: Myo-inositol metabolism in diabetes mellitus: effect of insulin treatment. Diabetes, 26:215, 1977.

15. Clementson, C.A.B.: Histamine and ascorbic acid in human blood. J. Nutr., 110:662, 1980.

16. Committee on Nutrition: Commentary on breast-feeding and infant formulas including proposed standards for formulas. Pediatrics, 57:278, 1976.

17. Coronary Drug Project Research Group: Clofibrate and niacin in coronary heart disease. JAMA, 231:360, 1975.

18. Corrigan, J.J., and Marcus, F.I.: Coagulopathy associated with vitamin E ingestion. JAMA, 230:1300, 1974.

19. Corrigan, J.J., Jr., and Ulfers, L.L.: Effect of vitamin E on prothrombin levels in warfarin-induced vitamin K deficiency. Am. J. Clin. Nutr., 34:1701, 1981.

20. Coulehan, J.L., et al.: Vitamin C and acute illness in Navaho children. N. Engl. J. Med., 295:973, 1976.

21. Coulehan, J.L., et al.: Vitamin C prophylaxis in a boarding school. N. Engl. J. Med., 290:6, 1974.

22. Essays on the History of Nutrition and Dietetics. Chicago, American Dietetic Association, 1967.

23. Farrell, P.M., and Bieri, J.G.: Megavitamin E supplementation in man. Am. J. Clin. Nutr., 28:1381, 1975.

24. Food and Nutrition Board, National Research Council: Recommended Dietary Allowances. 9th ed. Washington, D.C., National Academy of Sciences, 1980.

25. Fukuma, M., et al.: An alteration in internodal myelin membrane structure in large sciatic nerve fibers in rats with acute streptozotocin diabetes and impaired nerve conduction velocity. Diabetologia, 15:65, 1978.

26. Geol, K.M., et al.: Florid and subclinical rickets among immigrant children in Glasgow. Lancet, 1:1141, 1976.

27. Gunther, S.: Vitamin A acid: clinical investigation with 405 patients. Cutis, 17:287, 1976.

28. Haeger, K.: Long-time treatment of intermittent claudication with vitamin E. Am. J. Clin. Nutr., 27:1179, 1974.

29. Hauschka, P.V.: Vitamin K-dependent α-carboxyglutamic acid formation by kidney microsomes in vitro. Biochem. Biophys. Res. Commun., 71:1207, 1976.

30. Hollis, B.W., et al.: Occurrence of vitamin D sulfate in human milk whey. J. Nutr., 109:384, 1981.

31. Hollis, B.W., et al.: Vitamin D and its metabolites in human and bovine milk. J. Nutr., 111:1240, 1981.

32. Horowitz, I., Fabry, E.M., and Gerson, C.D.: Bioavailability of ascorbic acid in orange juice. JAMA, 235:2624, 1976.

33. Horwitt, M.K., Harper, A.E., and Henderson, L.M.: Niacin-trypothan relationships for evaluating niacin equivalents. Am. J. Clin. Nutr., 34:423, 1981.

34. Howard, L., et al.: Reversible neurological symptoms caused by vitamin E deficiency in a patient with short bowel syndrome. Am. J. Clin. Nutr., 36:1243, 1982.

35. Hypervitaminosis E and coagulation. Nutr. Rev., 33:269, 1975.

36. Innis, S.M., and Allardyce, D.B.: Possible biotin deficiency in adults receiving long-term total parenteral nutrition. Am. J. Clin. Nutr., 37:185, 1983.

37. Jägerstad, M., Lindstrand, K., and Westesson, A.K.: Hydrolysis of conjugated folic acid by pancreatic "conjugase." Scand. J. Gastroenterol., 7:593, 1972.

38. Jusko, W.J., and Levy, G.: Absorption, protein binding, and elimination of riboflavin. In Rivlin, R.S. (ed.): Riboflavin. New York, Plenum Press, 1975.

39. Kesavan, V., and Noronha, J.M.: Folate malabsorption in aged rats related to low levels of pancreatic folyl conjugase. Am. J. Clin. Nutr., 37:262, 1983.

40. Kinsman, R.A., and Hood, J.: Some behavioral effects of ascorbic acid deficiency. Am. J. Clin. Nutr., 24:455, 1971.

41. Kühnau, J.: Flavonoids. A class of semi-essential food components: their role in human nutrition. World Rev. Nutr. Diet., 24:117, 1976.

42. Lakdawala, D.R., and Widdowson, E.M.: Vitamin D in human milk. Lancet, 1:167, 1977.

43. Lamden, N.: Dangers of massive vitamin C intake. N. Engl. J. Med., 284:336, 1971.

44. Logan, W.S.: Vitamin A and keratinization. Arch. Dermatol., 105:748, 1972.

45. Loomis, W.F.: Skin-pigment regulation of vitamin-D biosynthesis in man. Science, 157:501, 1967.

46. Lowenberg, M.E., et al.: Food and Man. 3rd ed. New York, John Wiley & Sons, Inc., 1983.

47. MacKenzie, J.F., and Russell, R.I.: The effect of pH on folic acid absorption in man. Clin. Sci. Mol. Med., 51:363, 1976.

48. Masek, J.: Contribution to the problem of vitamin C requirement in adults. Rev. Czech. Med., 12:54, 1966.

49. McClain, C.J., Baker, H., and Onstad, G.R.: Biotin deficiency in an adult during home parenteral nutrition. JAMA, 247:3116, 1982.

50. McCollum, E.V.: A History of Nutrition. Boston, Houghton-Mifflin Company, 1957.

51. Miller, J.Z., et al.: Therapeutic effect of vitamin C. A co-twin control study. JAMA, 237:248, 1977.

52. Muralidhara, K.S., and Hollander, D.: Intestinal absorption of α-tocopherol. The influence of luminal constituents on the absorptive process. J. Lab. Clin. Med., 90:88, 1977.

53. Oberleas, D.: Phytates. In Toxicants Occurring Naturally in Foods. Washington, D.C., National Academy of Sciences, 1973, pp. 363–371.

54. Olson, R.E.: Vitamin K. In Goodhart, R.S., and Shils, M.E. (eds.): Modern Nutrition in Health and Disease. 6th ed. Philadelphia, Lea & Febiger, 1980.

55. Olson, R.E., and Suttie, J.W.: Vitamin K and carboxyglutamate biosynthesis. Vit. Horm., 35:59, 1977.

56. Pauling, L.: Vitamin C and the Common Cold. San Francisco, W.H. Freeman & Co., 1970.

57. Pauling, L.: Vitamin C, the Common Cold and the Flu. San Francisco, W.H. Freeman & Co., 1976.

58. Pelletier, O.: Cigarette smoking and vitamin C. Nutr. Today, 5:12, 1970.

59. Plaitakis, A., et al.: Effect of thiamin deficiency on brain neurotransmitter systems. Ann. N.Y. Acad. Sci., 378:367, 1982.

60. Prasad, A.S., et al.: Effect of oral contraceptive agents on nutrients. II. Vitamins. Am. J. Clin. Nutr., 28:385, 1975.

61. Reeve, L.E., DeLuca, H.F., and Schnoes, H.K.: Synthesis and biological activity of vitamin D₃ sulfate. J. Biol. Chem., 256:823, 1981.

62. Rizvi, S.N.A., and Vaishnava, H.: Secondary hyperparathyroidism in nutritional osteomalacia. J. Indian Med. Assoc., 64:199, 1975.

63. Roberts, H.J.: Perspective on vitamin E as therapy. JAMA, 246:129, 1981.

64. Rodriguez, M.S., and Irwin, M.I.: A conspectus of research on vitamin A requirements of man. J. Nutr., 102:909, 1972.

65. Rudolf, M., Arulanantham, K., and Greenstein, R.M.: Unsuspected nutritional rickets. Pediatrics, 66:72, 1980.

66. Russell, R.M., and Boyer, J.L.: Hepatic injury from chronic hypervitaminosis A resulting in portal hypertension and ascites. N. Engl. J. Med., 291:435, 1974.

67. Salway, J.G., et al.: Effect of myo-inositol on peripheral-nerve function in diabetes. Lancet, 2:1282, 1978.

68. Schmidt, K.H., et al.: Urinary oxalate excretion after large intakes of ascorbic acid in man. Am. J. Clin. Nutr., 34:305, 1981.

69. Shearer, M.J., et al.: Plasma vitamin K in mothers and their newborn babies. Lancet, 2:460, 1982.

70. Solomons, N.W., and Russel, R.M.: The interaction of vitamin A and zinc: implications for human nutrition. Am. J. Clin. Nutr., 33:2031, 1980.

71. Spector, R., Cancilla, P., and Damasio, A.: Is idiopathic dementia a regional vitamin deficiency state? Med. Hypotheses, 5:763, 1979.

72. Stephens, W.P., et al.: Observations on the natural history of vitamin D deficiency amongst Asian immigrants. Quart. J. Med., 51(202):171, 1982.

73. Stone, I.: The healing factor: vitamin C against disease. New York, Grosset & Dunlap, Inc., 1972.

74. Sydenstricker, V.P., et al.: Observations on the "egg-white injury" in man and its cure with a biotin concentrate. JAMA, 118:1199, 1942.

75. Symposium: Vitamin D in health and disease. Ann. Int. Med., 96:674, 1982.

76. Ten-State Nutrition Survey, 1968–70. Department of Health, Education and Welfare Publ. No. (HSM) 72–8134, 1972.

77. The vitamin D activity of milk. Nutr. Rev., 40:27, 1982.

78. Tsai, A.C., et al.: Study on the effect of megavitamin E supplementation in man. Am. J. Clin. Nutr., 31:831, 1978.

79. Vilter, R.W., et al.: The effect of vitamin B_6 deficiency induced by desoxypyridoxine in human beings. J. Lab. Clin. Med., 42:335, 1953.

80. Vitamin D and insulin. Nutr. Rev., 40:221, 1982.

81. Wald, G.: The interconversion of the retinenes and vitamin A in vitro. Biochem. Biophys. Acta, 4:215, 1950.

82. Wason, S.: Vitamin A toxicity (letter). Am. J. Dis. Child., 136:174, 1982.

83. Weber, F.L., et al.: Reversible hepatotoxicity associated with hepatic vitamin A accumulation in a protein-deficient patient. Gastroenterology, 82:118, 1982.

84. Williams, R.J.: Biochemical individuality. The basis for the genotrophic concept. Austin, Texas, University of Texas Press, 1956.

85. Wilson, C.W., and Loh, H.S.: Common cold and vitamin C. Lancet, 1:638, 1973.

86. Yagi, N., and Itokawa, Y.: Cleavage of thiamine by chlorine in tap water. J. Nutr. Sci. Vitaminol., 25:281, 1979.

Additional References

GENERAL

Barker, B.M., and Bender, D.A.: Vitamins in Medicine. Vol. 1. London, William Heinemann Medical Books, Ltd., 1980.

Composition of Foods. Agriculture Handbooks No. 8:1–9, Consumer and Food Economics Institute. Washington, D.C., U.S. Department of Agriculture, 1976–1982.

Goodhart, R.S., and Shils, M.E. (eds.): Modern Nutrition in Health and Disease. 6th ed. Philadelphia, Lea & Febiger, 1980.

Hardinge, M.G., and Crooks, H.: Lesser known vitamins in foods. J. Am. Diet. Assoc., 38:240, 1961.

Holub, B.J.: The nutritional significance, metabolism and function of myoinositol and phosphatidyl-inositol in health and disease. In Draper, H.H. (ed.): Advances in Nutritional Research. Vol. 4. New York, Plenum Press, 1982.

Nutrients in Processed Foods, Vitamins and Minerals. American Medical Association. Acton, Mass., Publishing Sciences Group, Inc., 1974.

Orr, M.L.: Pantothenic Acid, Vitamin B_6 and Vitamin B_{12} in Foods. Home Economics Research Report No. 36, Washington, D.C., Agricultural Research Service, U.S. Department of Agriculture, 1969.

Preliminary Findings of the First Health and Nutrition Examination Survey, United States, 1971–72, Dietary Intake and Biochemical Findings. Washington, D.C., Department of Health, Education and Welfare Publ. No. (HRA) 74–1219–1, 1974.

Sauberlich, H.E., Skala, J.H., and Dowdy, R.P.: Laboratory Tests for the Assessment of Nutritional Status. Cleveland, Ohio, CRC Press, 1974.

Worthington-Roberts, B.S.: Contemporary Developments in Nutrition. St. Louis, C. V. Mosby Company, 1981, Chapters 6 and 7.

VITAMIN A

Baum, J.L., and Rao, G.: Keratomalacia in the cachectic hospitalized patient. Am. J. Ophthamol., 82:435, 1976.

Goodwin, T.W.: Nature and distribution of carotenoids. Food Chem., 5:3, 1980.

Mori, S.: Primary changes in eyes of rats that result from deficiency of fat soluble A. JAMA, 79:197, 1922.

Pereira, S.M., et al.: Vitamin A therapy in children with kwashiorkor. Am. J. Clin. Nutr., 20:297, 1967.

Simpson, K.L., and Chichester, C.O.: Metabolism and nutritional significance of carotenoids. In Darby, W.J. (ed.): Annual Review of Nutrition. Vol. 1. Palo Alto, Calif., Annual Reviews, Inc., 1981.

The pathophysiological basis of vitamin A toxicity. Nutr. Rev., 40:272, 1982.

The therapeutic use of vitamin A acid. Acta Derm. Venereol. (Suppl.), 55:74, 1976.

Wolf, G.: Is dietary β-carotene an anti-cancer agent? Nutr. Rev., 40:257, 1982.

VITAMIN D

Blunt, J.W., De Luca, H.F., and Schnoes, H.K.: 25-hydroxycholecalciferol: a biologically active metabolite of vitamin D_3. Biochem., 7:3317, 1968.

De Luca, H.F.: Vitamin D endocrinology. Ann. Int. Med., 85:367, 1976.

De Luca, H.F.: Metabolism and molecular mechanism of action of vitamin D: 1981. Biochem. Soc. Transactions, 10:147, 1982.

Food and Nutrition Board, NRC/NAS: Hazards of overdose of vitamin D. Am. J. Clin. Nutr., 28:512, 1975.

Fraser, D.R., and Kodicek, E.: Unique biosynthesis by kidney of a biologically active vitamin D metabolite. Nature, 228:764, 1970.

Holick, M.F., et al.: Isolation and identification of 1,25-dihydroxycholecalciferol. A metabolite of vitamin D active in intestine. Biochem., 10:2799, 1971.

Lawson, D.E., et al.: Identification of 1,25-dihydroxycholecalciferol, a new kidney hormone controlling calcium metabolism. Nature, 230:228, 1971.

VITAMIN E

Bieri, J.G., Corash, L., and Hubbard, V.S.: Medical Uses of vitamin E. N. Engl. J. Med. 308:1063, 1983.

Effect of vitamin E on prostanoid biosynthesis. Nutr. Rev., 39:317, 1981.

Horwitt, M.K.: Vitamin E: a reexamination. Am. J. Clin. Nutr., 29:569, 1976.

Horwitt, M.K., et al.: Polyunsaturated lipids and tocopherol requirements. J. Am. Diet. Assoc., 38:231, 1961.

Lubin, B., and Machlin, L.J.: Vitamin E: biochemical, hematological and clinical aspects. Ann. N.Y. Acad. Sci., Vol. 393, 1982.

Machlin, L.J. (ed.): Vitamin E. A comprehensive treatise. New York, Marcel Dekker, Inc., 1980.

Oski, F.A., and Barnes, L.A.: Vitamin E deficiency: a previously unrecognized cause of hemolytic anemia in the premature infant. J. Pediatr., 70:211, 1967.

Prostaglandin metabolism as related to vitamin E and zinc status. Nutr. Rev., 40:338, 1982.

VITAMIN K

Cross, V.M., et al.: Kernicterus and prematurity. Arch. Dis. Child., *30*:501, 1955.

Suttie, J.W.: Vitamin K and prothrombin synthesis. Nutr. Rev., *31*:105, 1973.

Udall, J.A.: Human sources and absorption of vitamin K in relation to anticoagulation stability. JAMA, *194*:127, 1965.

Vietti, T.J., Stephens, J.C., and Bennett, K.R.: Vitamin K₁ prophylaxis in the newborn. JAMA, *176*:791, 1961.

RIBOFLAVIN

Rivlin, R.S. (ed.): Riboflavin. New York, Plenum Press, 1975.

NIACIN

Roe, D.A.: A Plague of Corn: The Social History of Pellagra. Ithaca, New York, Cornell University Press, 1973.

VITAMIN B₆

Dakshinamurti, K.: Neurobiology of pyridoxine. In Draper, H.H. (ed.): Advances in Nutritional Research. Vol. 4. New York, Plenum Press, 1982.

Jacobs, F.A.: Role of vitamin B₆ in intestinal absorption of amino acids in situ. JAMA, *179*:523, 1962.

Miller, L.T., and Linkswiler, H.M.: Effect of protein intake on the development of abnormal tryptophan metabolism by men during vitamin B₆ depletion. J. Nutr., *93*: 53, 1967.

Vitamin B₆ deficiency and immune responses. Nutr. Rev., *34*: 188, 1976.

PANTOTHENIC ACID

Walsh, J.H., Wyse, B.W., and Hansen, R.G.: Pantothenic acid content of 75 processed and cooked foods. J. Am. Diet. Assoc., *78*:140, 1981.

Wirtschafter, Z.T., and Walsh, J.R.: Hepatocellular lipoid changes in pantothenic acid deficiency. Am. J. Clin. Nutr., *10*:525, 1962.

FOLACIN

Rodriguez, M.S.: A conspectus of research on folacin requirements of man. J. Nutr., *108*:1983, 1978.

Streiff, R.R., and Little, A.B.: Folic acid deficiency in pregnancy. N. Engl. J. Med., *276*:776, 1967.

VITAMIN B₁₂

Drapanas, T., et al.: Role of the ileum in the absorption of vitamin B₁₂ and intrinsic factor (IF). JAMA, *184*:337, 1963.

Herbert, V., et al.: Folic acid and vitamin B₁₂. In Goodhart, R.S., and Shils, M.E. (eds.): Modern Nutrition in Health and Disease. 6th ed. Lea & Febiger, 1980.

Hines, J.D.: Megaloblastic anemia in adult vegan. Am. J. Clin. Nutr., *19*:260, 1966.

VITAMIN C

Hodges, R.E.: The effect of stress on ascorbic acid metabolism in man. Nutr. Today, *5*:11, 1970.

Hodges, R.E., et al.: Experimental scurvy in man. Am. J. Clin. Nutr., *22*:535, 1969.

Schwartz, F.W.: Ascorbic acid in wound healing—a review. J. Am. Diet. Assoc., *56*:497, 1970.

Sherlock, P., and Rothchild, E.O.: Zen diets and scurvy. JAMA, *199*:794, 1967.

Stevenson, N.R.: Active transport of L-ascorbic acid in the human ileum. Gastroenterology, *67*:952, 1974.

Vitamin C toxicity. Nutr. Rev., *34*:236, 1976.

CHAPTER 7

Minerals

DORICE M. CZAJKA-NARINS, Ph.D.

DEFINITION. The term *minerals* means the elements in their simple inorganic form. In nutrition they are commonly referred to as *mineral elements* or, in the case of those present or required in small amounts, *trace elements* or *trace minerals.*

Mineral Composition of the Body

The 22 mineral elements known to be essential in nutrition are listed in Table 7–1. Although the analysis of mineral ash shows the presence of more, for purposes of nutrition the minerals of the body are classified as follows: *macronutrient* elements (> 0.005 per cent body weight: calcium, chloride, magnesium, phosphorus, potassium, sulfur and sodium) and *micronutrient* elements (< 0.005 per cent body weight: arsenic, chromium, cobalt, copper, fluoride, iodine, iron, manganese, molybdenum, nickel, selenium, silicon, tin, vanadium and zinc). There are also traces of barium, bromine, strontium, gold, silver, aluminum, bismuth, gallium and others. Mineral elements exist both in the body and in food in organic and inorganic combinations.

Collectively, about 4 to 5 per cent of body weight is in the form of minerals, compared with approximately 14 to 16 per cent protein and 12 to 20 per cent fat. For a man weighing 70 kg., there are approximately 2.8 kg. of minerals.

Table 7–1. MINERAL ELEMENTS IN HUMAN NUTRITION

(Known or Believed to Be Essential)

I. Macronutrients essential at levels of 100 mg. or more per day

MINERAL	LOCATION IN BODY AND SOME BIOLOGICAL FUNCTIONS	RDA or ESADDI* FOR ADULTS	FOOD SOURCES	COMMENTS ON LIKELIHOOD OF A DEFICIENCY
Calcium	99% in bones and teeth. Ionic calcium in body fluids essential for ion transport across cell membranes. Calcium is also bound to protein, citrate or inorganic acids.	800 mg.	Milk and milk products, sardines, clams, oysters, kale, turnip greens, mustard greens, broccoli.	Dietary surveys indicate that many diets do not meet recommended dietary allowances for calcium. Since bone serves as a homeostatic mechanism to maintain calcium level in blood, many essential functions are maintained, regardless of diet. Long-term dietary deficiency is probably one of the factors responsible for making osteoporosis (bone-thinning) a significant clinical problem.
Phosphorus	About 80% in inorganic phase of bones and teeth. Phosphorus is a component of every cell and of highly important metabolites, including DNA, RNA, ATP (high energy compound), and phospholipids. Important to pH regulation.	800 mg.	Cheese, egg yolk, milk, meat, fish, poultry, whole-grain cereals, legumes, nuts.	Dietary inadequacy not likely to occur if protein and calcium intake is adequate. However, increased need for phosphorus is postulated with diet leading to acid urine and during prolonged therapy with certain antacids.
Magnesium	About 50% in bone. Remaining 50% is almost entirely inside body cells with only about 1% in extracellular fluid. Ionic Mg functions as an activator of many enzymes and must influence almost all processes.	350 mg. for male, 300 mg for female	Whole-grain cereals, nuts, meat, milk, green vegetables, legumes.	Dietary inadequacy considered unlikely, but conditioned deficiency is often seen in clinical medicine, associated with surgery, alcoholism, malabsorption, loss of body fluids, certain hormone and renal diseases, etc. Magnesium deficiency has a profound effect on other animals.
Sodium	30 to 45% in bone. Major cation of extracellular fluid and only a small amount is inside cell. Regulates body fluid osmolarity, pH and body fluid volume.	1100–3300 mg.	Common table salt, seafoods, animal foods, milk, eggs. Abundant in most foods except fruit.	Dietary inadequacy probably never occurs, although low blood sodium requires treatment in certain clinical disorders. Evidence is accumulating that requirements increase during pregnancy. Sodium restriction is practiced in certain cardiovascular disorders.
Chloride	Major anion of extracellular fluid, functioning in combination with sodium; serves as a buffer, enzyme activator; component of gastric hydrochloric acid. Mostly present in extracellular fluid; less than 15% inside cells.	1700–5100 mg.	Common table salt, seafoods, milk, meat, eggs.	In most cases dietary intake is of little significance except in presence of vomiting, diarrhea or profuse sweating, when a deficiency may develop.

Table continued on the following page

145

Table 7-1. MINERAL ELEMENTS IN HUMAN NUTRITION (*Continued*)

(*Known or Believed to Be Essential*)

MINERAL	LOCATION IN BODY AND SOME BIOLOGICAL FUNCTIONS	RDA or ESADDI* FOR ADULTS	FOOD SOURCES	COMMENTS ON LIKELIHOOD OF A DEFICIENCY
I. Macronutrients essential at levels of 100 mg. or more per day (*Continued*)				
Potassium	Major cation of intracellular fluid, with only small amounts in extracellular fluid. Functions in regulating pH and osmolarity, and cell membrane transfer. Ion is necessary for carbohydrate and protein metabolism.	1875–5625 mg.	Fruits, milk, meat, cereals, vegetables, legumes.	Dietary inadequacy unlikely, but conditioned deficiency may be found in kidney disease, diabetic acidosis, excessive vomiting or diarrhea, hyperfunction of adrenal cortex, etc. Potassium excess may be a problem in renal failure and severe acidosis.
Sulfur	Bulk of dietary sulfur is present in sulfur-containing amino acids needed for synthesis of essential metabolites; functions in oxidation-reduction reactions. Sulfur also functions in thiamin and biotin, and as inorganic sulfur.	Need for sulfur is satisfied by essential sulfur-containing amino acids.	Protein foods (meat, fish, poultry, eggs, milk, cheese, legumes, nuts).	Dietary intake is chiefly from sulfur-containing amino acids and adequacy is related to protein intake.
II. Micronutrients essential at levels of a few milligrams				
Iron	About 70% is in hemoglobin; about 26% stored in liver, spleen and bone. Iron is a component of hemoglobin and myoglobin, important in oxygen transfer; also present in serum transferrin and certain enzymes. Almost none in ionic form.	10 mg. for male, 18 mg for female	Liver, meat, egg yolk, legumes, whole or enriched grains, dark green vegetables, dark molasses, shrimp, oysters.	Iron-deficiency anemia occurs in women in reproductive years and in infants and preschool children. May be associated in some cases with unusual blood loss, parasites, and malabsorption.
Zinc	Present in most tissues, with higher amounts in liver, voluntary muscle and bone. Constituent of many enzymes and insulin; of importance in nucleic acid metabolism.	15 mg.	Milk, liver, shellfish, herring, wheat bran (widely distributed).	Extent of dietary inadequacy in this country not known. Conditioned deficiency may be seen in systemic childhood illnesses and in patients who are nutritionally depleted or have been subjected to severe stress, such as surgery.
Copper	Found in all body tissues; larger amounts in liver, brain, heart and kidney. Constituent of enzymes and of ceruloplasmin and erythrocuprein in blood. May be integral part of DNA or RNA molecule.	2–3 mg.	Liver, shellfish, whole grains, cherries, legumes, kidney, poultry, oysters, chocolate, nuts.	No evidence that specific deficiencies of copper occur in the human.

Mineral	Function	Sources	Amount	Comments
Iodine	Constituent of thyroxine and related compounds synthesized by thyroid gland. Thyroxine functions in control of reactions involving cellular energy.	Iodized table salt, seafoods, water and vegetables in nongoitrous regions.	150 µg.	Iodization of table salt is recommended especially in areas where food is low in iodine.
Manganese	Highest concentration is in bone; also relatively high concentrations in pituitary, liver, pancreas and gastrointestinal tissue. Constituent of essential enzyme systems; rich in mitochondria of liver cells.	Beet greens, blueberries, whole grains, nuts, legumes, fruit, tea.	2.5–5.0 mg.	Unlikely that deficiency occurs in humans.
Fluoride	Present in bone. In optimal amounts in water and diet, reduces dental caries and may minimize bone loss.	Drinking water (1 ppm. F1), tea, coffee, rice, soybeans, spinach, gelatin, onions, lettuce.	1.5–4.0 mg.	In areas where fluoride content of water is low, fluoridation of water (1 ppm.) has been found beneficial in reducing incidence of dental caries.
Molybdenum	Constituent of an essential enzyme xanthine oxidase and of flavoproteins.	Legumes, cereal grains, dark green leafy vegetables, organs.	0.15–0.5 mg.	No information.
Cobalt	Constituent of cyanocobalamin (vitamin B_{12}), occurring bound to protein in foods of animal origin. Essential to normal function of all cells, particularly cells of bone marrow, nervous system and gastrointestinal system.	Liver, kidney, oysters, clams, poultry, milk; variable in vegetables and grains—depends upon selenium content of soil.	3.0 µg. of vitamin B_{12}	Primary dietary inadequacy is rare except when no animal products are consumed. Deficiency may be found in such conditions as lack of gastric intrinsic factor, gastrectomy and malabsorption syndromes.
Selenium	Associated with fat metabolism and vitamin E.	Grains, onions, meats, milk, vegetables variable—depends upon selenium content of soil.	0.05–0.2 mg.	No known deficiency disease seen in man.
Chromium	Associated with glucose metabolism.	Corn oil, clams, wholegrain cereals, meats, drinking water variable.	0.05–0.2 mg.	Deficiency found in severe malnutrition, diabetes and cardiovascular diseases.
Arsenic Tin Nickel Vanadium Silicon	Now known to be essential but no RDA or ESADDI established.			

*RDA = Recommended Dietary Allowances.
ESADDI = Estimated Safe and Adequate Daily Dietary Intakes.

CLASSIFICATION

The minerals are found in the body and in food chiefly in their ionic form. Metals form positive ions (cations); non-metals form negative ions (anions). Sodium, potassium and calcium are cations. Non-metals forming anions include chlorine, sulfur (as sulfate) and phosphorus (as phosphate). Sodium chloride and calcium phosphate are typical salts. In bones and teeth the minerals are found as the fixed salts, primarily of calcium and phosphorus. In solution the salts dissociate and are found in body fluids as Na^+, K^+, Ca^{++}, Cl^- and $H_2PO_4^-$.

The minerals are also organic compounds such as phosphoproteins, phospholipids and hemoglobin. The hormone thyroxine contains four atoms of iodine. Phosphorus has been shown to occur in carbohydrates, fats and proteins; and sulfur has been shown to be an integral part of some amino acids and enzymes.

FUNCTIONS

Mineral elements have many essential roles, both in their ionic forms in solution in body fluids and as constituents of essential compounds. The balance of mineral ions in body fluids regulates the metabolism of many enzymes, maintains acid-base balance and osmotic pressure, facilitates membrane transfer of essential compounds, and maintains nerve and muscular irritability, and in some cases mineral ions are building constituents of body tissue. Indirectly many minerals are involved in the growth process.

Although the various minerals will be discussed individually, nutrients cannot be considered separately with respect to their utilization and requirement since they influence each other.

REQUIREMENTS

The requirements for mineral elements vary greatly. Some elements, such as calcium and phosphorus, are required in amounts exceeding 100 mg. per day. Others, such as iron and zinc, are required in amounts less than 20 mg. per day.

The importance of many minerals has long been established and appreciated; however, new functions have been identified for some of these minerals. The role of other minerals, particularly some of the more recently recognized trace minerals, is not clear, and since even the number of required minerals is not known, there is much need for additional work.

Special care must be taken to assure that individuals in high-risk populations, such as children under two years of age and pregnant women, meet their increased need for minerals during these periods. Times of stress, trauma, surgery and multiple drug administration also require special attention to mineral needs.

The Food and Nutrition Board of the National Research Council has established recommended intakes for calcium, chloride, potassium, phosphorus, sodium, sulfur, iodine, iron, magnesium and zinc. For chromium, copper, fluoride, manganese, molybdenum and selenium, safe and adequate dietary intakes have been estimated and are given in Table 7–1. Specific recommendations are not yet established for the other minerals because of the lack of sufficient information upon which to base the recommendation. A varied or mixed diet of animal and vegetable products that meets energy and protein needs will also furnish adequate intake of minerals with well-understood functions as well as of those whose functions are not known. In those circumstances in which oral intake is diminished or nil, such as during extended periods of total parenteral nutrition (see Chapter 35), there is great potential for mineral deficiency.

SOURCES

Most minerals are obtained from foods in which they exist as salts and organic compounds. The exception is sodium chloride (table salt), which is used as a condiment or a preservative. Highly processed foods and foods such as sugar contain few minerals. The mineral content of food is determined by first destroying the organic matter with heat and/or acid and analyzing the ash by flame photometry or atomic absorption spectroscopy.

Macronutrients Essential at Levels of 100 Milligrams or More per Day for Adult Humans

CALCIUM AND PHOSPHORUS

Calcium and phosphorus are frequently considered together because they are so closely related in the body. They are discussed here separately to emphasize their independent roles as well as their association in the way they function together in the body. The normal metabolism of calcium and phosphorus is maintained by a number of physiological mechanisms.

Calcium

The body needs calcium throughout life, but especially during periods of growth, pregnancy and lactation. According to the data obtained during the Public Health Services Health and Nutrition Examination Surveys (HANES I and II) and illustrated in Figure 7–1, males of all ages have higher intakes of calcium than females.[11] Between ages 18 and 35, 60 to 70 per cent of the males surveyed had intakes exceeding the RDA and 75 per cent consumed at least 500 mg. per day. For women the picture is not as good. Half the women over age 15 consumed less than the RDA; by age 35 the proportion of women consuming less than the RDA had increased to 75 per cent.

Calcium is the most abundant mineral in the body. The average adult male has about 1200 grams of calcium and the average adult female 1000 grams. It makes up about 1.5 to 2.0 per cent of the body weight and 39 per cent of the total minerals present; 99 per cent of it is in the hard tissues, bones and teeth. The other 1 per cent is present in the blood and extracellular fluids and within the cells of soft tissues where it regulates many important metabolic functions.

In the bones, calcium occurs in the form of salts. *Hydroxyapatite,* composed of calcium phosphate and calcium carbonate arranged in a characteristic crystal structure around a framework of softer protein material (organic matrix), provides strength and rigidity to the soft matrix. Many other ions are also present in this crystal complex, including fluoride, magnesium, zinc and sodium. Blood vessels, lymph vessels, nerves and bone marrow pass through the matrix and between the crystal structures. The mineral ions diffuse into the extracellular fluid, bathing the crystals and permitting deposition of new mineral or its absorption from bones.

The same type of crystals are present in the enamel and dentin of teeth; however, the crystals are larger. There is little turnover of calcium in teeth; i.e., the calcium or phosphate is not readily available during periods of deprivation.

In the skeleton calcium exists in two chemically and physically distinct forms: a relatively *non-exchangeable* calcium component not available for short-term regulation of calcium homeostasis, and a rapidly *exchangeable* component used for metabolic activities. This calcium is part of the most recently deposited surface bone, which together with the calcium entering from the diet helps to maintain the serum levels within a defined range. The rapidly exchangeable component of the bone may be considered a reserve that may be built up when the dietary provides an adequate intake of calcium. This reserve is stored, especially in the trabeculae, the ends of the long bones. This calcium may be mobilized to meet the body's increased need (growth, pregnancy, lactation), if

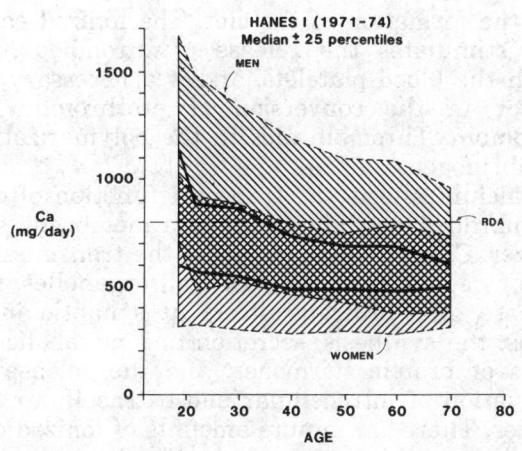

Figure 7–1. Median calcium intake of men and women ages 18 to 70. Values were derived from HANES I survey. Shaded areas represent the 25th to 75th percentiles. HANES II and Food Consumption Surveys show similar patterns. (From Heaney, R. P., et al.: Calcium nutrition and bone health in the elderly. Am. J. Clin. Nutr., *36*:986, 1982.)

calcium is not supplied in adequate amounts by the food intake. If there is no reserve, the calcium must be drawn from the more stable bone substance itself, which must be broken down before calcium is liberated. This results in a deficiency in the bone structure following prolonged inadequate intake. As it is with most components in the body, bone is constantly being synthesized and resorbed. Depending upon the physiological state or age of the individual, one aspect of the process may predominate. In children, for example, bone synthesis is greater than the destruction of bone. In the normal adult these processes are in balance; approximately 600 to 700 mg. of calcium enter and leave the bones every day. In later adult life bone is lost as resorption predominates. Adult bone loss begins during the fifth decade in both sexes, but progresses more rapidly in the female as discussed on page 153 and in Chapter 33. Sixty per cent of serum calcium is ionized and physiologically active. Forty per cent is non-ionized and physiologically inert—35 per cent bound to protein, and 5 per cent as the calcium salts of citrate, bicarbonate and phosphate. A significant increase in serum calcium can cause cardiac or respiratory failure and a decrease causes tetany. Circadian rhythms of ionized calcium concentration have been demonstrated in human blood.

FUNCTIONS. In addition to the major function of calcium to build and maintain bones and teeth, it is also important metabolically for the activity of certain enzymes, notably adenosine triphosphatase in the release of energy for muscular contraction, and for the activity of cyclic AMP. In the blood clotting process, calcium must be present to initiate the changes needed for the formation of the clot. The ionized calcium stimulates the release of thromboplastin from the blood platelets, and is a necessary cofactor in the conversion of prothrombin to thrombin. Thrombin aids in the polymerization of fibrinogen to fibrin.

Calcium affects the transport function of cell membranes, possibly acting as a membrane stabilizer. Calcium also influences the transmission of ions across membranes of cell organelles, the release of neurotransmitters at synaptic junctions, the synthesis, secretion and metabolic effects of protein hormones, and the release or activation of intracellular and extracellular enzymes. There are minute amounts of ionized calcium as a phosphate salt in the mitochondria and endoplasmic reticulum.

Calcium is required in nerve transmission and regulation of heart beat. The proper balance of calcium, sodium, potassium and magnesium ions maintains muscle tone and controls irritability.

ABSORPTION AND UTILIZATION. Usually only 20 to 30 per cent of ingested calcium, and sometimes as little as 10 per cent, is absorbed. Calcium is absorbed mainly in the duodenum in an acid medium, and its absorption is much reduced in the lower part of the intestinal tract when the food content becomes alkaline. However, evidence is accumulating to suggest that absorption of calcium is not limited to the small intestine. The fibrous plant cell wall contains calcium that becomes available only when the structure is digested by microbial fermentation in the colon and the calcium is changed into an available form. Calcium is absorbed by active transport requiring energy and by passive diffusion. The amount absorbed depends largely upon the nature of the diet. Calcium will be absorbed only if it is present in a water-soluble form in the intestine and is not precipitated by another dietary constituent. Unabsorbed calcium is excreted in the feces. Many factors influence the actual amount of calcium absorbed.

Factors That Increase Calcium Absorption

VITAMIN D Vitamin D in its active form $1,25(OH)_2D_3$ stimulates intestinal absorption of calcium through a complex series of steps including transfer of calcium across the mucosal bruch border.

ACIDITY OF GASTRIC JUICES. The hydrochloric acid secreted in the stomach lowers the pH of the contents of the digestive tract in the small intestine and favors calcium absorption.

LACTOSE. In humans with normal lactase, calcium absorption is enhanced by lactose. Although the exact mode of action is unknown, one hypothesis suggests that a relatively high ratio of lactose to calcium permits the formation of a sugar-calcium complex in the intestine that keeps the calcium in the form in which it can be transported to and across the intestinal mucosa.[2] Alternatively, the lactose-calcium complex may possibly prevent the precipitation of an insoluble calcium complex as the contents of the intestinal tract change from acid to alkaline. In humans with lactase deficiency, lactose inhibits calcium absorption.

FAT. When fat is present in moderate amounts, transit time through the digestive tract increases, allowing more time for mineral absorption.

PROTEIN INTAKE. When the intake of protein is high, a greater percentage of calcium is absorbed than when the intake of protein is low. The action of certain amino acids upon intestinal pH and upon the formation of the soluble complex with calcium facilitates calcium absorption.

PHYSIOLOGICAL STATE. The body absorbs more effectively when in need. The greater the need and the smaller the dietary supply, the more efficient the absorption. During periods of growth, absorption is increased. Efficiency of absorption decreases after middle age owing in part to a drop in circulating levels of $1,25(OH)_2D_3$. In elderly individuals, the adaptive response of increased absorption of calcium to decreased intake is blunted.

Factors That Decrease Calcium Absorption

VITAMIN D DEFICIENCY. Lack of or insufficient amount of vitamin D in its active form $1,25(OH)_2D_3$ decreases or prevents the absorption of calcium.

FATS. The excretion of large amounts of calcium in the feces of patients with steatorrhea suggests that diets high in fat might affect calcium absorption. Studies in humans and animals have produced conflicting data. The effect may depend on the kind of fat in the diet.[49]

OXALIC ACID. The calcium availability from some fruits and vegetables depends upon the amount of oxalic acid they contain. In the digestive tract oxalic acid combines with calcium to form an insoluble compound, calcium oxalate, so that the calcium is not absorbed. Rhubarb, spinach, chard and beet greens contain oxalic acid in appreciable amounts.

PHYTIC ACID. Phytic acid, a phosphorus-containing compound found principally in the outer husks of cereal grains (especially oatmeal), combines with calcium to form calcium phytate, which is insoluble and is not absorbed from the intestines.

FIBER. There is some evidence that fiber itself, not just the phytate associated with it, may decrease calcium absorption from the small intestine.

ALKALINE MEDIUM. In an alkaline medium, calcium (and phosphorus) will form insoluble and non-absorbable calcium phosphate.

GASTROINTESTINAL MOTILITY. When the food passes through the intestinal tract too rapidly, calcium absorption is decreased.

IMMOBILIZATION. Lack of exercise and lack of weight-bearing on the legs cause a decrease in the ability to absorb calcium.

STRESS. Emotional instability may influence the efficiency of calcium absorption. Mental stress tends to decrease absorption and increase excretion of calcium. Under distress, emotional or physical, a higher intake of calcium is required to maintain calcium equilibrium. Whether increased calcium intake during times of stress will prevent losses has not been clearly shown.

DRUGS. Long-term use of thiazide diuretics results in decreased calcium absorption, which may be due to decreased plasma calcitriol levels.[11] Aluminum-containing drugs result in hypercalciuria and bone resorption, which may contribute to bone disease.[50]

CALCIUM-PHOSPHORUS RATIO. High levels of phosphorus in the diet or at least a high ratio of phosphorus to calcium has been suggested as a factor that contributes to the development of osteoporosis. However, the importance of either the level of phosphorus or the ratio of phosphorus to calcium is not clear at this time. Consumption of 2.0 gm. or less of phosphorus daily does not appear to affect bone or calcium metabolism provided the intake of calcium is adequate. Unfortunately, adequate intake of calcium, particularly for women, is not now well defined.

MAINTENANCE OF SERUM CALCIUM LEVEL. Calcium is transported by the blood to the fluids bathing the tissues of the body and to the cells wherever needed. Most of the calcium is used in the bones. The calcium in the bones is in equilibrium with calcium in the blood. *Parathormone*, the hormone secreted by the parathyroid gland, and *calcitonin*, secreted chiefly by the thyroid gland, keep the serum calcium at a normal concentration of about 10 mg. per 100 ml. of blood serum. When it falls below this level, parathormone causes a transfer of exchangeable calcium from the bone into the blood. At the same time the parathyroid causes the kidney to reabsorb calcium that normally might be excreted in the urine and it stimulates more absorption of calcium from the intestines. When the blood calcium level is above normal, calcitonin acts to lower it by inhibiting further bone resorption, and since the processes of renal ex-

cretion and endogenous fecal secretion continue, the net effect is to lower serum calcium.

EXCRETION. Normally most of the ingested calcium (65 to 75 per cent) is excreted in the feces and urine. Fecal calcium correlates with intake. Consumption of high-protein diets appears to impair the ability of the kidney to reabsorb calcium. Urinary calcium 2 to 4 hours after the meal was significantly higher in subjects fed meals containing 54 gm. of protein than in subjects fed 18 gm. of protein.[1] One proposed mechanism of this effect is a change in acid-base balance that would necessitate the use of bone calcium as a buffering agent.[15, 55]

There are also some dermal losses—1 to 2 per cent—of which one third is from body fluids and two thirds from the skin itself. The loss of calcium in sweat is about 15 mg. per day. Strenuous physical activity will increase loss even in persons on a low intake. In cases of excessive urine excretion of calcium, calcium kidney stones may develop.

DIETARY SOURCES. Milk and milk products are the best sources of calcium; 8 ounces of milk (whole or non-fat) supplies about 288 to 298 mg. of calcium. It is difficult to meet the RDA for calcium without milk or milk products. Dark green leafy vegetables such as kale, turnip greens, mustard greens and broccoli, and sardines, clams and oysters are good sources of calcium.

Infants can easily meet the calcium intake because milk is their chief food. Children can best meet the requirement by including the amount of milk recommended for each age group (Table 10–8), or its equivalent, daily. Table 7–2 shows the calcium content of selected foods.

RECOMMENDED DIETARY ALLOWANCE. Most of the data regarding calcium requirements for man have been obtained from calcium balance studies. (A controversy exists regarding the interpretation of the data and the use of the balance studies as a basis for requirements.) These studies measure the intake and output of calcium over periods of time. To determine the minimum calcium requirement, the calcium intake is reduced until the person can no longer remain in balance (i.e., his excretion becomes greater than his intake). It is evident from these studies that man, if given time to adjust to changes in levels, can remain in calcium balance over a very wide range of calcium intakes. Man has been shown to adapt and maintain calcium balance on intakes as low as 200 to 400 mg. per day.

The 1980 revision of the RDA by the National Research Council recommends 800 mg. of calcium per day in view of the high levels of protein and phosphorus provided by the U.S. diet. This

Table 7–2. CALCIUM AND PHOSPHORUS CONTENT OF FOODS

FOOD	AVERAGE SERVING		
	APPROXI-MATE MEASURE	MILLIGRAMS OF CALCIUM	MILLIGRAMS OF PHOS-PHORUS
Peanuts, roasted, with skins	⅔ cup	69	391
Turkey, roasted, flesh only	3 oz.	7	213
Fish (halibut, broiled with butter or margarine)	4.5 oz.	20	310
Pork loin, broiled, med. fat	2 oz.	7	181
Milk, nonfat (skim), fluid	1 glass (8 oz.)	296	233
Milk, whole, fluid	1 glass (8 oz.)	288	227
Chicken, roasted	3⅓ oz.	12	242
Loin lamb chop, broiled	3⅓ oz.	9	163
Beef, hamburger, cooked (reg. ground)	3 oz.	10	196
Oysters, raw	6 oysters	81	123
Cheese, cheddar	1 oz.	213	136
Peas, cooked	⅔ cup	25	105
Egg, poached	1 large	51	121
Wheat cereal, flakes	1 cup	12	83
Sweet corn, canned, vacuum packed	⅔ cup	4	102
Spinach, cooked	½ cup, packed	89	34
Bread, white, enriched	1 slice	21	24

From Agriculture Handbook Number 456. U.S. Dept. of Agriculture, Washington D.C., 1975.

amount covers basic needs and allows for a margin of safety. These allowances are greater than those recommended by the FAO/WHO Expert Group, whose report concludes that intakes of 400 to 500 mg. per day would represent a suggested practical allowance for adults. The Committee felt that the usefulness of exceeding this has not been proved, and that this level can more readily be achieved by a larger segment of the world's population since sources of calcium are limited in the national food supply of many countries.

The National Research Council justifies the allowance of 800 mg. on the basis that calcium losses in metabolism amount to approximately 320 mg. per day. Since only 20 to 30 per cent of the dietary calcium is absorbed, 800 mg. would be required to maintain balance. Also, food sources of calcium are readily available to the population of the United States.

The need for calcium is increased during pregnancy and lactation. An increase in calcium is needed for the calcification of fetal bones and teeth and for the storage of calcium by the mother to meet the demands of lactation. The RDA includes an additional 400 mg. of calcium daily to meet the demands of the fetus and mother. Indications are that the pregnant woman may absorb up to 40 per cent of dietary calcium, depending on the need.

The amount needed by the lactating mother is 400 mg. daily over normal requirements in order to provide adequate calcium in milk without causing depletion of the mother's calcium reserve or a decrease in milk production. Since some women with a high production of milk may lose nearly 1 gm. per day of calcium directly via the milk, calcium intakes must be adjusted on the basis of individual milk secretion.

During these periods of increased dietary needs for calcium the growing fetus or nursing child will satisfy his need for calcium at the mother's expense. If her dietary intake is deficient, presumably the mother will lose bone calcium. However, decreased bone density has also been noted in newborn infants whose mothers had diets deficient in calcium (as well as energy and protein) during pregnancy.[24]

The calcium requirement of the infant is not precisely known. A breast-fed infant receives about 60 mg. of calcium per kilogram of body weight and retains about two thirds of this amount. An infant fed a standard cow's milk formula receives about three times this amount of calcium per kilogram of body weight, and retains 25 to 30 per cent. The National Research Council recommends 60 mg. of calcium per kilogram of body weight or 360 mg. for infants from birth to 6 months of age and 540 mg. for 6 months to a year of age. It is assumed that the calcium needs of the breast-fed infant have been met even though calcium intake is considerably less than that obtained from a diet of cow's milk.

Children from ages 1 to 10 years need 800 mg. of calcium daily. From 11 to 18 years of age the recommendation for males and females is 1200 mg. daily.

DEFICIENCY. Four clinical problems, rickets, osteomalacia, osteoporosis and scurvy, are characterized by abnormalities of calcium in structural bone. Rickets, osteomalacia and scurvy are discussed in detail in Chapter 6 under deficiencies of vitamins D and C. Two other clinical problems, tetany and hypertension, may be related to abnormalities of ionized calcium.

Calcium deficiency in children may lead to *rickets* with retarded growth or, more likely, continued body growth, but with abnormal development of bones resulting in bowed legs and other bone deformities. Deficiency of calcium in adults may result in *osteomalacia* (sometimes referred to as adult rickets), a failure to mineralize the bone matrix, resulting in a reduction in the mineral content of the bone. Usually, rickets and osteomalacia are associated with a concurrent lack of vitamin D and imbalance in the calcium-phosphorus intake. In scurvy, the lack of ascorbic acid prevents the formation of bone matrix and normal mineralization does not occur.

Osteoporosis. This is a metabolic disorder that may be defined as a reduction in the amount of bone without any changes in its chemical composition. With bone loss, skeletal strength cannot be maintained and fractures occur with minimal stress. Osteoporosis (deossification) is frequently confused with osteomalacia (demineralization). Whether deficient calcium intake is a factor in the etiology of osteoporosis is not clear. A person with osteoporosis is in negative calcium balance and may have a daily calcium loss as high as 90 mg./day.[35] Over a lifetime this could result in a significant loss of skeleton. Other factors, such as decreased calcium absorption with aging, level of protein intake, the dietary calcium: phosphorus ratio, impaired renal function with aging, exercise and estrogen level, are also important in the development of osteoporosis. These are discussed further on page 674.

Tetany. Extremely low levels of calcium in the blood may increase the irritability of nerve fibers and nerve centers and result in muscle spasms such as leg cramps, a condition known as *tetany*. It sometimes occurs in pregnant women who have received too little calcium in their diets or who have received too much phosphorus. (The latter is responsible for hastening the excretion of calcium during pregnancy.) The rise in serum phosphorus causes a compensatory decrease in serum calcium. Tetany sometimes occurs in newborn infants fed undiluted cow's milk, which contains more phosphorus than calcium. The kidneys of the infants cannot clear the excess phosphate.

Hypertension. Recently abnormalities of extracellular and intracellular calcium metabolism have been identified in both humans and animals with hypertension. Epidemiological studies indicate an inverse correlation between the calcium content of the drinking water and mean arterial pressure. Early studies of intake reveal that patients with hypertension consume as much fluid milk as normotensive patients, but much less of other dairy products.[29] Furthermore, high sodium intake is associated with calciuresis. Additional information is needed, but data suggest a note of caution regarding dietary restrictions and the hazards of linking a single nutrient to a complex problem. See page 558 for further discussion.

TOXICITY. A very high intake of calcium and the presence of a high intake of vitamin D such as may occur in children receiving supplements is a potential source of *hypercalcemia* (elevated blood calcium levels). This may lead to widespread excessive calcification not only in bone but also in the soft tissues such as kidneys.

Phosphorus

Phosphorus is one of the most essential elements, but it receives little attention from nutritionists since it is a universal cell component available in all foods. Second to calcium in abundance, it comprises 22 per cent of the total minerals in the body. The bulk of phosphorus (about 80 per cent) is present as insoluble calcium phosphate (apatite) crystals in bones and teeth. The other 20 per cent is very active metabolically and is distributed in every cell in the body and in the extracellular fluid in combination with carbohydrates, lipids, protein and a variety of other compounds.

The serum inorganic phosphorus is closely maintained at levels of 3 to 4 mg./100 ml. in adults. Levels in infants are somewhat higher.

FUNCTIONS. In addition to its structural role, phosphorus has numerous functions, more than any other mineral element. A complete discussion would require consideration of every metabolic process in the body. Phosphorus is an essential component of nucleic acids, and phospholipids are key components in the structure of cell membranes. Glucose is phosphorylated as the first step in its utilization and at other steps. High-energy phosphate compounds play a central role in many reactions, as does cyclic AMP. Phosphorus is part of some conjugated proteins, for example, casein from milk. Many of the B vitamins function as coenzymes only when in combination with phosphate. The phosphate buffer system is important particularly in intracellular fluid, where its concentration is much higher than in extracellular fluid, and in the tubular fluids of the kidney.

ABSORPTION. In older children and adults absorption from mixed diets varies between 50 and 70 per cent. Infants absorb more than 85 per cent from human milk and 65 to 75 per cent from cow's milk. Most favorable absorption of inorganic phosphate takes place when calcium and phosphorus are ingested in approximately equal amounts. This makes milk a good source since calcium and phosphorus are present in equal amounts, as shown in Table 7–2. As with calcium, the presence of vitamin D increases absorption. Simple phosphates such as calcium phosphate or potassium sodium phosphate are absorbed as such in the small intestine. In the digestion of complex compounds, phosphate is split off and absorbed. The factors that aid or deter the absorption of calcium act essentially in the same manner with regard to the absorption of phosphate. Phosphorus is present as phytic acid in some cereals and flours. If bread made from the flour is unleavened, the phytic acid can complex calcium, iron and zinc and depress their absorption. During the leavening process the phosphorus of phytic acid is converted to orthophosphate.

DIETARY SOURCES. In the U.S., the average daily intake of phosphorus by adults is approximately 1500 to 1600 mg. Meat, poultry, fish and eggs are excellent sources of phosphorus. Milk and milk products are good sources, as are nuts and legumes. Cereals and grains are good sources, but availability of the phosphorus as well as its effect on calcium absorption has been questioned because of the phytic acid, as explained previously. Table 7–2 shows the phosphorus content of average servings of various foods. Note that the good sources of protein are also good sources of phosphorus. Additives contribute about 20 to 30 per cent of the phosphorus consumed by the average adult. Some forms of polyphosphate additives are not hydrolyzed in the human gut. Therefore, orthophosphate and polyphosphate additives may differ in their biological effect.

RECOMMENDED DIETARY ALLOWANCE. The Food and Nutrition Board recommends that the daily intake of phosphorus approximately equal that of calcium for all age groups except the young infant. The phosphorus allowances for infants to one year of age are slightly less than those for calcium (see Table 10–1). Current evidence supports the recommendation that in infancy the calcium:phosphorus ratio in the diet be 1.15:1, decreasing to 1:1 at one year of age. Because phosphorus is so liberally distributed in foods, there is little possibility of a dietary inadequacy if the food intake contains adequate protein and calcium.

DEFICIENCY. Phosphorus depletion has long been recognized in animals, but only recently has it been described in man in various disease states. The widespread, severe and ultimately fatal consequences of phosphorus depletion result from its widespread function, and are primarily the result of a decrease in ATP synthesis and other organic phosphate compounds. There are neuromuscular, skeletal, hematological and renal manifestations. Clinical phosphate depletion and hypophosphatemia are associated with administration of glucose or total parenteral nutrition without sufficient phosphate, excessive use of phosphate-binding antacids, hyperparathyroidism, treatment of diabetic acidosis, alcoholism in patients with or without decompensated liver disease and other conditions.[25] Parenteral phosphate should be given for critically depleted patients; other patients can be given oral phosphate therapy. Premature infants weighing less than 1000 gm. who are fed human milk develop hypophosphatemia. Phosphorus supplementation resolves the abnormalities.[40]

SULFUR

Sulfur occurs principally as a constituent of the amino acids cystine, cysteine and methionine. It is present in all proteins but is most prevalent in the keratin of skin and hair (4 to 6 per cent sulfur) and in insulin (3.2 per cent sulfur). Glutathione, a tripeptide containing cysteine, is important in cellular reactions involving the sulfur amino acids in protein. Sulfur exists in a reduced form ($-SH$) in cysteine and in an oxidized form ($-S-S-$) as the double molecule, cystine. This is important in the specific configuration of some proteins and in the activity of some enzymes. Sulfur also occurs in carbohydrates such as heparin, an anticoagulant found in liver and some other tissues, and chondroitin sulfate in bone and cartilage. Two vitamins, thiamin and biotin, contain sulfur. The poisonous effects of arsenic are due to its ability to combine with sulfhydryl groups.

MAGNESIUM

The adult human contains approximately 20 to 28 grams of magnesium. Approximately 60 per cent is found in bone, 26 per cent in muscle, and the remainder in soft tissues and body fluids. Normal serum levels are usually in the range of 1.5 to 2.1 mEq. per liter. It is second to potassium as an intracellular cation. About half of the magnesium, including most in bone, is not exchangeable.

FUNCTIONS. Magnesium is essential for the production and transfer of energy for protein synthesis, for contractility of muscle and excitability in nerves, and as a cofactor in numerous enzyme systems related to other functions. Magnesium and calcium, having similar functions, may antagonize each other. An excess amount of magnesium will inhibit bone calcification. Calcium and magnesium also play antagonistic roles in normal muscle contraction, calcium acting as a stimulator and magnesium as a relaxer. An excessive amount of calcium may induce signs typical of magnesium deficiency.

A review of the role of magnesium in ischemic heart disease suggests that therapeutic use in the acute phase may be justified. Its usefulness is best explained by its metabolic effect within the cell, but the interrelationship with lipid metabolism and coagulation-fibrinolytic mechanisms may also be significant. The use of magnesium to inhibit atherogenesis or prevent ischemic heart disease or both requires further study.[46] It has also been shown that diets high in magnesium are partially effective in preventing the deposition of oxalate stones in the kidneys of rats deficient in vitamin B_6. This is discussed further on page 629.

ABSORPTION AND EXCRETION. The rate of absorption of magnesium ranges from 24 to 85 per cent. The factors that increase the absorption of magnesium from the upper intestine are similar to those governing calcium absorption, but vitamin D has no effect on magnesium absorption. The presence of fat, phytates, and calcium decreases magnesium absorption. As dietary calcium is reduced, magnesium absorption is increased.

The kidney conserves magnesium efficiently. Renal reabsorption tends to vary inversely with that of calcium.

DIETARY SOURCES. Magnesium intake varies widely. The average range for healthy adults in the United States and Western Europe is estimated to be 15 to 40 mEq. per day. The ordinary diet is generally believed to provide adequate amounts of magnesium, since it occurs abundantly in foods, particularly nuts, legumes, cereal grains and dark-green vegetables, where it is an essential constituent of chlorophyll. Other sources are seafood, cocoa and chocolate. High calcium, protein, vitamin D and alcohol intakes all function to increase the requirement (particularly in those on low magnesium intake). Physical or psychological stress can also increase magnesium needs.

RECOMMENDED DIETARY ALLOWANCE. Based on balance studies, the recommendation by the National Research Council (1980 revision) is 350 mg. per day for adult males and 300 mg. per day for adult females. For pregnant or lactating women the recommended allowance is 450 mg. per day. The recommended allowances for children have been estimated from the magnesium content of human milk (4 mg. per 100 ml.) and cow's milk (12 mg. per 100 ml.). Allowances for children and adolescents are only estimates, but they are intended to allow for increased needs during rapid bone growth. The allowances range from 50 to 250 mg. per day (see Table 10–1).

DEFICIENCY. Magnesium deficiency is clinically manifested by anorexia, growth failure, ECG changes and neuromuscular changes, and may develop under conditions of stress and in the course of disease. A deficiency may precipitate from any condition in which there is a decreased intake or increased loss of magnesium or a shift in electrolyte balance.

The hypomagnesemic tetany syndrome is reported to be almost identical to hypocalcemic tetany (see page 153) but can be differentiated chemically. Prominent signs are depression, muscular weakness, vertigo and tendency to convulsions. Administration of magnesium promptly relieves the symptoms. Patients observed with this syndrome all have a dietary inadequacy. In addition, one or more of the following factors are present: (1) excessive loss of magnesium from persistent vomiting or from removal of intestinal contents by mechanical suction, (2) intestinal malabsorption, or (3) administration of large amounts of magnesium-free parenteral fluids to postsurgical patients. Treatment with intramuscular magnesium sulfate promptly reverses the condition.

Conditions in which acute deficiencies may develop are renal disease, diuretic therapy, malabsorption, hyperthyroidism, acute alcoholism, kwashiorkor, diabetes, parathyroid gland disorders, postsurgical stress, and vitamin D–resistant rickets in patients who are receiving massive doses of the vitamin.[3]

SODIUM, CHLORINE AND POTASSIUM

These three indispensable dietary constituents are so intimately related in the body that it is most convenient to discuss them together. Sodium constitutes 2 per cent, potassium 5 per cent and chloride 3 per cent of the total mineral content of the body. They are distributed ubiquitously throughout all body fluids and tissues, but sodium and chloride are primarily extracellular elements, while potassium is mainly an intracellular element. Sodium, potassium, and chloride are involved in at least four important physiological functions of the body:

1. Maintenance of normal water balance and distribution.

2. Maintenance of normal osmotic equilibrium.

3. Maintenance of normal acid-base balance.

4. Maintenance of normal muscular irritability.

All three elements are readily absorbed through the intestinal tract and are excreted through the urine, feces and sweat. These minerals are widely found in nature and in the ordinary diet. In a healthy person there is little chance of an occurrence of deficiency, but there is a chance of excess, particularly of sodium.

Hormonal control of sodium, potassium and chloride balance is mediated through the adrenal cortex hormones and hormones of the anterior pituitary gland. An example of this important regulatory function is seen in Addison's disease, in which there is a decreased secretion of the adrenal cortex hormones with consequent sodium chloride loss and potassium retention by the body, causing weakness, muscle cramps, weight loss and other symptoms. The symptoms can be dramatically alleviated by giving sodium chloride alone or with adrenal cortex extract.

Because sodium, potassium and chloride primarily function as electrolytes, they will be discussed more completely in Chapter 8.

Micronutrients or Trace Elements

Certain elements, although present in minute amounts in the tissue, are as essential to optimal growth and development as those required in larger amounts. Inadequate intake may impair cellular and physiological function or cause illness. Trace elements were so named because they were not easily quantified by early analytical methods. The recent development of instruments with increased sensitivity has enabled investigators to study the role of these micronutrients or trace elements more carefully.

A broad definition of essential trace elements is widely accepted: "An element is essential when a deficient intake consistently results in an impairment of a function from optimal to suboptimal and when supplementation with physiological levels of this element, but not others, prevents or cures this impairment."[30] Essentiality must be demonstrated by more than one independent investigator and in more than one species before that trace mineral is generally accepted as essential.

Those elements fulfilling the requirements for essentiality are arsenic, chromium, cobalt, copper, fluoride, iodine, iron, manganese, molybdenum, nickel, selenium, silicon, tin, vanadium and zinc. Each element exhibits a spectrum of actions that depends on the dosage and nutritional state of the recipient with respect to the element. Increasing amounts evoke an increasing biological response until a plateau is reached. Larger intakes may produce pharmacological actions, and still larger intakes may produce toxic effects. For example, the toxic effects of fluoride and selenium were known before these elements were identified as essential nutrients.

The 1980 RDA includes a new table (Table 10–2) containing three vitamins and nine minerals that do not appear in Table 10–1 because allowances cannot be established on the basis of present knowledge. Ranges for appropriate intakes of the electrolytes sodium, potassium and chloride, and for trace elements copper, manganese, fluoride, chromium, selenium and molybdenum are given in Table 10–2. It is recommended that the upper limits of safe intake of the trace elements not be habitually exceeded, as this could lead to toxic effects.

FUNCTIONS OF MICRONUTRIENTS

Essential trace elements are constituents of or interact with larger molecules, such as enzymes or hormones. Many enzymes require a small amount of a trace metal for full activity. Metals function in enzymes by: (1) direct participation in catalysis; (2) combination with substrate to form a complex upon which the enzyme acts; (3) formation of a metalloenzyme that binds substrates; (4) combination with a reaction product; and (5) maintenance of quaternary structure. In vitro, one trace element can frequently replace another with little loss of enzyme activity. In vivo, there is high specificity possibly regulated by carriers with specific sites that transport a particular trace mineral to its own site of action.

The effect of essential trace elements is amplified by their interaction with the larger enzymes or hormone molecules that regulate masses of substrate. If, in turn, the substrate has some regulatory function, there is further amplification of the effect of the trace element. This is a mechanism by which the minute concentrations of trace minerals can affect the whole body.

ABSORPTION AND TRANSPORT

Absorption occurs in and is regulated at the mucosa of the small intestine. It occurs in three stages: the intraluminal stage, the translocation stage and the mobilization stage. The *intraluminal stage* consists of the chemical reactions and interactions in the stomach and intestines. These reactions are dominated by the pH of the luminal contents and the composition of the food entering from the stomach. Small anionic elements, such as fluoride, are essentially not influenced by either pH or the composition of the diet and are therefore absorbed quite freely. The cationic forms of the transition elements are, however, frequently affected by both pH and the composition of the diet. These cations are soluble in the acidic pH of the stomach, but form insoluble hydroxides when the chyme passes into the small intestine and the pH rises. These cations are frequently kept available for absorption by ligands that form coordination or chelation compounds with the elements. This is an important determinant in the concept of bioavailability. The coordination complexes or chelates may be absorbed directly or they may be cleaved at the surface of the mucosal cell just prior to absorption across the cell membrane. Amino acids and other organic acids and sugars are examples of important ligands.

The *translocation stage* involves diffusion or transport of the trace element across the membrane of the intestinal cell. For small anions the mechanism may be simple diffusion. For most cationic elements, the mechanism may be either facilitated diffusion or active transport, both of which are saturable. For at least one mineral, calcium, a hormone is involved in the translocation process. For some trace elements, more than one method of translocation may be operable depending on the concentration of that particular trace element in the intestinal contents. In the young of some animal species, trace minerals can be translocated by the process of pinocytosis (i.e., the cell membrane surrounds the mineral, which is then taken in as a vacuole).

The *mobilization stage* includes mobilization of the trace elements and their sequestration in the intestinal cells or transport across the serosal surfaces of the intestinal cells into the blood stream. This stage is not well defined in general, but specific mechanisms have been postulated for iron and zinc. These elements are bound within the cell to specific proteins or form part of the intracellular pool. Those ions which remain in the pool can be mobilized and transported across the serosal surface. The ions bound to the intracellular proteins can either be released to become part of the pool or remain bound and lost with the cell during desquamation.

The gastrointestinal tract is the site of important interactions between metals. Medication with iron may depress the absorption of copper. Copper in turn may lower iron and molybdenum absorption. Cobalt absorption is increased in patients with iron deficiency, but cobalt and iron compete and inhibit absorption of each other. These interactions probably reflect a lack of complete specificity of the absorption mechanisms.

For transport, the metals are bound to proteins. Carriers are either specific, such as transferrin, which binds with iron, or general, such as albumin. A fraction of the trace elements is also carried in the serum in the form of amino acid or peptide complexes. Specific protein carriers are usually undersaturated and the reserve capacity may be a buffer against excessive exposure. Toxicity from trace minerals usually results only after this buffering capacity is exceeded. Plasma concentrations of the micronutrients are regulated; concentration in plasma declines with low intake and increases with adequate intake. However, low plasma concentration may also result from shifts rather than deficiency.

EXCRETION

For chromium, selenium, fluoride and iodide, the major route of excretion is the urinary tract. For other minerals, the major route is the gut and losses in urine are negligible except during periods of stress, such as prolonged starvation. Losses of trace elements via sweat and breath may be important in hot climates.

DIETARY SOURCES

In general, foods of animal origin are superior sources of trace elements, since concentrations tend to be higher and the metals are more available for absorption. Manganese is an exception, being readily available from plant sources. Trace elements are not evenly distributed in the wheat grain. Milling technology removes the germ and outer layers which contain the most minerals. Although the mineral content of white flour is fairly low, however, those minerals left are more readily available since some of the metals in whole wheat flour are firmly complexed by phytate and fiber concentrations. Seafoods are usually rich in many micronutrients.

Micronutrients Essential at Levels No Higher than a Few Milligrams per Day for Adult Humans

IRON

Boussingault in the 1860's was the first to regard iron as an essential nutrient for animals. In the early 20th century there was great interest in iron absorption and excretion, even though the techniques used for analysis were tedious. By the 1920's, an animal model for the study of iron deficiency anemia was produced by feeding rats a milk diet. Interest in iron and iron deficiency anemia has continued to the present, and although there is more information on iron than on any of the other trace minerals, there are still unresolved questions and problems.

In a healthy adult there are 3 to 5 gm. of iron. An adult male has 40 to 50 mg. of iron per kilogram of body weight and the female 35 to 50 mg. per kg. of body weight. In the newborn there are 70 mg. of iron per kg. of body weight and a total of approximately 250 mg.

Sixty to 70 per cent of the iron in the body is classified as essential or functional iron, and 30 to 40 per cent as storage or non-essential iron. The *essential iron* is incorporated into hemoglobin, myoglobin and certain respiratory enzymes that catalyze oxidation-reduction processes within the cell. The approximate distribution of iron in the body, as shown in Figure 7–2, is as follows: 2.5 to 3.0 gm. is in the hemoglobin of erythrocytes; about 200 to 1500 mg. is stored in the liver, bone marrow and spleen as ferritin and hemosiderin; 150 mg. is in the muscles as myoglobin; 3 to 4 mg. is in the plasma bound to the protein transferrin; and 300 mg. is distributed among all of the cells in respiratory enzymes.

FUNCTIONS. Iron plays a role in the transport of oxygen from the lungs to the tissues, in the transport of CO_2 away from the cells to the lungs, and in the process of cellular respiration.

The first two of these functions are accomplished by hemoglobin in the erythrocytes or red blood cells. *Hemoglobin* is a metalloprotein with heme, an iron porphyrin, attached to the protein moiety. The iron combines with oxygen in the lungs, where the concentration is high, and releases the oxygen in the tissues where it is needed. *Myoglobin* within the muscle cell has a function similar to that of hemoglobin. The *cytochromes*, present in all cells, do not combine with oxygen, but function in the respiratory chain in the transfer of electrons and storage of energy through alternate oxidation and reduction of iron ($Fe^{++} \longleftrightarrow Fe^{+++}$).

In fetal life, the red blood cells are manufactured principally in the liver and the spleen. Fetal red blood cells contain a different form of hemoglobin, fetal hemoglobin, which has different association-disassociation characteristics. In the adult, red blood cells are formed chiefly in the bone marrow. The erythrocytes begin as erythroblasts (immature cells). As they mature in the bone marrow, heme is synthesized from glycine and iron in the presence of pyridoxine and combined with the globin. Adequate amounts of amino acids must be available for the simultaneous synthesis of globin. Copper and vitamin C are also essential for the synthesis of hemoglobin.

Since they are non-nucleated, red blood cells live only as long as the enzymes present at maturity remain functional. As cells age and approach the end of their life span (120 days), they become more fragile. Old cells are removed from circulation by the cells of the reticuloendothelial system. The iron is released from the porphyrin, taken up by the transferrin, and either returned to the bone marrow for the production of new blood cells or stored in the liver and spleen, as shown in Figure 7–2. Without

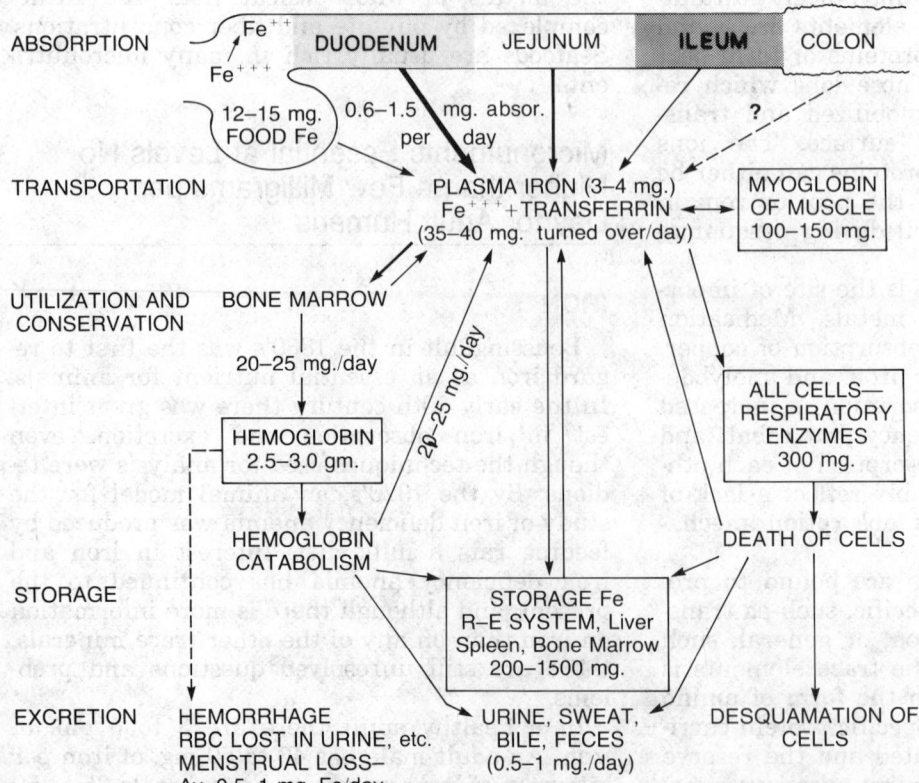

Figure 7–2. Schematic outline of iron metabolism in adults.

this effective conservation it would be impossible to provide the iron needed from dietary sources. The iron-free porphyrin is converted to bilirubin and carried to the liver for excretion in the bile. Deficiencies of ascorbic acid, vitamin E, folic acid, and vitamin B_{12} accelerate the rate of destruction of the red blood cells.

The respiratory enzymes function in oxidation-reduction at the cellular level. There is evidence from animal studies that with a deficiency of iron the concentration of these enzymes may drop before the hemoglobin level in the blood drops.[28] Although these enzymes represent only a small part of the total iron, a drop in the cellular concentration of these vital enzymes can still have a long-range effect.

Several other functions have been proposed for iron on the basis of the association of some changes noted in animals or humans with iron deficiency anemia. There has been a great deal of interest in two areas in particular, the role of iron in the immune function and the role of iron in cognitive performance. Iron deficiency has been shown to impair the resistance of animals to infection. In one group of children with iron deficiency, there were immunological changes that were corrected with iron treatment.[4] In another study, other coexisting forms of malnutrition were carefully excluded and T-cell immunity was still slightly impaired in children with iron deficiency.[23] Once again oral iron therapy corrected these changes. These data and others from studies of children with protein-energy malnutrition and iron deficiency anemia suggest that iron does function in the immune response by a mechanism not yet determined.

Investigators have also found differences between the scholastic performance, sensorimotor competence, attention, learning and memory of anemic children and control subjects.[36] Deficits in the ability of anemic animals to transfer a learned association have also been observed, further suggesting an impairment.[28] Definitive answers are not available on the basis of present information, but there are enough suggestive data to increase the interest in the prevention of iron deficiency anemia in the world population.

ABSORPTION. There are two forms of dietary iron, *heme* iron in the form of hemoglobin and myoglobin, and *non-heme* iron. Heme iron is absorbed into the mucosal cells as the intact porphyrin complex and is little affected by the composition of the meal and gastrointestinal secretions, but is affected by iron deficiency. Heme iron represents 5 to 10 per cent of the dietary iron, but in the individual with iron stores of approximately 500 mg., absorption is about 25 per cent as compared with 5 per cent for non-heme iron. Non-heme iron is affected by the composition of the meal, as well as other factors. This "two-pool" concept is central to understanding the luminal phase of iron absorption. Once in the mucosal cell, both types of iron form a common pool.

To be absorbed, non-heme iron must be present in the duodenum and upper jejunum in a soluble form. In the luminal stage, non-heme iron must first be ionized by the acid gastric juice. As the chyme passes from the stomach to the duodenum, the pH increases to 7 because of the addition of duodenal secretions. Unless chelated, most ferric iron is precipitated. Ferrous iron is significantly more soluble at pH 7 and is therefore still available for absorption. When non-heme food items are ingested at the same meal, all of the iron mixes and forms a common luminal pool of non-heme iron.

The rate of iron absorption seems to be controlled by the amount accepted by the intestinal mucosa in response to the body's requirement for iron, which is reflected by the amount available from the blood to meet the needs of newly formed cells, as shown in Figure 7–3. There is no mechanism specifically for adjusting the rate

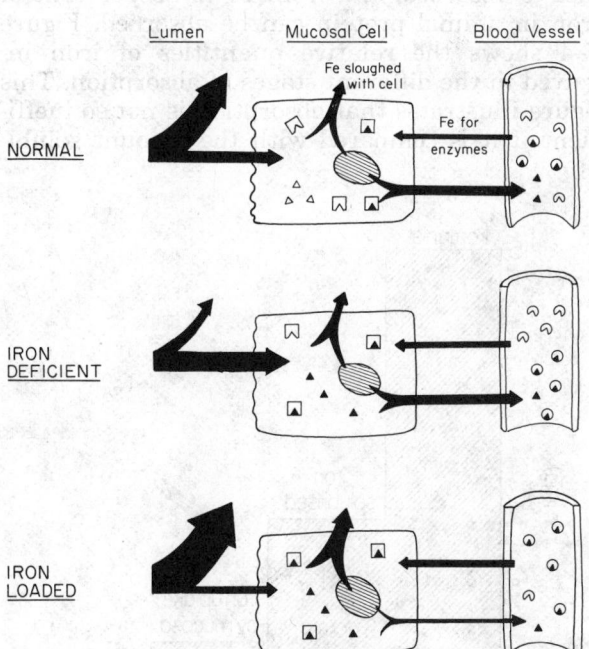

▲IRON ▣FERRITIN ▨APOFERRITIN ◍TRANSFERRITIN

Figure 7–3. Iron equilibrium in the intestinal mucosa. In normal subjects, mucosal cells contain iron supplied from body stores. The amount of iron that enters the cells is regulated, within limits, by the amount in the cells or the amount circulating bound to transferrin. In iron-deficient subjects, little iron is incorporated into the mucosal cells and less is present bound to transferrin. Therefore, iron absorption is increased and excretion is decreased. In iron-loaded subjects, both the mucosal cells and transferrin are saturated. This limits absorption and increases excretion.

of excretion of iron; therefore, the iron content of the body is regulated by the rate of absorption. Within the mucosal cell the iron may combine with *apoferritin* to form *ferritin,* the form in which iron is temporarily stored in the mucosal cells.

Transfer from mucosal cells to the body is slower than uptake and is affected by the size of the body stores and the quantity of iron in the diet. The rate at which the iron is released from the mucosal cells into general circulation may be regulated by the amount and saturation of *transferrin.* Transferrin is usually saturated to about one third of its *total iron-binding capacity* (TIBC). If iron is not needed, transferrin remains saturated, less is absorbed from the mucosal cells, and that remaining in the cells is sloughed with the cells at the end of their 2- to 3-day life. If iron is needed, the transferrin is less saturated when it reaches the intestinal mucosal cells and more iron passes from the mucosal cell to the transferrin.

It is estimated that only 5 to 15 per cent of the iron in food is absorbed by adults with normal hemoglobin values, although absorption can be as high as 50 per cent in an iron-deficient person. From 2 to 10 per cent of iron in vegetables is absorbed, and from 10 to 30 per cent of iron in animal protein can be absorbed. Figure 7–4 shows the relative quantities of iron involved in the different stages of absorption. This figure illustrates that absorption is not so inefficient if it is compared with the amount solubilized rather than with the total amount in the diet.

Factors That Enhance Absorption

ASCORBIC ACID. Dietary ascorbic acid is the most potent enhancer of iron absorption known. Ascorbic acid forms a soluble chelate at low pH that remains soluble at the higher pH of the small intestine. The effect of ascorbic acid is so well accepted that it is now recommended that total iron intake be corrected for intake of ascorbic acid as well as for intake of meat, fish and poultry.[31] Foods kept on warming tables lose substantial ascorbate in the first hour.[8] This may have an important impact on the iron status of persons eating a high proportion of their meals from large scale catering units. Caution should be used in increasing the amount of ascorbic acid greatly over the recommendation since the amount in the diet may affect absorption of other minerals.

ANIMAL PROTEINS. Not all animal proteins increase non-heme iron absorption. Cellular proteins, such as beef, pork, veal, lamb, liver, fish and chicken, enhance absorption; cow's milk, cheese and eggs do not. The exact factor responsible for the enhancement of absorption is not known, but is referred to as an *MFP (meat, fish, poultry) factor.*

HUMAN MILK. Infants retain more iron from human milk than from cow's milk or infant formulas. Data from several laboratories using different techniques confirm this observation. Whether the increased retention from human milk results from the form in which the iron is present or other factors is not known at the present time (see page 274).

ACID MEDIUM. The degree of gastric acidity influences solubility and availability of iron in food.

CALCIUM. The presence of an adequate amount of calcium helps to remove phosphate, oxalate and phytate that would combine with iron and inhibit its absorption.

INTRINSIC FACTOR. Besides hydrochloric acid, gastric secretions include intrinsic factor and ascorbate. Intrinsic factor increases absorption of heme iron because of the structural similarity of heme and vitamin B_{12}.

PHYSIOLOGICAL STATE. During periods of increased rate of formation of blood, such as pregnancy and growth, absorption is increased. People with deficiency also absorb more iron.

Factors That Decrease Absorption

ALKALINE MEDIUM. The lack of hydrochloric acid in the stomach or the administration of alkaline substances such as antacids interferes with iron absorption.

COMPLEXING AGENTS. Phytates, oxalates and phosphates form insoluble iron complexes, reducing absorption.

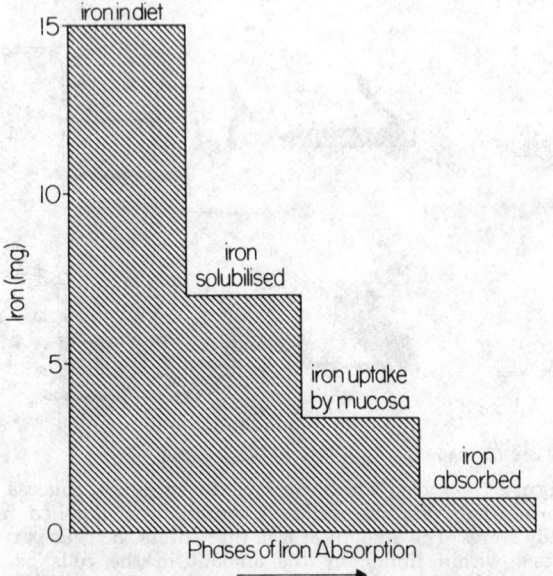

Figure 7–4. Relative quantities of iron involved in different phases of iron absorption. Note that the greatest effect is solubilization of the iron in the diet. (From Bothwell, T. H., et al: Iron Metabolism in Man. Oxford, Blackwell Scientific Publications, 1979, p. 283.)

INTESTINAL MOTILITY. Increased motility decreases absorption by decreasing the contact time.

STEATORRHEA. Maldigestion of fat leading to steatorrhea decreases absorption.

CHEMICAL FORM OF IRON. Studies have also indicated wide differences in the availability of iron from various compounds used for enrichment or supplementation, as shown in Figure 7–5. Ferrous lactate, fumarate, glycinesulfate, succinate and glutamate are absorbed as well as ferrous sulfate. Ferrous citrate, tartrate and pyrophosphate are poorly absorbed.

When abnormally large amounts of iron are present as a result of long-term ingestion of extremely high amounts, or excessive blood transfusions, the apoferritin in the liver becomes saturated and hemosiderin appears in large quantities. *Hemosiderin* is similar to ferritin but contains more iron and is very insoluble. Certain individuals with a genetic defect absorb more than an ordinary amount of iron and develop an iron storage condition, which is called *hemosiderosis*. If the hemosiderosis is associated with tissue damage, it is called *hemochromatosis*, which is discussed further in Chapter 29.

STORAGE. About 200 to 1500 mg. of iron are stored in the body as ferritin and hemosiderin; 30 per cent is in the liver, 30 per cent in the bone marrow and the rest in the spleen and muscles. Up to 50 mg. per day can be mobilized from storage iron. About 20 mg. of iron is used daily in hemoglobin synthesis. Iron is used very conservatively in the body. Approximately 90 per cent is conserved and used over and over again. Minute amounts of serum ferritin can be detected in normal human serum using sensitive immunoassay techniques. This circulating ferritin is closely correlated with body iron stores.[5] Measurement of serum ferritin has proved to be an invaluable tool for evaluating iron status clinically, as discussed in Chapter 9.

EXCRETION. Only very small amounts of iron are normally excreted from the body. The bulk of the iron lost in the feces consists of that not absorbed from food intake. The remainder is iron contained in exfoliated cells from the gastrointestinal epithelium, and the excretion of bile. Normal exfoliation of the cells of the skin and bleeding are additional sources of iron loss. Virtually no iron is excreted in the urine and sweat.

The normal male loses about 1.0 mg. of iron daily. In the female, there is the additional loss of iron accompanying menstruation, which averages about 0.5 mg. per day—the amount of iron in the menstrual blood flow averaged over one month. Wide variations exist among individuals, and menstrual losses of over 1.4 mg. of iron per day have been reported in about 5 per cent of normal women.

METABOLISM. Figure 7–2 contains a schematic outline of the essential steps in the metabolism of iron in adults.

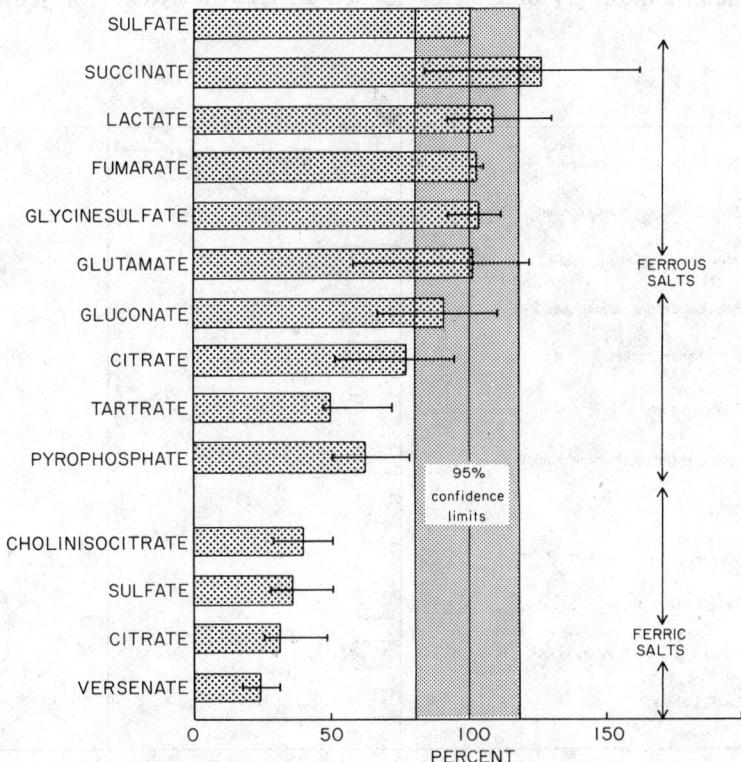

Figure 7–5. Absorption of iron from dose equivalent to 30 mg. of elemental iron. Mean indicated by bar, range indicated by line.

DIETARY SOURCES. By far the best source of dietary iron is liver, with oysters, shellfish, kidney, heart, lean meat, poultry and fish as second choices. Dried beans and vegetables are the best plant sources. Some other foods that add iron are egg yolks, dried fruits, dark molasses, whole grain and enriched breads, wines and cereals. Milk and milk products are practically devoid of iron. Foods high in iron content are shown in Figure 7–6. A more complete table is given in the Appendix Table 11.

The size of the average serving of food and the availability of the iron present in the food must be taken into account when thinking of sources of dietary iron. For example, only half or less of the iron in whole grain cereals and some green leaves is available in utilizable form. Raisins, though popularly thought to be a good source of iron, really do not contribute a significant amount to the diet on a percentage basis because even though iron content may be good, the average serving is relatively small. Iron fortification of cereals, flours and bread has added significantly to the total iron intake. Fortified infant cereal is a substantial source of iron for children up to 12 months of age.[39] However, controversy surrounds iron fortification of foods. It has been suggested that iron fortification will cause more hemosiderosis in susceptible people. On the other hand, iron supplementation of more foods might prevent iron deficiency among the high-risk population.

RECOMMENDED DIETARY ALLOWANCE. A sufficient quantity of iron is needed in the diet to prevent the development of iron deficiency anemia. Iron requirements are determined by the demands for tissue growth and hemoglobin accretion and by replacement needs for iron lost in the urine, feces and sweat and in the female in menstruation, pregnancy and lactation. Recommendations of the Food and Nutrition Board are for a daily intake of 10 mg. of iron for men and older women. An intake of 18 mg. per day is recommended for women during child-bearing years. This amount is required to cover menstrual losses and the demands of pregnancy and lactation.

An otherwise adequate diet frequently contains no more than 6 mg. of iron per 1000 kilocalories. The average female consuming 2300 kilocalories would consume only approximately 13.8 mg. of iron, or approximately 75 per cent of the RDA. Since the RDA can be met by dietary intake only with difficulty and with good planning, there is a controversy whether it is set too high. Table 7-3 shows the average daily iron intake of Americans as reported in HANES II.[27]

The infant is born with a reserve supply of iron and is apparently unable to utilize additional iron over and above that furnished by reduction of its hemoglobin mass shortly after birth. The recommended allowance for a normal term infant is based on an average need of 1.5 mg. per kg. of weight per day during the first year of life. Premature infants have limited iron stores, since most of the iron is transferred during the last trimester of pregnancy. The need for iron to support rapid growth in premature

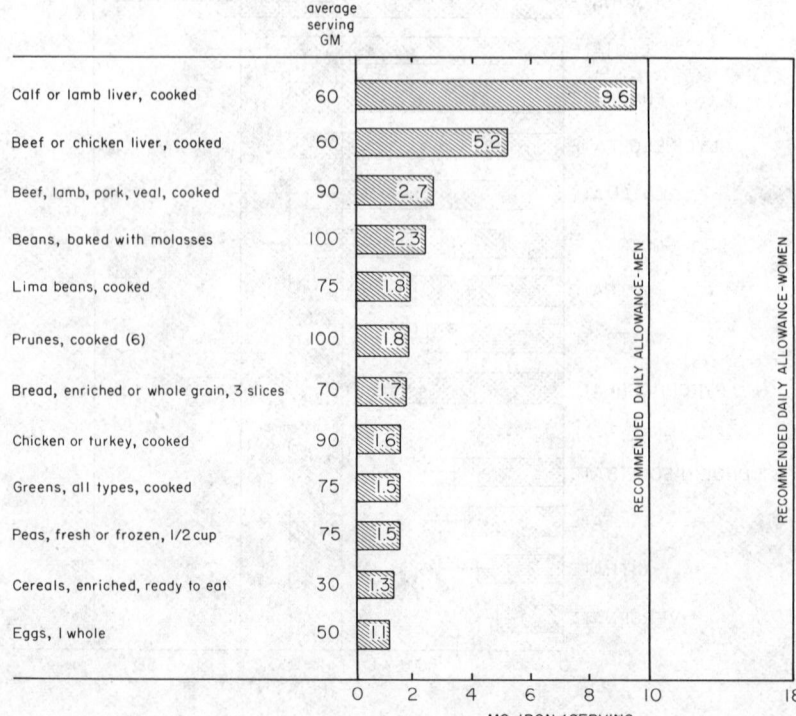

Figure 7–6. Iron in average servings of food compared with the RDA for men and women.

Table 7–3. AVERAGE DAILY IRON INTAKE AS REPORTED IN HANES II*

	MALES		FEMALES	
AGE	*mg.*	*mg./1000 kcal.*	*mg.*	*mg./1000 kcal.*
6–11 mos.	12.8	12.8	12.9	13.0
1–2 yrs.	8.7	6.6	8.5	6.7
3–5 yrs.	10.5	6.5	9.5	6.3
12–14 yrs.	15.9	6.5	10.8	5.9
25–34 yrs.	17.3	6.3	10.9	6.6
55–64 yrs.	14.8	7.1	10.7	7.6

*Intakes by both sexes were somewhat lower in HANES I.
(Adapted from Lynch, S. R., et al.: Iron status of elderly Americans. Am. J. Clin. Nutr., 36:1032, 1982.)

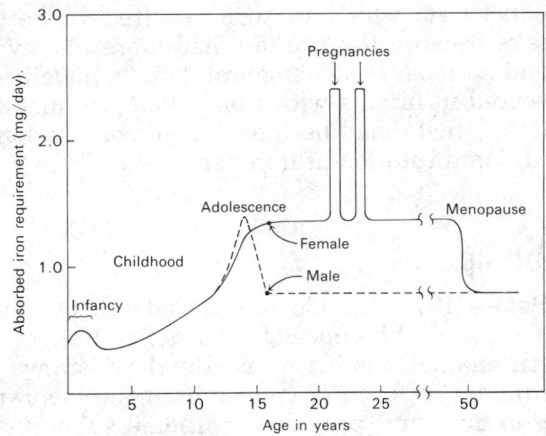

Figure 7–7. The absorbed iron requirement in males and females of various ages. The greatest requirements in relation to food intake occur during infancy. During childhood, requirements are the same for both sexes. During the adolescent growth spurt there is an increase in iron needs—more in the male than in the female. Because of menstruation, the female's requirement remains high, while the requirement for the male decreases after adolescence. (From Wintrobe, M. S., et al.: Clinical Hematology. 7th ed. Philadelphia, Lea & Febiger, 1974.)

infants becomes apparent at approximately 2 to 3 months of age and is discussed in Chapter 37. The recommended allowance for the period from birth to 6 months is 10 mg.; for children 6 months to 3 years it is 15 mg.; for children aged 4 to 10 years it is 10 mg. The daily need for boys aged 11 to 18 years is 18 mg., dropping to 10 mg. for men 19 to 50 years and older. For girls and women aged 10 to 50, the RDA is 18 mg.; for women 50 years of age and older, it is 10 mg.

IRON REQUIREMENT IN RELATION TO AGE. Figure 7–7 shows the absorbed requirement in relation to age. The requirement during infancy is the greatest in relation to food intake. The adolescent growth spurt is another period of increased requirement, higher in the male than in the female, even with the onset of menstruation in the female. However, the male's requirement decreases after adolescence, while the female's remains high.

Because of individual variation in absorptive capacity, the differences among foods in the availability of their iron for absorption, and the ability of the body to increase iron absorption during periods of deficiency, it is difficult to convert physiological requirements for iron into dietary allowances. Hence the RDA and the recommendations of the Joint FAO/WHO Expert Group differ, although they are based on the same considerations.

DEFICIENCY. A deficiency of iron has been cited as the commonest of all deficiency diseases in humans in both developing and developed countries. Groups considered most frequently at risk are infants under two years of age, teenage girls, pregnant women and the elderly. Pregnant teenagers are frequently at very high risk. In some developing countries, iron deficiency has been found in 30 to 50 per cent of the entire population. In the United States, similar percentages of some high-risk groups have been found to be affected. Iron deficiency manifests itself ultimately by the development of an anemia *(hypochromic microcytic anemia)*, which is

corrected by giving diets rich in absorbable iron and by providing iron supplements in the form of ferrous sulfate or ferrous gluconate. Iron deficiency can be caused by illness (for example, blood loss due to hookworms or gastrointestinal diseases that interfere with iron absorption), injury or hemorrhage and is aggravated by a poorly balanced diet that is often deficient in dietary iron, protein and the vitamins folate, B_{12}, B_6 and C. Iron deficiency is manifested by hematological and non-hematological changes. Iron deficiency anemia may develop on a purely nutritional basis as a result of an inadequate diet or faulty absorption of iron.

The sequence of events in the development of iron deficiency anemia is: desaturation of tissue stores, diminished levels of certain enzymes, decreased serum iron levels, increased TIBC, and finally decreased hemoglobin and hematocrit (see Fig. 29–1). Clinical symptoms develop slowly and frequently are not perceived by the patient. In severe anemia, cardiac symptoms develop. Iron deficiency anemia is discussed in detail in Chapter 29.

During iron depletion, organs with rapid cell turnover become rapidly depleted of iron-dependent enzymes; in organs with slow turnover, enzymes may remain unaltered.[7] These non-hematological changes are receiving more attention now than previously. Nutrition surveys done in the United States and internationally have identified iron deficiency anemia as a major impairment of health and working capacity in adults and as a consequence of this an economic loss to the individual and the country. Supplementation has been shown to increase productivity, which in turn resulted in better intake because the workers had more money to spend on food. Developmental deficits have been observed in infants with iron deficiency anemia. These deficits may be the most important long-term manifestation of iron deficiency.

FLUORIDE

Before 1972 fluoride was considered by some to be essential because of its beneficial effect on tooth enamel, conferring maximal resistance to dental caries. In 1972 studies from the laboratories of Schwarz[43] provided additional support for fluoride as an essential trace element.

The skeleton of the average man contains 2.6 gm. of fluoride. The average daily intake of fluoride by adults is approximately 4.4 mg. Of greatest importance is the amount ingested in drinking water. The fluoride content of food varies according to the content of the soil in which it is grown. Table 7–4 lists the fluoride content of selected foods.

Dental fluorosis may occur at fluoride concentrations of 2 to 7 ppm. and *osteosclerosis* at 8 to 20 ppm. To produce symptoms of chronic toxicity, daily intakes of 20 to 80 mg. or more must be consumed for years. In parts of the western United States the water sometimes contains 10 to 45 ppm. of fluoride and tooth mottling as shown in Figure 7–8 is endemic. In other areas such as parts of Michigan and New York where fluoride is deficient, the incidence of dental decay is quite high. One mg. of fluoride per liter of drinking water produces a 60 to 70 per cent reduction in dental caries. For maximal effect, the fluoride must be used in the early years when teeth are forming. Approximately 10,000 communities in which the fluoride content of water is low have added this amount to water supplies serving over 100 million people. This practice is recognized as an important public health measure (see Chapter 33). Studies have demonstrated that the hydroxyapatite crystals in bone are larger and more nearly perfect when the fluoride content of the diet is adequate. Bone containing fluoride is more stable and more resistant to degeneration. A further benefit may be a reduction in the incidence of osteoporosis in areas where fluoride intake is adequate.

There has also been a decline in caries prevalence in communities without fluoridated water. The causes of this are still a matter of speculation, but may be related to increased use of fluorides in the food chain, especially from the use of fluoridated water in food processing, and the unintentional ingestion of toothpaste.[26] Mild fluorosis, probably not discernible by the layman, is increasing.[26] A redefinition of optimum con-

Table 7–4. FLUORIDE CONTENT OF SELECTED FOODS

FOOD	FLUORIDE CONTENT (PPM.)
Meats	
Beef liver	5.20–5.80
Chicken	1.40
Beef	2.00
Pork chops	1.0
Lamb	1.2
Veal	0.9
Fish	
Mackerel, fresh	26.89
Salmon, canned	4.5
Sardines, in olive oil	16.1
Eggs	
Whole	1.2
Yolk	0.6
Milk, whole	0.07–0.22
Cereals and cereal products	0.54
Vegetables	0.1–0.2
Fruits	0.1–0.2

(Adapted from Bell, M. E., et al.: The Supply of Fluorine to Man in Fluorides and Human Health, WHO Monograph No. 59, Geneva, Switzerland, WHO, 1970.)

centration of fluoride may be necessary. The 1980 RDA (Table 10–2) lists the safe range of recommended intake of fluoride for all ages.

ZINC

Zinc has been known to be essential for microorganisms for approximately 100 years, and for rats for approximately 50, but deficiency was first demonstrated in man only approximately 20 years ago.[9,38] Zinc deficiency was manifested by severe iron deficiency anemia, hepatosplenomegaly, short stature, marked

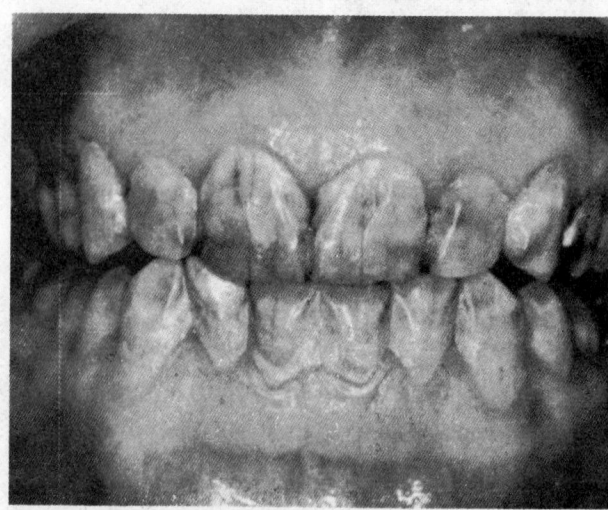

Figure 7–8. Mottled enamel caused by excess fluoride in water. (From Nizel, A.: Nutrition in Preventive Dentistry: Science and Practice. 2nd edition. Philadelphia, W. B. Saunders Company, 1981.)

hypogonadism and a history of geophagia (clay eating), a form of pica. There is now evidence not only that zinc deficiency disease can be found in malnourished populations, but also that marginal deficiency may be widespread in the United States and that disease and physical injury can alter zinc metabolism and excretion.

Zinc is ubiquitous in plants, microorganisms and animals. There are 1.4 to 2.3 grams of zinc in the body of an adult. The liver, pancreas, kidney, bone and voluntary muscles have the largest concentration. Other tissues with high concentrations include various parts of the eye, prostate gland and spermatozoa, skin, hair, fingernails and toenails.

FUNCTIONS. Many questions regarding the biological role of zinc in man are as yet unanswered; however, it is clear that zinc plays a role in a number of metabolic activities. There is a family of 70 or more metalloenzymes that require zinc to function. These include carbonic anhydrase, alkaline phosphatase, lactic dehydrogenase and carboxypeptidase, which participate in a variety of functions. Many of the zinc-containing enzymes decrease in activity during zinc depletion. In the preclinical stages of zinc deficiency, some enzymes, such as alkaline phosphatase and carboxypeptidase A, decrease in activity due to a decrease in apoenzyme. Zinc functions by maintaining spatial and configurational relationships necessary for enzymatic action. In this role it helps to bind enzymes to substrates and may modify the molecular shape of enzymes by simultaneously combining with amino acids at different places on the protein, thus affecting secondary, tertiary and quaternary protein structure. Zinc-dependent enzymes are not all affected equally in all tissues in zinc-deficient animals. Those enzymes that bind zinc with high affinity are still fully active even during severe deficiency.

In addition to its function in enzymes, zinc participates in the metabolism of nucleic acids and the synthesis of proteins. Although its role is not completely understood, zinc appears to be an integral part of the RNA molecule of a number of species and is thought to help maintain stable molecular configuration. Zinc may also have an important role in cell division since zinc deficiency causes adverse effects on the incorporation of thymidine into the DNA of rats. Zinc is required for DNA synthesis, and the DNA-dependent RNA polymerase is a zinc-dependent enzyme, as is thymidine kinase.

There are also several other possible functions of zinc. Early studies in animals suggest a specific effect of zinc on the testes through alteration of testicular steroidogenesis. Reduced resistance to infection is seen in patients with acrodermatitis enteropathica and is normalized by zinc replacement. This and other data suggest a possible action on the cell membrane.

ABSORPTION. Zinc absorption is affected by body size, the level of zinc in the diet and the presence of interfering substances. Zinc is most available as zinc sulfate. The exact site of zinc absorption has not been determined but data suggest the ileum as the primary site. Figure 7–9 describes what is presently felt to be the regulatory pathway of dietary zinc absorption. In the lumen, the zinc appears to be associated with a low-molecular-weight ligand. The binding ligand may be citric acid, picolinic acid or an as yet undetermined compound. Zinc is translocated across the cell membrane against a concentration gradient by a carrier-mediated system and enters the intracellular zinc pool. Prostaglandin E_2 binds zinc and may facilitate transport in animals. From the pool the ion may be incorporated into a zinc-requiring function within the cell, be stored bound to the protein metallothionein, or be transferred across the serosal border into the blood stream. There is also enteric circulation of zinc from the gastrointestinal secretions.

When zinc is given as an aqueous solution,

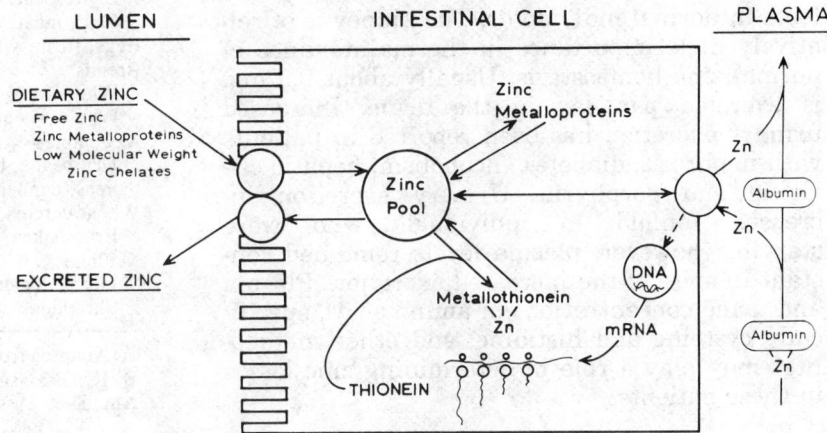

Figure 7–9. Regulatory pathway of dietary zinc absorption by intestinal cells. (Dashed line denotes induction of metallothionein mRNA. Thionein is metal-free metallothionein.) (From Cousins, R. J.: Regulatory aspects of zinc metabolism in liver and intestine. Nutr. Rev., *37*:98, 1979.)

mean absorption ranges from 43 to 69 per cent. When the isotope is consumed with food, the range of absorption drops to about 14 to 42 per cent.

Inhibiting Factors. Scientific arguments as to whether the fiber or phytate in foods is responsible for the decrease in zinc absorption are academic since phytate and fiber frequently occur in the same foods. Other complexing agents, such as tannins, oxalates, ascorbic acid and sodium metaphosphatase, apparently do not affect zinc absorption. Copper will inhibit zinc absorption if given in high enough concentration. However, the biological importance of this observation is questionable since the concentration of copper in the diet does not reach the levels needed. There is also competition between zinc and iron for access to the absorption channels through the intestinal cells. Ratios of iron to zinc of 2:1 or 3:1 result in a significant reduction in zinc uptake.[47] Care should be taken in selecting vitamin-mineral mixtures in supplements. Many preparations contain an iron to zinc ratio greater than 3:1.

Enhancing Factors. In animals, glucose or lactose will increase zinc absorption. Red table wine will also increase zinc absorption, probably owing to the congeners present.[48] White wine has not been studied. In animals, soy protein alone or mixed with beef will enhance zinc absorption. Zinc is better absorbed from human milk than from cow's milk.

TRANSPORT. Serum or plasma concentrations of zinc in normal subjects are 70 to 130 μg./ml. Red cell zinc concentrations vary from 10 to 14 μg./ml. of red cells. The concentration in serum or plasma is lower in females than in males, and there is a small decrease in males with age. Albumin is the major transport protein for zinc. Other proteins, such as transferrin, ceruloplasmin and gamma globulin, also bind significant amounts of zinc. A small proportion exists mostly bound to amino acids and a still smaller fraction as ionic zinc.

EXCRETION. Excretion is almost solely via the feces in normal individuals. The kidney is of relatively little importance in the maintenance of normal zinc homeostasis. Usually about 0.5 mg. is excreted per day in the urine. Increased urinary excretion has been reported in patients with nephrosis, diabetes, alcoholism, hepatic cirrhosis and porphyria. Urinary excretion increased tenfold in individuals who were starving; however, plasma levels remained constant in spite of the increased excretion. Plasma and urine concentrations of amino acids, specifically cysteine and histidine, and other metabolites may play a role in determining zinc losses in these patients.

DIETARY SOURCES. Zinc should come from a balanced diet that contains sufficient animal protein. Meat, liver, eggs and seafood (particularly oysters) are good sources of available zinc. Table 7–5 lists the actual zinc content of selected foods; a more complete list is included in Appendix Table 12. The zinc content of most drinking water is negligible. Human milk contains 20 mg./liter in colostrum and approximately 2 mg./liter in mature milk.

RECOMMENDED DIETARY ALLOWANCE. In healthy adults, metabolic studies indicate positive zinc balance with intakes of 12.5 mg. per day from a mixed diet. Therefore, the RDA for 1980 was set at 15 mg. per day for adolescents and adults, plus 5 mg. additional during pregnancy and 10 mg. during lactation. For preadolescents the requirement is estimated at 6 mg. per day but there are greater dermal losses and more variation, so the RDA has been set at 10 mg. There is limited information on the zinc requirements of infants. The RDA is tentatively set at 3 mg. per day for the first six months of life and increases to 5 mg. from age six months to one year.

The American adult consuming a mixed diet has an average intake of 10 to 15 mg. For children one to three years of age, the intake has been estimated at 5 mg., increasing to 13 mg. for adolescents.

Table 7–5. ZINC CONTENT OF SELECTED FOODS

FOOD	ZINC MG./100 GM.
Meat	
Beef, separable lean, cooked	6.2
Liver, calf, cooked	6.1
Pork loin, separable lean, cooked	3.1
Sausages and cold cuts	
Bologna, beef	1.8
Braunschweiger	2.8
Beef and pork frankfurters	1.6
Turkey	
Light meat, cooked, dry heat	2.1
Dark meat, cooked, dry heat	4.4
Eggs, fresh, whole	1.0
Breads	
White	0.6
Whole wheat	1.8
Vegetables	
Dry beans, boiled, drained	1.0
Peas, canned, drained solids	0.8
Wheat cereals, ready-to-eat	
Bran flakes, 40%	3.6
Flakes	2.3
Germ, toasted	15.4
Shredded	2.8

(Adapted from Murphy, E. W., Willis, B. W., and Watt, B. K.: Provisional tables on the zinc content of foods. J. Am. Diet. Assoc., 66:345, 1975.)

DEFICIENCY. The teratogenic effect of zinc deficiency in humans has not been demonstrated; however, there is a wealth of evidence demonstrating the effect in animals. Ingestion of a zinc-deficient diet by rats during pregnancy results in a number of congenital anomalies.[14] There is sufficient circumstantial evidence suggesting a relationship between maternal zinc status and congenital anomalies to urge further careful study of this problem. In one study, eight children born to alcoholic mothers had multiple congenital anomalies reminiscent of those seen in the progeny of zinc-deficient rats. Low serum zinc and hyperzincuria have been noted in other alcoholics, and with the added stress of pregnancy and poor diet, these women may have been zinc deficient.[16]

Zinc therapy improves healing in patients with zinc deficiency. However, there is no conclusive evidence that zinc stimulates healing in the individual with an adequate zinc nutriture.

Deficiency of zinc has been associated with alterations in taste. Treatment with zinc, nickel or copper results in an improvement in taste perception. Children with low zinc content in the hair and poor growth, who also had loss of taste and smell, showed reversal of the abnormalities following zinc supplementation. The diets of these children had consisted of very little meat and a great deal of milk, a poor source of zinc.[10]

Symptoms. The clinical entity was first described in young males in Iran and Egypt and was characterized by short stature, hypogo-nadism, mild anemia and low plasma zinc levels, as shown in Figure 7–10. After supplementation with zinc sulfate the boys began to grow and pubertal changes occurred. The anemia may have been due to a coexisting protein and/or iron deficiency. Additional symptoms such as *hypogeusia* (decreased taste acuity), delayed wound healing, alopecia, and a dermatitis called *acrodermatitis enteropathica* have also been found to be part of the zinc deficiency syndrome.

Etiology and Incidence. The deficiency described in young males in Iran and Egypt was caused by the high phytate or fiber content of the diet from unrefined cereal and unleavened bread. The phytate or fiber in the intestine chelates with zinc and prevents its absorption, which results in a conditional deficiency.

In 1974 Moynahan described *acrodermatitis enteropathica*, an inherited zinc deficiency that results in eczematoid skin lesions, alopecia, diarrhea, low plasma zinc levels, poor growth and development, malnutrition, intercurrent bacterial and yeast infections and eventually death if left untreated.[32] It usually shows up in infancy upon changing from breast milk to cow's milk. It has been postulated that cow's milk contains a peptide that children with this disease cannot digest and that chelates with zinc and prevents its absorption. The treatment is to provide zinc sulfate in amounts large enough to overcome this chelation effect and allow zinc absorption. Neldner and Hambidge found that zinc supplementation at a level of 22 mg. of elemental zinc

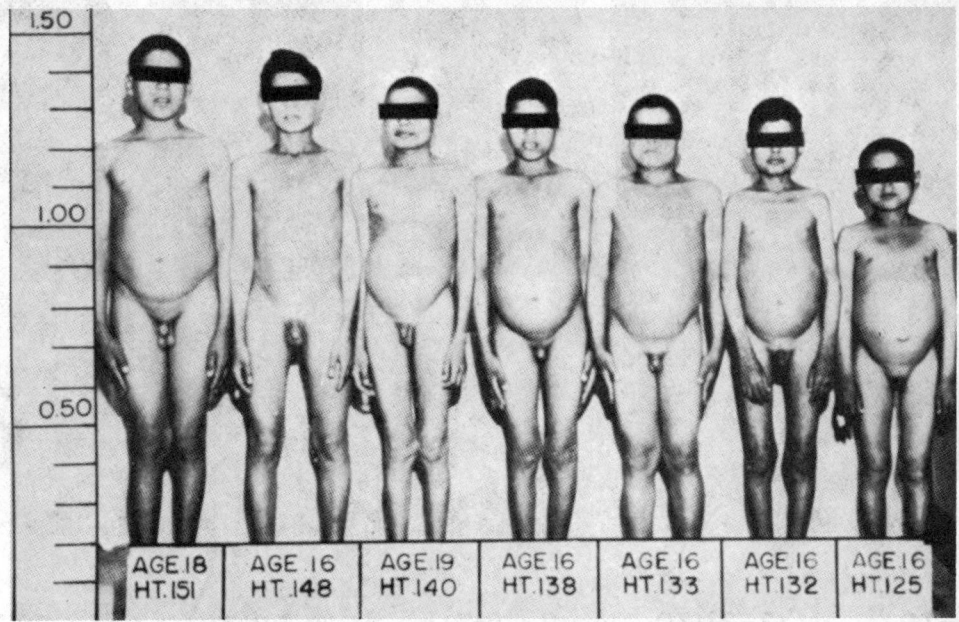

Figure 7–10. Zinc deficiency in dwarfs. (From: Prasad, A. S., et al.: Zinc metabolism in patients with the syndrome of iron deficiency anemia, hepatosplenomegaly, dwarfism and hypogonadism. J. Lab. Clin. Med., *61*:537, 1963.)

was enough to cause remission of the disease in an adult.[33]

Acute zinc deficiency has recently been reported in patients receiving total parenteral nutrition (TPN). Urinary zinc losses can be very high in these patients because of the high rate of catabolism. However, plasma zinc does not fall until there is sustained anabolism and weight gain, which increases the requirement for zinc for the process of building tissue. Four of 37 adult patients who had low plasma zinc also had a syndrome characterized by diarrhea, mental depression, paranoia, oral and perioral dermatitis and alopecia. Response to zinc therapy was rapid except for regrowth of hair, which took longer.[17] A single case of acquired zinc deficiency of such severity as to cause the cutaneous manifestations of *acrodermatitis enteropathica* has also been reported.[52]

Based on the similarities between patients with sickle cell anemia and zinc deficiency, the possibility of a secondary zinc deficiency in people with sickle cell anemia has been suggested. This is discussed further in Chapter 29.

Other cases of low serum zinc levels as a result of chronic illness, malabsorption or long-term zinc-free parenteral feedings have also been reported. The case in Figure 7–11 is an example. In addition several investigators have demonstrated an accelerated healing of wounds in patients receiving zinc sulfate.

Treatment and Prevention. Treatment is alleviation of the situation causing the reduced zinc absorption and supplementation with zinc sulfate. The patient should eat a diet high in foods containing zinc, such as meat, liver, wheat germ and nuts. A particularly good source is oysters. See Appendix Table 12 for the zinc content of various foods.

After studying human zinc requirements and the level of zinc in the U.S. diet, Sandstead has suggested that a significant portion of the population, particularly those subsisting on low-income diets, may have a marginal zinc intake.[41] These people may be adversely affected by this marginal zinc intake, especially if they are subjected to stress or trauma.[52]

TOXICITY. Taken in amounts of 2 gm. or more per day, zinc sulfate can cause gastrointestinal irritation and vomiting. Chronic consumption of high levels of zinc may also aggravate marginal copper deficiency.

COPPER

An adult human body weighing 70 kg. contains 80 to 120 mg. of copper. Concentrations are highest in brain, liver, heart and kidney. Bone and muscle have lower concentrations but contain one half of the total because of their large mass.

The concentration of copper is greatest in the

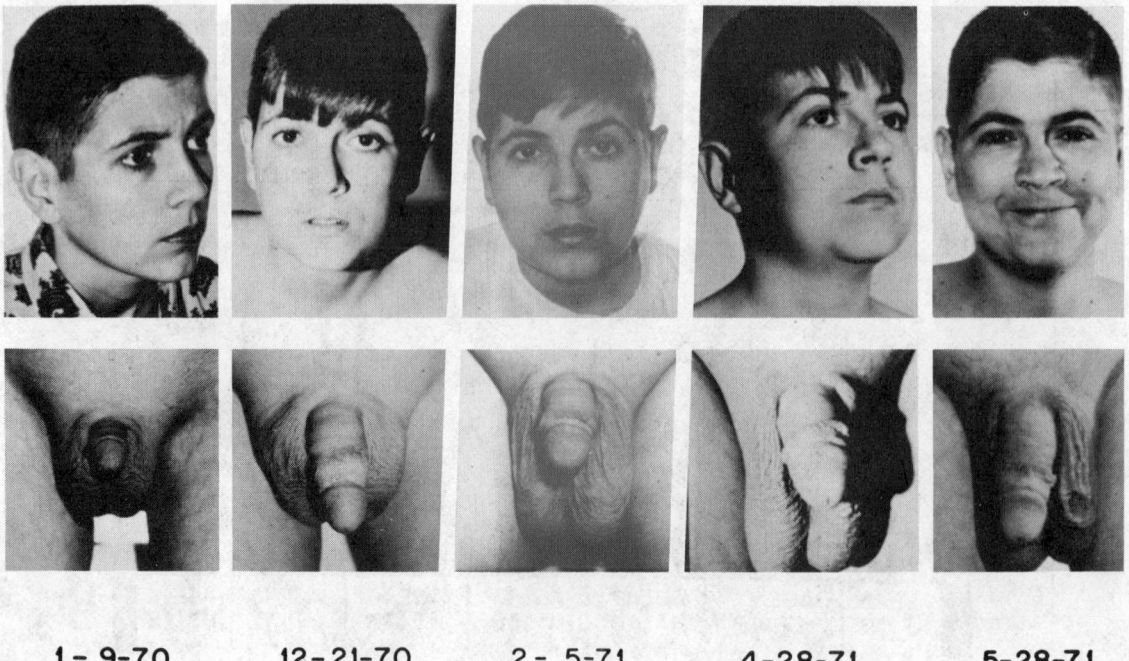

1- 9-70　　12-21-70　　2- 5-71　　4-28-71　　5-28-71

Figure 7–11. Zinc deficiency from malabsorption and after treatment with zinc sulfate. Note the physical maturation and growth that result from zinc supplementation. (From: Sandstead, H. H.: Zinc as an unrecognized limiting nutrient. Am. J. Clin. Nutr., *26*:790, 1973.)

newborn, decreasing during the first year of life. Infants have an exceptional requirement of about 0.08 mg./kg. of body weight. Older children need only half this amount, and for adults 0.03 mg./kg. is sufficient.

Copper concentrations are higher in serum than in plasma, and values depend on copper intakes. Average plasma values for women range from 87 to 153 mg./dl. with a mean value of 120 mg./dl.; for men the range is 89 to 137 mg./dl. with a mean of 109 mg./dl. Approximately 90 per cent of the copper in the plasma is incorporated into *ceruloplasmin*; the rest is loosely bound to albumin and amino acids.

FUNCTIONS. Copper is a component of many enzymes and there are at least three functional areas of prime importance. It is involved in the development and maintenance of (1) cardiovascular and skeletal integrity, (2) central nervous system structure and function, (3) erythropoietic function and (4) hair keratinization and pigmentation. There are numerous amine oxidases that are copper and pyridoxal phosphate dependent. Several *cuproenzymes* have well-defined functions; however, a specific pathologic sign cannot be identified with each enzyme function. On the other hand, there are cuproenzymes associated with specific pathological signs. The bones of copper-deficient chicks contain a higher than normal proportion of soluble collagen, and collagen crosslinking is impaired with resulting bone fragility. The radiographic similarity of bones that are copper deficient and bones that are ascorbic acid deficient suggests a metabolic link between the two. For example, plant ascorbate oxidase is a copper enzyme. No mammalian ascorbate oxidase has been isolated, but copper itself can also be catalytic for ascorbic acid oxidation. Cardiac failure, reported in animals raised on a copper-deficient diet, may also result from failure of collagen and elastin crosslinking or from an as yet undefined muscular defect.[18] Many of the enzymes involved with the developing central nervous system are copper dependent. Menkes' kinky hair syndrome, described on page 170, may result if copper is not properly absorbed.

In animals with pigmented hair, wool or feathers, copper deficiency results in a failure of *melanin* formation. Tyrosinase, a cuproenzyme, catalyzes the hydroxylation of tyrosine to DOPA (3,4-dihydroxyphenylalanine), and the oxidation of DOPA to a quinone gives rise to melanin.

ABSORPTION, TRANSPORT AND EXCRETION. Copper is absorbed from the stomach and upper gut by at least two mechanisms. One mechanism, facilitated by L-amino acids, is an energy-dependent process and may represent the absorption of copper complexes of amino acids. A smaller portion is absorbed by this mechanism. The bulk of the copper is absorbed by the second mechanism involving binding to two protein fractions in the small intestine.

Zinc interferes with copper absorption. High dietary zinc stimulates the intestinal cells to produce more metallothionein. Metallothionein also participates in copper absorption and in fact binds the copper more avidly than it binds the zinc. With more metallothionein binding more copper very tightly there is less transported across the serosal surface for transport to the rest of the body. More of this copper bound to metallothionein is lost with the intestinal cells. The net effect is that less copper is absorbed.

Cadmium, molybdenum and sulfate also alter or interfere with copper absorption. High dietary ascorbic acid causes copper deficiency in several species, but has not been demonstrated to be important in man. Copper forms stable complexes with phytate; therefore, a high intake of dietary fiber may result in depressed copper retention.

Small amounts of copper are present in urine, sweat and menstrual flow. Unabsorbed copper is found in the feces.

DIETARY SOURCES. Copper is widely distributed and most diets provide about 2 mg. per day. Foods high in copper are liver, kidney, oysters, chocolate, nuts, dried legumes, cereals, dried fruits, poultry, shellfish and animal tissues. Milk is as poor in copper as it is in iron, containing 0.015 to 0.18 mg./liter. Human milk content ranges from 0.15 to 1.05 mg./liter.

Analysis of diets revealed values lower than calculated from standard sources (3.6 mg. vs 1.27 mg.).[22] If the lower values are confirmed more attention must be paid to factors that might affect copper absorption.

RECOMMENDED INTAKE. While sufficient data are not available to set an RDA, the 1980 revision recommends a daily intake of 2 to 3 mg. for adults, and 0.08 mg./kg. per day for infants and children. See Table 10–2 for the range of estimated safe intakes.

DEFICIENCY. The signs of copper deficiency in order of appearance are: fall in serum copper and ceruloplasmin levels, failure of iron absorption, neutropenia, leukopenia, bone demineralization, failure of erythropoiesis and finally death. Neutropenia and leukopenia are the best early indications of copper deficiency in children.

Copper deficiency has not been reported in humans consuming a varied diet. Copper is stored in the liver in appreciable quantities; therefore, deficiency develops slowly. Low serum copper values have been reported in patients receiving total parenteral nutrition without copper supplementation. Low serum copper and ceruloplasmin provide supportive evidence of copper deficiency. With the resumption of oral feeding, serum copper rises rapidly. Bone changes including osteoporosis, metaphyseal spur formation and soft tissue calcification have been seen in infants receiving prolonged TPN.

Three deficiency syndromes have been recognized in infants. One is manifested by moderate to severe *anemia* in infants whose diet is based on cow's milk. The anemia of copper deficiency is probably due to a disruption of iron metabolism. Ceruloplasmin may aid the mobilization of iron from ferritin in the liver and other iron storage sites. For complete recovery, therapy with both copper and iron is required since serum levels of both are low. This disorder is discussed in Chapter 29.

The second syndrome is associated with *chronic malnutrition and diarrhea*. The use of modified cow's milk to alleviate the malnutrition contributed in some cases to the development of anemia.

The third syndrome, *Menkes' kinky hair syndrome*, is a sex-linked recessive defect of copper absorption. The infants have retarded growth, defective keratinization and pigmentation of the hair, hypothermia, degenerative changes in aortic elastin, abnormalities of the metaphyses of long bone and progressive mental deterioration. Brain tissue is practically devoid of cytochrome *c* oxidase, a cuproenzyme, and there is a marked accumulation of copper in the intestinal mucosa. Parenteral administration of copper results in transient improvement.

Decreased plasma copper is seen in patients with several malabsorption diseases such as celiac sprue, tropical sprue, protein-losing enteropathies and nephrotic syndrome.

It has been hypothesized that a metabolic imbalance produced by a high ratio of zinc to copper or an absolute deficiency of copper results in hypercholesterolemia, which in turn leads to coronary heart disease.[21] Additional studies are needed to provide evidence to confirm or deny this hypothesis (see Chapter 28).

TOXICITY

Hypercupremia. Ceruloplasmin concentrations increase during pregnancy and in women taking oral contraceptives. Serum copper concentrations in pregnant women are approximately twice the values of non-pregnant women.[54] Serum copper concentration is increased in some patients with acute and chronic infections, patients with liver disease and patients with pellagra. The physiological significance of these elevations is not known.

Wilson's Disease (Hepatolenticular Degeneration). At birth the child with Wilson's disease is indistinguishable from normal neonates. However, the physiologic increase in serum ceruloplasmin and decrease in hepatic copper do not occur. Hepatic copper continues to accumulate with age, producing fatty deposition, necrosis of cells, pigmentary changes and an excess of fibrous tissue. The central nervous system is also adversely affected. Copper deposits in the cornea, *Kayser-Fleischer rings*, do not interfere with vision and are of no pathologic significance. The clinical symptoms of Wilson's disease vary depending on which organs are most seriously affected. Patients are treated with a low-copper diet and with penicillamine, which chelates the copper and allows it to be excreted in the urine.

IODINE

The only known function of iodine is as an integral part of thyroid hormones. These hormones regulate a large number of activities which include (1) energy transformation through an effect on oxygen consumption and heat production, (2) growth, (3) reproduction, (4) neuromuscular function, (5) skin and hair growth and (6) cellular metabolism.

The body normally contains 20 to 30 mg. of iodine. About 60 per cent of it is in the thyroid gland and the rest is diffused throughout all tissues, especially in the ovaries, muscles and blood.

FUNCTIONS. Iodine metabolism and thyroid hormone production are under neuroendocrine control. *A thyrotropin releasing hormone* (TRH) secreted by the hypothalamus stimulates the secretion of *thyrotropin* by the adenohypophysis. This hormone acts on the thyroid, causing it to increase the entrapment of iodide and production of *triiodotyrosine* (T_3) and *thyroxine* (T_4). Increasing levels of circulating T_3 and T_4 inhibit the release of additional TRH and thyrotropin and so provide a negative feedback control on the concentration of the hormones in the circulation.

ABSORPTION AND EXCRETION. Iodides are readily absorbed from the intestinal tract and rapidly transported in the blood stream to the thyroid gland, where they are oxidized to iodine and utilized in the production of the hormones. About one third of the absorbed iodine is utilized by the thyroid gland, while two thirds is excreted in the urine. Iodine in the feces comes mainly from the bile.

DIETARY SOURCES. Iodine occurs in extremely variable amounts in food and drinking water. Seafoods, such as clams, lobsters, oysters, sardines and other fish, are rich sources of iodine. Saltwater fish contain 300 to 3000 μg./kg. of flesh; freshwater fish contain 20 to 40 μg./kg.

The iodine content of cow's milk and of eggs is determined by the iodides available in the diet of the animal, and the iodides in vegetables vary according to the amount in the soil in which they are grown.

The best way to obtain an adequate intake of iodine is to use iodized salt (76 μg. iodine per gram of salt) in the cooking of food. Only about 50 per cent of the table salt sold in the United States is iodized. Mandatory iodization has been adopted by many nations. In Europe 10 μg./gm. of salt is used. The importance of iodized salt should still be emphasized in certain areas to prevent goiter. Other methods of increasing iodine intake (adding iodine to water supply and use of iodide tablets) have been tried in the iodine-deficient areas and were found to be impractical.

Iodine also enters the food chain through the use of *iodophores* as disinfectants, coloring agents and dough conditioners. The Food and Nutrition Board of the National Academy of Sciences states that the present intake is safe, but that additional intake must be viewed with concern and the adventitious sources of iodine should be removed.

RECOMMENDED DIETARY ALLOWANCE. The National Research Council has suggested that an intake of 150 μg. per day is sufficient for all adults and adolescents. Pregnant or lactating women need more and therefore the RDA for these groups is increased 25 μg. and 50 μg. respectively.

DEFICIENCY. Lack of iodine intake is associated with the development of a type of thyroid gland dysfunction known as *endemic* or *simple goiter*. Simple goiter is a state of enlargement of the thyroid gland which develops through a deficiency of ingested iodine. The deficiency may be absolute, especially in areas of subnormal iodine intake, or relative, subsequent to various demands of the body which increase the need for thyroid secretion in the female during adolescence, pregnancy and lactation. Chapter 26 contains a discussion of iodine deficiency and goiter.

Incidence. The highest incidence of goiter in areas where the disorder is endemic usually occurs in females 12 to 18 years of age and males 9 to 13 years. The incidence of goiter can be correlated with the iodine intake from the water and food of a specific region. Figure 7–12 shows the regions known as the "goiter belt" in the United States and other areas worldwide where the soil is iodine-poor, producing iodine-poor food. The WHO has estimated that there are approximately 200 million goitrous individuals in the world today, and few countries are exempt. In some countries goiter is so common that it is

regarded as a normal physical feature, as shown in Figure 7–13.

Food iodine is an important factor determining the incidence of goiter in a region. Nutritional iodine is derived essentially from the food and to a lesser degree from supplemented salt or water. The amount of iodine in the local drinking water may be regarded as a measure of the iodine content of the soil and, consequently, of the iodine content of the fruits, grasses and vegetables grown in the region. However, the iodine content of water is not important as a source of nutritional iodine except in unusual circumstances.

Goitrogens in food can also cause goiter. These are natural inhibitors of the thyroid gland. Some foods containing goitrogens are cabbage, turnips, rapeseeds, mustard seeds, groundnuts, cassava and soybeans. Cooking inactivates goitrogens.

Other studies suggest that local water may contain goitrogenic substances from geological origin or possibly from *Escherichia coli* in the water.[6] This may explain the prevalence of goiter in some areas where it does not seem dependent on iodine deficiency alone.

Prevention and Treatment. Simple goiter can be prevented and frequently cured by the administration of iodine. To supply the needed iodine, the use of iodized salt is advised. People residing along the seacoast may obtain iodine from fresh shellfish (rich in iodine) and foods grown in iodine-rich soil. People living in the goiter belt who consume local produce especially should be urged to use iodized salt. With the rapid interstate transportation of food, the regular use of iodized salts and iodized fertilizers, iodine deficiency is unlikely in the United States.

Endemic goiter is still widespread in the underdeveloped areas. The international agencies, particularly WHO and ICNND, have addressed a great deal of attention toward effective salt iodization.

TOXICITY. Data on 35,999 persons in the Ten-State Nutrition Survey revealed a 3.1 per cent prevalence of thyroid enlargement. However, urinary excretion of iodine was also high. Two other surveys confirm high levels of urinary iodine excretion by the U.S. population, thus reflecting high iodine intake. A study of dietary frequency histories from 754 children, ages 9 to 16 years, revealed that milk processed in equipment cleaned with iodates, bread made with iodine dough conditioners, and iodized salt are significant dietary sources of iodine.[20] Accumulating evidence of increased iodine intake has caused concern that the population's iodine intake may be too high. However, at this point, adverse reaction to iodine in foods is not a sig-

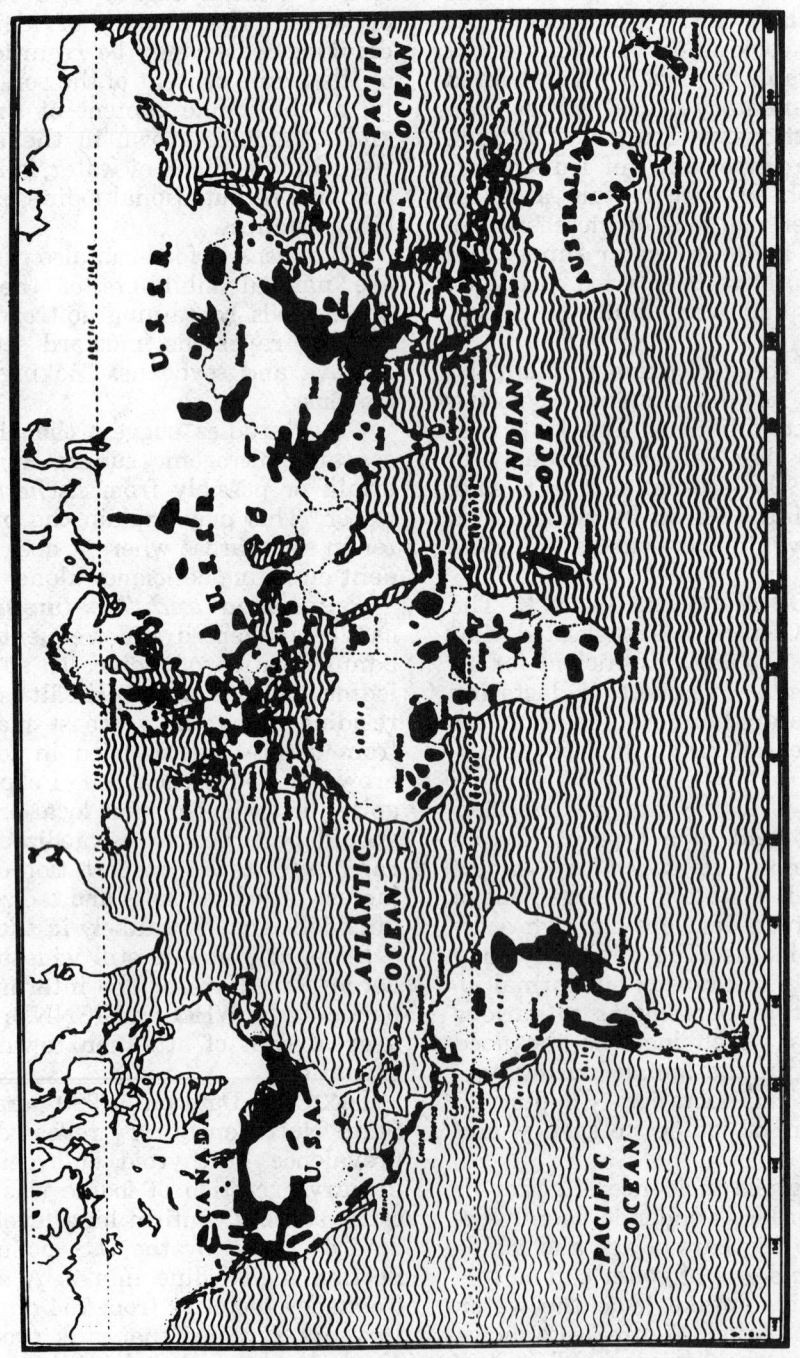

Figure 7–12. Goiter areas of the world. (From Volume III, Agriculture. Science, Technology, and Development. U.S. papers prepared for the United Nations Conference on the application of Science and Technology for the Benefit of the Less Developed Areas, 1962.)

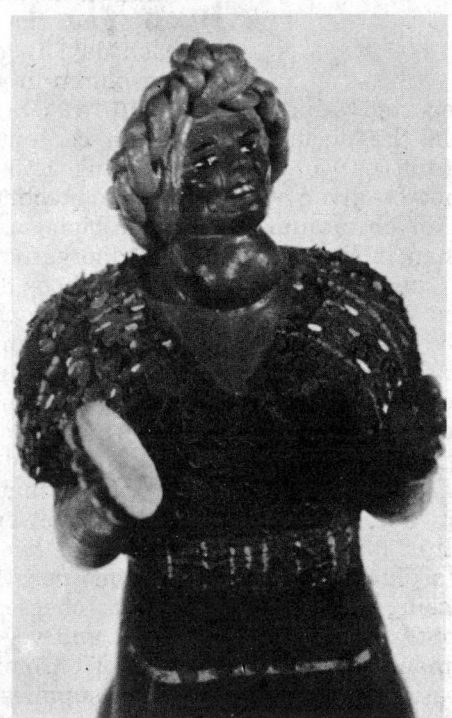

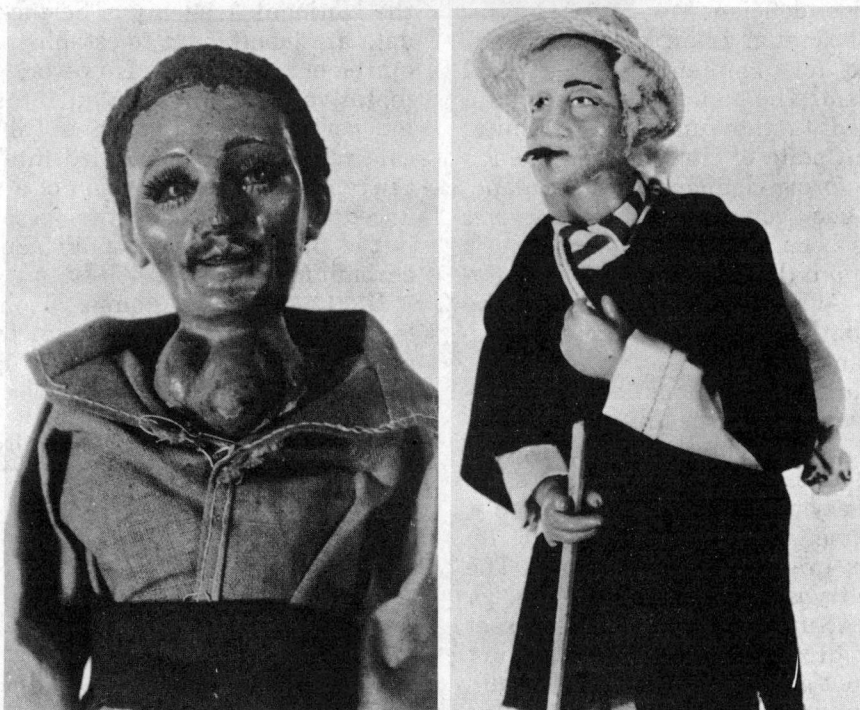

Figure 7–13. Dolls with goiter from the goitrous belt of Middle America. *Above,* figure of village woman making tortillas, made in local village and purchased in Guatemala City market; *lower left,* old religious statue from Antigua, Guatemala; *lower right,* doll of more recent date manufactured in village in Colombia. All illustrate the acceptance of goiter as a normal physical feature. (From Volume III, Agriculture. Science, Technology, and Development. U.S. papers prepared for the United Nations Conference on the application of Science and Technology for the Benefit of the Less Developed Areas, 1962.)

nificant clinical or public health problem in the United States.

CHROMIUM

Over the past two decades reported values for the chromium concentration in the plasma of normal subjects has ranged from 0.075 to 13 ng./ml. A reliable range cannot be given with full confidence. Concentration of chromium in the hair is ten times higher than in blood, and hair concentration has been suggested as a means of assessing chromium status.

In both man and animals the concentration of chromium in tissues is higher during the newborn period than later in life. The chromium concentration of most tissues decreases steadily with increasing age. In pregnant women the fasting plasma chromium level is lower than in non-pregnant women. Further, women in late pregnancy do not show any fall in plasma chromium concentration following a glucose load as do non-pregnant women. Increasing impairment of glucose tolerance throughout normal pregnancy has been amply documented, and the changes in chromium concentration in the plasma may reflect decreased glucose tolerance or may actually reflect deficiency.

FUNCTIONS. Chromium is an essential trace element required for maintenance of normal glucose metabolism. The function of chromium is directly related to the function of insulin. Only the trivalent state of chromium is biologically active and forms complexes with organic compounds. One such complex, *glucose tolerance factor (GTF)*, has been identified from brewer's yeast as a chromium (III) dinicotinic acid–glutathione complex. GTF not only potentiates the effect of insulin but also results in decreased serum cholesterol and triglycerides.

Insulin–chromium interactions are not restricted to glucose metabolism. In animal studies, chromium stimulated amino acid transport and protein synthesis. In vitro, chromium stimulates several enzyme systems, for example, succinic–cytochrome *c* dehydrogenase, and inhibits others, for example, glucuronidase. The digestive enzyme trypsin contains chromium.

ABSORPTION AND EXCRETION. The exact mechanism of chromium absorption is not known, but it is not simple diffusion. Chromium is transported in the plasma in combination with transferrin. Plasma chromium does not reflect chromium status. Unlike other metals, once chromium is absorbed it is almost entirely excreted in the urine. Therefore, urine chromium is a rough estimate of status. Mean 24-hour chromium excretion has been reported as 0.8 ± 0.4 μg. and the range as 0.4 to 1.8 μg. Inorganic chromium is poorly absorbed. The average intake of 50 to 100 μg. per day of inorganic chromium from food and water supplies only 0.25 to 0.5 μg. of the 7 to 10 μg. excreted in the urine each day. In contrast, 10 to 25 per cent of the chromium in yeast extracts is absorbed.

DIETARY SOURCES. Table 7–6 shows the chromium content of selected foods. Human milk contains 1.55 to 18.5 ng./ml. At the present state of technology, it is not possible to distinguish biologically available GTF from chromium and inorganic chromium. Total chromium content of foods does not correlate well with biological effectiveness. Ethanol extracts of foodstuffs correlate significantly with GTF activity and may be useful in assessing dietary chromium status. Refining whole wheat removes most of the chromium, since it is largely contained in the germ and the bran. Refining sugar results in a fractionation of the chromium into the molasses. Brewer's yeast, oysters, potatoes with skins and liver have a high chromium concentration per 1000 kcalories. Seafoods, whole grains, cheeses, chicken, meats, bran, and fresh fruits and vegetables have an intermediate content of chromium per 1000 kcalories. Drinking water supplies variable amounts.

RECOMMENDED INTAKE. Expert committees of the National Academy of Science and WHO feel data are insufficient to establish a chromium requirement for man. However, the 1980 RDA tentatively recommends an intake of 50 to 200 μg. per day for adults. See Table 10–2 for the safe range of recommended intake for all ages. Currently, the consumption of a varied diet, balanced with regard to other essential nutrients, is the best assurance of an adequate and safe chromium intake.

DEFICIENCY. In humans, chromium deficiency is characterized by glucose intolerance, impaired growth, peripheral neuropathy, negative

Table 7–6. CHROMIUM IN FOODS

FOOD	μG./GM.	μG./100 KCAL.
Vegetable oils		
Margarine, corn oil	0.23	2.56
Corn oil	0.12	0.33
Cotton seed oil	0.05	1.0
Safflower oil	0.07	0.8
Butter, unsalted	0.21	2.3
Grains		
Buckwheat	0.38	11.0
Wheat	0.03	0.8
Cereal Products		
All bran	0.25	8.1
Puffed rice	0.71	18.2
Wheat germ	0.07	2.0
Molasses	0.22	10.0

(Schroeder, H. A., Nason, A. P., and Tipton, I. H.: Chromium deficiency as a factor in atherosclerosis. J. Chronic Dis. *23*:123, 1970.)

nitrogen balance and decreased respiratory quotient. Frank deficiency has been reported only in patients maintained on total parenteral nutrition for prolonged periods of time. Marginal deficiency may appear in pregnant or elderly persons as well as in malnourished children or patients with diabetes or early coronary heart disease.

One study showed abnormal glucose tolerance in 77 per cent of normal elderly subjects over 70 years of age. Supplementation of the diet with chromium resulted in improved glucose tolerance in 50 per cent of middle-aged subjects. Four of ten elderly subjects had improved glucose tolerance; the remaining six who did not improve originally had more severe impairment.[42]

COBALT

Cobalt is unique in that it must be supplied entirely in its physiologically active form, *vitamin B₁₂*. Vitamin B_{12} is essential for the maturation of red blood cells and normal functioning of all cells. This is the only known biological function of cobalt.

ABSORPTION AND EXCRETION. Although earlier it was thought to be poorly absorbed, cobalt is now known to be well absorbed. Cobalt absorption is increased in patients with iron deficiency, portal cirrhosis with iron overload, and idiopathic hemochromatosis. Cobalt may share at least part of the same intestinal transport mechanism with iron. The major route of excretion is the urine, with small amounts excreted in the feces, sweat and hair. Most of the cobalt in the body is found in the liver, the main storage organ, with some found in the spleen, kidneys and pancreas. About 1 μg. per 100 ml. is found in the blood plasma.

DIETARY SOURCES. Organ meats, such as liver and kidneys which contain 0.15 to 0.25 ppm. of cobalt on a dry weight basis, are excellent sources. Muscle meats contain approximately half that amount. Oysters and clams are also excellent sources. Fruits, vegetables and cereals contain none of their cobalt as vitamin B_{12}. Strict vegetarians, who avoid all animal products, are known to become deficient; however, it may take 3 to 6 years for the deficiency to develop.

RECOMMENDED DIETARY ALLOWANCE. The dietary requirement for cobalt is 3 μg. per day in the form of vitamin B_{12}. There is not sufficient information upon which to base the requirement for cobalt itself. Neither animals nor plants can synthesize vitamin B_{12}. Ruminants are dependent upon the symbiotic relationship with the microorganisms of their gastrointestinal tract, which synthesize vitamin B_{12}. The microorganisms of monogastric species, such as

man, have an extremely limited capacity for synthesis in areas where the vitamin can be absorbed; therefore, humans get their B_{12} from animal foods.

DEFICIENCY. Deficiency of vitamin B_{12} produces a macrocytic anemia or *pernicious anemia*. However, in the case of pernicious anemia, deficiency results from a genetic defect, failure of the gastric mucosa to form a mucoprotein necessary for absorption of the vitamin, rather than a dietary inadequacy.

TOXICITY. A high intake of inorganic cobalt in animal diets has been shown to produce *polycythemia* (overproduction of red blood cells), hyperplasia of bone marrow, reticulocytosis and increased blood volume. In view of the levels of cobalt required, this should be regarded as a pharmacological rather than a physiological effect.

Essential Micronutrients—Amounts Needed for Humans Cannot Be Estimated at Present

SILICON

During the last decade, silicon has been recognized as an essential trace element.[43] Early studies suggested a role for silicon in growth and bone formation. The primary role of silicon appears to be in the formation of bone matrix, although it has a role in the mineralization process independent of vitamin D. In animals with silicon deficiency, the bone matrix is more transparent and less calcified. Silicon deficiency results in decreased bone collagen, skull deformity and long bone abnormalities. Silicon has been shown to be the major anion of osteogenic cells with a concentration in the same range as calcium, magnesium and phosphorus.

The highest concentration of silicon in the body is in the epidermis and connective tissue. There is a trend toward decreasing concentration with age in the dermis and aorta. In patients with atherosclerosis, the concentration of silicon in some tissues remains high instead of decreasing with age.

As is relatively common among the trace elements, there is come evidence suggesting a silicon–molybdenum interaction. The nature of this interaction has not been established.

Silicon, as *silicic acid,* is absorbed readily and excreted in the urine. Age, sex and some hormones affect the concentration in tissues and blood. The concentration in plasma averages 0.5 mg./liter.

DIETARY SOURCES. Animal foods, with the exception of chicken skin, are poor sources of silicon; plant foods, particularly unrefined grains, contain large amounts of silicon. The most concentrated source of silicon is beer, which contains 1200 μg./gm.[34]

VANADIUM

Data from four laboratories on studies of two different species have established vanadium as an essential nutrient. Vanadium deficiency in rats and chicks produced reduced growth, poor reproductive performance, changes in hematological parameters, bone defects and alterations of lipid metabolism.

Very little is known about the function of vanadium, but an important role for humans may be in lipid metabolism either directly in the control of an enzymatic function or as part of a lipid-soluble molecule with high biological activity.[13] Vanadium is found mainly in the fat of animals. Vanadium-deficient chicks have high plasma cholesterol and triglyceride concentrations. It is most likely that vanadium functions as an oxidation-reduction catalyst. Human intake has been established to be 2 mg. daily in a "well-balanced diet" for a person weighing 75 kg. Little information is available on vanadium requirements.

DIETARY SOURCES. Good sources of vanadium are bread, some grains and nuts, vegetable oils and a few root vegetables. The amounts vary from less than 0.1 ng./gm. in peas, beets, carrots and peas to 52 ng./gram in radishes. Liver, fish and meat contain up to 10 ng./gram. A diet could contain very low amounts, less than 50 ng. of vanadium per gram of diet, if intake were exclusively milk, meat and certain vegetables.

TIN

Until recently, the presence of tin in tissues was attributed to environmental contamination. However, the accuracy of early quantitative data is questionable because of the considerable loss of the metal during analytical procedures— a loss that has been noted only recently. Careful work by Schwarz and colleagues[44] demonstrated that tin produced an acceleration of growth in rats and met the standards for essentiality. As a member of the fourth main chemical group of elements, tin has many chemical and physical properties similar to those of carbon, silicon, germanium and lead. Tin is similar to carbon in its tendency to form truly covalent linkages. A large proportion of tin is found in the lipid-extractable portion of commercial fats. Recently, tin has been shown to exert a potent induction effect on heme oxygenase, enhancing heme breakdown in the kidney and impairing heme-dependent cellular functions, such as drug biotransformation mediated by cytochrome P–450.

SELENIUM

Although toxic in high doses, selenium is an essential nutrient for some species. Selenium prevents the development of exudative diathesis in chicks and muscular dystrophy in lambs and calves, as well as a number of other diseases. Some of the disorders also respond to vitamin E (tocopherol), thus establishing a relationship between it and selenium. Other disorders are not corrected by tocopherol, showing there is a separate need for selenium.

There is little information available on the concentration of selenium in various human tissues. Based on limited information, it appears that the highest concentration is in the kidney; the next highest is in the liver. Concentration in the blood depends on intake and varies widely. Selenium values in people living in selenious areas may be tenfold higher than those of people living in a region where the soil is low in selenium.

FUNCTIONS. Selenium is an important constituent of *glutathione peroxidase* in erythrocytes; this enzyme protects against accumulation of hydrogen peroxide. The antioxidant effects of selenium and vitamin E may reinforce each other by overlap of remedial action. Selenium functions with tocopherol to protect cell and organelle membranes from oxidative damage, to facilitate union between oxygen and hydrogen at the end of the metabolic chain, to transfer ions across cell membranes and to aid in immunoglobulin and ubiquinone synthesis.

Patients with cancer have lowered plasma selenium levels. Statistical analysis of data has shown lower cancer mortality in those states with higher levels of selenium in forage crops and grains. Another hypothesis suggests that human heart disease is due in part to dietary inadequacy of selenium and vitamin E.

Work in New Zealand and China has shown beneficial effects of small quantities of selenium. In New Zealand, selenium was added to the intravenous feeding solutions reversing severe muscular discomfort.[53] In China, *Keshan's disease,* a cardiomyopathy affecting mainly children, was prevented in a four-year feeding trial of 12,000 children.[19] Although there may be other factors involved, selenium was still shown to be important.

DIETARY SOURCES. The selenium content of foods is dependent on the amount in the soil. A study of four composite diets from three Canadian cities showed they contained 191, 220, 113 and 115 μg. of selenium.[51]

Cereals contain the most selenium, with meat, poultry and fish, and dairy products following in decreasing concentration. Selenium may be lost from foods by washing, cooking and storing.

RECOMMENDED INTAKE. The 1980 RDA recommends a range of 50 to 200 μg. per day as adequate and safe for adults. See Table 10–2 for the safe range of suggested intakes for all ages. The requirements may increase as the unsaturated fatty acid content of the diet increases.

DEFICIENCY. Reported manifestations of selenium deficiency include myalgia, muscle tenderness, cardiac myopathy, increased red blood cell fragility and pancreatic degeneration.

MANGANESE

In 1972 the first report of manganese deficiency in man appeared.[12] Until that time there was doubt that manganese deficiency could occur in humans. The symptoms were weight loss, transient dermatitis, occasional nausea and vomiting, changes in hair and beard color, and slow growth of hair and beard. Studies of manganese deficiency in animals revealed effects on reproductive capacity, pancreatic function and other aspects of carbohydrate metabolism which may relate to its role with pyruvate carboxylase. There are 10 to 20 μg. of manganese in the adult human body. The concentration of manganese tends to be high in tissues rich in mitochondria. Serum concentration is reported to range from 1 to 200 μg./liter.

FUNCTIONS. The manganous ion is known to be an activator of many enzymes. However, it is not possible at this time to correlate effects on dependent enzymes with the deficiency state. Manganese appears to be essential for sulfomucopolysaccharide biosynthesis. Abnormalities of cellular ultrastructure include an increase in the vascular portion of the cell, abnormal mitochondria, enlargement of the Golgi apparatus and disorganization of the rough endoplasmic reticulum. Changes in the latter two organelles are particularly significant since they are felt to be the sites of mucopolysaccharide synthesis. Information regarding the relationship between manganese and various hormones, nucleic acids and therapeutic applications is just beginning to be studied.

ABSORPTION AND EXCRETION. Mechanisms of absorption from the gastrointestinal tract are unknown, but there is a specific manganese-carrying plasma protein, *transmanganin*. Absorbed manganese appears rapidly in the bile and is excreted in the feces. Selective excretion rather than selective absorption appears to regulate tissue levels.

DIETARY SOURCES. The manganese content of foods also varies greatly. The richest sources are blueberries, wheat bran, dried legumes, nuts, lettuce, beet tops and pineapple. Animal tissues, seafood and dairy products are poor sources. Instant coffee and tea have relatively high amounts. Human milk is relatively deficient in manganese. The most recent reported median value for the concentration of manganese in human milk is 5.9 μg./liter.

RECOMMENDED INTAKE. The 1980 RDA recommends that in order to include an extra margin of safety, the manganese intake of adults over long periods of time should be in the range of 2.5 to 5 mg. per day. See Table 10–2 for the safe ranges of recommended intake for all ages.

DEFICIENCY. Animal studies have established the essentiality of manganese for reproduction: deficiency results in sterility in both sexes. The most striking effects of manganese deficiency are the skeletal abnormalities and ataxia of the offspring of deficient mothers.

TOXICITY. Manganese toxicity has been seen in miners as a result of absorption of manganese through the respiratory tract after prolonged exposure to dust. The excess accumulates in the liver and central nervous system. Symptoms resemble those found in Parkinson's and Wilson's diseases.

NICKEL

In 1974, nickel was found to be an essential nutrient for the chick.[34] Since that time the essentiality of nickel has been demonstrated in rats, miniature pigs and goats.

Nickel is present in human blood, lung, pancreas, adrenal glands, brain, teeth, bone, kidney, aorta and skin. Nickel has been shown to be consistently present in ribonucleic acids (RNA). Increased amounts of nickel are present in several pathological conditions. Patients with cancer, myocardial infarction or thyrotoxicosis have increased blood levels. Increased blood and skin levels are seen in individuals with psoriasis, photodermatitis and several forms of eczema. There is a decrease in blood nickel in patients with vitamin B_{12} deficiency, cirrhosis of the liver, chronic uremia or renal insufficiency. The reasons for changes in the circulating level of nickel in these, as well as other conditions, are not known.

FUNCTIONS. The most likely roles for nickel are in some aspect of hormonal, membrane or enzyme activity. Excessive levels of nickel cause an increase in the release of prolactin-inhibiting factor, which in turn decreases the *in vitro* release of prolactin from bovine and rat pituitary glands. Increased and deficient intakes of nickel are both associated with reduced litter size in animals. Nickel deficiency results in changes in the livers of animal species studied thus far. Rats maintained on a nickel-deficient diet develop anemia associated with a reduction in iron absorption. Dietary nickel enhances the absorption of ferric iron (the relatively unavailable form) when the supply is only slightly less than optimal. Nickel deficiency also results in parakeratotic skin lesions.

DIETARY SOURCES. Grains and vegetables appear to be good sources of dietary nickel; however, there is the possibility that some of the nickel in these foods may not be bioavailable. Foods of animal origin contain relatively little nickel. It would appear that diets high in foods of animal origin or fats might be low in nickel.

MOLYBDENUM

Molybdenum has been shown to be an integral part of xanthine oxidase and has been implicated in aldehyde oxidase and sulfite oxidase activities. *Xanthine oxidase,* which also contains iron, is involved in the formation of uric acid from the purine xanthine and is important in the mobilization of ferritin iron from liver reserves. An interrelationship between molybdenum, copper and sulfate absorption has been demonstrated in livestock. Copper and molybdenum each prevent the uptake of excessive amounts of the other, but these actions require the presence of inorganic sulfate. Seelig suggests that the high copper intake of people in the United States lowers molybdenum and iron absorption.[45] Molybdenum is found in minute amounts in the body, is readily absorbed from the gastrointestinal tract and is excreted mainly in the urine. The daily requirement is not known. However, the 1980 RDA recommends 0.15 to 0.5 mg. per day as a safe intake for adults. The recommendations for other age groups are listed in Table 10–2. It is widely distributed in commonly used foods such as legumes, whole-grain cereals, dark-green leafy vegetables, milk and liver.

TOXICITY. An excessive intake of 10 to 15 mg. per day is associated with a high incidence of goutlike syndrome.

ADDITIONAL TRACE ELEMENTS

Arsenic has been recently reported to be an essential trace element, but little is known about its function. In addition, other minerals may have specific essential physiological functions. Research and interest is ever growing. *Cadmium* may play a role in control of blood pressure. High levels have been found in the kidneys of patients with hypertension. In contrast to other non-essential trace elements, cadmium has a specific pattern of distribution. The kidney has ten times the concentration of the liver, which has five times more than any other organ. There are no known functions or needs for *aluminum, boron* or *bromine,* although these elements are found in animal and plant tissues.

They seem to be harmless for man in their naturally occurring concentrations.

Problems and Suggested Topics for Discussion

1. Keep a record of your food intake for 24 hours and evaluate the intake for foods high in iron, zinc and calcium. Make suggestions for improvement in selection.
2. Plan a diet for yourself, omitting milk and milk products, and check for adequacy of calcium.
3. What are the functions of (a) iodine, (b) zinc, (c) copper, (d) chromium, (e) selenium and (f) magnesium?
4. Describe the effects of deficiency of each of the minerals listed in question 3.
5. Which nutrients are involved in the synthesis of hemoglobin?
6. Survey the literature and report on a mineral now under investigation for its importance to human nutrition.
7. Discuss absorption of iron and zinc. Include in your discussion factors and compounds that enhance or inhibit absorption.

Cited References

1. Allen, L.H., Bartlett, R.S., and Block, G.D.: Reduction of renal calcium reabsorption in man by consumption of dietary protein. J. Nutr., *109*:1345, 1979.
2. Alvioli, V.: Intestinal absorption of calcium. Arch. Intern. Med., *129*:345, 1971.
3. Caddell, J.L.: Magnesium in the nutrition of the child. Clin. Pediatr., *13*:263, 1974.
4. Chandra, R.K., and Saraya, A.K.: Impaired immunocompetence associated with iron deficiency. J. Pediatr., *86*:899, 1975.
5. Cook, J.D., and Skikne, B.S.: Serum ferritin: a possible model for the assessment of nutrient stores. Am. J. Clin. Nutr., *35*:1180, 1982.
6. Endemic goiter and antithyroid agents. Nutr. Rev., *33*: 171, 1975.
7. Hagler, L., et al.: Influence of dietary iron deficiency on hemoglobin, myoglobin, their respective reductases and skeletal muscle mitochondrial respiration. Am. J. Clin. Nutr., *34*:2169, 1981.
8. Hallberg, L., et al.: Deleterious effects of prolonged warming of meals on ascorbic acid content and iron absorption. Am. J. Clin. Nutr., *36*:846, 1982.
9. Halsted, J.A., et al.: Zinc deficiency in man—the Shivaz experiment. Am. J. Med., *53*:277, 1972.
10. Hambidge, K.M., et al.: Low levels of zinc in hair, anorexia, poor growth and hypogeusia in children. Pediatr. Res., *6*:868, 1972.
11. Heaney, R.P., et al.: Calcium nutrition and bone health in the elderly. Am. J. Clin. Nutr., *36*:986, 1982.
12. Henkin, R.I.: Trace metals in endocrinology. Med. Clin. North Am., *60*:779, 1976.
13. Hopkins, L.L., and Mohr, H.E.: Vanadium as an essential nutrient. Fed. Proc., *33*:1773, 1974.
14. Hurley, L.S.: Trace elements and teratogenesis. Med. Clin. North Am., *60*:771, 1976.
15. Johnson, N.E., Alcantara, E.N., and Linksweiler, H.: Effect of level of protein intake on urinary and fecal calcium and calcium retention of young adult males. J. Nutr., *100*:1425, 1970.
16. Jones, K.L., et al.: Pattern of malformation of offspring of chronic alcoholic mothers. Lancet, *1*:1267, 1973.
17. Kay, R.G., et al.: A syndrome of acute zinc deficiency during total parenteral alimentation in man. Ann. Surg., *183*:331, 1976.

18. Kelley, W.A., Kesterson, J.W., and Carleton, W.W.: Myocardial lesions in the offspring of female rats fed a copper deficient diet. Exp. Mol. Pathol., 20:40, 1974.
19. Keshan Disease Research Group. Chinese Med. J., 92:471 and 92:477, 1979.
20. Kidd, P.S., et al.: Sources of dietary iodine. J. Am. Diet. Assoc., 65:420, 1974.
21. Klevay, L.M.: The ratio of zinc to copper of diets in the United States. Nutr. Reports Int., 11:237, 1975.
22. Klevay, L.M., et al.: The human requirement for copper. I. Healthy men fed conventional American diets. Am. J. Clin. Nutr., 33:482, 1980.
23. Krantman, H.J., et al.: Immune function in pure iron deficiency. Am. J. Dis. Child., 136:840, 1982.
24. Krishnamachari, K.A.V.R., and Iyengar, L.: Effect of maternal malnutrition on the bone density of the neonate. Am. J. Clin. Nutr., 33:482, 1975.
25. Lee, D.B., and Kleeman, C.R.: Phosphorus in man. McGaw Clinical Digest 5, No. 3, 1976.
26. Leverett, D.H.: Fluorides and the changing prevalence of dental caries. Science, 217:26, 1982.
27. Lynch, S.R., et al.: Iron status of elderly Americans. Am. J. Clin. Nutr., 36:1032, 1982.
28. Massaro, T.F., and Widmayer, P.: The effect of iron deficiency on cognitive performance in the rat. Am. J. Clin. Nutr., 34:864, 1981.
29. McCarron, D.A., Morris, C.D., and Cole, C.: Dietary calcium in human hypertension. Science, 217:267, 1982.
30. Mertz, W.: The essential trace elements. Science, 213:1332, 1981.
31. Monsen, E.R., et al.: Estimation of available dietary iron. Am. J. Clin. Nutr., 31:134, 1978.
32. Moynahan, E.J.: Acrodermatitis enteropathica: a lethal inherited human zinc deficiency. Lancet, 2:399, 1974.
33. Neldner, K.H. and Hambidge, K.M.: Zinc therapy of acrodermatitis enteropathica. N. Engl. J. Med., 292:879, 1975.
34. Nielsen, F.H., and Sandstead, H.H.: Are nickel, vanadium, silicon, fluoride and tin essential for man? A review. Am. J. Clin. Nutr., 27:515, 1974.
35. Nordin, B.E.C.: Metabolic bone and bone disease. Baltimore, Williams & Wilkins Co., 1973.
36. Pollitt, E., Greenfield, D., and Leibel, R.L.: Behavioral effects of iron deficiency among preschool children in Cambridge, MA. Fed. Proc., 37:487, 1976.
37. Prasad, A.S.: Clinical biochemical and pharmacologic roles of zinc. Ann. Rev. Pharmacol. Toxicol., 20:393, 1979.
38. Prasad, A.S., et al.: Zinc metabolism in patients with the syndrome of iron deficiency anemia, hepatosplenomegaly, dwarfism and hypogonadism. J. Lab. Clin. Med., 61:537, 1963.
39. Purvis, G.A.: What nutrients do our infants really get? Nutr. Today, 8:29, 1973.
40. Rowe, J.C., et al.: Nutritional hypophosphatemic rickets in a premature infant fed breast milk. N. Engl. J. Med., 300:293, 1979.
41. Sandstead, H.: Zinc nutrition in the United States. Am. J. Clin. Nutr., 26:1251, 1973.
42. Saner, G. (ed.): Chromium in Nutrition and Disease. New York, Alan R. Liss, Inc., 1980.
43. Schwarz, K.: Recent dietary trace element research exemplified by tin, fluorine and silicon. Fed. Proc., 33:1748, 1974.
44. Schwarz, K., Milne, D.B., and Vinyard, E.: Growth effect of tin compounds in rats maintained in a trace element controlled environment. Biochem. Biophys. Res. Commun., 40:22, 1970.
45. Seelig, M.S.: Review: relation of copper and molybdenum to iron metabolism. Am. J. Clin. Nutr., 25:1022, 1972.
46. Seelig, M.S., and Heggtveit, H.A.: Magnesium interrelationships in ischemic heart disease: a review. Am. J. Clin. Nutr., 27:59, 1974.
47. Solomons, N.W., and Jacob, R.A.: Studies on the bioavailability of zinc in humans. Effect of heme and nonheme iron in the absorption of zinc. Am. J. Clin. Nutr., 34:474, 1981.
48. Solomons, N.W.: Biological availability of zinc to humans. Am. J. Clin. Nutr., 35:1048, 1982.
49. Speckman, E.W., and Brink, M.F.: Relationship between fat and mineral metabolism—a review. J. Am. Diet. Assoc., 51:517, 1974.
50. Spencer, H., and Lender, M.: Adverse effects of aluminium-containing antacids on mineral metabolism. Gastroenterology, 76:603, 1979.
51. Thompson, J.M., Erdoby, P., and Smith, D.C.: Selenium content of food consumed by Canadians. J. Nutr., 105:274, 1975.
52. Tucker, S.B., et al.: Acquired zinc deficiency. Cutaneous manifestations typical of acrodermatitis enteropathica. JAMA, 235:2399, 1976.
53. Van Rij, A.M., et al.: Selenium deficiency in total parenteral nutrition. Am. J. Clin. Nutr., 32:2076, 1979.
54. Vir, S.C., et al.: Serum and hair concentrations of copper during pregnancy. Am. J. Clin. Nutr., 34:2382, 1981.
55. Walker, R.M., and Linkswiler, H.: Calcium retention in the adult male as affected by protein intake. J. Nutr., 102:1297, 1972.

Additional References

GENERAL

Alfin-Slater, R.B., and Kritchevsky, D.: Human Nutrition. A Comprehensive Treatise. New York, Plenum Press, 1979.
Bronner, F., and Cobrun, J.W.: Disorders of Mineral Metabolism. New York, Academic Press, 1981.
Burch, R.E., and Sullivan, J.F. (eds.): Trace Elements. Med. Clin. North Am., 60(4), 1976.
Davidson, S., et al.: Human Nutrition and Dietetics. 7th ed. Edinburgh, Churchill Livingstone, 1979.
Food and Nutrition Board, National Research Council: Recommended Dietary Allowances. 9th ed. Washington, D.C., National Academy of Sciences, 1980.
Goodhart, R.E., and Shils, M.E. (eds.): Modern Nutrition in Health and Disease. 6th ed. Philadelphia, Lea & Febiger, 1980.
Mertz, W., and Cornatzer, W.E. (eds.): Newer Trace Elements in Nutrition. New York, Marcel Dekker, 1971.
Prasad, A.S., and Oberleas, D. (eds.): Trace Elements in Health and Disease. Vols. I and II. New York, Academic Press, 1976.
Randolph, P.M., and Dennison, C.I.: Diet Nutrition and Dentistry. St. Louis, C. V. Mosby, 1981.
The Ten-State Nutrition Survey 1968–1970. U.S. Department of Health, Education and Welfare, Publication No. HSM 72–8130–4.
Underwood, E.J.: Trace Elements in Human and Animal Nutrition. 4th ed. New York, Academic Press, 1977.

CALCIUM, PHOSPHORUS AND MAGNESIUM

Altchuler, S.I.: Dietary protein and calcium loss: a review. Nutr. Res., 2:193, 1982.
Braulbar, N., et al.: Intestinal absorption of calcium: role of dietary phosphate and vitamin D. Am. J. Physiol., 241:G49, 1981.
Spencer, H.: Osteoporosis: goals of therapy. Hospital Practice 37:131, 1982.

Tsang, R.C., Donovan, E.F., and Steichen, J.J.: Calcium physiology and pathology in the neonate. Pediatr. Clin. North Am., 23:611, 1976.

IRON

Bothwell, T.H., et al. (eds.): Iron Metabolism in Man. London, Blackwell Scientific Publ., 1979.

Cook, J.D. (ed): Iron. New York, Churchill-Livingstone, 1980.

Jacobs, A., and Worwood, M.: Iron in Biochemistry and Medicine II. London, Academic Press, 1980.

Muller-Eberhard, U., Miescher, P.A., and Jaffe, E.R.: Iron Excess—Aberrations of Iron and Porphyrins. New York, Grune & Stratton, 1977.

FLUORIDE

Bell, M.E., et al.: The Supply of Fluorine to Man in Fluorides and Human Health. WHO Monograph, No. 59, Geneva, Switzerland, 1970.

Maheshwari, U.R., et al.: Fluoride balance studies in ambulatory healthy men with and without supplements. Am. J. Clin. Nutr. 34:2679, 1981.

Reinhold, J.G.: Trace elements—a selective survey. Clin. Chem., 21:476, 1975.

OTHER TRACE MINERALS

Carlisle, E.M.: In vivo requirement for silicon in articular cartilage and connective tissue formation in the chick. J. Nutr., 106:478, 1976.

Fowden, L., Garton, G.A., and Mills, C.F.: Metabolic and physiological consequences of trace element deficiency in animals and man. Phil. Trans. R. Soc. Lond. B, 294:1, 1981.

Golden, M.H.N., and Golden, B.E.: Trace elements. Potential importance in human nutrition with particular reference to zinc and vanadium. Brit. Med. Bull., 37:31, 1981.

Hafey, Y., and Kratzer, F.H.: The effect of dietary vanadium on fatty acid and cholesterol synthesis and turnover in the chick. J. Nutr., 106:249, 1976.

Kirchebner, M., Reichlmeyr-Lais, A.M., and Schwarz, F.J.: Interactions of trace elements in human metabolism. XII International Congress of Nutrition. New York, 1981.

Mena, I.: The role of manganese in human disease. Ann. Clin. Lab. Sci., 4:487, 1974.

Mills, C.F.: Biochemical roles of trace elements. In Harper, A. E., and Davis, G.K. (eds.): Nutrition in Health and Disease and International Development: Symposia from the XII International Congress of Nutrition. New York, Alan R. Liss, Inc. 1981.

Sandstead, H.H.: Copper bioavailability and requirements. Am. J. Clin. Nutr., 35:809, 1982.

Thauer, R.K., et al.: Biological role of nickel. Trends Biochem. Sci., 5:304, 1980.

Young, V.R., et al.: Selenium bioavailability with reference to human nutrition. Am. J. Clin. Nutr., 35:1076, 1982.

CHAPTER 8

Water and Electrolytes

DORICE M. CZAJKA-NARINS, PH.D.

Water, an essential and major component of all living matter, is closer to being a universal solvent than any other material. Water is, however, more than a passive solvent; it also participates actively in reactions and provides form to the cells.

Electrolytes are those substances or compounds which when dissolved in water dissociate into positively and negatively charged ions. Electrolytes can be simple inorganic salts of sodium, potassium or magnesium or complex organic molecules.

Acid-base balance is the dynamic state of equilibrium with regard to hydrogen ion concentration. Marked alterations in rates of chemical reactions can occur with only slight changes in hydrogen ion concentration. Illness, trauma or surgery can cause an alteration in the amount and composition of tissue fluids which if not corrected can result in dehydration, shock and death.

Total Body Water

Water is the largest single component of the body. Metabolically active cells of the muscle and viscera have the highest concentration of water and the skeletal cells the lowest. Total body water as a percentage body weight decreases significantly with age. Body water is a higher percentage of weight in athletes than in non-athletes.

Dehydration (water loss) will kill far quicker than starvation. In moderate weather, adults can live up to ten days without water; children up to five. In contrast, a person can live without food for several weeks.

A man can lose most of his fat and glycogen and half his protein (40 per cent loss of body weight) and survive, but a 20 per cent loss of body water may cause death, and a loss of only 10 per cent of water causes severe disorders.

Life goes on in a milieu of water. Water is an essential component of all protoplasm and plays a major role in cellular metabolism. Water is classified as intracellular and extracellular water. *Intracellular* water (ICW) is within the cells of the body. *Extracellular* water (ECW) includes the water in the plasma, lymph, spinal fluid and secretions, and the *intercellular* or *interstitial* water that is found between and around the cells.

More than 99 per cent of the interstitial water is held in a gel in the interstitial spaces and communicates continually with the plasma through pores in the capillaries. Capillaries are porous enough to allow water and most dissolved substances to diffuse freely, but movement of protein is minimized by colloid osmotic pressure exerted by plasma proteins. Edema results when there is an abnormal accumulation of fluid in the intercellular tissue spaces or body cavities.

Figure 8–1 compares the water content as a percentage of total weight of individuals at different ages. Total body water and extracellular body water decrease with age, but intracellular water increases with increased body cell mass. Clinically extracellular water is commonly estimated as 20 per cent of body weight. The distribution of body water can vary under different circumstances, but the total amount in the body remains relatively constant.

Functions of Water

Water serves many functions in the body. Water is the solvent in which many solutes available for cell function are dissolved and is the medium for all reactions. It serves as a building material for growth and repair of the body. Water functions in digestion, absorption, circulation and excretion. It acts as a transport medium for nutrients and all body substances. Metabolic waste products generated in the cells are transported via the plasma to the kidneys, from which the wastes are excreted in the urine. Cellulose and hemicellulose in foods absorb water and swell, thus increasing the fecal weight and aiding in elimination. Water maintains the physical and chemical constancy of intracellular and extracellular fluids. Water plays a role in the maintenance of body temperature. Perspiration during warm weather and in fevers keeps the skin moist; by evaporation of perspiration the body is cooled. Substances containing water act as lubricants in the body. Special water-soluble substances in saliva make foodstuffs slippery, and others around bones lubricate the joints.

Water Balance

The water content of the fat-free body weight remains fairly constant by homeostatic regulation resulting from interactions among antidi-

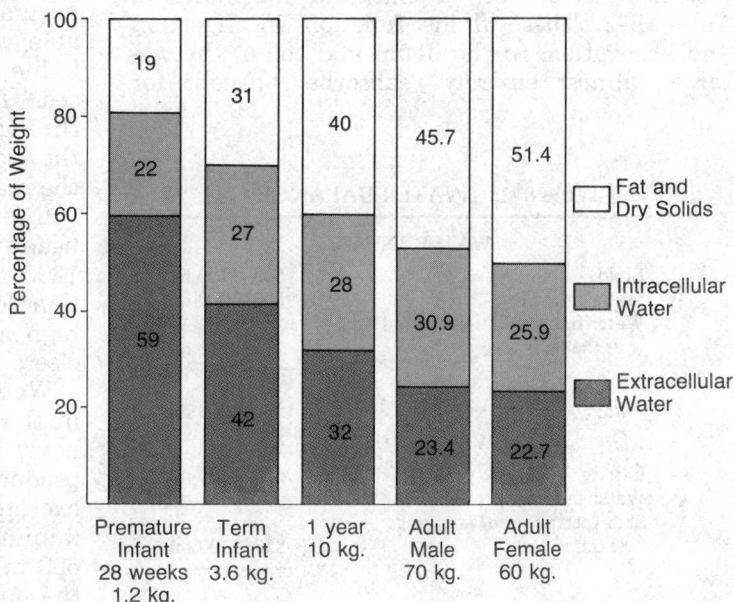

Figure 8–1. Body water as percentage of body weight with approximate distribution between intracellular water and extracellular water. (Data from Foman, S. J., et al.: Body composition of reference children, birth to age ten years. Am. J. Clin. Nutr., *35*:1169, 1982; and Moore, F. D., et al.: Body Cell Mass and Its Supporting Environment. Philadelphia, W. B. Saunders Company, 1963.)

uretic hormone (ADH), the gastrointestinal tract, the kidneys and the brain. That is, the amount of water taken in daily is approximately equivalent to the amount of water loss, as summarized in Table 8–1.

WATER INTAKE

In healthy individuals water intake is controlled largely by thirst sensations. The thirst control centers are located in the ventromedial and anterior hypothalamus, in close relationship to the centers that regulate ADH. Thirst is stimulated when osmolarity increases with a change in volume or when extracellular volume decreases. The brain may also receive information on body water volume from receptors in the walls of the great vessels and atria, but this is a less sensitive mechanism. The sensation of thirst serves as a signal to seek fluids.

Water is ingested as such and as part of ingested food. Most adults in the United States consume 1.5 to 2.0 liters of fluids daily in drinks and food. The main source of preformed water for infants is human milk or infant formula.

In addition to the water contained in ingested foods and liquids, the oxidation of these foods in the body also produces water as an end product, *metabolic water*. The oxidation of 100 gm. of fat, carbohydrate or protein yields 107, 55 and 41 gm. of water, respectively. The amount of water that results from the oxidation of food is 10 to 14 grams per 100 kcalories, or approximately 200 to 300 ml. per day.

In addition to water taken into the digestive tract by mouth, 7 to 9 liters of extracellular fluid are secreted daily into the stomach and intestines. The sources of this fluid are shown in Table 8–2. These fluids function in digestion and absorption. In the ileum and colon, the water is almost entirely reabsorbed, except for

Table 8–2. SOURCES OF WATER IN THE DIGESTIVE JUICES*

Saliva	1500 ml.
Gastric secretions	2500 ml.
Bile	500 ml.
Pancreatic secretions	700 ml.
Intestinal mucosa secretions	3000 ml.
Total	8200 ml.

*Gamble, J. L.: Chemical Anatomy, Physiology and Pathology of Extracellular Fluids. Cambridge, Harvard University Press, 1954.

about 100 ml. that is excreted in the feces. Because this volume of reabsorbed fluid is about twice that of the blood plasma the loss of large amounts from the gastrointestinal tract (diarrhea) may be of serious consequence to the individual.

Water is absorbed rapidly from the digestive tract into the blood and lymph because it moves freely by diffusion through membranes. The movement of water is controlled mostly by osmotic forces generated by the inorganic ions found in solution in the body.

When water cannot be taken orally, it may be given intravenously, subcutaneously or rectally in the form of salt (saline) solutions that resemble closely the fluids of the body. Water also may be given intravenously as glucose solutions or as blood, plasma or protein hydrolysate mixtures.

WATER ELIMINATION

There are four avenues by which the body normally eliminates water. *Sensible* or measurable water is lost from the body through the kidneys as urine and through the bowel in feces. *Insensible*, unmeasurable water is lost through the lungs with expired air, and through the skin as perspiration. The kidney is by far the main regulator of water loss.

Insensible water loss goes on constantly and usually unconsciously, and amounts to 850 to 1200 ml. daily in normal conditions. Perspiration losses are quite variable and may be as high as 5000 ml. during prolonged heavy exercise.

Water is lost from the lungs as tiny droplets in the expired air. Water loss through the kidneys, perspiration and feces carries out waste products and minerals with it. Normally adults excrete 600 to 1600 ml. of urine each day. The minimal urine volume in young adults is 400 to 600 ml. per day. In patients with renal disease, the minimal volume to clear a given solute load is higher because of the decreased ability of the

Table 8–1. WATER BALANCE

WATER INTAKE

Fluids	500–1700 ml.
Water in food	800–1000 ml.
Water from oxidation of food in the body	200–300 ml.
Total	1500–3000 ml.

WATER OUTPUT

Urine	600–1600 ml.
Water in feces	50–200 ml.
Skin (perspiration) and lungs (expired air)	850–1200 ml.
Total	1500–3000 ml.

kidney to concentrate urine. The neonate is not able to excrete a water load as well as an adult, but the ability to handle a water load improves rapidly to adult levels in the first month of life. Neonates can dilute urine to the same degree as adults but are not able to respond to dehydration or hypertonic solute loading by concentrating the urine as an adult would.

Abnormal losses of water occur through vomiting, diarrhea, hemorrhages, draining fistulas, exuding of burns, nasogastric tubes, draining surgical tubes and the ingestion of diuretics. When water intake is insufficient or water loss occurs, the kidney attempts to compensate by conserving water and thereby excretes a more concentrated urine. Concentration of urine is measured by *specific gravity*, normally between 1.010 and 1.030. During dehydration the specific gravity is increased. ADH regulates water and water excretion by stimulating the renal tubules to increase the reabsorption of water.

Water balance is directly related to the homeostatic functioning of the internal environment. Body fluids contain water and electrolytes; variations in the water balance affect electrolyte concentration, and vice versa. When excess water is lost, changes in electrolyte balance occur. The interaction between the electrolytes sodium and potassium in maintaining water balance will be discussed later.

The body has no place to store water. Water held in the bladder is of no metabolic use. Therefore, the amount lost every 24 hours must be replaced to maintain health and efficiency.

Water in Foods

Foods range from 4 to 98 per cent water. Vegetables and fruits contain approximately 90 per cent water, as shown in Table 8–3. Milk is 87 per cent water, meat 60 to 75 per cent water. Even dried foods such as figs and raisins contain about 20 per cent water. Only truly dried foods, the commercially dehydrated foods, do not contain water.

Recommended Allowance of Water

The water requirement depends upon the losses through the various routes—sensible and insensible. The Food and Nutrition Board in 1980 stated that the multitude of factors determining water loss precludes the setting of a general value for minimal water requirement. Under ordinary circumstances, a reasonable al-

Table 8–3. PERCENTAGES OF WATER IN SOME COMMON FOODS

Lettuce (iceberg)	96
Snapbeans, radishes, celery	94
Watermelon	93
Cabbage (raw)	92
Broccoli, carrots, beets, collards	91
Orange	88
Milk	87
Cereals (cooked)	87
Apples	85
Potatoes (boiled)	80
Bananas	76
Eggs	74
Corn	74
Chicken (boiled)	71
Fish (baked)	68
Prunes (cooked)	66
Beef (lean)	60
Cheese	40
Bread	36
Cake (sponge)	32
Butter	16
Nuts	5
Soda crackers, dry cereals	4
Sugar (white)	trace
Oils	0

From Nutritive Value of Foods, U.S. Department of Agriculture. Home Garden Bull. No. 72, revised 1964. Appendix Table 1.

lowance based on recommended caloric intake is 1 ml./kcal. for adults and 1.5 ml./kcal. for infants. A suitable daily allowance for adults in most instances is 2.5 liters or approximately 2.5 to 3 quarts. A large percentage of this is contained in prepared foods. Diets such as the Zen macrobiotic diet, which recommends severely restricted intakes of water and other fluids, or very high-protein weight reduction diets that require a very high intake of water to excrete the catabolic products of protein metabolism can be extremely dangerous. During lactation the need for water is greatly increased because of the high additional losses in the milk produced.

Thirst is usually an adequate guide for water intake except in infants and the sick. In cases of extreme heat or excessive sweating thirst may not keep pace with the actual water requirement. Anyone sick enough to be hospitalized, regardless of diagnosis, is at risk of water and electrolyte imbalance. Special attention to water needs should be given to infants on high-protein formulas; to individuals who are consuming high-protein diets; to comatose patients; to those individuals with fever, excessive urine loss or diarrhea; and to all persons in hot environments.

Dehydration by excess sweating or fluid restriction has frequently been used by young wrestlers trying to "make weight." This is a harmful practice and can adversely affect performance.

Electrolytes

SODIUM CHLORIDE

The need for salt has been known ever since man and animals started living on this planet. Carnivores do not have an urge for salt because animal foods and milk contain sufficient salt, but the herbivorous animals and people on basically vegetarian diets demand salt because it is scant or lacking in cereals, grains, fruits and vegetables.

The mean intake of sodium chloride is 10 to 12 gm. per person per day in Western societies. Approximately 3 gm. occurs naturally in foods, 3 to 5 gm. is added during processing and 4 gm. is added by the person when he prepares and eats his food. Present evidence indicates that 0.6 to 3.5 gm. is an adequate daily intake, much less than many Americans consume. Salt is 40 per cent sodium and 60 per cent chloride.

LOW SALT SYNDROME. Deficiency of sodium chloride occurs mainly during hot weather or as a result of heavy work in a hot climate when excessive sweating takes place. Water intoxication can occur if a large quantity of water is given either by mouth or intravenously without added salt. The simple provision of extra salt in food or in salt tablets will prevent or correct this condition for people working in a hot climate. Fifteen to 20 gm. daily, or even more, may be needed until acclimatization to heat is established. However, it is best to increase salt intake by salting food rather than taking salt tablets.

Adrenal cortical insufficiency, or certain conditions such as marked vomiting and diarrhea, burns, surgical procedures with marked loss of blood, and long-term and overly vigorous treatment of heart failure or kidney disease with very low salt (sodium) diets are some instances that may produce the "low salt syndrome." Signs of salt depletion are given on page 555.

SODIUM

The average adult male contains 52 to 60 milliequivalents (mEq.) per kg. of sodium; the average adult female 48 to 55 mEq. per kg. (Milliequivalents are explained in Appendix Table 40.) For a 70-kg. male this would be 83 to 97 grams of sodium. Thirty-five to 40 per cent of the sodium is in the skeleton. Most of this sodium is unexchangeable or only slowly exchangeable with that in body fluids. Sodium is the major cation of extracellular fluid. Various intestinal secretions, such as bile and pancreatic juice, contain substantial amounts of sodium.

FUNCTIONS. Sodium has several important functions in the body. As the dominant ion of extracellular fluid, sodium regulates the size of this compartment as well as plasma volume. Sodium also aids in conduction of nerve impulses and control of muscle contraction.

ABSORPTION AND EXCRETION. Sodium is readily absorbed in the intestine and carried by the blood to the kidneys, where it is filtered out and returned to the blood in the amounts needed to maintain blood levels required by the body. The greater the sodium intake, the greater the amount absorbed.

Sodium excretion is maintained by a mechanism that involves glomerular filtration rate, the cells of the juxtaglomerular apparatus of the kidneys, the renin-aldosterone system, the sympathetic nervous system, circulating catecholamines and blood pressure. About 90 to 95 per cent of normal body sodium loss is via the urine and the rest is lost in perspiration and in the feces. Normally the quantity of sodium excreted daily equals the amount ingested, so that a state of sodium balance prevails.

Aldosterone, a mineralocorticoid secreted by the adrenal cortex, controls the regulation of sodium balance. When blood sodium levels rise, the thirst receptors in the hypothalamus stimulate the thirst sensation. When blood levels are low, the excretion of sodium through the urine decreases. The levels of sodium in the urine reflect the dietary intake.

DIETARY SOURCES. In addition to salt (sodium chloride) used in cooking, in processing and as seasoning, sodium is present in most foods in varying amounts, as listed in Appendix Table 10. Generally more sodium is present in the protein foods than in vegetables and grains. Fruits contain little or no sodium. The sodium added to these foods in their preparation could be many times that found in them naturally. The sodium content of the water supply varies considerably and in some areas of the country, the amount of sodium in water is of a sufficient quantity to be of significance in the total daily intake. Many non-prescription over-the-counter drugs contain significant amounts of sodium. For example, over-the-counter antacids supply from 500 to 1000 mg. per dose.

RECOMMENDED INTAKE. Daily requirements for sodium are not known. However, the 1980 RDA gives the safe range of recommended intake for all ages, as listed in Table 10–2. Deficiencies are rarely encountered under normal conditions, and the body functions on a wide range of intakes through its mechanisms that conserve or excrete sodium. The sodium intake of Americans has been estimated to be 4.0 to 4.8 gm. of sodium per day (10 to 12 gm. of sodium chloride). Estimates of human requirements are as low as 200 mg. per day.

Sodium intake is frequently restricted in order to control the excessive retention of body water in various pathological states, particularly hypertension. The exact role of sodium in the etiology of hypertension is not clear-cut, but susceptibility to salt-induced hypertension appears to be genetic. Several federal agencies as well as the AMA recommend that Americans reduce their sodium intake in order to reduce the chances of developing hypertension. Hypertension is discussed in Chapter 28.

CHLORINE

Chlorine is widely distributed throughout the body as chloride. It is the principal anion of the extracellular fluids. Together with sodium it helps to maintain water balance and osmotic pressure. The highest concentration is in the cerebrospinal fluid and in the gastric and pancreatic juices of the gastrointestinal tract. In the gastric juice, chloride is secreted as hydrochloric acid, which is necessary to maintain normal acidity of the stomach. Chloride is present in relatively small amounts in the alkaline pancreatic juice. Along with phosphate and sulfate, chloride helps to maintain acid-base balance in the body fluids. Chloride ions participate in the chloride-bicarbonate shift by having the ability to move in and out of the red blood cells and blood plasma, and to maintain osmotic equilibrium in the face of changing levels of carbon dioxide as bicarbonate in the plasma and red blood cells.

Chloride is almost completely absorbed in the intestine and is excreted in urine and sweat. Most of the chloride ingested in the diet occurs as sodium chloride, and the amount in food and added table salt provides approximately 3 to 9 gm. daily. The 1980 RDA gives the safe range of chloride intake for all ages, as listed in Table 10–2. Whenever there are excessive losses of sodium, as in vomiting, diarrhea and profuse sweating, there are losses of chloride ions.

DEFICIENCY. For years chloride had been considered necessary only to neutralize the basic cation sodium. More recently, extra chloride has been found to be necessary for the correction of the metabolic alkalosis that results from disease or the use of diuretics, and a syndrome of chloride deficiency has been described. Chloride deficiency developed in infants fed almost exclusively on a chloride-deficient formula. The syndrome is characterized by loss of appetite, failure to thrive, muscle weakness, lethargy and severe hypokalemic metabolic alkalosis.[1]

POTASSIUM

Potassium constitutes 5 per cent of the total mineral content of the body. It is the major cation of the intracellular fluid, and there is also a small amount in the extracellular fluid.

FUNCTIONS. Along with sodium, potassium is involved in the maintenance of normal water balance, osmotic equilibrium and acid-base balance. It is important along with calcium in the regulation of neuromuscular activity. Potassium also promotes cellular growth. Any considerable increase or decrease of potassium in the extracellular fluid may be regarded as evidence of serious disturbances in muscle biochemistry, since the change in the extracellular fluid occurs late in the process.

ABSORPTION AND EXCRETION. Potassium is readily absorbed from the small intestine. Eighty to 90 per cent of the potassium ingested is excreted in the urine. Ten to 20 per cent is lost in the feces. The kidney maintains normal serum levels through its ability to filter, reabsorb and excrete potassium. The adrenal cortex hormone, *aldosterone*, influences potassium excretion. It conserves sodium, and ionized potassium is excreted in place of ionized sodium by means of the exchange mechanism in the renal tubules.

Potassium level in muscle is related to muscle mass; therefore, if muscle is being formed, an adequate supply of potassium is essential. The same applies to glycogen storage.

RECOMMENDED INTAKE. A potassium deficiency from inadequate intake is not likely to happen in healthy individuals, since potassium is widely distributed in foods. No requirement has been established, but the 1980 RDA listing of the safe range of recommended intakes for all ages is given in Table 10–2. The average intake is estimated to range from 0.8 to 1.5 gm. of potassium per 1000 kcalories. An adequate intake of milk, meats, cereals, vegetables and fruits will provide ample potassium. Appendix Table 10 lists the potassium content of various foods.

DEFICIENCY. Excessive loss of extracellular fluid may result in potassium deficiency. The loss may be due to vomiting, diarrhea, excessive diuresis or prolonged malnutrition. These are conditions in which potassium from the intracellular fluid is transferred to the extracellular fluid. The serum potassium level is low and ionized potassium excretion is increased. The chief features of deficiency are muscular weakness and mental apathy. In hypokalemia cardiac failure can result from depletion of ionized potassium in heart muscle. Any condition giving rise to acidosis is liable to cause potassium loss. The acidotic patient has usually lost large quantities of water, potassium, sodium and accompanying anions owing to osmotic diuresis. Diabetic acidosis requires replacement of potassium when insulin and glucose are given. Insulin is more effective if blood pH is normal and there is adequate renal blood flow to assure excretion of acid metabolites.

Intravenous feedings may lack sufficient potassium. Certain diuretics and adrenal cortical hormones may cause potassium depletion if efforts are not made to replace potassium in the diet.[2]

TOXICITY. In hyperkalemia, the serum level is elevated, resulting from kidney failure to clear ionized potassium. The symptoms are mental confusion, numbness of extremities, poor respiration and weakening of heart action.

Water and Electrolytes

When a salt, acid or base is dissolved in water it dissociates into its constituent ions. Because these charged particles can conduct an electric current they are known as *electrolytes*. Glucose, alcohols, urea and protein, along with many other substances involved in metabolism that do not separate into charged particles, are called *non-electrolytes* because these molecules do not ionize.

Some major differences in the electrolyte composition of extracellular and intracellular fluids are shown in Figure 8–2. The composition of the extracellular fluid is well known because blood, the main extracellular fluid, is readily available for study. Obtaining representative samples of intracellular fluids for analysis is no easy task. Thus the data on their composition are less reliable than that of extracellular fluids. The substances present in the fluid between the cells (interstitial fluid) closely resemble those found in blood plasma except that the concentration of proteins is lower.

Electrolytes are of importance in relation to their concentration (number of particles per unit volume) and because of their number of charges. Electrolyte concentrations are conventionally expressed in terms of *milliequivalents* (mEq.) When the concentrations of each ionic constituent of extracellular or intracellular fluids are expressed in terms of milliequivalents per liter, the sum of all the positively charged ions (*cations*) exactly equals the sum of all the negatively charged ions (*anions*). Thus, every positively charged ion is exactly balanced by a negatively charged ion. The average sum of the concentration of all the cations in serum is about 150 mEq. per liter. This is balanced by 150 mEq. per liter of anions to make a total serum osmolarity of about 300 mEq. per liter.

Osmolality and osmolarity are defined on page 716. Serum *osmolarity* can be generally determined using the following formula:

$$\text{Serum osmolarity (mOsm./liter)} =$$
$$\text{serum sodium (mEq./liter)} \times 2$$
$$+ \frac{\text{blood urea nitrogen (mg./100 ml.)}}{3}$$
$$+ \frac{\text{glucose (mg./100 ml.)}}{20}$$

Normal osmolarity is equal to 275 to 298 mOsm. per liter in adults and 270 to 285 mOsm. per liter in children.

OSMOTIC PRESSURE

The body seeks to equalize the total salt concentrations (in milliequivalents) of the intracellular and extracellular fluids. Reference is being made to total cation and anion concentrations and not the concentrations of individual ions because it has already been noted that sodium and potassium, for example, are normally distributed in quite a different manner between intracellular and extracellular fluid.

In an effort to maintain these equal concentrations, small shifts of water may take place. These shifts are due to a force called *osmotic pressure*, which is directly proportional to the number of particles in solution. If the salt content of the tissues (intracellular fluid) gets too high, water passes from the surrounding fluid (extracellular fluid) into the cell and thus reduces the salt concentration in the cell and also increases the concentration of salt in the extracellular fluid. If, on the other hand, the salt concentration in the intracellular fluid is too low, water passes out of the cells into the extracellular fluid. It is convenient (although not entirely accurate) to consider the osmotic pressure of the intracellular fluid as a function of its content of potassium, which is the predominant cation in the intracellular fluid, whereas the osmotic pressure of the extracellular fluid may be conveniently considered to relate to its content of sodium, which is the major cation present in the intracellular fluid. Shifts in the distribution of these ions are the principal cause of shifts of water between the various fluid compartments, although chloride and PO_4 can also influence H_2O balance.

Proteins, non-diffusible because of their size, also play an important part in maintaining osmotic equilibrium. Their presence in the plasma exerts a colloidal osmotic pressure that helps to retain water within the blood vessel lumen and thereby prevents the leakage of water from the plasma into the interstitial fluid. In some disease states, such as protein-energy malnutrition, when the protein content of plasma is exceptionally low, water does leak into the interstitial fluids, resulting in edema.

WATER AND SODIUM BALANCE AND IMBALANCE

Water and sodium imbalances are either osmolar or volume imbalances. *Osmolar imbalance* is caused by a gain or loss of water relative to solute or a gain or loss of solute relative to water. *Volume imbalance* occurs when sodium,

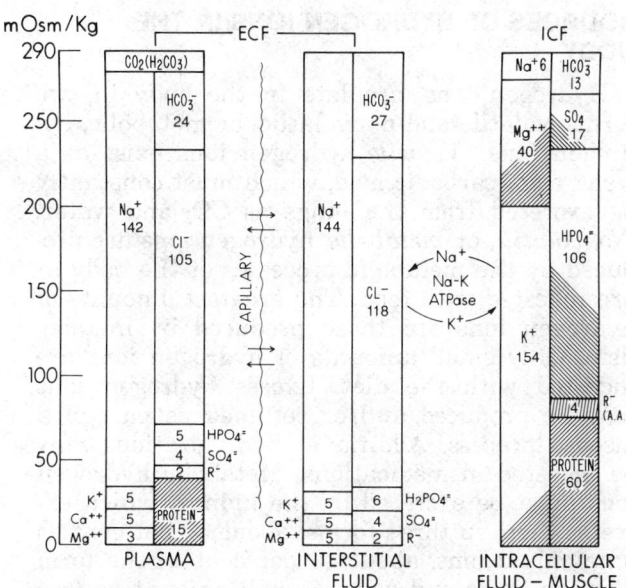

Figure 8-2. Electrolyte composition of the three principal body fluid compartments. These diagrams are arranged to stress electroneutrality. All have the same osmolality in spite of differences in the total charges. Shading indicates large molecules or bound ions whose osmolal contribution is less than their electric charge, but which are important to the distribution of ions because of their impermeability. (From Finberg, L., Kravath, R. E.: and Fleischman, A. R.: Water and Electrolytes in Pediatrics. Philadelphia, W. B. Saunders Company, 1982.)

chloride and water are either gained or lost together.

Sodium and potassium concentrations are of major influence in directing the movement of water from one body compartment to another, and these two cations are in control of total hydration of the body. The shifts in water from one compartment to another are due to changes occurring in the extracellular concentrations of electrolytes. When water loss exceeds electrolyte loss, the extracellular fluid becomes *hypertonic* to the intracellular fluid (i.e., the osmotic pressure of the extracellular fluid is higher than the osmotic pressure of the intracellular fluid) and water shifts from the cells to the extracellular space to compensate. When water enters the extracellular fluid with the electrolytes in amounts insufficient to maintain normal density of the solutions, the extracellular fluid becomes *hypotonic* to the intracellular fluid (i.e., the osmotic pressure of the extracellular fluid is lower than the osmotic pressure of the intracellular fluid) and water shifts from the extracellular space into the cell. The reduction of the extracellular fluid continues until osmotic equilibrium between intracellular and extracellular fluids is reestablished. When the body is unable to maintain osmotic equilibrium, dehydration or edema may result. *Dehydration* can result from decreased water intake, excessive water output or heavy solute load. *Edema* can result when there is a decrease in plasma proteins and plasma oncotic pressure secondary to malnutrition or other causes. Note that oncotic pressure is not the same as osmotic pressure. *Oncotic pressure* or *colloid osmotic pressure* is the pressure at the capillary membrane due to dissolved proteins in the plasma and interstitial fluids. *Osmotic pressure* or total osmotic pressure is the pressure at the cell membrane and is due to all dissolved substances of the body fluids.

Volume imbalances are characterized by changes in extracellular fluid volume. Circulatory collapse can occur if the extracellular fluid volume decreases. Circulatory overload and edema can result when extracellular fluid volume increases. Excess volume is treated with diuretics and sodium restriction. However, the use of diuretics can cause depletion of other minerals.

Acid-Base Balance

The regulation of the acid-base balance in the body actually means regulation of the hydrogen ion (H^+) concentration of the body fluids. The symbol pH is used to express this ion concentration and is related as follows:

$$pH = \log \frac{1}{H^+ \, conc.} = -\log H^+ conc.$$

The acidity of the body is closely regulated within a narrow range by complex homeostatic mechanisms. The pH of blood is usually 7.36 to 7.44; below pH 7.30 the person has acidosis, and at a blood pH above 7.44 the person has alkalosis. Only blood pH values between 6.8 and 7.8 are compatible with life. Intracellular pH measured indirectly usually ranges between 6.0 and 7.4. A rapid rate of metabolism or poor blood flow cause increased carbon dioxide accumulation and decreased blood pH.

In contrast, the pH of body secretions and excretions are more variable, ranging from 1.0 in gastric juice to 8.2 in pancreatic juice.

SOURCES OF HYDROGEN IONS IN THE BODY

Hydrogen ions circulate in the body in two forms, volatile and nonvolatile, or metabolic, hydrogen ions. *Volatile* hydrogen ions exist as a weak acid, carbonic acid, which must constantly be excreted from the lungs as CO_2 and water. *Nonvolatile*, or *metabolic*, hydrogen ions are produced by the metabolic processes of the body or are ingested with food. The greatest amounts of hydrogen ions are those produced by metabolism. Only small amounts of hydrogen ions are ingested with the diet. Excess hydrogen ions may be produced and/or retained as part of a disease process. Additional hydrogen ions may be ingested in medications. Metabolic hydrogen ions must be excreted by the kidney, which excretes them in three forms: about 60 per cent as ammonium ions, about 40 per cent in the form of weak acids and a very small amount as free hydrogen ion. The latter ions determine the pH of the urine.

Hydrogen ion concentration, or pH, is regulated by dilution, buffering, respiratory control of volatile hydrogen ion concentration and renal control of nonvolatile hydrogen ions. Buffer systems react to readjust hydrogen ion concentration in fractions of a second. The respiratory system reacts in minutes and the kidneys take from an hour to as much as one to three days.

BUFFER SYSTEMS IN THE BODY

There are three major buffer systems in the body: bicarbonate, phosphate and protein. Only five of every million hydrogen ions are not handled by the buffer systems of the body. These five are handled by the lungs or kidneys. Buffers function by reacting with strong acids or bases to produce weaker acids or bases. Strong acids and bases hydrolyze in solution, whereas weak acids and bases do not to the same extent. This effectively binds the hydrogen ion and prevents it from altering the pH of the solution.

Of the three buffer systems, the most important in the extracellular fluid is *bicarbonate*, which buffers up to 90 per cent of the hydrogen ions in the fluid. About 70 mEq. of acid are produced daily. Considering all the different acids together as HA (total body acid) the body protects itself from wide shifts of pH by the reaction of the acid with sodium bicarbonate as follows:

$$HA + NaHCO_3 \rightarrow NaA + H_2CO_3$$

acid   sodium   salt   carbonic
bicarbonate   acid

H_2CO_3 is excreted by the lungs, and the $NaHCO_3$ supply is regenerated by the kidney. The ratio of H_2CO_3 to $NaHCO_3$ is more important than the absolute amount of each. Normally the extracellular fluid contains one part of carbonic acid (H_2CO_3) to 20 parts of $NaHCO_3$ (1.37 mEq./liter H_2CO_3 to 27 mEq./liter $NaHCO_3$). If this ratio is disturbed, an imbalance occurs.

The *phosphate buffer* system is more important within the cells than in the extracellular fluid because the concentration of phosphate in the cells is higher. The phosphate buffer system is also important in the kidney tubules. Phosphate becomes concentrated in the tubules and as the tubular fluid becomes more acidic than the extracellular fluid the efficiency of the system increases.

The *protein buffer* system is important because it can function as either an acid or a base because of the unique structures of the amino acids in protein. Hemoglobin alone provides nearly 75 per cent of the buffering power of this system in body fluids.

RESPIRATORY CONTROL IN HYDROGEN ION BALANCE

During metabolic processes oxygen is being constantly used by the tissues and carbon dioxide being produced. A respiratory control center in the medulla controls H_2CO_3 excretion from the lungs by means of a feedback system. Because of their large surface area, the lungs are a vital part of the system controlling hydrogen ion concentration. Three factors affect respiration, pCO_2, pH and pO_2. The partial pressure of carbon dioxide in the blood, pCO_2, has the most pronounced effect on the rate of respiration. Next is the pH of the blood and least important the partial pressure of oxygen in the blood, pO_2. When pCO_2 increases, pH drops and respiration is stimulated. When pCO_2 decreases, respiration slows. CO_2 is actually present as H_2CO_3 because the expired air is moist. Hydrogen ion increases result in a drop in pH and an increase in respiration. Increases in pO_2 have very little effect; decreases stimulate respiration and CO_2 is excreted. Elimination of CO_2 functions as a negative feedback for the control of H_2CO_3. Respiratory control is only 50 to 75 per cent effective in returning the pH to normal because as the pH returns toward normal the stimulus for the change will be dampened. This system alone cannot return the body to a normal pH. However, one to ten times as much acid or base can be buffered by the respiratory system as by the protein system.

RENAL CONTROL IN HYDROGEN ION BALANCE

The $NaHCO_3$ part of the bicarbonate buffer system is regulated by the kidneys. The kidney excretes metabolic hydrogen ions. Although it is slow, the kidney is powerful and efficient at neutralizing hydrogen ion imbalance by altering the rate of excretion of hydrogen ions, sodium ions and potassium ions and the concentration of bicarbonate ions in body fluids.

Several tubular mechanisms that help regulate hydrogen ion concentration of body fluids are shown in Figure 8–3. Hydrogen ions are secreted into the tubular fluids by cells of the proximal and distal tubules and collecting ducts. The hydrogen ions result from the reaction of CO_2 and water to form carbonic acid, which dissociates into hydrogen and bicarbonate ions. Hydrogen ions will be secreted into the tubules until the pH of the fluids drop to about 4.5. The greater the concentration of CO_2 in the extracellular fluids, the more rapid the reaction and the greater the rate of hydrogen ion secretion will be. Hydrogen ion concentration is regulated by the concentration of CO_2 in the extracellular fluids. Hydrogen ions in the tubular cell combine with HCO_3^- to form H_2CO_3, which promptly dissociates into CO_2 and H_2O. The CO_2 diffuses through the cell and into the extracellular fluid to form more bicarbonates. Secondly, the sodium released in the tubule also moves through the cell and into the extracellular fluid.

Under normal conditions the quantities of hydrogen ion and bicarbonate entering the tubules are almost equivalent and in a sense "titrate" each other. Usually there is a slight excess of hydrogen ion from metabolic processes. Only rarely are bicarbonate ions in excess. The basic mechanism to correct acidosis or alkalosis is by incomplete titration of hydrogen ions against bicarbonate ions. These ions pass into the urine and are removed from extracellular fluid. The carbonic acid formed in the proximal tubules is split very rapidly because the luminal brush border surface has a large amount of attached carbonic anhydrase.

Two other buffer systems, phosphate and ammonia, are of major importance in the renal tubules (there are also a number of minor buffer systems such as urate and citrate). Phosphates become more concentrated because of their relatively poor absorption and because of the removal of water from the tubular fluid. Phosphate reactions in the buffer system are also shown in Figure 8–3. The net effect is the absorption of sodium and re-formation of bicarbonate in the extracellular fluid.

Ammonia is formed in the tubular epithelium by the breakdown of some amino acids. Sixty per cent is derived from glutamine catabolism and 40 per cent from different amino acids, particularly glycine and alanine. The net effect of the ammonia buffer system (Figure 8–3) is once again to increase bicarbonate concentration of the extracellular fluids. The ammonia buffer system can increase tenfold to handle greatly increased loads of acids needing to be excreted.

As stated earlier, the renal system is the slowest mechanism for maintaining hydrogen ion balance; its action often takes one to three days to complete. However, it continues to function until the pH is almost exactly normal. In order to adjust the hydrogen ion concentration of the extracellular fluid the urine produced can have a pH as low as 4.5 or as high as 8.0.

ACIDS AND BASES

Clinically the term base is frequently applied to the cations (Na^+, K^+, Mg^{++}, Ca^{++}) of the body fluids and the term acid is commonly applied to the anions (Cl^-, HCO_3^-, $SO_4^=$, $HPO_4^{\equiv}$). The term "total base" is frequently used in reference to the sum of the cations.

The term *alkali reserve* is frequently used by clinicians to refer to plasma bicarbonate concentration. This anion is available to neutralize acids that might enter the plasma. The term alkali reserve should really refer to all the relatively strong buffer bases of the body fluids, such as HCO_3^-, $H_2PO_4^=$, $HPO_4^{\equiv}$, and protein, but under ordinary conditions the bicarbonate levels will reflect the condition of the entire buffer complex.

HYDROGEN ION IMBALANCES

Imbalances are of two types, acidosis and alkalosis. In the condition of *acidosis* the hydrogen ion concentration is above normal or the

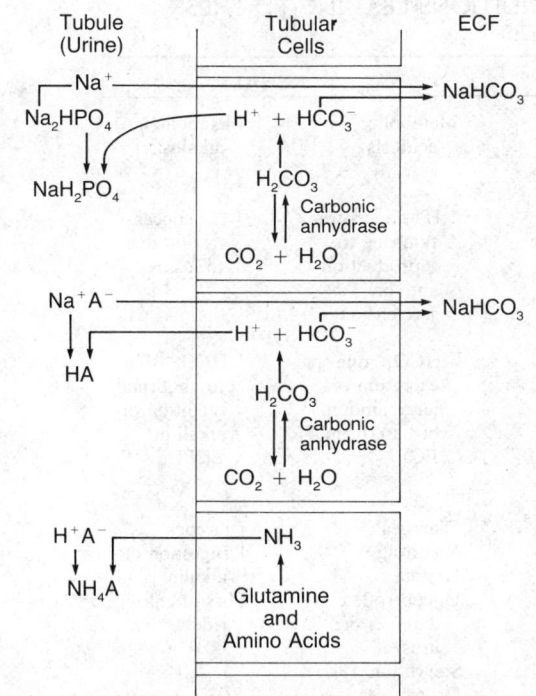

Tubule (Urine)	Tubular Cells	ECF

Figure 8–3 Generation of $NaHCO_3$ and clearance of H^+ by the three buffer systems that function in the kidney. HA = any acid in the body; ECF = extracellular fluid.

alkali reserve (bicarbonate) is below normal. In the condition of *alkalosis* the hydrogen ion concentration is below normal or the body base is above normal. If the basic failure of the regulatory system is pulmonary the condition is called *respiratory* and if the basic regulatory failure is renal the condition is called *metabolic*. The conditions causing these hydrogen ion imbalances are shown in Table 8–4. These underlying conditions must be corrected before the imbalance can be corrected. The immediate causes are due to changes in concentration of carbonic acid, hydrogen ion or base. Imbalances may also be grouped as primary, secondary or mixed. *Primary imbalances* arise either from acid or base overload or from a disease of the kidneys or lungs. *Secondary imbalances* occur in response to an attempt to compensate. *Mixed imbalances* result from distinct diseases and their complications and are both primary and secondary imbalances.

POTASSIUM IMBALANCES

Hypokalemia is potentially deadly. Causes are inadequate intake, increased utilization or excessive loss. Extreme dieting is one of the reasons for inadequate intake, and acute alcoholism is another. Losses of potassium can also result from drug therapy, conditions of the GI tract such as ulcerative colitis, metabolic disorders and renal disorders. *Hypokalemia* affects cellular metabolism, which in turn affects several systems including the neurological, cardiovascular, gastrointestinal, respiratory and renal systems. *Hyperkalemia* can result from potassium retention in patients in renal failure, postoperative patients with poor renal output and those with adrenocortical insufficiency. A second cause is an excessive release of potassium from cells damaged by trauma.

OTHER ELECTROLYTE IMBALANCES

Imbalances of calcium and magnesium are discussed in Chapter 7.

EFFECTS OF DIET

In starving patients there are changes in body composition resulting from major changes in both water and electrolyte balance. Initial weight loss in starving patients is largely water and salt. The sodium losses exceed those seen in patients eating a diet restricted in sodium. As sodium and water are lost and the extracellular fluid volume decreases, blood volume changes can be detected. Decreases in blood volume can be minimized by giving the fasting patients 90 mEq. of sodium per day as sodium chloride. So-

Table 8–4. CLASSIFICATION OF THE FOUR MAJOR HYDROGEN ION IMBALANCES AND SOME OF THE CONDITIONS LEADING TO THESE IMBALANCES

	PULMONARY		RENAL	
Nature of failure	Respiratory acidosis	Respiratory alkalosis	Metabolic acidosis	Metabolic alkalosis
Imbalance	↑ H_2CO_3 due to retention of CO_2	↓ H_2CO_3 due to excessive expiration of CO_2 and H_2O	↑ H^+ concentration due to ↑ production and/or ↑ retention OR ↓ HCO_3^- due to excretion of large amounts of base from ECF	↓ H^+ concentration due to losses ↑ HCO_3^- due to abnormal retention of alkali in ECF
Diseases that may cause	Conditions of ↓ lung surface area, such as emphysema	Aftermath of severe exercise Anxiety reaction	Diarrhea Vomiting Uremia Uncontrolled diabetes mellitus Starvation Drugs High-fat or low-CHO diet	Diuretics ↑ Ingestion of alkali Loss of chloride

dium loss is due to abrupt decrease in dietary carbohydrate. Adding small amounts of carbohydrate results in sodium and water retention. Eating a high-fat, low-carbohydrate diet results in a shift in the water content of the body. Urine volume increases when carbohydrate is first omitted and decreases again when carbohydrate is added back.

Summary

Acid-base balance and maintenance of proper body fluid concentration involves primary homeostatic mechanisms basic to survival. Because it is so important, the mechanisms are complicated and have many checks, balances and feedback controls. Fortunately this regulating capacity allows the human to function in a wide range of environments and to eat a variety of diets.

Problems and Suggested Topics for Discussion

1. Keep a record of your water and fluid intake for a period of 24 hours. Evaluate it.
2. Select references from the list of Additional References pertaining to water and salt relationship for either an oral or written report.
3. What are the routes of water elimination from the body?
4. What is insensible water loss? What is the usual amount? When would it be increased? Decreased?
5. List the functions of water in the body.
6. List the conditions that affect water balance in the body.
7. What is meant by the acid-base regulation of the body?
8. List two causes of each of the hydrogen ion imbalances.
9. Describe changes in acid-base balance that result from starvation or from consumption of a high-fat diet.

Cited References

1. Grossman, H., et al.: The dietary chloride deficiency syndrome. Pediatrics *66*:366, 1980.
2. Meneely, G.R., and Battarbee, H.D.: Sodium and potassium. Nutr. Rev., *34*:225, 1976.

Additional References

Altschul, A.M., and Grommet, J.K.: Sodium intake and sodium sensitivity. Nutr. Rev., *38*:393, 1980.

Burke, S.R.: The Composition and Function of Body Fluids. 3rd ed. St. Louis, C.V. Mosby Company, 1980.

Carroll, H.J., and Oh, M.S.: Water, Electrolytes and Acid-Base Metabolism. Philadelphia, J.B. Lippincott, 1978.

Food and Nutrition Board, National Research Council, Recommended Dietary Allowances. 9th ed. Washington, D.C., National Academy of Sciences, 1980.

Gamble, J.L.: Chemical Anatomy, Physiology and Pathology of Extracellular Fluid. 6th ed. Cambridge, Harvard University Press, 1954.

Goodhart, R.S., and Shils, M.E. (eds.): Modern Nutrition in Health and Disease. 6th ed. Philadelphia, Lea & Febiger, 1980, Chapter 8, Water, electrolytes and acid-base balance.

Groer, M.E.: Physiology and Pathophysiology of Body Fluids. St Louis, C.V. Mosby Company, 1981.

Guyton, A.C.: Textbook of Medical Physiology, 6th ed. Philadelphia, W.B. Saunders Company, 1981.

Luckmann, J., and Sorensen, K.C.: Medical-Surgical Nursing. 2nd ed. Philadelphia, W.B. Saunders Company, 1980, Chapter 12, Fluid and electrolyte imbalances.

Moses, C. (ed.): Sodium in Medicine and Health. Baltimore, Reese Press, Inc., 1980.

Simopoulos, A.P., and Bartter, F.C.: The metabolic consequences of chloride deficiency. Nutr. Rev. *38*:201, 1980.

Stoot, V., Lee, C., and Schaper, C.A.: Fluids and Electrolytes: A Practical Approach. Philadelphia, F.A. Davis, 1977.

Vanatta, J.C., and Fogelman, M.J.: Moyer's Fluid Balance—A Clinical Manual, 3rd ed. Chicago, Year Book Medical Publishers, Inc., 1982.

NUTRITIONAL STATUS OF THE INDIVIDUAL

The Assessment of Nutritional Status

The influence of nutrition on the health of the individual is measured through assessment of nutritional status. Within the past decade, there has been a tremendous interest in nutritional status, especially that of hospitalized patients, and in developing methods to assess it. This chapter will discuss the methods currently used to evaluate nutritional status, and how these findings are put together to develop a clinically relevant picture.

Definitions

An individual's *nutritional status* is the measurement of the degree to which the individual's physiological need for nutrients is being met. It is the state of balance in the individual between the nutrient intake and the nutrient expenditure or need. Many factors influence this balance, as shown in Figure 9–1. The individual's nutritional status has an effect on his or her well-being, performance, resistance to disease and growth.

Evaluation of nutritional status involves examination of the individual's physical condition, growth and development, the function of various organ systems, behavior, the urinary blood or tissue levels of nutrients, and the quality and quantity of the nutrient intake. Information on medication, stress or chronic illness, economic situation, knowledge about nutrition, cultural patterns and living conditions is also useful because these factors influence nutritional intake and sometimes nutritional requirements, and thus nutritional status. In a thorough *nutrition-*

al status assessment, all of the following aspects are considered:

1. Dietary history and intake data
2. Biochemical data
3. Clinical examination and pertinent health history
4. Anthropometric data
5. Psychosocial data

Besides adding to the assessment of health, this information will give the health professional information for *anticipating* problems and preventing poor nutrition before it develops.

In situations of limited time, money, or professional staff, less information can be gathered, and of necessity the assessment must be abbreviated. The minimal nutritional screening, especially for the hospitalized patient, includes measurement of height and weight, non-volitional weight loss, change in appetite and serum albumin, all of which can be easily measured in the hospital. This identifies patients at nutritional risk. With regard to all aspects of nutritional status assessment, a finding below the standard means only that the individual is *likely* to have a deficiency. The individual is thus "at risk" of developing a clinical nutritional deficiency, which should be verified by a clinical examination.

Development of Nutritional Deficiency

Nutritional deficiency is a progressive phenomenon, and different techniques of assessment detect different stages of nutritional adequacy or deficiency. Obviously, the ideal

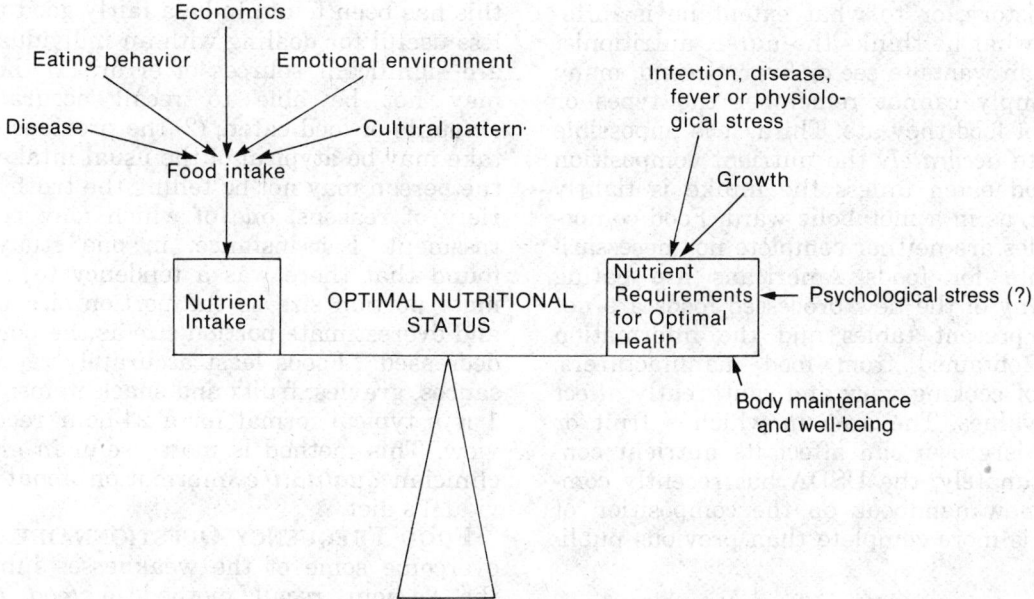

Figure 9–1. Optimal nutritional status as a balance between nutrient intake and nutrient requirements.

methods are those which detect nutritional deficiency in its early stages of development so that dietary intake can be improved through nutritional support and nutritional counseling before the more severe deficiency lesion appears.

The early stage of a nutritional deficiency is characterized by body adaptation to the decreased intake and less than optimal amounts of the nutrient present in the blood and tissues. For example, plasma vitamin A will be less, or urinary riboflavin excretion will fall. A more severe or prolonged nutritional deficiency will result in a biochemical "lesion" or a tissue enzyme deficiency or malfunction, as shown in Figure 9–2. By using biochemical tests, the clinician attempts to detect a nutritional deficiency in these early stages. Some nutritional deficiency states are reflected in changes in the functions of organs (e.g., maladaptation of the eyes to darkness in vitamin A deficiency). These

stages are detected by clinical examination. If well designed, functional tests of nutritional status may be very useful because they are usually non-invasive and clinically relevant.

Somewhere between the initial stage of deficiency development and the biochemical lesion is the effect of nutritional deficiency on growth and anthropometric data; this is the reason these measurements are used in nutritional assessment, especially in children.

Purposes of Nutritional Assessment

The purposes of the nutritional assessment are (1) to identify a subset of patients in need of further nutritional determinations, (2) to establish baseline values for evaluating the efficacy of nutritional regimens and (3) to provide a system for early recognition of the probability of health risk due to nutritional factors.

Components of Nutritional Assessment

DIETARY INTAKE

The accurate recording and evaluation of the dietary intake of an individual is the most difficult and frustrating aspect of nutritional assessment. First, it is difficult to record a person's food intake without influencing it. When people are watched, questioned about what they eat, or asked to write down what they eat, eating patterns tend to change. The extent of change depends on how well the person understands the

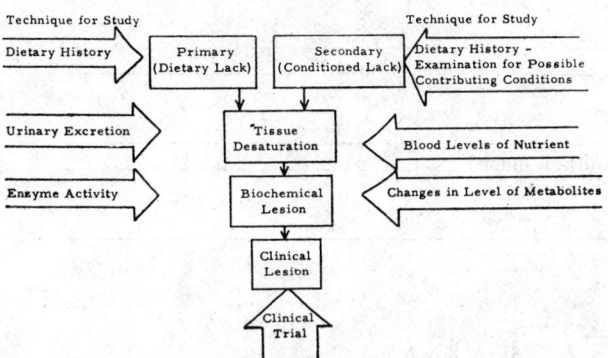

Figure 9–2. Sequence of events leading to clinical nutrition lesion. (From Pearson, W. N.: Biochemical appraisal of the vitamin nutritional status in man. JAMA, 180:49–55, 1962.)

dietary history, or to what extent he is influenced by what he thinks the nurse, nutritionist or physician wants to see or hear. Second, many people simply cannot remember the types or amounts of food they ate. Third, it is impossible to evaluate *accurately* the nutrient composition of the food eaten unless the intake is tightly controlled, as in a metabolic ward. Food composition tables are neither complete nor necessarily accurate for foods Americans are eating today. Many of the new processed foods are not listed in present tables and the information must be obtained from food manufacturers. Methods of cooking vary and can greatly affect nutrient values. The area in which a fruit or vegetable is grown can affect its nutrient content. Fortunately, the USDA has recently completed a new handbook on the composition of food that is more complete than previous publications.[8]

Methods for Obtaining Dietary Information

24-HOUR RECALL. The most popular and easiest method for obtaining an idea of a person's dietary intake is the 24-*hour recall*. The individual completes a questionnaire or is interviewed by a dietitian/nutritionist or nurse experienced in dietary interviewing and is asked to recall everything eaten within the last 24 hours, or the previous day. In surveys of population groups this has been found to be a fairly good tool; it is less useful for dealing with an individual. There are significant sources of error: (1) the person may not be able to recall accurately the amounts of food eaten; (2) the previous day's intake may be atypical of the usual intake; and (3) the person may not be telling the truth for a variety of reasons, one of which may be embarrassment. For instance, in one study Young found that there was a tendency to underestimate portion size as the portion size increased and overestimate portion size as the portion size decreased.[39] Foods least accurately reported are sauces, gravies, fruits and snack items. Table 9–1 is a typical format for a 24-hour recall interview. This method is most useful in giving the clinician *qualitative* information about an individual's diet.

FOOD FREQUENCY QUESTIONNAIRE. To help overcome some of the weaknesses inherent in the 24-hour recall method, a *food frequency questionnaire* may also be completed. Using this tool, the health professional can collect information on how many times per day, week or month the individual eats particular foods. This information can aid in validating the accuracy of the 24-hour recall data and clarify the picture of the person's real food consumption pattern. The food frequency questionnaire may be selective, with questions about foods suspected of being deficient or excessive in the diet, or general, with questions concerning all foods

Table 9–1. 24-HOUR RECALL FORM AND FOOD GROUP EVALUATION

The following question pattern may be used for conducting the 24-hour recall. The information should then be recorded in the chart at the end.

"In order to get a more complete picture of your health. I need to know more about your eating habits. Would by please tell me everything you ate or drank, all day yesterday. Let's begin with:"

1. What time did you go to bed the night before last? _____ (typical versus atypical day)
   Was this the usual time? _____
2. What time did you get up yesterday? _____
   Was this the usual time? _____
3. When was the first time you had anything to eat or drink? _____ What did you have and how much?

   _____

4. When did you eat again? _____ Where? _____ What and how much?_____

   _____

5. When did you eat next?_____ What did you eat and how much?_____

   _____

6. Did you eat or drink anything else? _____
   a. Anything from 1st to 2nd "meal?" _____
   b. Anything from 2nd to 3rd "meal?" _____
   c. Anything from 3rd "meal" to bedtime? _____
7. Was this day's food intake different from usual? _____ If so, how? _____
8. Is weekend eating different? _____ If so, how?_____

Table 9–1.   24-HOUR RECALL FORM AND FOOD GROUP EVALUATION (*Continued*)

FOOD AND FLUID INTAKE FROM TIME OF AWAKENING UNTIL
THE NEXT MORNING—24-HOUR RECALL

TIME	FOOD AND DRINK CONSUMED		NUMBER OF SERVINGS IN THE FOOD GROUPS							
	Name and Type	*Amount*	*Milk Grp.*	*Meat Grp.*	*Vit A Grp.*	*Vit C Grp.*	*Other F & V*	*Bread & Cereal*	*Butter, Fat, Oil*	*Miscellaneous (Candy, alcohol, etc.)*
TOTALS										
		Amount	*Milk Grp.*	*Meat Grp.*	*Vit A Grp.*	*Vit C Grp.*	*Other F & V*	*Bread & Cereal*	*Butter Fat, Oil*	*Miscellaneous (Candy, etc.)*
Recommended No. of Servings Daily										
Children 6 or under			2–3 c.	2	3/wk	1	2	4	2 TBSP.*	†
Adolescent			4 c.	2	3/wk	1	2	4	2TBSP.	
Adult			2 c.	2	3/wk	1	2	4	2 TBSP.	
Pregnant or Lactating			4 c.	2	3/wk	1	2	4	2 TBSP.	
			Milk Grp.	Meat Grp.	Vit A Grp.	Vit C Grp.	Other F&V	Bread & Cereal	Butter, Fat, Oil	Miscellaneous (Candy, etc.)
Evaluation L = Low A = Adequate E = Excessive										

*2 Tbsp./day recommended to meet calorie and essential fatty acid needs. Excessive amounts in this group usually mean excessive caloric intake.

†Servings of high calorie, low nutrient items such as sugar, candy, soda pop. Excessive amounts in this group usually mean excessive caloric intake and possibly dental caries.

Table 9–2. A GENERAL FOOD FREQUENCY QUESTIONNAIRE

For the frequency of food use, the following pattern of questions may be useful. However, you may have to modify questions after learning some information from the 24-hour recall. For instance, if the patient has said he had a glass of milk yesterday, you wouldn't ask "Do you drink milk?", but rather "How much milk do you drink?" Record answers as 1/day, 1/wk., 3/mo., for example, or as accurately as possible. It may just have to be noted as "occasionally" or "rarely."

1. Do you drink milk? If so, how much? _____ What kind? Whole _____ Skim _____
2. Do you use fat? If so, what kind? _____ How much? _____
3. How many times do you eat meat? _____ eggs _____ cheese _____ beans _____
4. Do you eat snack foods? If so, which ones? _____ How often? _____ How much? _____
5. What vegetables do you eat? (in each group) How often?
   a. Broccoli _____ greenpeppers _____ cooked greens _____ carrots _____ sweet potato _____
   b. Tomatoes _____ raw cabbage _____
   c. Asparagus _____ beets _____ cauliflower _____ corn _____ cooked cabbage _____ celery _____ peas _____ lettuce _____
6. What fruits and how often?
   a. Apples or applesauce _____ apricots _____ banana _____ berries _____ cherries _____ grapes or grape juice _____ peaches _____ pears _____ pineapple _____ plums _____ prunes _____ raisins _____
   b. Oranges _____ orange juice _____ grapefruit _____ grapefruit juice _____
7. Bread and cereal products
   a. How much bread do you usually eat with each meal? _____ between meals _____
   b. Do you eat cereal (daily, weekly) cooked _____ dry _____
   c. How often do you eat foods such as macaroni, spaghetti, noodles, etc. _____
8. Do you use salt? _____ Do you salt your food before tasting it? _____ Do you cook with salt? _____ Do you "crave" salt or salty foods? _____
9. How many tsp. of sugar do you use/day (1 packet = 1 tsp.)? _____ (Be sure and ask patient about sugar on cereal, fruit, toast and in coffee, tea, etc.)
10. Do you drink water? _____ How often during the day? _____ How much each time? _____ How much would you say you drink each day? _____
11. Do you drink alcohol? _____ How often? _____ How much? _____ Beer, wine, liquor? _____

likely to be eaten. Table 9–2 is a general food frequency questionnaire. Table 9–3 is a selective food frequency questionnaire.

The problems with the food frequency questionnaire are: (1) it does not give quantitative data on intake and (2) it usually relies on the person's memory for determining how often a food is eaten.

DIETARY HISTORY. The dietary history is more complete than either the 24-hour recall or food frequency questionnaire, and it usually includes both of these sources. The dietary history

Table 9–3. SELECTIVE FOOD FREQUENCY QUESTIONNAIRE FOR INQUIRING ABOUT CHOLESTEROL, FAT, SODIUM, IRON OR SUGAR INTAKE

FREQUENCY OF FOOD USE: RECORD AS TIMES/WK. OR DAY OR N = NEVER, R = RARE

High or Moderately High in:	Use of		High or Moderately High in:		
CHOLESTEROL:	Eggs	_____	UNSATURATED FAT:	Soft margarine	_____
	Liver	_____		Vegetable oils	_____
	Shellfish	_____			
	Beef	_____	SODIUM:	Prepared frozen foods	_____
	Pork	_____		Sausages or franks	_____
				Snack foods, e.g.,	
SATURATED FAT:	Beef	_____		pretzels, potato chips,	
	Pork	_____		salted peanuts	_____
	Butter	_____		Softened water	_____
	Whole milk	_____		Olives, pickles	_____
	Cream	_____		Smoked fish; canned fish	_____
	Pastries	_____		Ham & other canned	
	Gravies	_____		meat	_____
	Ice cream	_____			
			IRON:	Iron supplements	_____
SUGAR:	Cakes	_____		Dark green leafy veg.	_____
	Pastries	_____		Enriched cereals	_____
	Cookies	_____		Dried beans	_____
	Coke	_____		Meat, fish, or poultry	_____
	Soda pop	_____		Eggs	_____
	Candy	_____			

contains the additional information given in Table 9–4.

Remember that dietary habits are personal and an individual may be unwilling to talk about them, especially if he or she perceives the interviewer as being judgmental. This is one of the problems with the dietary interview. It is necessary to be as objective as possible when interviewing in order to gain a complete and accurate insight into a person's eating patterns. A second problem is that the dietary history takes a fair amount of time and requires an experienced interviewer. However, it is possible to save some time by putting the dietary history into a questionnaire format that can be filled out by the patient. The reader is also referred to one of the many good books on interviewing. Interviewing regarding dietary patterns is discussed further in Chapter 18.

FOOD DIARY OR RECORD. This method requires more time, understanding, and motivation on the part of the patient or client. The subject is asked to write down everything he or she eats or drinks for a certain time period. Three days, particularly two week days and one weekend day, has been found to be a representative time period for most people.[34] The length of time that the food diary must be kept in order to accurately reflect usual nutrient intake depends on whether the person has a regular food pattern. A daily food pattern requires fewer days of recording than a random, haphazard eating style. The nutrient contribution for each food is calculated; the total day's intake for each nutrient is totaled and then divided by the number of days to give an average daily intake.

The health practitioner can gain information about lifestyle, companions, and meal eating atmosphere by asking the person to also note the time, place and people with whom he or she eats. Recall can be combined with the food diary method when the nutrition counselor goes over the food record with the patient and asks the patient to supply additional information regarding amounts and types of preparation of the food. This is a very good way to get to know a person's lifestyle, since food habits are an intimate part of that lifestyle. A food diary is most complete and accurate if the patient is instructed to record it immediately after eating.

The difficulties with the food diary are (1) patient non-compliance, (2) inaccuracy because not everything is recorded and (3) the intake on the recorded days may not be typical.

OBSERVATION OF FOOD INTAKE. Observation of food intake is the most accurate method of dietary intake assessment, but also the most time consuming, expensive and difficult. Observation must be non-intrusive and is most easily done when the person's meals are provided for him, as in the case of a hospitalized person, nursing

Table 9–4. INFORMATION OBTAINED FROM A DIETARY HISTORY

1. Economics
   a. income—frequency and steadiness of employment
   b. amount of money for food each week or month and individual's perception of its adequacy for meeting food needs
   c. eligibility for food stamps and cost of stamps
   d. public aid recipient?
2. Physical activity
   a. occupation—type, hours/week, shift, energy expenditure
   b. exercise—type, amount, frequency (seasonal?)
   c. sleep—hours/day (uninterrupted?)
   d. handicaps
3. Ethnic or cultural background
   a. influence on eating habits
   b. religion
   c. education
4. Homelife and meal patterns
   a. number in household (eat together?)
   b. person who does shopping
   c. person who does cooking
   d. food storage and cooking facilities (stove, refrigerator)
   e. type of housing (home, apartment, room, etc.)
   f. ability to shop and prepare food
5. Appetite
   a. good, poor, any changes
   b. factors that affect appetite
   c. taste and smell perception and any changes
6. Allergies, intolerances or food avoidances
   a. foods avoided and reason
   b. length of time of avoidance
   c. description of problems caused by foods
7. Dental and oral health
   a. problems with eating
   b. foods that cannot be eaten
   c. problems with swallowing, salivation, food sticking
8. Gastrointestinal
   a. problems with heartburn, bloating, gas, diarrhea, vomiting, constipation, distention
   b. frequency of problems
   c. home remedies
   d. antacid, laxative or other drug use
9. Chronic disease
   a. treatment
   b. length of time of treatment
   c. dietary modification—physician prescription?, date of modification, education, compliance with diet
10. Medication
   a. vitamin and/or mineral supplements—frequency, type, amount
   b. medications—type, amount, frequency, length of time on medication
11. Recent weight change
   a. loss or gain
   b. how many pounds, over what length of time
   c. intentional or non-volitional
12. Dietary or nutritional problems (as perceived by patient)

home resident or child at a boarding school. It requires knowing the amount and kind of food presented to the person and a record of the amount actually eaten. The ultimate in a controlled situation is that in a metabolic unit when a weighed amount of food is presented, the amount of uneaten food is reweighed, and the difference is recorded as the amount eaten.

The problems with this method are the time,

the expense and the difficulty of obtaining patient compliance.

HOUSEHOLD FOOD CONSUMPTION. This method involves visiting a household periodically and recording the amounts and types of food purchased for that household and the disappearance of that food. The food unaccounted for is assumed to be that consumed by the family. It is most commonly used in large population surveys and is not a good evaluation of individual intake, because of food wastage and lack of a record of the individual household members' consumption. Another problem with this method is patient compliance.

However, in attempting to gain insight into the nutrition situation in the community, this information can be very valuable. It can be traced backward from the food in the household to the income of the household, to the food available in the market, and so on, as shown in Figure 9–3. This flow chart would apply more to a rural or less developed economy, where climate and food transportation have more effect on the food available in the market than in a developed country. However, the "food available in the market" could be significant in the case of the inner city dweller, such as an elderly person who is trapped into shopping at the corner market that might not carry certain needed items such as bran flakes, diet soda, salt-free crackers or good fresh fruits. Depending on the situation, different factors in the food chain should be scrutinized.

METHODS FOR EVALUATING DIETARY INFORMATION

There are basically two methods by which food intake information is evaluated for adequacy—the food group methods and the nutrient composition method.

The intakes of vitamins A and C and folic acid are the most variable intakes in the majority of U.S. diets. Because they are not widely present in foods, except for particular fruits and vegetables that are concentrated sources, the intake of these vitamins is greatly influenced by specific food choices during a day. Second, the intake of these nutrients frequently is seasonal, with a higher intake in the summer and fall when abundant amounts of fresh fruits and vegetables are more available because they are cheaper, or because the family has a fruit and vegetable garden. Riboflavin, calcium and vitamin D intakes are largely dependent on the intake of milk and milk products. The dietary intake of thiamin, niacin, protein, phosphorus, calories, iron and vitamins E, B_6 and B_{12}, which are present in a wide variety of foods, is more consistent each day.

EVALUATION BY FOOD GROUP METHOD. The simplest, fastest, yet crudest way to evaluate food intake data is to determine how many servings from each of the four food groups were consumed during the recorded day. The number of servings from each group is then compared with the number of servings suggested in the Basic Four Food Groups, as shown in Table 9–1. Gross deficiencies of protein, iron, calcium, riboflavin, vitamin A and vitamin C in the diet can be detected in this way. It becomes more difficult to use this method if the diet has many food mixtures or unusual cultural foods that do not fit into one of the food groups.

A more accurate assessment of the calories, protein and fat in the diet can be derived by quantifying the food intake in terms of diabetic exchanges (see Table 25–8.) These figures can then be compared with the recommended daily allowances (RDA, Table 10–1) for the individual. For nutrients usually consumed in excess (fat, cholesterol, sodium and sugar), the Dietary Goals or the recommendations of the Food and Nutrition Board can be used. These are given in Tables 17–7 and 17–10.

EVALUATION BY NUTRIENT COMPOSITION. The dietary intake can be evaluated more accurately by calculating the amounts of each nutrient in each food consumed, which can be done by hand or with the use of a computer, as explained in Chapter 20. The nutrient values for foods can be obtained from several publications[1, 8, 31] and from nutrition labels and food manufacturers' information on the nutrient composition of the food.

After recording the nutrient composition for the various foods in the diet, the nutrient composition of the total diet can be determined.

A more accurate, yet far more difficult and expensive method is to prepare a total day's food intake identical to that taken by the patient and have it chemically analyzed for its nutrient content. Again, this is usually done in a metabolic unit where extreme accuracy is essential.

Standard for Evaluation of Nutrient Intake—the RDA

Once the nutrient composition is determined it can be used as such or compared with the RDA as listed in Chapter 10. Although the RDA are frequently used to evaluate an *individual's* diet, this is theoretically an *improper* use of them. The RDA are set at a level above the requirement in order to include all those individuals within the population who might have an increased need for a particular vitamin or mineral above the mean requirement of the population. Because the RDA include this "safety fac-

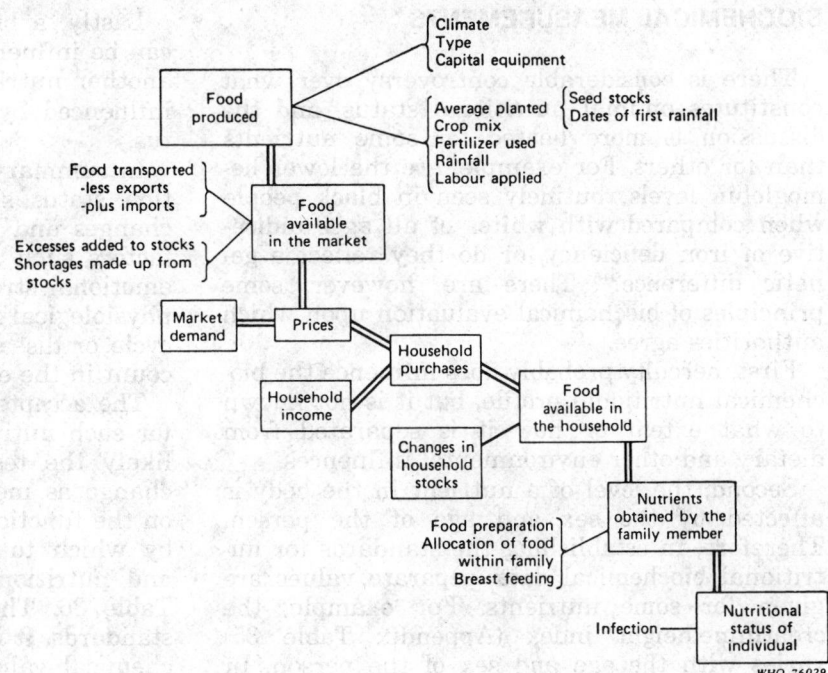

Figure 9–3. Flow chart for household food consumption: a food chain. (Adapted from Methodology of Nutritional Surveillance. Joint FAO/UNICEF/WHO Expert Committee. Geneva, WHO, 1976.)

tor," they are probably higher than a typical individual's requirement. The reader is referred to Chapter 10 for further discussion of the RDA.

Energy and protein intake should be evaluated on the basis of body weight, or in the case of the underweight or overweight, on the basis of height. This increases the usefulness of the RDA in individual assessment, especially with children, who at any particular age, may differ greatly in size. Table 9–5 shows how the RDA are interpreted on the basis of height and how an individual's intake is compared with the RDA.

An additional shortcoming of the RDA is that they are not meant to be applied to sick individuals, whose requirements may be very different from those of healthy individuals. At present, however, there are no established nutrient requirements for various disease states. With these limitations in mind as well as those presented in Chapter 10, the nutritionist can use the RDA to evaluate in a general manner the dietary intake of an individual.

Interpretation of Dietary Intake Data

The intakes of most nutrients are interdependent. Guthrie postulates that for U.S. preschool children, the intakes of iron and energy are as indicative of the adequacy of the dietary intake as a more complete evaluation.[17] In other words, only the caloric and iron content of the diet would need to be calculated. If these were adequate, one could assume that the diet would be adequate for the rest of the nutrients needed by

healthy children 12 to 72 months of age. Others have also developed similar abbreviated systems.

It is impossible and inaccurate to judge the adequacy of a person's intake of a nutrient by looking at dietary intake alone. The practitioner must also evaluate serum and tissue levels of the nutrient, examine the person for clinical signs of a deficiency and take a thorough history. For example, one cannot assume that if the vitamin A intake of Joyce, age 20, is only 1000 I.U. per day, she is deficient in vitamin A. Measurement of the serum levels of vitamin A and retinol-binding protein and the liver stores of vitamin A and examination for clinical signs such as night blindness and follicular hyperkeratosis would complete the assessment.

Table 9–5. APPLICATION OF RECOMMENDED DIETARY ALLOWANCES TO INDIVIDUAL INTAKE

RDA for energy based on size
   19–22-year-old-female: 2100 kcal.
   The height of the reference female for this age in the RDA is
      163 cm.
$$\frac{2100}{163} = 12.8 \text{ kcal/cm} = \text{the RDA for kcalories based on height}$$
Dietary intake of 21-year-old female shows 2080 kcal./day. This
   woman is 155 cm. tall. The caloric intake based on her height
   is 13.4 kcal./cm./day.
This woman's intake is higher than the RDA of 12.8
   kcal./cm./day. However, the RDA has a range of energy
   intakes (10.4 to 14.7 kcal./cm./day) which should also be
   considered.

BIOCHEMICAL MEASUREMENTS

There is considerable controversy over what constitutes optimal nutritional status, and the discussion is more heated for some nutrients than for others. For example, are the lower hemoglobin levels routinely seen in black people when compared with whites of all ages indicative of iron deficiency, or do they reflect a genetic difference?[15] There are, however, some principles of biochemical evaluation upon which authorities agree.

First, heredity probably does influence the biochemical nutritional profile, but it is not known to what extent or how it is separated from dietary and other environmental influences.

Second, the level of a nutrient in the body is affected by the sex and age of the person. Therefore, in establishing the standards for nutritional biochemical data, separate values are given for some nutrients. For example, the creatinine:height index (Appendix Table 35) varies with the age and sex of the person. In others, knowledge is not complete enough to allow standards to be set that are specific for sex and age.

Third, there is not a definite value for a biochemical test that clearly delineates the deficient person from the non-deficient person. It is difficult to know when a "deficient" level is due to actual lack of nutrients and when it is due to metabolic alteration of body composition and function, especially in illness. For this reason, standards are somewhat arbitrary and are usually given as ranges. Being deficient implies less than optimal growth, health or performance, and this must be defined by clinical examination.

Fourth, some tests, such as measurement of urinary excretion of riboflavin, reflect the end point of metabolism of the nutrient. Such tests are not as useful in detecting actual risk of deficiency as are tests that measure the nutrient at the functional level, such as the test for ascorbic acid in leukocytes.

Fifth, some biochemical values reflect immediate nutrient intake, whereas others reflect past or long-term intake. For example, levels of carotene and triglycerides in plasma reflect immediate intake, since these nutrients are quickly transported by the blood to other tissues.

Sixth, the sensitivity of a test to changes in the status of a particular nutrient is important. For example, serum thyroxine–binding prealbumin seems to be more sensitive to protein nutriture than serum transferrin. Yet serum transferrin is more sensitive than serum albumin. This is due to the fact that the half-life of albumin is 14 days, that of transferrin is 8 to 10 days and that of prealbumin is 2 to 3 days.

Lastly, a biochemical value for one nutrient can be influenced by the intake or body level of another nutrient. For example, serum folate is influenced by the individual's vitamin B_{12} status.

In summary, a good biochemical test of nutrition status should be sensitive to nutritional changes and be minimally influenced by other factors such as exercise, infection, physical or emotional stress, or trauma. If it is affected by physiological factors such as age, sex, menstrual cycle or disease, these should be taken into account in the evaluation.

The accepted tests for biochemical evaluation for each nutrient are listed in Table 9–6. Most likely the tests and the accepted values will change as more information becomes available on the functions of the nutrients. The standards by which to judge biochemical measurements and nutritional status are given in Appendix Table 36. These are average, widely accepted standards. It is still important to evaluate a biochemical value based on the normal range as stated by the laboratory performing the analysis.

Biochemical data regarding nutritional status can be obtained from examination of plasma, red blood cells, white blood cells, urine or tissues such as liver, bone, hair and fingernails. Obviously the latter two tissues are much easier to obtain, and more information on the biochemical nature of these tissues as reflections of nutrient intake would be very useful.

Hair Analysis

Clinicians and researchers are beginning to analyze hair root samples in order to evaluate zinc and other trace mineral status. This method gives a measure of long-term status of the mineral and could be very useful in determining cumulative intakes, as in the case of heavy toxic metals. However, the clinical use in some cases is exceeding its reliability. It is being used to make judgments on nutritional status or mineral toxicity beyond what is reasonable.

A careful examination of the use of hair analysis reveals some problems that must be kept in mind. First, concentrations of metals in hair can be correlated with the amount of exposure of an individual to that metal. For example, the concentration of lead in hair has been found to be lowest in rural population groups, higher in urban groups and highest in individuals who live close to lead smelters.[25] Air, tobacco, smoke, water, sweat, shampoos and hair sprays can deposit trace elements on the surface of the hair.

Second, there is little agreement about precisely what constitutes normal concentrations of trace elements in hair, and until there is more

Table 9–6. BIOCHEMICAL MEASUREMENTS OF NUTRITIONAL STATUS

NUTRIENT	MORE SENSITIVE	LESS SENSITIVE
Protein	Plasma amino acids Serum thyroxine–binding pre-albumin Urinary creatinine:height index Urinary hydroxyproline Serum retinol–binding protein Serum transferrin	Total serum protein Serum albumin
Lipids	Serum cholesterol—HDL and LDL Serum triglycerides Lipoproteins	
Vitamin A	Serum carotene Serum retinol Liver retinol stores Serum retinol–binding protein	Blood leukocytes
Vitamin D	Serum 25OHD$_3$ Serum 1,25(OH)$_2$D$_3$ Serum alkaline phosphatase	Urinary calcium Serum phosphorus Serum parathormone Serum calcium
Vitamin E	Hydrogen peroxide erythrocyte hemolysis test Serum or plasma vitamin E Erythrocyte vitamin E	Platelet assessment
Vitamin K	Plasma clotting factors II, VII, IX, X	Prothrombin time
Thiamin	Erythrocyte transketolase activity Thiamin pyrophosphate effect (TPPE)	Blood pyruvate Urinary thiamin
Riboflavin	Plasma riboflavin Erythrocyte glutathione reductase Erythrocyte riboflavin	Urinary riboflavin
Nicotinic acid	Urinary N^1-methylnicotinamide Urinary 2-pyridone/ N-methylnicotinamide ratio Erythrocyte nicotinamide mononucleotide	Urinary 2-pyridone
Vitamin B$_6$	Tryptophan load test (mg. xanthurenic and kynurenic acids excreted in urine are measured after tryptophan load) Plasma and erythrocyte pyridoxal phosphate Erythrocyte transaminase-SGOT and SGPT	Urinary pyridoxine excretion (µg./gm. creatinine)
Folic Acid*	Red cell folate	Serum folate Bone marrow film Urinary FIGLU excretion Mean corpuscular volume (MCV)
Vitamin B$_{12}$	Serum B$_{12}$ Erythrocyte B$_{12}$ Serum thimidylate synthetase Urinary methylmalonic acid*	Bone marrow film Thin blood film Schilling test
Pantothenic Acid	Blood pantothenic acid	Urinary pantothenic acid
Biotin	Serum biotin	Urinary biotin
Vitamin C	Serum ascorbic acid Leukocyte ascorbic acid Vitamin C saturation	Urinary ascorbic acid
Iron	Iron deposits in bone marrow % saturation of transferrin Serum ferritin Protoporphyrin heme	Mean corpuscular volume (MCV) Hemoglobin Hematocrit Thin blood film Serum iron Mean corpuscular hemoglobin concentration (MCHC)
Iodine	Serum protein–bound iodine (PBI) Radioiodine uptake	Urinary iodine Tests for thyroid function
Calcium	Serum alkaline phosphatase	
Phosphorous		Serum phosphorus
Zinc	Serum and plasma zinc	Hair zinc
Magnesium	Serum magnesium	Urinary magnesium
Copper	Serum copper	

*Tests of folate status do not distinguish between folate and B$_{12}$ deficiency except in the case of urine methylmalonic acid, which will distinguish between the two.

information, any hair analysis must be looked at with a very critical eye.

Third, different laboratories use different procedures to remove contaminants and different proportions of trace elements, and this is a major source of inconsistency. Although measurements made in any laboratory today can generally be assumed to be accurate, comparisons of data obtained from different laboratories often show large variations in absolute values. The actual techniques of analysis vary between the laboratories and, at present, there are no standard reference materials with which to calibrate instruments. Fortunately, the International Atomic Energy Agency is particularly interested in nuclear techniques for hair analysis and is attempting to develop some standards.

Hair analysis should not be the sole basis for assessment of nutritional status with regard to any mineral. Assessment, even for zinc, for which hair analysis is most highly developed, should include additional biochemical or functional evaluation for the mineral.

Immunological Measurements

Data indicative of immunological function can also be valuable. Malnutrition is associated with depressed immune competence,[3,4,37] so total white blood cell count, lymphocyte count and delayed cutaneous hypersensitivity (DCH) indicate the status of the immunocompetence and thus indicate nutriture.

Delayed cutaneous hypersensitivity (DCH) usually consists of the response to five recall antigens, usually *Candida*, streptokinase-streptodornase (SK-SD), coccidioidin, mumps and purified protein derivative (PPD). The size of the induration is measured to give the clinician a measure of the body's ability to mount an immune response. However, a wide variety of metabolic abnormalities, including edema, can interfere with skin reactions of this nature. The primary question regarding the use of the skin test to measure protein-energy nutriture is whether the absence of the DCH response represents a protein-energy depletion defect or the effect of a variety of other unrelated parameters, such as trauma, sepsis, malignancy, chemotherapy or radiation therapy.[9] There is no question that absent DCH response identifies a patient who is at risk for the development of infection, but the utility of skin testing in nutritional assessment remains unproven.[36]

It has been suggested that present biochemical measurements are static and thus not very useful. Future studies must concentrate on measurement of function because nutritional status is dynamic. An example of a functional test is measurement of taste acuity to assess zinc sta-

tus. Table 9–7 gives some functional tests of nutritional status.

CLINICAL EXAMINATION

Clinical examination includes a complete physical examination and a medical history. In the clinical examination special attention should be given to the skin, hair, teeth, gums, lips, tongue and eyes, and in men the genitalia, since these are areas that show signs of nutritional deficiencies. Hair, skin and mouth are susceptible because of the rapid cell turnover of epithelial and mucosal tissue. Early ramifications may also be reflected in the gastrointestinal tract, such as diarrhea because of GI mucosal changes.

The medical history should include questions about mastication and swallowing. Are the teeth painful? Are teeth missing? Does the patient wear dentures, and if so, do they fit well? Any dryness of mouth or throat owing to decreased salivation? Does this prevent eating certain foods? Appetite, food avoidances or preferences, and digestion problems should be delved into thoroughly. These habits or problems all affect food intake, and thus nutritional status.

Through the history one can also learn of any behavioral or functional *changes* in gastrointestinal, neuromuscular or cardiovascular systems that may not be apparent to the clinician but are remarkable to the patient or the patient's family.

The clinical examination for nutritional assessment in many hospitals now includes assessment of energy expenditure of the patient through measurement of O_2 consumption and CO_2 production. This assessment—indirect calorimetry—is further discussed on page 12.

Table 9–8 gives the clinical signs of possible nutritional significance in the examination of the patient. A description of the clinical terms in this table is included in Appendix 37. Very few of these signs are diagnostic for specific nutritional deficiencies (although some are more reliable than others), which means that other causes such as environmental factors or underlying disease must be ruled out. Clinical signs of nutritional deficiency should always be confirmed with biochemical and dietary data. A clinical symptom can and usually does reflect the presence of more than one nutritional deficiency.

ANTHROPOMETRY

An important part of the clinical examination, especially in infants, children, adolescents and pregnant women, is measurement and evaluation of growth and development. The lack of

Table 9–7.   A SYSTEMS CLASSIFICATION OF PRESENT AND POTENTIAL
FUNCTIONAL INDICES OF NUTRITIONAL STATUS

SYSTEM	NUTRIENTS
Structural integrity	
Erythrocyte fragility	Vitamin E, Se
Capillary fragility	Vitamin C
Tensile strength of skin	Cu
Experimental wound-healing	Zn
Collagen accumulation in implant sponge	Zn
Lipoprotein peroxidation (breath ethane/pentane)	Vitamin E, Se
Host Defense	
Leukocyte chemotaxis	P/E,* Zn
Leukocyte phagocytic activity	P/E, Fe
Leukocyte bactericidal capacity	P/E, Fe, Se
Leukocyte metabolism (glycolysis, iodination, etc.)	P/E
Serum opsonic activity	P/E
White cell interferon production	P/E
Lymphocyte (T-cell) blastogenesis	P/E, Zn
Delayed cutaneous hypersensitivity	P/E, Zn
Rebuck skin window	P/E
Transport	
i) Intestinal absorption:	
Iron absorption	Fe
Cobalt absorption	Fe
ii) Plasma/tissue transport:	
^{65}Zn uptake by erythrocyte	Zn
^{75}Se uptake by erythrocyte	Se
Retinol relative-dose-response	Vitamin A
Post-glucose plasma chromium response	Cr
Post-glucose urine chromium response	Cr
Thyroid radioiodine uptake	I
Hemostasis	
Prothrombin time	Vitamin K
Platelet aggregation	Vitamin E, Zn
Reproduction	
Sperm count	Energy, Zn
Nerve Function	
Dark adaptation	Vitamin A, Zn
Color discrimination	Vitamin A
Central scotoma	Vitamin A
Olfactory acuity	Vitamins A & B_{12}, Zn
Taste acuity	Vitamin A, Zn
Nerve conduction	P/E, Vitamins B_1 & B_{12}
Skin conductivity	P/E
Abducens (VI cranial nerve) function	Vitamin B_1
Electroencephalography	P/E
Sleep pattern	P/E
Work Capacity/Hemodynamics	
Task performance/endurance	P/E, Vitamins B_1, B_2 & B_6, Fe
VO$_2$ max	P/E, Fe
VO$_2$ submax	P/E, Fe
Heart rate (cumulative)	P/E, Fe
Vasopressor response	Vitamin C
Unclassified	
d-Uridine suppression test	Vitamin B_{12}, Folic Acid

From Solomons, N. W., and Allen, L. H.: The functional assessment of nutritional status: principles, practice and potential. Am. J. Clin. Nutr., *41*:33, 1983.

* P/E = protein-energy nutriture.

Tests of pathways in intermediary metabolism and those of the whole individual have not been included in this classification system.

Table 9–8. PHYSICAL SIGNS INDICATIVE OR SUGGESTIVE OF MALNUTRITION

	NORMAL APPEARANCE	SIGNS ASSOCIATED WITH MALNUTRITION	POSSIBLE DISORDER OR NUTRIENT DEFICIENCY	POSSIBLE NON-NUTRITIONAL PROBLEM
Hair	Shiny; firm; not easily plucked	Lack of natural shine; dull and dry Thin and sparse Silky and straight; fine Dyspigmented Flag sign Easily plucked (no pain)	Kwashiorkor and, less commonly, marasmus	Excessive bleaching of hair Alopecia
Face	Skin color uniform; smooth, pink, healthy appearance; not swollen	Nasolabial seborrhea (scaling of skin around nostrils) Swollen face (moon face) Paleness	Riboflavin Iron Kwashiorkor	Acne vulgaris
Eyes	Bright, clear, shiny; no sores at corners of eyelids; membranes a healthy pink and moist; no prominent blood vessels or mound of tissue or sclera	Pale conjunctiva Red membranes Bitot's spots Conjunctival xerosis (dryness) Corneal xerosis (dullness) Keratomalacia (softening of cornea) Redness and fissuring of eyelid corners Corneal arcus (white ring around eye) Xanthelasma (small yellowish lumps around eyes)	Anemia (e.g., iron) Vitamin A Riboflavin, pyridoxine Hyperlipidemia	Bloodshot eyes from exposure to weather, lack of sleep, smoke or alcohol
Lips	Smooth, not chapped or swollen	Angular stomatitis (white or pink lesions at corners of mouth) Angular scars Cheilosis (redness or swelling of lips and mouth)	Riboflavin	Excessive salivation from improper fitting dentures
Tongue	Deep red in appearance; not swollen or smooth	Scarlet and raw tongue Magenta tongue (purplish) Swollen tongue Filiform papillae atrophy or hypertrophy	Nicotinic acid Riboflavin Niacin Folic acid Vitamin B_{12}	Leucoplakia
Teeth	No cavities; no pain; bright	Mottled enamel Caries (cavities) Missing teeth	Fluorosis Excessive sugar	Malocclusion Periodontal disease Health habits
Gums	Healthy; red; do not bleed; not swollen	Spongy, bleeding Receding gums	Vitamin C	Periodontal disease
Glands	Face not swollen	Thyroid enlargement (front of neck swollen) Parotid enlargement (cheeks become swollen)	Iodine Starvation	Allergic or inflammatory enlargement of thyroid

Table 9–8. PHYSICAL SIGNS INDICATIVE OR SUGGESTIVE OF MALNUTRITION
(*Continued*)

	NORMAL APPEARANCE	SIGNS ASSOCIATED WITH MALNUTRITION	POSSIBLE DIS-ORDER OR NUTRIENT DEFICIENCY	POSSIBLE NON-NUTRITIONAL PROBLEM
Skin	No signs of rashes, swellings, dark or light spots	Xerosis (dryness)	Vitamin A	Environmental exposure
		Follicular hyperkeratosis (sandpaper feel to skin)		
		Petechiae (small skin hemorrhages)	Vitamin C	
		Pellagrous dermatosis (red swollen pigmentation of areas exposed to sunlight)	Nicotinic acid	
		Excessive bruising	Vitamin K	Physical abuse
		Flaky paint dermatosis	Kwashiorkor	
		Scrotal and vulval dermatosis	Riboflavin	
		Xanthomas (fat deposits under skin around joints)	Hyperlipidemia	
Nails	Firm; pink	Koilonychia (spoon-shaped)	Iron	
		Brittle; ridged		
Subcutaneous tissue	Normal amount of fat	Edema	Kwashiorkor	
		Fat below standard	Starvation; marasmus	
		Fat above standard	Obesity	
Muscular and skeletal systems	Good muscle tone; some fat under skin; can walk or run without pain	Muscle wasting	Starvation, marasmus, Kwashiorkor	
		Craniotabes (thin, soft skull bones in infant)	Vitamin D	
		Frontal and parietal bossing (round swelling of front and side of head)		
		Epiphyseal enlargement (swelling of ends of bones)		
		Persistently open anterior fontanelle (soft area on head closes late)		
		Knock knees or bow legs		
		Musculoskeletal hemorrhages	Vitamin C	
		Calf muscle tenderness	Thiamin	
		Thoracic rosary	Vitamin D; Vitamin C	
		Fractures in elderly	Osteoporosis	
Cardiovascular system	Normal heart rate and rhythm; no murmurs or abnormal rhythms; normal blood pressure for age	Cardiac enlargement	Thiamin	
		Tachycardia		
		Elevated blood pressure	Sodium?	
Gastrointestinal system	No palpable organs or masses (in children, however, liver edge may be palpable)	Hepato-splenomegaly	Kwashiorkor	

Table continued on the following page

Table 9–8. PHYSICAL SIGNS INDICATIVE OR SUGGESTIVE OF MALNUTRITION
(*Continued*)

	NORMAL APPEARANCE	SIGNS ASSOCIATED WITH MALNUTRITION	POSSIBLE DIS-ORDER OR NUTRIENT DEFICIENCY	POSSIBLE NON-NUTRITIONAL PROBLEM
Nervous system	Psychological stability; normal reflexes	Psychomotor changes	Kwashiorkor	
		Mental confusion	Nicotinic acid; thiamin	
		Depression	Pyridoxine; vitamin B_{12}	
		Sensory loss		
		Motor weakness		
		Loss of position sense		
		Loss of vibration	Thiamin	
		Loss of ankle and knee jerks		
		Burning and tingling of hands and feet (paresthesia)		

(Adapted from Jelliffe, D. B.: The Assessment of the Nutritional Status of the Community. WHO Monograph No. 53, Geneva, 1966.

McLaren, D. S.: Nutritional assessment. In McLaren, D. S., and Burman, D.: Textbook of Pediatric Nutrition. Edinburgh, Churchill Livingstone, 1976, pp. 91–102.

Christakis, G. (ed.): Nutritional Assessment in Health Programs, Washington, D.C., Am. Pub. Health Assoc., Inc., 1973.)

proper growth is usually an early sign noticed by the clinician and should immediately arouse suspicion that nutrition may be at fault. This information is most valuable when obtained over a *period of time* with regular, accurate and consistent recording of anthropometric data and development. Physical measurements reflect the total nutritional status over a lifetime. Some measurements, such as height and head circumference, reflect past nutrition or chronic nutritional status. Others such as mid-arm circumference, weight and skinfold thickness reflect present nutritional status and are used to assess the skeletal energy reserves both as fat and as protein.

Height and Weight

Height and weight are the most common measurements made, but because their significance and importance are not appreciated, they are frequently measured sloppily, incorrectly or inconsistently. Height is a measure of chronic nutrition or undernutrition and should be measured as accurately as possible. Children less than 36 months should be measured in the recumbent position (crown–heel length) and the length plotted on the chart for children 1 to 36 months of age. For young children the recumbent length is generally greater than stature by about 2 cm. or almost 1 inch. After 4 or 5 years the difference is closer to 1 cm. In any case, when the child can stand, the measurements should be *consistent*. Figure 9–4 shows a child being measured and gives guidelines for proper

measurement of crown–heel length. Measuring the child by holding a tape measure at the child's head and stretching it to the heel does not give an accurate measurement of length. See cited references 29 and 35 for further discussion of techniques for measuring infants and children.

Weight in children is a sensitive measure of growth and can be an early clue to growth problems and nutritional inadequacy. It reflects more recent nutrition of the child or adult than does length or height. In adults regular weight measurements are particularly important when there is chronic illness. By documenting weight loss in a previously normal-weight individual, one verifies the inability of that individual to meet nutritional requirements.

Height and weight are properly measured in the following manner:

Height

1. The person should be barefoot or wearing only socks or stockings.

2. The person's feet should be together with the heels against the wall or measuring board.

3. The person should be standing erect, neither slumped nor stretching, looking straight ahead, without tipping the head up or down. The top of the ear and outer corner of the eye should be in a line parallel to the floor—called the *Frankfort plane*.

4. A horizontal bar, a rectangular block of wood, or the top of the statiometer then should be lowered to rest flat on the top of the head.

5. Read the height to the nearest 1/4 in. or 0.5 cm.

Figure 9–4. Measurement of length of an infant. Crown-heel length should be measured in children 36 months and younger in the following manner: (1) The child is laid on a ruled board that has an attached piece of wood at one end and a movable piece at the other. (2) Make sure that the child is stretched out on the board to give the most accurate measurement. This usually requires two people. The top of the child's head is placed against the immovable end. (3) The movable end is placed so that it is flat against the bottom of the child's foot, and the length is read from the side of the board. (From Jelliffe, D. B.: The Assessment of the Nutritional Status of the Community. WHO Monograph No. 53. Geneva, WHO, 1966.)

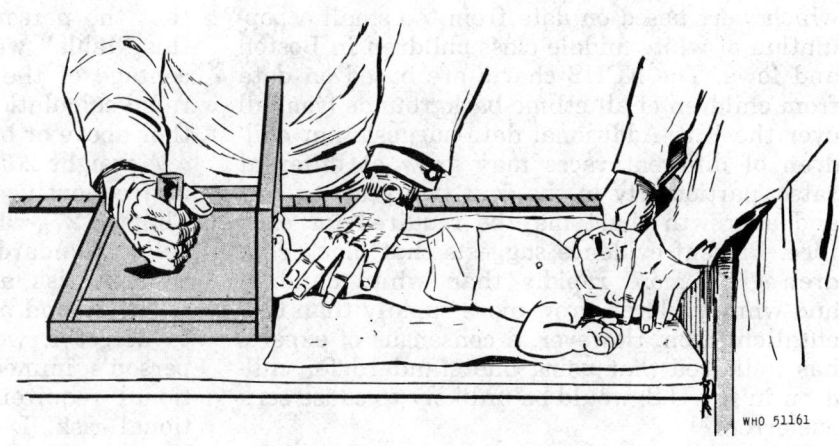

WHO 51161

Weight

1. Use a beam balance scale, not a spring scale, whenever possible.

2. Periodically calibrate the scale for accuracy, using known weights.

3. The person should be weighed in light clothing without shoes.

4. Record weight to the nearest 1/2 lb. or 0.2 kg. for adults, and 1/4 lb. or 0.1 kg. for infants.

INTERPRETATION OF HEIGHT AND WEIGHT. The height and weight measurements are evaluated by comparing them to various norms. For children, the height and weight are recorded as a percentile, which reflects the percentage of the total population of children of the same sex at or below that height or weight at that age, and the child's growth at each age, or growth "curve," can be followed. This is done using Appendix Tables 15 and 17 for infants and Appendix Tables 19 and 21 for children and adolescents.

Children whose measurements are between the 25th and 75th percentiles are likely to represent normal growth. Crossing a percentile with advancing age is not unusual unless it reflects a progressively upward or downward trend. Many children cross percentiles during the first two years—it often takes two years for a child to "find his growth channel." Measurements between the 10th and 25th or between the 75th and 90th may or may not be normal, depending on previous and subsequent measurements and on genetic and environmental factors. Measurements above the 90th or below the 10th should be checked for accuracy, and further evaluation may be necessary. Measurements below the 5th percentile or above the 95th percentile warrant further medical and nutritional evaluation.

Two measurements at different times that reflect a markedly different percentile ranking (25 percentiles or greater) should be checked for accuracy. The child may be having a change in growth velocity that is physiologically normal or may have a medically or nutritionally related cause. Evaluation of weight and height measurements and growth in pregnancy, prematurity, infancy, childhood and adolescence is further discussed in Chapters 11, 37, 12, 13 and 14 respectively.

Weight and height can also be compared with each other in an evaluation of growth by using the weight for standard length curve for prepubescent children only (males less than 11.5 years of age and no more than 145 cm. [57 inches] in height, and females less than 10 years of age and no more than 137 cm. [54 inches] in height). For most children a weight for height between the 25th and 75th percentiles is appropriate. Children whose weight for height percentile is above or below this should be evaluated further by using skinfold measurements or other anthropometry. Use of this weight for height table gives the clinician a method for evaluating whether a child's weight is appropriate. In addition, it has the advantage that one does not need to know the child's exact age. When height for age is above the 10th percentile but weight for height is less than the 5th percentile it is suggestive of acute or chronic illness or nutritional deficiency.[12] (See Appendices 16, 18, 20 and 22.)

Unfortunately, a similar curve is not available for pubescent children, and they should not be plotted on this weight for height curve even if their height can be registered on the curve. The problem of determining whether the adolescent is of appropriate weight for height is discussed in Chapter 14.

The National Center for Health Statistics (NCHS) growth charts presented in the Appendix are more acceptable than previous charts, which were based on data from too small a population of white middle class children in Boston and Iowa. The NCHS charts are based on data from children of all ethnic backgrounds from all over the U.S. Additional data suggest that children of different races may grow at different rates, particularly in the first two years of life, and a growth chart may be required for each race. Present evidence suggests that black children grow more rapidly than white children and white children grow more rapidly than Oriental children. However, a consensus of experts has indicated that using one standard for children in the U.S. would be unlikely to cause serious errors.[33]

Height and weight measurements in adults are also useful in determining nutritional status. The same applies to techniques of measurment, with the caution that adults' heights should always be measured, not just recorded from history. Men frequently exaggerate their height, and in older people there is frequently a decrease from young adulthood height. Weight should always be measured also. An adult's weight is taken for two reasons: (1) to determine whether weight is appropriate for height and (2) to determine whether there has been a change in weight.

To determine whether an adult's weight is appropriate for height, the weight is usually compared with one of two sets of charts that give the weights for heights for males and females. The first of these, and certainly the most common, are the Metropolitan Life Insurance (MLI) Tables. The most recent edition of these tables, published in 1983, can be found in Appendix Table 25. The tables give weight ranges for men and women at 1-inch increments of height for three body frame sizes. The problems with using these tables to determine appropriate body weight are: (1) the stated weight ranges merely reflect the weights of those with lowest mortality of *insured* persons, which may not reflect the U.S. population, (2) weight ranges for lowest mortality do not necessarily reflect optimal weight for height for health, and (3) it is often not clear whether the body frame size is small, medium or large. However, the method used to determine body frame size for the new 1983 MLI Tables is described in Appendix Table 26.[14] These problems in determining ideal body weight are further discussed in Chapter 27.

The second set of tables frequently used came out of the 1973 Fogarty conference.[5] This Table (Appendix Table 27) gives one weight for each height for men and women that is the median weight for the medium frame from 1959 Metropolitan Life Insurance Tables. There are many disadvantages to using a single number as an ideal weight for height, but the advantage is

that the person's present weight in relation to this "table" weight can be expressed as a percentage of the "table" weight. This allows for rapid calculation of difference from standard (either above or below) and the consequent risk.

A weight 20 per cent or more above standard is frequently cited as reflecting obesity (see Chapter 27), while a weight 20 per cent or more below standard is frequently equated with nutritional risk, as has been discussed.

The second purpose of weight measurement is to detect a weight change which reflects the person's immediate ability to meet his nutritional requirements, and this indicates nutritional risk. Determination of per cent weight loss

$$\frac{\text{usual weight} - \text{present weight}}{\text{usual weight}} \times 100$$

is highly reflective of the extent of illness. Another useful calculation is present weight as a percentage of usual weight.

Besides just comparing the measurements with appropriate tables, several researches have related weight and height to each other in an attempt to develop a ratio that indicates appropriate weight for height. The most common and well accepted is the *body mass index* (BMI) (Table 27–1). This index:

$$\frac{\text{weight (in kilograms)}}{\text{height}^2 \text{(in meters)}}$$

has been found to have the least correlation with body height and high correlation with body fatness.[22,23] A body mass index of 27 or greater indicates obesity.[6]

Arm Span Length

In situations in which height is difficult to measure, such as in elderly persons with severe skeletal changes or children with cerebral palsy, scoliosis or muscular dystrophy, arm span is being correlated with height and being used clinically to determine height.[16, 28]

Head Circumference

The measurment of head circumference is somewhat useful in children, especially in those under the age of three, because it reflects brain growth, which is very rapid in the first two years of life. Head circumference grossly inappropriate for the size of the child is significant, but usually reflects non-nutritional abnormalities rather than nutritional abnormalities.

APPROPRIATE WEIGHT   OBESE

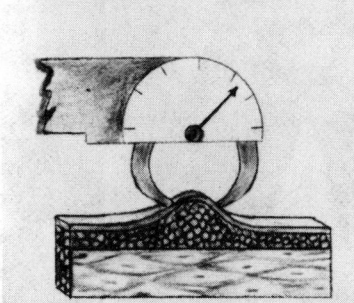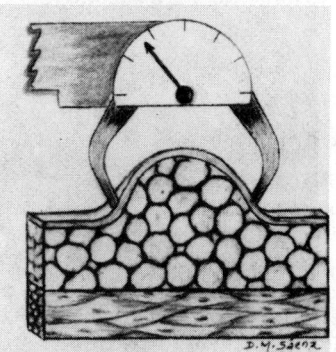

Figure 9–5. Skinfold calipers measure in mm. the thickness of the subcutaneous fat tissue. This gives a rough measurement of adiposity. (Diagram courtesy of Dr. Dorice Czajka-Narins.)

Body Composition

SKINFOLD THICKNESS. Skinfold thickness, as shown in Figure 9–5, is a measurement of subcutaneous fat that is coming into greater use as health practitioners become more concerned with assessing body fatness and muscle protein reserves. The measurement is usually taken over the triceps or biceps muscle, below the scapula (subscapular) or above the iliac crest (suprailiac), although other sites can be used. It is generally agreed that the triceps and scapular measurements are the most useful because the most complete standards and methods of evaluation have been developed for these sites. Figures 9–6 and 9–7 show the measurement of the skinfold thickness at these sites and the description of the method.[21] The amount of body fatness and the presence of excess body fat can be determined since the amount of subcutaneous fat is related to the amount of body fat. The population averages for triceps skinfold thickness are given in Appendix Tables 30 and 31. Because the amount of fat located subcutaneously varies with age and sex, it is important that tables used to evaluate skinfold measurements are age- and sex-appropriate.

OTHER ANTHROPOMETRIC DATA. If more complete information on actual body composition is needed, additional anthropometric data can be obtained. These usually include additional skinfold measurements and mid upper arm circumference.

Mid upper arm circumference, as shown in Figure 9–8, is measured halfway between the acromion process of the scapula and the tip of the elbow. Standards for arm circumference are given in Appendix Table 32.

When the mid upper arm circumference is combined with the triceps skinfold thickness measurement, an even better assessment of protein and energy nutriture can be made. It becomes possible to determine indirectly the arm *muscle* area and arm *fat* area, which of course would be impossible to measure directly. Figure 9–9 gives the method of calculating the arm muscle and fat areas. The arm muscle area is a good indication of the lean body mass and thus the skeletal protein reserves. This is important in growing children and is especially valuable in evaluating the person who may be protein-energy-malnourished from chronic illness, stress, multiple surgeries or inadequate diet. Nomograms for determining arm muscle and fat areas for children and adults appear in Appendices 28 and 29. With these nomograms determinations can be made without lengthy calculations. Norms for arm muscle and arm fat areas are given in Appendix Table 33.

Recently Heymsfield has reported that the present methods shown in Figure 9–8 for determining arm muscle area (AMA) tend to overestimate the AMA by 20 to 25 per cent because of the inclusion of some subcutaneous fat, the neu-

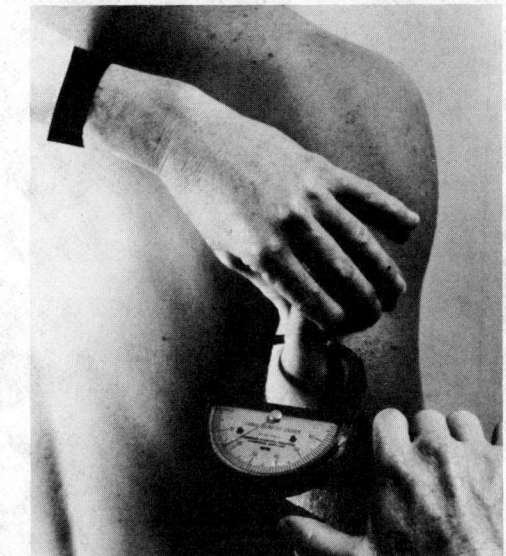

Figure 9–6. The triceps skinfold measurement is made at a point over the triceps muscle midway between the acromion and olecranon processes on the posterior aspect of the arm; the arm is held vertically, with the skinfold running parallel to the length of the arm.

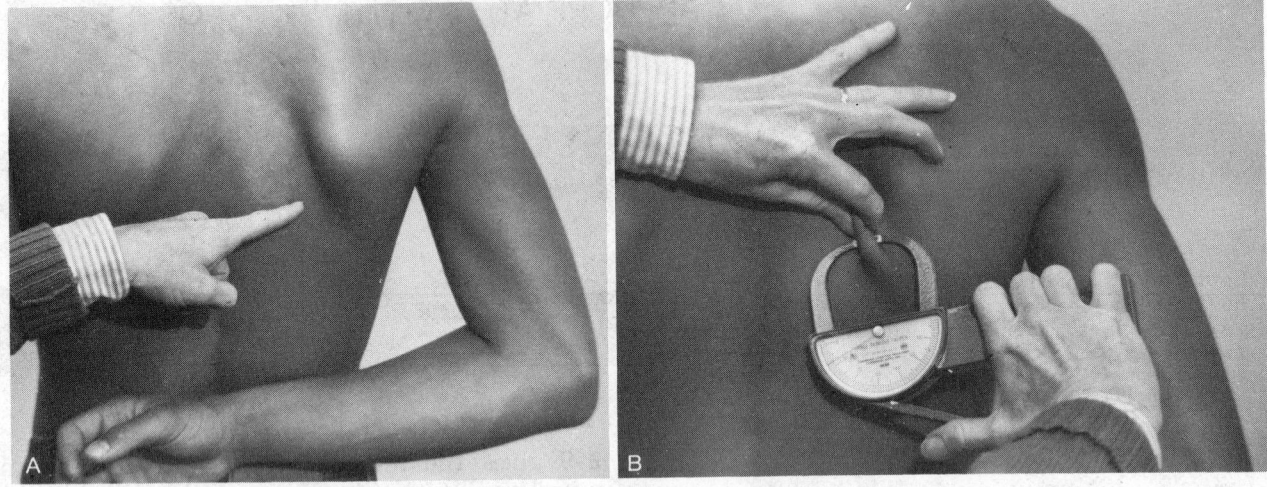

Figure 9–7. Measurement of the subscapular skinfold thickness.

romuscular sheath and bone.[19] He presented new formulas for calculating *corrected AMA* for men and women from mid-arm circumference (MAC) and triceps skinfold (TSF) measurements:

$$\text{AMA (men)} = \frac{(\text{MAC} - \pi \times \text{TSF})^2}{4\pi} - 10$$

$$\text{AMA (women)} = \frac{(\text{MAC} - \pi \times \text{TSF})^2}{4\pi} - 6.5$$

These equations calculate AMA with an average error of 7.7 per cent when compared with computerized tomography assessment of arm muscle area. Heymsfield goes on to suggest that a minimum AMA for survival is 9 to 11 cm.² in adults 152 to 168 cm. in height. *Available AMA* is the corrected AMA minus 9 cm.² Average corrected AMA values for healthy subjects aged 20 to 70 years were 51 cm.² for men (range 35 to 68 cm.²) and 28 cm² for women (range 17 to 39 cm.²), and the available AMA were 42 and 19 cm.² respectively.

Several formulas have also been developed for determining body fatness as a percentage of body weight using anthropometric data. In adults, the most widely used method is that of Durnin and Wormersly,[11] which uses four

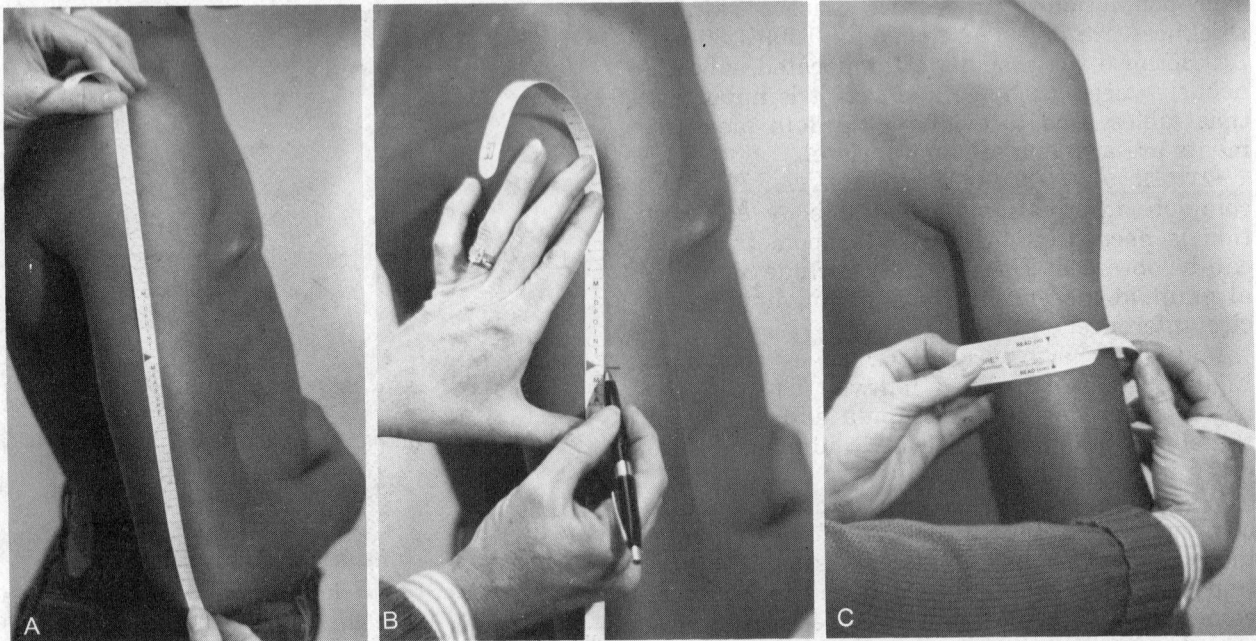

Figure 9–8. *A,* Measurement of midpoint between acromion process at shoulder and olecranon process at elbow. *B,* Marking of midpoint. *C,* Measurement of arm circumference in cm. at midpoint.

Figure 9–9. Upper arm area (A), upper arm muscle area (M) and upper arm fat area (F) are derived from measures of upper arm circumference. (C_1) and triceps skinfold (T) in mm.

$$A \ (mm.^2) = \frac{\pi}{4} \times d_1^2 \text{ where } d_1 = \frac{C_1}{\pi}$$

$$M \ (mm.^2) = \frac{(C_1 - \pi T)^2}{4\pi} = \frac{(C_1 - \pi T)^2}{12.56}$$

$$F \ (mm.^2) = A - M$$

Arm area and muscle area can also be determined using the nomograms in Appendix Tables 28 and 29.

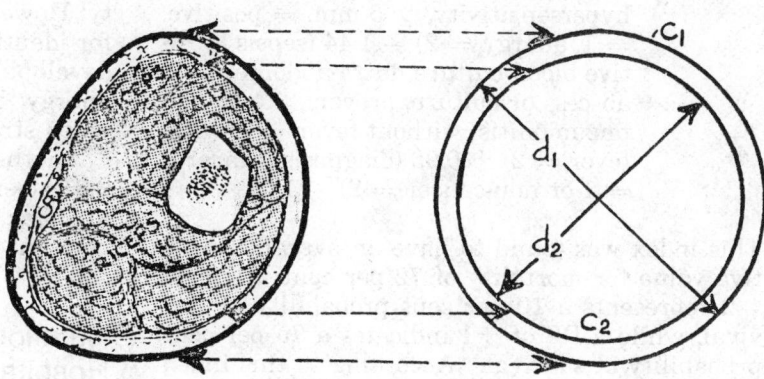

skinfold sites, (Appendix 34), the biceps, triceps, subscapular and suprailiac. Cited references 10, 13 and 30 describe methods for use with adolescents and children. An actual percentage of body fatness is most often desired as part of a fitness assessment, as discussed in Chapter 14.

More exact methods for determining body fatness are hydrostatic (underwater) weighing, total body potassium and total body water. These methods are usually reserved for research purposes.

The *creatinine:height index* has been used to assess the amount of skeletal muscle mass, which indicates muscle protein reserves, but the parameter is fraught with problems. Collection of a 24-hour urine sample is difficult, the creatinine excretion is affected by the amount of meat in the diet, other factors such as stress affect the excretion, and the precision and variability of the creatinine equivalence figures are questionable. However, Heymsfield concludes that it could be useful in selected patients, if several measurements of urinary creatinine are performed.[20]

BEHAVIOR EVALUATION

Behavior and changes in behavior are an elusive, hard to quantify aspect of the clinical examination. It is difficult to separate nutritional influence from the social and psychological environment. Some neurological and behavioral changes from vitamin deficiencies are given in Table 32–1. Unfortunately, there are no accepted criteria for this area, but the overall appearance of an adult or child can give an impression of nutritional status. The reader is referred to Chapter 32 as well as to other detailed references.[26, 38] Listlessness is very apparent in severe protein-energy malnutrition; the person is apathetic, withdrawn and uninterested in the surroundings.

The Nutritional Status Assessment and Prognosis

Now that the nutritional markers have been discussed, it is important to combine these in a useful system of evaluation. It is important to identify, quantify and validate the clinical importance and relevance of these markers individually and when integrated together. For example, a biochemical indicator of protein-energy malnutrition (PEM) that has no clinical impact in terms of morbidity and mortality would have minor importance compared with another marker that portends an increase of morbidity and mortality secondary to PEM. It is important to try to define *clinically relevant malnutrition* and a system of integrating the components of assessment is necessary.

One group in attempting to relate nutritional parameters to risk of operative complications has developed the *prognostic nutritional index* (PNI), which gives a percentage of risk of operative complications:[7, 27]

PNI = 158 − 16.6 (serum albumin [gm./dl.]) − 0.78 (triceps skinfold [mm.]) − 0.2 (serum transferrin [mg./dl.]) − 5.8 (delayed hypersensitivity, graded 0 = non-reactive, 1 = <5 mm. reactivity, 2 = >5 mm reactivity)

The higher the PNI, the greater the risk of operative complications due to nutritional factors that could be reduced by appropriate nutritional support.

Another group has developed a similar *hospital prognostic index* to predict subsequent hospital outcome. This index is:

discriminant function (DF) = 0.91 (serum albumin [gm./dl.]) − 1.00 (delayed hypersensitivity, ≥ 5 mm. = positive = 1, anergy = 2) − 1.44 (sepsis [positive blood culture, intra-abdominal abscess or culture, proven pneumonitis] without fever = 1, with fever = 2) + 0.98 (diagnosis, cancer = 1 or non-cancer = 2) − 1.09

This index was found to have an overall predictive value for mortality of 72 per cent. A DF of −2 represents a 10 per cent probability of survival, while a DF of +1 indicates a 75 per cent probability of survival.[18] According to this index delayed hypersensitivity, serum albumin and the presence or absence of sepsis or cancer provide a useful objective index to identify high-risk patients and to predict the outcome of their hospital course. Estimation of peripheral energy stores (fat and skeletal muscle as represented by weight for height, TSF and AMA) did not correlate with immune function, infection or mortality. However, anthropometric data are important for identifying those patients at greatest risk for developing significant hypoalbuminemia and anergy in the absence of nutritional support when stress is superimposed.

Another equation is 1.2 (serum albumin) + 0.013 (serum transferrin) − 6.43. This nutritional index was effective in predicting outcome 88 per cent of the time.[32]

Nutritional Assessment for Hospitalized and Stressed Patients

Table 9–9 presents the likely nutritional indicators for the physically stressed, ill or traumatized patient. This assessment focuses on protein-energy nutrition, which seems at this

Table 9–9. NUTRITIONAL AND METABOLIC VARIABLES COMMONLY USED IN ASSESSING PROTEIN-ENERGY MALNUTRITION

ANTHROPOMETRY		COMMENTS
Height	—	
Weight	—	
Usual weight	—	
Sex	—	
Ideal body weight (IBW)	—	Determined from Appendix Table 24, 25, or 27
Weight as % IBW	—	
Weight as % usual weight	—	
Triceps skinfold (mm.)	—	
Triceps skinfold as percentile of norms	—	Determined from Appendix Table 30 or 31
Arm circumference (cm.)	—	
Arm muscle area (mm.²)	—	Calculated from Figure 9–9
Arm muscle area as percentile of norms	—	Determined from Appendix Table 32
BIOCHEMICAL/IMMUNOLOGICAL		
Serum albumin (gm./dl.)	—	3 gm./dl. acceptable < 3 gm./dl. deficient
Total iron-binding capacity (TIBC) μg/100 ml.	—	
Serum transferrin mg./100 ml.	—	Calculated from TIBC: transferrin = (0.8 × TIBC) − 43	170 gm./dl. acceptable < 170 gm./dl. deficient
Serum thyroxine–binding prealbumin (mg./dl.)	—		Consult laboratory
White blood cell count (no./mm.³)	—	
Lymphocytes as % of WBC	—	
Total lymphocyte count (TLC) (no./mm.³)	—	Calculated as follows: TLC = WBC × % lymphocytes	1200/mm.³ acceptable < 1200/mm.³ low
24-hour urinary creatinine (mg.)	—	
*Creatinine:height index %	—	Determined as follows: $\dfrac{\text{24-hour urinary creatinine (mg.)}}{\text{expected 24-hour urinary creatinine (mg.)}}$	60% standard† < 60% standard
Skin test results	—	

* Creatinine: height index is appropriate to use in a limited number of patients in whom the meat content of the diet is constant, 24-hour urine collections are complete, and emotional stress and physical activity are kept to a minimum. The creatine equivalence (mg. creatinine excreted/kg. body weight) is 20 for children, 23 for adult males and 17 for adult females.

†Standards for adults are given in Appendix Table 35 and for children in Viteri, F., and Alvarado, J.: The creatinine height index: its use in the estimation of the degree of protein depletion and repletion in protein calorie malnourished children, Pediatrics, 46:696, 1970.

point to be most indicative of risk of developing anergy, sepsis and poor outcome from surgery or major illness in the hospital. It assesses the three body energy stores: skeletal muscle (arm muscle area and creatinine:height index), visceral protein (serum albumin and transferrin) and total body fat (triceps skinfold, weight).

Use of the Nutritional Status Assessment

An assessment of nutritional status should be done routinely for all persons in a health care system, although it is usually done in greater depth for those people in whom a nutritional problem is suspected. The information in the nutritional assessment is usually used as the basis for designing the nutritional care plan, as discussed in Chapter 19. A thorough nutritional assessment makes the planning of nutritional support, nutrition education or counseling more effective.

Problems and Suggested Topics for Discussion

1. Is it accurate to say, based solely on dietary data, that a person is deficient in a nutrient? Explain.
2. Perform a complete nutritional status assessment on a patient in your care.
   a. What problems did you have in collecting data?
   b. Are you missing necessary data?
   c. Were clinical findings confirmed by biochemical and dietary data?
   d. From the nutritional assessment, state the nutritional problems of your patient.
3. Evaluate a patient with a below normal nutritional biochemical finding. What does this indicate about his or her nutritional status? What additional information would be helpful?
4. Which anthropometric parameters are helpful in assessing the nutritional status of an individual? Explain. What are the inherent weaknesses in the use of these measurements?
5. Use one of the prognostic indexes developed from nutritional assessment to predict the outcome of one of your patients. What type of nutritional support could change this?

Cited References

1. Adams, C.F.: Nutritive Value of American Foods. Agricultural Research Service, Agricultural Handbook No. 456. Washington D.C., U.S. Government Printing Office, 1975.
2. Bistrian, B.R.: Nutritional assessment and therapy of protein-calorie malnutrition in hospital. J. Am. Diet. Assoc., 71:393, 1977.
3. Bistrian, B.R., et al.: Cellular immunity in adult marasmus. Arch. Int. Med., 137:1408, 1977.
4. Bistrian, B.R., et al.: Cellular immunity in semi-starved states in hospitalized adults. Am. J. Clin. Nutr., 28:1148, 1975.
5. Bray, G.A. (ed.): Obesity in America. NIH Publ. No. 79–359. Washington, D.C., U.S. Department of Health and Human Services, 1979.
6. Bray, G.A., Jordan, H.A., and Sims, E.A.H.: Evaluation of the obese patient. I. An algorithm. JAMA, 235:1487, 1976.
7. Buzby, G.P., et al.: Prognostic nutritional index in gastrointestinal surgery. Am. J. Surg., 134:160, 1980.
8. Composition of Foods. Agricultural Handbooks No. 8:1–9. Consumer and Food Economics Institute. Washington, D.C., U.S. Department of Agriculture, 1976–1982.
9. Daly, J.M., Dudrick, S.J., and Copeland, E.M.: Intravenous hyperalimentation: effect of delayed cutaneous hypersensitivity in cancer patients. Ann. Surg., 192:587, 1980.
10. Dugdale, A.E., and Griffiths, M.: Estimating body fat mass from anthropometric data, Am. J. Clin. Nutr., 32:2400, 1979.
11. Durnin, J.V.G.A., and Wormersley, J.: Body fat assessed from total body density and its estimation from skinfold thickness: measurements on 481 men and women aged from 16–72 years. Br. J. Nutr., 32:77, 1974.
12. Foman, S.J.: Nutritional disorders of children. DHEW Publication No. (HSA) 77–5104. Rockville, Md., U.S. Department of Health, Education and Welfare, 1977.
13. Frerichs, R.R., Hasha, D.W., Berenson, G.S.: Equations for estimating percentage body fat in children 10–14 years old. Pediatr. Res., 13:170, 1979.
14. Frisancho, A.R., and Flegel, P.N.: Elbow breadth as a measure of frame size for US males and females. Am. J. Clin. Nutr., 37:311, 1983.
15. Garn, S.M., Smith, N.J., and Clark, D.C.: The magnitude and the implication of apparent race differences in hemoglobin values. Am. J. Clin. Nutr., 28:563, 1975.
16. Gleason, C.: Nutritional assessment of boys with physical deformities: stature estimation (abstract). Fed. Proc., 42:1044, 1983.
17. Guthrie, H.A., Owen, G.M., and Guthrie, G.M.: Factor analysis of measures of nutritional status of preschool children. Am. J. Clin. Nutr., 26:497, 1973.
18. Harvey, K.B., et al.: Biological measures for the formulation of hospital prognostic index. Am. J. Clin. Nutr., 34:2013, 1981.
19. Heymsfield, S.B., et al.: Anthropometric measurement of muscle mass: revised equations for calculating bone-free arm muscle area. Am. J. Clin. Nutr., 36:680, 1982.
20. Heymsfield, S.B., et al.: Measurement of muscle mass in humans: validity of the 24 hour urinary creatinine method. Am. J. Clin. Nutr., 37:478, 1983.
21. Keys, A.: Committee on Nutritional Anthropometry. Food and Nutrition Board: Recommendations concerning body measurements for characterization of nutritional status. Human Biol., 28:11, 1956.
22. Keys, A., et al.: Indices of relative weight and obesity. J. Chron. Dis., 25:329, 1972.
23. Khosla, T., and Lowe, C.R.: Indices of obesity derived from body weight and height. Br. J. Prev. Soc. Med., 21:122, 1967.
24. Laker, M.: On determining trace element levels in man: the uses of blood and hair. Lancet, 1:260, 1982.
25. Maugh, T.H.: Hair: a diagnostic tool to complement blood serum and urine. Science, 202:1271, 1978.
26. Miller, S.A. (ed.): Nutrition and the Brain. Philadelphia, The Franklin Institute Press, 1981.
27. Mullen, J.L., et al.: Reduction of operative morbidity and mortality by combined preoperative and postoperative nutritional support. Ann. Surg., 192:604, 1980.
28. Mitchell, C.O., and Lipschitz, D.A.: Arm length measurement as an alterative to height in nutritional assessment of the elderly. JPEN, 6:226, 1982.
29. Murphy, S., and Trahms, C.M.: Assessment of Children: A Guide for Weighing and Measuring. Seattle,

Wash., Child Development and Mental Retardation Center, 1981.

30. Parizkova, J.: Total body fat and skinfold thickness in children. Metabolism, *10*:794, 1961.

31. Pennington, J.A.T., and Church, H.N.: Bowes and Church's Food Values of Portions Commonly Used. 13th ed. Philadelphia, J.B. Lippincott Company, 1980.

32. Rainey-MacDonald, C.G., et al.: Validity of a two-variable nutritional index for use in selecting candidates for nutritional support. JPEN, *7*:15, 1983.

33. Roche, A.F., and McKigney, J.I.: Physical growth of ethnic groups comprising the U.S. population. Am. J. Dis. Child., *130*:62, 1976.

34. Stuff, J.E., et al.: A comparison of dietary methods in nutritional studies, Am. J. Clin. Nutr., *37*:300, 1983.

35. Trahms, C.M.: Rate Yourself Measurement Techniques. Seattle, Wash., Child Development and Mental Retardation Center, 1982.

36. Twomey, P., Ziegler, D., and Rombeau, J.: Utility of skin testing in nutritional assessment: a critical review. JPEN, *6*:50, 1982.

37. WHO Scientific Group: Cell-mediated immunity and resistance to infection. Geneva, WHO Tech. Rep. Ser., 519, 1973.

38. Wurtman, R.J., and Wurtman, J.J. (eds.): Nutrition and the Brain. Vol. 1. New York, Raven Press, 1977.

39. Young, C.M.: Subjects' estimation of food intake and calculated nutritive value of the diet. J. Am. Diet. Assoc., *29*:1216, 1953.

Additional References

Baker, J.P., et al.: Nutritional assessment. A comparison of clinical judgement and objective measurements. N. Engl. J. Med., *306*:969, 1982.

Beal, V.A.: The nutritional history in longitudinal research. J. Am. Diet. Assoc., *51*:426, 1967.

Blackburn, G.L. et al.: Nutritional and metabolic assessment of the hospitalized patient, JPEN, *1*:11, 1977.

Burk, M.C., and Pao, E.M.: Methodology for Largescale Surveys of Household and Individual Diets. Home Economics Research Report No. 40, Agriculture Research Service, Washington, D.C., U.S. Government Printing Office, 1976.

Burke, B.S.: The dietary history as a tool in research. J. Am. Diet. Assoc., *23*:1041, 1947.

Christakis, G. (ed.): Nutritional Assessment in Health Programs. Washington, D.C., American Public Health Association, 1973.

Frisancho, A.R.: New norms of upper limb fat and muscle areas for assessment of nutritional status. Am. J. Clin. Nutr., *34*:2540, 1981.

Frisancho, A.R., and Flegel, P.N.: Relative merits of old and new indices of body mass with reference to skinfold thickness. Am. J. Clin. Nutr., *36*:697, 1982.

Grant, A.: Nutritional Assessment Guidelines. 2nd ed., 1979. Available from Anne Grant, Box 25057, Northgate Station, Seattle, Wash., 98125.

Hamill, P.V., and Moore, W.M.: Contemporary growth charts: needs, construction and application. Dietetic Currents, *3*(5), 1976.

Heymsfield, S.B., et al.: Muscle mass: reliable indicator of protein-energy malnutrition severity and outcome. Am. J. Clin. Nutr., *35*:1192, 1982.

Jelliffe, D.B.: The Assessment of the Nutritional Status of the Community. WHO Monograph No. 53. Geneva, World Health Organization, 1966.

Katch, V.L., and Freedson, P.S.: Body size and shape: derivation of the "HAT" frame size model. Am. J. Clin. Nutr., *36*:669, 1982.

Krantzler, N.J., et al.: Methods of food intake assessment—an annotated bibliography. J. Nutr. Educ., *14*:108, 1982.

Lopes, J., et al.: Skeletal muscle function in malnutrition. Am. J. Clin. Nutr., *36*:602, 1982.

McLaren, D.S.: Nutritional assessment. In McLaren, D.S., and Burman, D.: Textbook of Paediatric Nutrition. Edinburgh, Churchill Livingstone, 1976.

Meakins, J.L., et al.: Delayed hypersensitivity: indicator of acquired failure of host defenses in sepsis and trauma, Ann. Surg., *186*:241, 1977.

Methodology of Nutritional Surveillance. Joint FAO/UNICEF WHO Expert Committee, WHO Tech. Rep. No. 593. Geneva, World Health Organization, 1976.

Nutritional Assessment—Present Status, Future Directions and Prospects. Report of the Second Ross Conference on Medical Research. Columbus, Ohio, Ross Laboratories, 1981.

Pietsch, J.B., Meakins, J.L., and MacLean, L.D.: The delayed hypersensitivity response: application in clinical surgery. Surgery, *82*:349, 1977.

Sauberlich, H.E., Skala, J.H., and Dowdy, R.P.: Laboratory Tests for the Assessment of Nutritional Status. Cleveland, CRC Press, Inc., 1974.

Shelty, P.S., et al.: Rapid-turnover transport proteins: an index of subclinical protein-energy malnutrition. Lancet, *1*: 230, 1979.

Simopoulos, A.P. (ed.): Assessment of nutritional status. Am. J. Clin. Nutr., *35*(Suppl.)(5), 1982.

Ten-State Nutrition Survey, 1968–70. U.S. Department of Health, Education and Welfare Publ. No. (HSM) 72–8130–33. Washington, D.C., U.S. Government Printing Office, 1972.

Todd, K.S., Hudes, M., and Calloway, D.H.: Food intake measurement: problems and approaches. Am. J. Clin. Nutr., *37*:139, 1983.

Recommended Dietary Allowances and the Adequate Diet

Interpretation of an Adequate Diet

An adequate diet is composed of the various nutrients that the body needs for maintenance, repair, the living processes, and growth or development. It is a diet that meets in full all the nutritional needs of the person. There is no *ideal* diet, since such a diet is a matter of individual requirement.

In the preceding chapters the various nutrients needed by the body have been discussed. In this chapter, these principles of nutrition will be translated into the selection of an adequate diet.

Besides nutrition principles, the adequate diet will also reflect the availability of foods, socioeconomic conditions, taste preferences, food habits, age of the family members, storage and preparation facilities, and cooking skills.

Dietary Interrelationships

All studies of the interaction of nutrients indicate the need for a balanced diet. Clinical reports show that often when an individual is found deficient in one nutrient, such as a vitamin, deficiencies in others are also found. It is an established fact that the presence or absence of one essential nutrient may affect the availability, absorption, metabolism or dietary need for others.

Interrelationships exist not only among the vitamins but among the minerals. Vitamins interact with minerals just as both vitamins and minerals are related to fat, protein and carbohydrate functions and requirements. Numerous experiments have extended understanding of the broad nutritional import of interrelationships or "balance" among nutrients. While certain interrelationships have long been known, the recognition of the large number of them reemphasizes the basic soundness of the principle of maintaining variety in foods in order to provide the most complete diet. Much current research is being devoted to dietary interrelationships.

Defining Nutritional Needs of Humans

The dietary standards set up by the Food and Nutrition Board (FNB) of the National Research Council of the National Academy of Sciences are listed in Tables 10–1, 10–2 and 10–3. These standards are universally accepted as the guide or yardstick for planning and evaluating diets and food supplies for population groups and individuals in the United States. FAO/WHO has established standards for people in developing countries and several other countries have their own standards for human nutrient requirements. These standards represent years of research by many workers on both animals and human beings. The U.S. standards, revised in 1980 (ninth revision; original edition published in 1943), represent the latest U.S. interpretation of human nutritional needs by a large number of nutrition authorities.

RECOMMENDED DIETARY ALLOWANCES (RDA)

The purposes and the applicability of the recommended dietary allowances can best be explained by quoting from the 1980 revised publication.[5]

Recommended Dietary Allowances (RDA) are the levels of intake of essential nutrients considered, in the judgment of the Committee on Dietary Allowances of the Food and Nutrition Board on the basis of available scientific knowledge, to be adequate to meet the known nutritional needs of practically all healthy persons.

RDA are recommendations for the average daily amounts of nutrients that *population groups* should consume over a period of time. RDA should not be confused with requirements for a specific individual. Differences in the nutrient requirements of individuals are ordinarily unknown. Therefore, RDA (except for energy) are estimated to exceed the requirements of most individuals and thereby to ensure that the needs of nearly all in the population are met. Intakes below the recommended allowance for a nutrient are not necessarily inadequate, but the risk of having an

Table 10–1. FOOD AND NUTRITION BOARD, NATIONAL ACADEMY OF SCIENCES–NATIONAL RESEARCH COUNCIL RECOMMENDED DAILY DIETARY ALLOWANCES,[a] Revised 1980

Designed for the maintenance of good nutrition of practically all healthy people in the U.S.A.

	AGE (years)	WEIGHT (kg.)	WEIGHT (lb.)	HEIGHT (cm.)	HEIGHT (in.)	PROTEIN (g.)	FAT-SOLUBLE VITAMINS Vitamin A (μg. RE)[b]	Vitamin D (μg.)[c]	Vitamin E (mg. α-TE)[d]
Infants	0.0–0.5	6	13	60	24	kg. × 2.2	420	10	3
	0.5–1.0	9	20	71	28	kg. × 2.0	400	10	4
Children	1–3	13	29	90	35	23	400	10	5
	4–6	20	44	112	44	30	500	10	6
	7–10	28	62	132	52	34	700	10	7
Males	11–14	45	99	157	62	45	1000	10	8
	15–18	66	145	176	69	56	1000	10	10
	19–22	70	154	177	70	56	1000	7.5	10
	23–50	70	154	178	70	56	1000	5	10
	51+	70	154	178	70	56	1000	5	10
Females	11–14	46	101	157	62	46	800	10	8
	15–18	55	120	163	64	46	800	10	8
	19–22	55	120	163	64	44	800	7.5	8
	23–50	55	120	163	64	44	800	5	8
	51+	55	120	163	64	44	800	5	8
Pregnant						+30	+200	+5	+2
Lactating						+20	+400	+5	+3

[a]The allowances are intended to provide for individual variations among most normal persons as they live in the United States under usual environmental stresses. Diets should be based on a variety of common foods in order to provide other nutrients for which human requirements have been less well defined. See reference 5 for detailed discussion of allowances and of nutrients not tabulated.

[b]Retinol equivalents. 1 retinol equivalent = 1 μg. retinol or 6 μg. β carotene. See page 104 for calculation of vitamin A activity of diets as retinol equivalents.

[c]As cholecalciferol. 10 μg. cholecalciferol = 400 IU of vitamin D.

[d]α-tocopherol equivalents. 1 mg d-α tocopherol = 1 α-TE. See page 114 for variation in allowances and calculation of vitamin E activity of the diet as α-tocopherol equivalents.

[e]1 NE (niacin equivalent) is equal to 1 mg of niacin or 60 mg of dietary tryptophan.

inadequate intake increases to the extent that intake is less than the level recommended as safe.

RDA are recommendations established for *healthy* populations. Special needs for nutrients arising from such problems as premature birth, inherited metabolic disorders, infections, chronic diseases, and the use of medications require special dietary and therapeutic measures. These conditions are not covered by the RDA.

RDA are intended to be met by a diet of a wide variety of foods rather than by supplementation or by extensive fortification of single foods. RDA have not been set for all recognized nutrients. (Estimated safe and adequate intakes have been set for some nutrients in this edition.) Therefore diets should be composed of a *variety* of foods that are acceptable, palatable, and economically attainable by the consumer using the RDA as a guide to assessment of their nutritional adequacy.

The RDA are stated as the amounts of nutrients to be consumed. They do not take into account the nutrient losses that occur during processing and preparation of food.

The RDA have been used as guides in planning nutritionally adequate diets for groups. They are used in the interpretation of the adequacy of nutrient intakes of groups in dietary surveys. They are to be used as a reference. Any deviations of the individual intakes from the recommended nutrient allowances should be regarded as significant only in terms of the individual's total health status. The nutritional status is the sum total of the food consumption: present and past nutrient intake, clinical signs and symptoms, growth and development, biochemical data and excretory levels of nutrients, as explained in Chapter 9.

It would be a mistake to assume that individuals whose diets do not meet the RDA are necessarily suffering from malnutrition, since the RDA allow for a margin of safety for individual variations. Equally invalid are statements to the effect that "the average intake of a population meets the RDA; therefore there is no problem of nutritional inadequacy as applied to individuals." In most cases this may be true, but there should be individual assessment.

The recommended allowances are designed for the population of the United States and are revised periodically in order to include new research findings. Nutritional surveys are also needed periodically to determine the nature, causes and location of malnutrition in the United States.

Table 10–1. FOOD AND NUTRITION BOARD, NATIONAL ACADEMY OF SCIENCES–NATIONAL RESEARCH COUNCIL RECOMMENDED DAILY DIETARY ALLOWANCES,[a] Revised 1980 (*Continued*)

Designed for the maintenance of good nutrition of practically all healthy people in the U.S.A.

WATER-SOLUBLE VITAMINS							MINERALS					
Vitamin C (mg.)	Thiamin (mg.)	Riboflavin (mg.)	Niacin (mg. NE)[e]	Vitamin B_6 (mg.)	Folacin[f] (µg.)	Vitamin B_{12} (µg.)	Calcium (mg.)	Phosphorus (mg.)	Magnesium (mg.)	Iron (mg.)	Zinc (mg.)	Iodine (µg.)
35	0.3	0.4	6	0.3	30	0.5[g]	360	240	50	10	3	40
35	0.5	0.6	8	0.6	45	1.5	540	360	70	15	5	50
45	0.7	0.8	9	0.9	100	2.0	800	800	150	15	10	70
45	0.9	1.0	11	1.3	200	2.5	800	800	200	10	10	90
45	1.2	1.4	16	1.6	300	3.0	800	800	250	10	10	120
50	1.4	1.6	18	1.8	400	3.0	1200	1200	350	18	15	150
60	1.4	1.7	18	2.0	400	3.0	1200	1200	400	18	15	150
60	1.5	1.7	19	2.2	400	3.0	800	800	350	10	15	150
60	1.4	1.6	18	2.2	400	3.0	800	800	350	10	15	150
60	1.2	1.4	16	2.2	400	3.0	800	800	350	10	15	150
50	1.1	1.3	15	1.8	400	3.0	1200	1200	300	18	15	150
60	1.1	1.3	14	2.0	400	3.0	1200	1200	300	18	15	150
60	1.1	1.3	14	2.0	400	3.0	800	800	300	18	15	150
60	1.0	1.2	13	2.0	400	3.0	800	800	300	18	15	150
60	1.0	1.2	13	2.0	400	3.0	800	800	300	10	15	150
+20	+0.4	+0.3	+2	+0.6	+400	+1.0	+400	+400	+150	h	+5	+25
+40	+0.5	+0.5	+5	+0.5	+100	+1.0	+400	+400	+150	h	+10	+50

[f] The folacin allowances refer to dietary sources as determined by *Lactobacillus casei* assay after treatment with enzymes (conjugases) to make polyglutamyl forms of the vitamin available to the test organism.

[g] The recommended dietary allowance for vitamin B_{12} in infants is based on average concentration of the vitamin in human milk. The allowances after weaning are based on energy intake (as recommended by the American Academy of Pediatrics) and consideration of other factors, such as intestinal absorption; see reference 5.

[h] The increased requirement during pregnancy cannot be met by the iron content of habitual American diets nor by the existing scores of many women; therefore the use of 30–60 mg of supplemental iron is recommended. Iron needs during lactation are not substantially different from those of nonpregnant women, but continued supplementation of the mother for 2–3 months after parturition is advisable in order to replenish stores depleted by pregnancy.

A history of the development of the RDA is given in Table 10–4. In the 1968 revision recommended allowances were added for vitamins E, B_6, B_{12} and folacin and for the minerals iodine, magnesium and phosphorus. The 1974 revision added allowances for zinc. The 1980 revision added a new table (Table 10–2), a compilation of safe and adequate intakes for three vitamins and nine minerals for which RDA cannot be established on the basis of present knowledge. Ranges are given for appropriate intakes of vitamins K, biotin and pantothenic acid; of electrolytes sodium, potassium and chloride; and of trace elements copper, manganese, fluoride, chromium, selenium and molybdenum. Calling these ranges safe intakes draws attention to the fact that there are upper limits for the safe use of many nutrients. The ranges for the trace elements emphasize that consumption of excessive amounts of these could lead to the buildup of toxic amounts in the body.[14]

The age and sex groupings include two periods of infancy up to one year, three age groupings for children and seven age groups of males and females from 11 to 51 years of age and beyond. The average man (weight 154 lb. or 70 kg., height 70 in. or 178 cm.) and average woman (weight 120 lb. or 55 kg., height 64 in. or 163 cm.) are used for the age groups 23 to 50 years of age and 51+ years of age. They are presumed to live in an environment with a mean temperature of 70°F. (20°C.). Their physical activity is considered "light" (neither sedentary nor heavy physical activity).

Certain of the 1980 RDA require comments:

ENERGY. Because of the concern over the fact that a considerable segment of the American population is overweight, and the belief that the average adult exerts much less energy than was allowed for in the 1958 and 1964 RDA, the 1968, 1974 and 1980 calorie allowances are lower and reflect the lowest energy intake thought to be compatible with health for males and females in certain age groups. The factor of 4.2 kjoules per kcalorie has been included for conversion of kcalories to kjoules.

An innovation of the revised 1980 RDA is the presentation of energy (calorie) allowances in a separate table (Table 10–3), together with a table of desirable body weights (Appendix Table 27). This focuses attention on maintenance of desirable body weight. Ranges are given for body weights and for average calorie intakes. The energy allowances for young adults are for

Table 10–2. ESTIMATED SAFE AND ADEQUATE DAILY DIETARY INTAKES OF SELECTED VITAMINS AND MINERALS[a]

	AGE (years)	VITAMINS Vitamin K (μg.)	Biotin (μg.)	Pantothenic Acid (mg.)
Infants	0–0.5	12	35	2
	0.5–1	10–20	50	3
Children	1–3	15–30	65	3
and Adolescents	4–6	20–40	85	3–4
	7–10	30–60	120	4–5
	11+	50–100	100–200	4–7
Adults		70–140	100–200	4–7

	AGE (years)	TRACE ELEMENTS[b] Copper (mg.)	Manganese (mg.)	Fluoride (mg.)	Chromium (mg.)	Selenium (mg.)	Molybdenum (mg.)
Infants	0–0.5	0.5–0.7	0.5–0.7	0.1–0.5	0.01–0.04	0.01–0.04	0.03–0.06
	0.5–1	0.7–1.0	0.7–1.0	0.2–1.0	0.02–0.06	0.02–0.06	0.04–0.08
Children	1–3	1.0–1.5	1.0–1.5	0.5–1.5	0.02–0.08	0.02–0.08	0.05–0.1
and Adolescents	4–6	1.5–2.0	1.5–2.0	1.0–2.5	0.03–0.12	0.03–0.12	0.06–0.15
	7–10	2.0–2.5	2.0–3.0	1.5–2.5	0.05–0.2	0.05–0.2	0.10–0.3
	11+	2.0–3.0	2.5–5.0	1.5–2.5	0.05–0.2	0.05–0.2	0.15–0.5
Adults		2.0–3.0	2.5–5.0	1.5–4.0	0.05–0.2	0.05–0.2	0.15–0.5

	AGE (years)	ELECTROLYTES Sodium (mg.)	Potassium (mg.)	Chloride (mg.)
Infants	0–0.5	115–350	350–925	275–700
	0.5–1	250–750	425–1275	400–1200
Children	1–3	325–975	550–1650	500–1500
and Adolescents	4–6	450–1350	775–2325	700–2100
	7–10	600–1800	1000–3000	925–2775
	11+	900–2700	1525–4575	1400–4200
Adults		1100–3300	1875–5625	1700–5100

[a]Because there is less information on which to base allowances, these figures are provided here in the form of ranges of recommended intakes.

[b]Since the toxic levels for many trace elements may be only several times usual intakes, the upper levels for the trace elements given in this table should not be habitually exceeded.

(From Food and Nutrition Board, National Research Council: Recommended Dietary Allowances. 9th ed. Washington, D.C., National Academy of Sciences, 1980.)

men and women living in a temperate climate and doing light work. Thus, for example, the daily energy expenditure for a man aged 19 to 22 weighing 70 kg. would average 2900 kcal. (12,200 KJ.), and for a woman the same age weighing 55 kg. the daily energy expenditure would average 2100 kcal. (8,800 KJ.), based on energy needs. Allowances are given for three age groups after age 22: those aged 23 to 50 years, those aged 51 to 75 years, and those over age 75. These allowances are based on an average 2 per cent decrease in basal metabolism per decade and a reduction in activity of 200 kcal. per day for men and women between 51 and 75 years, 500 kcal. for men over 75 years, and 400 kcal. for women over 75 years.

Energy intake must be adjusted for variations in physical activity, body size and rarely for climate so that an individual maintains ideal weight. Since the RDA energy allowances for adults are set for persons doing light or sedentary activities, those for persons with moderate activity might be increased by adding 300 kcal. per day, and those who are very active may need to add 600 to 900 kcal. per day. Chapter 1 describes energy requirements in detail. Energy intake for infants is discussed in Chapter 12 and for children in Chapter 13.

Children or adults who gain excessive weight while habitually consuming the recommended number of kcalories should be encouraged to increase their activity to achieve the desired

Table 10–3. MEAN HEIGHTS AND WEIGHTS AND RECOMMENDED ENERGY INTAKE[a]

CATEGORY	AGE (years)	WEIGHT (kg.)	WEIGHT (lb.)	HEIGHT (cm.)	HEIGHT (in.)	ENERGY NEEDS (WITH RANGE) (kcal.)		ENERGY NEEDS (WITH RANGE) (MJ.)
Infants	0.0–0.5	6	13	60	24	kg × 115	(95–145)	kg × 0.48
	0.5–1.0	9	20	71	28	kg × 105	(80–135)	kg × 0.44
Children	1–3	13	29	90	35	1300	(900–1800)	5.5
	4–6	20	44	112	44	1700	(1300–2300)	7.1
	7–10	28	62	132	52	2400	(1650–3300)	10.1
Males	11–14	45	99	157	62	2700	(2000–3700)	11.3
	15–18	66	145	176	69	2800	(2100–3900)	11.8
	19–22	70	154	177	70	2900	(2500–3300)	12.2
	23–50	70	154	178	70	2700	(2300–3100)	11.3
	51–75	70	154	178	70	2400	(2000–2800)	10.1
	76+	70	154	178	70	2050	(1650–2450)	8.6
Females	11–14	46	101	157	62	2200	(1500–3000)	9.2
	15–18	55	120	163	64	2100	(1200–3000)	8.8
	19–22	55	120	163	64	2100	(1700–2500)	8.8
	23–50	55	120	163	64	2000	(1600–2400)	8.4
	51–75	55	120	163	64	1800	(1400–2200)	7.6
	76+	55	120	163	64	1600	(1200–2000)	6.7
Pregnancy						+300		
Lactation						+500		

[a]The data in this table have been assembled from the observed median heights and weights of children shown in Appendix Tables 15, 17, 19 and 21, together with desirable weights for adults given in Appendix Table 27 for the mean heights of men (70 in.) and women (64 in.) between the ages of 18 and 34 years as surveyed in the U.S. population (HEW/NCHS data).

The energy allowances for the young adults are for men and women doing light work. The allowances for the two older age groups represent mean energy needs over these age spans, allowing for a 2-percent decrease in basal (resting) metabolic rate per decade and a reduction in activity of 200 kcal./day for men and women between 51 and 75 years, 500 kcal. for men over 75 years, and 400 kcal. for women over 75 years. The customary range of daily energy output is shown in parentheses for adults and is based on a variation in energy needs of ±400 kcal. at any one age, emphasizing the wide range of energy intakes appropriate for any group of people.

Energy allowances for children through age 18 are based on median energy intakes of children of these ages followed in longitudinal growth studies. The values in parentheses are 10th and 90th percentiles of energy intake, to indicate the range of energy consumption among children of these ages.

(From Food and Nutrition Board, National Research Council: Recommended Dietary Allowances. 9th ed. Washington, D.C., National Academy of Sciences, 1980.)

weight, rather than decrease their energy intake to below the RDA. It is difficult to obtain adequate intakes of all the other nutrients when the energy intake is much below the RDA, unless sugar, alcohol and fats are greatly restricted, which is not the habit in most American families. These foods are of low nutrient density, contributing many kcalories but few nutrients.

PROTEIN. Knowledge regarding human protein requirements is not complete. This is evidenced by the fact that adult protein requirements were decreased from 1.0 gm./kg./day in 1963 to 0.9 gm./kg./day in 1968 and to 0.8 gm./kg./day in 1974 and 1980. These allowances were established to cover the needs of most people who encounter the stresses of normal living. Allowances are increased for pregnancy, lactation and growth and may also need to be increased during stress.

Since high protein foods are also good sources of vitamins B_6, B_{12} and trace elements not included in the RDA but still essential, there has been some concern that the intake of these nutrients will be inadequate on the low protein intake being recommended. The protein intakes of Americans, however, are generally larger than those recommended. Protein is discussed further in Chapter 4.

VITAMIN E. It is interesting to note that the 1974 RDA for vitamin E, 15 I.U. for the reference male and 12 I.U. for the female, are about half those stated in 1968 and are expressed as mg. alpha-tocopherol equivalents in 1980. They reflect the incomplete knowledge regarding the functions of vitamin E in the human and the level of optimal tissue saturation and intake. Vitamin E is further discussed on page 113.

ASCORBIC ACID. This vitamin is another good example of the controversy that exists about the optimal level of intake of a nutrient. The optimal amount can be assessed as the daily intake required to prevent scurvy (10 mg. per day), on the one extreme, or the amount required to maintain maximum tissue concentration and body stores (80 mg. per day)[12] at the other extreme. Which is optimal? The 1980 RDA place the allowance for vitamin C for adults at 60 mg.

Table 10–4. NUTRIENTS KNOWN TO BE ESSENTIAL FOR THE HUMAN BEING

Protein Vitamin A Vitamin D Vitamin C Thiamin Riboflavin Niacin Calcium Iron	RDA first established in 1963 or earlier
Vitamin E Folacin Vitamin B$_6$ Vitamin B$_{12}$ Phosphorus Magnesium Iodine	RDA first established in 1968
Zinc	RDA first established in 1974
Vitamin K Pantothenic acid Biotin Sodium Potassium Chloride Copper Fluoride Chromium Manganese Molybdenum Selenium	No RDA established, but estimated safe and adequate daily dietary intakes (ESADDI) established in 1980
Essential fatty acids Carbohydrate Choline Other trace minerals	No RDA or ESADDI yet established

per day, an increase of 15 mg. per day over the 1974 RDA. In comparison, the Canadian (Table 10–5) and British recommendations are for 30 mg. per day.

CALCIUM. The calcium allowance illustrates how the interaction between a mineral and protein must be considered when setting the RDA. The FNB set the RDA for calcium at 800 mg. per day, considerably above the FAO/WHO allowance of 400 to 500 mg. per day.[2] This is based on evidence that calcium excretion is increased by a high protein intake and that Americans have a known high protein intake.[13]

IRON. Because of the wide individual variability in its absorption and availability in various foods, iron is the most problematic nutrient. Absorbability is assumed to be about 10 per cent of the food intake of iron. For males the 10 mg. per day recommended may be attained readily from the average American diet, but the RDA of 18 mg. per day for females on 2000 kcal. per day may be difficult to obtain from the dietary sources. Iron is discussed in Chapter 7 and in Chapter 29.

ZINC. A recommended allowance for this nutrient was first established in 1974 after accumulation of enough data to give an estimate of human requirements. The RDA for adults has been set at 15 mg. per day. This recommendation will probably undergo many refinements in the ensuing revisions of the RDA.

See Table 10–2 for nutrients known to be essential, but for which there is not enough data to define an average human requirement. Since the recommended allowance is derived from the average human requirement, there are no RDA for these nutrients, but estimated safe and adequate intakes are listed.

The RDA for a 70-kg. man are summarized in Figure 10–1. About 9 gm. of nitrogen is present in the 56 gm. of protein required. Leucine and tryptophan are shown in the figures to represent the extremes of essential amino acid need.

The scientific bases for the Recommended Dietary Allowances are described in full in the publication. For proper and intelligent use of this table, it is strongly recommended that the report be read in its entirety.[5]

Table 10–5. DIETARY STANDARD FOR CANADA—RECOMMENDED DAILY NUTRIENT INTAKE—REVISED 1975

									WATER-SOLUBLE VITAMINS			
Age	Sex	Weight (kg.)	Height (cm.)	Energy[a] (kcal.)	(M.J.)[b]	Protein (g.)	Thiamin (mg.)	Niacin (NE.)	Ribo-flavin (mg.)	Vita-min B6[g] (mg.)	Folate[h] (μg.)
0–6 mo	Both	6	—	kg × 117	kg × 0.49	kg × 2.2(2.0)[e]	0.3	5	0.4	0.3	40
7–11 mo	Both	9	—	kg × 108	kg × 0.45	kg × 1.4	0.5	6	0.6	0.4	60
1–3 yrs	Both	13	90	1400	5.9	22	0.7	9	0.8	0.8	100
4–6 yrs	Both	19	110	1800	7.5	27	0.9	12	1.1	1.3	100
7–9 yrs	M	27	129	2200	9.2	33	1.1	14	1.3	1.6	100
	F	27	128	2000	8.4	33	1.0	13	1.2	1.4	100
10–12 yrs	M	36	144	2500	10.5	41	1.2	17	1.5	1.8	100
	F	38	145	2300	9.6	40	1.1	15	1.4	1.5	100
13–15 yrs	M	51	162	2800	11.7	52	1.4	19	1.7	2.0	200
	F	49	159	2200	9.2	43	1.1	15	1.4	1.5	200
16–18 yrs	M	64	172	3200	13.4	54	1.6	21	2.0	2.0	200
	F	54	161	2100	8.8	43	1.1	14	1.3	1.5	200
19–35 yrs	M	70	176	3000	12.6	56	1.5	20	1.8	2.0	200
	F	56	161	2100	8.8	41	1.1	14	1.3	1.5	200
36–50 yrs	M	70	176	2700	11.3	56	1.4	18	1.7	2.0	200
	F	56	161	1900	7.9	41	1.0	13	1.2	1.5	200
51+ yrs	M	70	176	2300[c]	9.6[c]	56	1.4	18	1.7	2.0	200
	F	56	161	1800[c]	7.5[c]	41	1.0	13	1.2	1.5	200
Pregnancy				+300[d]	1.3[d]	+20	+0.2	+2	+0.3	+0.5	+50
Lactation				+500	2.1	+24	+0.4	+7	+0.6	+0.6	+50

[a] Recommendations assume characteristic activity pattern for each age group.

[b] Megajoules (10^6 joules). Calculated from the relation 1 kilocalorie = 4.184 kilojoules and rounded to 1 decimal place.

[c] Recommended energy intake for age 66+ years reduced to 2000 kcal. (8.4 M.J.) for men and 1500 kcal. (6.3 M.J.) for women.

[d] Increased energy intake recommended during 2nd and 3rd trimesters. An increase of 100 kcal. (418.4 kJ.) per day is recommended during the 1st trimester.

[e] Recommended protein intake of 2.2 gm./kg. body wt. for infants age 0–2 mo. and 2.0 gm./kg. body wt. for those age 3–5 mo. Protein recommendation for infants 0–11 mo. assumes consumption of breast milk or protein of equivalent quality.

[f] 1 N.E. (niacin equivalent) is equal to 1 mg. of niacin or 60 mg. of tryptophan.

[g] Recommendations are based on estimated average daily protein intake of Canadians.

[h] Recommendation given in terms of free folate.

Table continued on following page

Essentials of an Adequate Diet

The task of planning nutritious meals centers on the inclusion of the essential nutrients in optimal amounts along with adequate energy. Because some of the essential nutrients do not have established RDA, and others may not even be known, we must continue to rely on the principle of consumption of a wide variety of foods to provide for these unknowns. In addition, there must be attention to the palatability, cultural appropriateness and feasibility of the diet. People do not eat solely for nutrition, and these other factors are very important when planning an acceptable diet. Cultural factors are discussed in Chapter 16.

PROTEIN. Animal proteins are furnished through meats (muscle and organs), fish, fowl, eggs, milk and products made from milk, such as cheese. Vegetable proteins are furnished through nuts, legumes, grains, and some of the vegetables and fruits. A blend of the two types

Table 10–5. DIETARY STANDARD FOR CANADA—RECOMMENDED DAILY NUTRIENT INTAKE—REVISED 1975 (*Continued*)

WATER-SOLUBLE VITAMINS (*Continued*)		FAT-SOLUBLE VITAMINS			MINERALS					
Vitamin B$_{12}$ (µg.)	Vitamin C (mg.)	Vitamin A (R.E.)[j]	Vitamin D (µg. cholecalciferol)[k]	Vitamin E (mg. d-α-tocopherol)	Calcium (mg.)	Phosphorus (mg.)	Magnesium (mg.)	Iodine (µg.)	Iron (mg.)	Zinc (mg.)
0.3	20[i]	400	10	3	500[m]	250[m]	50[m]	35[m]	7[m]	4[m]
0.3	20	400	10	3	500	400	50	50	7	5
0.9	20	400	10	4	500	500	75	70	8	5
1.5	20	500	5	5	500	500	100	90	9	6
1.5	30	700	2.5[l]	6	700	700	150	110	10	7
1.5	30	700	2.5[l]	6	700	700	150	100	10	7
3.0	30	800	2.5[l]	7	900	900	175	130	11	8
3.0	30	800	2.5[l]	7	1000	1000	200	120	11	9
3.0	30	1000	2.5[l]	9	1200	1200	250	140	13	10
3.0	30	800	2.5[l]	7	800	800	250	110	14	10
3.0	30	1000	2.5[l]	10	1000	1000	300	160	14	12
3.0	30	800	2.5[l]	6	700	700	250	110	14	11
3.0	30	1000	2.5[l]	9	800	800	300	150	10	10
3.0	30	800	2.5[l]	6	700	700	250	110	14	9
3.0	30	1000	2.5[l]	8	800	800	300	140	10	10
3.0	30	800	2.5[l]	6	700	700	250	100	14	9
3.0	30	1000	2.5[l]	8	800	800	300	140	10	10
3.0	30	800	2.5[l]	6	700	700	250	100	9	9
+1.0	+20	+100	+2.5[l]	+1	+500	+500	+25	+15	+1[n]	+3
+0.5	+30	+400	+2.5[l]	+2	+500	+500	+75	+25	+1[n]	+7

[i] Considerably higher levels may be prudent for infants during the first week of life to guard against neonatal tyrosinemia.

[j] R.E. (retinol equivalent) corresponds to a biological activity in humans equal to 1 µg. retinol (3.33 I.U.) or 6 µg. β-carotene (10 I.U.).

[k] One µg. cholecalciferol is equivalent to 1 µg. ergocalciferol (40 I.U. vitamin D activity).

[l] Most older children and adults receive vitamin D from irradiation but 2.5 µg. daily is recommended. This intake should be increased to 5.0 µg. daily during pregnancy and lactation and for those confined indoors or otherwise deprived of sunlight for extended periods.

[m] The intake of breast-fed infants may be less than the recommendation but is considered to be adequate.

[n] A recommended total intake of 15 mg. daily during pregnancy and lactation assumes the presence of adequate stores of iron. If stores are suspected of being inadequate, additional iron as a supplement is recommended.

of proteins is needed to provide the essential amino acids.

CARBOHYDRATE. Carbohydrates are supplied through grains, fruits, vegetables, starches, sugars, and milk and milk products.

FAT. Fats are furnished through the "invisible" fat content of meats, eggs, cheese, and nuts, and the "visible" fats, such as butter, fortified margarine, oil, cream, and products made from cream. Saturated fats are found in animal products and rare vegetable oils such as coconut oil, while unsaturated fats are found in vegetables and vegetable products.

VITAMINS AND MINERALS. Vitamins and minerals are supplied through meats, fish, fowl, eggs, milk and products made from milk, and through nuts, legumes, grains, and some of the fruits and vegetables. Some foods have higher vitamin and mineral content than others. The food values given in the Appendix Tables are used as guides.

FIBER. Cellulose or fiber is furnished through the skins, peelings and pulp of fruits and vegetables, and the hulls of grains.

WATER. Water is supplied as such, and through the water content of foods and liquids.

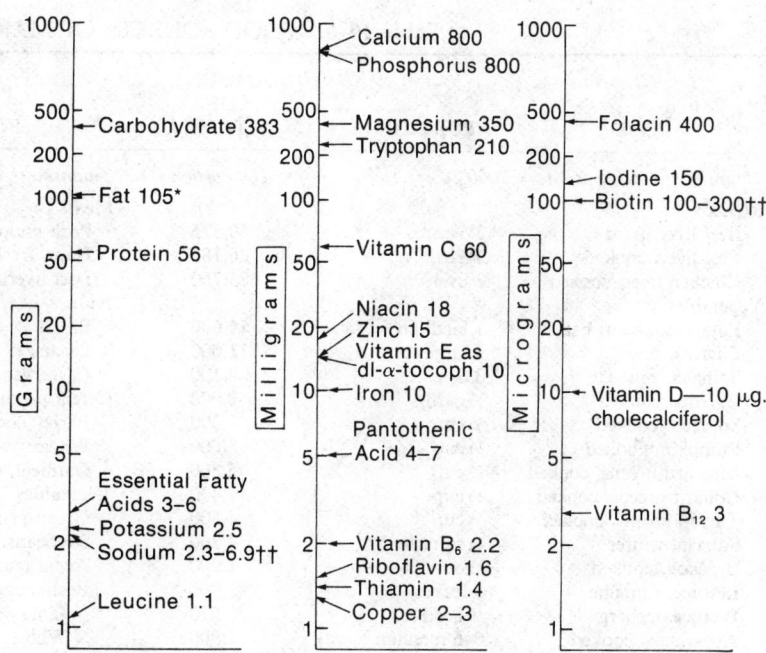

Figure 10–1. Summary of the 1980 Recommended Dietary Allowances and Estimated Safe and Adequate Daily Dietary Intakes for a 70-kg., 178-cm. man consuming 2700 kcal. daily.

*Based on Am. Heart Assoc. recommendation of 35% of kcal from fat.

†Based on best estimates that 1–2% of kcal should be from EFA.

††Based on reports of present daily intake.

Application of Dietary Allowances

In the previous discussion and chapters the physiological necessities for specific nutrients have been presented. The various quantities of nutrients recommended as allowances may generally be obtained from usual portions of commonly available foods in the United States. As previously pointed out, variety in foods is of considerable advantage in the selection of an adequate diet, since it offers the potential of affording many essential nutrients in natural proportions. Some foods are unique because of their important contributions to the diet. For example, milk is an important source of calcium, protein, and riboflavin; citrus fruits and tomatoes provide relatively large amounts of ascorbic acid. These foods known to be high in necessary nutrients are called "protective" foods, because when they are included regularly as the basis for a diet, they protect against certain vitamin and mineral deficiencies. Tables 10–6 and 10–7 list foods especially high in various nutrients. Table 10–8 offers a guide to the foods that should be included daily in meals. Table 10–9 presents a daily food guide for an ovo-lacto vegetarian. The vegan would require more servings from the vegetable protein foods and the bread and cereal group. Table 10–10 should also be helpful. It has been recommended that the vegan should get 60 per cent of his or her protein from grains, 35 per cent from legumes and 5 per cent from leafy greens.[3] The various types of vegetarian diets are described on page 342.

DAILY FOOD GUIDE

This basic pattern forms a *foundation* for a good diet providing the essential nutrients. It will supply the adult with approximately one half to two thirds of the energy allowance, and all the protein, vitamin A, riboflavin, ascorbic acid, calcium and phosphorus needed. Almost all the thiamin and niacin allowances are provided, but the iron supply is about half that needed by the female adult. The zinc intake does not usually meet the RDA either. Other foods are added, as necessary, to meet the energy requirement, to meet unknown trace mineral requirements, to increase the mineral content and to add palatability. These may be more of the same foods listed above, or others. Since butter, margarine, other fats, oils, sugars, and refined cereal foods are usually combined with other specified foods, they are not included in the food plan. See Table 10–11 for an evaluation of the foundation of an adequate diet for an adult.

Table 10–6. FOOD SOURCES OF MAJOR VITAMINS

FOOD	PORTION SIZE	AMOUNT OF VITAMIN	FOOD	PORTION SIZE	AMOUNT OF VITAMIN
Vitamin A—Adult RDA = 5000 IU		IU/Portion	*Thiamin—Adult RDA = 1.0–1.5 mg.*		mg./Portion
Meats			Meats		
Beef liver, fried	3½ oz.	50,375	Pork chops, cooked	3½ oz.	0.96
Calf liver, cooked	3½ oz.	26,782	Ham, fresh, cooked	3½ oz.	0.58
Chicken liver, cooked	2 livers	25,760	Beef liver, fried	3½ oz.	0.24
Vegetables			Nuts		
Potatoes, sweet, baked	1 medium	14,600	Brazil	¼ cup	0.82
Carrots, raw	1 large	11,000	Pecans	¼ cup	0.18
Spinach, raw	3½ oz.	8,100	Cashews	¼ cup	0.11
Carrots, cooked	½ cup	8,000	Cereal products		
Spinach, cooked	½ cup	7,300	Barley cereals	½ cup	0.65
Pumpkin, cooked	½ cup	8,000	Wheat germ	1 tbsp.	0.20
Mustard greens, cooked	½ cup	5,800	Oatmeal, cooked	½ cup	0.11
Collard greens, cooked	½ cup	5,400	Vegetables		
Turnip greens, cooked	½ cup	4,800	Green peas, cooked	½ cup	0.21
Squash, winter	½ squash	4,200	Soybeans, cooked	½ cup	0.21
Broccoli, cooked	½ cup	1,900	Asparagus, cooked	5–6 medium	0.16
Lettuce, romaine	4 leaves	1,900	Beans, cooked		
Lettuce, iceberg	¼ head	970	Lima	½ cup	0.14
Asparagus, cooked	5–6 medium	900	White	½ cup	0.14
Tomatoes, raw	1 small	900	Kidney	½ cup	0.14
Fruits			Corn on cob, cooked	4-in. ear	0.12
Watermelon	1/16 melon (10 x 16 in.)	5,310	Miscellaneous		
Cantaloupe	¼ melon	3,400	Brewer's yeast	1 tbsp.	1.25
Apricots, dried	4 halves	2,275			
Apricots, raw	2–3 medium	2,700	*Vitamin C—Adult RDA = 60 mg.*		mg./Portion
Papaya, raw	1/3 medium	1,750	Vegetables		
Nectarines, raw	1 medium	1,650	Green pepper, raw	1 large	128
			Broccoli, cooked	½ cup	68
			Brussels sprouts, cooked	½ cup	66
			Spinach, raw	3½ oz.	51
			Mustard greens, cooked	½ cup	48
			Cabbage, raw	1 cup	47
			Collard greens, cooked	½ cup	46
Riboflavin—Adult RDA = 1.2–1.7 mg.		mg./Portion	Parsley, raw	2 tbsp.	34
Meats			Spinach, cooked	½ cup	25
Beef liver, fried	3½ oz.	3.46	Tomatoes	1 small	23
Calf liver, cooked	3½ oz.	3.34	Potatoes, white, baked	1 small	20
Chicken liver, cooked	2 livers	1.77	Fruits		
Veal roast, cooked	3½ oz.	0.25	Acerola	3½ oz.	1,300
Beef, ground, cooked	3½ oz.	0.21	Oranges	1 medium	80
Egg, boiled	1 medium	0.13	Strawberries	10 large	59
Cereal products			Papayas, raw	1/3 medium	56
Barley cereals	½ cup	0.49	Lemons, peeled	1 medium	53
Dairy products			Grapefruit	½ medium	38
Milk, whole	1 cup	0.42	Limes, peeled	1 medium	37
Cheese			Kumquats, raw	5–6 medium	36
Cottage, creamed	1/3 cup	0.25	Cantaloupe	¼ medium	33
Blue or Roquefort	1 oz.	0.17	Tangerines	1 large	31
Brick	1 oz.	0.13	Honeydew melon	¼ small	23
Cheddar	1 oz.	0.13			
Ice cream	½ cup (1 scoop)	0.14	*Niacin—Adult RDA = 13–19 mg.*		mg./Portion
Vegetables			Meats		
Collard greens, cooked	½ cup	0.20	Calf liver, cooked	3½ oz.	15.8
Spinach, raw	3½ oz.	0.20	Beef liver, fried	3½ oz.	13.7
Broccoli, cooked	½ cup	0.15	Chicken liver, cooked	2 livers	9.4
Asparagus, cooked	5–6 medium	0.18	Chicken, cooked	3½ oz.	8.8
Brussels sprouts, cooked	½ cup	0.11	Beef, ground, cooked	3½ oz.	5.4
Mustard greens, cooked	½ cup	0.14	Haddock, cooked	3½ oz.	3.2
Spinach, cooked	½ cup	0.13			
Miscellaneous					
Brewer's yeast	1 tbsp.	0.34			

Table 10–6. FOOD SOURCES OF MAJOR VITAMINS (*Continued*)

FOOD	PORTION SIZE	AMOUNT OF VITAMIN	FOOD	PORTION SIZE	AMOUNT OF VITAMIN
Niacin—Adult RDA = 13–19 mg.—cont.		*mg./Portion*	*Vitamin B₆ — Adult RDA = 2.0–2.2 mg.—cont.*		*mg./Portion*
Nuts			Chicken, dark	3½ oz.	0.3
Peanuts, roasted	3 tbsp.	7.5	Halibut	3½ oz.	0.4
Peanut butter	2 tbsp.	4.8	Tuna	3½ oz.	0.4
Vegetables			Vegetables		
Green peas, cooked	½ cup	1.7	Beans, dry		
Potatoes, white, baked	1 small	1.7	soy	½ cup	0.8
Asparagus, cooked	5–6 medium	1.4	navy	½ cup	0.6
Corn on cob, cooked	4-in. ear	1.4	lentils	½ cup	0.6
Black-eyed peas	3½ oz.	1.4	garbanzo	½ cup	0.5
Lima beans, cooked	½ cup	1.0	black eyed peas	½ cup	0.5
Collard greens, cooked	½ cup	1.2	Potatoes	1 cup, diced	0.4
Miscellaneous			Spinach, raw	4 oz.	0.3
Brewer's yeast	1 tbsp.	3.0	Kale, raw	4 oz.	0.3
			Tomato juice	1 cup	0.5
Folic Acid—Adult RDA = 400 μg.		*μg./Portion*	Broccoli, raw	3 stalks	0.9
Meats			Asparagus, raw	12–14 spears	0.3
Beef liver	3½ oz.	290	Corn, canned, cooked	1 cup	0.4
Chicken liver	2 livers	230	Cereals		
Vegetables			Rice bran	¼ cup	0.8
Asparagus	5–6 medium	89–140	Wheat germ	¼ cup	0.3
Turnip greens	½ cup	63	Brewer's yeast	1 tbsp.	0.2
Spinach	½ cup	49–110	Whole wheat bread	1 slice	0.04
Kale	½ cup	34	Dairy products		
Endive	20 long leaves	27–63	Milk, whole	1 cup	0.1
Broccoli	½ cup	26	Cottage cheese	1 cup	0.1
Escarole	4 large leaves	26	Fruits		
Okra	8–9 pods	24	Avocado	½ medium	0.45
Brussels sprouts	½ cup	20	Banana	1 medium	0.61
Mustard greens	½ cup	17–38	Raisins	1 cup	0.35
Cauliflower	½ cup	16	Nuts		
Acorn squash	½ cup	17	Walnuts	4–7 halves	0.1
Nuts					
Walnuts	8–10 halves	12	*Vitamin B₁₂—Adult RDA = 3.0 μg.*		*μg./Portion*
Filberts	10–12 nuts	10	Meats		
Peanuts	1 tbsp.	9	Beef liver	3½ oz.	31–120
Almonds	12–15 nuts	7	Beef round	3½ oz.	3.4–4.5
Pecans	12 halves	4	Ham	3½ oz.	0.9–1.6
			Haddock	3½ oz.	0.6
Vitamin B₆— Adult RDA = 2.0–2.2 mg.		*mg./Portion*	Egg, whole	1 egg	0.2
Meats			Dairy products		
Beef liver	3½ oz.	0.8	Milk, whole	1 cup	0.7–1.2
Pork	3½ oz.	0.5	Cheese		
Beef round	3½ oz.	0.4	Swiss	1 oz.	0.3
Chicken, light	3½ oz.	0.7	American	1 oz.	0.2

Using the basic four food groups is not the only way to obtain a good diet. For example, a vegetarian can avoid meat and all foods in the milk group and still obtain an adequate diet if vegetables high in iron and calcium (such as kale) are included regularly. A person can avoid all fruits and still obtain adequate amounts of vitamin C if vegetables known to be good vitamin C sources such as cabbage and broccoli are included frequently.

On the other hand, an individual can follow the basic four food pattern and still have iron, zinc, magnesium, folic acid, vitamin E and vitamin B₆ intakes less than the RDA, depending on the foods selected in each group.[6, 9] It is important to look at the individual diet. The Basic Four Food Groups, however, can still serve as a practical guide in planning meals.

The Milk Group is counted on to provide most of the calcium requirement. In addition, it provides riboflavin, high quality protein, other vitamins and minerals, carbohydrate, and fat.

The Meat Group provides generous amounts of protein of high quality. In addition, iron, thi-

Table 10–7. FOOD SOURCES OF MAJOR MINERALS

FOOD	PORTION SIZE	AMOUNT OF MINERAL	FOOD	PORTION SIZE	AMOUNT OF MINERAL
Calcium—Adult RDA = 800 mg.		mg./Portion	*Phosphorus—Adult RDA = 800 mg.*		mg./Portion
Dairy products			Meats		
Milk, whole	1 cup	288	Calf liver, cooked	3½ oz.	537
Cheese			Cod, broiled	3½ oz.	274
Swiss	1 oz.	248	Beef, lean round, cooked	3½ oz.	250
Cheddar	1 oz.	211	Pork, lean, cooked	3½ oz.	249
Brick	1 oz.	204	Halibut, broiled	3½ oz.	248
Cottage, creamed	1/3 cup	94	Dairy products		
Blue or Roquefort	1 oz.	88	Milk, whole	1 cup	227
Ice cream	½ cup (1 scoop)	84	Cheese		
Vegetables			Swiss	1 oz.	158
Collard greens, cooked	½ cup	152	Cottage, creamed	1/3 cup	152
Turnip greens, cooked	½ cup	140	Cheddar	1 oz.	134
Mustard greens, cooked	½ cup	138	Brick	1 oz.	127
Spinach, cooked	½ cup	83	Blue or Roquefort	1 oz.	95
Broccoli, cooked	½ cup	67	Nuts		
White beans, cooked	½ cup	50	Peanuts, roasted	3 tbsp.	180
Cabbage, raw	1 cup	49	Brazil	4 nuts	104
Kidney beans, cooked	½ cup	48	Peanut butter	1 tbsp.	59
Lima beans, cooked	½ cup	38	Vegetables		
Carrots, raw	1 large	37	Beans, cooked		
Fruits			Kidney	½ cup	175
Prunes	8 large	90	White	½ cup	148
Oranges	1 medium	62	Lima	½ cup	97
Tangerines	1 large	40	Green peas, fresh, cooked	½ cup	75
			Artichokes, cooked	1 bud	69
Iron—Adult RDA = 10–18 mg.		mg./Portion	Potatoes, white, baked	1 small	65
Meats			Brussels sprouts, cooked	½ cup	55
Calf liver, cooked	3½ oz.	12.4	Miscellaneous		
Beef liver, cooked	3½ oz.	7.8	Carbonated drinks	10 oz.	2–47
Chicken liver, cooked	2 livers	6.0			
Beef, lean round, cooked	3½ oz.	3.5			
Chicken, cooked, no bone	3½ oz.	2.1			
Egg, boiled	1 medium	1.1	*Zinc—Adult RDA = 15 mg.*		mg./Portion
Fruits			Meats		
Watermelon	1/16 melon (10 x 16 in.)	4.5	Oysters, Atlantic, raw	5–8 medium	160
Prunes	8 large	4.4	Oysters, Pacific, raw	6–9 medium	31
Dates, dried	¼ cup	1.4	Beef liver	3½ oz.	3.0–8.5
Apricots, dried	4 halves	1.4	Eggs	1 egg	2.8
Raisins	¼ cup	1.3	Beef	3½ oz.	2–5
Blueberries, raw	1 cup	1.0	Clams	4 large/9 small	2.0
Strawberries, raw	10 large	1.0	Vegetables		
Vegetables			Corn	½ cup	3.1
Spinach, raw	3½ oz.	3.1	Beets	2 beets	2.8
Beans, cooked			Peas	½ cup	2.3–3.8
Kidney	½ cup	3.0	Carrots	½ cup	0.4–2.1
White	½ cup	2.7	Spinach	½ cup	0.3–0.8
Lima	½ cup	2.0	Cabbage	½ cup	0.1–0.8
Asparagus, canned	5–6 medium	2.0	Lettuce	¼ head	0.1–0.7
Lettuce, iceberg	¼ head	2.0	Cereal products		
Spinach, cooked	½ cup	2.0	Barley	½ cup	0.6
Mustard greens, cooked	½ cup	1.8	Bread, whole wheat	1 slice	0.7–1.0
Green peas, cooked	½ cup	1.4	Bread, rye	1 slice	0.5
Cauliflower, raw	1 cup	1.1	Fruits		
Miscellaneous			Cherries, canned	½ cup	1.6–2.2
Molasses, medium	1 tbsp.	1.2	Pears, canned	2 small halves	1.5–1.8

Table 10–8. FOUNDATION OF AN ADEQUATE DIET—DAILY FOOD GUIDE

SERVINGS RECOMMENDED	SERVING RECOMMENDATIONS
MEAT GROUP 2 or more	2 to 3 ounces of lean cooked meat, poultry or fish. As alternates: 1 egg, ½ cup cooked dry beans or peas, or 2 tablespoons of peanut butter may replace ½ serving of meat.
MILK GROUP CHILD, under 9 .... 2 to 3 CHILD, 9 to 12 .... 3 or more TEENAGER .... 4 or more ADULT........................ 2 or more PREGNANT WOMAN .... 3 or more NURSING WOMAN .... 4 or more	One 8-ounce cup of fluid milk: whole, skim, buttermilk or evaporated or dry milk, reconstituted. As alternates: 1⅓ ounces cheddar-type cheese, or 1⅓ cups cottage cheese, 1⅔ cups ice cream, 1 cup yogurt.
VEGETABLE–FRUIT GROUP 4 or more, including:	½ cup of vegetable or fruit; or a portion, for example, 1 medium apple, banana, or potato, half a medium grapefruit or cantaloupe.
1 good or 2 fair sources of vitamin C	Good sources: Grapefruit or grapefruit juice, orange or orange juice, cantaloupe, guava, mango, papaya, raw strawberries, broccoli, Brussels sprouts, green pepper, sweet red pepper. Fair sources: Honeydew melon, lemon, tangerine or tangerine juice, watermelon, asparagus, cabbage, cauliflower, collards, garden cress, kale, kohlrabi, mustard greens, potatoes and sweet potatoes cooked in the jacket, rutabagas, spinach, tomatoes or tomato juice, turnip greens.
1 good source of vitamin A—at least every other day	Good sources: Dark-green and deep-yellow vegetables and a few fruits, namely: apricots, broccoli, cantaloupe, carrots, chard, collards, cress, kale, mango, persimmon, pumpkin, spinach, sweet potatoes, turnip greens and other dark green leaves, winter squash.
BREAD–CEREAL GROUP 4 or more	COUNT ONLY IF WHOLE-GRAIN OR ENRICHED. 1 slice of bread or similar serving of baked goods made with whole-grain or enriched flour, 1 ounce ready-to-eat cereal, ½ to ¾ cup cooked cereal, cornmeal, grits, spaghetti, macaroni, noodles or rice.
OTHER WHOLESOME FOODS AS NEEDED To round out meals and meet energy requirements.	

amin, riboflavin, niacin, vitamins B_6 and B_{12}, phosphorus, zinc and other trace minerals are supplied.

There are several non-meat alternatives that provide the same nutrients as animal flesh. In addition, the complete vegetarian can combine incomplete proteins to meet the complete or high quality protein requirement, as shown in Table 10–10 and Figure 10–2.

The Bread and Cereal Group furnishes protein, carbohydrate, fiber, thiamin, niacin, iron, zinc and other trace minerals at a relatively low cost. The enrichment of breads and cereals with iron, thiamin, riboflavin, and niacin substantially contributes additional amounts of these nutrients to the diet. Table 40–4 gives enrichment levels for breads and flours.

The Vegetable and Fruit Group is an important supplier of fiber, vitamins and minerals, particularly vitamins A and C. Dark green and deep yellow vegetables are especially valuable for carotene, a precursor of vitamin A, and citrus fruits for vitamin C. Folic acid is found in the dark leafy vegetables and other fresh vegetables.

Criticism

When the daily food guide was designed in the mid-1950's, certain nutrients, such as phosphorus, zinc, iodine, vitamins B_6, B_{12}, E and K, folacin, pantothenic acid, biotin and trace minerals, were not considered in the calculations. However, since most of these nutrients are found in many foods, the intake of a variety of foods within the four food groups will probably provide the needed amounts.

Table 10–9. FOOD GUIDE FOR AN OVO-LACTO VEGETARIAN

FOOD GROUPS (servings per day)	SIZE OF SERVING	FOOD SOURCES OR EXCHANGES
I. Milk Group (2 or more servings)	1 c. milk	½ c. evaporated milk 1 c. yogurt 1 c. skim milk 1 oz. cheese ¼ c. cottage cheese 1 c. soymilk 4 T. powdered soymilk
II. Vegetable Protein Foods (2 or more servings)	1 c. legumes (beans, garbanzos, lentils, peas) 2–3 oz. meat analogs	4 T. peanut butter 20–30 gm. dry textured vegetable proteins 4 oz. soy "cheese" or curd 1½ T. nuts or oil seeds
III. Fruits and Vegetables (4 or more servings)	½ c. cooked vegetables and/or fruits 1 c. raw vegetables ½ c. juice	1 serving vitamin C rich foods: citrus, cabbage and tomatoes, melon, green pepper, strawberries 1–2 servings of green leafy vegetables and yellow vegetables and fruits (carotene-rich)
IV. Bread and Cereals (4 or more servings)	1 slice of whole wheat or enriched bread ½–¾ c. cooked cereal, whole grain ¾–1 c. dry cereal	½–¾ c. enriched or whole rice ½–¾ c. enriched noodles, macaroni, or spaghetti ½ c. granola ½ hamburger bun Crackers: graham (2) saltines (5) wheat thins (8)
V. Other Foods Eggs (3–4 per week) Fats (1 T. per day)	1 egg 1 t. oil 1 t. soft margarine	

(From Vyhmeister, I.B., Register, U. D., and Sonnenberg, L. M.: Safe vegetarian diets for children. Pediatr. Clin. North Am., *24*:203, 1977.)

At present there is a great deal of criticism of the use of the Four Food Groups as a basis for nutrition education for the public.[11] The main arguments against its use are:

1. An individual can eat the proper number of servings from the four food groups and still not be getting an adequate intake of some vitamins and minerals, iron in particular.

2. Following the food guide can result in a diet high in saturated fat, cholesterol and sodium and low in fiber that many authorities feel does not constitute the optimal diet for health. Table 10–12 presents a modification of the Daily Food Guide that considers fat, cholesterol, sodium and sugar intake. However, it has not been validated for educational effectiveness. The U.S. Department of Agriculture has also published a similar guide.[4]

3. The additional assumption by educators using the guide that persons eating a wide variety of foods will meet other unknown requirements is fallacious since "a wide variety of foods" is ill defined in our society.

This last point is especially frustrating for the person trying to apply nutrition principles and select and prepare an adequate diet. The "wide variety" could be a variety of snack foods and drinks that add calories and no nutrients, or a variety of vegetables and fruits that add large amounts of nutrients and few calories.

For the nutrition professional trying to guide and educate the public it is equally frustrating. At present there is no adequate yet simple system that has been tested for effectiveness. Many are suggested.[10, 17]

NUTRIENT DENSITY

The problem of selecting an adequate diet becomes especially difficult when in the presence

Table 10–10. EXAMPLES OF COMPLEMENTARY PROTEINS

COMBINATIONS	SUGGESTED RECIPE EXAMPLES
1. Rice + Legumes	a) Hopping John
	b) Roman Rice and Beans
	c) Crusty Soybean Casserole
2. Rice + Wheat + Soy	a) Mexican Grains
3. Rice + Sesame Seed	a) Sesame Vegetable Rice
4. Rice + Milk	a) Con Queso Rice
	b) Spinach Casserole
	c) Spinach Rice Loaf
5. Wheat Products + Milk	a) Lasagna
	b) French Fondue
	c) Macaroni and Cheese Puff
6. Wheat + Beans	a) Tabouili
7. Cornmeal + Beans	a) Mexican Pan Bread
8. Beans + Milk	a) Bean Chowder
9. Peanuts + Milk	a) Peanut Butter Sandwich and Milk

(From Goodwin, M. T.: Better Living Through Better Eating. 2nd ed. Montgomery County Health Department, Maryland. 1974. p. 19.)

of tremendous variety and abundance there are the constraints of calories and money. In situations of limited calories (due to concern regarding overweight) and limited financial resources, the food selections must have a high nutrient:energy (calorie) ratio. The protective foods such as milk, liver, dark green and yellow vegetables, high vitamin C fruits and whole grain or enriched breads and cereals have high nutrient:calorie ratios, whereas most snack foods, such as cola drinks, cookies, cakes, candy and other heavily processed foods, have low ratios and less nutrient density. Because these low nutrient density foods add cost and calories to a diet, it is important to counsel people regarding their use.

Hansen and associates[7, 18] have designed an index of food quality based on nutrient density. They converted the RDA for each nutrient into an allowance per 1000 kcal. by dividing each RDA by the average caloric allowance and then multiplying by 1000.[8] This establishes a single-value nutrient allowance based on the nutrient requirements of those in the age and sex categories who also have the lowest energy requirements. These single-value nutrient allowances are given in Table 10–13. The method is applied in diet planning by giving each food an *index of nutritional quality* (INQ) based on its nutrient density. For example, bananas provide 6.1 mg. of vitamin B_6 per 1000 kcal. The single-value allowance for vitamin B_6 per 1000 kcal. is 1.0 mg. The resultant INQ for banana B_6 is 6.1 (6.1/1.0), making it a good source of vitamin B_6. By using

the INQ an assessment of food combinations or meals to meet dietary allowances becomes possible, and it is easy to see the nutrient contributions of various foods. They can be examined for their nutrient contribution relative to their energy contribution.

NUTRITION LABELING

The U.S. RDA

To aid in the translation of nutritional requirements into foods and meals, the FDA in 1973 developed a system of nutrition labeling of foods to replace the old system using MDR—minimum daily requirements. A standard was defined to be used in nutrition labeling—the *U.S. RDA*. This is not to be confused with the NRC-RDA discussed earlier in this chapter, although the U.S. RDA is derived from the 1968 RDA with additional figures for zinc, copper, biotin and pantothenic acid.

In general the U.S. RDA is the highest value recommended for the nutrient in any age category in the RDA. Unlike the RDA, the U.S. RDA has only three categories constituting three U.S. RDA standards: (1) adults and children over 4 years of age (the standard used in most nutrition labeling of foods), (2) infants and children under 4 years of age (the standard used on baby foods and vitamin-mineral supplements for infants and small children) and (3) pregnant or lactating women (the standard used on vitamin-mineral supplements for this group of women). Table 10–14 gives the U.S. RDA, which can be compared with the 1980 RDA in Table 10–1.

HOW NUTRITION LABELING CAN HELP IN FOOD SELECTION AND MEAL PLANNING. Nutrition labels express the nutrient composition of the food in terms of the U.S. RDA. The label as shown in Figure 10–3 must state (1) the serving size, (2) the percentage of the U.S. RDA that the serving meets for protein, five vitamins, iron and calcium, (3) the amount of protein, carbohydrate and fat in grams and (4) the calories from protein, carbohydrate and fat. Listing of the percentage of the U.S. RDA for 12 other vitamins and minerals is optional. Cholesterol, polyunsaturated and saturated fat and sodium content may also be given.

Since the nutrient contribution of each food serving is stated on the label, except in the case of unpackaged fresh produce, meat and some other products, it is possible to compose an adequate daily intake by adding the percentages for the nutrients contributed by the servings of food throughout the day. A booklet and educational tool have been devised by the USDA to explain the nutrition label.[15, 16] Table 10–15

Table 10-11. EVALUATION OF THE FOUNDATION OF AN ADEQUATE DIET FOR AN ADULT

FOOD	AVERAGE SERVING Household Measure	AVERAGE SERVING Weight Gm.	KILO-CAL-ORIES	PRO-TEIN Gm.	FAT Gm.	CAR-BOHY-DRATE Gm.	MINERALS Calcium Mg.	MINERALS Iron Mg.	VITAMINS A. (I.U.)	VITAMINS Ascorbic Acid Mg.	VITAMINS Thiamin Mg.	VITAMINS Ribo-flavin Mg.	VITAMINS Niacin Mg.
Milk, whole (or equivalent)	1 pt.	488	320	18.0	18	24	576	.2	700	4	.16	.84	.2
Meat group													
Eggs	1	50	80	6.0	6	tr.	27	1.1	590	—	.05	.15	tr.
Meat, poultry, fish[1]	3 oz. (cooked)	85	237	23.0	15	0	10	2.4	10	—	.09	.21	4.7
Vegetable—fruit group													
Vegetables:													
Deep green or yellow[2]	1 salad or cooked	50 raw or 75 cooked	27	1.4	tr.	6	36.7	.6	3016	20.5	.046	.08	.4
Other, cooked[3]	½ cup	80	41	2.5	tr.	7.7	15	.93	225	11	.12	.06	1.5
Potato, peeled, boiled	1 medium	122	80	2.0	tr.	18	7	.6	tr.	20	.11	.04	1.4
Fruits:													
Citrus[4]	1 serving	125	57	.8	tr.	14	28	.35	302	58	.09	.03	.36
Other (fresh and canned)[5]	1 serving	150	92	.5	tr.	24	8	.5	164	5	.03	.04	.4
Bread-cereal group													
Cereal (whole grain and enriched)[6]	½ cup cooked	28 (dry)	88	2.2	1	17.7	7.7	.6	—	—	.11	.02	.3
Bread (whole grain and enriched)	3 slices	69	180	6.0	3	36	57	1.8	tr.	tr.	.18	.15	1.8
Totals[7]			1202 (5000 kJ.)	62.4	43	147.4	772.4	9.1[8]	5007[8]	118.5	.986[9]	1.62	11.6[10]

Recommended Dietary Allowances*

			KILO-CAL-ORIES	PRO-TEIN Gm.			Calcium Mg.	Iron Mg.	A. (I.U.)	Ascorbic Acid Mg.	Thiamin Mg.	Ribo-flavin Mg.	Niacin Mg.
Man (age 23–50, wt., 70 kg., ht., 178 cm.)			2700	56			800	10	5000	45	1.4	1.6	18[11]
Woman (age 23–50, wt., 55 kg., ht., 163 cm.)			2000	46			800	18	4000	45	1.0	1.2	13[11]

Evaluation based on Table 1 in the Appendix.

[1]Evaluation based on figures for cooked (lean and fat) beef, lamb, and veal.

[2]Evaluation based on lettuce, cooked carrots, green beans, winter squash and broccoli.

[3]Evaluation based on average for cooked peas and beets.

[4]Evaluation based on Florida orange and white and pink grapefruit: whole and juice.

[5]Evaluation based on canned peaches, applesauce, raw pears, apples and bananas.

[6]Evaluation based on oatmeal and cornflakes.

[7]With the addition of more of the same foods, or other foods, to meet calorie requirement, the totals will be increased.

[8]With the use of liver this figure will be markedly increased.

[9]With the use of pork, legumes and liver this figure will be markedly increased.

[10]The average diet in the United States, which contains a generous amount of protein, provides enough tryptophan to increase the niacin value by about a third.

[11]These figures are expressed as niacin equivalents, which include dietary sources of the preformed vitamin and the precursor, tryptophan.

*Recommended Dietary Allowances, Washington, D.C., National Research Council, 1980.

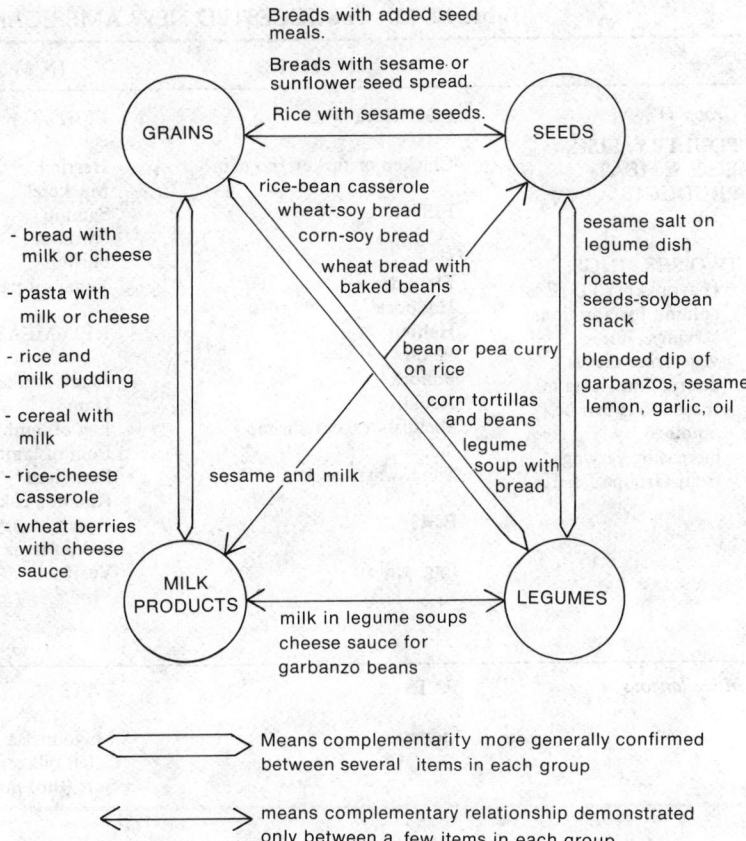

Figure 10–2. Summary of complementary protein relationships. (From: Lappé, F. M.: Diet for a Small Planet. New York, Ballantine Books, 1971.)

Table 10–12.   A SUGGESTED NEW AMERICAN EATING GUIDE

	ANYTIME	IN MODERATION	NOW AND THEN
Group I BEANS, GRAINS & NUTS FOUR OR MORE SERVINGS/DAY	Barley Beans Bread & rolls (whole grain) Bulghur Lentils Oatmeal Pasta Rice Whole grain cereal (except granola)	Granola cereals Nuts Peanut butter Soybeans White bread and cereals	
Group II FRUITS & VEGETABLES FOUR OR MORE SERVINGS/DAY	All fruits and vegetables except those listed on right Unsweetened fruit juices Unsalted vegetable juices Potatoes, white or sweet	Avocado Fruits canned in syrup Salted vegetable juices Sweetened fruit juice Vegetables canned with salt	French fries Olives Pickles
Group III MILK PRODUCTS CHILDREN: 3 TO 4 SERVINGS OR EQUIVALENT ADULTS: 2 SERVINGS (Favor ANYTIME column for additional servings)	Buttermilk Farmer or pot cheese Lowfat cottage cheese Lowfat milk with 1% milkfat Skim milk ricotta Skim milk	Frozen lowfat yogurt Ice milk Lowfat milk with 2% milkfat Lowfat (2%) yogurt, plain or sweetened Regular cottage cheese (4% milkfat)	Hard cheeses: blue, brick, camembert, cheddar (note: part-skim mozarella and part-skim ricotta are preferable but still rich in fat) Ice cream Processed cheeses Whole milk Whole milk yogurt

Table continued on the following page

Table 10–12. A SUGGESTED NEW AMERICAN EATING GUIDE (*Continued*)

	ANYTIME	IN MODERATION	NOW AND THEN
Group IV POULTRY, FISH, EGG & MEAT PRODUCTS TWO SERVINGS: (Favor ANYTIME column for additional servings. If a vegetarian diet is desired, nutrients in these foods can be obtained by increasing servings from Groups I & III.)	POULTRY Chicken or turkey (no skin) FISH Cod Flounder Haddock Halibut Perch Pollock Rockfish Shellfish, except shrimp Sole Tuna, water-packed EGG Egg whites	FISH Herring Mackerel Salmon Sardines Shrimp Tuna, oil-packed RED MEATS Flank steak Ham* Leg of lamb* Loin of lamb* Plate beef* Round steak* Rump roast* Sirloin steak* Veal*	POULTRY & FISH Deep fried and breaded fish or poultry RED MEATS Bacon Corned beef Ground beef Hot dogs Liver Liverwurst Pork, loin Pork, Boston butt Salami Sausage Spareribs Untrimmed meats EGG Egg yolk or whole egg
Miscellaneous	FATS (none)	FATS Mayonnaise Salad oils Soft (tub) margarines	FATS Butter Cream Cream cheese Lard Sour cream
NOTE: Snack foods should not be used freely, but the middle column suggests some of the better choices.	SNACK FOODS (none)	SNACK FOODS Angel food cake Animal crackers Fig bars Gingerbread Ginger snaps Graham crackers Popcorn (small amounts of fat and salt) Sherbet	SNACK FOODS Chocolate Coconut Commercial pies, pastries and doughnuts Potato chips Soda pop

*Trim all outside fat.
"Anytime" foods contain less than 30 percent of calories from fat and are usually low in salt and sugar. Most of the "now and then" foods contain at least 50 percent of calories from fat—*and* a large amount of saturated fat. Foods to eat "in moderation" have medium amounts of total fat and low to moderate amounts of saturated fat *or* large amounts of total fat that is mostly unsaturated. Foods meeting the standards for fat, but containing large amounts of salt or sugar, are usually moved into a more restricted category, as are refined cereal products. For example, pickles have little fat, but are so high in sodium that they fall in the "now and then" category.

Important:
To cut down on salt intake, choose varieties of the foods listed here that do not have added salt, such as no-salt cottage cheese, rather than the regular varieties. This guide is not appropriate for individuals needing very low-salt diets.
(From Center for Science in the Public Interest, 1755 S St. N.W., Washington, D.C. 20009, 1979.)

shows how a typical day's intake for a 25-year-old woman is expressed as a percentage of the U.S. RDA. The contributions from all foods are totaled and the day's intake is compared with the U.S. RDA.

The U.S. RDA provides for a margin of safety sometimes even higher than that of the RDA; so the fact that the diet does not meet the U.S. RDA does not necessarily mean that it is inadequate. For example, the niacin intake of the 25-year-old woman mentioned in Table 10–15 is only 71 per cent of the U.S. RDA (20 mg.). But since the NRC-RDA for niacin for a 25-year-old woman is only 13 mg., the woman only has to meet 65 per cent of the U.S. RDA to have an adequate intake.

Table 10–13.   SINGLE-VALUE NUTRIENT ALLOWANCES PER 1000 KILOCALORIES

NUTRIENT	AMOUNT	NUTRIENT	AMOUNT
Vitamin A	400 μg. RE	Zinc	8 mg.
Vitamin D	4 μg.	Iodine	75 μg.
Vitamin E	4 mg. α-T.E.	Copper	1 mg.
Vitamin C	30 mg.	Manganese	1.5 mg.
Thiamin	0.5 mg.	Fluoride[a]	1 mg./L. H_2O
Riboflavin	0.6 mg.	Chromium	0.03 mg.
Niacin	7 mg. NE	Selenium	0.035 mg.
Vitamin B_6	1.0 mg.	Molybdenum	0.08 mg.
Folacin	200 μg.	Sodium	1500 mg.
Vitamin B_{12}	1.5 μg.	Potassium	2500 mg.
Vitamin K	30 μg.	Chloride	1500 mg.
Biotin	50 μg.	Protein[b]	25 gm.
Pantothenic acid	2 mg.	Carbohydrate[b]	137.5 gm.
Calcium	450 mg.	Fat[b]	39 gm.
Phosphorous	450 mg.	Oleic acid[c]	12.25 gm.
Magnesium	150 mg.	Linoleic acid[c]	10 gm.
Iron	8 mg.	Saturated fatty acids[c]	14.25 gm.

[a]Based on amount of fluoride found in fluoridated water supplies so stated as mg./liter of water.

[b]Based on arbitrary standard of 35 per cent of kcalories from fat, 10 per cent of kcalories from protein and 55 per cent of kcalories from carbohydrate.

[c]Allowances for fatty acids are based on a P:S ratio of 0.7.

(Adapted from Hansen, R. G., and Wyse, B. W.: Expression of nutrient allowances per 1,000 kilocalories. J. Am. Diet. Assoc., 76:223, 1980.)

FAMILY MEAL PLANNING AND SAMPLE MENUS

The suggested basic pattern for meals applies to the entire family group. Serving size and number can be changed to meet the requirements of children, adolescents, pregnant women, lactating mothers or elderly people in the family. Changes can also be made for activity, disease, or food preferences. For example, a lactating mother can have 4 cups of milk instead of 2 and fulfill her increased requirements for calcium, phosphorous, riboflavin and protein.

Table 10–14.   U.S. RECOMMENDED DAILY ALLOWANCES (U.S. RDA)

VITAMINS AND MINERALS	UNIT OF MEASUREMENT	ADULTS AND CHILDREN 4 OR MORE YEARS OF AGE*	INFANTS AND CHILDREN UNDER 4 YEARS OF AGE	PREGNANT OR LACTATING WOMEN
Protein	Grams	65[a]	28	[b]
Vitamin A	International Units	5,000	2,500	8,000
Vitamin D	"	400	400	400
Vitamin E	"	30	10	30
Vitamin C	Milligrams	60	40	60
Folic Acid	"	0.4	0.2	0.8
Thiamin	"	1.5	0.7	1.7
Riboflavin	"	1.7	0.8	2.0
Niacin	"	20	9.0	20
Vitamin B_6	"	2.0	0.7	2.5
Vitamin B_{12}	Micrograms	6	3	8
Biotin	Milligrams	0.3	0.15	0.3
Pantothenic Acid	"	10	5.0	10
Calcium	Grams	1.0	0.8	1.3
Phosphorus	"	1.0	0.8	1.3
Iodine	Micrograms	150	70	150
Iron	Milligrams	18	10	18
Magnesium	"	400	200	450
Copper	"	2.0	1.0	2.0
Zinc	"	15	8.0	15

*These U.S. RDA values are on most nutrition labels

[a]If protein efficiency ratio of protein is equal to or better than that of casein, U.S. RDA is 45 gm. for adults and 20 gm. for infants.

[b]Not specified because this U.S. RDA used only in vitamin and mineral supplements for pregnant or lactating females.

[c]Presence optional for adults and children 4 or more years of age in vitamin and mineral supplements.

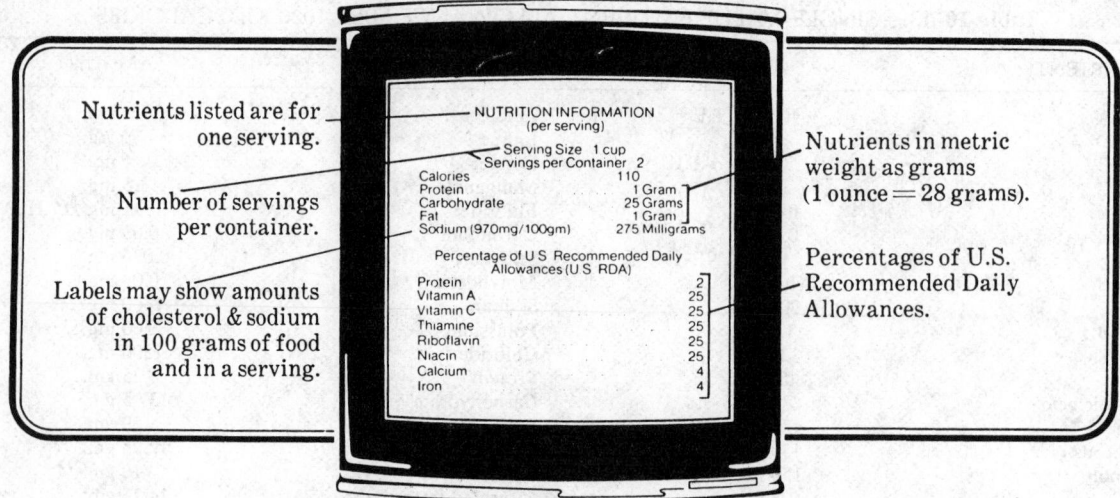

Figure 10–3. Example and explanation of a nutritional label.

There are many choices of food around the world that will provide adequate meals for the day. From the nutrition point of view, a meal should contain a complete protein or two or more complementary proteins, sufficient calories for energy needs and a good percentage of the vitamin and mineral requirements. Table 10–16 gives sample menus at three energy levels using the Daily Food Guide.

OMITTING A MEAL. If any meal is omitted or neglected, there is too much nutritional load put on the remaining meals and snacks in a day's intake. For example, if breakfast is omitted, the intake of nutrients for the day is inade-

Table 10–15. EVALUATION OF DIET USING THE U.S. RDA

FOOD FOR A DAY, WOMAN, 25 YEARS OLD

Food	Amount eaten	Calories	Percentage of U.S. RDA							
			Protein	Vita-min A	Vita-min C	Thia-min	Ribo-flavin	Niacin	Cal-cium	Iron
Ready-to-eat cereal	1 ounce	110	4	20	20	25	25	20	—	20
Milk	½ cup	80	10	3	2	2	12	—	15	—
Orange juice	½ cup	60	1	5	100	8	1	2	1	1
Peanut butter	2 tbsp.	180	16	—	—	4	1	2	1	1
Bread	2 slices	160	8	—	—	8	8	8	4	8
Jelly	1 tbsp.	50	—	—	2	—	—	—	—	2
Margarine	1 pat	35	—	4	—	—	—	—	—	—
Banana	1	100	2	4	20	4	4	4	—	4
Milk	1 cup	160	20	6	4	4	25	—	30	—
Ham	1 ounce	180	60	—	—	35	15	25	2	20
Mashed potatoes	¾ cup	150	4	6	22	9	4	8	3	3
Spinach	½ cup	20	4	145	40	4	8	2	8	10
Applesauce	½ cup	115	—	1	2	2	1	—	—	4
Brownie	1	100	2	—	—	2	2	—	—	2
Iced tea	1 glass	—	—	—	—	—	—	—	—	—
Ice cream	½ cup	130	8	6	1	2	8	—	10	—
Total:		1630	139	200	213	109	114	71	74	75
Goal for a 25-year-old woman*		2000	67	80	100	67	70	65	80	100

Evaluation: The day's food provided less calcium and iron than recommended for a 25-year-old woman. The food provided fewer calories than many women need to maintain their weight, but may have provided enough for this woman.

*Goals are the percentages of the U.S. RDA that must be reached in order to meet age- and sex-appropriate NRC-RDA.

Table 10–16. SAMPLE MENUS AT THREE LEVELS OF ENERGY INTAKE BASED ON THE DAILY FOOD GUIDE

1200 CALORIES	1800 CALORIES	2400 CALORIES
Breakfast		
Orange juice, 1/2 cup	Orange juice, 3/4 cup	Orange juice, 1 cup
Bran flakes with raisins, 1/2 cup	Bran flakes with raisins, 1/2 cup	Bran flakes with raisins, 1/2 cup
Milk, whole, 1/2 cup	Milk, whole, 1/2 cup	Milk, whole, 1/2 cup
Whole-wheat toast, 1 slice	Whole-wheat toast, 1 slice	Whole-wheat toast, 1 slice
Coffee/Tea	Jelly, 2 tsp.	Jelly, 1 tbsp.
	Coffee/Tea	Coffee/Tea
Lunch		
Sandwich:	Sandwich:	Sandwich:
Ham, 2 ounces	Ham, 2 ounces	Ham, 2 ounces
Cheese, 1 slice (1 oz.)	Cheese, 1 slice (1 oz.)	Cheese, 1 slice (1 oz.)
Lettuce	Lettuce	Lettuce
Tomato, 1/2 medium	Tomato, 1/2 medium	Tomato, 1/2 medium
Enriched bread, 2 slices	Enriched bread, 2 slices	Enriched bread, 2 slices
Apple, 1 medium	Salad dressing, 2 tsp.	Salad dressing, 2 tsp.
Coffee/Tea	Apple, 1 medium	Apple, 1 medium
	Coffee/Tea	Plain cookies, 4
		Coffee/Tea
Dinner		
Beef roast, 3 ounces	Beef roast, 4 ounces	Beef roast, 5 ounces
Baked potato, 1 medium	Baked potato, 1 medium	Baked potato, 1 medium
Broccoli, 1/2 cup	Broccoli, 1/2 cup	Broccoli, 1/2 cup
Milk, skim, 1 cup	Roll, 1	Roll, 1
	Margarine, 1 tsp.	Margarine, 2 tsp.
	Milk, lowfat (1%), 1 cup	Milk, lowfat (2%), 1 cup
	Angel food cake (1/16), with strawberries, 1/2 cup	Angel food cake (1/12), with strawberries, 1/2 cup and ice milk, 1/3 cup
Snacks		
Cucumber slices, 1 small cucumber	Peach, fresh, 1 medium	Peach, fresh, 1 medium
Carrot sticks, 3–4 strips (2-1/2" to 3" long)		Fruit-flavored yogurt, 1 cup
		Banana, 1 small

From Food, Home and Garden Bulletin No. 228, Washington, D.C., U.S. Department of Agriculture, 1979.

The menus above illustrate how different foods can be added to a 1,200-calorie diet for an adult (the average calorie level provided by the suggested servings of the first four food groups) to increase the calorie level to 1,800 and 2,400 calories.

Note that in all diets both lowfat and whole milk are used. As the calorie level increases, larger or additional servings from each of the groups are added. For example, while the amount of meat and cheese remains the same for lunch at the three calorie levels, the amount of meat at dinner is increased. Strawberries and angel food cake are added to dinner in the 1,800-calorie menu and ice milk enhances this dessert in the 2400 calorie menu. More snacks are included at the highest calorie level. These snacks, of course, can be eaten any time.

quate, or one's food intake is concentrated later in the day instead of being divided throughout the 24 hours. Many times poor snacks, which are mainly "empty" calorie foods and drinks, compose the entire day's food if there is only snacking and no meals.

The neglect of breakfast is more common in cities than in rural areas and does not seem to be related to income. Eating breakfast has been found essential for maximum efficiency—both physical and mental—during the morning hours. Skipping or slighting breakfast results in decreased output and decreased mental alertness, especially in children.[1, 19]

Sometimes five or six small meals are preferable to the usual three meals, in which case the milk and/or fruit allowance could be taken between meals.

COST COMPARISON. To determine the economy of a choice of food, it is helpful to make a cost comparison. For example, to decide the form of milk which is most economical for the family food budget, the following cost analysis for the equivalent of 7 quarts of milk could be made:

Whole milk: 7 quarts at . . . cents a quart would cost . . .

Evaporated milk: 7 tall (14½ oz.) cans at . . . cents a can would cost . . .

Skim milk: 7 quarts at . . . cents a quart would cost . . .

Dry whole milk: 23 ounces at . . . cents an ounce would cost . . .

Dry skim milk: 23 ounces at . . . cents an ounce would cost . . .

For food values, Appendix Table 1 should be consulted.

The same procedure may be followed to determine the most economical source of the other foods and nutrients. For example, vitamin C, to fit the family budget can be purchased as orange juice, canned or frozen grapefruit juice, canned tomatoes, fresh strawberries, raw cabbage, raw turnips or rutabagas.

The Optimal Diet for Health

The optimal diet for the best health is an individual practice that is tempered by the genetic makeup and the environment of the individual. Because it is so complex, and because much of nutrition is not completely understood, authorities do not agree on the optimal diet, although they would agree on the foundations of an adequate diet as already described. The optimal diet would be the one that allowed the development of an individual to his or her fullest potential, promoted the best mental and physical performance, afforded the greatest resistance to infection and disease, and did not accelerate the aging process. Many feel that this means saturated fat and cholesterol should be limited, sodium reduced, sugar omitted or protein limited. Others would say food additives and colorings should be reduced, or fiber and vitamin C increased. At this point there is not enough information to design the optimal diet for each person's biological individuality, but it is possible to state which basics should be included in the adequate diet for most people.

Many professional groups have published statements on the goals for dietary intake for optimal health for the U.S. population. These are discussed in Chapter 17.

Problems and Suggested Topics for Discussion

1. List your food intake for a week and compare with the basic food pattern in Table 10–8. List any necessary adjustments for improvement.
2. Compare the daily recommended allowances suggested for each member of the following family as determined from Table 10–1: Mother, age 35, overweight 30 pounds, who does own housework; father, age 40, who works as a mason and carries his lunch; girls, ages 3 and 6; active boy, age 12, 10 pounds underweight, who goes to school and comes home for lunch.
3. Compare costs of different sources of milk to meet the daily calcium allowance. Follow the same procedure to compare costs of foods containing ascorbic acid; iron.
4. Define what you think your optimal diet should be. What improvements would you need to make to achieve it? Why is this your optimal diet?
5. Keep a record of your intake for two days in terms of percentage of U.S. RDA from the labels of foods you eat. What are some difficulties in this method? How does your total day's intake compare to the U.S. RDA and to the RDA?
6. Evaluate your diet using a nutrient density approach. Which foods are major contributors of nutrients in your diet?

Cited References

1. Arvedson, I., Sterky, G., and Tjernstrom, K.: Breakfast habits of Swedish school children. J. Am. Dietet. Assoc., 55:257, 1969.
2. Calcium Requirements. FAO/WHO Expert Committee on Calcium Requirements, WHO Tech. Rep. Series 230. Rome, FAO, 1962.
3. Calloway D., as quoted in Robertson, L., Flinders, C., and Godfrey, B.: Laurel's Kitchen. Berkeley, Calif., Nilgiri Press, 1976.
4. Food. Home and Garden Bulletin No. 228. Washington D.C., U.S. Department of Agriculture, 1979.
5. Food and Nutrition Board, National Research Council: Recommended Dietary Allowances, 9th ed. Washington D.C., National Academy of Sciences, 1980.
6. Guthrie, H.A., and Scheer, J.C.: Nutritional adequacy of self-selected diets that satisfy the four food groups guide. J. Nutr. Educ., 13:46, 1981.
7. Hansen R.G.: An index of food quality. Nutr. Rev., 31: 1, 1973.
8. Hansen R.G., and Wyse B.W.: Expression of nutrient allowances per 1000 kilocalories. J. Am. Diet. Assoc., 76:223, 1980.
9. King, J.C. et al.: Evaluation and modification of the basic four food guide. J. Nutr. Educ., 10:27, 1978.
10. Lachance, P.A.: A suggestion on food guides and dietary guidelines. J. Nutr. Educ., 13:56, 1981.
11. Light, L., and Cronin, F.J.: Food guidance revisited. J. Nutr. Educ., 13:57, 1981.
12. Lowry, O.H., et al.: The interrelationship of dietary serum white blood cell and total ascorbic acid. J. Biol. Chem., 166:111, 1946.
13. Margen, S., et al.: Studies in calcium metabolism. I. The calciuretic effect of dietary protein. Am. J. Clin. Nutr., 27:584, 1974.
14. Mertz, W.: The new RDAs: estimated adequate and safe intake of trace elements and calculation of available iron. J. Am. Diet. Assoc., 76:128, 1980.
15. Nutrimeter. Student's Guide and Teacher's Guide. U.S. Department of Agriculture, Agricultural Research Service, Consumer and Food Economics Institute, Washington, D.C., May, 1975.

16. Nutrition Labeling. Tools for Its Use. U.S. Department of Agriculture, Agricultural Information Bulletin No. 382. Washington, D.C., U.S. Government Printing Office, 1975.

17. Pennington, J.A.T.: Considerations for a new food guide. J. Nutr. Educ., *13*:53, 1981.

18. Sorensen, A.W., and Hansen, R.G.: Index of food quality. J. Nutr. Educ., *7*:53, 1975.

19. Tuttle, W.W., et al.: Effect on school boys of omitting breakfast: psychologic responses, attitudes and scholastic achievements. J. Am. Diet. Assoc., *30*:674, 1954.

Additional References

Adams, C.F.: Nutritive Values of American Foods in Common Units. Agricultural Handbook No. 456. Washington, D.C., U.S. Department of Agriculture, Agricultural Research Service, 1975.

Adams, C.F., and Richardson, M.: Nutritive Value of Foods. Home and Garden Bulletin No. 72. Washington, D.C., U.S. Department of Agriculture, 1981.

Bieri, J.G.: An overview of the RDAs for vitamins. J. Am. Diet. Assoc., *76*:134, 1980.

Buss, D.H.: Some consequences of the new U.K. "recommended daily amounts of food energy and nutrients" for evaluating food consumption surveys. J. Hum. Nutr., *33*:325, 1979.

Composition of Foods. Agricultural Handbooks No. 8–1 to 8–9. Washington, D.C:, Consumer and Food Economics Institute, U.S. Department of Agriculture, 1976–1982.

Conserving the Nutritive Values in Foods. Home and Garden Bulletin Number 90. Washington, D.C., U.S. Department of Agriculture, 1963.

Deutsch, R.: Nutrition Labeling—How It Can Work For You. Chicago, The Nutrition Consortium, American Dietetic Association, 1976.

Dietary Standard for Canada. Bureau of Nutritional Sciences, Food Directorate, Information Canada, 171 Slater St., Ottawa, Ontario, 1975.

Family Fare: A Guide to Good Nutrition. Home and Garden Bulletin Number 1. Washington, D.C., U.S. Department of Agriculture. Revised, 1970.

Food for Fitness—A Daily Food Guide. Washington, D.C., U.S. Department of Agriculture, 1958. Rev. ed., Leaflet No. 424, 1977.

Food for the Young Couple. Home and Garden Bulletin No. 85. Washington, D.C., U.S. Department of Agriculture, 1967.

Goodwin, M.T.: Better Living Through Better Eating. 2nd ed. Rockville, Maryland, Montgomery County Health Department, 1974.

Leverton, R.M.: The RDAs are not for amateurs. J. Am. Diet. Assoc., *66*:9, 1975.

Ohlson, M.A., and Hart, B.P.: Influence of breakfast on total day's food intake. J. Am. Diet. Assoc., *47*:282, 1965.

Pennington, J.A.T., and Church, H.N.: Bowes and Church's Food Values of Portions Commonly Used. 13th ed. Philadelphia, J.B. Lippincott Co., 1980.

The Food Group Approach to Good Eating. Dairy Council Digest, *52*(6):1, 1981.

The Recommended Dietary Allowances. Nutr. Today, *14*(5):6, 1979.

Vegetables in Family Meals: A Guide for Consumers. Home and Garden Bulletin No. 105, Washington, D.C., U.S. Department of Agriculture, Revised, 1975.

Williams, R.J.: We abnormal normals. Nutrition Today, *2*: 19, 1967.

NUTRITION IN THE LIFE CYCLE

Nutrition During Pregnancy and Lactation

BONNIE S. WORTHINGTON-ROBERTS, Ph.D.

Pregnancy

Introduction

Numerous factors interact to determine the progress and outcome of pregnancy. These factors have been studied for a number of years and among the most influential are: (1) inherited characteristics conducive to poor reproductive success, (2) trauma or illness during pregnancy, (3) infection during pregnancy, (4) smoking or drinking excessively during pregnancy, (5) exposure to harmful chemicals, including drugs, (6) simultaneous development of more than one fetus in utero, (7) age of the mother, (8) adverse delivery circumstances, (9) inappropriate care of the infant immediately after birth and (10) poor nutrition before and/or during pregnancy.

Research related to nutrition and pregnancy has been extensively pursued with animal models. In addition, human subjects have been examined within the confines of normal daily circumstances. Although much remains to be learned about the role of nutrition in modifying pregnancy course and outcome in humans, it is reasonable to suggest that women should try to optimize their reproductive experience. While many inherited problems or perinatal insults cannot be prevented effectively, malnutrition is one important variable that a woman is in a position to prevent. Not only should the pregnant woman choose to provide herself with a proper diet and supplements *during* pregnancy, but she should prepare herself for reproduction by assuring that good nutritional status exists *at the time of conception.*

HISTORICAL OBSERVATIONS

Both World War I and World War II led to famine in several parts of Europe, and the effects of undernutrition (and the accompanying stress) on previously well-nourished populations can be explored. In all situations thus far examined, the incidence of amenorrhea increased significantly. Such a phenomenon should be viewed as protective in that amenorrheic women often are nutritionally unprepared for pregnancy and/or other stresses may be undesirably great. With increased amenorrhea came reduced birth rates, and in many cases the viable offspring showed lower birth weight than was traditional for their locale.

In Germany during both world wars, undernutrition was very common. In the winter of 1916–1917 during the blockade of Germany, food deprivation was especially severe. The birth rate was markedly reduced, with the smallest decline in fertility being among those who lived in rural areas or had priority access to food rations. While birth weight was not markedly reduced, descriptions of newborns suggest less than normal "vitality."[23]

During and after World War II in parts of Germany, low-birth-weight premature delivery

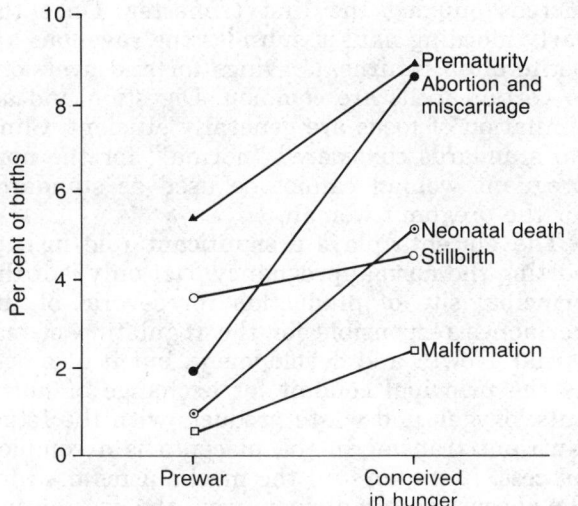

Figure 11–1. Pregnancy outcome in Rotterdam, Holland, before and during World War II.

was more common. In Wuppertal, Germany, average recorded birth weights in 1945 were 185 gm. below the prewar level. As living conditions improved in this area, mean birth weight rose steadily, returning to normal by 1948. After the war, while food supplies and other conditions were still poor, the incidence of malformations, especially involving the central nervous system, was significantly higher than usual.[23]

In Holland and Leningrad during part of World War II, food supplies were extremely low, and one clear result of the deprivation was that fertility of the women was greatly decreased. In Holland, 50 per cent of the female population stopped menstruating and only about 30 per cent had normal menstrual cycles. This circumstance of "war amenorrhea" was associated with reduction in birth rate to one third of the normal level. In addition, when prewar births were compared with those that were the result of conception during the famine, it was seen that miscarriages and abortions, stillbirths, neonatal deaths and malformations were all increased in infants conceived during famine, as indicated in Figure 11–1. Surviving infants showed a significant reduction in mean birth weights and birth lengths. Among those women who experienced the famine during the last two trimesters, mean birth weight fell by 327 gm., or 9 per cent.[23]

While the consequences of severe nutritional deficiency on pregnancy course and outcome are appreciated, the impact of marginal nutritional imbalances during this time is less well understood. One of the best controlled efforts to study this relationship was initiated by Burke and colleagues,[4] who compared the quality of maternal diet with the condition of the baby at birth. As is evident in Figure 11–2, better maternal dietary quality was associated with better condition of the offspring. Such studies are difficult to execute, however, and an assortment of conflicting results have been reported. Overall, however, the consensus now indicates that the diet of pregnant women can affect the development of the fetus.

SUPPLEMENTATION STUDIES

A number of efforts have been made over the years to improve the outcome of pregnancy in poorly nourished women. Various approaches

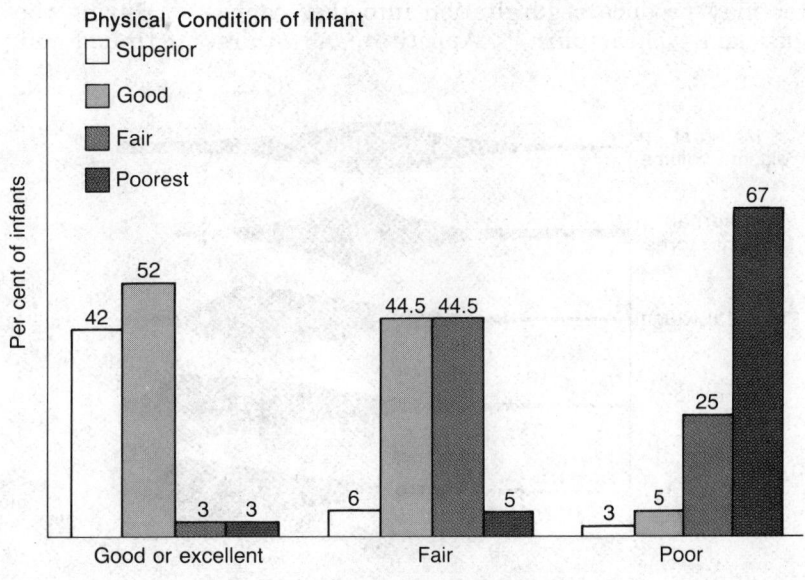

Figure 11–2. Correlation of prenatal nutrition of mother with condition of the infant at birth. (Adapted from Burke, B.S., et al.: The influence of nutrition upon the condition of the infant at birth. J. Nutr., 26:569, 1943.)

have been used in these trials including diet counseling, nutrition education and provision of extra foods or supplements; in many cases a combination of interventions was employed. The results of these investigations have been somewhat contradictory in that clear beneficial effects of food or nutrient supplements have been demonstrated in only some of the trials. Overall, however, the findings appear to suggest that *the worse the nutritional condition of the mother entering pregnancy, the more valuable the prenatal diet and/or nutritional supplement will be in improving the course and outcome of her pregnancy.*

PHYSIOLOGICAL CHANGES DURING PREGNANCY

Many physical and biochemical changes occur in normal pregnancy. The timing of some of these changes is shown in Figure 11–3. As the blood volume increases, concentration of hemoglobin is reduced. Plasma albumin falls. Amino acids may be excreted in the urine. Edema is sometimes present. Changes occur in cardiac and pulmonary functions. Serum alkaline phosphatase may rise markedly and other enzymes increase in amount. Most plasma lipid fractions rise during pregnancy. The thyroid gland often enlarges because of the loss of inorganic iodine in the urine. A renal loss of folate occurs in some individuals. During late pregnancy, the ability to excrete a water load is below normal and the water may pool in the lower limbs. This fluid retention is normal. The stomach shows signs of depressed function. (Histamine is depressed and pepsin production is reduced.) Reduced motility of the gastrointestinal tract can result in constipation. A relaxed cardiac sphincter may produce regurgitation into the esophagus and "heartburn." Appetite and thirst increase during the first trimester. Once the early morning nausea subsides the ravenous appetite often returns. Cravings for and aversions to certain foods are common. Digestion and assimilation of foods are generally efficient. Clinical standards considered "normal" for the nonpregnant woman cannot be used as standards for the pregnant woman.

The placenta plays a significant role in supporting the normal pregnancy. Not only is it the principal site of production for several of the hormones responsible for the regulation of maternal growth and development, but it also acts as the principal conduit for exchange of nutrients, oxygen and waste products with the fetus. Nutrient transfer in the placenta is a complex process. It employs all the mechanisms used for the absorption of nutrients from the gastrointestinal tract: simple diffusion, facilitated diffusion, active transport and pinocytosis. The difference, however, is that in the placenta two completely separate blood supplies are maintained. Any damage done to the placenta during the course of pregnancy will compromise its ability to nourish the fetus; infarction is one such insult of significance, but other reasons for placental insufficiency exist.

MATERNAL WEIGHT GAIN AND PREPREGNANCY WEIGHT

While good maternal diet has long been appreciated as important to the developing fetus, attitudes have varied over the years about desirable weight gain and adverse consequences of overeating and excessive weight gain. Several centuries ago it was felt that overeating might be associated with abortion, "fetal outgrowth of the womb" and a variety of other disorders. During the nineteenth century this theme continued and pregnant women were encouraged to

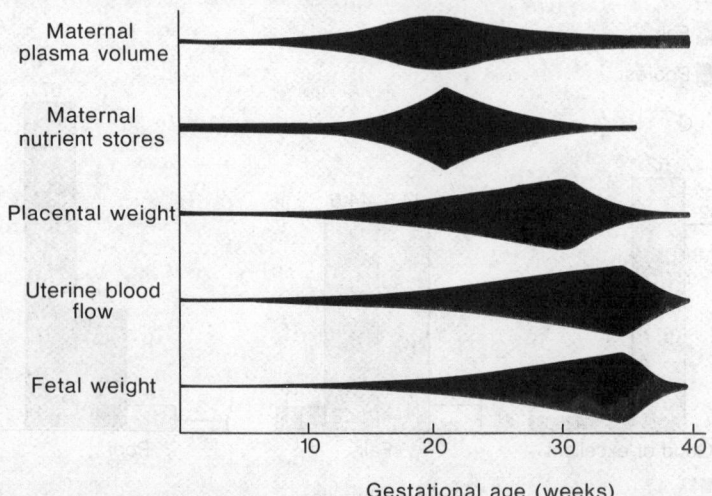

Figure 11–3. Gestational changes in maternal plasma volume, maternal nutrient stores, placental weight, uterine blood flow and fetal weight in normal human pregnancy. The thickness of each bar represents the degree of change at specific times during pregnancy.

eat in moderation, select light meals and restrict their use of carbohydrate. The prevalent idea that evolved at this time was that overeating led to the development of larger babies, which complicated the process of labor and delivery. As cesarean sections were rarely done and maternal mortality was high, restriction of fetal size seemed justifiable. Prochownik reported in 1901 that birth weight of infants could be successfully limited through restricted diet during pregnancy. In his study, 48 offspring of women who had followed this routine showed an average birth weight of 2906 gm. for males and 2735 gm. for females. The normal birth weights for this population were 3333 gm. and 3250 gm. for males and females, respectively.[40]

The general philosophy of weight gain restriction prevailed into the 1960's and is still espoused by a minority of clinicians. Interestingly, however, in 1916, Smith[52] reported that poor maternal nutritional status had a profound influence on birth weight and outcome of pregnancy. Based on evaluations of diet, height-weight status and physical condition, women were grouped according to nutritional status. Women considered to have poor nutritional status had a higher incidence of stillbirth, prematurity, and term babies weighing less than six pounds. In a later study of 150 women, birth weight was found to increase with increasing pregnancy weight gain and with few exceptions this observation has been corroborated by the majority of subsequent studies. One of the largest of these later studies was conducted in Baltimore in 1968 and included 6675 white and 5236 black women. The data clearly showed that (1) an increase in weight gain during pregnancy is associated with a parallel increase in birth weight and a progressive decrease in the number of low-birth-weight infants, and (2) increased prepregnancy weight is also associated with increased birth weight and reduced incidence of very small babies.[12]

Over the years, observations have confirmed that both weight gain during pregnancy and prepregnancy weight are directly related to birth weight of the infant. It appears, in fact, that these variables are independent, so that when varied in the same direction their effects are additive, whereas when change is in opposite directions they tend to neutralize each other. Largest babies are thus frequently found when both prepregnancy weight and weight gain during pregnancy are high; smallest infants conversely derive most frequently from thin mothers with low pregnancy weight gain.

International surveys support the view that "normal" patients gain an average of 24 lb. during the course of a "typical" 40-week pregnancy. A typical grid to evaluate weight gain is given in Figure 11–4. The normal composition of weight gain is illustrated in Figure 11–5. Less than half the total weight gain resides in the fetus, placenta and amniotic fluid; the remainder is found in maternal reproductive tissues, fluid, blood and "stores." The weight component labeled "maternal stores" is largely composed of body fat. The action of progesterone in the pregnant woman dictates that a fat pad be produced to serve as an energy reserve for both pregnancy and lactation. Fatfold measurements from 10 to 30 weeks of gestation have shown gradual increases in subcutaneous fat at the abdomen, back and upper thigh. The pregnant woman who attempts to restrict weight gain to avoid development of the fat pad may do so but will simultaneously affect to some degree normal development of the other products of pregnancy.

While a weight gain of 24 to 28 lb. is recommended for pregnant women in developed countries, this recommendation does not fully consider the status of maternal nutritional reserves. With this in mind, Naeye reevaluated weight gain data of over 53,000 women from 12 United States hospitals who were followed between 1959 and 1966.[35] Weight gain was compared with prepregnancy body weight and perinatal mortality. The results of the study are expressed diagrammatically in Figure 11–6. Mothers who were overweight at the start of pregnancy had the fewest fetal and neonatal deaths with a 16-lb. weight gain at term. The optimal weight gain for normally proportioned mothers was 20 lb. and for underweight mothers 30 lb. For all three groups perinatal mortality rates increased with weight gains less or more than these optimal values. While the results of this study do not dictate that all overweight mothers gain 16 lb., normal weight mothers 20 lb. and underweight mothers 30 lb., they do suggest a range of desirable weight gains during pregnancy that relates in part to prepregnancy weight status.

With regard to prepregnancy weight of the mother, underweight status has been shown to be associated with higher risk of adverse outcome. This relationship has been known for quite some time, and was confirmed by Edwards and colleagues in a study of the obstetric performance and pregnancy outcome of 354 underweight patients and matched controls of normal prepregnancy weight, and the growth patterns of their infants.[14] The underweight women had significantly higher rates of cardiac and respiratory problems, anemia, premature rupture of membranes and endometritis. Prematurity and low Apgar scores were significantly more frequent in the infants of underweight women. Although no difference was found in the frequency of intrauterine growth retardation and in peri-

Prenatal Gain In Weight

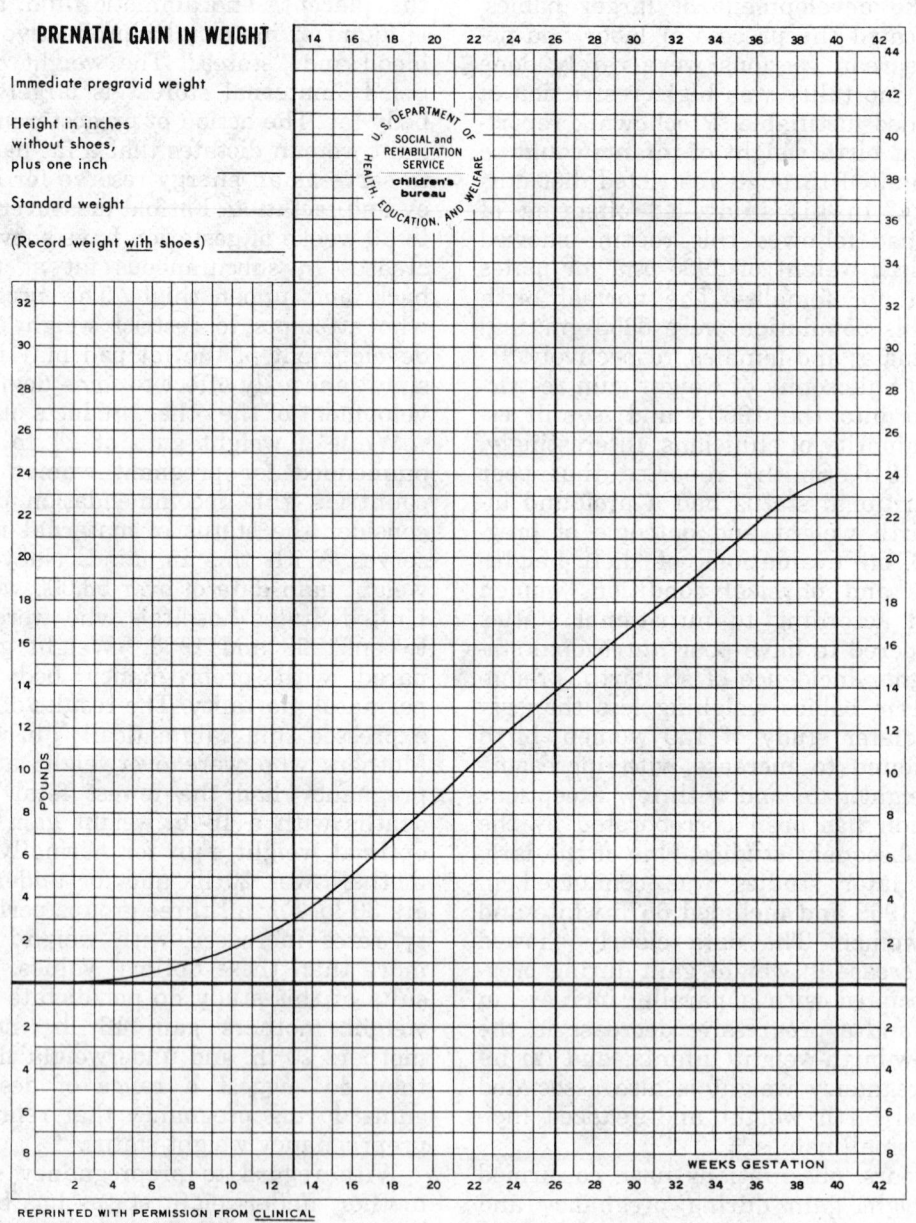

PRENATAL GAIN IN WEIGHT

Immediate pregravid weight _____

Height in inches
without shoes,
plus one inch _____

Standard weight _____

(Record weight with shoes) _____

U. S. DEPARTMENT OF
SOCIAL and
REHABILITATION
SERVICE
HEALTH, EDUCATION, AND WELFARE
children's
bureau

WEEKS GESTATION

POUNDS

REPRINTED WITH PERMISSION FROM CLINICAL
OBSTETRICS 1953, J. B. LIPPINCOTT AND CO.

Figure 11–4. Curve of normal weight gain during pregnancy.

natal mortality rates, the mean birthweight of the infants of underweight women was 231 gm. less than that of infants of control subjects. Incidence of low birth weight was higher in children of underweight mothers, especially if the mothers were anemic; this was true even when the mothers achieved adequate weight gain. Observations of the infants during the first year of life showed that those whose weight was appropriate for gestational age were more likely to be below the 25th percentile for weight correlated

with length at 12 months of age if their mothers were underweight prior to pregnancy; limited data also suggested delayed neurological development in these babies.

Several studies have confirmed that obese women have a higher incidence of obstetric complications.[13] Nearly two thirds of 48 massively obese patients studied developed obstetric complications.[61] These included a sevenfold increase in toxemia, fivefold increase in pyelonephritis and tenfold increase in diabetes.

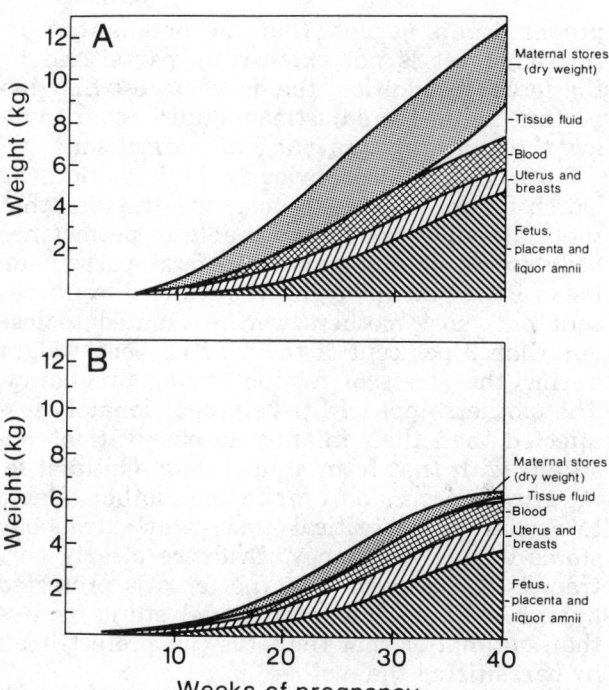

Figure 11–5. Estimated composition of weight gain during pregnancy for a normal, healthy Northern European woman *(A)* and a poor, underfed woman from India *(B)*. (Adapted from Hurley, L.S.: Developmental Nutrition. Englewood Cliffs, N.J., Prentice-Hall, Inc., 1980. After Committee on Maternal Nutrition, National Research Council: Maternal Nutrition and the Course of Pregnancy. Washington, D.C., National Academy of Sciences, 1970.)

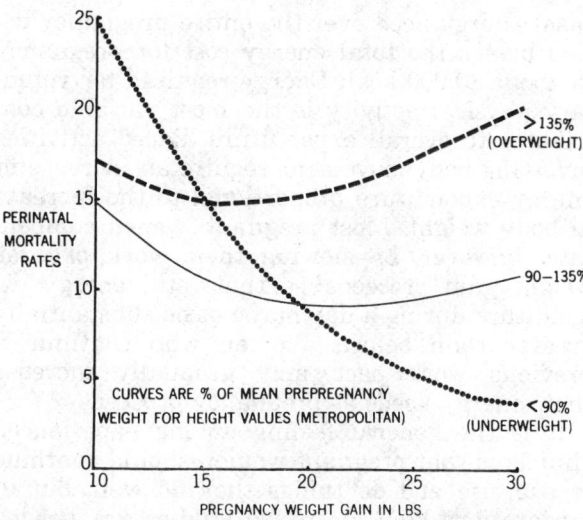

Figure 11–6. Perinatal mortality rates related to weight gain of mother during pregnancy. Dashed line indicates overweight mothers, with prepregnancy weight greater than 135 per cent of ideal weight; solid line indicates normal weight mothers, with prepregnancy weight 90 to 135 per cent of ideal weight; dotted line indicates underweight mothers, with prepregnancy weight less than 90 per cent of ideal weight. (From Naeye, R.L.: Weight gain and the outcome of pregnancy. Am. J. Obstet. Gynecol., *135*:3, 1979.)

Complications were more likely to develop in obese women, including hypertension, diabetes, wound complications and thromboembolism. In a ten-year review of the maternal mortality rate in Minnesota, 12 per cent of the mothers who died but only 2 per cent of a control group had a prepregnancy weight in excess of 200 pounds.[33] The leading cause of death was pulmonary embolus. The risk of death from this complication was more than twice as high in the obese as in the non-obese.

Obese women are known to be inclined toward delivery of larger than average babies. Interestingly enough, this phenomenon often occurs even when maternal weight gain and/or energy consumption is below average.[13] The mean birth weight of the infants of obese women was 209 gm. greater than that of infants of the control subjects and a significantly increased number of the obese patients were delivered of high-birth-weight infants. Massively obese women demonstrated a significantly increased incidence of "inadequate weight gain" but at the same time delivered significantly larger babies and more excessively large infants. Maternal stores are obviously used to provide for some of the nutritional needs of the offspring in utero. The incidence of obesity in infants of obese women was not significantly increased at birth or 6 months of age. By 12 months of age, however, these infants were significantly more obese than the control infants. This latter findings suggests that the familial tendency toward obesity is not obvious at birth but begins to be manifested by the end of the first year of life. Whether or not this delayed onset of obesity indicates that an improved obesity prognosis may be achievable through preventive nutrition counseling and weight monitoring remains to be established. It may very well be that a nutritious diet *moderately* restricted in calories is justifiable for many of these obese women.

ENERGY REQUIREMENTS

In order to support optimal weight gain during pregnancy, sufficient energy must be consumed. Energy is required for (1) the deposition of new tissue associated with pregnancy, (2) the increased metabolic expenditure to maintain the new tissue and (3) the increased energy needed to move the pregnant body around. The total fat and protein deposits represent a need for about 41,000 kcal. during the course of pregnancy. If basal energy needs increase from 0.9 to about 1.1 kcal. per minute, the increased energy needed for metabolism totals about 300 kcal. per day. Extrapolation of this increased basal energy need over the entire pregnancy period brings the total energy cost for pregnancy to about 80,000 kcal. Energy required for voluntary physical activity is the most variable contributor to overall expenditure. Paced activities involving body movement require an increase in energy expenditure proportional to the increase in body weight. Most pregnant women compensate, however, by slowing their work pace as weight gain proceeds[2] so that total energy expenditure during a day may not be substantially greater than before. Women who continue a previous work pace may gradually increase their energy needs as pregnancy proceeds.

It is the general feeling among experienced clinicians that pregnant women should continue to exercise and do things they do well, but in moderation. Well-controlled studies are needed in this area.

In general, with regard to energy requirements, the Recommended Dietary Allowances (RDA) state that pregnant women need an additional 300 kcal. per day or at least *36 kcal. per kg. body weight*. This recommendation accounts for the increase in basal metabolism and is considered the minimal increased need during pregnancy. Regular participation in weight-bearing activities will augment energy needs further; since individuals vary considerably in level and intensity of activity, it is best to advise women to eat enough to support physiologic appetite and to support a gain of about 0.4 kg. (14 oz.) per week during the last 30 weeks of pregnancy.[10]

Actual energy intakes of pregnant women reveal several basic features in populations studied. First, intake is often less than recommended; this may be due to omissions in recalls or records, extremely sedentary lifestyles, or purposeful restriction of weight gain. Women from countries in which obsession with body weight is not as great as it is in the United States often report higher levels of daily energy intake. Second, energy intakes often remain rather constant throughout the last two trimesters. It is suspected that energy intake is greater early in pregnancy when maternal stores are being deposited, and that as pregnancy continues, gradual use is made of the maternal stores.

DIETING, FASTING AND FOOD RESTRICTION

The degree to which the mother is parasitized by the fetus has been the subject of much debate for many decades. Although it is known that the fetus can draw on maternal stores when maternal dietary input is limited, the extent and duration of this process is unknown. Recent studies on the effect of food restriction on the body composition of pregnant and non-

pregnant rats suggest that the pregnant, food-restricted rat is not extensively parasitized by the fetus. In addition, the data suggest that important metabolic adjustments must occur to allow the mother to prevent fetal parasitism.

Human data are obviously limited, but the Dutch famine experience supports the idea that the malnourished mother is able to protect her body stores of nutrients from fetal parasitism. Mean infant birth weight was reduced by 10 per cent but most mothers were estimated to lose less than 3 per cent of their initial body weight during the stress of famine during pregnancy. The mothers appeared to be proportionately less affected than their infants, an observation consistent with that from animal data. Optimal fetal growth occurs only when the mother is able to accumulate a critical amount of extra body stores during pregnancy. Evidence clearly contradicts the concept that the fetus is protected by the mother when nutritional status is less than optimal or that the fetus can protect itself by parasitizing the mother.

The fact that nature protects the mother more than the fetus seems reasonable from the point of view of survival of the species. During a famine caused by a serious drought, for example, a normal-sized newborn delivered by a nutritionally depleted mother would have little chance to survive if the mother could not initiate lactation, protect herself and her young, and cover enough ground during the day to secure food. A stronger or healthier mother that produces a small baby or few offspring probably has a better chance to survive and conceive again in the future.

One recognized consequence of energy restriction is the increased production of ketone bodies and their ultimate spillage into the urine. Although it is known that the fetus can metabolize ketone bodies to some degree, the consequences of maternal ketosis are incompletely understood. Severe ketoacidosis, as occurs in diabetics, is appreciated as harmful to the fetus, but the short-term and long-term effects of maternal acetonuria are unclear. Churchill and associates first reported that children whose diabetic and non-diabetic mothers had acetonuria during pregnancy had lower mental and motor scores at 8 months and lower IQ values at 4 years of age than children not so exposed.[7] Stebhens and colleagues later examined offspring of diabetic women and found a significant association of gestational acetonuria with lower IQ values at 5 years of age.[57] Reports by Naeye and associates in the past few years, have not confirmed these earlier reports; maternal acetonuria was not related to results of mental and motor tests administered to offspring at 4 to 7 years of age.[35, 36]

Data collected from both animals and humans indicate that ketone bodies are probably normally presented to the fetal brain at various times during pregnancy. After an overnight fast, maternal ketone body concentrations are about threefold greater in pregnant than in non-pregnant women and ketonuria will often be seen.[9, 15] A recent study found that urine concentrations of ketone bodies may abruptly increase in the presence of less than a twofold increase in blood concentrations; in addition, blood levels generally fall within the upper limit of the normal range.[10] These investigators concluded that acetonuria in normal pregnancy "probably does not usually signify that any abnormality is present." More serious conditions of ketoacidosis should likely be viewed as more hazardous.

PROTEIN REQUIREMENTS

Additional protein is obviously needed during pregnancy to support the synthesis of maternal and fetal tissues. Needs increase as pregnancy proceeds, so that greatest demands occur during the second and third trimesters. Considerable uncertainty still exists, however, as to the magnitude of the extra need.

Currently the RDA for pregnant women includes 30 gm. of extra protein per day along with satisfactory energy intake. On the basis of nitrogen balance research, however, this recommended level of protein consumption is higher than necessary for the healthy pregnant woman in the first trimester.

Adverse consequences of protein deficiency during pregnancy are difficult to separate from the effects of energy deficiency in clinical situations. Almost all cases of limited protein intake are accompanied by limitation in availability of energy; under such circumstances decreased birth weight and greater incidence of preeclampsia have been reported. Suggestions have been made by several investigators that protein deficiency may be the cause of toxemia of pregnancy. This is discussed further on page 261.

Adverse effects of excessive protein during pregnancy are poorly understood at the present time. A supplementation study conducted in New York City has provoked much discussion of this issue, since use of the high-protein supplement was associated with an increased number of very prematurely born infants and excessive neonatal deaths.[48] Analysis of a number of other supplementation studies in human populations has suggested that providing a supplement with more than 20 per cent of the calories from protein is associated with retarded fetal growth, while supplements providing less than 20 per cent of calories from protein yield increments in birthweight of offspring.[49] While these data suggest that too much protein (presented in an unbalanced nutritional package) may have negative effects on pregnancy course and outcome, data are limited and the debate continues about the relevance of these observations.

Table 11–1.   RECOMMENDED DIETARY ALLOWANCES

	NON-PREGNANT FEMALES				PREG- NAN- CY	LACTA- TION
	11–14 yr.*	15–18 yr.†	19–22 yr.†	23–50 yr.†		
Energy (kcal.)	2200 (1500–3000)	2100 (1200–3000)	2100 (1700–2500)	2000 (1600–2400)	+ 300	+ 500
Protein (gm.)	46	46	44	44	+ 30	+ 20
Vitamin A (µg. RE)	800	800	800	800	+ 200	+ 400
Vitamin D (µg.)	10	10	7.5	5	+ 5	+ 5
Vitamin E (mg. α-TE)	8	8	8	8	+ 2	+ 3
Ascorbic acid (mg.)	50	60	60	60	+ 20	+ 40
Folacin (µg.)	400	400	400	400	+ 400	+ 100
Niacin (mg.)	15	14	14	13	+ 2	+ 5
Riboflavin (mg.)	1.3	1.3	1.3	1.2	+ 0.3	+ 0.5
Thiamin (mg.)	1.1	1.1	1.1	1.0	+ 0.4	+ 0.5
Vitamin B$_6$ (mg.)	1.8	2.0	2.0	2.0	+ 0.6	+ 0.5
Vitamin B$_{12}$ (µg.)	3	3	3	3	+ 1	+ 1
Calcium (mg.)	1200	1200	800	800	+ 400	+ 400
Phosphorus (mg.)	1200	1200	800	800	+ 400	+ 400
Iodine (µg.)	150	150	150	150	+ 25	+ 50
Iron (mg.)	18	18	18	18	‡	‡
Magnesium (mg.)	300	300	300	300	+ 150	+ 150
Zinc (mg.)	15	15	15	15	+ 5	+ 10

(From Food and Nutrition Board, National Research Council: Recommended Dietary Allowances. 9th ed. Washington, D.C., National Academy of Sciences, 1980.)

*Weight 46 kg. (101 lb.), height 157 cm. (62 in.).

†Weight 55 kg. (120 lb.), height 163 cm. (64 in.).

‡The increased requirements of pregnancy cannot usually be met by ordinary diets; therefore, the use of 30 to 60 mg. of supplemental iron is recommended. Continued supplementation for two to three months after parturition is advisable.

Table 11–2. FAT-SOLUBLE VITAMIN DEFICIENCIES AND EXCESSES AND OBSERVATIONS OF HUMAN PREGNANCY OUTCOME

VITAMIN	DEFICIENCY	EXCESS	VITAMIN	DEFICIENCY	EXCESS
Vitamin A	Indian woman, blind from vitamin A deficiency, gave birth to premature infant with microcephaly and anophthalmia. Prenatal vitamin A deficiency has been related in several instances to eye abnormalities and impaired vision in children.	One case: congenital renal anomalies in offspring of woman who consumed high doses of vitamin A during pregnancy. One case: multiple malformations, especially involving the central nervous system, in infant of woman who consumed 150,000 I.U. of vitamin A from day 19 through day 40 of pregnancy. Higher concentrations of vitamin A were found in blood of mothers bearing babies with CNS abnormalities as compared with mothers of normal infants; liver vitamin A levels from abortuses and/or malformed fetuses found to be higher than in fetal liver from normal samples.	Vitamin D— Cont.	Vitamin D supplementation of pregnant Asian women was associated with improved maternal weight gain, normal 25-OHD$_3$ levels in mothers and infants at term, reduced incidence of SGA babies and fewer babies with neonatal hypocalcemia. Neonatal hypocalcemia is reportedly more common during months of the year when daily sunlight is least.	nosis with elfin facies and mental retardation appeared in Gottingen, Germany, where rickets prophylaxis (consisting of huges doses of vitamin D) was begun.
Vitamin D	Case of fetal rickets: mother had low serum vitamin D and developed osteomalacia some months after delivery of her infant. Case of neonatal rickets: mother suffered from osteomalacia during pregnancy. Low levels of 25-OHD$_3$ seen in hypocalcemic premature infants and their mothers. Enamel hypoplasia of the teeth seen in infants with neonatal tetany; maternal vitamin D deficiency was associated.	Women treated with high doses of vitamin D for hypoparathyroidism show no evidence of cardiovascular or craniofacial abnormalities in their offspring. These mothers do not develop characteristic hypercalcemia. It has been hypothesized that excessive intake of vitamin D or unusual sensitivity to the vitamin might be related to mild idiopathic hypercalcemia in infants. Supravalvular aortic ste-	Vitamin E	Positive correlation noted between birth weight and cord blood levels of vitamin E, but gestational age and other variables were not controlled for.	Comparison of 50 spontaneously aborting women with 50 women whose pregnancies terminated uneventfully showed a significantly higher percentage of aborting women with serum alpha-tocopherol above normal limits; a causal association was not proposed.
			Vitamin K	Some evidence that use of dicumarol during pregnancy is associated with increased fetal mortality and morbidity. A number of cases have been reported of fetal abnormalities in infants of mothers treated with anticoagulants. Prenatal vitamin K deficiency caused by dicumarol drugs is known to produce the coumadin syndrome unless dosage is properly controlled.	Parenteral administration of menadione to the mother has been associated with hyperbilirubinemia and kernicterus of premature infants and severe hyperbilirubinemia in term infants.

VITAMINS AND MINERALS

Maintenance of health during the course of pregnancy obviously requires an adequate supply of vitamins and minerals. Precise requirements for each of these nutrients have not been established, but the 1980 RDA have been de-

vised on the basis of available evidence and are listed in Table 11–1. The consequences of vitamin and mineral deficiency and excess are only partially understood. A number of animal experiments have been completed during the past 30 years, but data from humans largely represent only fortuitous observations of natural events in individual women. Tables 11–2, 11–3 and 11–4 summarize basic information on the consequences of vitamin and mineral deficiencies and excesses in humans. In the following paragraphs, comments relate to nutritional requirements for selected vitamins and minerals.

IRON. As the maternal blood supply increases markedly during pregnancy, the demand for iron obviously is great. Total erythrocyte volume increases by 20 to 30 per cent in accord with the availability of dietary or supplemental iron. An active bone marrow may utilize an extra 500 mg. of elemental iron during pregnancy, and the term fetus and placenta accumulate 250 to 300 mg. of elemental iron. Overall, the pregnant woman must have between 700 and 800 mg. of extra iron, the majority of which is needed during the last half of pregnancy, when the heaviest maternal and fetal demands occur.

This amounts to a daily increment of 5 to 6 mg., but diet typically provides only 1 to 2 mg. each day unless aggressive attention to selection of iron-rich foods is maintained. While some women may possess available iron stores, rarely are these sufficient to cover all needs without compromising maternal well-being.

Iron supplementation is thus often acknowledged as a necessary means of preventing iron deficiency anemia. Simple ferrous salts are recommended in the 1980 RDA in amounts of 30 to 60 mg. of iron daily for prophylaxis. Larger amounts of iron occasionally may be prescribed for treatment of established iron deficiency. The elemental iron content varies among supplements, but in general all forms are viewed as acceptable. See Chapter 29 for ways to enhance iron absorption.

Maternal anemia is the major clinical consequence of iron deficiency, but its effects on the

Table 11–3. WATER-SOLUBLE VITAMIN DEFICIENCIES AND EXCESSES AND OBSERVATIONS OF HUMAN PREGNANCY OUTCOME

VITAMIN	DEFICIENCY	EXCESS	VITAMIN	DEFICIENCY	EXCESS
Thiamin	If deficiency is severe, congenital beriberi. If deficiency is mild to moderate, no reported complications.	None reported	Ascorbic acid— *Cont.*	and serum vitamin C; frequency of congenital malformations was no higher in the women with the lowest serum levels but increased frequency of premature births occurred in the women with the lowest intake; these women also had the lowest serum concentrations of vitamin C of the group.	of ascorbic acid to terminate suspected pregnancies; each had shown a 10- to 15-day delay in onset of their menstrual period. In 16 of the 20 women, menstrual bleeding occurred within 1 to 3 days after starting the treatment. The results were interpreted as indicating that the large doses of ascorbic acid terminated the pregnancies. Since the pregnancies were not initially confirmed, this conclusion must be questioned.
Riboflavin	One study of 900 pregnant women showed that 190 were riboflavin deficient. These women demonstrated a higher incidence of vomiting during pregnancy, premature delivery and stillbirths. No increased incidence of malformations was seen. Unsuccessful lactation was more common. Among middle-class European women, biochemical evidence of riboflavin deficiency was not associated with abortion, hydramnios, preeclampsia, stillbirth or low birth weight.	None reported		Several reports indicate that low serum vitamin C levels were associated with threatened abortion or history of previous abortions; other studies found no relation.	Several infants have been reported to develop "conditioned scurvy" in the neonatal period owing to excessive ascorbic acid catabolism following high prenatal ascorbic acid exposure.
Niacin	None reported	None reported			
Ascorbic acid	The Vanderbilt study of over 2000 pregnant women assessed diet	In one study, women took large doses (6 gm./day for 3 days)			*Table continued on the following page*

Table 11–3. WATER-SOLUBLE VITAMIN DEFICIENCIES AND EXCESSES AND OBSERVATIONS OF HUMAN PREGNANCY OUTCOME (*Continued*)

VITAMIN	DEFICIENCY	EXCESS	VITAMIN	DEFICIENCY	EXCESS
Folic acid	Humans treated with folate antagonists (methotrexate, aminopterin, chlorambucil) during early pregnancy often suffer spontaneous abortion, and some cases of severe congenital anomalies in term infants have been reported. While naturally occurring folate deficiency in pregnant women has not been *proved* to have an adverse effect on pregnancy outcome, correlations have been reported between red cell folate level and incidence of congenital malformations, small for gestational age (SGA) babies and third trimester bleeding. This observation has been questioned by others, and the relationship between folate deficiency and abruptio placentae is equally controversial. Most folate-supplementation studies report no effect on pregnancy outcome, but several reports from Africa and India indicated that the rate of prematurity was significantly reduced. One prospective study of 800 women indicated that low red cell folate level was associated with increased incidence of SGA infants and congenital malformations. Another large prospective study showed significantly lower levels of red cell folate in mothers who subsequently gave birth to babies with neural tube defects as compared with controls. A report from northern Europe showed that women who had previously delivered	None reported	Folic acid— *Cont.*	babies with neural tube defects showed reduced incidence of the same problem when multiple-vitamin supplementation (rich in folic acid) was provided instead of no supplement at all. This report has been highly controversial and is currently being replicated in Europe.	
			Vitamin B$_{12}$	Pernicious anemia is rare in women of child-bearing age, but it generally is accompanied by infertility.	A human fetus with vitamin B$_{12}$ dependency has been successfully treated by feeding high doses of vitamin B$_{12}$ to the mother.
			Pantothenic acid	None reported	None reported
			Biotin	None reported	None reported
			Vitamin B$_6$	Low maternal blood levels of B$_6$ have not generally been associated with neonatal clinical sequelae. One study reported, however, that women with low dietary and/or serum levels of B$_6$ produced a greater number of babies with low Apgar scores at 1 minute than comparable mothers with good B$_6$ status. Supplementation of pregnant women with B$_6$ has not been found to reduce any clinical complication of pregnancy except "poor appetite" and pregnancy sickness. In one study, maternal serum levels of B$_6$ were inversely correlated with degree of pure pregnancy depression. Pregnant women in a low socioeconomic group showed biochemical evidence of vitamin B$_6$ deficiency and orolingual lesions (e.g., glossitis, angular stomatitis); both responded positively to vitamin B$_6$ supplementation.	None reported

Table 11–4. SOME MINERAL DEFICIENCIES AND EXCESSES AND OBSERVATIONS OF HUMAN PREGNANCY OUTCOME

MINERAL	DEFICIENCY	EXCESS	MINERAL	DEFICIENCY	EXCESS
Iron	Mean hemoglobin level of the fetus is unaffected by maternal iron levels, unless deficiency is severe. Infants of anemic mothers showed reduced iron stores and greater tendency to develop anemia in the first year of life. Effect of maternal iron deficiency on birthweight of infant is controversial. Increased incidence of prematurity has been reported with maternal iron deficiency. No evidence links iron deficiency with congenital malformations.	None reported	Iodine— Cont.	tinism and goiter dramatically. New Guinea reported the most recent outbreak of cretinism, related to substituting local iodine-rich salt with imported rock salt low in iodine. Intramuscular iodized oil injections to women prior to pregnancy was later shown to markedly reduce the incidence of cretinism. In addition, offspring of injected women were significantly faster and more accurate in tests of manual function than children without cretinism from noninjected mothers.	
Calcium	Mean bone densities of malnourished mothers and their neonates were lower than those of well-nourished counterparts. One study of Indian women with low daily calcium intake (~400 mg./day) indicated that daily calcium supplementation during the third trimester was associated with increased bone density in the offspring. Calcium deficiency has been proposed to be the major etiological factor in toxemia of pregnancy.	None reported	Magnesium Sodium	None reported Hyponatremia has been reported in offspring of women who rigorously restricted sodium during pregnancy. Sodium restriction does not help prevent or alleviate toxemia of pregnancy.	None reported None reported
			Potassium	Human embryonic kidney development in culture is abnormal. Suggests that potassium insufficiency in fetal plasma may cause abnormal development of the kidney in humans.	None reported
Iodine	Cretinism was first described in the 16th century. Its association with goiter was recognized in the 19th century, although endemic cretinism does not always occur where there is a high incidence of endemic goiter. The cretinous child shows mental and physical retardation with potbelly, large tongue and facial characteristics like those of children with Down's syndrome. Iodine prophylaxis has reduced the incidence of cre-	Women provided large amounts of iodides during pregnancy (often as treatment for asthma or bronchitis) have given birth to abnormal infants with congenital goiter and hypothyroidism. Neonatal mortality was high and many survivors were mentally retarded. Use of radioactive sodium iodide during pregnancy is associated with the same outcome.	Manganese Copper	None reported Menkes' kinky hair syndrome demonstrates the impact of prenatal copper deficiency in humans. Abnormalities are seen in development of the brain, hair, bones and blood vessels. One case: a young woman treated with penicillamine during pregnancy gave birth to a child with connective tissue defects including lax skin, hyperflexibility of the joints, fragility of the veins, varicosities, and impairment of wound healing. Copper deficiency is proposed to be of possible etiological importance.	None reported Small amounts of metallic copper from intrauterine devices can prevent mammalian embryogenesis, but teratogenicity has not been established.

Table continued on the following page

Table 11–4. SOME MINERAL DEFICIENCIES AND EXCESSES AND OBSERVATIONS OF HUMAN PREGNANCY OUTCOME (*Continued*)

MINERAL	DEFICIENCY	EXCESS	MINERAL	DEFICIENCY	EXCESS
Zinc	Epidemiological data may support a relationship between zinc deficiency and CNS malformations; significant zinc deficiency has been found in Egypt, Turkey and Iran, where high rates of CNS anomalies are seen. Women with acrodermatitis enteropathica (a genetic disorder of zinc metabolism now treated with supplemental zinc) have shown very poor pregnancy outcome in the past when zinc therapy was not used; miscarriage and malformations were much higher than in the general population. Alcohol-abusing mothers show reduced serum levels of zinc and are known to demonstrate a higher than normal incidence of poor pregnancy outcome. A relationship has been proposed but not proved. Among 272 pregnant adolescent women, those experiencing hypertension/toxemia had significantly lower plasma zinc levels; mothers of infants with congenital defects had plasma zinc levels well below the mean. Among 60 pregnant women in Belfast, 2 aborted spontaneously; these 2 women had serum zinc levels in the lower range and hair zinc values in the higher range. Leukocyte zinc levels were significantly lower in mothers giving birth to babies who were small for gestational age as compared with mothers of normal babies or mothers of infants who were small but	In one report, zinc supplements were given to pregnant women (100 mg. zinc sulfate, 3 times daily) during the third trimester; in four consecutive subjects, three delivered prematurely and one gave birth to a stillborn infant.	Zinc — *Cont.* Selenium Chromium Fluoride Mercury	appropriate for gestational age. Plasma zinc concentrations were significantly lower in the maternal blood of 54 women giving birth to congenitally abnormal babies when compared with control mothers. None reported None reported None known, although one report suggests that prenatal fluoride supplements were associated with reduced incidence of dental caries in offspring. None reported	 None reported None reported Mothers using well water containing 12 to 18 ppm fluorine produced offspring with significant mottling of the deciduous teeth. An epidemic of cerebral palsy and microcephaly occurred in Minamata, Japan, and the cause was felt to be maternal ingestion of fish contaminated with methylmercury. Severe central nervous system damage was seen in one infant whose mother ate meat from a pig contaminated by a mercury-containing grain diet; ingestion occurred during the third gestational month. Studies on 15 mother-child pairs in Iraq were reported; mothers ingested homemade bread prepared from wheat treated with methylmercury fungicide. In all cases but one, the infant's blood level was higher than the mother's. Six of the infants were severely impaired in their mental and motor development. Cerebral palsy occurred even when exposure was in the third trimester. Milder cases showed developmental retardation and exaggerated tendon reflexes and pathological extensor plantar reflexes.

outcome of pregnancy are poorly understood. Anemia is considered present when the hematocrit is less than 32 per cent and the hemoglobin level is less than 11 gm./dl.; this situation is commonly seen in one third to one half of pregnant women who do not use iron supplements. An anemic woman is clearly less able to tolerate hemorrhage with delivery, and she is more prone to develop puerperal infection. Data suggest that the fetal effects of maternal iron deficiency are relatively mild, but several reports suggest that pregnancy outcome may be compromised. Observations in India in the early 1970's showed that moderate to severe anemia in pregnant women was associated with increased incidence of spontaneous abortion, premature delivery, low-birth-weight delivery, stillbirth and perinatal death. It might be hypothesized that poor iron consumption leads to poor hemoglobin production, followed by compromised delivery of oxygen to the uterus, placenta and developing fetus, as shown in Figure 11–7. If maternal cardiac output increases to accommodate the insufficiency in hemoglobin content per red cell, the added work load undertaken by the heart could unduly stress maternal systems.

The pregnant woman with iron deficiency anemia should be treated for a finite period with iron supplements containing 100 mg. or more iron per tablet. In a large proportion of anemic women treated in this fashion, an upward shift in hematocrit can be achieved easily. However, 15 or 20 per cent of such women will not respond to typical iron therapy by obvious improvement in hematocrit level; this group is suspected to represent individuals in whom expanded plasma volume is significantly greater than normal. This phenomenon is reportedly common in situations of multiple pregnancy. Supplementation with iron in excess of need has not been evaluated through critical research; one report, however, suggested that unnecessary use of iron supplements led to macrocytosis in a small number of pregnant women.[60]

FOLACIN. Folacin needs increase during pregnancy, specifically because of the demands of maternal erythropoiesis and fetal-placental growth. Requirements are estimated to approximately double, so the RDA is 800 rather than 400 μg. daily.[17] In the presence of folic acid deficiency, there is a reduction in the rate of DNA synthesis and a delay in mitotic activity of individual cells. A typical picture of dysplastic cell maturation develops, and this state is recognized by the megaloblast in the bone marrow because of the exceptionally high fetal and maternal demands. It most frequently appears as anemia during the third trimester, but preliminary morphological and biochemical signs of deficiency may precede this state.

Low serum folates may be found, however, in as many as 20 per cent of women with otherwise normal pregnancies. The clinical significance of this preanemic state is the subject of much speculation and debate. Maternal folic acid deficiency in experimental animals is associated with increased incidence of problems related to pregnancy as well as increased delivery of abnormal offspring.[20] Some evidence in hu-

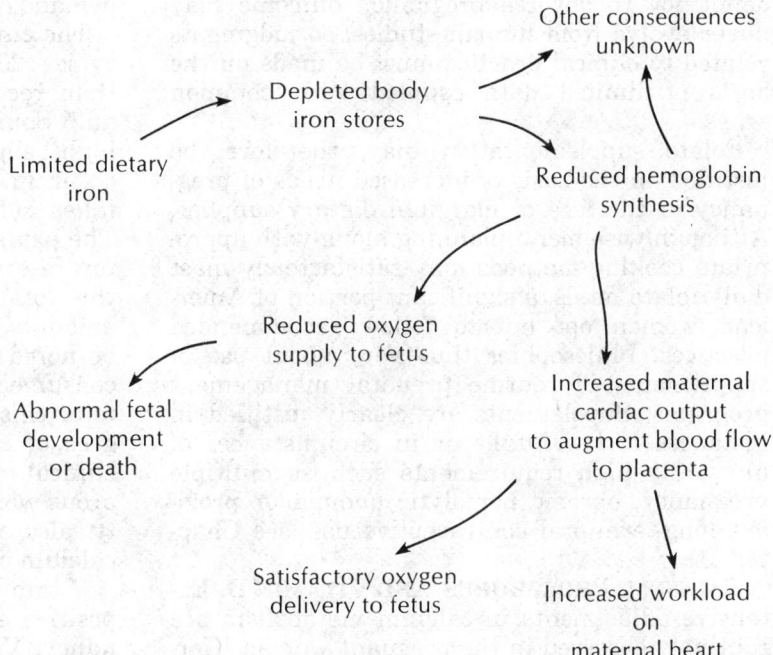

Figure 11–7. Hypothetical consequences of iron deficiency anemia on pregnancy course and outcome. (Adapted from Worthington-Roberts, B.S.: Contemporary Developments in Nutrition. St. Louis, C. V. Mosby Company, 1981.)

mans suggests that deficiency of this vitamin may be associated with abruptio placentae, spontaneous abortion, preeclampsia, fetal malformations and subnormal infant development; such reports, however, are by no means direct proof of association.[53]

In one study of over 900 women, both serum and red-cell folate were assessed during the first trimester of pregnancy, and the outcome of pregnancy was later reported. In six women who gave birth to infants with neural tube defects, red-cell folates recorded in the first trimester were significantly lower than in controls (141 ng./ml. versus 228 ng./ml.). The researchers suggested that these observations are compatible with the hypothesis that folic acid deficiency causes congenital defects in the neural tube of developing humans.[53] This theory has recently gained limited recognition in reports of the positive value of vitamin supplementation[27, 54, 55] or dietary counseling[28] for women with a history of delivering infants with neural tube defects. Smithells and colleagues reported that preconceptional and prenatal vitamin supplementation of mothers who had previously delivered babies with neural tube defects was associated with a significant decrease in incidence of these same defects in their next offspring.[54, 55] Laurence and coworkers found that basic nutritional counseling including guidelines for healthful eating was associated with reduced incidence of neural tube defects among babies of mothers with previous delivery of neural tube defect infants.[28]

Other studies, however, have not demonstrated any association between low folate status and malformation.[19, 51] Solid proof relating folic acid deficiency to adverse pregnancy outcome may never evolve from human studies, so judgments related to clinical practice must be made on the basis of limited data coupled with common sense.

Folate supplementation may, therefore, be justified on the basis of increased needs of pregnancy in the face of marginal dietary supplies. Although wise menu planning along with appropriate cooking methods may satisfactorily meet daily folate needs, a significant portion of American women opt not to follow recommended practices. Philosophies thus vary about use of supplements in routine prenatal management programs. Supplements are clearly justified in instances of low intake or in circumstances of unusually high requirements such as multiple pregnancy, chronic hemolytic anemia or previous long-term oral contraceptive use (see Chapter 21).

CALCIUM, PHOSPHORUS, AND VITAMIN D. Extensive adjustments in calcium metabolism are routinely observed in the pregnant woman. Hormonal factors are largely responsible, with the following consequences known to occur:

1. Human chorionic somatomammotropin (from the placenta)—increases the rate of bone turnover progressively through pregnancy.

2. Estrogen (largely from the placenta)—inhibits bone resorption and thus provokes a compensatory release of parathyroid hormone, which maintains the serum calcium level while enhancing intestinal calcium absorption and decreasing its urinary excretion.

The net effect of these changes is the promotion of progressive calcium retention. The prenatal changes begin well ahead of the time when fetal skeletal mineralization ensues. It thus appears that anticipatory adjustments ready the maternal organism for the increased calcium demands later on. Mineralization of the fetal skeleton is ultimately stimulated, largely through active placental calcium transport leading to fetal hypercalcemia and subsequent endocrine adjustments. Vitamin D and its metabolites also cross the placenta and appear in fetal blood in the same concentration as found in maternal circulation.

Approximately 30 gm. of calcium is accumulated during pregnancy, almost all of it in the fetal skeleton. Most of the accretion occurs during the latter part of pregnancy, with an estimated average of 300 mg. deposited daily during the last trimester. It is suspected, however, from calcium balance studies that calcium retention occurs in the maternal organism as well. Storage of calcium in the maternal skeleton may occur under the hormonal stimuli previously defined. Such a phenomenon might be readily supported as preparative for the extensive calcium demands of lactation.

The current RDA for calcium during pregnancy is 1200 mg. daily—a level 400 mg. higher than recommended for the non-pregnant woman.[17] Some argue that this allowance is set too high, since apparently successful pregnancies occur in many other cultures with calcium intakes substantially below those recommended. The explanation likely relates to the large calcium reservoir in the maternal skeleton, of which the total requirement of pregnancy (30 gm.) amounts to about 2.5 per cent.[39] It should also be noted that in many other cultures, diets are consumed that contain less phosphorus and protein; this factor might serve to reduce the degree of calcium loss in the urine. Evidence of clinical manifestation of osteomalacia in multiparous women is available.[16] Neonatal bone density also may relate to adequacy of maternal calcium consumption during pregnancy.[43]

Vitamin D has long been appreciated for its positive effects on calcium balance during pregnancy. Vitamin D may be involved in neonatal calcium homeostasis. Observations in Great Britain indicate that the peak season for neonatal hypocalcemia coincides with the time of least sunlight.[44] Additionally, serum vitamin D levels are often low in such infants, suggesting that some cases of neonatal hypocalcemia and/or enamel hypoplasia may relate to maternal vitamin D deficiency and subsequent limitation in placental transport of vitamin D to the fetus.[42] In pregnant Asian women it was shown that vitamin D supplementation during the third trimester was associated with improved rate of maternal weight gain, higher maternal and newborn serum 25-OHD$_3$ levels at term, reduced incidence of symptomatic hypocalcemia in newborns and lower percentage of small-for-gestational-age infants.[3] Excessive amounts of vitamin D may be harmful during gestation, however; severe infantile hypercalcemia and associated problems have been reported in newborn animals and in human infants, as listed in Table 11–2.

Calcium-phosphorus balance frequently is discussed in relation to maintenance of neuromuscular normality. Twenty years ago, several clinicians suggested that sudden clonic or tonic contractions of the gastrocnemius muscle (often at night) are caused by a decline in serum calcium. Prevention or relief of these leg cramps was reported to be obtained through reduction in intake of milk (a high-phosphorus, high-calcium beverage). Supplementation with non-phosphate calcium salts was also recommended, along with regular ingestion of aluminum hydroxide to promote formation of insoluble aluminum phosphate salts in the gut. Several studies confirmed the benefit of these measures in the total serum calcium level in affected women. It is clear, however, that the clinical correlation of these observations is far from perfect, since some controlled and double-blind studies have failed to indicate a correlation between leg cramps and either intake of dairy products or type of calcium supplement employed.

SODIUM. Sodium metabolism is altered during pregnancy under the stimulus of a modified hormonal milieu. Glomerular filtration increases markedly over time in order to "clean up" the increased maternal blood volume. An additional filtered sodium load of 5000 to 10,000 mEq. daily is typically seen during pregnancy. Compensatory mechanisms come into play to maintain fluid and electrolyte balance.

Restriction of dietary sodium has been common in the past among pregnant women suffering from edema, but moderate edema is normal during pregnancy and should not be combatted with diuretics or low-sodium diets. The increased fluid retained normally during pregnancy actually increases somewhat the body's demand for sodium. Rigorous sodium restriction in pregnant animals stresses the renin-angiotensin-aldosterone system to the point of breakdown; such animals tend to develop water intoxication along with renal and adrenal tissue degeneration.[38] Restricted mothers deliver smaller litters, fewer live births and more stillbirths per litter than controls; nursing offspring also show a markedly reduced rate of survival.[5] Neonatal hyponatremia (low blood sodium) has been observed in offspring of women who unduly restricted sodium intake before delivery. While moderation in use of salt and other sodium-rich foods is appropriate for all people, aggressive restriction is unwarranted during pregnancy, when *no less than 2 to 3 gm.* of sodium should be consumed on a daily basis.

VITAMIN A. Both vitamin A and carotene cross the placenta, and fetal storage of vitamin A accounts in part for the 1980 RDA for pregnant women of an extra 200 R.E. (1000 I.U.) of this vitamin daily. An intake of this level can be readily provided by dietary sources, and there appears to be no need for routine supplementation. Vitamin A deficiency is teratogenic in lower animals, but confirmatory evidence of its teratogenicity in humans is lacking.

Excessive vitamin A consumption is believed to be teratogenic in humans, as indicated by the limited evidence mentioned in Table 11–2, but most scientific evidence describes developmental anomalies in animals.

VITAMIN E. Vitamin E needs are believed to increase somewhat during pregnancy, but deficiency in humans rarely occurs and has not been linked with either damage to offspring or reduced fertility. However, the 1980 RDA recommends an increase of 2 mg. α-TE daily to compensate for the amount deposited in the fetus. Since vitamin E deficiency in experimental animals has long been associated with spontaneous abortion, there has been interest in the use of vitamin E for prevention of abortion in humans. In general, however, studies in humans have not supported this as a preventive measure.

Although the vitamin E level in the infant at birth is significantly less than in the mother, the infant's level has been shown to correlate directly with the maternal concentration. Attempts to raise the fetal level by supplementing the mother with vitamin E during the last trimester have confirmed the direct correlation of fetal and maternal vitamin E concentrations, but also have indicated the great difficulty encountered by the administration of tocopherol to the mother. Therefore, it has been concluded that parenteral vitamin E administration to the mother prior to delivery is not enough to prevent an infant from having the hemolytic anemia of vitamin E deficiency. Since this problem develops six weeks after birth, it can probably be prevented best by oral supplementation of the infant during the postnatal time interval.

VITAMIN K. Interest in vitamin K largely centers on hemorrhagic disease of the newborn due to vitamin K deficiency. Parenteral vitamin K is often administered to parturient women, since the newborn has a sterile gut and bacterial synthesis of vitamin K is thus an unreliable source in the neonatal period. Some authorities object to this practice because of the increased tendency in the infant toward hyperbilirubinemia, which results from excessive dosage. Treatment of the newborn with natural vitamin K_1 has been alternatively recommended; oral administration of K_1 during about the last week of pregnancy also may be both safe and beneficial.

VITAMIN B_6. Much attention has recently been devoted to the vitamin B_6 status of pregnant women. The current RDA for vitamin B_6 is 2.6 mg. daily during pregnancy, 0.6 mg. more than is recommended for the non-pregnant woman.[17] Just how much vitamin B_6 is needed to meet fetal requirements is unknown. Some evidence suggests, however, that a significant number of pregnant women on presumably normal diets develop biochemical abnormalities suggestive of vitamin B_6 deficiency.[1] The depth of pure pregnancy depression has been correlated negatively with serum B_6 concentrations.[41] Administration of vitamin B_6 supplements corrects the biochemical deficit, and dosages amounting to 10 mg. daily have been recommended by several investigators.

Another report suggests that supplements of 5 to 10 mg. per day (pyridoxine hydrochloride) are needed to maintain plasma pyridoxal phosphate levels of pregnant women who have not used oral contraceptives but ≥ 15 mg. are needed by long-term oral contraceptive users.[46] Others have reported relief of symptoms of pregnancy sickness and mental depression by administration of pyridoxine supplements.[64] Whether or not this practice is justified remains to be determined by additional observations in human subjects. The tendency at the moment is to regard the apparent alterations in B_6 status as indicative of some poorly understood physiological adjustment to pregnancy. Supplementation is therefore not routine. But one new observation of considerable interest involved assessment of babies born of mothers with varying vitamin B_6 status. Vitamin B_6 levels were measured in maternal serum at 5 and 7 months gestation and at delivery, in cord serum, and in milk at 3 and 14 days postpartum. Mothers whose infants had unsatisfactory Apgar scores (less than 7) at one minute had significantly lower intakes of vitamin B_6 and lower levels of the vitamin in both serum and milk than mothers whose infants had satisfactory scores.[45] Later work suggested the same thing.[50] Further study is obviously needed to clarify the impact of moderate B_6 deficiency on both mothers and offspring.

ASCORBIC ACID. Ascorbic acid deficiency has not been shown to affect the course or outcome of pregnancy in humans. However, because low plasma levels of vitamin C have been reported to be associated with premature rupture of the membranes as well as preeclampsia, questions have arisen about its possible association with these conditions. An extra 20 mg. of vitamin C is recommended daily for the pregnant woman; this total recommendation of 80 mg. daily is easily met by the American diet. Massive intake of vitamin C supplements may adversely influence fetal metabolism. Metabolic dependency on high doses may develop in the offspring such that scurvy may arise in the neonatal period.[8, 37]

IODINE. For many years it has been understood that maternal iodine deficiency leads to cretinism in offspring. Recent data also suggest that suboptimal iodine nutrition of the mother may compromise development of her fetus even when cretinism does not occur.[11] Findings indicate that iodine deficiency may lead to a spectrum of subclinical deficits that place the children at a developmental disadvantage.

ZINC. The effect of zinc deficiency on the course and outcome of pregnancy is of considerable interest. Zinc deficiency is highly teratogenic in rats and leads to the development of a variety of congenital malformations. Non-human primates also are affected and abnormal brain development and behavior have been described in offspring of zinc deficient monkeys.

Unfortunately, it seems that a zinc-deficient diet does not effectively lead to the mobilization of zinc stored in maternal bones. This storage pool appears somewhat unavailable, so that dietary deficiency can impact quickly upon the mineral balance of the maternal organism. Recent evidence from human populations suggests that the malformation rate and other poor pregnancy outcomes may be higher in populations where zinc deficiency has been recognized.[6, 24, 55, 61] Jameson, for example, observed in Scandinavia that women with low serum levels of zinc demonstrated higher incidence of abnormal deliveries, including congenital malformations.[24]

Studies in animals suggest that adequate zinc intake may be important in protecting the fetus from harm from a noxious or foreign agent.[18, 24]

The potential hazard of prenatal zinc supplementation has not been determined in human populations. Modest zinc supplements provided to pregnant rats produced an increased number of fetal resorptions.[26] Additionally, of four pregnant women with marginal zinc status who were provided 100 mg. of zinc sulfate three times daily during the third trimester, three delivered prematurely and the fourth delivered a stillborn infant.[26] Whether or not the supplements were directly related to the adverse pregnancy outcomes remains to be seen. Haphazard use of nutritional supplements, however, has no role in prenatal care. The 1980 RDA for zinc is an additional 5 mg. over that for the non-gravid woman.

COPPER. Hurley and colleagues have been instrumental in defining the consequences of prenatal copper deficiency. In both experimental and field animals, copper deficiency has been found to be teratogenic. Lambs, rats, guinea pigs and mice have been examined. It is also possible that copper deficiency may compromise pregnancy outcome in humans. One case has been reported of a young woman treated with D-penicillamine (a copper-chelating medication) during pregnancy who gave birth to an abnormal child.[22] The child had a connective tissue defect including lax skin, hyperflexibility of the joints, fragility of the veins, varicosities and impairment of wound healing; some of these features have been recognized previously as associated with copper deficiency.

It is presently unknown whether moderate dietary copper deficiency is of consequence to the developing human fetus. A study of copper and zinc balance in 20 pregnant women on self-selected diets showed that a positive balance of copper was achieved in these subjects only if a copper supplement was consumed.[59] The authors suggest that the diets of many pregnant women may have only a marginal copper content. Should these findings be confirmed and adverse consequences to the fetus suspected, copper supplementation may someday be advisable for selected women.

FLUORIDE. The role of fluoride in prenatal development is poorly understood at the present time. Some question has existed over the past 50 years as to the degree of fluoride transport across the placenta. Should it cross the placenta, further question still remains about its value in the development of caries-resistant permanent teeth. Glenn examined nearly 500 women (and their offspring) who were provided varying levels of fluoride during the last two trimesters of their pregnancies. About half of the women received fluoridated water only while the others not only received fluoridated water but also took a sodium fluoride supplement that provided 1 mg. of fluoride daily. When the offspring were examined at five to nine years of age, those whose mothers had received the sodium fluoride supplement averaged 0.17 ± 0.07 decayed or filled surfaces, and 97 per cent were caries-free; those whose mothers had not received the sodium fluoride supplement averaged 8.7 ± 0.6 decayed or filled surfaces, and 15 per cent were caries-free.[21]

Development of the primary dentition begins at 10 to 12 weeks of pregnancy; from the sixth to the ninth month of pregnancy, the first four permanent molars and eight of the permanent incisor teeth begin formation. Thus, 32 of the ultimate teeth are forming and developing during human pregnancy. Since there is no indication that color of the teeth is adversely affected and some evidence that caries-resistance and morphological characteristics are improved, prenatal fluoride supplementation may be justified.

FOOD ALLOWANCES FOR THE NORMAL PREGNANT WOMAN

To meet the increased requirements of pregnancy, the adequate diet pattern discussed in Chapter 10 is used, with a few important changes and additions as listed in Table 11–5.

Four cups of milk per day are recommended. This will provide the additional 30 gm. of high-quality protein needed, will increase the calcium intake to 1.2 gm. and will provide an additional 320 kcal. from skim milk or 640 kcal. from whole milk. A number of choices are available: whole milk, skim milk, fluid and non-fat powdered milk, buttermilk, acidophilus milk, evaporated milk, yogurt and cheese. Those who find drinking milk disagreeable may utilize the required amount in soups, custards, puddings, ice cream or flavored beverages. The use of non-fat skim powder is an inconspicuous and acceptable way to add milk to the diet as a dry ingredient in the preparation of meatloaf, soups, scrambled eggs, mashed and scalloped potatoes, sandwich spreads, cooked cereals, homemade breads, cookies or pastries. Approximately 1.5 ounces (5 tablespoons) of dried skim milk will equal 1 cup of fluid milk. Milk can be made richer in calcium, protein and calories by adding 2 tablespoons of dried non-fat milk to a glass of fluid milk.

For women who have lactose intolerance, which is present in a large percentage of the black, Oriental and Mexican-American populations, cheese, which contains very minute quantities of lactose, may be used. A small amount of milk may be beneficial in preventing or treating constipation. Commercial calcium preparations such as calcium lactate or carbonate may have to be prescribed.

The daily consumption of whole-grain or enriched bread and cereals, leafy green and yellow vegetables and fresh and dried fruits should be encouraged to provide additional minerals, vitamins and fiber. Careful attention to the selection of foods that are good sources of iron and folic acid (see Tables 10-6 and 10-7) is

Table 11–5. DAILY FOOD PATTERN TO ENSURE OPTIMAL NUTRITION DURING PREGNANCY

FOOD	AMOUNT	PROTEIN (gm.)
Milk, whole	3 or 4 8-oz. glasses.	24 to 32
Meat (lean), poultry, fish, liver is desirable at least once each week, cheese	2 servings/day, in all at least 4 oz. or equivalent in grams of protein.	28
Egg	One	7
Fruit	At least 2 servings. Two servings of citrus fruit or equivalent should be eaten. (1 serving equals 4 oz. of orange juice, 1 med. orange, 8 oz. of tomato juice, or ½ med. grapefruit.)	1
Potato	1 med. (150 gm.), preferably cooked in skin.	3
Other vegetables cooked and/or raw	2 or more servings. (1 serving equals ½ cup.) Dark green leafy or deep yellow vegetables often.	4
Bread and cereal	3 to 4 servings. (1 serving equals 1 slice of bread or ½ cup of cereal.) Whole grain or enriched.	6 to 8
Vegetable oil or special margarine, butter or fortified margarine	1 tablespoon	
Vitamin D	Increased by the addition of 5 µg. (200 I.U.) to the non-pregnant allowance. Vitamin D–fortified milk (1 qt.) will supply 10 µg. (400 I.U.).	0
Total		73 to 83

stressed to provide as much dietary iron and folic acid as possible.

Three to four cups of milk fortified with vitamin D provide 7.5 to 10 µg. of cholecalciferol (300 to 400 I.U.). If milk is used in limited amounts, a vitamin D supplement may be necessary, especially if the woman has very little or no exposure to sunlight.

Table 11–6 gives an example of a menu that meets the needs of the normal pregnant woman.

TOTAL FLUIDS. The drinking of six to eight glasses (2 liters) of water daily is encouraged. Intestinal stasis is often encountered as a result of the necessary restrictions of activities and the pressure of the enlarging uterus. However, for most individuals the bulky content of the protective diet plus the suggested amount of water will counteract any difficulty. Mineral oil is discouraged, since it may interfere with the absorption of the fat-soluble vitamins.

NUTRITION EDUCATION

Usually the prospective mother is anxious to have a normal, healthy baby and seeks obstetric care early. Well-presented advice about nutrition is more apt to be accepted at this time than at any other stage or period in life (Fig. 11–8). Methods of educating patients about nutrition are discussed in Chapter 18. The special nutritional needs of the pregnant woman are summarized in Table 11–7. However, unless such advice is based on previous food habits, customs and food budget, it may not be followed. Any improvement in food pattern depends upon how the person perceives the task of change. With few exceptions, a woman whose diet is poor during pregnancy can be considered as having been on a poor diet prior to conception.

Full discussion of individual needs with involvement of the person in planning for the nec-

Table 11–6. SAMPLE MENU FOR PREGNANCY*

BREAKFAST
Orange juice, 4 oz.
Oatmeal, ½ cup
Soft cooked egg
Whole grain or enriched toast, 1 slice
Butter or fortified margarine, 1 pat
Coffee or tea

MID-MORNING
Orange juice, 4 oz.
Wheaties, ¾ cup
Milk, 4 to 8 oz.

LUNCH
Meat or cheese sandwich with rye or whole-grain bread and 1 pat butter
Lettuce and tomato salad
Grapefruit, half
Milk, 8 oz.

MIDAFTERNOON
Milk, 8 oz.

DINNER
Broiled beef liver, 4 oz.
Baked potato with 1 pat butter or fortified margarine
Peas and carrots
Crisp celery
Baked custard

BEDTIME
Hot or cold milk, or cocoa, 8 oz.

*Kcalories are adjusted for desired weight. If the gravid individual is an adolescent, additional milk, fresh fruits or vegetables, whole-grain bread and butter or margarine are suggested.

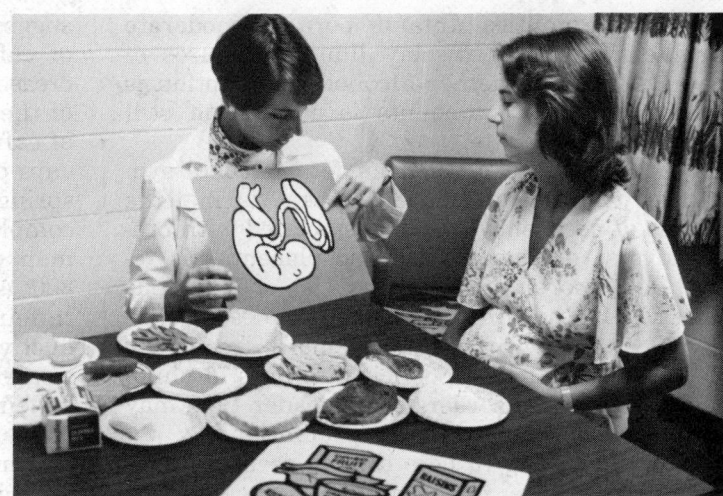

Figure 11–8. A pregnant woman learning about food in relation to her pregnancy. (Photograph courtesy of Nutrition Department, Lutheran General Hospital, Park Ridge, Illinois.)

essary changes is the only effective approach. Even then the results may be disappointing, since some women do not take their nutritional supplements or do not change their eating habits after intensive counseling.

To gain cooperation for dietary improvement from the prospective mother, a discussion of the dietary habits of the prospective father and any other members of the family is also necessary. A prospective father, convinced that it is an essential part of his duties as a parent, will join in improving the family's food pattern and food habits. The counselor utilizes this interest and helps the parents to move in the direction of changes needed to provide an adequate diet. If each parent tends to watch the other's diet, both will improve their food habits. Thus, if both parents adopt an adequate diet, another family is started with good nutritional habits.

ALCOHOL

Abundant evidence has accumulated on the teratogenicity of alcohol in mammals. Animal studies, as well as human experiences, show that "heavy drinking" during pregnancy is asso-

ciated with considerable risk of fetal damage. A pattern of abnormalities has been identified in affected offspring and labeled the *fetal alcohol syndrome* (FAS) (Figure 11–9).[58] Some features associated with this syndrome are prenatal and postnatal growth failure, developmental delay, microcephaly, eye changes including the epicanthal fold, facial abnormalities and skeletal-

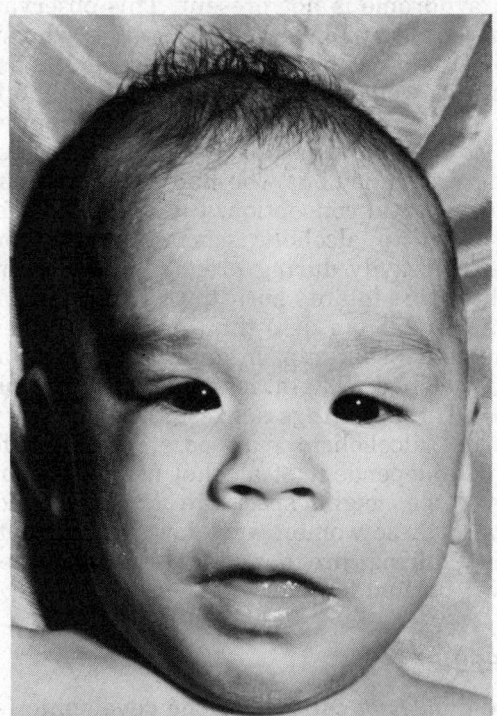

Figure 11–9. A child with the classic features of fetal alcohol syndrome as seen at eight months of age. Observable craniofacial features include small head circumference, short palpebral fissures, flat mid-face, long and indistinct philtrum and thin upper lip. This child was diagnosed at birth and most recently evaluated at five years of age, at which time his IQ was estimated to be about 45. (Photograph courtesy of Dr. Ann Streissguth and colleagues, University of Washington.)

Table 11–7. SUMMARY OF NUTRITIONAL CARE FOR THE PREGNANT WOMAN

1. Energy to meet nutritional needs and allow for about a 0.4 kg. (14 oz.) gain per week during the last 30 weeks of pregnancy.
2. Protein to meet nutritional needs—about an additional 30 gm. per day.
3. Sodium should not be excessive, but should be no less than 2 gm. per day.
4. Minerals and vitamins to meet the RDA. For iron and folate this may necessitate supplementation.
5. Alcohol should be omitted or at least restricted to very small amounts infrequently.
6. Caffeine should be reduced to less than 500 mg./day, the equivalent of 4 cups of coffee.

joint abnormalities. Infants born to moderate drinkers also may display limited features of the syndrome. Whether alcohol consumption is harmful in small amounts is a question still open to much debate.

Aside from the problem of fetal alcohol syndrome, significant alcohol intake during the course of pregnancy may be associated with other adverse outcomes. Abruptio placentae is reportedly more common, as is spontaneous abortion in the first and second trimester. Surviving infants without FAS more frequently demonstrate attention deficit disorders in childhood. Learning disorders of a broader type may also be more common in this population.[58]

It is interesting to note that in several observations, decrease in normal drinking activity has been recorded among women during the course of pregnancy. The decrease in consumption appears to be related primarily to the adverse physiological effect of alcohol during pregnancy and only secondarily to concern for fetal welfare. This change in drinking habits has been hypothesized to be a signal of a biological regulatory mechanism protecting the fetus.

In alcoholic women who cease drinking during pregnancy, fetal growth retardation may be evident in their offspring even though fetal alcohol syndrome is not present. This observation was reported by Little and colleagues, who studied 50 infants of non-drinking mothers and 100 infants of women with a history of alcoholism. Fifty of the infants in the latter group were born to women who reported total abstinence during pregnancy but who had a history of alcoholism prior to conception; the other 50 infants were born to alcoholic women who reported drinking heavily during pregnancy. Mean birth weight of the infants born to the abstinent alcoholics was 258 gm. less than mean birth weight of the control infants. Infants of drinking alcoholics weighed 493 gm. less than the control infants.[32] These findings suggest that a history of maternal alcoholism may pose a risk to fetal growth independent of alcohol use during pregnancy. One might speculate that nutritional stores in these women were low or that dietary quality during pregnancy was inadequate to support normal fetal growth.

CAFFEINE

The danger of caffeine to the developing fetus has been studied in several animal models. Massive doses appear to be teratogenic in mice, but the effects of smaller quantities have not been satisfactorily examined. Epidemiological investigations have produced limited evidence of caffeine-induced birth defects in humans. A recent report from the Food and Drug Administration suggests, however, that rather modest amounts of caffeine provided to pregnant rats may increase the incidence of defects in development of the digits. Pregnant rats provided an amount of caffeine (per unit size) equivalent to about 30 cups of coffee per day for humans, produced offspring with an increased incidence of partial or complete absence of the digits of the paws. Human data are very limited, but one survey of 800 American households suggests that heavy caffeine use is associated with increased reproductive loss and pregnancy complications; of 16 women who consumed more than 600 mg. of caffeine daily, five delivered stillborn babies, eight spontaneously aborted, two delivered prematurely and one achieved a normal pregnancy and delivery.[63] While this study succeeded in provoking interest in caffeine, recent observations of human populations do not support a role of *moderate* (< 500 mg. per day) caffeine exposure in adverse pregnancy course or outcome.[27, 31, 47] Still, a general warning has been voiced to the public to avoid unnecessary caffeine consumption during pregnancy.

OTHER NON-NUTRITIONAL SUBSTANCES IN FOOD

A number of "contaminants" are found in food, and some of these may adversely affect the course and outcome of pregnancy if consumed in sufficient amounts. Most heavy metals are embryotoxic but only mercury, lead, cadmium and possibly nickel and selenium have been implicated in this regard. Lead toxicity has long been known to be associated with abortion and menstrual disorders. Evidence as to whether lead is teratogenic is conflicting; some authors report a correlation between atmospheric lead levels and congenital malformations, while others deny these associations.

BELIEFS, AVOIDANCES, CRAVINGS AND AVERSIONS

Most women change their diets during the course of pregnancy. Some changes are based on medical advice, others on folk medical beliefs, and others on changes in preference and appetite which may be idiosyncratic or culturally patterned. Since those which are culturally sanctioned will affect a woman's willingness to follow prescribed dietary regimes, the health care provider should be sensitized to their existence.

Another important group of beliefs surrounds dietary means by which the mother can ensure an easier delivery. Most important of these, from the biomedical viewpoint, are beliefs that lead a woman to avoid animal protein foods or to avoid "excessive" weight gain. Most lay people know very well that a smaller weight gain during pregnancy produces a smaller fetus; since a smaller baby may be "easier to deliver," low weight gain has been proposed as desirable, especially since it is commonly believed that the baby can "catch up" after birth.

Food avoidances are the mother's conscious choices not to consume certain foods during her pregnancy, usually for a reason she can articulate and that seems reasonable to her. The four most commonly avoided foods are sources of animal protein: milk, lean meats, pork and liver. Cravings and aversions are powerful urges toward or away from foods, including foods about which women experience no unusual attitudes outside of pregnancy. The most commonly reported craved foods are sweets and dairy products. The most common aversions are reported to be alcohol, caffeinated drinks and meats. However, cravings and aversions are not limited to any particular foods or food groups.

The nutritional significance of these food-related behaviors is difficult to evaluate, since information about them has often been collected in an anecdotal or one-sided manner. The nutritional importance of such practices cannot be assessed without reference to the rest of the individual's diet. Overall, however, most cravings result in increased intake of calcium and energy, while aversions often result in decreased intake of alcohol and caffeine but also decreased intake of animal protein. Cravings and aversions are not necessarily deleterious.

PICA

Pica refers to the compulsion for persistent ingestion of unsuitable substances having little or no nutritional value. Pica of pregnancy most often involves consumption of dirt or clay (geophagia) or starch (amylophagia). However, compulsive ingestion of a variety of non-food substances has been noted, e.g., ice, burnt matches, hair, stone or gravel, charcoal, soot, cigarette ashes, mothballs, antacid tablets, milk of magnesia, baking soda, coffee grounds and tire inner tubes. The practice of pica is not new nor is it limited to any one geographic area, race, creed, culture, sex or status within a culture.

The medical implications of pica are not well understood, although several speculations have been put forward. Non-food substances could displace nutritious foods in the diet, leading to inadequate intakes of essential nutrients. Alternatively, substances that provide calories, such as starch, could lead to obesity if ingested in amounts above the usual dietary intakes. Some substances ingested by those with pica may con-

tain toxic compounds, and others interfere with the absorption of certain mineral elements (e.g., iron). Other less commonly reported complications of pica include (1) congenital lead poisoning secondary to maternal pica for wall plaster, (2) tender, irritable uterus with dystocia associated with fecal impaction from clay ingestion, (3) fetal hemolytic anemia due to maternal pica for mothballs and toilet air fresheners, (4) parotid enlargement and gastric and small bowel obstruction from ingestion of excessive laundry starch, and (5) parasitic infection from ingestion of contaminated soil or clay.

The etiology of pica is poorly understood, although several proposals have been put forth. One theory suggests that the ingestion of non-food substances relieves nausea and vomiting. The example of the dog that will eat dirt or grass during illness is often used to illustrate this theory. Recent research indicates that pica is a normal behavorial response to gastrointestinal upset in rats. It has also been hypothesized that a deficiency of an essential nutrient such as calcium or iron results in the eating of non-food substances that contain these nutrients. When prenatal patients are questioned concerning the reasons for pica, a variety of answers are given, including a taste for clay or the pleasantness of chewing clay and starch; relief of nervous tension or hunger pains; beliefs that clay keeps the baby from being marked at birth, that starch makes the baby lighter in color or that starch makes the baby "slide out" more easily during delivery; and social approval of pica. Many of these reasons are based on superstitions, customs and traditions that are often passed from mother to daughter.

COMPLICATIONS OF PREGNANCY IN WHICH DIET IS A FACTOR

NAUSEA AND VOMITING IN PREGNANCY. Morning sickness or nausea is common during the early months of pregnancy, and the condition usually disappears just as spontaneously as it appears. However, when early pregnancy is characterized by excessive vomiting, an acute protein and energy deficit and the loss of minerals, vitamins and electrolytes may result.

In cases of *pernicious vomiting*, many obstetricians achieve benefits for women by advising the withholding of fluids from one to two hours before and following meals, in addition to the prescription of a dry diet. Frequent small meals consisting of such foods as thickly cooked cereal, Melba toast with jelly, saltines and baked potato, served at two-hour intervals, usually are well tolerated initially. If the food is retained, fluids may be tried one hour before and after the serving of food. A dry, soft diet may be given as soon as all fluids and foods are retained. Fats are often a problem. A low-fat diet should be followed until fats can be tolerated. Fats and fluids, as tolerated, are gradually added to the meals.

The pregnant woman should be told of the importance of eating during this period and be encouraged to eat as much as possible when she is not nauseated. She can be told about ways to include concentrated sources of calories in her diet, which are discussed in Chapter 27. As mentioned on page 254, vitamin B₆ has been proposed as useful in relieving nausea of pregnancy, but this is not recommended routinely.[64]

HEARTBURN. During the latter part of pregnancy, women often complain of heartburn. In most cases this results from the pressure of the enlarged uterus on the stomach, which causes occasional regurgitation of stomach contents. This can usually be relieved by limiting the amount of food consumed at one time.

CONSTIPATION. Pregnant women often develop constipation, most frequently during the latter stages of pregnancy. Causes of this problem include reduced gut motility, physical inactivity and the pressure exerted on the bowel by the enlarged uterus. Increased consumption of fluid and fiber-rich foods eliminates this problem for some women (page 441), but others sometimes find it necessary to use commercial laxatives as well.

CHRONIC HYPERTENSIVE DISEASE. About 30 per cent of women with hypertension during pregnancy will remain hypertensive when pregnancy is over. This chronic hypertension, is frequently confused with toxemia of pregnancy because it is often first diagnosed in a prenatal visit. Difficult decisions must be made in these cases, since therapy differs between them. When chronic renal disease exists, urinary protein losses may be high; dietary supplements usually are not necessary, however, because the urinary losses comprise only about 5 to 7 per cent of the usual protein intake. The general dietary recommendations would include a well-balanced diet containing a mixture of essential nutrients. Sodium restriction to about 2000 mg per day may be indicated in essential hypertension. If diuretics are being used, it should be recognized that potassium as well as sodium will be lost in the urine; for this reason the patient should be counseled as to good dietary sources of potassium, which may be found in Appendix Table 10.

CARDIAC DISEASE. Cardiac diseases during pregnancy are treated in much the same fashion as in the non-pregnant state. Dietary regulation in pregnant cardiac patients is concerned mainly with obesity and vascular congestion as contributory causes of failure, as discussed in Chapter 28. Overweight must be avoided to minimize the work of the heart, and adequate rest is essential.

Sodium and Fluids. The relation of vascular congestion to fluid balance is discussed in Chapter 28. Since sodium and fluids are frequently restricted in certain cardiac diseases, the diet of the pregnant woman requires careful, supervised planning. It must also be kept in mind that sodium retention and intravascular volume expansion are normal in the pregnant woman.

Cholesterol. With the current emphasis on the influence of cholesterol as a cause of vascular sclerosis, it seems appropriate to mention that serum cholesterol values may rise to as high as 350 to 400 mg./dl. during the last trimester of *normal* pregnancy. (The normal serum cholesterol range is approximately 150 to 250 mg./dl., with an average of 180 mg./dl. in the non-pregnant state.)

DIABETES. The diet of the pregnant diabetic woman must be adequate to meet maternal and fetal nutritional needs. Statistics reveal that pregnancy may aggravate uncontrolled cases or may initiate imbalance in controlled ones. Diabetes may exist only during the stress of pregnancy and resolve itself after delivery, a condition called "gestational diabetes." The etiology of "gestational diabetes" is not understood, but it usually can be controlled by diet alone. In the diabetic who is pregnant the instance of toxemia is high, and fetal morbidity and mortality are significantly greater than in normal pregnancy. For instance, respiratory distress symptoms are five to six times more likely to develop in infants of diabetic mothers than in infants of non-diabetic mothers. Successful pregnancy depends upon adequate dietary and insulin management to meet the growth needs of the fetus and to prevent depletion of the mother's nutritional stores. Needs for increased intake go hand in hand with needs for increased insulin. The demands of pregnancy may impose a need for insulin in a diabetic gravid woman whose condition was adequately controlled by diet alone in the non-pregnant state.

There is no fixed rule to determine the amount of insulin administered during pregnancy. Insulin requirements usually increase, but only temporarily. The increase occurs rather abruptly during the fifth month and may last through the ninth month. Frequent changes in the diet and the insulin dosage may be necessary.

Infants born to diabetics are, as a rule, larger than those of non-diabetics. The reason for this is most likely the exposure of the infant in utero to supernormal levels of its own insulin, which in fact is a growth hormone. High insulin levels are caused by the hyperglycemia of the mother; this causes high levels of glucose to cross the placenta. Infants of diabetic mothers also tend to become hypoglycemic shortly after birth. The probability of the infant's becoming hypoglycemic is directly related to the maternal glucose intolerance.

The hazards of labor are increased and in many cases cesarean section is advised. It must be emphasized that unfavorable effects are in proportion to the care the mother receives. Early prenatal care is an important factor.

A major goal in the prenatal period is to avoid large fluctuations in blood sugar during the day, and the appropriate nutritional care is discussed in Chapter 25.

Experience has shown that individualized, expert care is needed for the nutritional management of the pregnant diabetic. On the basis of nutritional history and assessment early in pregnancy, an individually adapted dietary plan should be developed by a skilled nutritionist as part of the health care team.

TOXEMIA (PREECLAMPSIA AND ECLAMPSIA). Toxemia, or pregnancy-induced hypertension, is a syndrome characterized by hypertension, edema, and protein spillage in the urine. It affects about 7 to 8 per cent of the obstetric population, particularly those who are young, pregnant for the first time and of low socioeconomic status. The disease usually develops in the third trimester.

Moderate edema of the lower extremities is fairly common in pregnancy and is not indicative of toxemia. This extravascular fluid is often mobilized in the evening when the woman is lying down, and this results in a tendency to urinate during the night. The swelling of the lower extremities may be caused by the pressure of the enlarging uterus on the veins returning fluid from the legs. When the edema is generalized, however, it would indicate that the kidneys are reabsorbing large amounts of sodium and the control of the extracellular fluid volume has been lost. With generalized edema, there appears to be an increased sensitivity to renin, and some hypertension can be expected to develop.

The etiology of toxemia is still unknown. Nutritional deficiencies, including protein deficiency and calcium deficiency, genetic predisposition and immunologic factors, have been suggested as causes. Most researchers agree that it is associated with a decreased uterine blood flow leading to a reduction in fetal nourishment. Of the nutritional causes, protein deficiency has been linked most frequently to toxemia. However, one study showed that women with toxemia ate more protein than controls.[65] In addition, low protein intakes are often associated with poverty, poor health, poor eating and health habits

and emotional stress, and it may be that in many patients toxemia and protein deficiency occur together because they both result from the same problem. Therefore, the link between protein intake and toxemia is not clear, and evidence of the benefit of a high-protein diet in preventing the disorder is inconclusive.

In years past, attempts to treat toxemia have focused on three nutritional therapies—sodium restriction, diuretics and dieting. Sodium restriction has failed to significantly alter blood pressure, weight gain or proteinuria in gravid women and seems to have no place in treatment or prevention of toxemia. The same can be said for diuretics; use of such drugs does not lower the incidence of toxemia or aid in its management. In fact, it may be dangerous to recommend diuretics for the woman with toxemia since she is known to have a subnormal intravascular volume due to peripheral vasoconstriction. Diuretics would restrict intravascular volume even further through forced kidney diuresis of sodium and water. As with diuretics and sodium restriction, restricted energy intake has not been found to prevent toxemia in pregnant women with high weight gain.

A direct role for nutrition (or malnutrition) in the development of toxemia is still uncertain, but continued observations may confirm a relationship in the future. Since a variety of different nutritional deficiencies have been reported to occur in toxemic women, a complex combination of nutritional deficiencies very possibly could be involved. The increased incidence of toxemia among women of low socioeconomic groups (and theoretically less adequate food supplies) supports this notion, but clearly other factors may play an equally important role. Still, supplementing diets with vitamins and minerals and correcting dietary errors reduces the incidence of toxemia.

MULTIPLE PREGNANCY. The nutritional needs of the woman with more than one fetus theoretically should be greater to support the extra blood volume and placental and fetal tissue. Since no formal evaluation of needs has been reported, specific guidelines cannot be provided. In making recommendations to the woman in this situation, it should be pointed out that her needs are not likely to be twice those of the woman with one fetus but are likely to exceed them by some unknown degree. The energy demand for activity in the third trimester will be sizable, so the level of activity engaged in at this time will impact significantly upon daily energy requirements.

ADOLESCENT PREGNANCY. The overall incidence of adolescent pregnancy has increased steadily in the past several decades despite a declining birth rate in the general population.

Pregnancy among teenagers is a serious public health problem with medical, social, psychological and vocational implications for the mother and baby. Prolonged labor and low-birth-weight infants are more common among adolescents, especially those 14 years old or younger. Adolescents who conceive shortly after menarche seem to be at particular risk. These difficulties probably result from the complex interaction among biological, social and nutritional problems experienced by the pregnant adolescent rather than from one single factor.

Very few good studies on the nutritional requirements of pregnant adolescents have been reported. It is likely, however, that the nutritional needs of the adolescent who conceives before her longitudinal growth is complete are greater than those of girls who are four or more years past the age of menarche. If the growth of the adolescent continues during pregnancy, higher protein intakes are recommended. The needs for energy, vitamins and minerals are also increased for younger pregnant adolescents. The nutritional needs of the younger pregnant woman are discussed on page 312 and can be estimated by using Table 14–5.

FOOD INTAKE DURING LABOR

Patients who are in early labor frequently make the mistake of eating a hearty meal before entering the hospital. They believe erroneously that large amounts of food are required to give strength for parturition.

It has been demonstrated that during labor the stomach does not readily empty itself. It is not uncommon for patients at delivery to vomit food that was ingested 24 to 48 hours previously.

The pregnant patient should be warned against ingestion of solid foods or liquids once labor has commenced. Food particles may remain in the stomach and later on be vomited and aspirated if the woman is anesthetized, thereby causing serious obstructive reactions of the respiratory tract. Suffocation and massive atelectasis may result.

The work of Mendelson,[34a] which showed the possibility of aspiration of liquid stomach contents during anesthesia, has resulted in the hospital practice of omitting all oral feedings during the first stages of labor. If the patient has ingested solid or liquid food recently, he suggests the alkalinization and emptying of the stomach contents prior to the administration of general anesthesia, if the woman has elected to have it during delivery. Should fluid and calorie balance be disturbed in the event of prolonged labor, parenteral feedings may be given.

Breast-feeding

Interest in breast-feeding has increased significantly since the beginning of the 1970's. Prior to that time, formulas were preferred and in many areas were considered the "modern" method of infant feeding. As information about the apparent superiority of human milk has accumulated, enthusiasm for breast-feeding has mounted. Currently more than 50 per cent of U.S. mothers leave the hospital nursing and planning to continue the practice well into the first year of their infants' lives. More than 15 per cent of infants continue to breast-feed well beyond six months of age.[34] While the advantages of nursing vary among mother-infant pairs, those features of breast-feeding that are typically viewed as superior to formula-feeding are defined in Table 11–8. The composition of human milk is discussed in Chapter 12.

The mammary glands prepare for lactation through a series of developmental steps that occur during adolescence and pregnancy. Hormonal changes that take place prior to and during puberty markedly increase breast, areola and nipple size. The major changes involve an increase in connective tissue and fat with limited development of the duct system and alveolar cells. The principal feature of mammary growth in pregnancy is a great increase in ducts and alveoli under the influence of many hormones. Late in pregnancy, the lobules of the alveolar system are maximally developed and small amounts of colostrum may be released for several months prior to delivery. Anatomical features of the human mammary gland are illustrated in Figure 11–10.

With delivery of the infant a dramatic change occurs in the hormonal pattern of the mother. A sudden drop in circulating levels of estrogen and progesterone accompanies a rapid rise in secretion of prolactin. These and other changes set the stage for the formal onset of lactation.

The typical stimulus for milk production and

Table 11–8. PROPOSED ADVANTAGES OF BREAST-FEEDING

1. Breast milk is nutritionally superior to any alternative.
2. Breast milk is bacteriologically safe and always fresh.
3. Breast milk contains a variety of anti-infectious factors and immune cells.
4. Breast milk is the least allergenic of any infant food.
5. Breast-fed babies are least likely to be overfed.
6. Breast-feeding promotes good jaw and tooth development.
7. Breast-feeding generally costs less than the commercial infant formulas currently available.
8. Breast-feeding automatically promotes close mother-child contact.
9. Breast-feeding is generally more convenient once the process is established.

secretion is the suck of the infant at the mother's breast. Nerves beneath the skin of the areola carry a nervous message to the spinal cord, which transmits it to the hypothalamus; from the hypothalamus a message is sent to the pituitary gland where both the anterior and posterior areas are stimulated to release their respective hormones. Prolactin is released from the anterior pituitary for ultimate stimulation of milk production by alveolar cells in the mammary tissue, as shown in Figure 11–11. Oxytocin is released from the posterior pituitary for action on the myoepithelial cells of the mammary gland; these cells are stimulated to contract, causing movement of milk through the duct system and lactiferous sinuses for ultimate arrival in the mouth of the infant. This latter process is referred to as "let-down" and is accompanied in the woman by a distinct sensation described as a "tingling feeling." Since oxytocin also stimulates the muscle cells of the uterus to contract, lactation immediately following delivery is considered useful in assisting in rapid shutdown of bleeding from this tissue.

The process of let-down appears to be sensitive to small changes in circulating oxytocin levels; minor emotional disturbances or environmental stresses may influence the ease with which breast milk is provided to the infant. The

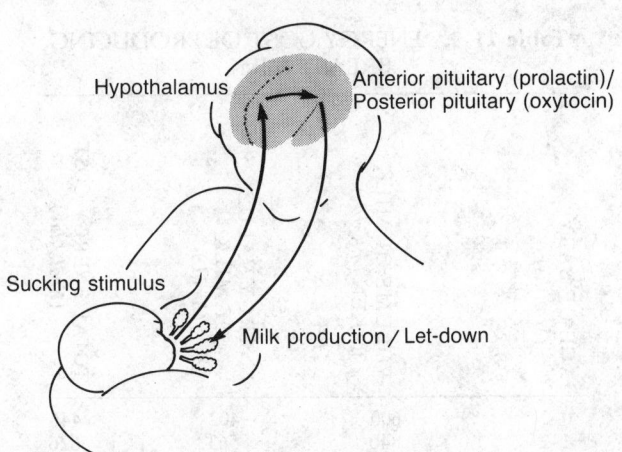

Figure 11–11. Diagrammatic representation of the basic physiological features of milk production and the "let-down" reflex. The sucking stimulus provided by the baby sends a message to the hypothalamus. The hypothalamus stimulates the anterior pituitary to release prolactin, the hormone that promotes milk production by alveolar cells of the mammary glands. The hypothalamus also promotes the release of oxytocin from the posterior pituitary. Oxytocin stimulates the contraction of the myoepithelial cells around the alveoli in the mammary glands. Contraction of these muscle-like cells causes the milk to be propelled through the duct system and into the lactiferous sinuses, where it becomes available to the nursing infant.

attitude of the mother toward the process of breast-feeding is a powerful factor in determining her success at lactation. The support of her husband, physician, nurse, extended family and friends is also an important determinant of the degree of satisfaction and success derived from the breast-feeding experience.

MATERNAL NUTRITIONAL NEEDS

The process of lactation is nutritionally demanding, especially for the woman who fully nurses for a number of months. Increased intake of all nutrients is reasonably advised, as is indicated in Table 11–1. Energy requirements vary in accord with the amount of milk produced, as shown in Table 11–9. A typical woman synthesizing enough milk to meet all nutritional needs of an 11–lb. infant must secrete about 850 ml. of milk providing about 600 kcal. daily. Since human milk is produced with close to 80 per cent efficiency, the requirement for lactation is about 750 kcal. per day. During the early months of lactation, the maternal fat stores accumulated during pregnancy may be drawn upon to satisfy about one third of the daily energy needs for lactation; the RDA for lactation is 500 kcal. per day over the allowance for the non-lactating woman. When the maternal fat pad has been depleted, dietary energy support for lactation must be increased if the mother in-

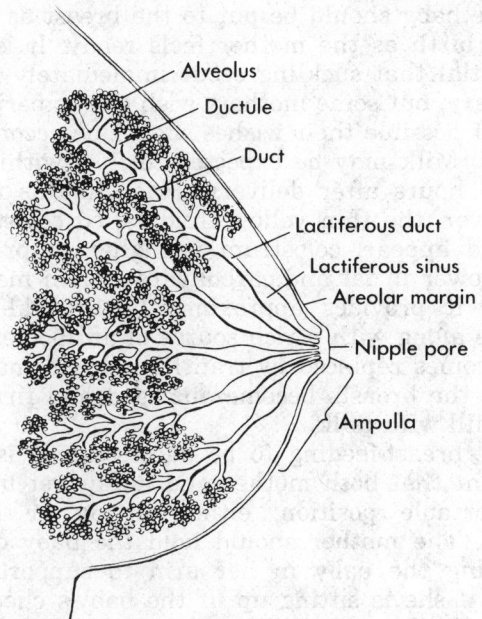

Figure 11–10. Detailed structural features of the human mammary gland showing the terminal glandular (alveolar) tissue of each lobule leading into the duct system, which eventually enlarges into the lactiferous duct and lactiferous sinus. The lactiferous sinuses rest beneath the areola and converge at the nipple pore. (From Worthington-Roberts, B. S., Vermeersch, J., and Williams, S.R.: Nutrition in Pregnancy and Lactation. St. Louis, C. V. Mosby Company, 1981.)

Table 11–9. ENERGY COST OF PRODUCING BREAST MILK

AGE OF BABY (Months)	VOLUME OF MILK TAKEN (ml./day)	ENERGY VALUE OF MILK (Kcal.)	TOTAL ENERGY COST* (Kcal./day)
0–1	600	402	446
1–2	840	563	626
2–3	930	623	692
3–4	960	643	714
4–5	1010	677	752
5–6	1100	737	819

(From Winick, M.: Nutritional disorders of American women. Nutrition Today, *10*:26, 1975.)

*Assuming 90% efficiency.

tends to provide all or most of her infant's nutrition through breast milk alone.

The increased recommended intakes of specific nutrients in the diet largely represent the need to replace in the mother what is lost in her milk. With regard to protein, however, conversion of dietary protein to milk protein is not a process with 100 per cent efficiency; thus, intake of dietary protein must exceed the amount found in the daily milk supply. The RDA for protein for the lactating woman is an additional 30 gm. over that for the non-lactating woman.

IMPACT OF MATERNAL DIET ON MILK COMPOSITION

The influence of maternal diet on the composition of human milk reflects in part the nutritional status of the mother. If the mother's nutritional stores are substantial, consumption of a poor-quality diet for a period of time may have limited impact on the *quality* of the milk she produces; she will draw from her stores if her diet is suboptimal. However, this utilization of maternal stores has obvious limits; this is especially true for water-soluble vitamins, which typically are found in low levels in human milk if the maternal diet is low in these nutrients.

The major effect on lactation of maternal undernutrition is the production of reduced *quantity* of milk each day. Such a consequence may be seen in the nursing mother who takes on a rigorous weight reduction diet while attempting to breast-feed her young infant. Suboptimal *quantity* of milk production may also result from inadequate fluid intake on the part of the mother. Breast-feeding mothers should be dis-

couraged from dieting and encouraged to consume 3 to 4 quarts of fluid daily. They should also be advised that use of oral contraceptives may suppress lactation, especially in the first six to ten weeks.[66]

COUNSELING THE BREAST-FEEDING MOTHER

Preparation

Positive emphasis on the advantages of breast-feeding should be presented early in pregnancy. Women should be encouraged to express their opinions and feelings so that they can be discussed and any misinformation can be corrected. During the last months of pregnancy, counseling on the process of lactation should be made available to women who have decided to breast-feed.[30] Fathers should be encouraged to participate in counseling sessions, since their encouragement and emotional support contribute to successful lactation. Many mothers have never seen a woman nursing an infant; they therefore find it especially helpful to have a woman who has successfully nursed an infant available to answer questions and provide positive reinforcement.

The Technique

The baby should be put to the breast as soon after birth as the mother feels ready. It is not essential that suckling occur immediately after delivery, but some mothers wish this experience and if possible their wishes should be accommodated. Milk may be expected to flow within 48 to 96 hours after delivery. Prior to this time, however, the thin yellow fluid called colostrum should appear; colostrum is higher in protein and lower in fat and carbohydrate than mature milk; it provides approximately 15 kcal. per ounce along with a rich source of antibodies. As it becomes replaced by transitional and mature milk, the breasts become enlarged and firm as they fill with milk.

For breast-feeding to be successful, it is important that both mother and infant get into a comfortable position, either sitting or lying down. The mother should hold the baby close, cradling the baby in her arm to support the head if she is sitting up. If the baby's cheek is touched, the baby will turn toward that side (the rooting reflex). The mother should hold her breast so that the areola and nipple are in the baby's mouth as much as possible, as shown in Figure 11–12. If the breast is very full, it helps to press the breast gently away from the baby's nose so that the infant can breathe more easily. Alternatively, if may be helpful for the mother

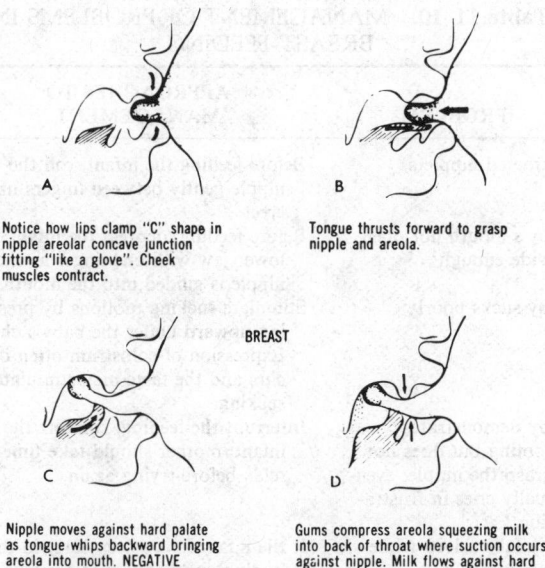

Notice how lips clamp "C" shape in nipple areolar concave junction fitting "like a glove". Cheek muscles contract.

Tongue thrusts forward to grasp nipple and areola.

BREAST

Nipple moves against hard palate as tongue whips backward bringing areola into mouth. NEGATIVE pressure is created by tongue and cheeks against nipple. Suction effect is created.

Gums compress areola squeezing milk into back of throat where suction occurs against nipple. Milk flows against hard palate from high pressure system to negative pressure at back of throat.

Figure 11–12. How the infant breast-feeds.

to express a little milk before letting the baby nurse. The baby should be allowed to nurse from five to ten minutes on each side initially, then longer if both wish. The let-down reflex is detected by a tingling sensation, which is often accompanied by dripping from the opposite nipple and occasionally by uterine cramps. It may take some time for the let-down reflex to become fully functional and conditioned. Some women never feel the let-down, but swallowing by the baby is a definite sign that it has occurred. Rest or a hot shower before nursing may help the let-down reflex. If the woman has too much milk, the baby may need to nurse on only one side at a feeding for a while. This will reduce overall stimulation and reduce the milk supply. This could also be a good time to express milk from the other breast for storage for a future feeding when the mother needs to be away.

To remove the baby from the breast, a finger is placed in the corner of the baby's mouth until the suction is broken. The breast can then be comfortably removed. Most babies need to be burped before feeding from the second breast; the need for burping, however, is highly individual among babies.

Since breast milk is more easily digested than other infant feeds, breast-fed infants may wish to be fed more often than formula-fed babies. If the baby wants to nurse, there is no reason not to let him or her do so; breast-fed babies consume what they need and no more. Breast-feeding whenever the baby is hungry is easy to do because the milk is always ready. Some babies may be hungry as frequently as every hour or two on some days, whereas others may at times not become hungry until four hours after the previous feeding. The more often the baby nurses, the more milk the breasts produce; thus, whenever a woman's supply is low (for example, during or after an illness, provided that there is no risk that the baby will contract the disease through breast-feeding), she should nurse more often.

Parents should realize that crying does not always mean that the baby is hungry. He may be physically uncomfortable or just want to be held, burped or changed. Parents usually learn to distinguish the different needs of their infants.

Feeding time is perfectly suited for establishing and maintaining close mother-child interactions, as shown in Figure 11–13. The mother, however, need not be tied to her infant all of the time. On occasions when she wants or needs to be away from her infant at the usual time of feeding, a bottle can be given. The bottle might contain formula or breast milk that has been expressed earlier. It is best to avoid supplemental bottles other than water until the woman is satisfied that her milk supply is well established and regulated, usually around six weeks postpartum. She should consider taking the baby with her instead. Whenever she wishes to nurse in a public place, she can do it unobtrusively if she is wearing an overblouse or sweater that can be pulled up and a nursing bra with a front opening.

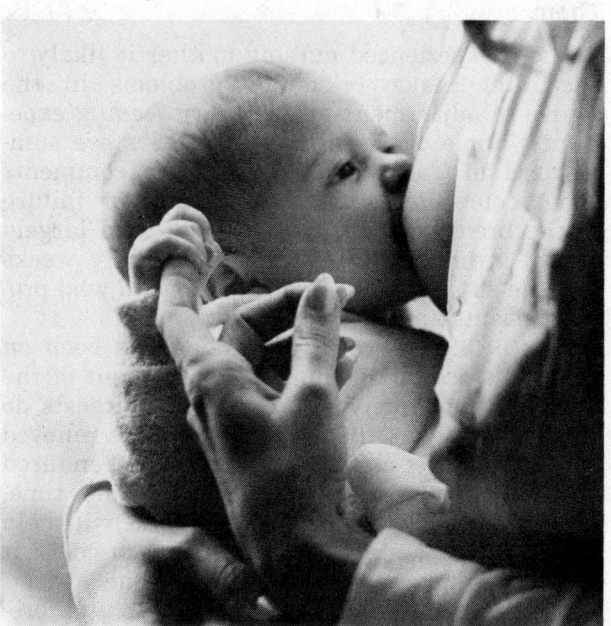

Figure 11–13. A mother and her baby enjoying the close physical contact while nursing. (Photograph copyright Kathryn Abbe, New York.)

Duration of Breast-feeding

The length of time a woman breast-feeds her infant will depend on her own feelings and situation. If she is working, she can continue to breast-feed, using bottles if necessary. Milk will continue to be produced as long as there is demand for it and it is taken from the breast, although a breast may not be emptied at any given feeding.

Some mothers prefer to breast-feed until the baby can be weaned to a cup (thus avoiding bottles altogether); this can be accomplished when the baby is about nine to ten months of age. Some mothers choose to breast-feed much longer—for several years—letting the baby decide when to be weaned. There is a wide variability in ease of weaning, depending on the baby's overall interest in nursing, the relationship between mother and child and the use of bottles. Babies who have had frequent supplemental bottles from birth are likely to wean themselves at an early age.

When a mother decides to wean her baby, it should be done gradually over a period of several weeks. At first, one feeding can be omitted for several days; two feedings may then be skipped until the baby is down to one feeding a day (usually the night or early morning feeding). Eventually this last feeding can be discontinued. Weaning in this gradual manner will be easier on the mother, avoiding engorgement of her breasts, and easier for the baby to adjust to the new routine.

Common Problems and How to Avoid Them

The inexperienced nursing mother is likely to encounter major or minor problems in the course of adjustment to the breast-feeding experience. Some of the initial difficulties are summarized in Table 11–10 along with comments about counseling strategies. Success or failure at the breast-feeding effort may depend largely on the availability of help in the early weeks and the support of a clinician or friend who provides useful tips.

ENGORGED BREASTS. If nursing has been on demand since birth, painful engorgement of the breasts is not likely to occur. If the breasts do become engorged, the discomfort can be relieved by applying wet cloths as hot as can be endured to the whole breast and, at the same time, expressing milk from the nipple. This will help to relieve discomfort. As the wet cloth cools, it should be replaced with another hot one.

To express milk by hand, the thumb and forefinger are placed on opposite sides of the breast just outside the areola, pressed into the rib cage and then squeezed together and downward; the

Table 11–10. MANAGEMENT OF PROBLEMS IN BREAST-FEEDING

PROBLEM	APPROACHES TO MANAGEMENT
Retracted nipple(s)	Before feeding the infant, roll the nipple gently between fingers until erect.
Baby's mouth not open wide enough	Before feeding, depress the infant's lower jaw with one finger as the nipple is guided into the mouth.
Baby sucks poorly	Stimulate sucking motions by pressing upward under the baby's chin. Expression of colostrum often occurs and the taste may stimulate sucking.
Baby demonstrates rooting but does not grasp the nipple; eventually cries in frustration	Interrupt the feeding, comfort the infant; mother should take time to relax before trying again.
Baby falls asleep while nursing	If the infant falls asleep early in the feeding, mother should awaken the infant by holding him upright, rubbing his back, talking to him, or providing similar quiet stimuli; another effort can then be made. If the baby falls asleep again, the feeding should be postponed.

nipple should not be pulled outward. The procedure is repeated, moving the thumb and forefinger around the nipple until as much as desired has been expressed. Sometimes it helps to do breast massage before expressing the milk; this is done by putting the thumbs together on top of the breast and the remaining fingers under the breast. Gentle traction is then exerted from around the breast toward the nipple. If the milk is to be used later, it should be expressed into a sterile bottle and refrigerated. Milk expression is not easy for some women at first, but persistence usually brings success if the mother takes the time.

SORE NIPPLES. The nipples may become sore at the beginning of breast-feeding. This problem may be minimized if the woman toughens the skin of the nipple and surrounding area by massage during the latter months of pregnancy. Nipple rolling is sometimes practiced, or alternatively frequent massage with a bath towel may be useful. During the early days of nursing, soreness may be limited by utilizing a correct nursing position, avoiding undue breast engorgement and gradually increasing the length of time the baby is allowed to nurse. If soreness occurs, it is always temporary and occurs until the nipples become accustomed to the baby's sucking. One of the best ways to relieve the soreness is to expose the nipples to the air. This is done by removing the bra and wearing a loose cotton blouse or shirt. It is also helpful to briefly expose the bare nipples to a sunlamp or the sun. It may also help to apply a soothing oint-ment like lanolin. Persistence in breast-feeding is important because the soreness will be gone in several days. Until soreness subsides, nursing should be initiated on the side that feels the best. Limiting sucking leads to engorgement and increased soreness. However, nursing should be limited to 10 to 15 minutes per side while the soreness persists.

INVERTED (RETRACTED) AND FLAT NIPPLES. Most nipples protrude a bit from the surround-ing areola. Sometimes, however, they look flat, or even go inward partially or completely, as shown in Figure 11–14. These are called invert-ed or "turned in" nipples. Careful examination will determine whether these nipples are truly inverted or not.

Truly inverted nipples can cause serious diffi-culties, but they are very rare. Most of these nipples are just flat and, with patience and care during pregnancy and the first part of breast-feeding, will become normal. If the nipple is pulled out (protracted) but slips away as if it is fastened to the tissues beneath the skin, it is po-tentially functional. If it is truly inverted, it may not be protracted at all. Usually it is possi-ble to pull the nipple out a short way, and such a nipple will stretch when the baby sucks from it. Some flat-looking nipples protract very well.

A truly inverted (non-protractible) nipple can be quite difficult to manage but must be treated if breast-feeding is to be attempted. The first step is to obtain plastic "Woolwich breast shells" as shown in Figure 11–15 or something similar to wear inside the bra. The woman should wear these shells daily over her nipples from the seventh month of pregnancy until term. She must also do the "pulling exercise"— repeatedly pulling the nipple away from the areola. Also, during the early days of feeding she may wish to use a nipple shield. Some wom-

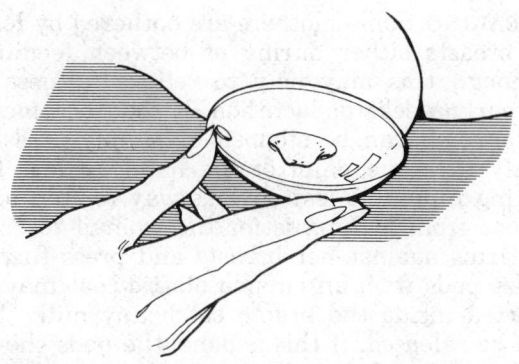

Figure 11–15. Breast shell fitted over the nipple (From Worthington-Roberts, B.S. Vermeersch, J., and Williams, S.R.: Nutrition in Pregnancy and Lactation. St. Louis, C. V. Mosby Company, 1981).

en with flat but protractible nipples may also need to use nipple shells and shields.

PLUGGED DUCTS. Occasionally a milk duct will become plugged, creating a tender spot on the breast which may even appear lumpy and hot. This might result from inadequate empty-ing of the milk ducts or from wearing a bra that is too tight. Should a plugged duct develop, the following approaches might be taken:

1. Offer the sore breast first to the baby so that it will be emptied more completely.

2. Nurse longer and more often; if the breast gets too full, the plugged duct becomes worse and infection may develop.

3. Change positions at every feeding so that the pressure of the nursing will be applied to different places on the breast.

4. Apply warm compresses to the breasts be-tween feedings to reduce the risk of infection.

INFECTION. If breast tenderness is accompa-nied by fever and a general flulike feeling, a breast infection is probably present. Treatment involves bed rest, continued nursing (offering the sore breast first), application of heat with a hot water bottle or heating pad, supporting the breasts with a firm bra and consulting a physi-cian.

There is generally no danger from the baby becoming ill from nursing the infected breast. The same bacteria as those responsible for the infection of the mother are usually already present in the baby's nose and throat. Breast in-fections are sometimes complicated by localized pus accumulation; this is referred to as a breast abscess and may require surgical opening and draining in addition to antibiotics. Women are advised not to nurse on the affected side until the abscess heals. During the interval when the woman is not nursing, the milk should be fre-quently expressed by hand from the affected breast.

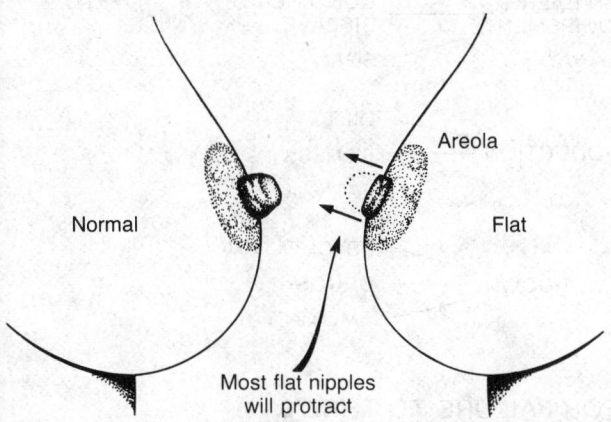

Figure 11–14. Typical appearance of normal and flat nip-ples.

LEAKING. Some mothers are bothered by leaking breasts either during or between feedings. Although this may help to relieve fullness in the early weeks of lactation, it soon becomes a nuisance. It can be stopped by simply pressing firmly with the palm of the hand against the leaking nipple. A less obvious way to stop both breasts from leaking is for the woman to cross her arms against her breasts and press firmly. Gauze pads with an outside plastic coat may be inserted inside the bra to catch any milk that may be released. If this is done, the pads should be changed at frequent intervals.

FAILURE TO THRIVE IN THE BREAST-FEEDING INFANT. Insufficient milk supply is rarely a problem for the well-fed mother. Since sucking stimulates the flow of milk, feeding on demand for adequate duration should supply ample amounts of milk. If the baby continues steadily to gain weight and length, has at least six wet diapers daily and normal stools, the milk supply is probably adequate.

Occasionally, however, an infant will fail to thrive while seemingly nursing properly. A variety of circumstances can be explored as likely bases for the unsatisfactory breast-feeding experience.[30] Figure 11–16 illustrates diagrammatically potential problems in the mother or in the infant that should be investigated during the

course of evaluation. If the cause of the problem cannot be identified or the defined problem cannot be corrected, it may be necessary to encourage the mother to turn to commercial infant formula for at least partial nutritional support of the infant.

RELACTATION AND INDUCED LACTATION. Occasionally a mother starts breast-feeding late or discontinues nursing but decides at a much later date that she would like to begin again. She can attempt "relactation" through providing the infant substantial opportunities to suck at the breast. With much sucking stimulus over several days time, many patient and persistent women can initiate the lactation process late or once again. Their volume of milk production may be less than the infant demands, in which case a supplemental feeding following nursing may be necessary. Alternatively, some women find that the Lact-aid Nursing Trainer* nicely complements their own milk production. While the baby sucks at the breast, he also obtains milk via suction through a small tube leading to a bag of fresh formula that is clipped to the mother's bra. While the baby sucks, he simultaneous-

---

*Lact-aid Nursing Trainer. Available from Resources in Human Nurturing International, 3885 Forest St., P.O. Box 6861, Denver, Colorado 80206.

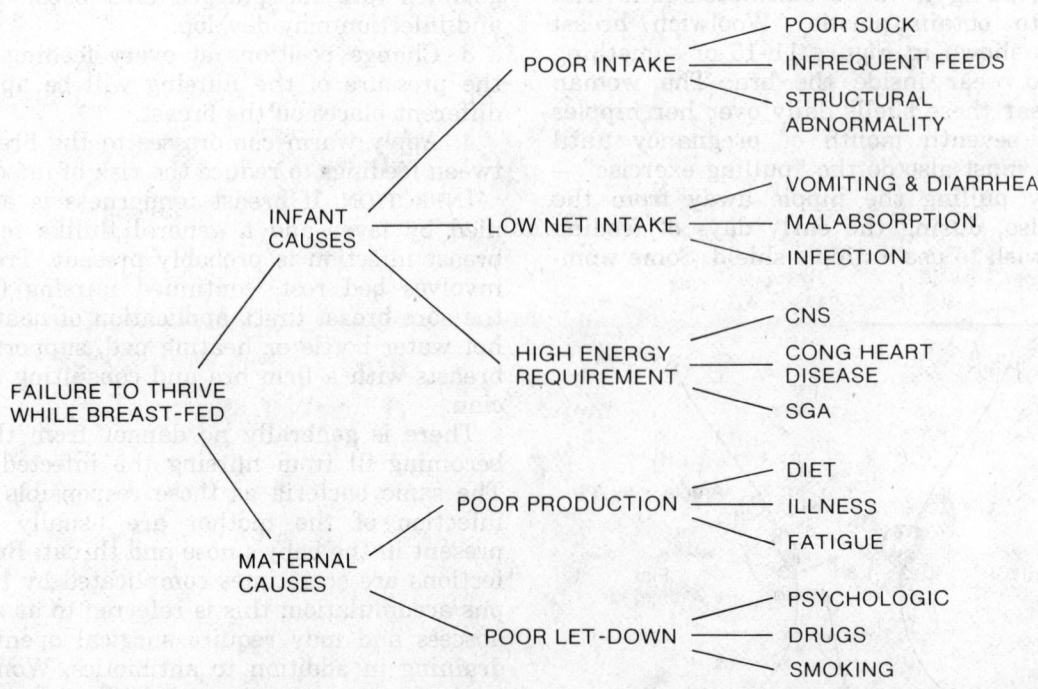

DIAGNOSTIC FLOW CHART FOR FAILURE TO THRIVE

Figure 11–16. Diagnostic flow chart for failure to thrive. CNS = central nervous system problems; SGA = small for gestational age. (From Lawrence, R.: Breast-feeding: A Guide for the Medical Profession, St. Louis, C. V. Mosby Company, 1980.)

ly builds up the mother's milk supply but receives adequate nutrition through the Lact-aid feeding device.

After adopting an infant, a minority of women decide to attempt lactation. Some of these women have never done so before, and others have breast-fed a previous baby of their own. With much sucking stimulus, lactation can be induced, but only with great perseverance and in most cases only if a woman has once carried a pregnancy well into the second trimester. Since the mammary glands complete their development for lactation during the first six months of pregnancy, a woman who has never been pregnant or never carried a pregnancy beyond the first trimester is a poor candidate for successful induction of lactation.

BREAST PUMPING. Mothers may wish to remove milk from their breasts for a number of reasons, for example, to save it for a later feeding, take it to their hospitalized neonate, or donate it to a milk bank. Under such circumstances, some women find it satisfactory to express milk by hand. For many women, however, a manual or electric breast pump provides a better stimulus for milk flow and a more efficient mode of milk collection.* Instructions for use of these pumps accompany each apparatus, but individual counseling by a skilled clinician or experienced nursing mother can greatly simplify the process of learning to pump.

Contraindications to Breast-feeding

The vast majority of women nurse their babies with the knowledge that both of them will profit from the experience. Circumstances exist, however, in which breast-feeding should be discouraged. Usually there is need to consider the details of the individual case. It may be appropriate, however, to discourage nursing in the following situations:

1. The infant has galactosemia. In this case, it is vital that the infant receive an alternative to breast milk, since exposure to galactose (from the lactose in human milk) will lead to serious mental retardation, cataracts and liver damage.

2. The infant has phenylketonuria (PKU). Such infants need a diet low in phenylalanine. Since breast milk contains phenylalanine in higher concentration than is found in the special formula Lofenalac, breast-feeding, if undertaken, should be accompanied by careful monitoring of the infant's blood phenylalanine concentration.

3. The mother must take a drug that passes into her milk and is known or suspected to harm the infant. Table 11–11 lists types of drugs that are excreted in human milk. The mother should check with her physician about the safety in breast-feeding of any drugs she is receiving.

4. The mother has a serious psychiatric disorder or chronic disease.

5. The mother has cancer and is being treated with anti-cancer agents.

6. The mother's food or water supply has been contaminated with "pollutants" such that her milk may be especially high in these compounds and potentially harmful to her infant.

7. The mother honestly does not want to breast-feed but opts to do so to protect herself from suspected scorn from others. Such women should know that infants in the United States can thrive on commercial infant formulas and that they need not feel guilty about choosing this source of nutrition for their infants.

Nutritional Implications of Oral Contraceptives

Millions of women take oral conceptives as a convenient way to extend the period between pregnancies, prevent unwanted pregnancies or delay the starting of a family. Oral contraceptives appear to increase the requirement for several nutrients, in particular folic acid and vitamin B_6, and to a lesser extent riboflavin, thiamin and ascorbic acid. Clinical evidence of deficiency is rare, although vitamin B_6–responsive depression and folate-responsive megaloblastic anemia have been reported. Subclinical deficiency, identified as lowered serum levels of these nutrients, is more common. Table 11–12 lists laboratory and clinical findings that indicate nutritional disturbances caused by use of oral contraceptives.

On the other hand, plasma levels of some nutrients, such as vitamin A, iron and copper, increase. The implications for nutritional requirements in women taking oral contraceptives are unclear. Serum iron may increase because of decreased iron loss that accompanies reduced menstrual flow, commonly associated with oral contraceptive use. Additional discussion of the processes involved in the effects of these drugs on nutritional status can be found in Chapter 21.

The period between pregnancies should be a time of good nutrition not only to offset the effects of oral contraceptives, but also to maintain lactation with no nutritional cost to the mother and to replace any calcium, iron, protein or vi-

---

*A good breast pump is the Kaneson Breast Pump, available from Happy Family Products, 12300 Venice Blvd., Los Angeles, California 90066 and other infant supply stores.

Table 11–11. DRUGS EXCRETED IN HUMAN MILK

DRUG	IMPLICATION FOR MOTHER	IMPLICATION FOR NURSING INFANT
Antibiotics (broad- and medium-spectrum)	Mother should not take certain ones	Sensitization of baby may occur, especially with penicillin Anemia, shock, death Hepatotoxic
Anticoagulants	Mother should not take	Infant can develop serious hemorrhage
Anticonvulsants	No problem except with primidone (Mysoline)	Drowsiness in infant
Antimigraine agents, e.g. ergotamine (Cafergot)	Mother should not take	May cause vomiting, diarrhea, shock and hypertension
Antitumor drugs	Mother should not take	May harm infant's developing cells
Antispasmodics and anti- cholinergics, e.g., trihexyphenidyl (Artane) and nylidrin (Arlidin)	Mother should not take	Diminish lactation and may cause heart irregularities in baby
Aspirin, phenacetin and combinations	Mother should not take	May cause bleeding in infant May cause a macular rash
Hypotensives in combina- tion with diuretics	Mother should not take; may cause galactor- rhea	Hazardous to infant because may cause increased respiratory tract secre- tions, cyanosis, and anorexia
Isoniazid	Mother should not take	Causes mental retardation in infant
Laxatives	Present in milk	Can cause diarrhea in baby
Propanol	Mother should not take	May cause bronchospasm, brady- cardia, hypotension, congestive heart failure and hypoglycemia in baby
Psychotropic drugs	Mother should not take	Drowsiness, other unknown effects in infant
Radioactive iodine	Mother should not be given	Suppresses infant's thyroid
Steroids	Mother should not take; decrease lactation	Decrease lactation and thus infant growth Cause gynecomastia in baby
Thiazide diuretics	Present in milk	May cause dehydration in infant
Urinary anti-infectives	Present in milk; mother should not take sul- fonamides	May be noxious to infant if taken by mother continuously Sulfonamides noxious to infants less than 2 months old.
Vaginal medications (Flagyl vaginal inserts, AVC cream, other sul- fonamides)	Mother should not use	Cause jaundice of newborn

(Adapted from Rothermel, P.C., and Faber, M.M.: Drugs in breastmilk—a consumer's guide. Birth Fam. J., *2*:76, 1975.)

tamin stores that may have been reduced dur- ing pregnancy. An equally important reason is to provide good nutrition for the entire family and to initiate good eating habits in the new family member.

Problems and Suggested Topics for Discussion

1. What are the special nutritional needs during preg- nancy? What kinds and amounts of food supply these needs?
2. Why are diet and good nutrition important during the prenatal period? During lactation?
3. Visit a patient in the prenatal clinic and obtain an av- erage dietary intake for a day. Check diet for nutri- tional adequacy. How does it need to be nutritionally improved?
4. Interview a pregnant woman and learn about her

physical activity. Has it changed, and if so, how? What will this mean for her energy requirements?
5. Visit a patient in the postnatal clinic and obtain an average dietary intake for a day. Check diet for nutri- tional adequacy. Is her weight normal? Help her with the necessary corrections.
6. Visit a patient in your hospital who has toxemia com- plications in her pregnancy. Obtain a listing of her typical dietary intake. Calculate it to determine ade- quacy of protein and other nutrients. Follow the prog- ress of the patient.
7. Assess the nutritional status of a pregnant woman with diabetes. How does her diet need to be modified to handle her situation?
8. How does the diet during lactation differ from that of a non-lactating woman? Take a diet history of a lac- tating woman and assist her with the changes she needs to make in her dietary pattern.
9. Observe a woman nursing her infant. Did she have any problems in early lactation? What were they and how did she handle them?

Table 11–12. NUTRITIONAL ABERRATIONS ATTRIBUTED TO CONTRACEPTIVE STEROIDS

NUTRIENT	EFFECTS OF CONTRACEPTIVES
Folacin	Serum level ↓ Erythrocyte level ↓ Megaloblastic anemia (rare)
Vitamin B_{12}	Serum level ↓
Riboflavin	Erythrocyte level ↓ Glossitis (rare)
Vitamin B_6	Disturbed tryptophan metabolism Plasma PLP ↓ Depression
Ascorbic acid	Leukocyte content ↓ Platelet level ↓
Vitamin A	Plasma level ↑
Iron	Serum level ↑ TIBC ↑
Copper	Plasma copper ↑ Ceruloplasmin ↑
Zinc	Plasma zinc ↓

Cited References

1. Bapurao, S., Raman, L., and Tulpule, P.G.: Biochemical assessment of vitamin B_6 nutritional status in pregnant women with orolingual manifestations. Am. J. Clin. Nutr., 36:581, 1982.
2. Blackburn, M.W., and Calloway, D.H.: Basal metabolic rate and work energy expenditure of mature pregnant women. J. Am. Diet. Assoc., 69:24, 1976.
3. Brookes, O.G., et al.: Vitamin D supplements in pregnant Asian women: effects on calcium status and fetal growth. Brit. Med. J., 1:751, 1980.
4. Burke, B.S., et al.: The influence of nutrition upon the condition of the infant at birth. J. Nutr., 26:569, 1943.
5. Bursey, R.G., and Watson, M.L.: The effect of sodium restriction during gestation on offspring brain development in rats. Am. J. Clin. Nutr., 37:43, 1983.
6. Cavdar, A.O., et al.: Effect of nutrition on serum zinc concentration during pregnancy in Turkish women. Am. J. Clin. Nutr., 33:542, 1980.
7. Churchill, J.A., and Berendes, H.W.: Intelligence of children whose mothers had acetonuria during pregnancy. In Perinatal Factors Affecting Human Development. Scientific Rev. No. 185, Washington, D.C., Pan American Health Organization, 1969, p. 30.
8. Cochrane, W.A.: Overnutrition in prenatal and neonatal life: a problem? Canad. Med. Assoc. J., 93:893, 1965.
9. Coetzee, E.J., Jackson, W.P.U., and Berman, P.A.: Ketonuria in pregnancy with special reference to caloric-restricted food intake in obese diabetics. Diabetes, 29:177, 1980.
10. Committee on Maternal Nutrition, Food and Nutrition Board, National Research Council: Maternal Nutrition and the Course of Pregnancy. Washington, D.C., National Academy of Sciences, 1970.
11. Connolly, K.J., Pharoah, P.O.D., and Hetzel, B.S.: Fe-

tal iodine deficiency and motor performance during childhood. Lancet, 2:1149, 1979.
12. Eastman, N.J., and Jackson, E.: Weight relationship in pregnancy. 1. The bearing of maternal weight gain and prepregnancy weight on birth weight in full term pregnancies. Obstet. Gynecol., 23:1002, 1968.
13. Edwards, L.E., et al.: Pregnancy in the massively obese: course, outcome and obesity prognosis of the infant. Am. J. Obstet. Gynecol., 131:479, 1978.
14. Edwards, L.E., et al.: Pregnancy in the underweight woman: course, outcome and growth patterns of the infant. Am. J. Obstet. Gynecol., 135:297, 1979.
15. Felig, P., and Lynch, V.: Starvation in human pregnancy: hypoglycemia, hypoinsulinemia and hyperketonemia. Science, 170:990, 1970.
16. Felton, D.J.C., and Stone, W.D.: Osteomalacia in Asian immigrants during pregnancy. Brit. Med. J., 1:1521, 1966.
17. Food and Nutrition Board, National Research Council: Recommended Dietary Allowances. 9th ed. Washington, D.C., National Academy of Sciences, 1980.
18. Fratta, I.D., et al.: Fetal death from nicotinamide-deficient diet and its prevention by chlorpromazine and imipramine. Science, 145:1429, 1964.
19. Giles, C.: An account of 335 cases of megaloblastic anemia of pregnancy and the puerperium. J. Clin. Pathol., 19:1, 1966.
20. Giroud, A.: Nutrition requirements of the embryo. World Rev. Nutr. Diet., 18:195, 1973.
21. Glenn, F.B., Glenn, W.D., and Duncan, R.C.: Fluoride tablet supplementation during pregnancy for caries immunity: a study of the offspring produced. Am. J. Obstet. Gynecol., 143:560, 1982.
22. Hurley, L.S.: Developmental Nutrition. Englewood Cliffs, N.J., Prentice-Hall, Inc., 1979.
23. Hytton, F.E., and Leitch, I.: The Physiology of Human Pregnancy. 2nd ed. Oxford, Blackwell Scientific Publications, 1971.
24. Jackson, A.J., and Schumacher, H.J.: The teratogenic activity of a thalidomide analogue EM_{12} in rats on a low zinc diet. Teratology, 19:341, 1979.
25. Jameson, S.: Effects of zinc deficiency in human reproduction. Acta Med. Scand. (Suppl.), 593:1, 1976.
26. Kumar, S.: Effect of zinc supplementation on rats during pregnancy. Nutr. Rep. Intern., 13:33, 1976.
27. Kurppa, K., et al.: Coffee consumption during pregnancy. N. Engl. J. Med., 306:1548, 1982.
28. Laurence, K.M., et al.: Increased risk of recurrence of pregnancies complicated by fetal neural tube defects in mothers receiving poor diets and possible benefit of dietary counselling. Brit. Med. J., 281:1592, 1980.
29. Laurence, K.M., et al.: Double-blind randomised controlled trial of folate treatment before conception to prevent recurrence of neural-tube defects. Brit. Med. J., 282:1509, 1981.
30. Lawrence, R.: Breast-feeding: a guide for the medical profession. St. Louis, C. V. Mosby Company, 1980.
31. Linn, S., et al.: No association between coffee consumption and adverse outcomes of pregnancy. N. Engl. J. Med., 306:141, 1982.
32. Little, R.E., et al.: Decreased birthweight in infants of alcoholic women who abstained during pregnancy. J. Pediatr., 96:974, 1980.
33. Maeder, E.C., Barno, A., and Mecklenburg, F.: Obesity: a maternal high risk factor. Obstet. Gynecol., 45:669, 1975.
34. Martinez, G.A., and Nalenzienski, J.P.: The recent trend in breastfeeding. Pediatrics, 64:686, 1979.
34a. Mendelson, C. L.: The aspiration of stomach contents into the lung during obstetric anesthesia. Am. J. Obstet. Gynecol., 52:191, 1946.
35. Naeye, R.L.: Weight gain and the outcome of pregnancy. Am. J. Obstet. Gynecol., 135:3, 1979.

36. Naeye, R.L., and Chez, R.A.: Effects of maternal acetonuria and low pregnancy weight gain on children's psychomotor development. Am. J. Obstet. Gynecol., *139*:189, 1981.

37. Norkus, E.P., and Rosso, R.: Effects of maternal intake of ascorbic acid on the postnatal metabolism of this vitamin in the guinea pig. J. Nutr., *111*:624, 1981.

38. Pike, R., Miles, J.E., and Wardlaw, J.M.: Juxtaglomerular degranulation and zona glomerulosa exhaustion in pregnant rats induced by low sodium intakes and reversed by sodium load. Am. J. Obstet. Gynecol., *95*:604, 1966.

39. Pitkin, R.M.: Vitamins and minerals in pregnancy: a review. Am. J. Obstet. Gynecol., *121*:724, 1975.

40. Prochownik, M.O.: Über Ernährungscuren in der Schwangerschaft. Ter. Monat., *15*:446, 1901.

41. Pulkkinen, M.O., Salminen, J., and Virtanen, S.: Serum vitamin B_6 in pure pregnancy depression. Acta Obstet. Scand., *57*:471, 1978.

42. Purvis, R.J., et al.: Enamel hypoplasia of the teeth associated with neonatal tetany: a manifestation of maternal vitamin D deficiency. Lancet, *2*:811, 1973.

43. Ramon, L., et al.: Effects of calcium supplementation to undernourished mothers during pregnancy on the bone density of the neonates. Am. J. Clin. Nutr., *31*:231, 1969.

44. Roberts, R.A., Cohan, M.D., and Forfar, J.O.: Antenatal factors in neonatal hypocalcemic convulsions. Lancet, *2*:809, 1973.

45. Roepke, J.L.B., and Kirksey, A.: Vitamin B_6 nutriture during pregnancy and lactation. I. Vitamin B_6 intake levels of the vitamin in biological fluids and condition of the infant at birth. Am. J. Clin. Nutr., *32*:2249, 1979.

46. Roepke, J.L.B., and Kirksey, A.: Effects of vitamin B_6 supplementation during pregnancy on the vitamin B_6 nutriture of previous long term oral contraceptive users and nonusers. Fed. Proc., *40*:863, 1981.

47. Rosenberg, L., et al.: Selected birth defects in relation to caffeine-containing beverages. J.A.M.A., *247*:1429, 1982.

48. Rush, D., Stein, Z., and Susser, M.: A randomized controlled trial of prenatal supplementation in New York City. Pediatrics, *65*:683, 1980.

49. Rush, D., Stein, Z., and Susser, M.: Controlled trial of prenatal nutritional supplementation defended. Pediatrics, *66*:656, 1980.

50. Schuster, K., Bailey, L.B., and Mahan, C.S.: Vitamin B_6 status of low income adolescent and adult pregnant women and the condition of their infant at birth. Am. J. Clin. Nutr., *34*:1731, 1981.

51. Scott, D.E., Whalley, P.J., and Pritchard, D.J.A.: Maternal folate deficiency and pregnancy wastage. II. Fetal malformations. Obstet. Gynecol., *36*:26, 1970.

52. Smith, G.F.D.: Effects of the state of nutrition of the mother during pregnancy and labour on the condition of the child at birth and for the first few days of life. Lancet, *2*:54, 1916.

53. Smithells, R.W., Sheppard, S., and Schorah, C.J.: Vitamin deficiencies and neural tube defects. Arch. Dis. Child., *51*:944, 1976.

54. Smithells, R.W., et al.: Possible prevention of neural-tube defects by periconceptional vitamin supplementation. Lancet, *1*:339, 1980.

55. Smithells, R.W., et al.: Apparent prevention of neural tube defects by periconstitutional vitamin supplementation. Arch. Dis. Child., *56*:911, 1981.

56. Soltan, M.H., and Jenkins, M.H.: Maternal and fetal plasma zinc concentration and fetal abnormality. Brit. J. Obstet. Gynecol., *89*:56, 1982.

57. Stebhens, J.A., Baker, G.I., and Kitchell, M.: Outcome at ages 1, 3, and 5 years of children born to diabetic mothers. Am. J. Obstet. Gynecol., *127*:408, 1977.

58. Streissguth, A.P., et al.: Teratogenic effects of alcohol in humans and laboratory animals. Science, *209*:353, 1980.

59. Taper, L.J., et al.: Zinc and copper retention in pregnant women. Fed. Proc., *40*:855, 1981.

60. Taylor, D.J., and Lind, T.: Haematological changes during normal pregnancy: iron-induced macrocytosis. Brit. J. Obstet. Gynecol., *83*:760, 1976.

61. Tracy, T.A., and Miller, G.L.: Obstetric problems of the massively obese. Obstet. Gynecol., *33*:204, 1969.

62. Vir, S.C., Love, A.H.G., and Thompson, W.: Zinc concentration in hair and serum of pregnant women in Belfast. Am. J. Clin. Nutr., *34*:2800, 1981.

63. Weathersbee, P.S., Olsen, L.K., and Lodge, J.R.: Caffeine and pregnancy: a retrospective study, Postgrad. Med., *62*:64, 1977.

64. Wheatley, D.: Treatment of pregnancy sickness. Brit. J. Obstet. Gynecol., *84*:444, 1977.

65. Williams, C., Highley, W., and Ma, W.: Protein, amino acid and caloric intakes of selected pregnant women. J. Am. Diet. Assoc., *78*:28, 1981.

66. Worthington-Roberts, B.S., Vermeersch, J., and Williams, S.R.: Nutrition in Pregnancy and Lactation. 2nd ed. St. Louis, C.V. Mosby Company, 1981.

Additional References

Chung, R., et al.: Diet-related toxemia in pregnancy. 1. Fat, fatty acids, and cholesterol. Am. J. Clin. Nutr., *32*:1902, 1979.

Critical weight loss in breast fed infants. Nutr. Rev., *40*:53, 1983.

Hambridge, K.M., et al.: Zinc nutritional status during pregnancy: a longitudinal study. Am. J. Clin. Nutr., *37*:429, 1983.

James, N., Laurence, K.M., and Miller, M.: Diet as a factor in aetiology of neural tube defects. Z. Kinderchir., *31*:302, 1980.

Lu, J.Y., et al.: Intakes of vitamins and minerals by pregnant women with selected clinical symptoms. J. Am. Diet. Assoc., *78*:477, 1981.

Meadows, N.J., et al.: Zinc and small babies. Lancet, *2*:1135, 1981.

Naeye, R.L.: Teenaged and pre-teenaged pregnancies: consequences of the fetal-maternal competition for nutrients. Pediatrics, *67*:146, 1981.

Rees, J.M., and Worthington-Roberts, B.S.: Adolescence, nutrition, and pregnancy: interrelationships. In Mahan, L.K., and Rees, J.M. (eds.): Nutrition in Adolescence. St. Louis, C.V. Mosby Company, 1984.

The nutritional value of breast milk from non-pregnant mothers. Nutr. Rev., *39*:308, 1981.

Pritchard, J.A., and McDonald, P.C.: Williams' Obstetrics. 15th ed. New York, Appleton-Century-Crofts, 1976.

Suggestions for Patient Education

Brewster, D.P.: You Can Breastfeed Your Baby. Emmaus, Pa., Rodale Press, 1979.

Brown, J.E.: Nutrition for Your Pregnancy. Minneapolis, University of Minnesota Press, 1983.

Eiger, M.S., and Olds, S.W.: The Complete Book of Breastfeeding. New York, Bantam Books, 1973.

La Leche League International: The Womanly Art of Breastfeeding. Franklin Park, Ill., 1981.

Nutrition in Infancy

PEGGY L. PIPES, M.P.H., R.D.

The first two years of life, characterized by rapid physical and social growth and development, are years in which many changes that affect feeding and nutrient intake occur. Also, the adequacy of infants' nutrient intakes affects their interaction with their environment. Healthy, well-nourished infants have the energy to respond to and learn from the stimuli in their environment and to interact with their parents in a manner which encourages bonding and attachment.

GROWTH AND BODY COMPOSITION

During the first few days of life infants lose weight, but birth weight is usually regained by the seventh to the tenth day of life. Thereafter growth proceeds at a rapid but decelerating rate. Infants usually double their birth weight by four months and triple it by one year of age. The number of pounds gained during the second year approximates the birth weight. Infants increase their length by 50 per cent during the first year of life and double it by four years of age.

Changes occur not only in height and weight but also in the components of tissue. The nitrogen content of the body increases from 2 per cent of body weight at birth to 3 per cent by age four years. Total body fat increases rapidly during the first nine months, but the increments in fat gain show a steady decrease throughout the rest of childhood. Total body water decreases from 70 per cent of body weight at birth to 60 per cent at one year. The reduction is almost entirely in extracellular water, which decreases from 42 to 32 per cent.[11]

DIGESTION AND ABSORPTION

The stomach capacity of infants increases from 10 to 20 ml. at birth to 200 ml. by 12 months, enabling infants to consume more food at a time and at less frequent intervals as they grow older. The rate of emptying depends on the size and composition of the meals. During the first weeks after birth, gastric acidity decreases; for the first few months it is lower than that of adults.

Tryptic activity of duodenal fluids is less in infants than in older children. However, the enzymatic action is sufficient to digest the milk protein ingested by normal infants.

Newborns absorb 85 to 90 per cent of human milk fat, but they sometimes absorb less than 70 per cent of cow's milk fat. However, the fat in infant formulas is modified so that it is absorbed almost as well as that of human milk. Fat digestion is influenced by the placement of the fatty acids on the triglyceride molecule, the length of the fatty acid chains and the degree of saturation, as discussed in Chapter 3. The fatty acid stearic acid is poorly absorbed. Palmitic acid hydrolyzed from the first and third positions on the glycerol moiety are poorly absorbed, while palmitic acid in the second position appears to be well absorbed.[8] Human milk fat has a greater proportion of palmitic acid in the second position than in the first and third. This is thought to be one factor that explains its high absorbability.

The bile acid pool of the infant per unit of body surface area is about one half that of the adult.[26] The absorption of fat begins to reach adult levels between 6 and 9 months of age.

The activity of the enzymes maltase, isomaltase, and sucrase reaches adult levels by 28 to 32 weeks of gestation. Lactase activity increases near term and reaches adult levels by birth. Pancreatic amylase, which digests starch, continues to remain low during the first 6 months after birth. However, if starch is fed before this time, there is usually compensation by an increased activity of salivary amylase.[7] Though usually not of clinical importance, the early introduction of cereal has been known to cause diarrhea in some infants.

RENAL FUNCTION

The newborn has a functionally immature kidney. The concentrating capacity is limited to as little as 700 mOsm./liter in some infants. Others have the concentrating capacity of adults—1200 to 1400 mOsm./liter.[22]

DEVELOPMENT OF FEEDING SKILLS

Infants at birth coordinate sucking, breathing and swallowing, and are prepared to suck or suckle liquids, but not foods with texture. During the first year normal infants develop head control, the ability to move into and sustain a sitting posture, and the ability to grasp, first with a palmar grasp and then with a refined pincer grasp. They develop a mature suck and rotary chewing, progress from being fed to finger feeding. In the second year they learn to independently feed themselves with a spoon. They learn to crawl and then to walk and seek food for themselves.

PSYCHOSOCIAL DEVELOPMENT

Social and psychological development also occurs. Infants form attachments with tactile stimulation, cuddling and loving care. They bond with their parents and learn to interact with other individuals in their environment, and as a result they acquire a sense of self. Their sense of security is optimized when their needs are met in a prompt and loving manner.

Milk for Infants

Human milk is unquestionably the food of choice for the infant. Its composition is designed to provide the necessary energy and nutrients in appropriate amounts. It contains factors that provide protection against certain bacteriological infections. Allergic reactions to human milk are minimal. Many also feel that since parents have no knowledge of how much the child consumes, overfeeding is often avoided when the infant is breast fed. In addition, the closeness of the mother and infant during feeding facilitates attachment and bonding.

Unmodified cow's milk is inappropriate for infants. The tough hard curd is difficult for young infants to digest, and the absorption of cow's milk fat is less than that of human milk, as mentioned on page 273. Cow's milk has a much higher protein and ash content than human milk; this results in a higher renal solute load, which is the excess amount of nitrogenous waste and minerals that must be excreted by the kidney.

Proprietary formulas made from heat-treated non-fat milk are designed so that they provide necessary nutrients in a well-absorbed form for normal infants. Infants allergic to cow's milk may consume a formula prepared from a soy-protein isolate, a casein hydrolysate, or a meat base formula. A variety of other formula and electrolyte replacement solutions are available for infants who have special problems, as shown in Table 12–1.

COMPOSITION OF HUMAN AND COW'S MILK

Human and cow's milk each provide 20 kcal./oz.; however, the nutrient source of the calories is different. Protein provides 6 to 7 per cent of the calories in human milk and 20 per cent of the calories in cow's milk. Sixty per cent of human milk protein is *lactalbumin (whey)*. *Casein* is the main protein in cow's milk, accounting for 80 per cent of its total protein. Casein forms a tough, hard-to-digest curd in the infant's stomach; lactalbumin forms soft, flocculent, easy-to-digest curds. The amino acids taurine and cystine are present in higher concentrations in human milk than in cow's milk. These amino acids may be essential for premature infants.[1]

The carbohydrate lactose provides 42 per cent of calories in human milk and only 30 per cent of the calories in cow's milk.

Lipids provide 50 per cent of the calories in both human and cow's milk. The fatty acid composition of human milk depends on the fatty acids consumed by the lactating mother. There is a smaller proportion of unsaturated fatty acids in cow's milk than in human milk. Monounsaturated oleic acid is the predominant fatty acid in both milks. Linoleic acid, the essential fatty acid, provides 4 per cent of calories in human milk and only 1 per cent in cow's milk. The cholesterol content of human milk is 7 to 47 mg./dl. and is 10 to 35 mg./dl. for cow's milk. Milk from all species contains a serum-stimulated lipoprotein lipase in the cream fraction. This enzyme is inhibited by bile salts. Human milk contains an additional lipase which is found in the non-fat fraction. This enzyme is stimulated by bile salts and it contributes significantly to the hydrolysis of milk triglycerides.

All of the water-soluble vitamins in human milk reflect maternal intake. Cow's milk contains adequate quantities of the B complex vitamins but very little vitamin C. Both milks provide sufficient vitamin A. Human milk, providing 2 IU per liter, is a richer source of vitamin E than cow's milk. Human milk contains five metabolites of vitamin D providing 40 to 50 IU/liter of vitamin D activity.[23] Human milk provides calcium and phosphorus to neonates in a utilizable form. However, the need for additional vitamin D becomes progressively more important with age. Cow's milk is usually fortified with 400 IU per liter.

The quantity of iron in human and cow's milk is small, 0.3 mg./liter. Forty-nine per cent of iron in human milk but less than 1 per cent of iron in cow's milk is absorbed.[18] The bioavailability of zinc in human milk is thought to be 59.2 per cent, compared with 43 to 53.9 per cent

Table 12–1. COMPOSITION OF INFANT FORMULAS PER LITER

MILK OR FORMULA	KCAL.	PROTEIN (gm.)	FAT (gm.)	CHO (gm.)	ASH (gm.)	CALCIUM (mg.)	PHOSPHORUS (mg.)	SODIUM (mg.)	SODIUM (mEq.)	POTASSIUM (mg.)	POTASSIUM (mEq.)	IRON (mg.)	PROTEIN SOURCE	FAT SOURCE	CHO SOURCE	COMMENT
Human milk	750	11	45	70	2.0	340	140	161	7	570	15	0.2	Lactalbumin, casein	Human	Lactose	Protein readily digested; adequate in all nutrients except vitamin D and fluoride
Proprietary Formulas																
Similac	680	15.5	36	72	3.3	510	390	250	11	1200	31	tr.*	Casein	Soy, coconut and corn oil	Lactose	Vitamins and minerals added
Similac with Whey	670	15	36	72	3.4	400	300	240	10	750	19	12	Lactalbumin, casein	Soy and coconut oil	Lactose	Vitamins and minerals added; whey predominant formula for normal infants; vitamins and minerals added
Enfamil	670	15	38	69	3.0	460	345	210	9	680	17	1*	Reduced whey, casein	Mineral, coconut, and soy oils	Lactose	Whey predominant formula for normal infants; vitamins and minerals added
SMA	670	15	36	72	2.5	445	330	150	7	560	14	13	Casein, demineralized whey	Oleo, soybean, safflower and coconut oils	Lactose	Whey predominant formula for normal infants; vitamins and minerals added
Advance	540	20	27	55	3.8	510	390	300	13	1100	28	12	Casein, soy protein	Soy and corn oils	Corn syrup solids	Formula for infants over 6 months of age

Table continued on the following page

Table 12–1. COMPOSITION OF INFANT FORMULAS PER LITER (*Continued*)

MILK OR FORMULA	KCAL.	PROTEIN (gm.)	FAT (gm.)	CHO (gm.)	ASH (gm.)	CALCIUM (mg.)	PHOSPHORUS (mg.)	SODIUM (mg.)	SODIUM (mEq.)	POTASSIUM (mg.)	POTASSIUM (mEq.)	IRON (mg.)	PROTEIN SOURCE	FAT SOURCE	CHO SOURCE	COMMENT
Cow's milk																
Evaporated milk formula†	715	29	32	65	7.0	1027	845	481	20	1235	32	tr.	Casein	Butterfat	Lactose, sucrose	Inadequate in iron and vitamin C
Skim	360	36	1	51	7.0	1210	950	520	23	1450	37	tr.	Casein	None	Lactose	Inappropriate for infants
2%	590	42	20	60	8.0	1430	1120	610	27	1750	45	tr.	Casein	Butterfat	Lactose	Inappropriate for infants
Whole	670	36	36	49	7.0	1220	960	498	22	1440	37	tr.	Casein	Butterfat	Lactose	Inappropriate for infants less than 6 months of age
Special Formulas																
ProSobee	675	20	36	68	4.0	634	502	290	13	824	21	12.6	Soy protein	Soy oil	Corn syrup solids	Vitamins and minerals added; for infants allergic to cow's milk; lactose and sucrose free
Isomil	680	20	36	68	3.8	700	500	300	13	710	18	12	Soy protein	Coconut and soy oils	Sucrose, corn syrup solids	Vitamins and minerals added; for infants allergic to cow's milk
Meat base formula	655	26	32	62	4.5	980	655	268	12	530	14	13	Beef hearts	Sesame oil	Modified tapioca, sucrose	Vitamins and minerals added; for infants allergic to milk and soy protein

Nutramigen	670	22	26	88	5.6	635	475	315	14	685	18	12.6	Casein hydrolysate	Corn oil	Modified tapioca, sucrose	Hydrolyzed casein; lactose-free; vitamins and minerals added; infants allergic to soy and cow's milk may tolerate
Similac PM 60/40	670	15	35	75	2.2	400	200	161	7	580	15	2.6	Casein, demineralized whey	Coconut and corn oils	Lactose	Vitamins and minerals added; for infants in the lower range of homeostatic capacity
Pregestimil	670	22	28	88	6.0	630	470	315	14	680	17	12.6	Casein hydrolysate	MCT† oil, corn oil	Dextrose, modified tapioca	Vitamins and minerals added; protein and fat easily digested; hydrolyzed casein; infants allergic to soy and cow's milk may tolerate; used in malabsorption

*Available with iron supplement (12–13 mg./liter).
†Formula: 13 oz. evaporated milk
2 tbsp. corn syrup
18 oz. water
32 oz. formula total
‡MCT, medium chain triglyceride.

in cow's milk.[14] Cow's milk contains three times as much calcium and six times as much phosphorus as does human milk. The fluoride concentration of cow's milk is twice that of human milk. The fluoride concentration of milk from women living in areas where the water supply contains little fluoride is similar to that of women living in areas where the water is fluoridated.[19] Thus, most of the fluoride in the mother's diet does not pass into her milk in large enough quantities and the diet of the breast-fed infant needs to be supplemented.

The sodium and potassium concentrations of human milk are about one third that of cow's milk. The osmolality of human milk averages 286 mOsm./kg., whereas the osmolality of cow's milk is 400 mOsm./kg.[21]

ANTI-INFECTIVE FACTORS

Human milk and colostrum contain antibodies and anti-infective factors that are not present in cow's milk. Secretory IgA is the predominant immunoglobin in human milk and plays a role in protecting the infant's immature gut from infection.

The iron-binding protein lactoferrin in human milk deprives bacteria of iron and thus slows their growth. Lysozymes, bacteriolytic enzymes found in human milk, destroy bacteria cell membranes after they have been inactivated by the peroxides and ascorbic acid also present in human milk. The growth of the bacterium *Lactobacillus bifidus* is enhanced by breast milk and produces an acidic gastrointestinal environment, which interferes with the growth of certain pathogenic organisms. Because of these anti-infective factors, the incidence of infections is less in breast-fed than in bottle-fed babies.

COW'S MILK–BASED FORMULAS

Infants whose mothers are unwilling or unable to breast feed will usually be fed a cow's milk–based formula or a soy-based product. Those who have special requirements will receive specially designed products.

The Committee on Nutrition of the American Academy of Pediatrics, concerned about the composition of proprietary infant formulas, made a policy statement on standards for these products.[5] These standards are based on the composition of milk from a healthy mother and are shown in Table 12–2. The minimum amount for each nutrient is close to that in human milk and thus is the preferable quantity. The maximum amount is given for formulas intended for low-birth-weight or sick infants who take less formula and, therefore, need the higher nutrient content.

Three formulas made from non-fat milk are available for normal infants. Some formulas have been modified in order to provide a whey:casein ratio similar to that of human milk. These are Enfamil, Similac with Whey, and SMA. Another popular formula, Similac, is made by heat treatment, which reduces the curd tension. Vegetable oils are added so that fat absorption is similar to that from human milk. Vitamins and minerals are re-added to the milk to meet the recommended intake for infants. Formulas are available with and without additional iron.

Evaporated milk formula is used by a few parents for economic reasons. It is made by mixing 3 oz. of evaporated milk, 4.5 oz. of water and 2 tsp. of corn syrup.

One manufacturer markets a formula for the older infant providing fewer kcal./oz. than others but still fortified with all necessary vitamins and minerals (including iron). Table 12–1 shows the composition of various formulas and human milk.

SOY-BASED FORMULAS

A variety of products are available for infants who do not tolerate cow's milk. Soy products designed to meet all the nutrient needs of infants are most often used for infants allergic to cow's milk.

Infants intolerant to soy products also may be fed a formula made from hydrolyzed casein (Nutramigen) or a meat base formula commercially available or prepared at home. Other formulas are available for children with specific problems such as malabsorption or phenylketonuria.

FORMULA PREPARATION

The formulas are available in ready-to-feed forms requiring no preparation, in concentrates prepared by mixing with equal parts of water, and in powders made by mixing 2 oz. of water with each level tablespoon of the powder.

In most households that maintain a reasonable level of sanitation, sterilization of formula is seldom practiced. However, since terminal sterilization is not effective in controlling growth of microorganisms, preparation of one feeding at a time is generally recommended when sterilization is necessary.

All equipment to be used in the formula preparation, including bottles, nipples, mixers and the top of the can of milk, should be thoroughly washed. The infant should be fed immediately after the formula is prepared, and any milk not consumed at that feeding should be discarded. Any open cans of formula should be covered and refrigerated.

Table 12–2. NUTRIENT LEVELS OF INFANT FORMULAS (PER 100 KCAL.)

NUTRIENT	CON 1976 RECOMMENDATIONS			
	Minimum		*Maximum*	
Protein (gm.)	1.8		4.5	
Fat				
(gm.)	3.3		6.0	
(% cal.)	30.0		54.0	
Essential fatty acid (linoleate)				
(% cal.)	3.0		—	
(mg.)	300.0		—	
Vitamins				
A (IU)	250.0	(75 µg.)*	750.0	(225. µg.)*
D (IU)	40.0		100.0	
K (µg.)	4.0		—	
E (IU)	0.3	(with 0.7 IU/gm.	—	
C (ascorbic acid) (mg.)	8.0	linoleic acid)	—	
B$_1$ (thiamine) (µg.)	40.0		—	
B$_2$ (riboflavin) (µg.)	60.0		—	
B$_6$ (pyridoxine) (µg.)	35.0	(with 15 µg./gm. of protein in formula)	—	
B$_{12}$ (µg.)	0.15		—	
Niacin				
(µg.)	250.0		—	
(µg. equiv.)	—		—	
Folic acid (µg.)	4.0		—	
Pantothenic acid (µg.)	300.0		—	
Biotin (µg.)	1.5		—	
Choline (mg.)	7.0		—	
Inositol (mg.)	4.0		—	
Minerals				
Calcium (mg.)	50.0†		—	
Phosphorus (mg.)	25.0†		—	
Magnesium (mg.)	6.0		—	
Iron (mg.)	0.15		—	
Iodine (µg.)	5.0		—	
Zinc (mg.)	0.5		—	
Copper (µg.)	60.0		—	
Manganese (µg.)	5.0		—	
Sodium (mg.)	20.0	(6 mEq.)‡	60.0	(17 mEq.)‡
Potassium (mg.)	80.0	(14 mEq.)‡	200.0	(34 mEq.)‡
Chloride (mg.)	55.0	(11 mEq.)‡	150.0	(29 mEq.)‡

*Retinol equivalents.
†Calcium to phosphorus ratio must be not less than 1.1 nor more than 2.0.
‡Millequivalents for 670 kcal./liter of formula.
From Committee on Nutrition, American Academy of Pediatrics: Commentary on breast feeding and infant formulas, including proposed standards for formulas. Pediatrics, *57*:279, 1976.

Foods for Infants

A variety of commercially prepared foods are available for infants. In fact, there are over 400 different strained and junior foods on the market. However, many mothers prefer to make their own.

There are wide ranges of nutrient values between the food groups and among the foods within the groups, as shown in Table 12–3. Ready-to-serve dry infant cereals are fortified with electrolytically reduced iron, and 10 per cent of this iron is absorbed. Three level tablespoons of cereal mixed with liquid will provide 7 mg. of iron, over half the amount the infant requires. Therefore, cereal is usually the first food added to the infant's diet. Cereal and fruit mixtures in jars are fortified with 5 mg. of ferrous sulfate per 4.5 oz. jar.

Strained and junior vegetables and fruits provide carbohydrate and variable amounts of vitamins A and C. Vitamin C is added to a number of fruits and all of the fruit juices. Several fruits, including apricots, have sugar added and are marketed as fruit desserts. Tapioca is added to a number of the fruits. Milk is added to creamed vegetables and wheat is incorporated into the mixed vegetables.

Strained and junior meats and egg yolk are prepared with only water, except for lamb, which has lemon juice added. The strained meats have the highest caloric density of any of

Table 12–3.   AVERAGE VALUES OF SELECTED NUTRIENTS IN INFANT FOOD
PER 100 GRAMS*

	CALORIES	PROTEIN gm.	IRON mg.	VITAMIN A IU	VITAMIN C mg.
Infant cereals, dry (tbsp.)[†]					
Mixed	13.6	0.57	1.7	—	—
Rice cereal w/bananas	14.0	0.32	1.7	—	—
Strained fruits (per 100 grams [7 tbsp.])					
Pears & pineapple	53	0.4	0.1	29	12.3
Prunes with tapioca	72	0.6	0.3	279	5.1
Strained vegetables					
Green beans	24	1.3	0.5	313	4.1
Sweet potatoes	60	1.2	0.2	7050	9.9
Strained meat					
Beef	94	13.4	1.4	68	2.2
Chicken	140	14.4	1.0	53	2.1
Strained egg yolk	196	9.7	3.1	581	2.3
Strained vegetables and meat					
Vegetables & chicken	48	2.3	0.4	1170	1.2
Macaroni & cheese	63	2.8	0.3	38	1.2
Strained high meat dinners					
Ham with vegetables	78	6.6	0.5	509	1.9
Strained desserts					
Fruit dessert	68	.3	.1	351	1.0
Vanilla custard pudding	82	1.3	0.2	65	0.7

*Except where specified otherwise.
[†]3.55 gm. = 1 tbsp.
From Nutrient Values of Gerber Baby Foods. Fremont, Michigan, Gerber Products Company, 1981. Reprinted with permission.

the commercial baby foods. They are an excellent source of high-quality protein and heme iron.

Water is the most abundant ingredient in vegetable and meat combinations and high meat dinners, and these dinners have a lower caloric density than the pure strained meats or vegetables. The meat and vegetable combinations include a wide variety of ingredients. The introduction of these products should be delayed until it has been ascertained that an infant has no allergic reactions to any of the ingredients in the products.

A number of dessert items are also marketed, including puddings and fruit desserts. All include sugar and modified corn or tapioca starch. The nutrient composition of these products vary, but vitamin A is the major nutrient contributed.

Mothers who wish to make their own baby food can easily do so, as explained in Table 12–4. Home prepared foods generally are more concentrated in nutrients than commercially prepared ones. Parents should be careful to use only fresh foods rather than canned foods to avoid the possibility of lead poisoning. Salt should not be added to foods prepared for infants, and sugar should be added sparingly.

Nutrient Needs of Infants

Nutrient needs of infants reflect rates of growth, energy expended in activity, basal metabolic needs and the interaction of nutrients

Table 12–4.   DIRECTIONS FOR HOME PREPARATION OF INFANT FOODS

1. Select fresh, high quality fruits, vegetables or meats.
2. Be sure all utensils, including cutting boards, grinder, knives, etc., are thoroughly clean.
3. Wash hands before preparing the food.
4. Clean, wash and trim the food in as little water as possible.
5. Cook the foods until tender in as little water as possible. Avoid overcooking, which may destroy heat-sensitive nutrients.
6. Do not add salt. Add sugar sparingly. Do not add honey to food for infants less than 1 year of age.*
7. Add enough water so that the food has a consistency that is easily puréed.
8. Strain or purée the food using an electric blender, a food mill, a baby food grinder or a kitchen strainer.
9. Pour purée into ice cube tray and freeze.
10. When food is frozen hard, remove the cubes and store in freezer bags.
11. Unfreeze and heat in serving container the amount of food that will be consumed at a single feeding (in water bath or microwave oven).

*Botulism spores have been reported in honey and young infants do not have the immune capacity to resist this infection.

consumed. Balance studies have defined minimal acceptable levels of intakes for a few nutrients, but for most nutrients the suggested intakes have been extrapolated from intakes of normal thriving infants. The Recommended Dietary Allowances (RDA) for infants are shown in Table 12–5.

ENERGY

The RDA suggest an energy intake for infants of 115 kcal./kg. in the first six months, 105 kcal./kg. in the second six months, and 100 kcal./kg. for ages one to three years. Normal infants who are breast fed to satiety and infants fed a standard 20 kcal./oz. formula whose mothers are sensitive to their cues of hunger and satiety will generally adjust their intake to meet their energy needs.

The best way to determine the adequacy of infants' energy intakes is to carefully monitor their gain in height and weight. When these values are plotted on the growth grids shown in Appendix Tables 15 and 17, one can visualize if their energy intakes are supporting an appropriate weight gain for linear growth. It is important to recognize that during the first year one may see "catch up" or "lag down" in growth. Infants who are genetically determined to be larger than indicated by their birth weight will shift channels of growth in the first three to six months of life. Those whose genotypes are for smaller size tend to grow at their fetal rate and a growth "lag down" becomes evident. They may be 13 months old before their appropriate growth channel is evident.[25] This is demonstrated in Figure 12–1.

Growth in height and weight should proceed at approximately the same rate. If an infant begins to reduce his rate of weight gain, does not gain weight, or loses weight, the energy and nutrient intake should be carefully monitored. If the rate of growth in height is reduced or ceases, the probability of malnutrition and/or undetected disease should be thoroughly investigated. If weight gain proceeds at a much more rapid rate than growth in height, investigation should be made regarding the calorie concentration of the formula, the quantity of formula consumed and the amount and type of semisolids and table food offered the baby.

Difficulties in achieving adequate intake or concerns about excessive intake may occur when the infant is fed a calorically dilute or concentrated milk or formula. Infants fed a calorically dilute milk such as non-fat milk, or formula to which more water than instructions indicate has been added, will increase their intake of milk but not enough to insure an adequate intake of nutrients, and adequate weight gain will not occur.

Excessive weight gain may occur when the baby is fed a concentrated formula. If the formula is concentrated because insufficient water has been added to the powder concentrate, infants will become thirsty and cry. Parents may think that their infant is crying for food and offer more of the concentrated formula. This will result in an inadequate intake of water and an excessive energy intake and weight gain.

Studies have shown that the type of feeding— breast or bottle—and the age at which semisolid foods are introduced are not etiological factors in infantile obesity.[27] Factors that appear to be important in obesity are the family attitudes toward feeding, parental recognition of cues of hunger and satiety, and the mother's confidence in her own parenting skills and bonding with the baby. Signs of satiety are listed in Table 12–6.

PROTEIN

Protein requirements during infancy, when there is rapid growth, are higher on a per kilogram basis than those of the adult or older child. Nitrogen from protein must be provided for the formation of new tissue, the maturation of tissue, and the maintenance of tissue.

The efficiency of utilization of the protein of mother's milk by the infant is assumed to be 100 per cent. Based on the composition of human milk (Table 12–1), the requirements for

Table 12–5.   RECOMMENDED DAILY ALLOWANCES FOR CHILDREN, BIRTH TO AGE 3 YEARS

AGE (YEARS)	0.0–0.5	0.5–1.0	1–3
Energy needs (kcal.)	kg. × 115	kg. × 105	1300
Protein (gm.)	kg. × 2.2	kg. × 2.0	23
Vitamin A (μg. RE)*	420	400	400
Vitamin D (μg.)†	10	10	10
Vitamin E (mg.)‡	3	4	5
Vitamin C (mg.)	35	35	45
Thiamin (mg.)	0.3	0.5	0.7
Riboflavin (mg.)	0.4	0.6	0.8
Niacin (mg.)	6	8	9
Vitamin B_6 (mg.)	0.3	0.6	0.9
Folacin (μg.)	30	45	100
Vitamin B_{12} (μg.)	0.5	1.5	2.0
Calcium (mg.)	360	540	800
Phosphorus (mg.)	240	360	800
Magnesium (mg.)	50	70	150
Iron (mg.)	10	15	15
Zinc (mg.)	3	5	10
Iodine (μg.)	40	50	70

*Retinol equivalents. 1 retinol equivalent = 1 μg. retinol or 6 μg. β-carotene.

†As cholecalciferol. 10 μg. cholecalciferol = 400 IU of vitamin D.

‡α-Tocopherol equivalents. 1 mg. d,α-tocopherol = 1 α TE.

From Food and Nutrition Board, National Research Council: Recommended Dietary Allowances. 9th ed. Washington, D.C., National Academy of Sciences, 1980.

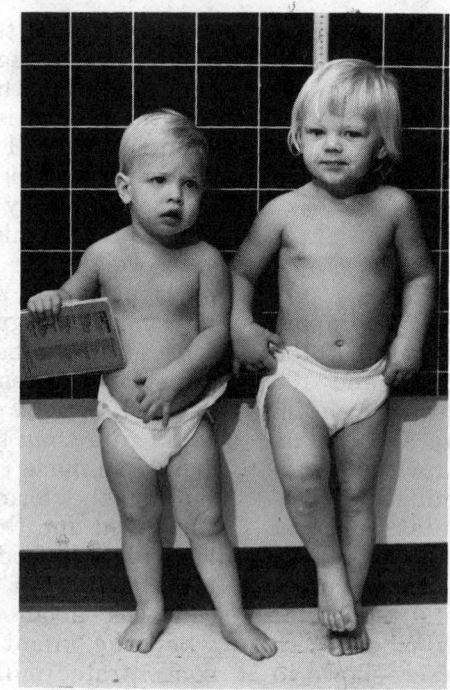

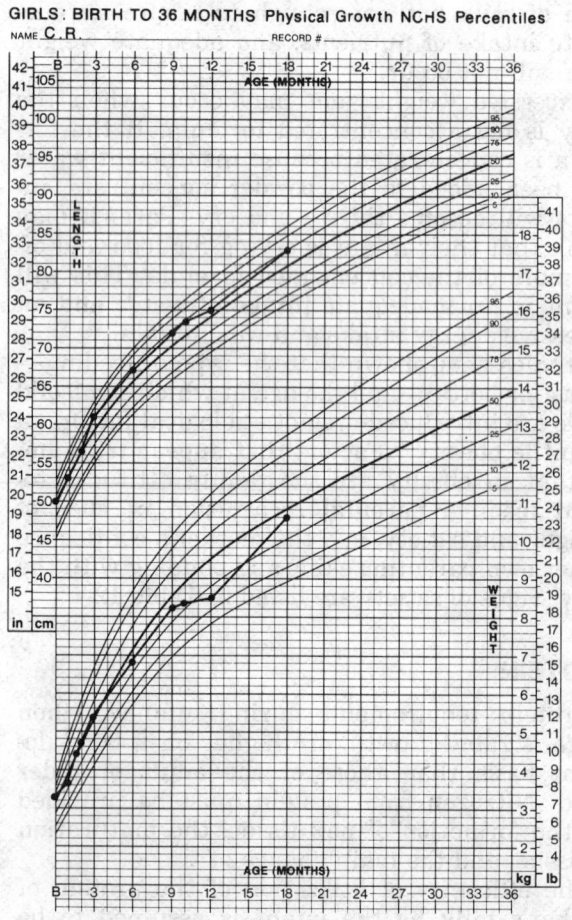

GIRLS: BIRTH TO 36 MONTHS Physical Growth NCHS Percentiles

NAME C.R. _____ RECORD # _____

Provided as a service of Ross Laboratories

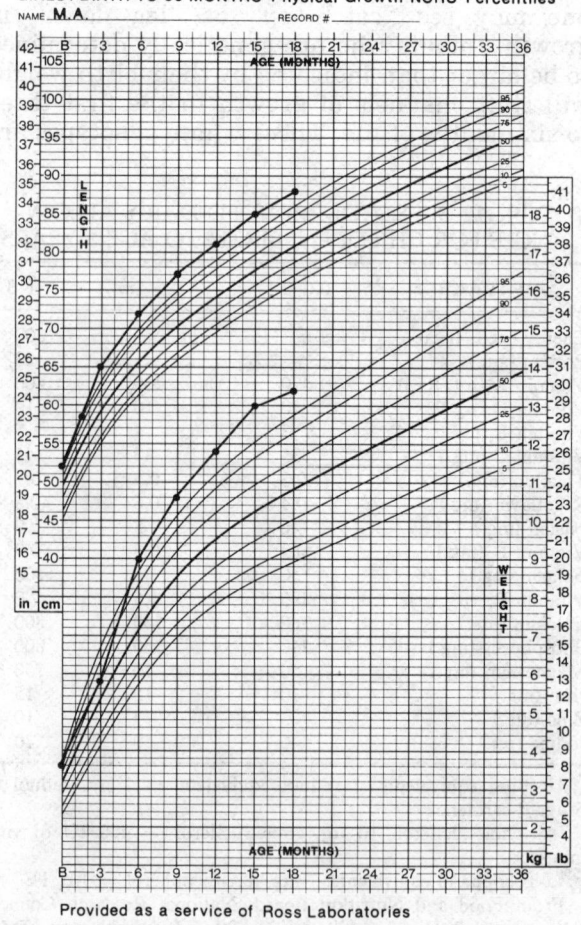

GIRLS: BIRTH TO 36 MONTHS Physical Growth NCHS Percentiles

NAME M.A. _____ RECORD # _____

Provided as a service of Ross Laboratories

Figure 12–1. *See legend on opposite page*

Table 12–6. SATIETY BEHAVIORS IN INFANTS

4–12 weeks	Draws head away from the nipple
	Falls asleep
	When nipple reinserted, closes lips tightly
	Bites nipple, purses lips, or smiles and lets go
16–24 weeks	Releases nipple and withdraws head
	Fusses or cries
	Obstructs mouth with hands
	Increased attention to surroundings
	Bites nipple
28–36 weeks	Changes posture
	Keeps mouth tightly closed
	Shakes head as if to say "no"
	Plays with utensils
	Hands become more active
	Throws utensils
40–52 weeks	Behaviors of above period
	Sputters with tongue and lips
	Hands bottle or cup to mother

Adapted from Gesell, A., and Ilg, F. L.: Feeding Behavior of Infants. Philadelphia, J. B. Lippincott Company, 1937. Reprinted with permission from Pipes, P. L.: Health care professionals. In Garwood, G., and Fewell, R.: Educating Handicapped Infants. Rockville, Maryland, Aspen Systems, 1982.

protein are 1.6 gm. per 100 kcal. from birth to age 4 months, 1.4 gm./100 kcal. from 4 to 12 months of age, and 1.2 gm./kg./day from 12 to 36 months of age.[10] The RDA on the basis of body weight for the first 6 months is 2.2 gm./kg. and from 6 months to 1 year of age 2.0 gm./kg. *Histidine,* an essential amino acid for the infant, is needed in addition to the eight amino acids required by the adult. The minimum requirement is 34 mg./kg./day and is amply supplied by human or cow's milk as well as by the standard formulas. *Tyrosine* and *cystine* may also be essential for the premature infant.[1] To allow for proteins of lower biological value than those of human milk as in infant formulas, the advisable intakes of protein are 1.9 gm./100 kcal. for infants 0 to 4 months of age, 1.7 gm./100 kcal. for infants 4 to 12 months of age and 1.4 gm./kg./day for infants 12 to 36 months of age.[9]

Human milk or formula provides the major portion of protein ingested during the first year of life. Although there is much less protein in human milk than in formula, the amount in human milk is perfectly adequate for the first six months. Parents of breast-fed infants should add additional sources of high-quality protein such as cereal mixed with milk, egg yolk or strained meats to their infants' diets in the last six months of the first year.

Kwashiorkor (protein-energy malnutrition) has been described in infancy and the early preschool years in families who experience extreme poverty. Other reasons for inadequate intakes are varied and include excessive dilution of formula, continuation of a regimen designed to treat diarrhea after an enteric illness, and extreme vegetarian food patterns.[4, 24] See Chapter 4 for further discussion.

LIPID

It is recommended that infants consume a minimum of 3.8 gm./100 kcal. and a maximum of 6.0 gm./100 kcal. of fat (30 to 54 per cent of calories).[9] This quantity is present in human milk and all formulas prepared for infants. If the fat intake is significantly less than this, as in the case of skim milk feedings, the infant may have a deficient intake of calories. He or she may try to make up the caloric deficit by increasing the volume of milk, but usually cannot make up the entire amount. Even if the infant can take the increased volume needed to make up the calories, he or she may become dehydrated because of the high renal solute load resulting from excessive protein, calcium and phosphorus intake from skim milk.

On the other hand, a high fat intake (40 per cent or more of the calories), particularly from poorly absorbed butterfat, will also result in an inadequate caloric intake. The infant unable to digest the excessive amounts of fat will lose the calories from the unabsorbed fat. This typically happens in the infant who at an early age (less than six months), is fed only homogenized milk or evaporated milk without added carbohydrate.

Linoleic acid is essential for growth and dermal integrity. Young infants lacking this fatty acid in their diet have been reported to develop thickening and dryness of the skin, oozing in the body folds and eruptions in the diaper region as shown in Figure 3–4. Three per cent of the total calories should be provided by linoleic acid. Five per cent of calories in human milk and 10 per cent of calories in most infant formula are derived from linoleic acid.

Controversy exists as to whether infants should consume unsaturated in preference to saturated fats and whether their intakes of cholesterol should be limited in order to prevent atherosclerosis. Human milk is a relatively rich source of cholesterol, and some therefore believe

Figure 12–1. These two little girls, born just one month apart with only a one-pound difference in birthweight, show a marked difference in rates of growth and appearance. Note the early catch-up growth shown in the growth grid for M.A. to above the 95th percentile in height and weight prior to 3 months of age. Also note the effect of illness on both weight gain and linear growth in C. R. at age 12 months and the subsequent catch-up growth. The photograph shows the two girls at approximately 20 months of age. (Growth grids adapted from National Center for Health Statistics: NCHS Growth Charts, 1976. Monthly Vital Statistics Report. Vol. 25, No. 3, Supp. (NRA) 76–1120. Health Resources Administration, Rockville, Maryland, June, 1976. Data from The Fels Research Institute, Yellow Springs, Ohio. Courtesy of Ross Laboratories, Columbus, Ohio.)

it may be essential in infancy and that a cholesterol challenge in the first year might be necessary to initiate a cholesterol degrading mechanism. This has not been proved. Infants who receive commercial formula that is very low in cholesterol have been found to have cholesterol levels at the ages of four and seven years that reflect their dietary intake.[12]

CARBOHYDRATE

Carbohydrate should supply 30 to 60 per cent of the energy intake during infancy. Thirty-seven per cent of the calories in human milk and 40 to 50 per cent of the calories in proprietary formulas are derived from lactose or other carbohydrates. A rare infant may not tolerate lactase and a special diet would be required, as discussed in Chapter 39. Eighty per cent of the calories in commercially prepared baby foods selected by the typical parent are from carbohydrate.

Honey, which is sometimes used in home-prepared foods, has been identified as the only food source of *Clostridium botulinum* spores in infants' diets. These spores are extremely resistant to heat treatment and are not destroyed by present methods of processing honey. Botulism in infancy is caused by ingestion of these spores, which germinate and produce toxin in the lumen of the bowel. Honey should not be fed to infants less than one year of age because they do not have the immunity to resist the botulism spore development.[2]

WATER

The water requirement is determined by the amount lost from the skin and lungs and in the feces and urine. In addition, a small amount of water is needed for growth. The National Research Council recommends an intake of 1.5 ml./kcal./day. Water requirements per kilogram are shown in Table 12-7.

Infants have a relatively greater demand for water than adults. The renal concentrating capacity of the young infant may be less than that of older children and adults; therefore, the infant is vulnerable to water imbalance. Human milk and properly prepared formula supply adequate water and under ordinary conditions additional water is not needed. During very hot, humid conditions the infant may require additional water. When a formula is boiled the water evaporates and the solutes become concentrated. Therefore, boiled milk or formulas are inappropriate for infants. When other than renal losses of water are high, as in cases of vomiting and diarrhea, infants should be carefully monitored for both fluid and electrolyte balance.

Table 12-7. WATER REQUIREMENTS OF INFANTS AND CHILDREN

	AMOUNT OF WATER
AGE	(ml./kg./day)
1 week	80–100
2 weeks	125–150
3 months	140–160
6 months	130–155
9 months	125–145
1 year	120–135
2 years	115–125

Adapted from: Vaughan, V. C., McKay, R. J., and Behrman, R. E. (eds.): Nelson Textbook of Pediatrics. 11th ed. Philadelphia, W. B. Saunders Company, 1979.

Water intoxication, which occurs when excessive quantities are fed to infants, results in hyponatremia, restlessness, nausea, vomiting, diarrhea, and polyuria or oliguria. Convulsions can result. This may happen if water is fed as a replacement for milk or if the formula is excessively diluted.[20]

MINERALS

CALCIUM. Recommendations for intakes of calcium have been planned to meet the needs of infants fed cow's milk–based formula who retain approximately 25 to 30 per cent of their intake. Breast-fed infants will retain approximately two thirds of their intake of calcium. The recommended intake of 360 to 540 mg./day is not applicable to breast-fed infants, whose calcium needs are fully met on lower intakes than this.

It is recommended that the calcium:phosphorus ratio in the infant's diet be 1.5:1, decreasing to 1:1 by one year of age. The ratio of calcium to phosphorus in human milk is 2:1, and in cow's milk 1.2:1.

IRON. Normal infants have adequate stores of iron for growth up to a doubling of their birth weight. This occurs at approximately four months of age in full-term infants, and at a much earlier age in prematurely born infants. Recommended intakes of iron increase from 10 mg. per day in the first six months to 15 mg. per day until three years of age. The high bioavailability of iron in human milk makes it an asset during infancy. However, both breast-fed infants and those fed formula should receive an additional source of iron by four to six months of age. Iron-fortified formula and cereals are the most commonly used food sources.

Fresh cow's milk has been shown to be associated with a small but chronic gastrointestinal blood loss that can lead to anemia. Therefore, fresh cow's milk should not be used before the child is six months of age and preferably not until after the first year of life. Daily intake should not exceed 24 to 32 oz. per day when the child is six months to one year old.

ZINC. Normal newborns have no reserves of zinc but are born with tissue concentrations that approximate those of adults. They are therefore immediately dependent on a dietary source of zinc. Although there are not sufficient data to determine the zinc requirements for the human infant, the RDA has been set at 3 mg. per day for the first six months of life and 5 mg. per day for the second six months. For the second year, the RDA is increased to 10 mg. and remains at this level throughout childhood. Human milk and infant formulas provide adequate zinc for the first year of life, and other foods should provide most of the zinc required during the second year.

FLUORIDE. The importance of fluoride in the prevention of dental caries has been well documented. Human milk contains little fluoride, and commercially prepared formulas are made with non-fluoridated water. Therefore infants who are breast-fed, those who consume ready-to-feed formula and those whose formulas are prepared with non-fluoridated water should receive supplemental fluoride. Suggested dosages are shown in Table 12–8.

VITAMINS

Milk from an adequately fed lactating mother will supply all the vitamins that the term infant needs except for vitamin D. Breast-fed infants should receive a vitamin D supplement or be regularly exposed to sunlight. Commercially prepared infant formulas are fortified with all necessary vitamins. Both evaporated and homogenized cow's milk are fortified with vitamin D but have very little vitamin C. Fresh goat's milk is deficient in vitamin D, vitamin C and folate.

A number of vitamin deficiencies have been reported in infants fed formula products in which nutrients were destroyed or omitted during processing. In addition, symptoms of vitamin deficiency have been found in infants fed

products deficient in a specific vitamin who were not given supplements and in infants who were fed by a lactating mother whose diet was inadequate and who was not taking appropriate vitamin supplements.

In the early 1950's infants fed a formula autoclaved during manufacture were found to be pyridoxine-deficient. It was later found that vitamin B_6 was destroyed during processing.[6] A similar incident was reported again in the early 1980's when a manufacturer neglected to add vitamin B_6 during manufacturing of the formula. Fortunately there are very few such instances; however, when formula-fed infants are noted to have symptoms of vitamin deficiency such errors must be considered.

Most infants can tolerate cow's milk or soy formulas. However, a small number who have been intolerant to cow's milk and soy milk and have had multiple food intolerances have been able to tolerate goat's milk as their only food for long periods in infancy. When their diets have not been supplemented with folate these infants have failed to thrive.

The fact that human milk contains only 40 to 50 IU/liter of vitamin D activity makes it important to supplement breast-fed infants with this nutrient. Cases of rickets have often been diagnosed in breast-fed infants with dark skin and little exposure to sunlight.[3]

Milk from lactating mothers who follow a strict vegan diet may be vitamin B_{12} deficient, especially if the mother has followed the regimen for a long time prior to and during the pregnancy. Also, vitamin B_{12} deficiency has been diagnosed in an infant breast fed by a mother with pernicious anemia.[13, 15]

The vitamin K nutriture of the newborn requires special attention. A deficiency may develop and result in bleeding or "hemorrhagic disease of the newborn." This is more common in breast-fed infants because breast milk contains only 15 μg. of vitamin K per liter, while cow's milk and cow's milk formulas contain approximately four times that amount. Breast-fed infants consume less milk during the first few days of life than do formula-fed infants, which also accounts for their low vitamin K intake. It is recommended that all formulas contain a minimum of 4 μg. vitamin K per 100 kcal. of formula. The suggested intake of 12 μg. per day can be supplied by mature breast milk (15 μg./liter), although perhaps not during the first few days to one week of life. Vitamin K supplementation may be necessary during that time.

Vitamin and mineral supplements should be prescribed after careful evaluation of the infant's intake and exposure to sunlight. Infants fed commercially prepared formula rarely need supplements. Breast-fed infants need additional vitamin D by two months of age. Infants fed ho-

Table 12–8. SUPPLEMENTAL FLUORIDE DOSAGE SCHEDULE (mg./day*)

AGE	CONCENTRATION OF FLUORIDE IN DRINKING WATER (ppm.)		
	< .3	0.3–0.7	> 0.7
2 weeks to 2 years	0.25	0	0
2 to 3 years	0.50	0.25	0
3 to 16 years	1.00	0.50	0

*2.2 mg. of sodium fluoride contains 1 mg. of fluoride.

From Committee on Nutrition: Fluoride supplementation: revised dosage schedule. Pediatrics, 63:150, 1979.

mogenized milk or an evaporated milk formula need a food source or supplement of vitamin C, and those who receive goat's milk need a food source or supplement of vitamin C, vitamin D and folate. Chapter 37 discusses the feeding of premature or high-risk infants and their special needs.

Feeding the Infant

Because human milk from a mother who consumes an adequate diet is uniquely designed to meet the needs of the human infant, breast feeding for the first six months is strongly recommended. Many mothers find the experience a very pleasing one because it offers an opportunity for skin to skin contact with their babies. This is obvious in Figure 12–2. The fact that milk is always available and at the right temperature is also felt to be an advantage.

There are few contraindications to breast feeding. Most chronic medical conditions do not contraindicate breast feeding. However, infectious diseases of the mother that require isolation from others may be a contraindication to breast feeding. Maternal breast cancer does contraindicate breast feeding because treatment for the cancer should begin immediately.

Some mothers view breast feeding as inconve-

nient or as having other disadvantages. It is more confining because mothers must feed their babies or express milk from their breasts at regular intervals. The very modest woman may find breast feeding embarrassing. Other reasons women may elect not to breast feed include concern that breasts will enlarge, a need to return to work, and concern that the infant will not sleep through the night as soon as he otherwise might.

A mother should be encouraged to nurse her infant immediately after birth. She may need help in establishing lactation and finding a comfortable position for herself and her infant. Those who care for and counsel parents during the first postpartum days should acquaint themselves with ways in which they can be supportive. Ideally counseling and preparation start in the last few months or weeks of pregnancy, as is discussed in Chapter 11.

During the first few days the baby will receive *colostrum,* a yellowish transparent fluid. This liquid, constructed to meet the needs of the infant during the first week, contains more protein but less fat and carbohydrate than mature milk. It has greater concentrations of sodium, potassium and chloride than later milk.

Infants who are bottle fed will most likely receive ready-to-feed formula in the hospital. Since these products are stored at room temperature they are generally fed at this temperature. When infants are at home, products that have been refrigerated, such as concentrated formula, should be mixed with warm water or heated to body temperature in a water bath. Refrigerated ready-to-feed formula will need to be warmed also.

Regardless of whether the infant is breast fed or bottle fed, the baby should be held and cuddled during feeding, as shown in Fig. 12–3. Once a feeding rhythm is established, infants will become fussy or cry to indicate hunger; often they will smile and fall asleep when they are satiated. Infants, not adults, should establish their feeding schedules. Most will initially feed at intervals of two to three hours, and by two weeks of age the majority of infants will have extended the intervals between feedings to four hours. By age two months sufficient maturation has occurred that most infants omit the night feeding.

A pattern of tooth decay that involves the upper and sometimes lower posterior teeth is common among infants and children who are given sugar-sweetened beverages or fruit juice in a bottle at bedtime. When infants suck these liquids as they go to sleep, the fluid remains in the mouth a long time, allowing bacteria to grow, and dental caries are often the result. Infants should be fed, burped and put to bed without food.

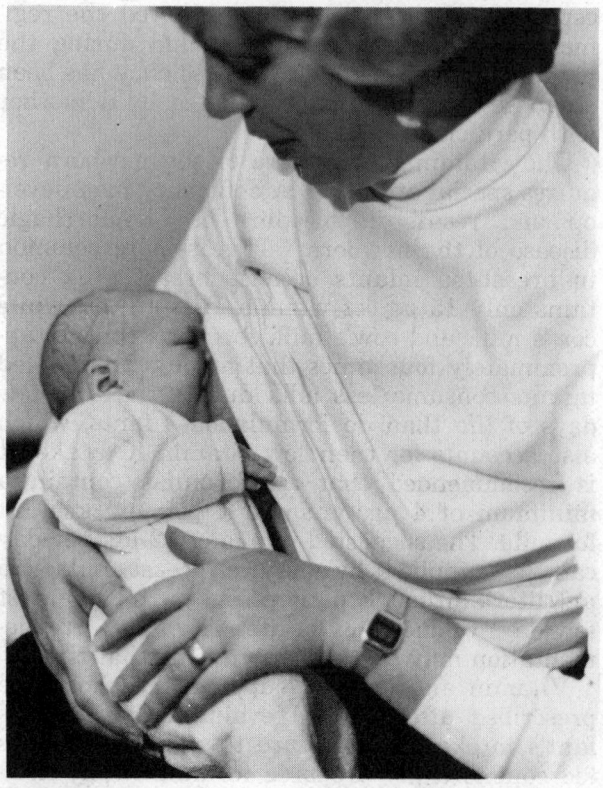

Figure 12–2. A mother and baby both enjoy breast-feeding.

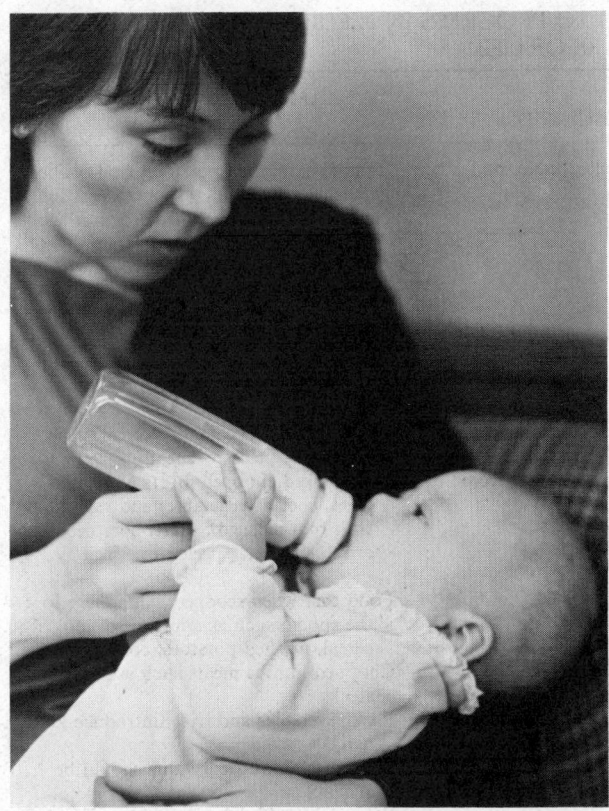

Figure 12–3 Feeding is a time of much interaction between mother and baby.

Although it is generally recommended that infants receive human milk or iron-fortified formula for the first year, many parents make the transition from formula to fresh cow's milk when the infant is between five and nine months of age. If there is concern about a very rapid weight gain, infants may be offered a formula prepared for the older infant that provides only 54 kcal./100 ml. or about 16 kcal./oz., as shown in Table 12–1. Low-fat (2 per cent) and non-fat milk are inappropriate feedings for the first year of life.

THE ADDITION OF SEMISOLID FOODS

That infants can and do consume pureed foods during the first few weeks of life and thrive was proven by the increasingly early ages that semisolids were introduced to infants between 1950 and 1970. Recommended ages for the introduction of foods ranged from three days to four months. In the last decade a more reasonable approach to the introduction of semisolid foods has been taken using developmental readiness as well as nutrient needs as criteria for the addition of various foods. Table 12–9 lists developmental landmarks and their indica-

tions for progression in semisolid and table food introduction. In terms of ages, the first four months are marked by postural maturation so that the infant attains head and neck control and can remain sitting if placed there. Oral motor patterns change from a suck to a suckling to beginnings of a mature sucking pattern. During this phase of development, the infant is prepared to suck and suckle liquids. If pureed foods are fed they are consumed in the same manner as liquids, with each suckle followed by a tongue thrust swallow.

Between four and six months of age, the mature suck is refined and munching movements (up and down chopping motions) begin. Infant cereal is usually introduced first because it offers a good source of iron. Thereafter, a variety of commercially or home prepared foods may be offered. The sequence in which these foods are introduced is not important. What is important is that only one food, e.g., peaches rather than peach cobbler with many ingredients, be introduced at a time.

As oral-motor maturation proceeds, infants' rotary chewing develops, indicating a readiness for more textured foods. Many foods from the family menu, such as well-cooked mashed vegetables, casseroles and pasta, can be successfully consumed. At the same time, babies have learned to grasp first with a palmar grasp, then an inferior and finally a refined pincer grasp. This indicates a readiness for finger foods such as oven-dried toast, arrowroot biscuits or cheese sticks. Table 12–10 gives recommendations for adding foods to the infant's diet.

During the last quarter of the first year, babies can approximate their lips to the rim of the cup. This makes it possible for them to drink from a cup if it is held by their parents.

During the second year they gain the ability to rotate their wrists and elevate their elbows. They feed very messily at first, but by two years most normal infants are skillful self-feeders, as shown in Figure 12–4.

FEEDING THE OLDER INFANT

Most young infants grow rapidly, have an excellent appetite, and parents or grandparents find it a delight to feed them, as is obvious in Figure 12–5. However, as maturation proceeds and the rate of growth slows down, infants' interest in and approach to food change. Between 9 and 18 months most reduce their milk intake. They become finicky about what and how much they will eat. They may go on food jags and learn from the models set for them. Parents need to become sensitive to their baby's stage of growth and development and to create an envi-

Table 12–9. DEVELOPMENTAL STAGES OF READINESS TO PROGRESS IN FEEDING BEHAVIORS DURING FIRST TWO YEARS OF LIFE.

DEVELOPMENTAL LANDMARKS	CHANGE INDICATED	EXAMPLES OF APPROPRIATE FOODS
Tongue laterally transfers food in the mouth Voluntary and independent movements of the tongue and lips Sitting posture can be sustained Beginning of chewing movements (up and down movements of the jaw)	Introduction of soft, mashed table food	Tuna fish; mashed potatoes; well-cooked mashed vegetables; ground meats in gravy and sauces; soft diced fruit such as bananas, peaches, pears, etc.; liverwurst; flavored yogurt
Reaches for and grasps objects with scissor grasp Brings hand to mouth	Finger feeding (large pieces of food)	Oven-dried toast, teething biscuits, cheese sticks, peeled Vienna sausage (food should be soluble in the mouth to prevent choking)
Voluntary release (refined digital grasp)	Finger feeding (small pieces of food)	Bits of cottage cheese, dry cereal, peas, etc., small pieces of meat
Rotary chewing pattern	Introduction of more textured food from family menu	Well-cooked chopped meats and casseroles, cooked vegetables and canned fruit (not mashed), toast, potatoes, macaroni, spaghetti, peeled ripe fruit
Approximates lips to rim of the cup	Introduction of cup	
Understands relationship of container and contained	Beginning self-feeding (messiness should be expected)	Food that when scooped will adhere to the spoon, such as applesauce, cooked cereal, mashed potatoes, cottage cheese
Increased rotary movements of the jaw	More skilled at cup and spoon feeding	Chopped fibrous meats such as roast and steak
Ulnar deviation of wrist develops		Raw vegetables and fruit (introduce gradually)
Walks alone	May seek food and get food independently	Food of high nutrient value should be available
Names food, expresses preferences; prefers unmixed foods Goes on good jags Appetite appears to decrease		Balanced food intake should be offered (child should be permitted to develop food preferences without parents being concerned that they will last forever)

From Pipes, P.: Nutrition in Infancy and Childhood. St. Louis, C. V. Mosby Company, 1981.

Table 12–10. SUGGESTED AGES FOR THE INTRODUCTION OF JUICE, SEMISOLID FOODS AND TABLE FOODS

FOOD	AGE (MONTHS)		
	4 to 6	6 to 8	9 to 12
Iron-fortified cereals for infants	Add		
Vegetables		Add strained	Gradually delete strained foods, introduce table foods
Fruits		Add strained	Gradually delete strained foods, introduce chopped well-cooked or canned foods
Meats		Add strained or finely chopped table meats	Decrease the use of strained meats, increase the varieties of table meats
Finger foods such as arrowroot biscuits, oven-dried toast		Add those that can be secured with a palmar grasp	Increase the use of small-sized finger foods as the pincer grasp develops
Well-cooked mashed or chopped table foods, prepared without added salt or sugar			Add
Juice or formula by cup			Add

From Pipes, P.: Nutrition in Infancy and Childhood. St. Louis, C. V. Mosby Company, 1981.

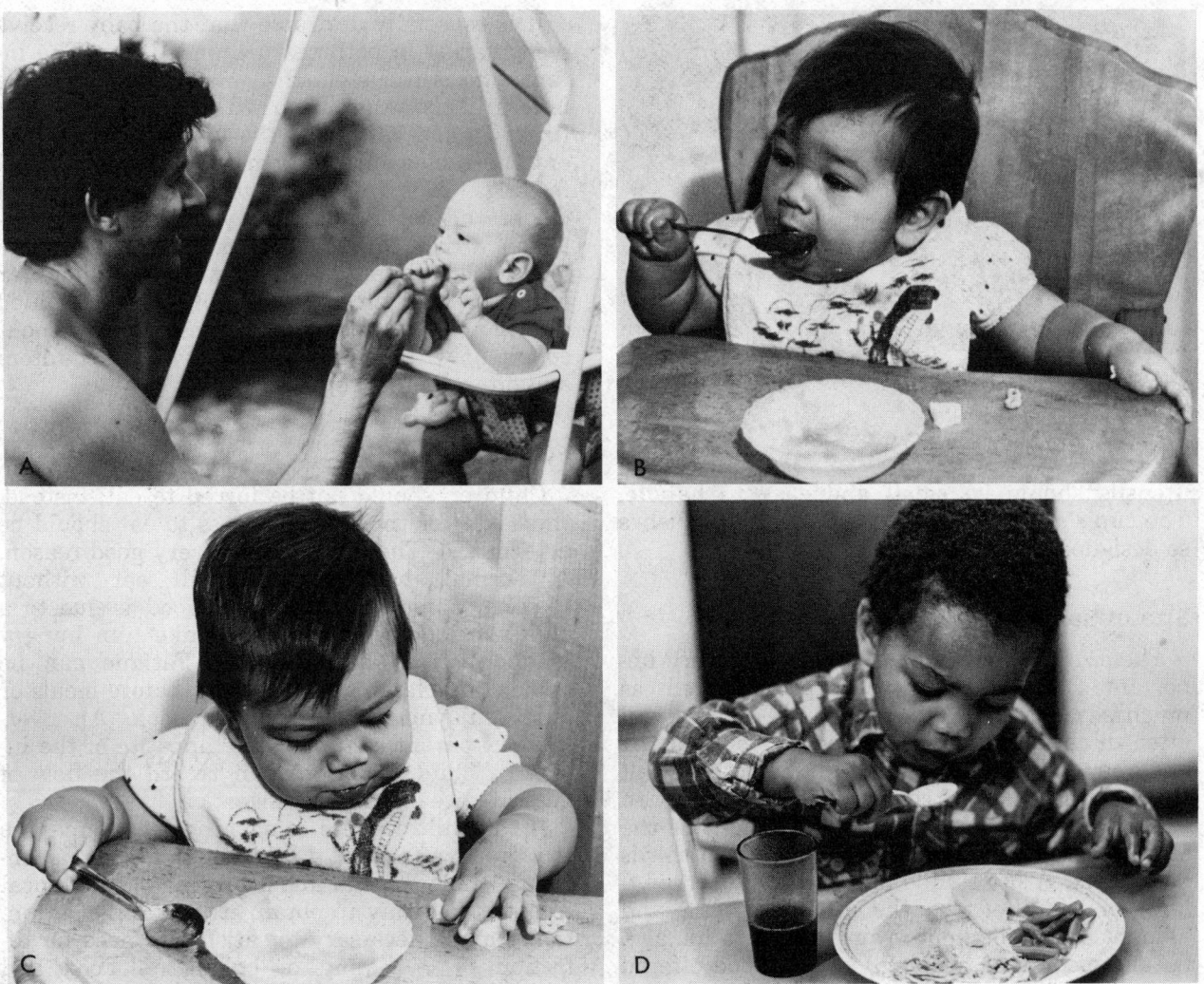

Figure 12–4. Development of feeding skills in infants and toddlers. *A,* At seven months this child shows beginning involvement with feeding and is reaching for the spoon. *B,* At nine months this little girl is beginning to use her spoon independently, although she is not yet able to keep food on it. *C,* Here the nine-month-old shows a refined pincer grasp to pick up food. *D,* The two-year-old is much more skillful at self-feeding, with the ability to both rotate the wrist and elevate the elbow to keep food on the spoon.

ronment in which he can develop sound and satisfying food habits.

In the weaning stage, infants have to learn many manipulative skills, including chewing and swallowing solid food and learning to use utensils. They learn to eat a variety of textures and flavors of food, to finger feed and then to feed themselves. Very young children should be encouraged to feed themselves. They will spill and scatter the food at first but should be encouraged to keep on trying (see Table 12–9). Too much help and attention from the mother or health care professional will slow down the child's efforts because he dislikes being interfered with and will build up his resistance to eating. Eating will cease to be fun.

At the beginning of a meal, the child is hungry and should be allowed to feed himself; when he becomes tired, he can quietly be helped. Emphasis on table manners and the fine points of eating should be left until later when he has matured and developed enough to be ready for it. If he wants to eat with his fingers instead of the spoon—let him! But if he plays with the food, just squeezing it or daubing it on himself and furniture, it should be put out of reach.

The food should be in a form that is easy to handle and eat. Meat should be cut into bite-sized pieces, potatoes and vegetables mashed so that a spoon can be used easily. Raw fruits and vegetables should be in sizes that can be picked up in the hands. In addition, the dishes and

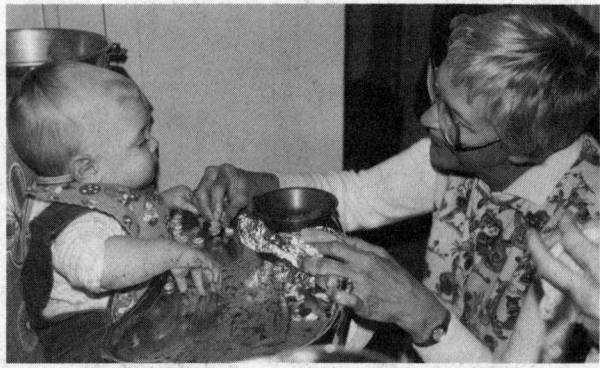

Figure 12–5. Grandparents and relatives often enjoy feeding the infant.

utensils should be small and easy to handle. The cup should be easy to hold and other dishes so designed that they do not tip over easily.

Size of Servings

The size of servings offered a child is very important. Children cannot be expected to eat as much as an adult. A large serving of food will often discourage the dainty, fastidious eater. At one year, babies will eat one third to one half the amount an adult consumes. This proportion rises to one half or a little more by the time the child reaches age three and to about two thirds by age six. A little child should not be served a large plate full of food; the size of the plate and amount should be kept in proportion to his age. A tablespoon (not heaping!) of each food offered for each year of age is a good guide to follow. Serving him less than you think or hope he will eat helps a child to eat successfully and happily. He will ask for more food if his appetite is not satisfied.

Type of Food

In general, children prefer simple, uncomplicated foods. Lowenberg found that a stew in which vegetables and meat were ground and cooked together was considerably more popular with young children than one with separate pieces of vegetables and meat.[16] It was found that children ages two to six years often prefer raw to cooked vegetables and fruits. Food from the meal planned for adult members of the family may be adapted for the child and served in child-size portions. Highly seasoned sauces should be omitted from the child's plate. Children under six years of age usually prefer mild-flavored foods. Because the young child's stomach is small, he may require a snack between meals. Fruit, cheese, crackers, fruit juices and milk contribute nutrients as well as energy.

It is especially desirable that the baby receive foods varied in both texture and flavor. The infant who is accustomed to many kinds of foods is less likely to grow up with definite food dislikes. To add variety to the infant's diet, different vegetables and fruits may be added to cereal feedings. It is important to offer a variety of dishes and not to allow the youngster to continue on a diet consisting of one or two favorite foods. Older infants generally reject unfamiliar foods the first time they are offered. Continued offering of small portions of these foods without comment will achieve familiarity with the item and often their acceptance.

FORCED FEEDING

Children should not be forced to eat; instead, the cause for the unwillingness to eat should be determined. They may have a very good reason. A normal, healthy child will eat without coaxing. Sometimes refusal of food is due to a child's being too inactive to make him hungry or too active and overtired. Fatigue can be avoided by planning a short rest before meals or quiet enjoyment of a picture book. An overanxious parent can affect the appetite of the infant or child. Emotions can retard the flow of gastric juice and inhibit digestion.

If the child refuses to eat, the reason may be too much attention. Children enjoy the attention of their parents and soon learn that refusal to eat is one way to obtain it. Seeking of attention may be necessary to satisfy the need for affection or a feeling of belonging. Food and eating contribute to cultural and emotional life as well as to physiological needs. Food contributes to the basic concepts infants and children form of the world in which they live, the people in it and their relationship to them.

If a child refuses to eat, the meal should be completed without comment and the child's plate removed. At the next mealtime he or she will be hungry enough to enjoy the food presented. The procedure is usually harder on the parent than on the child. However, the parent can display affection toward the child to prevent a feeling of not belonging.

WHERE THE CHILD SHOULD EAT

Children should eat their meals at the family table. They then have an opportunity to learn table manners while enjoying meals with a happy, well-established family group. Sharing the family fare strengthens ties and makes mealtime a pleasant period. However, if the adult meal is delayed or there are adult guests, the child should receive his meal at the usual time. If the child has young visitors, he may wish to

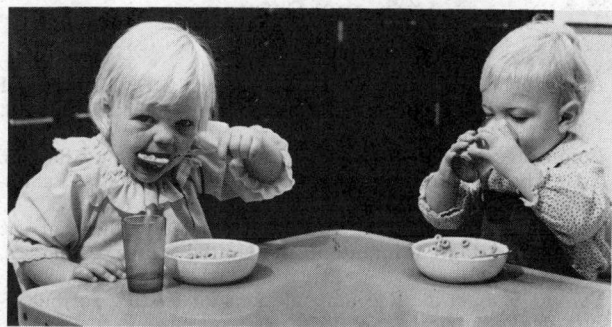

Figure 12–6. Eating with friends is enjoyable and often improves a child's intake.

entertain them at his own little table at the usual meal hour, as shown in Figure 12–6.

As the child eats with the family, everyone must be careful not to make unfavorable comments about any food. Children are great imitators of someone they admire, so if father turns up his nose at squash, for example, they are likely to do the same. Parents sometimes have to learn to eat what they want their infant to eat.

Developmental Growth

As the infant grows in height and weight, he is also making progress in what he does with his body and mind. He gains in understanding and body coordination. This is developmental growth. No two babies develop at the same rate; each sets his own pace. Each is influenced by his environment, to which he reacts according to his own capacities. However, all babies follow the same general pattern, as shown in Figure 12–4.

Infants should be encouraged to develop their natural desire to explore by being given surroundings and care that allow freedom for using their abilities. Let a baby finger and explore the food as much as he wishes. It is part of his development to find out the feel of scrambled eggs and oatmeal as well as their taste and smell. Food texture is important in forming likes and dislikes. It is possible that infants consider whether this or that food is worth chewing by feel and appearance, in much the same way that we look upon taste as a criterion in judging a meal.

Problems and Suggested Topics for Discussion

1. Make a survey of the formulas used for babies in your hospital. List the contents of the various formulas. What type of milk is used most frequently as the basis of the formula?
2. Observe for one week the feeding habits of a breast-fed and a bottle-fed newborn. How often is each infant fed? How much milk does the bottle-fed baby consume at a feeding?
3. List the benefits of breast-feeding over bottle-feeding.
4. Make a study of the following proprietary foods; dried milk, vegetable-protein formulas, liquid whole milk, and meat-base formula. Compare cost and food values. What are the major factors that determine the feeding used?
5. When are supplementary foods usually added to the infant's diet? List the order in which the various foods may be introduced and the reason for giving each.
6. What is meant by developmental growth? Do all infants develop at the same rate? Explain.

Cited References

1. Alfin-Slater, R. B., and Jelliffe D. B.: Nutritional requirements with special reference to infancy. Pediatr. Clin. N. Am. 24:3, 1977.
2. Arnon, S. S., et al.: Honey and other environmental risk factors for infant botulism. J. Pediatr. 94:331, 1979.
3. Bachrach, S., Fisher, J., and Parks, J. S.: An outbreak of vitamin D deficiency rickets in a susceptible population. Pediatrics 64:871, 1979.
4. Chase, H. P., et al.: Kwashiorkor in the United States. Pediatrics 66:972, 1980.
5. Committee on Nutrition, American Academy of Pediatrics: Commentary on breast feeding and infant formula including proposed standards for formulas. Pediatrics 57:279, 1976.
6. Coursin, D. B.: Convulsive seizures in infants with pyridoxine deficient diet. JAMA, 154:406, 1954.
7. Filer, L. J. (ed.): Dynamics of Infant Physiology and Nutrition. Bloomfield, New Jersey, Health Learning Systems, 1982.
8. Filer, L. J., Mattson, F. H., and Fomon, S. J.: Triglyceride configuration and fat absorption by the human infant. J. Nutr., 99:293, 1969.
9. Fomon, S. J.: Infant Nutrition. Philadelphia, W.B. Saunders Company, 1974.
10. Fomon, S. J., et al.: Requirements for protein and essential amino acids in early infancy. Acta Paediatr. Scand., 62:33, 1973.
11. Fomon, S. J., et al.: Body composition of reference children, birth to age 10 years. Am. J. Clin. Nutr., 35:1169, 1982.
12. Friedman, G., and Goldberg, S. J.: Concurrent and subsequent serum cholesterols of breast and formula-fed infants, Am. J. Clin. Nutr., 28:42, 1975.
13. Higgenbottom, L., Sweetman, L., and Nyhan, W. L.: A syndrome of megaloblastic anemia and neurological abnormalities of a vitamin B$_{12}$ deficient breast fed infant of a strict vegetarian. N. Engl. J. Med., 299:317, 1978.
14. Johnson, E. E., and Evans, G. W.: Relative zinc availability in human breast milk. Am. J. Clin. Nutr. 31:416, 1978.
15. Johnson, P. R., and Roloff, J. S.: Vitamin B$_{12}$ deficiency in an infant strictly breast-fed by a mother with latent pernicious anemia. J. Pediatr., 100:917, 1982.
16. Lowenberg, M.: The development of food patterns in young children. In Pipes, P. L.: Nutrition in Infancy and Childhood. St. Louis, C. V. Mosby Company, 1982.
17. Marlin, D. W., Picciano, M. F., and Livant, E. C.: Infant feeding practices. J. Amer. Diet. Assoc. 77:668, 1980.
18. McMillan, J. A., Landau, S. A., and Oski, F. A.: Iron

sufficiency in breast-fed infants and the availability of iron from human milk. Pediatrics, *58*:686, 1976.

19. Newbrun, E.: Dietary fluoride supplementation for the prevention of caries. Pediatrics, *62*:733, 1978.
20. Partridge, J. C., et al.: Water intoxication secondary to feeding mismanagement. Am. J. Dis. Child., *135*:38, 1981.
21. Paxon, C. L., Adcock, E. W., and Morris, F. N.: Osmolalities of infants formulas. Am. J. Dis. Child., *131*:139, 1977.
22. Polacek, E., et al.: The osmotic concentrating ability in healthy infants and children. Arch. Dis. Child., *40*:291, 1965.
23. Reeve, L. E., Chesney, R. W., and DeLuca, H. F.: Vitamin D of human milk: identification of biologically active forms. Am. J. Clin. Nutr. *36*:122, 1982.
24. Sinatra, F. R., and Merritt, R. J.: Iatrogenic kwashiorkor in infants. Am. J. Dis. Child., *135*:21, 1981.
25. Smith, D., et al.: Shifting linear growth during infancy: illustration of genetic factors in growth from fetal life through infancy. J. Pediatr., *89*:225, 1976.
26. Watkins, J. B.: Bile acid metabolism and fat absorption in newborn infants. Pediatr. Clin. N. Am., *21*:501, 1974.
27. Yeung, D. L., et al.: Infant fatness and feeding practices: a longitudinal assessment. J. Am. Diet. Assoc., *79*:531, 1981.

Additional References

Anderson, S. E., Chinn, H. I., and Fisher, K. D.: History and current status of infant formulas. Am. J. Clin. Nutr., *35*: 381, 1982.

Committee on Nutrition, American Academy of Pediatrics: On the feeding of supplemental foods to infants. Pediatrics, *65*:1178, 1980.

Committee on Nutrition, American Academy of Pediatrics: Sodium intake of infants in the United States. Pediatrics, *68*:444, 1981.

Fomon, S. J., et al.: Recommendations for feeding normal infants. Pediatrics, *63*:52, 1979.

Fomon, S. J., et al.: Cow milk feeding in infancy: gastrointestinal blood loss and iron nutritional status. J. Pediatr., *98*: 540, 1981.

Johnson, G. H., Purvis, G. A., and Wallace, R. D.: What nutrients do our infants really get? Nutrition Today, *16*:4, 1981.

Pipes, P.: When should semisolid foods be fed to infants? J. Nutr. Ed., *9*:57, 1977.

Pipes, P.: Nutrition in Infancy and Childhood. St. Louis, C. V. Mosby Company, 1981.

Pipes, P.: Feeding babies in the 1980's. In Worthington-Roberts, B. S.: Contemporary Developments in Nutrition. St. Louis, C. V. Mosby Company, 1981.

CHAPTER 13

Nutrition in Childhood

BETTY LUCAS, M.P.H., R.D.

The time from one year of age until puberty is often referred to as the "latent" or "quiescent" period of growth, in contrast to the dramatic changes in growth and development that occur in infancy and adolescence. These preschool and middle school years represent about half of the time period from birth to maturity but a time of tremendous acquisition of skills, abilities and knowledge. The one-year-old is just beginning to walk with a wide-based gait, has a few one-word utterances, and is dependent on adults to provide the basic necessities, in contrast to the ten-year-old youngster who can kick a soccer ball with agility and precision, work with a simple computer at school, and has an allowance from which snacks and toys are purchased. Although physical growth may be less remarkable and more steady than during the first year, there is significant growth in the social, cognitive and emotional areas.

Growth and Development

PHYSICAL GROWTH

The rate of growth slows considerably after the first year of life. In contrast to the tripling of birth weight in the first 12 months, another year passes before birth weight is quadrupled. Likewise, birth length is increased by 50 per cent in the first year but is not doubled until approximately the age of four. In general, growth is steady and slow during the preschool and school-age years, but it may be erratic in individual children. Some small children may be in an apparent "holding pattern" for several months or a year and then have a spurt in height and weight. Interestingly, these patterns usually parallel similar changes in appetite and food intake. For parents who are not knowledgeable about these trends (and even for some who are), periods of slow growth and poor appetite can cause anxiety, which may lead to mealtime struggles.

The actual increments in height and weight are small compared with those of infancy and adolescence. Weight increases an average of 2 to 3 kg. (4½–6½ lb.) per year until the child is nine or ten years old, when the rate increases, an initial sign of approaching puberty. Height increments average 6 to 8 cm. (2½–3½ in.) per year from age two until the pubertal acceleration.[35]

Body proportions of young children change significantly after the first year. There is little head growth, trunk growth slows substantially, and the limbs lengthen considerably to give a more mature body proportion. With increased physical activity and walking, the legs straighten, while the abdominal and back muscles tighten to support the now erect child. These changes are gradual and subtle, occurring over a period of years.

Body composition in preschool and school-age children remains relatively constant. Total body water is about 60 per cent, the average adult value. Sex differences begin early, with boys having more lean body mass per centimeter of height than girls. Fat gradually decreases during the childhood years, but an increase occurs before the pubertal growth spurt. Girls have a higher percentage of weight as fat, even in the early years, but these sex differences in lean body mass and fat do not become significant until adolescence.

Catch-up Growth

As a child recovers from an illness or undernutrition that has slowed or ceased growth, he or she will experience a greater than expected rate of growth. This is referred to as catch-up growth: the body strives to "catch up" to the child's normal growth curve. The degree of growth suppression is influenced by the timing, severity and duration of the insult; i.e., a severe illness or deprivation for an extended time during a period of rapid growth will have the most dramatic effect.

Early studies supported the thesis that malnourished infants who did not experience immediate catch-up growth would have permanent growth retardation. However, studies in developing countries of malnourished children who were subsequently treated, as well as reports of children malnourished because of chronic diseases such as celiac disease or cystic fibrosis, have demonstrated complete catch-up growth after the first year or two of life.[4, 17, 33] Although it is not possible to predict the degree of catch-up growth that a malnourished child will experience, it is clear that some will attain growth similar to that of their same-age peers.

Assessing Growth

Because children are constantly growing and changing, it becomes important for health-care professionals to assess their progress periodically. Any problems can thereby be detected early and treated. Clinics and physicians who serve young children usually offer well-child visits annually to preschool children and less frequently to older children. Because of attitudes regarding preventive health care and concerns about cost, however, many children are seen by health-care professionals only when they are ill, at which time growth and development may not be dealt with.

A complete assessment of nutritional status includes the collection of anthropometric data. This includes height and weight, weight for height (all with percentiles plotted on the National Center for Health Statistics [NCHS] growth grids), upper arm circumference, and triceps and subscapular fatfolds. The minimum measurements taken should be height and weight.

Growth measurements must be recorded at regular intervals in order to show the growth patterns of a child. Height and weight taken only once do not lend themselves to interpretation of growth status. Children generally maintain their heights and weights in the same channels during the preschool and early childhood years, although the channels are not well established until after age two. Individual children at times grow at faster or slower rates; nonetheless, they should follow along the same channels.

The height and weight of a child should be in proportion to one another; this can be assessed by plotting the weight for height. A gross assessment can also be made by noting the difference between the height and weight channels; a difference of more than two channels is suggestive of overweight or underweight and should be investigated further. Skinfold measurements also yield more specific information regarding the composition of the child's weight.

When children's growth is measured routinely, changes can be more quickly noted and problems corrected. Weight increasing at a rapid rate and crossing channels suggests the development of obesity. Lack of weight gain or loss of weight over a period of months may be a result of undernutrition, a severe acute illness, an undiagnosed chronic disease, or significant emotional or family problems. Figure 13–1 shows two cases that demonstrate these changes in growth parameters. Regular monitoring of growth enables these trends to be identified early and treatment to be given so that long-term growth is not compromised.

A thorough discussion of growth and nutritional assessment is found in Chapter 9.

DEVELOPMENTAL PROGRESS

A child's growth and development is dependent on more than food and nutrients. Emotional nurturing, learning experiences and socialization all play a part in the growth of a child's personality, abilities and uniqueness. The years between infancy and adolescence are marked by rapid growth in cognitive functioning, language acquisition and social skills. These changes are

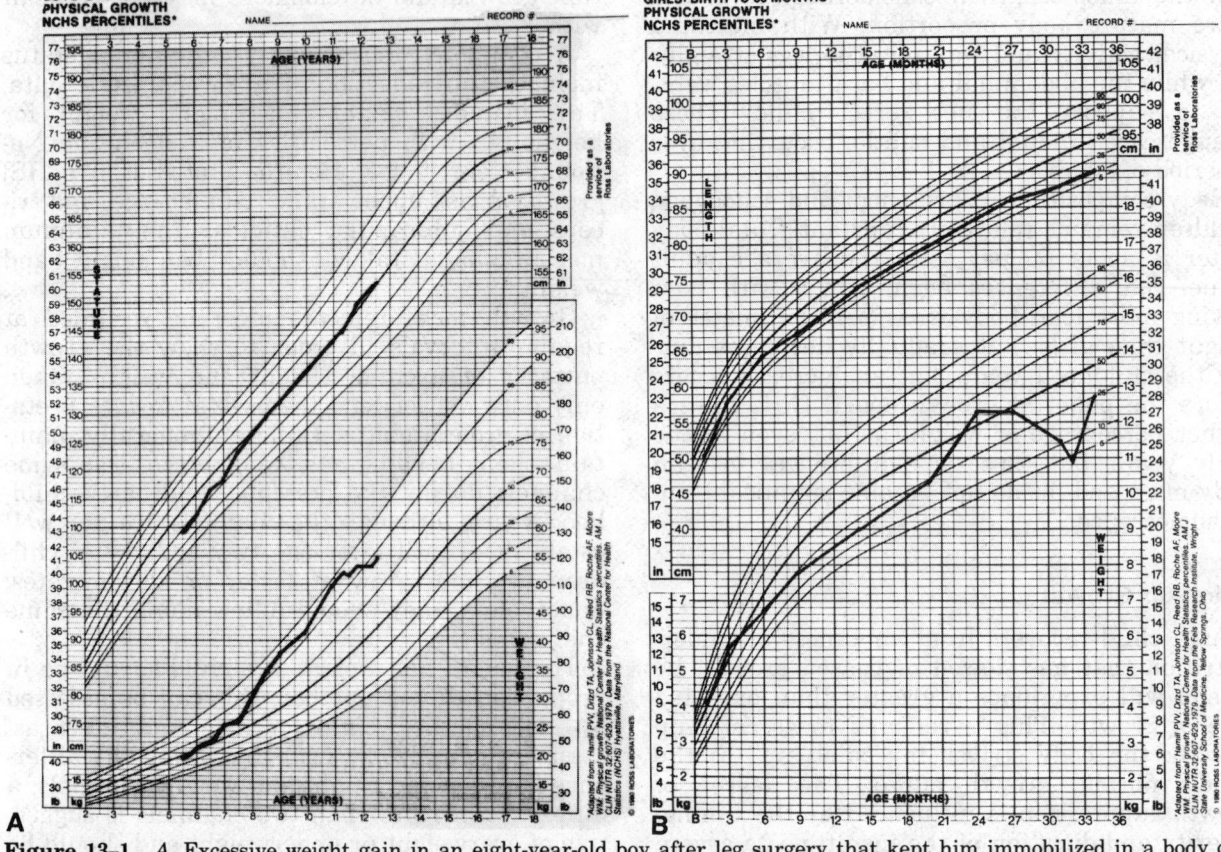

Figure 13–1. *A,* Excessive weight gain in an eight-year-old boy after leg surgery that kept him immobilized in a body cast for two months; this was followed by a long period of stress due to family problems. After age 11, he became involved in a weight management clinic. *B,* Significant weight loss in a two-year-old girl during a long period of diarrhea and feeding problems. After a diagnosis of celiac disease and the institution of a gluten-free diet, rebound weight gain was seen.

more dramatic in the preschool years and are marked by periods of equilibrium and disequilibrium. The term "terrible twos" is not without a rational basis.

Observations of children at various ages and stages can lead to identification of common characteristics. The toddler is striving toward independence and is aware of himself as a person; yet, he is still a baby wanting help and protection. He prefers activities involving the large muscles, and works hard at mastering his body as well as objects in his environment. The preschooler has explosive language development; maturation of gross and fine motor control is seen. Play, which is the child's work, takes on new dimensions—cooperative play, dramatic play, fantasy. The school-age years are a time of moving away from parents and toward peer relationships. There are more organized activities; games, rules and rituals become significant. It is a time of losing teeth and growing new ones.

There are many ways of interpreting and understanding child psychology and development. Piaget developed a theory of learning that acknowledges the input of physical maturation, experiences, and social transmission of knowledge.[31] In this theory, cognitive development is seen as a continuing process, each stage laying the groundwork for the next stage. Table 13–1 outlines the periods of Piaget's theory along with comments regarding commensurate progress in feeding and nutrition.

Nutrient Needs

Because children are growing and developing bones, teeth, muscles and blood, they need more nutritious food in proportion to their weight than do adults. They can become at risk for malnutrition when they have a prolonged poor appetite, accept a limited number of foods or dilute their diets with nutrient-poor foods.

The Recommended Dietary Allowances (RDA), established by the Food and Nutrition Board of the National Research Council—National Academy of Sciences, represent the current knowledge of nutrient intakes needed by children of different ages for optimal health (Table 13–2 and Table 10–1).[21] Most of the data for children

Table 13–1. PIAGET'S THEORY OF COGNITIVE DEVELOPMENT IN RELATION TO FEEDING AND NUTRITION

DEVELOPMENTAL PERIOD	COGNITIVE CHARACTERISTICS	RELATIONSHIPS TO FEEDING AND NUTRITION
Sensorimotor (Birth–2 years)	—progression from newborn with automatic reflexes to intentional interaction with the environment and the beginning use of symbols	—progression is made from sucking and rooting reflexes to the acquisition of self-feeding skills —food is used primarily to satisfy hunger, as a medium to explore the environment, and to practice fine motor skills
Preoperations (2–7 years)	—thought processes become internalized; they are unsystematic and intuitive —use of symbols increases —reasoning is based on appearances and happenstance —approach to classification is functional and unsystematic —child's world is viewed egocentrically	—eating becomes less the center of attention than social, language and cognitive growth —food is described by color, shape, and quantity but there is limited ability to classify food into "groups" —foods tend to be classed as "like" and "don't like" —foods can be identified as "good for you" but reasons are unknown or mistaken
Concrete operations (7–11 years)	—child can focus on several aspects of a situation simultaneously —cause/effect reasoning becomes more rational and systematic —ability to classify, reclassify and generalize emerges —decrease in egocentricism permits child to take another's view	—beginning realization that nutritious food has a positive effect on growth and health, but limited understanding of how or why this occurs —mealtimes take on a social significance —the expanding environment increases the opportunities for, and influences on food selection (peer influence rises)
Formal operations (11 years and beyond)	—hypothetical and abstract thought expand —understanding of scientific and theoretical processes deepens	—the concept of nutrients from food functioning at physiological and biochemical levels can be understood —conflicts in making food choices may be realized (knowledge of nutritious food vs. preferences and non-nutritive influences)

of these ages are interpolated values. Since they provide a margin of safety (except for energy) above the physiological requirement for most children in the United States, they cannot be applied appropriately to individual children. One cannot assume that a child is inadequately nourished if his or her intake falls below the recommended allowance (see Chapter 9). Another child's nutrient intake may come close to the RDA, and yet the child may be overweight.

ENERGY

The energy needs of a child are determined by his or her basal metabolism, rate of growth, body size, age and activity. Enough calories must be provided to ensure growth and to spare protein from being used as energy, yet they cannot be so excessive that obesity results. Of the total energy intake, a suggested proportion is 50 to 60 per cent as carbohydrate, 25 to 35 per cent as fat and 10 to 15 per cent as protein.

The most recent Recommended Dietary Allowances give a wide range of energy intake for each age group, a difference of up to 100 per cent from minimum to maximum (Table 13–2). This variability has been supported in studies that have shown large differences in energy intakes of healthy, growing children of the same age and sex. The age categories of the RDA limit their use for individuals. A one-year-old toddler has a different energy need for growth and activity than a child who is almost four years old; a 7-year-old boy and a 10½-year-old girl go-

Table 13–2. RECOMMENDED DIETARY ALLOWANCES OF ENERGY AND PROTEIN FOR CHILDREN

AGE (Years)	KCALORIES					GM. OF PROTEIN		PERCENTAGE OF KCALORIES FROM PROTEIN
	Daily Mean	Range	Per kg.	Per cm.	(Range)	Daily	Per kg.	
1–3	1300	900–1800	100	14.4	(10.0–20.0)	23	1.8	7.1
4–6	1700	1300–2300	85	15.2	(11.6–20.5)	30	1.5	7.1
7–10	2400	1650–3300	86	18.2	(12.5–25.0)	34	1.2	5.7

From Food and Nutrition Board, National Research Council: Recommended Dietary Allowances, 9th ed. Washington, D. C., National Academy of Sciences, 1980.

ing into puberty have significantly different factors determining their energy needs even though they are in the same RDA age-and-sex category.

Recent studies of food consumption have shown a reduced level of energy intake in children compared with the RDA. The 1977–1978 Nationwide Food Consumption Survey yielded lower caloric intakes for children, with 6- to 11-year-olds consuming more than 20 per cent below the mean RDA energy level.[20]

To estimate energy needs for an individual child, one must consider growth and activity patterns. Using kcalories per centimeter of height, as listed in Table 13–2, is a useful yardstick in assessing appropriate energy intake or planning a diet for a particular child.[7] Another indicator of adequate energy intake can be obtained by using the child's height, weight and general state of health.

PROTEIN

Children need an adequate protein intake to cover maintenance needs and to provide for optimal growth. The RDA indicate that the need for protein per kg. of body weight decreases from approximately 1.8 gm. in early childhood to 1.2 gm. in late childhood.[21]

Since there is not sufficient knowledge about the specific amino acid requirements of children after infancy, protein for this age group should be of high biological value. Milk and other dairy products contribute a significant amount of protein in the typical diets of most children. Meats and eggs are also important complete proteins, with the remaining protein coming from cereals, breads and vegetables.

Since 1958 the RDA for protein for children has decreased. The allowance for seven- to ten-year-olds has been reduced from 60 gm. to 34 gm. per day, a level that some authorities feel is too low to meet the needs of American children. This 34 gm. of protein represents only 5.7 per cent of the total average caloric intake for this age group, rather than 10 to 15 per cent, which is the usual recommendation. For the preschool age groups, the RDA for protein is 7.1 per cent of mean energy intake, as shown in Table 13–2. On the basis of nitrogen balance studies, Abernathy and Ritchey concluded that a more appropriate protein allowance for seven- to ten-year-old children would be 45 gm. or more daily.[1] Reported intakes from the Preschool Nutrition Survey, the Health and Nutrition Examination Survey, and the Child Research Council study have shown actual protein intakes to be in the higher range of 10 to 15 per cent of kcalories.[2, 7, 28] This seemingly lower proportion of protein kcalories in the RDA may in fact be an artifact of the higher energy allowances, which most children do not meet, as has been mentioned. When a child's diet is evaluated for adequacy, assessment should be made of the individual's protein needs in light of his or her appropriate energy intake.

Protein deficiency is uncommon in American children, partly because of our cultural emphasis on protein foods. Children most likely at risk for inadequate protein intake are those on strict vegan diets, those who have multiple food allergies or those who have limited food selection because of fad diets or behavior problems. In developing countries, however, lack of protein combined with inadequate energy consumption is a common nutritional problem, as discussed in Chapter 4.

MINERALS AND VITAMINS

Minerals and vitamins are necessary for normal growth and development. Insufficient intake can cause impaired growth and result in deficiency diseases, as described in Chapters 6 and 7. The RDA for different age groups are listed in Table 10–1.

The preschool child between one and three years of age is at high risk for iron deficiency anemia; thus, the RDA is set high at 15 mg. per day. This risk is due to the rapid growth period of infancy with its increase in hemoglobin mass and the continued need to maintain hemoglobin concentration as well as increase total iron mass during growth. In addition, the child's diet may not be rich in iron-containing foods.

The RDA for calcium is 800 mg. per day for children aged one through ten. Calcium is needed for adequate mineralization of growing bone and for its maintenance. Actual need for this nutrient is dependent upon individual absorption rates and dietary factors such as quantities of protein, vitamin D and phosphorus. A child who is receiving less than 800 mg. of calcium daily may not be in jeopardy. Since milk and other dairy products are the primary sources of calcium, children who consume none of these foods, or limited amounts of them, are at risk for calcium deficiency.

Vitamin D is needed for calcium metabolism and skeletal growth in children. Since this nutrient is also available from sunlight, the amount required from dietary sources is dependent on factors such as geographical location and time spent out of doors. Children living in tropical areas may need no dietary vitamin D or only up to 2.5 μg. (100 I.U.) for optimal utilization of calcium. In the temperate zones, however, some dietary source is needed, and the RDA is established at 10 μg. (400 I.U.) daily for children. Vitamin D–fortified milk is the main source of this nutrient, but other dairy products are not commonly made from fortified milk.

Zinc is essential for growth; a deficiency results in growth failure, poor appetite, decreased taste acuity and poor wound healing. Hambidge has reported marginal zinc deficiency in preschool and school-age children from both middle-income and low-income families.[22, 23] An allowance of 10 mg. zinc per day is recommended, but because the best sources of available zinc are meats and seafoods, some children may regularly have a reduced intake. Children in the United States are more likely to have marginal zinc nutriture than actual deficiency, but diagnosis may be difficult because of variations in laboratory methods and values. A child with symptoms and dietary intake suggesting zinc depletion should undergo analysis of plasma and hair zinc content. In some cases, a careful trial of zinc supplementation may be the only conclusive way to diagnose a problem.

Vitamin-Mineral Supplements

Parents frequently question health professionals about giving their children vitamin and/or mineral supplements. The use of supplements decreases after infancy, but approximately one half or more of preschool and school-age children take some vitamin and/or mineral preparation.[14, 15] Supplements do not necessarily fulfill nutrient needs, however. For instance, intakes of calcium and iron are often at lower levels, yet these two nutrients are not commonly supplemented. One study of school-age children reported that the use of supplements was significant in increasing the percentage of children whose dietary intakes of vitamins reached 67 per cent of the RDA.[14] The American Academy of Pediatrics does not support routine supplementation for normal children, except for fluoride in unfluoridated areas. It describes groups at nutritional risk to include (1) children from deprived families, (2) children with anorexia, poor appetites and poor eating habits and (3) children consuming vegetarian diets without adequate dairy products.[3] For parents who wish to give their children a standard multiple vitamin, however, no risk is involved if it is given in the appropriate amount. Megadoses should be avoided, particularly of the fat-soluble vitamins, large amounts of which can result in toxicity.

POSSIBLE NUTRIENT DEFICIENCIES

Studies of the dietary intakes of children have reported that calcium, iron, ascorbic acid and vitamin A are the nutrients most likely to be low or deficient. Clinical signs of malnutrition in American children, however, are rare. Popula-

tion studies of nutritional status have reported a higher frequency of low nutrient intakes and short stature in children from low-income families.[2, 12, 28] In addition, studies of certain geographical "poverty pockets" and ethnic groups such as blacks and American Indians have demonstrated a higher rate of biochemical and clinical signs of malnutrition as well as poor dietary intake.[27]

Providing an Adequate Diet

The fact that food and eating mean more than the provision of nutrients for body growth and maintenance is readily demonstrated in children. For the two-year-old, food may be the soothing of hunger pangs, a sign that Dad will soon be home from work or a tool to use in asserting independence. For the seven-year-old, food may be associated with the excitement of a birthday party, the sharing of the day's events with other family members at dinner or the satisfaction of preparing his own snack or part of a meal. Food and mealtime do not always signify pleasant associations; they may be negatively associated with struggles over the kind and amounts of food eaten, family tensions at meals or food that is boring, unpalatable or unappealing. Thus, there are many psychosocial parameters of food during the growing years.

PATTERNS OF INTAKE

Just as physical growth is not smooth and consistent, neither is food intake. Appetite, though a subjective assessment, usually follows the rate of growth and nutrient needs. From a "good" appetite in infancy, more "fair to poor" appetites are seen in young preschool children, a frequent cause of parental anxiety.[5]

Changes in food consumption are reflected in nutrient intakes. By the first birthday, milk consumption has declined and will continue to do so in the next year. There is a decrease in vegetable intake and an increase in desserts, starches and sweets. Ground beef and hot dogs are preferred to meats that are harder to chew such as roasts and steaks. Compared with nutrient intake in infancy, the early preschool years show a decrease in calcium, phosphorous, riboflavin, iron and vitamin A. Most other key nutrients remain relatively stable. During the early school years, a pattern of consistent and steady increases in all nutrients is seen until adolescence.

For any age and sex group, wide variability of nutrient intake is seen in healthy children. Beal has reported nutritional data from the Child Research Council longitudinal growth and development study. She found that at any age, the maximum intake of energy, carbohydrate, fat and protein was two to three times the minimum intake. Even wider ranges were noted in vitamin intakes; the maximum:minimum ratios were as high as 10:1 for ascorbic acid and 20:1 for carotene. The subjects were all healthy, well-growing children.[6]

FACTORS INFLUENCING FOOD INTAKE

Numerous influences, some obvious and some subtle, determine the food intake and habits of children. It is well known that habits, likes and dislikes are well grounded in the early years and carry through to adulthood, where change is often met with resistance and difficulty. The major influences on food intake in the developing years include family environment, the media, peers and illness or disease.

Family Environment

For the toddler and preschool child, the family is the primary influence in the development of food habits. Parents and older siblings are significant models for young children as they learn and imitate the individuals in their immediate environment. The father's role can be a significant influence because his likes and dislikes tend to be catered to.[11] Food attitudes of parents have been shown to be a strong predictor of food likes and dislikes as well as diet complexity in primary school children.[36] Birch, however, has suggested that although parental food preferences are related to children's preferences, the degree of correlation is no stronger

than that of other unrelated adults of a similar subcultural group.[8]

The atmosphere around food and mealtime is also an important aspect of attitudes toward food and eating. High expectations for a child's mealtime manners, with the threat of reprimand, can make dinner a dreaded time. Arguments and other emotional stress can also have a negative effect. Meals that are rushed create a hectic atmosphere and reinforce eating too fast. A more positive environment, such as that shown in Figure 13–2, allows enough time to eat, is tolerant of occasional spills and encourages conversation that includes all family members.

In recent decades, changes have occurred in the nuclear family, away from the traditional two-parent, one-income family. It is estimated that nearly half of all women are employed outside the home. Many children, therefore, eat one or more meals at babysitters' homes, day care centers and schools. Food purchasing and meal preparation routines are often modified by working parents because of time constraints. There may be more use of convenience foods or fast foods.

Another change has been the increase in single-parent households, often the result of divorce. Most single-parent homes are headed by women, which often means a lower income and thus less money for all expenses including food. Children whose parents are divorced may often be shuttled back and forth from one parent to another, and food may be used in inappropriate ways. Eating out and "treats" may help allay the divorced parent's guilt or may be used to win back a child's affection.

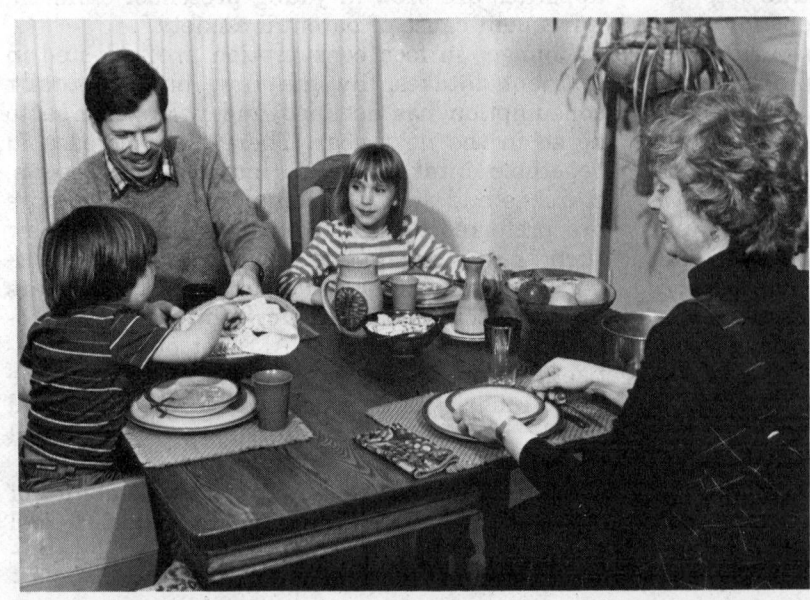

Figure 13–2. A pleasant mealtime atmosphere and appropriate adult models will have positive influences on children's food habits and attitudes.

Media

By the time the average American child has graduated from high school, he or she will have watched 15,000 hours of television and will have spent 11,000 hours in the classroom. No wonder television is considered by some to be a primary teacher. Aside from concerns about television's portrayal of violence, stereotyping and consumerism, it also has a negative effect on children's nutrition.

Nearly half of all commercials are for food, and the percentage is higher in programming for children. Most of the food commercials targeted to children are for cereal (primarily presweetened), candy and sweets, fast food establishments and snack foods. These foods are high in sugar, fat and/or sodium. One study found that food advertising made up 69 per cent of the commercials on children's programs, and that the food items were of poorer nutritional quality than foods advertised to adults. High-sugar cerals were advertised five times as often as those with less sugar.[10] The commercial message appeals to children to eat the food because it is "chocolatey" or "fun" or "gives you energy" rather than on any rational basis such as nutrient needs. In addition, there are rarely advertisements for foods such as fresh fruits, vegetables or whole-grain cereals and breads.

Preschool children are generally unable to distinguish commercial messages from the regular program, and in fact, often pay more attention to the former. As children get older, they become knowledgeable of the purpose of commercial advertising and become more critical of its validity.[9] However, they are still susceptible to the commercial message. Consumer groups such as Action for Children's Television monitor television's effect on children and encourage legislative or governmental action. The activity of this group is discussed in Chapter 17.

Television can also be detrimental to growth and development by encouraging inactivity and passive use of leisure time instead of engaging in sports, playing outdoors or doing creative work. A pattern of inactivity and watching television, along with multiple media cues to eat, may be a factor in excessive weight gain for children.

Other advertising also influences children's food habits through fast food promotions, box top and prize offers, and other non-nutritive means to increase the purchase and consumption of certain foods. Some promotions offer equipment and materials to schools in exchange for product labels or proofs of purchase. Although this is appealing to schools and PTA groups, it tends to encourage the purchase of food items (most of them highly processed) for reasons other than nutritional value, economy or food preference.

Peers

As children grow, their world expands and their social contacts take on more importance. The older they get, the more they are influenced by their peers, and this includes food attitudes and choices. This may be manifest in the child by a sudden refusal of a food or a request for a current "popular" food. Decisions on whether to participate in school lunch may be more a result of what friends do than of the menu offered. These behaviors usually represent a phase that will change. Positive aspects can be reinforced, such as trying new foods. For undesirable influences, parents need to set limits but to be realistic; struggles over food are self-defeating.

Illness or Disease

Children who are ill usually have a decreased appetite and food intake. Acute viral or bacterial illnesses are often of short duration but may require an increase in fluids, protein or other nutrients. Chronic conditions such as asthma, congenital heart disease and cystic fibrosis may make it difficult to obtain nutrients for optimal growth. Children with these types of disease are more likely to have behavior problems or family struggles around food. Children requiring special diets (such as those for diabetes or phenylketonuria) not only have to adjust to the limits of foods allowed but also have to deal with the issues of independence and peer acceptance as they grow older. It is not atypical to see some rebellion against the prescribed diet, especially as the child approaches puberty. Chapter 38 discusses nutritional care in chronic diseases for children.

FEEDING THE PRESCHOOL CHILD

The years from one to six are marked by vast development and acquisition of skills. The child learns to talk, run and become a social being. The one-year-old primarily uses fingers to eat and may need assistance with a cup. By age two, he or she can hold a cup in one hand and use a spoon well (Fig. 12–4), but hands may still be preferred at times. The six-year-old has refined skills and is beginning to use a knife for cutting as well as spreading.

Because growth is slower during these years, appetite also decreases, often causing parental concern. There is less interest in food and more interest in the world around them. Children develop "food jags" during this time, refusing previously accepted food or asking for one particular food at each meal. This behavior may be due to boredom with usual foods or may be a means of asserting newly discovered independence. In the survey of mothers summarized in Table 13–3, Eppright found that choosing a limited variety and dawdling with food were their major concerns, peaking when the children were three and four years old.[19] This is often a difficult time for parents, with their concern about the adequacy of diet and their frustration with their child's seemingly irrational food behavior. Struggles over control of the eating situation are fruitless—no child can be forced to eat. Parents need to understand that this period is developmental but temporary. They will still determine what foods are offered and will, as well, set limits on inappropriate behaviors. Neither rigid control nor a laissez-faire approach is likely to succeed. A variety of foods should continue to be offered, including the favorite ones, and substitutions for those refused should be made within the same food group. Young children usually respond positively when offered a choice of healthy foods.

Preschool children, because of their smaller capacity and variable appetites, do best with small servings of food offered several times a day. Portion sizes are small by adult standards. A general rule of thumb is to offer one tablespoon of each food for every year of age, initially, and to serve more according to appetite. Table 13–4 is a guide for food and portion sizes to provide an adequate diet for preschoolers.

Most children eat four to six times a day, making snacks as important as meals in contributing to the total day's nutrient intake. The most recent food consumption study showed that nearly 60 per cent of three- to five-year-olds eat more than three times a day.[20] Their snacks need to be carefully chosen so that they are dense in nutrients and are not limited to cookies, soda pop and chips. Likewise, foods least likely to promote dental caries should be selected. Wholesome snacks enjoyed by many young children include fresh fruit, cheese, hard-boiled or deviled eggs, raw vegetable sticks, milk, fruit juices, whole-grain crackers and peanut butter sandwiches.

Other senses in addition to taste play an important part in food acceptance by young children. Generally, extreme temperatures are avoided, and many children actually prefer their food lukewarm. Some foods may be rejected because of odor, e.g., overcooked cabbage, rather than taste. A sense of order in the food presentation is often required. Many children will not accept foods touching each other on the plate, and most casseroles and mixed dishes are not popular, except for spaghetti and pizza. It is not unusual for broken crackers to go uneaten or a sandwich to be refused because it is "cut the wrong way." Many young children are keenly sensitive to food palatability, and readily detect off-flavors or reject overcooked vegetables.

The physical setting of children's meals is as important as the emotional atmosphere. They should not be made to eat with feet dangling and arms reaching up to a table at chest height. Sturdy child-size tables and chairs are ideal; if children eat at a standard table with the family, a high chair, "booster chair" or other modification should be used to make them comfortable. Bowls, plates and cups should be non-breakable and heavy enough to resist spilling. A shallow bowl is better than a plate for younger children

Table 13–3. MOTHERS' CONCERNS ABOUT EATING BEHAVIOR OF PRESCHOOL CHILDREN

CONCERNS	0 TO 3 MO. (%)	3 TO 6 MO. (%)	6 TO 9 MO. (%)	9 MO. TO 1 YR. (%)	1 TO 1½ YR. (%)	1½ TO 2 YR. (%)	2 TO 3 YR. (%)	3 TO 4 YR. (%)	4 TO 5 YR. (%)	5 TO 6 YR. (%)	TOTAL (%)
Chooses limited variety	2.6	8.7	12.0	24.6	34.1	37.6	40.3	41.2	44.8	34.2	35.8
Dawdles with food	10.3	3.1	15.5	14.6	34.1	25.7	36.8	43.8	39.7	33.3	33.5
Eats too little fruits and vegetables	0.0	2.4	12.9	14.5	15.8	29.4	27.2	27.5	27.9	27.1	23.9
Eats too many sweets	0.0	0.0	0.0	1.4	4.7	7.8	26.3	28.9	27.9	26.4	20.7
Eats too little meat	0.9	4.7	7.2	22.5	22.6	30.3	22.3	21.6	24.0	17.7	20.5
Eats too little food	8.5	2.4	8.2	10.1	14.7	13.8	21.6	28.3	21.1	22.8	19.9
Drinks too little milk	0.0	3.9	4.8	10.9	10.8	16.5	20.1	18.6	18.7	18.5	16.3
Drinks too much milk	9.4	7.9	7.1	5.1	10.0	13.8	10.0	7.1	7.1	5.9	8.0
Eats too much food	7.7	4.7	8.2	8.7	5.1	3.7	2.7	3.1	5.4	6.4	4.9
Eats too much meat	0.0	0.0	0.0	0.0	1.4	5.0	3.5	4.4	4.3	5.9	3.7
Number of children	117	127	84	138	279	218	551	610	691	628	3444

From Eppright, E. S., et al.: Eating behavior of preschool children. J. Nutr. Ed., *1*:16, 1969. (This paper is published as Journal Paper No. J-5983 of the Iowa Agriculture and Home Economics Experiment Station, Ames, Iowa. Project No. 1532 contributing to North Central Regional Project No. 75.)

Table 13–4. FEEDING GUIDE FOR PRESCHOOL CHILDREN

The following is a guide to a basic diet. Fats, oils, sauces, desserts and snack foods will provide additional kcalories to meet the needs of a growing child. Foods can be selected from this pattern for both meals and snacks.

FOOD	2- to 3-YEAR-OLDS		4- to 6-YEAR-OLDS		COMMENTS
	Portion Size	Number of Servings	Portion Size	Number of Servings	
Milk and dairy products	1/2 cup (4 oz.)	4–5	1/2–3/4 cup (4–6 oz.)	3–4	The following may be substituted for 1/2 cup liquid milk: 1/2–3/4 oz. cheese, 1/2 cup yogurt, 2 1/2 tbsp. non-fat dry milk powder
Meat, fish, poultry or equivalent	1–2 oz.	2	1–2 oz.	2	The following may be substituted for 1 oz. meat, fish or poultry: 1 egg, 2 tbsp. peanut butter, 4–5 tbsp. cooked legumes
Fruits and vegetables		4–5		4–5	
Vegetables					Include one green leafy or yellow vegetable for vitamin A, such as spinach, carrots, broccoli, winter squash
Cooked	2–3 tbsp.		3–4 tbsp.		
Raw*	few pieces		few pieces		
Fruit					Include one vitamin C–rich fruit, vegetable or juice, such as citrus juices, orange, grapefruit sections, strawberries, melon in season, tomato, broccoli
Raw	1/2–1 small		1/2–1 small		
Canned	2–4 tbsp.		4–6 tbsp.		
Juice	3–4 oz.		4 oz.		
Bread and grain products		3		3	The following may be substituted for 1 slice of bread: 1/2 cup spaghetti, macaroni, noodles, or rice; 5 saltines
Whole grain or enriched bread	1/2–1 slice		1 slice		
Cooked cereal	1/4–1/2 cup		1/2 cup		
Dry cereal	1/2–1 cup		1 cup		

*Do not give to children until they can chew well.

Adapted from Lowenberg, M. E.: Development of food patterns in young children. In Pipes, P.: Nutrition in Infancy and Childhood. 2nd ed. St. Louis, C. V. Mosby Company, 1981.

to facilitate easier scooping. Thick, short-handled spoons and forks allow for an easier, less tiring grasp.

Young children usually do not eat well if they are fatigued, and this needs to be considered when meal and play times are scheduled. A quiet activity or rest immediately before eating is conducive to a relaxed, enjoyable meal. To stimulate a good appetite, however, children need active, large motor activity and time spent outside in the fresh air (Fig. 13–3).

Group Feeding

A generation ago the food experiences of preschool children centered on home and family. Today, because of changing family lifestyles, more children spend part or most of their days in day care centers, preschools, day care homes and Head Start programs. At such places, they may consume only a snack or as much as two meals and two snacks per day, depending on the time involved. For many children, therefore, more than half of their nutrients may be provided in these settings. They are likely to be exposed to a wider variety of foods, including ethnic foods.

Food service in group feeding settings such as day care centers and Head Start programs is regulated by federal and/or state guidelines, and some facilities may participate in USDA-sponsored food programs. The quality of meals and snacks can vary a great deal; parents should investigate this aspect when selecting a placement for their child. In addition to providing the child with optimal nutrients, a program should offer food that is appealing and safely prepared and consider cultural and developmental patterns in planning menus.

These group settings are ideal environments for nutrition education programs, both at mealtimes and in various learning activities. Experiencing new foods, participating in simple food preparation and planting a garden are all examples of activities that develop and enhance positive food habits and attitudes. To be effective, nutrition education efforts require the cooperation of food service personnel, teaching staff and nutrition consultants.

FEEDING THE SCHOOL-AGE CHILD

Growth during the school-age years (ages 6 to 12) is slow but steady, paralleled by a constant increase in food intake. In addition to being in school a greater part of the day, the child is also likely to begin participation in clubs and group activities, sports and recreational programs. The

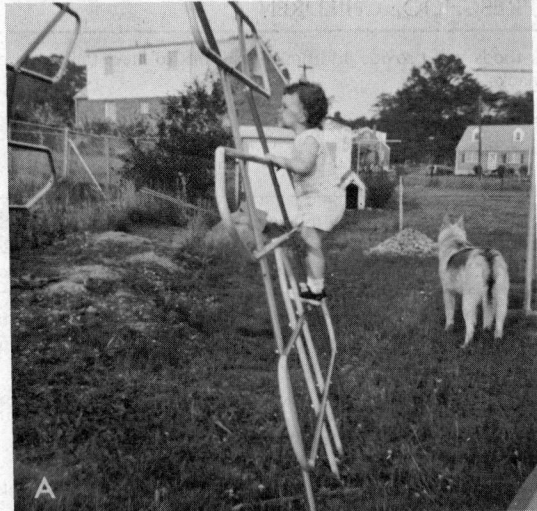

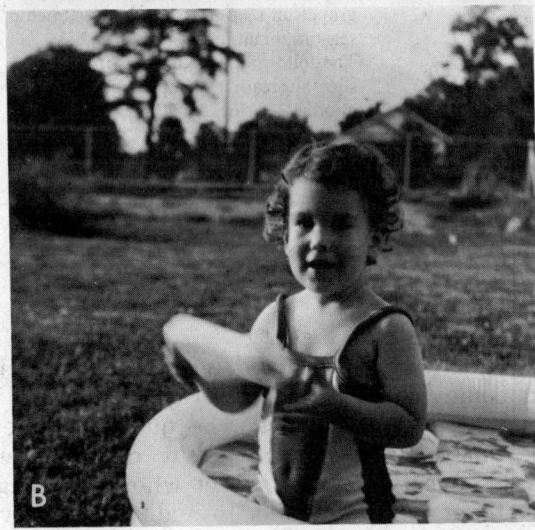

Figure 13–3. Along with a well-balanced, nutritious diet, this 23-month-old child enjoys ample outdoor play. Sun, air, water and fun all contribute toward a healthy body and a good appetite.

influence of peers and significant adults (e.g., teachers or sports idols) is greater. Friendships and other social contacts become more important. Except for severe cases, most behavioral problems connected with food have been resolved by this age, and the child enjoys eating to alleviate hunger and to obtain social satisfaction.

The school-age child may participate in the school lunch program or carry a lunch from home. The School Lunch Program supported by the Federal government provides approximately one third of the RDA for students. Children from low-income families are eligible for free or reduced-price meals. Some schools also offer a Special Milk Program or School Breakfast Program. These programs are discussed in Chapter 17. Recent years have seen changes in the school lunch to decrease plate waste and to be more responsive to students' needs. Popular items such as pizza, tacos and hamburgers appear more frequently on the menu, there is more choice of milks, and more fresh fruits are used instead of the traditional baked desserts. In an attempt to reduce waste, there is also more flexibility in what items the child must accept. Since the school lunch is nutritious only when it is consumed, these changes to make meals more appealing and wholesome are positive steps.

Reports as well as observations have shown that a lunch packed at home is likely to provide fewer nutrients than the school lunch meal.[18] Favorite foods tend to be packed and less variety is seen; limitations are set by choosing foods that travel well and do not need heating or refrigeration. Children needing diet modifications (low calorie, allergy, low sodium, etc.) will need to bring their lunches. A typical well-balanced lunch would include a sandwich with protein-rich filling (meat, egg, cheese, peanut butter), fresh fruit and/or vegetable, milk and an optional cookie or other whole-grain baked good. Children in elementary school can begin to prepare their own lunches if a variety of nutritious foods is available.

Because of changes in family lifestyles, many school children are responsible for preparing their own breakfasts. It is not uncommon for children to skip this meal altogether, even in the primary grades. The School Breakfast Program can aid in some situations, but it is not uniformly available in all school districts. A review of nutrition and school performance suggests that children who go to school without breakfast are likely to be more inattentive, lethargic and irritable, but there has not been strong documentation to support this association.[29] Pollitt studied 9- to 11-year-old children in a laboratory setting where problem solving, memory and attending abilities were measured after the children had been given or not been given breakfast. Although blood glucose levels were not significantly different between children fed or not fed, other biochemical parameters suggested a metabolic stress on those without breakfast. The children who had fasted made more errors on the problem-solving task but performed better on short-term memory recall. These results show that brief fasting can cause changes that affect cognitive function.[30]

Snacks are commonly consumed by school children, primarily after school and in the evening. Bakery products and soft drinks are the most frequently chosen snack foods.[20] As a child grows older and has money to spend, he or she consumes more snacks outside the home. Vending machines in schools or other public places tend to offer soft drinks, candy, packaged baked goods and chips. Similar snacks are also chosen at neighborhood groceries. Families can continue to offer wholesome snacks at home and support nutrition education efforts in the school (Fig. 13–4). In most instances, good eating habits established in the first few years will carry a child through this period of decision-making and responsibility.

Nutritional Concerns

OBESITY

Increasing overweight and obesity in childhood is usually not a benign condition, despite popular feelings that overweight children will "outgrow" their condition. Infant and childhood obesity has been linked to adult obesity but is by no means predictive of it. The longer a child has been overweight, however, the more likely he or she will continue in that state into adolescence and adulthood; by age six and beyond the overweight status does not usually spontaneously disappear.[37]

There is difficulty in determining obesity in growing children. Some excess fatness may occur at either end of this age spectrum; i.e., the one-year-old toddler and the prepubertal child may be heavier and fatter for developmental and physiological reasons, but this is not often permanent. Heights and weights alone do not allow for the highly muscled child. Other anthropometric methods such as skinfold measurements, however, are not commonly used. Children at risk for obesity should be monitored more frequently so that early intervention can

be provided. See Chapter 27 for more in-depth information about obesity.

Management of obesity in children should include nutrient needs for growth. More long-term success is likely with a program that includes family involvement, dietary modifications, activity planning and behavioral components. Depending on the child, goals for weight change may include a decrease in the rate of weight gain, a maintenance of weight, or, in severe cases, a slow weight loss.

UNDERWEIGHT

Weight loss or lack of weight gain can be caused by an acute or chronic illness, a restricted diet, a poor appetite, maternal deprivation or a simple lack of food. Careful assessment is critical and must include the social and emotional environment as well as physical findings. If the child also has short stature, the possibility of zinc deficiency should be investigated. The provision of adequate nutrients and nutrition education should be part of the management plan. Attempts should be made to increase appetite and modify the environment to assure an optimal intake.

IRON DEFICIENCY ANEMIA

This is one of the most common nutrient disorders of childhood, and it is especially prevalent in one- to three-year-olds. Certain low-income populations have shown a higher incidence of iron deficiency anemia, which is likely associated with factors such as parents' educational level and lack of medical care as well as dietary intake. In addition to growth and increased

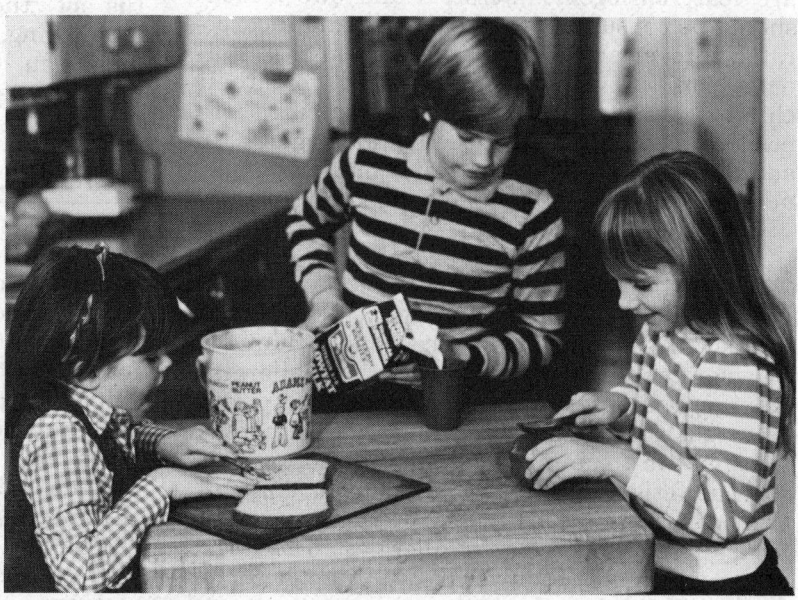

Figure 13–4. These elementary school children enjoy preparing their own after-school snacks. With a selection of nutritious foods available, this independence can be encouraged.

physiological need for iron, dietary factors also play a role. The average iron intake of children from one to three years of age is about one half the RDA.[15, 20] A one-year-old child may continue to consume a large quantity of milk to the exclusion of other foods, resulting in "milk anemia." Many young preschool children do not prefer meat, so that most of their iron is of the non-heme form, which is absorbed at a lower level as discussed in Chapter 29. Iron deficiency is less of a problem in older preschool and school-age children.

Attention to good dietary sources of iron can help prevent iron deficiency anemia. Some pediatric authorities recommend that iron-fortified infant cereals be offered until 18 months of age to ensure a good iron intake, but this is not commonly seen in practice yet. Since many young children consume more non-heme iron sources, education should be aimed at increasing the enhancing factors, such as ascorbic acid and meat, fish and poultry in the diet.

DENTAL CARIES

Nutrition and eating habits are important factors in dental health and disease. Optimal nutrient intake is needed to produce strong teeth and healthy gums. The composition of the diet and eating habits (i.e., amount of dietary sucrose, retentiveness of foods and frequency of eating) are significant factors in the development of dental caries. Infants and young children who drink sweetened liquids from a bottle at bedtime or frequently throughout the day are susceptible to nursing bottle syndrome, which is discussed in Chapter 33.

Since children tend to consume snacks regularly, emphasis should be placed on those which are least cariogenic. Desserts and sweet foods should be consumed less frequently and incorporated into meals to decrease cariogenicity. Parents can provide strong models for their children during this time, in practicing both positive food habits and good dental hygiene. In addition, fluoride from the water or as a supplement will help reduce the likelihood of caries.

ALLERGIES

Food allergies usually manifest themselves in infancy and childhood, and occur more frequently where there is a family history of allergies. Allergic responses most often include respiratory or gastrointestinal symptoms, and skin reactions, but in some instances may be more vague, such as fatigue, lethargy and behavior changes. Controversy exists as to a true definition of a food allergy, and tests for allergies to food are not specific and unequivocal. See Chapter 31 for further discussion of this topic.

HYPERACTIVITY

The hyperactive child syndrome, more a grouping of symptoms than a disease entity, usually presents itself in childhood. A diagnosis or label of hyperactivity most often occurs when a child is in a school setting, but is also seen less frequently in preschool children. Chapter 32 discusses this subject in depth.

DRUGS AND NUTRITION

Children who receive medication for chronic conditions may be at risk for nutrient deficiency or poor growth. Anticonvulsants used to control seizures can interfere with vitamin D and folate metabolism. Rickets have been reported in some of these children.[16, 26] Long-term use of these medications and multiple drug therapies tend to increase the risk of nutritional problems. Children receiving anticonvulsant therapy need to be monitored for dietary adequacy of vitamin D, calcium and folate. Some cases will require vitamin D supplementation which needs to be planned carefully in order to avoid toxicity.

Stimulant medication is an accepted therapy for the treatment of hyperactivity, but has been reported to retard the growth of children.[32] These drugs have a side effect of decreasing appetite and subsequently lowering energy intake.[25] The suppression of growth in these children seems to be temporary and does not necessarily affect adult stature. However, children may take in less energy and nutrients than required. The physical growth and dietary intake of these hyperactive children should be reviewed at regular intervals.

Children may also receive other drugs that cause nausea, gastric distress, vomiting or impaired nutrient absorption. The nutritional status of these individuals warrants periodic monitoring, especially if the drug regimen is long-term. Chapter 21 discusses drug–nutrient interactions in detail.

Nutrition Education

As children grow they acquire knowledge and assimilate concepts by leaps and bounds. These years are ideal for providing nutrition information and promoting positive attitudes about all foods. This learning can be informal and natural, as in the home, with parents as models and the provision of a diet from a wide variety of foods. Food can be used in everyday experiences for the toddler and preschooler and combined with development of language, cognition and self-help, i.e., labeling; describing size, shape and color; sorting; assisting in preparation; and tasting.

In more formal settings, nutrition education is provided in schools, preschools, Head Start programs, day care centers and children's clubs such as 4-H. Federal funds for nutrition education are provided to state education agencies in the NET program, as discussed in Chapter 17. A preliminary evaluation of these programs has shown positive effects on nutrition knowledge, with less consistent effects on food attitudes and habits, food preferences and plate waste.[34]

Attempts to teach children nutrition concepts and information should take into account their developmental level. The concept of nutrients is abstract and is lost on preschoolers and most primary school children. Contento suggests that some nutrition curricula are more sophisticated than children's ability to conceptualize, and that modification may be necessary to make the educational experiences meaningful.[13] Activities that concentrate on children's real-world relationship with food are more likely to yield positive results.

Since children of all ages benefit from a "hands-on" approach to learning, information about food and nutrition can be included in meals and snacks, food preparation and activities that also focus on cognitive learning. Parental involvement in nutrition education projects can also produce more positive outcomes and carry-over into the home.[24]

Summary

Children will grow and develop optimally when they are provided with adequate nutrition. Parents and others working with children need to be mindful of the importance of the social, emotional and psychological aspects of food and eating. For a child to achieve total well-being and a positive self-concept, he or she needs not only food but also love, support and appreciation of his or her own uniqueness.

Problems and Suggested Topics for Discussion

1. Check the children in your pediatric unit against the height-weight-age tables. Explain any variations.
2. What and how much are a one-year-old, a two-year-old and a six-year-old eating? Check their food records for nutritional adequacy.
3. Obtain a list of an average day's intake of food from a boy in the clinic who is ten years old. How does he rate his diet? How may it be improved?
4. Follow the same procedure suggested in problem 3 for a child who is three years old.
5. How does nutrition affect healthy growth and development? What are the visible signs of poor nutrition? How does a girl's growth and development differ from that of a boy? Give the general growth and development pattern of a child from ages 1 to 11.
6. What changes in eating habits take place from ages 1 to 11? Account for the changes.
7. Milk is a good food for children, but under what circumstances may it need to be limited?
8. Assess the eating behaviors of a four-year-old and explain how they reflect Piaget's concepts of development.
9. Why are adequate breakfasts and lunches of importance to the school child? What is a good breakfast? What is a good lunch?

Cited References

1. Abernathy, R.P., and Ritchey, S.J.: Position paper on RDA for protein for children. Adv. Exp. Med. Biol., 105:1, 1978.
2. Abraham, S., et al.: Dietary Intake Findings, United States, 1971–1974. DHEW Publication No. (HRA) 77–1647. Washington, D.C., U.S. Government Printing Office, 1977.
3. American Academy of Pediatrics, Committee on Nutrition: Vitamin and mineral supplementation needs in normal children in the United States. Pediatrics, 66: 1015, 1980.
4. Barr, D.G.D., Shmerling, D.H., and Prader, A.: Catch-up growth in malnutrition, studied in celiac disease after institution of gluten-free diet. Pediatr. Res., 6:521, 1972.
5. Beal, V.A.: On the acceptance of solid foods, and other food patterns of infants and children. Pediatrics, 20: 448, 1957.
6. Beal, V.A.: Dietary intake of individuals followed through infancy and childhood. Am. J. Pub. Health, 51:1107, 1961.
7. Beal, V.A.: Nutritional intake. In McCammon, R.W. (ed.): Human Growth and Development. Springfield, Ill., Charles C Thomas, 1970.
8. Birch, L.L.: The relationship between children's food preferences and those of their parents. J. Nutr. Ed., 12: 14, 1980.
9. Blatt, J., Spencer, L., and Ward, S.: A cognitive developmental study of children's reactions to television advertising. In Rubinstein, E.A., Comstock, G.A., and Murray, J.P. (eds.): Television and Social Behavior, Vol. 4, Television in Day to Day Life: Patterns of Use. Washington, D.C., U.S. Government Printing Office, 1972.
10. Brown, J.: Graduate students examine TV ads for food. J. Nutr. Ed., 9:120, 1977.
11. Bryan, M.S., and Lowenberg, M.E.: The father's influence on young children's food preferences. J. Am. Diet. Assoc., 34:30, 1958.
12. Center for Disease Control: Ten-State Nutrition Survey, 1968–70. DHEW Publication No. (HSM) 72–8130–34. Washington, D.C., U.S. Department of Health, Education and Welfare, Health Services and Mental Health Administration, 1972.
13. Contento, I.: Children's thinking about food and eating —a Piagetian-based study. J. Nutr. Ed., 13(Suppl.): 586, 1981.
14. Cook, C.C., and Payne, I.R.: Effect of supplements on the nutrient intake of children. J. Am. Diet. Assoc., 74: 130, 1979.
15. Crawford, P.B., Hankin, J.H., and Huenemann, R.L.: Environmental factors associated with preschool obesity. J. Am. Diet. Assoc., 72:589, 1978.
16. Crosley, C.J., Chee, C., and Berman, P.H.: Rickets associated with long-term anticonvulsant therapy in a pediatric outpatient population. Pediatrics, 56:52, 1975.
17. Ellis, C.E., and Hill, D.E.: Growth, intelligence, and school performance in children with cystic fibrosis who have had an episode of malnutrition during infancy. J. Pediatr., 87:565, 1975.
18. Emmons, L., Hayes, M., and Call, D.L.: A study of school feeding programs. II. Effects on children with

different economic and nutritional needs. J. Am. Diet. Assoc., *61*:268, 1972.

19. Eppright, E.S., et al.: Eating behavior of preschool children. J. Nutr. Ed., *1*:16, 1969.

20. Food and Nutrient Intakes of Individuals in 1 Day in the United States, Spring 1977. USDA Nationwide Food Consumption Survey, 1977–1978. Preliminary Report No. 2. Washington, D.C., Science and Education Administration, 1980.

21. Food and Nutrition Board, National Research Council: Recommended Dietary Allowances, 9th ed. Washington, D.C., National Academy of Sciences, 1980.

22. Hambidge, K.M., et al.: Low levels of zinc in hair, anorexia, poor growth, and hypogeusia in children. Pediatr. Res. *6*:868, 1972.

23. Hambidge, K.M., et al.: Zinc nutrition of preschool children in the Denver Head Start program. Am. J. Clin. Nutr., *29*:734, 1976.

24. Kirks, B.A., Hendricks, D.G., and Wyse, B.W.: Parent involvement in nutrition education for primary grade students. J. Nutr. Ed., *14*:137, 1982.

25. Lucas, B., and Sells, C.J.: Nutrient intake and stimulant drugs in hyperactive children. J. Am. Diet. Assoc., *70*:373, 1977.

26. Medlinsky, H.L.: Rickets associated with anticonvulsant medication. Pediatrics, *53*:91, 1974.

27. Owen, G., and Lippman, G.: Nutritional status of infants and young children: U.S.A. Pediatr. Clin. North Am., *24*:211, 1977.

28. Owen, G.M., et al.: A study of nutritional status of pre-school children in the United States, 1968–70. Pediatrics, *53*(Suppl.):597, 1974.

29. Pollitt, E., Gersovitz, M., and Gargiulo, M.: Educational benefits of the United States school feeding program: a critical review of the literature. Am. J. Pub. Health, *68*:477, 1978.

30. Pollitt, E., Leibel, R.L., and Greenfield, D.: Brief fasting, stress, and cognition in children. Am. J. Clin. Nutr., *34*:1526, 1981.

31. Robinson, N.M., and Robinson, H.B.: The Mentally Retarded Child, 2nd ed. St. Louis, McGraw-Hill Book Co., 1976.

32. Roche, A.E., et al.: The effects of stimulant medication on the growth of hyperkinetic children. Pediatrics, *63*:847, 1979.

33. Stoch, M.B., and Smythe, P.M.: 15-year developmental study of effects of severe undernutrition on subsequent physical growth and intellectual functioning. Arch. Dis. Child., *51*:327, 1976.

34. St. Pierre, R.G., and Rezmovic, V.: An overview of the National Nutrition Education and Training Program evaluation. J. Nutr. Ed., *14*:61, 1982.

35. Vaughan, V.C., McKay, R.J., and Behrman, R.E.: Nelson's Textbook of Pediatrics, 11th ed. Philadelphia, W.B. Saunders Co., 1979.

36. Yperman, A.M., and Vermeersch, J.A.: Factors associated with children's food habits. J. Nutr. Ed., *11*:72, 1979.

37. Zack, P.M., et al.: A longitudinal study of body fatness in childhood and adolescence. J. Pediatr., *95*:126, 1979.

Additional References

Birch, L.L., et al.: Mother-child interaction patterns and the degree of fatness in children. J. Nutr. Ed., *13*:17, 1981.

Burke, B.S., et al.: Relationships between animal protein, total protein, and total caloric intake in the diets of children one to eighteen years of age. Am. J. Clin. Nutr., *9*: 729, 1961.

Caliendo, M.A., et al.: Nutritional status of preschool children. J. Am. Diet. Assoc., *71*:20, 1977.

Dallman, P.R., Siimes, M.A., and Stekel, A.: Iron deficiency in infancy and childhood. Am. J. Clin. Nutr., *33*:86, 1980.

Dwyer, J.: Diets for children and adolescents that meet the dietary goals. Am. J. Dis. Child., *134*:1073, 1980.

Eppright, E.S., et al.: The North Central Regional study of diets of preschool children. II. Nutrition knowledge and attitudes of mothers. J. Home Econ., *62*:327, 1970.

Fomon, S.J.: Nutritional Disorders of Children. Prevention, Screening, and Follow-up. DHEW Publication No. (HSA) 76–5612. Washington, D.C., U.S. Department of Health, Education and Welfare, Public Health Service, 1976.

Gussow, J.: Counter-nutritional messages of TV ads aimed at children. J. Nutr. Ed., *4*:48, 1972.

Hertzler, A.A., and Vaughan, C.E.: The relationship of family structure and interaction to nutrition. J. Am. Diet. Assoc., *74*:23, 1979.

Huenemann, R.L: Environmental factors associated with preschool obesity. II. Obesity and food practices of children at successive age levels. J. Am. Diet. Assoc., *64*:489, 1974.

Juhas, L.: Nutrition education in day care programs. J. Am. Diet. Assoc., *63*:134, 1973.

Lowenberg, M.E.: Food preferences of young children, J. Am. Diet. Assoc., *24*:430, 1964.

Sims, L.S., and Morris, P.M.: Nutritional status of preschoolers. J. Am. Diet. Assoc., *64*:492, 1974.

Swanson-Ruud, J., et al.: Nutrition orientations of working mothers in the North Central Region. J. Nutr. Ed., *14*: 132, 1982.

CHAPTER 14

Nutrition in Adolescence

JANE MITCHELL REES, M.S., R.D.

Adolescence is one of the most challenging periods in human development. Because of the extent of the physical and psychological changes taking place, a number of important issues arise that influence the nutritional well-being of the teenager. A knowledge of the developmental process is a prerequisite to understanding the nutritional aspect of life in this period.

Growth and Development

PHYSIOLOGICAL CHANGES

Puberty, the process of physically developing from a child to an adult, is initiated by poorly understood physiological factors and includes maturation of the total body. Following a period

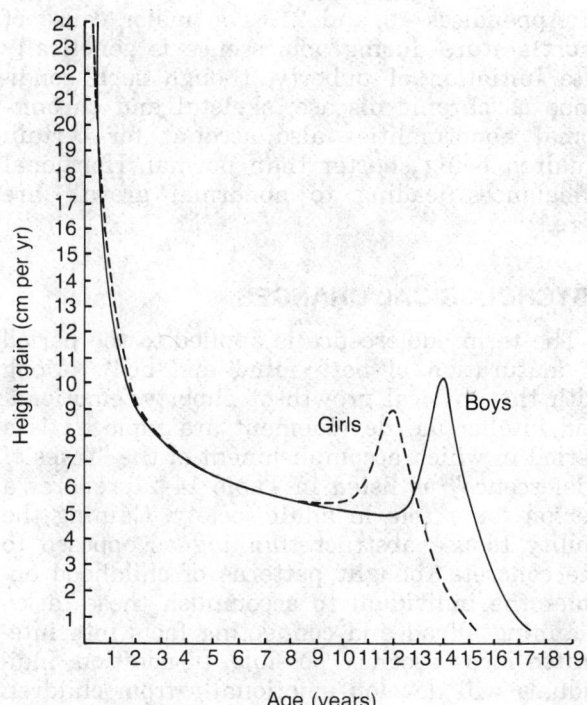

Figure 14–1. Typical individual velocity curves for supine length or height in boys and girls. The curves represent the velocity of growth of the typical boy and girl at any given age. (From Tanner, J. M.: Foetus into Man. Cambridge, Mass., Harvard University Press, 1978.)

of slow growth during late childhood, the change in adolescence is as rapid as that of early infancy. Figure 14–1 shows that the rate of linear growth during the teen years compares with that for the second year of life. The child will gain about 20 per cent of adult height and 50 per cent of weight during this period.[16]

This growth continues throughout the approximately 5 to 7 years of pubertal development, though a great percentage of height will be gained during the "growth spurt." This 18- to 24-month period of peak height gain velocity will occur at different ages for different individuals, as will the initiation of puberty. In general, it occurs earlier in life for girls than for boys. Factors known about the timing and milestones of pubertal development are summarized in Figure 14–2. Though growth slows following the achievement of sexual maturity, linear growth and weight acquisition continue. For rare females it will continue into the late teens and for males into the 20's. Most females will gain no more than 2 to 3 inches following the onset of menses, however.

In the process of total body maturation, the composition of the body changes. In the prepubertal period the proportion of fat and muscle in males and females tends to be similar, with body fat about 15 and 19 per cent respectively, and lean body mass varying similarly. During

puberty females gain more fat, so that adult females carry about 22 per cent body fat while males have about 15 per cent. Males during this time gain twice as much lean tissue as females.

Assessment of Growth

Weight can be plotted on a similar grid as height to determine whether or not an individual is keeping pace with peers, or exceeding them in total weight at a particular year. Because of the wide variation in weights seen in sample individuals (some of whom were obese) in the adolescent period the frequency distribution represented by the grid cannot be used for evaluation of weight in proportion to height as it can be for younger children. To evaluate the relationship between the weight and height of an individual one must turn to the detailed tables of the Health and Nutrition Examination Survey as shown in Appendix Table 24. For each 5-cm. increment of height at a particular year of age, a range of weights is given (5th to 95th percentiles). Weights for height for age and sex between the 25th and the 75th percentiles can be considered to be appropriate.[10] This range allows for the differences in body build of indi-

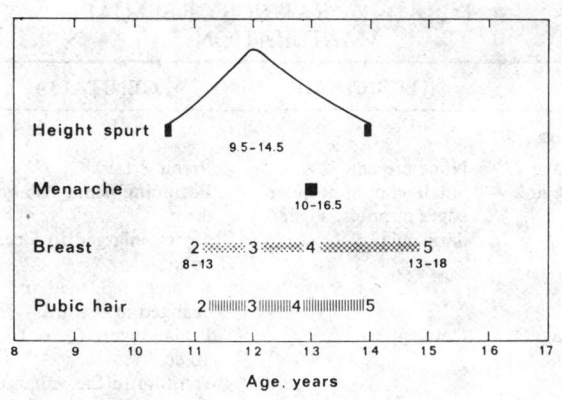

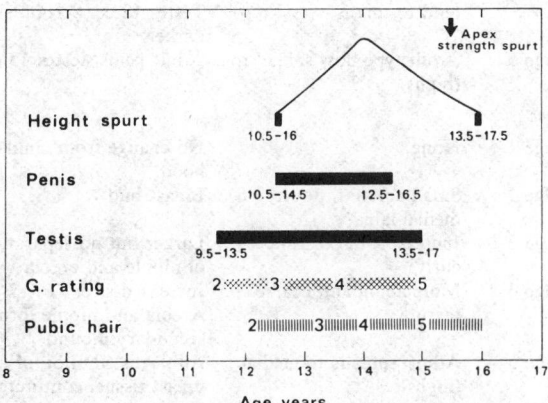

Figure 14–2. Diagram of sequence of events at puberty in girls (*above*) and boys (*below*). (From Marshall, W. A., and Tanner, J. M.: Variations in the pattern of pubertal changes in boys. Arch. Dis. Child., *45*:13, 1970.)

viduals. A skinfold evaluation in addition will yield a more precise assessment. For example, a low skinfold measurement in an individual above the 75th percentile weight for height indicates a state of being overweight but not overfat. An assessment of muscle and arm circumference will confirm the muscular composition. However, a skinfold at the 90th percentile or greater suggests obesity. Measurement of skinfolds is further discussed in Chapter 9.

Sexual Maturity Rating

Sexual development is a measurable indicator of the process of physical maturation. Use of weight and height tables and sexual maturity rating allows clinical monitoring of pubertal development. The sexual maturity ratings described in Table 14–1 outline the milestones of sexual maturation. Knowing the relationship between these milestones and physical growth will enable the clinician to assess the progress of growth in an adolescent at a particular time and give some indication of the extent of future growth.

Excessive or less than normal growth can be detected by plotting height changes on the grids in Appendices 19 and 21. The major cause of short stature during adolescence is genetically late initiation of puberty, though such conditions as chronic disease, skeletal and chromosomal abnormalities also account for certain children being shorter than normal. Hormonal imbalances leading to abnormal growth are rare.[16]

PSYCHOLOGICAL CHANGES

The term adolescence is applied to the period of maturation of both mind and body. Along with the physical growth of puberty, emotional and intellectual development are rapid. It is a period in which accomplishment of the "tasks of adolescence" as listed in Table 14–2 prepares a person for a role in adult society. Gaining the ability to use abstract thinking as opposed to the concrete thought patterns of childhood enables the individual to accomplish these tasks. Planning ahead and connecting facts into integrated ideas becomes possible. In addition, individuals will develop emotionally from children who need to have guidance and security provided for them, to a point where their emotional state must be mostly self-generated. The emotional turmoil during this process is an outstanding characteristic of the age which may affect adolescents' eating habits as well as the rest of their lives. The drive toward independence may result in their rejecting the dietary patterns of their family background, for example.

Many of the tasks of adolescence relate to the nutritional well-being of the individual. For example, emotional maturity allows teenagers to develop their own value system. As a result, they can choose foods that will enhance their state of health rather than responding to less healthful characteristics of foods as they may have done in childhood.[10]

Body Image

Developing an image of the physical self that includes an adult body is an intellectual and emotional task that is intertwined with nutritional issues. During the adolescent period individuals often feel uncomfortable with their rapidly changing bodies. At the same time, being very much affected by influences outside themselves, they want to be like their most perfect peers and the idols of their culture. Stereotypes in the mass media reinforce such images. They may derive their sense of worth from their feelings about their own physical attributes, a trait that causes them to be vulnerable to severe distortions if an eating disorder develops. Teenagers may wish certain body parts were

Table 14–1. RATINGS OF SEXUAL MATURATION

	PUBIC HAIR	GENITALIA
Boys		
Stage 1	None present	Prepubertal
Stage 2	Small amount at outer edges of pubis, slight darkening	Beginning penile enlargement. Testes enlarged to 5 cc. vol. Scrotum reddened and changed in texture.
Stage 3	Cover pubis	Penis longer, Testes to 8–10 cc. Scrotum further enlarged.
Stage 4	Adult type, does not extend to thighs	Penis wider and longer. Testes 12 cc. Scrotal skin darker.
Stage 5	Adult type now spread to thighs	Adult penis, testes 15 cc.
Girls		
Stage 1	None	No change from childhood.
Stage 2	Small amount, downy on medial labia	Breast bud
Stage 3	Increased, darker and curly	Larger but no separation of nipple and areola
Stage 4	More abundant, coarse texture	Increased size. Areola and nipple form secondary mound
Stage 5	Adult, spreads to medial thighs	Adult distribution of breast tissue, continuous outline

Adapted from Tanner, J.M.: Growth at Adolescence. 2nd ed. Oxford, Blackwell Scientific Publications, 1962.

Table 14–2. DEVELOPMENTAL TASKS IN ADOLESCENCE

DEVELOPMENTAL TASK (Havighurst, Thornburg)	HOW ADOLESCENTS MIGHT EXPRESS THE TASK	AGE 11 12 13 14 15 16 17 18 19 20 21 22 →
1. Forming more mature relationships with peers of both sexes	Exploring relationships with boyfriends/girlfriends	
2. Establishing a male or female social role	Learning a sex role	
3. Accepting one's physique and using one's body effectively	Looking great and becoming physically fit and less clumsy	
4. Becoming emancipated from parents and other adults	Cutting the apron strings	
5. Preparing for marriage and family life	Getting ready for marriage and family someday	
6. Choosing a vocation and preparing for that career	Choosing a career	
7. Developing standards and value systems as a guide to behavior	Organizing some values and achieving morality	
8. Developing social intelligence and a commitment to responsible citizenship	Getting along with others and following through with responsibilities	
9. Developing conceptual and problem-solving, decision-making skills	Developing intellectual skills	

From Mahan, L.K., and Rees, J.M.: Nutrition in Adolescence. St. Louis, C. V. Mosby Company, 1984. Adapted from Thornburg, H.: Contemporary Adolescence: Readings. 2nd ed. Monterey, Calif.: Brooks/Cole, 1975, p. 7.

larger and others were smaller than they are. They may want to grow faster or slower than they have. This can lead adolescents to try to change their bodies by manipulating their dietary consumption, a trait that certain commercial interests are quick to exploit. Rapid additions of weight connected with development of secondary sexual characteristics cause many young women who have not adopted a mature body image to unnecessarily restrict the amount of food they eat. Young men are tempted to use nutritional supplements, hoping to achieve the muscular appearance of adults.[5, 10]

Nutritional Requirements

The research base on which recommendations for fulfilling the nutritional needs of adolescents are made is small. Part of the difficulty lies in the fact that studies of requirements must take not only age but also stage of physical maturity into account. Since such studies are not available, the Recommended Dietary Allowances (RDA) are stated for three age groups as shown in Table 14–3. Adolescents at the peak of their growth velocity will need large quantities of nutrients. They have been shown to incorporate twice the amount of calcium, iron, zinc, magnesium and nitrogen into their bodies during the years of the growth spurt compared with other years. The highest levels of nutrients are recommended for the group assumed to be growing at the most rapid rate.

RECOMMENDATIONS TO SUPPORT GROWTH

To make the recommendations more specific for individuals, dividing the recommended quantity of a nutrient by the number of cm. of the RDA reference individual's height provides an amount of nutrient per cm. to apply to any size teen. For example, the RDA for protein for the 11- to 14-year old male is 45 gm. per day. The reference adolescent's height is 157 cm. Thus, 0.29 gm./cm. would be the recommended amount of protein. There will be great variation in size of teens, since they experience the growth spurt at different ages. Recommendations will come closest to meeting needs when the largest quantity of nutrient per cm. is suggested for those experiencing the growth spurt even if the age does not coincide with the age for which RDA are highest.

Energy

The recommended range of energy intake in the RDA for adolescence as shown in Table 14–4 reflects the differential needs of teenagers. Growth rate as well as level of exercise will need to be considered in determining the needs of the individual.

Protein

The protein requirements of adolescents have been least studied of all the age groups. On the basis of what is known, the recommendation is

Table 14–3. FOOD AND NUTRITION BOARD, NATIONAL ACADEMY OF SCIENCES–NATIONAL RESEARCH COUNCIL, RECOMMENDED DAILY DIETARY ALLOWANCES,[a] REVISED 1980

Designed for the maintenance of good nutrition of practically all healthy people in the U.S.A.

	AGE (years)	WEIGHT		HEIGHT		PROTEIN (g.)	FAT-SOLUBLE VITAMINS		
		(kg.)	(lb.)	(cm.)	(in.)		Vitamin A (μg. R.E.)[b]	Vitamin D (μg.)[c]	Vitamin E (mg. α-T.E.)[d]
Females	11–14	46	101	157	62	46	800	10	8
	15–18	55	120	163	64	46	800	10	8
	19–22	55	120	163	64	44	800	7.5	8
Males	11–14	45	99	157	62	45	1000	10	8
	15–18	66	145	176	69	56	1000	10	10
	19–22	70	154	177	70	56	1000	7.5	10

[a] The allowances are intended to provide for individual variations among most normal persons as they live in the United States under usual environmental stresses. Diets should be based on a variety of common foods in order to provide other nutrients for which human requirements have been less well defined.

[b] Retinol equivalents. 1 retinol equivalent = 1 μg. retinol or 6 μg. β carotene.

[c] As cholecalciferol. 10 μg. cholecalciferol = 400 I.U. of vitamin D.

that the energy value of the protein intake should make up 7 to 8 per cent of the total energy consumed. Sex, age, nutritional status and quality of the protein in the diet must be considered in estimating the amount an individual will need. The range of total protein will be from 44 to 56 gm. Protein consumption should not be overly emphasized; sufficient protein is usually obtained in the normal diet. In situations such as chronic illness in which nutritional depletion may be seen, protein stores of adolescents should be carefully monitored and supported so that physical development will not be impaired. Chapter 9 further discusses assessment of protein nutriture.

Minerals

The requirement for calcium in adolescence is based on needs for skeletal growth, 45 per cent of which occurs in this period. Therefore, the recommendations are higher for males than for females because of the larger skeleton males will achieve. Both males and females have high requirements for iron; males because the buildup of muscle mass is accompanied by greater blood volume and females because they will begin to lose iron monthly with the onset of menses. Zinc is known to be essential for growth and is therefore of great importance in adolescence. The retention of zinc increases especially during the growth spurt, leading to more efficient use of sources of this nutrient in the diet.

The role of other minerals in the nutriture of adolescents is not well studied, though, of course, magnesium, iodine, phosphorus, copper, chromium, cobalt and fluoride are important. The possibility of interactions between these nutrients cannot be overlooked. The recommenda-

tions for safe levels listed in Table 10–2 are made on the basis of the best data presently available and should be followed with moderation so that imbalances will not develop.

Vitamins

As to the need for vitamins in adolescence, high amounts of thiamin, riboflavin and niacin are recommended because of the high energy requirements. In most cases, because of increased energy intake, the intake of B vitamins will increase and be adequate. Vitamin D is especially needed for rapid skeletal growth. Recommended amounts of vitamins A, E, C, folic acid, and vitamin B_6 are the same as for adults. Often the amounts recommended are of necessity interpolated from studies in adults or children in order to provide a guide for meeting the nutrient needs of teenagers.[10]

NUTRITIONAL REQUIREMENTS LIKELY NOT TO BE MET

Surveys of nutrient intake have shown adolescents to be likely to obtain less vitamin A, thiamin, iron and calcium than recommended[19] and to ingest more fat, added sugar, protein and sodium than is currently thought to be optimal.[4] While concern has been expressed over the habit of snacking, teenagers may obtain substantial nourishment from foods eaten outside traditional meals. The choice of foods they make is of greater importance than the time or place of eating. Emphasis should be placed on fresh vegetables and fruit and whole grain products to compliment the foods high in energy value and protein which they commonly choose.[9, 17]

Table 14–3. FOOD AND NUTRITION BOARD, NATIONAL ACADEMY OF SCIENCES–NATIONAL RESEARCH COUNCIL RECOMMENDED DAILY DIETARY ALLOWANCES,[a] REVISED 1980 (*Continued*)

Designed for the maintenance of good nutrition of practically all healthy people in the U.S.A.

Vitamin C (mg.)	Thiamin (mg.)	Riboflavin (mg.)	Niacin (mg. N.E.)[e]	Vitamin B-6 (mg.)	Folacin[f] (µg.)	Vitamin B-12 (µg.)	Calcium (mg.)	Phosphorus (mg.)	Magnesium (mg.)	Iron (mg.)	Zinc (mg.)	Iodine (µg.)
50	1.1	1.3	15	1.8	400	3.0	1200	1200	300	18	15	150
60	1.1	1.3	14	2.0	400	3.0	1200	1200	300	18	15	150
60	1.1	1.3	14	2.0	400	3.0	800	800	300	18	15	150
50	1.4	1.6	18	1.8	400	3.0	1200	1200	350	18	15	150
60	1.4	1.7	18	2.0	400	3.0	1200	1200	400	18	15	150
60	1.5	1.7	19	2.2	400	3.0	800	800	350	10	15	150

Column group headers: **WATER-SOLUBLE VITAMINS** (Vitamin C through Vitamin B-12); **MINERALS** (Calcium through Iodine).

[d] α-tocopherol equivalents. 1 mg. *d*-α tocopherol = 1 α-T.E.

[e] 1 N.E. (niacin equivalent) is equal to 1 mg. of niacin or 60 mg. of dietary tryptophan.

[f] The folacin allowances refer to dietary sources as determined by *Lactobacillus casei* assay after treatment with enzymes (conjugases) to make polyglutamyl forms of the vitamin available to the test organism.

Influences on Food Habits

The growing independence of adolescents, increased participation in social life, and generally busy schedules influence their eating habits. They often eat rapidly and outside of the home. They are beginning to buy and prepare more food themselves.

The influences on eating behavior from outside the home in modern America are great. Television food commercials and the eating habits portrayed in program content have influenced people for more than a decade by the time they are adolescents. The average viewer will have watched over one hundred thousand food commercials, the majority of which are for products with a high concentration of sweetness and fat. For a more detailed discussion of the influence of television, see Chapters 13 and 17.

The ease of obtaining ready-to-eat food also influences the eating habits of teenagers. Through vending machines, at movies and sporting events, and at fast food outlets and convenience groceries, food is available at numerous times throughout the day. Figure 14–3 shows an example of a common eating place for an adolescent. During the time of their peak growth velocity, adolescents may need to eat often and in large amounts, and are able to use foods with a high concentration of energy. However, they will usually need to be more careful of amounts and frequency when growth has slowed. An imbalance in the consumption of nutrients may not appear to be a problem until a number of years have gone by, unless some specific problem, such as a chronic disease, exists. Ultimately, however, such overeating may contribute to a number of debilitating diseases.

Table 14–4. RECOMMENDED ENERGY INTAKES

	DAILY TOTAL		PER CM. HEIGHT	
	Median	*Range*	*Median*	*Range*
Children				
7–10 years	2400	1650–3300	18.2	14.8 –22.1 kcal
Males				
11–14 years	2700	2000–3700	17.2	15.1 –20.9 kcal
15–18 years	2800	2100–3900	15.9	13.5 –20.8 kcal
19–22 years	2900	2500–3300	16.4	15.8 –17.1 kcal
Females				
11–14 years	2200	1500–3000	14.0	11.2 –17.5 kcal
15–18 years	2100	1200–3000	12.9	7.9 –17.3 kcal
19–22 years	2100	1700–2500	12.9	11.6 –16.5 kcal

Median is the median energy intake of children of these ages followed in longitudinal growth studies. The values in range column are the 10th and 90th percentiles of energy intake of these children.

From Food and Nutrition Board, National Research Council: Recommended Dietary Allowances. 9th ed. Washington, D.C., National Academy of Sciences, 1980.

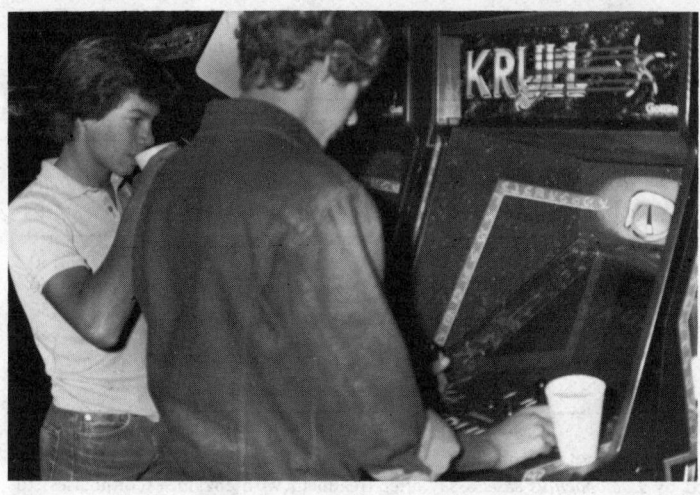

Figure 14-3. A typical eating place for teenagers.

Situations with Specialized Needs

PREGNANCY

The assumption that pregnant adolescents need a supply of nutrients to support their own growth along with the growing fetus has been questioned.[18] Because hormone levels are high in pregnancy, even the slower growth that usually follows the onset of menses may not occur. Whether or not actual growth continues for an adolescent who becomes pregnant, she will have experienced rapid growth more recently than her adult counterparts. She will have less time for storage of nutrients. It is suggested that there is a greater risk on physiological grounds to a woman who conceives soon after experiencing her first menstrual period.[21] The number of years between the onset of menses and the date of conception is calculated to determine the gynecological age. Those who are more sexually mature share a vulnerability to psychological stresses with adolescents of younger gynecological age but appear to have no more physically based complications than adult women.[2]

Pregnant adolescent women who are of young gynecological age or undernourished at the time of conception will have the greatest need for nutrients to support a pregnancy and themselves.[15] A list of recommended amounts of nutrients is provided in Table 14-5. It combines the same allowance for pregnancy in adult women with the amounts recommended for non-pregnant adolescents. A clinically practical way of assuring adequacy is to encourage the pregnant adolescent to gain the recommended amount of weight by consuming nutrient-rich foods. Sources of protein, calcium, iron, micronutrients and dietary fiber are especially important. Recommended gains during pregnancy may be somewhat higher for the teenager.[10] Most importantly, contact with health professionals during prenatal care provides the opportunity to teach adolescents about feeding themselves and their families.

The economic instability of the pregnant adolescent makes it impossible to assume that she will have an adequate food supply. The impact of economic and other stressful issues on the nutritional well-being of a young pregnant woman is great.

EATING DISORDERS

The terms defined in Table 32-5 are useful in studying these disorders. As depicted in Figure 14-4, the physical symptoms range on a spectrum from the extremely heavy to the extremely thin individual. The underlying psychological characteristics are similar across the spectrum. Because of the unique situation in adolescence and the standards of our culture, even those teenagers who become obese through physiological processes usually share in experiencing psychological problems such as distortions of body image and low self-esteem.[1]

Anorexia Nervosa

To cope with increasing demands of life as she reaches adolescence without having developed a sense of self, the anorectic adolescent defines success in terms of keeping herself thin. A distorted body image leads to choosing lower and lower goal weights. In addition to restricting the amount of energy she takes into her system she increases the output by exercising excessively and at times by self-initiated vomiting or use of laxatives or diuretics. The most critical time nutritionally will be when she has lost sufficient weight to be in a state of starvation. The psychological and developmental disturbance in anorexia thus brings about a state in which the anorectic cannot care for herself. Improvement

Table 14–5. RECOMMENDED DIETARY ALLOWANCES FOR PREGNANT ADOLESCENT FEMALES*

AGE REFERENCE HEIGHT	11–14 Yr. 157 cm.	per cm.	15–18 Yr. 163 cm.	per cm.
Energy (kcal.)	2500	15.9	2400	14.7
Protein (gm.)	76	0.48	76	0.47
Calcium (mg.)	1600	10.2	1600	9.8
Phosphorus (mg.)	1600	10.2	1600	9.8
Iron (mg.)	18[†]		18[†]	
Magnesium (mg.)	450	2.9	450	2.7
Iodine (μg.)	175	1.1	175	1.1
Zinc (mg.)	20	0.13	20	0.12
Vitamin A (μR.E.)	1000	6.4	1000	6.1
Vitamin D (μg.)	15	0.09	15	0.09
Vitamin E (mg. α-T.E.)	10	0.06	10	0.06
Ascorbic Acid (mg.)	70	0.45	80	0.49
Niacin (mg. N.E.)	17	0.11	16	0.10
Riboflavin (mg.)	1.6	0.01	1.6	0.01
Thiamine (mg.)	1.5	0.01	1.5	0.01
Folacin (μg.)	800	5.1	800	4.9
Vitamin B (mg.)	2.4	0.02	2.6	0.02
Vitamin B₁₂ (μg.)	4.0	0.03	4.0	0.02

* Second and third trimesters.
† Supplemental iron recommended.
From Mahan, L. K., and Rees, J. M.: Nutrition in Adolescence. St. Louis, C.V. Mosby Company, 1984.
Developed from Food and Nutrition Board, National Research Council: Recommended Dietary Allowance, Washington, D.C., National Academy of Sciences, 1980.

depends upon psychotherapeutic intervention to allow the anorectic to accept new ideas about her body, weight and food intake.[1] For further study of this disorder, see Chapter 32.

Bulimia

Bulimia does not often lead to the seriously depleted nutritional condition seen in anorexia nervosa. Bulimics generally maintain close to normal weight, periodically going on binges and vomiting, but not starving themselves. They usually have unrealistic ideas about food. In their personal definition a binge may consist of one cookie or a dozen. Their concepts of what is needed to sustain their bodies are equally distorted.[13]

Common physical problems in bulimia include (1) damage to the teeth, (2) irritation of the throat and (3) esophageal inflammation caused

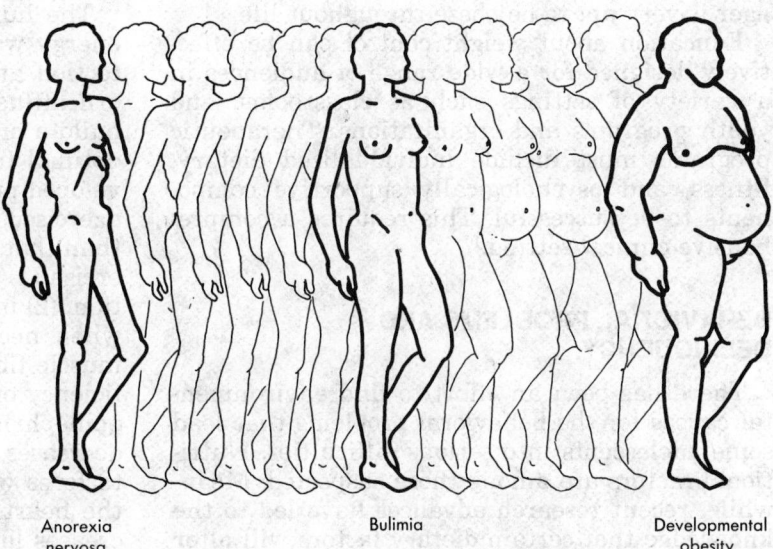

Anorexia nervosa

Bulimia

Developmental obesity

Figure 14–4. The spectrum of eating disorders. (From Mahan, L. K., and Rees, J. M.: Nutrition in Adolescence. St. Louis, C. V. Mosby Company, 1984.)

Underlying psychological characteristics are held in common while physical conditions vary across the spectrum by exposure of unprotected tissue to acidic vomitus; (4) swollen salivary glands caused by acidic reflux or constant stimulation; and (5) rectal bleeding as a result of the overuse of laxatives. More rare and serious are (6) fistulas or ruptures in the upper GI tract, and (7) fluid and electrolyte imbalances.

Many teenagers who do not have the psychological characteristics of the true bulimic use more casual vomiting as a means of weight control. It is a serious disorder when the habits are obsessional and interfere with normal education or employment.

Obesity

The obese teenager may have gained weight through a combination of psychological, physiological and cultural factors as discussed in Chapter 27. It appears that the longer teenagers have been obese for any reason, the greater the chance that their bodies will be subject to processes that tend to maintain the obese state. If not in childhood, by adolescence they will often adopt the restricted lifestyle characteristic of the obese. Commonly they will not want to be seen in settings requiring vigorous exercise and will be subject to real or imagined social rejection. They will be involved in fewer energy-expending and more energy-retaining pursuits.[7] Teenagers are vulnerable to unrealistic attitudes about the amount of time and effort necessary for effective weight management. Diet fads, drugs, and equipment appear to them to provide the quick remedy they seek.[5] Figure 27-7 gives some examples. Meanwhile, there is a scarcity of realistic educational and comprehensive therapeutic programs. Thus, the obese teenager is very apt to be obese throughout life.

Education about weight control can be effectively designed for a wide range of audiences in a variety of settings such as classrooms, and youth programs and organizations. Therapeutic programs must include individualized dietary, fitness, and psychologically supportive components to be successful. This requires a comprehensive clinical setting.[10]

BEHAVIORAL PROBLEMS AND DELINQUENCY

There has been an effort to find environmental causes for the behavioral problems that lead some adolescents into serious difficulties. Nutritional factors are among those suspected. Meanwhile, recent research advances have led to the knowledge that certain dietary factors will alter brain function or behavior.[20] However, at present these principles can be therapeutically applied only in a very limited number of rare neurological disorders. Theories that subclinical deficiencies of certain nutrients influence neurological function have centered on iron and the B vitamins, and have not yet led to clinically applicable intervention strategies.

The popular press has given widespread attention to untested theories about the effect of nutrition on behavior, leading to their acceptance among people who do not seek or have access to more in-depth information. Examples of these theories are that an abundance of sugar, intoxication with heavy metals, food additives and allergic reactions are responsible for behaviors ranging from shortened attention span to learning disorders and to the commission of crimes. The role of nutrition in behavior is discussed in more detail in Chapter 32.

There is a danger that educators and those responsible for juvenile detention facilities will expend public resources in ineffective programs if they accept untested theories. To demonstrate reasonable concern about nutrition, all institutions should support the teenagers they serve by making nourishing foods available to them. Such a policy will involve screening out less valuable foods that are tempting and commercially rewarding, such as those often sold in vending machines. Resulting improvements in nutritional health will contribute to the individual's physical well-being, but at this time it cannot be counted on to prevent criminal behavior, attention disorders or other behavioral problems.[10]

FITNESS AND ATHLETICS

Physiological Advantages of Fitness

The human body evolved in eras when great energy was expended in obtaining food, in protection and in surviving the elements. In modern affluent societies it is usually necessary to build a program of energy expenditure to assure optimal function for bodies that historically developed processes for such energy exchange. The exercised body is more likely to remain healthy than that which remains sedentary.[11] Regular exercise (1) helps maintain optimal body composition, (2) improves the possibility of losing weight when necessary, (3) increases the efficiency of muscle fibers to produce energy, (4) increases efficiency of hormones (insulin, lipoprotein lipase, epinephrine) to regulate energy metabolism, (5) decreases the production of lactic acid which interferes with energy production, (6) strengthens the heart, lungs, and circulatory system, (7) increases levels of HDL over LDL cholesterol and decreases serum triglycerides, (8) raises the rate of basal metabolism, and (9) helps control appetite.

Components of a Fitness Program

Elements of fitness which need to be considered are cardiorespiratory function and muscular strength, endurance and flexibility. Raising the heart rate to at least 50 per cent but no more than 75 per cent of maximum for 15 minutes with 5 minutes of warm up and cool down at least 3 days per week will maintain cardiorespiratory fitness. Stressful exercise is unnecessary. Continuous gradual improvement and maintenance is effective. A few well-chosen exercises will maintain muscular strength, flexibility and endurance. Adolescents participating in sports as well as those who do not should develop personal fitness programs. This will assure that fitness is maintained between seasonal participation in organized programs. All teenagers should be encouraged to increase their exercise in ways best suited to their lives.

Specialized Needs of Athletes

Adolescents who compete in athletics have specific nutritional needs. Foremost, there is a need to continue to support normal growth and physiological maturation. Energy is the pivotal factor in this process. The amount of additional energy that is needed will depend upon the type of exercise being done, the duration and the intensity. Table 14–6 gives the approximate energy expenditures of various sports and other activities.

Except for periods when weight gain (as muscle) is a goal, this energy is best utilized if it is supplied as carbohydrate. Six to 7 gm. of additional protein daily is sufficient in a muscle-building phase. Thereafter 2 to 3 gm. above the normal daily allowance will provide for body maintenance in most athletic endeavors. Higher than normal levels of protein are counterproductive, leading to water loss as the body rids itself of nitrogenous waste products.

Weight should be gained or lost following safe effective methods as described in Chapter 27. Long-term plans will be necessary to carry this out successfully. Any such goals must take the developmental pattern of linear growth and weight gain into consideration. Two dangers are seen in this area. Women who become too thin interrupt the menses, and men may stunt their growth. Anabolic steriods to increase weight in men also can cause stunting of growth and disturbed development of secondary sexual characteristics. Maintenance of 12 to 15 per cent body fat in athletic males and 18 to 20 percent in athletic females is recommended.

Of the vitamins and minerals, iron is particularly important to young athletes because anemia is associated with reduced oxygenation. The B vitamins are important in the production of energy. The increased total dietary intake should provide sufficient amounts of these and other nutrients, making supplements unnecessary. Available research has not demonstrated that taking supplements above recommended amounts results in benefits during competition.

SHORT-TERM EVENTS. An increase in the amount of carbohydrate combined with a light workout on at least one day prior to a short-term event will assure a supply of liver and muscle glycogen to support the athlete during that activity. On the day of the event the athlete is advised to eliminate roughage, fats, and gas-forming foods to avoid a heavy, long-lasting, flatus-producing residue. Additional carbohydrate during short-term events is necessary only if several are held in one day. Fluid replacement follows the principles discussed under long-term events.

LONG-TERM EVENTS. Prior to a long-term event, modified glucose loading as described in Table 14–7 on page 316 will increase muscle glycogen. After the event has begun, glucose ingestion is suggested in order to spare liver glycogen

Table 14–6. PHYSICAL ACTIVITY AND ENERGY EXPENDITURE FOR A 70-KG. ADOLESCENT

WORK INTENSITY	PULSE RATE	CALORIES (PER MIN.)	EXAMPLES
Light	Below 120	Under 5	Golf, bowling, walking, volleyball, most forms of work
Moderate*	120–150	5 to 10	Jogging, tennis, bike riding, handball, basketball, hiking, strenuous work
Heavy	Above 150	Above 10	Running, fast swimming, fast rowing, wrestling, football, handball, squash, other brief, intense efforts

* Preferred for weight control benefits.

From: Mahan, L. K., and Rees, J. M.: Nutrition in Adolescence, St. Louis, C. V. Mosby Company, 1984.

Adapted from: Sharkey, B. J.: Physiology of Fitness. Champaign, Illinois, Human Kinetics Publishers, 1979, p. 104.

Table 14–7.   MODIFIED GLYCOGEN LOADING REGIME

THIRD DAY PRIOR TO RACE* (e.g., Wednesday before Saturday event)

Exercise:	Run 12–15 miles or 1 1/2–2 hours hard work-out to deplete glycogen stores.
Eat:	After depletion exercise, eat predominantly low-fat, high-carbohydrate foods. Two or three *small* servings of protein/fat foods are O.K., but the majority (70–80%) of caloric intake should be carbohydrate. Minimize intake of salt and salty foods to avoid fluid imbalance and weight distortion.
Drink:	Drink 8 or more glasses (8 + oz.) of fluid; this can include both water and juices. Drink beyond thirst. If traveling, especially by plane, carry a bottle of water. Do not consume caffeine (coffee, tea, cola, cocoa, caffeine-containing medications), alcohol, or diuretic medications.
Weigh:	Weigh (nude) first thing in the morning, and before and after long run to assess fluid loss.

SECOND DAY PRIOR TO EVENT

Exercise:	Easy run of 3–4 miles or short, easy workout of 20–30 minutes.
Eat:	Same principles as previous day.
Drink:	Same principles as previous day.
Weigh:	Weigh (nude) first thing in the morning. If weight is down from yesterday morning, drink even more fluid today.

DAY PRIOR TO RACE

Exercise:	Easy run of 3–4 miles or short, easy workout of 20–30 minutes.
Eat:	Same principles as previous day. In addition, avoid foods high in fiber.
Drink:	Same principles as previous day. Decrease intake of solid food today, and obtain proportionately more calories from juice and other sweet beverages.
Weigh:	Same guidelines as yesterday. Possible weight gain due to the water retention associated with carbohydrate loading.

RACE DAY

Eat:	Eat no solid foods less than 2 1/2 hours prior to the start of the race. Food intake before this time should be light and carbohydrate, for example: juice, white toast, and jam or honey. (Quantity and frequency of food intake will depend on time of race start.)
Drink:	*Up until one hour prior to race start:* Drink at least 16 oz. of fluid per hour, preferably water and juice. No caffeine or alcohol.
	One hour (exactly) prior to race start: Drink 1–2 cups of coffee, tea, or the equivalent in No-Doz tablets (caffeine taken at this time has been shown to delay glycogen depletion, and therefore increase endurance). However, if significant adverse effects come from caffeine, omit this step.
	From one hour to 15 minutes prior to race start (i.e., 9:00–9:45 for 10:00 a.m. start): Drink *no* fluids.
	15 minutes prior to race start: Drink 1 1/2–2 eight oz. glasses of *water.* Drink *no* sugar-containing beverages.
	During Race: Drink frequently, preferably at every aid station. Considerations include heat, hills, and your ability to tolerate fluids. Remember thirst is not an adequate indicator of fluid need. Preferred beverages are water, replacement drinks, or very dilute juices.

AFTER THE EVENT

	Eat and drink whatever sounds good! Carbohydrate is essential to replace glycogen, but now that the race is over it isn't so critical to avoid fat, so enjoy favorite treats. Drink lots of fluid—at least 16 oz. per hour for the remainder of the day.

* It is possible that the glycogen loading regime could be used in preparation for endurance events other than running races.

From Mahan, L. K., and Rees, J. M.: Nutrition in Adolescence. St. Louis, C. V. Mosby Company, 1984.

Developed by Janet Edlefsen, M. S., Nutrition Counselor, formerly Nutrition Counselor, Sports Medicine Division, University of Washington, Seattle, Washington.

stores. Glucose immediately before an event will impair lipid mobilization and is therefore contraindicated.[11]

Fluid and electrolyte balance is of extreme importance during long-term events, and indeed throughout training and competition. Heat and the perspiration of exertion exacerbate shifts due to strenuous exercise. Water must be replaced at the level of one pint for each pound of body weight lost in any exercise or training session. Thus, fluid must be available to keep up with thirst during events and may have to be

Table 14–8. WATER AND ELECTROLYTE
REPLACEMENT DRINK

6 oz. orange juice concentrate (180 g.)*
6 oz. limeade or lemonade concentrate (180 g.)
3 T lime or lemon juice (45 ml.)
2 T honey or sugar (30 ml.)
Pinch of salt
2 quarts cold water (2 liters)

* This drink is designed to meet the recommendations of the American College of Sports Medicine for
fluid, electrolyte and glucose replacement.

From Peterson, M. S., and Martinsen, C. S.: The
Athlete's Cookbook. Seattle, Smuggler's Cove Publishing, 1980.

replaced at levels beyond thirst in the period after the event. Electrolytes and additional glucose can be obtained by using natural juices and
fluids made to specified concentrations as listed
in Table 14–8. Need for the latter will vary according to event and climate.

As in many other situations, maintenance of
appropriate weight for height is a good guide to
adequacy of the diet as long as the foods eaten
to maintain that weight are nutrient-rich. For
teenage athletes whose days may be filled from
early morning to late evening with practices as
well as classes and other activities, obtaining
sufficient food may prove difficult. Parents,
coaches and school officials may have to help
teenagers plan specifically to assure that adequate acceptable foods are available at the time
they can eat.[10]

ACNE

Acne is a normal characteristic of adolescent
development which occurs in varying degrees of
severity in individual teenagers. As many as 50
per cent of adolescent contacts with health professionals may be accounted for by dermatological complaints. Acne is initiated by the
influence of hormones on the sebaceous gland
and mediated by other factors such as stress,
stage of menstrual cycle, and makeup of the affected tissues in the individual. Dietary factors
have traditionally been blamed, but studies
have shown no correlation between the ingestion of foods and the appearance or degree of
acne.[10] Teenagers should be supported in their
efforts to deal with acne by discussion of the
physiological basis for its development and control. Certain medications have been shown to be
effective, such as systemic antibiotics given orally and topical applications of benzoyl peroxide
and tretinoin.[3]
The nutrients (zinc and vitamin A derivatives) that have been suggested as useful by research are used in sufficiently high levels that
they function as drugs. However, in one study
low levels of serum zinc have been found in

those suffering most from acne, suggesting that
zinc deficiency exacerbates the condition.[12] Although no research data are available to confirm the effect, it would seem that the optimally
nourished body, in the general sense, will be
best able to cope with the development of acne.

Strategies for Improving Nutritional Well-Being

PREREQUISITES FOR CHANGE

Especially because of the growing independence of adolescents, any attempt to help them
improve their nutritional status will need to be
planned carefully. The nutritional counselor
must be knowledgeable about adolescents and
ways to communicate with them. The adolescent will have to be in favor of making change
before a plan can succeed. In fact, a great
amount of attention usually must be given to
encouraging the adolescent to want to change.[8]
Knowledge, attitude and behavior must be addressed when guiding adolescents in the acquisition of healthful food habits. Providing
knowledge or teaching can be done in a variety
of settings from the classroom to a hospital bedside. Altering attitudes is much more difficult
and usually demands an individualized experience. Facilitating the adoption of new behaviors
is even more difficult and requires a lengthy period of time. A clinician will need to understand
the change process and communicate that in a
meaningful way to guide the adolescent. Because of the special situation of the adolescent,
parents must be included in the process. They
should be helped to be supportive but not intru-
sive as the adolescent makes changes.[10]

TECHNIQUES FOR FACILITATING CHANGE

Imparting knowledge can be accomplished in
a variety of ways, many of which allow a certain distance to exist between the educator and
the individual. Such techniques are useful then
in reaching large numbers of people as well as
an individual. Printed materials, audiovisual
presentations and lectures are common methods
of transmitting information. A one-to-one teaching session may be a simple exchange of information or grow into a conversation that can
include stimulants to attitudinal and behavioral
change also. While attitudes have a cognitive element, they are usually formed and changed by
the influence of others and the environment.[14]
Modeling by others, attitudes held by peers, actual experience and validation by respected people help to mold attitudes. Audiovisuals,
organized peer groups, demonstrations, and

guided experiences can provide this influence. Chapter 18 contains further discussion of nutrition education.

Counseling on an individual basis is also effective in changing attitudes. In the counseling relationship all aspects can be pulled together, motives examined and support given for change. The counseling techniques developed by the social sciences will be needed to accomplish the therapeutic goals in most nutritional disorders of adolescents.[6] In fact, helping teenagers improve their nutritional status is one of the most exciting challenges to nutrition professionals today.

Problems and Suggested Topics for Discussion

1. What are the main differences in adolescent growth in males and females? How do these influence nutritional requirements?
2. Measure and weigh a teenager in your clinic. Using the appropriate appendices, determine his or her percentile height for age. What percentile is his or her weight for age? Using Appendix Table 24, determine the percentile weight for height for age.
3. Describe what you remember about your body image during your adolescent years. Has it changed, and if so, how?
4. Interview and measure an adolescent female in your clinic and determine her recommended energy intake. Is her actual intake appropriate in view of this energy recommendation? Are there any consequences?
5. Which nutrients are likely to be low in teenagers' diets? Why do you think that this occurs?
6. How are eating disorders related to developmental stages in adolescence?
7. Interview a teenage athlete. Describe his or her typical daily activity and eating pattern. Is his or her diet adequate? If not, what would you recommend?

Cited References

1. Bruch, H.: Eating Disorders. New York, Basic Books, 1973.
2. Committee on Adolescence, American Academy of Pediatrics: Statement on teenage pregnancy. Pediatrics, *63*:795, 1979.
3. Cunliffe, W.: Dermatology, acne vulgaris. Brit. J. Hosp. Med., *20*:24, 1978.
4. Dwyer, J.P.: Diets for children and adolescents that meet the dietary goals. Am. J. Dis. Child., *134*:1073, 1980.
5. Dwyer, J.P., and Mayer, J.: The dismal condition: Problems faced by obese adolescent girls in American society. In Bray, G.A. (ed.): Obesity in Perspective. Vol. II, Part 1 and Part 2. Washington, D.C., U.S. Government Printing Office, 1973.
6. Hackney, H., and Cormier, L.S.: Counseling strategies and objectives. Englewood Cliffs, N.J., Prentice-Hall, Inc., 1979.
7. Hammar, S.L.: The obese adolescent. J. School Health, *35*:246, 1965.
8. Hammar, S.L., and Holterman, V.: Interviewing and counseling adolescent patients. Clin. Ped., *9*:47, 1970.
9. Leverton, R.M.: The paradox of teenage nutrition. J. Am. Diet. Assoc., *56*:116, 1968.
10. Mahan, L.K., and Rees, J.M.: Nutrition in Adolescence. St. Louis, C.V. Mosby Company, 1984.
11. McArdle, W.D., Katch, F.I., and Katch, V.L.: Exercise Physiology: Energy, Nutrition and Human Performance. Philadelphia, Lea & Febiger, 1981.
12. Michaelson, G., et al.: Effects of oral zinc and vitamin A in acne. Arch. Dermatol., *113*:31, 1977.
13. Pyle, R., Mitchell, J.E., and Eckert, E.D.: Bulimia, a report of 34 cases. J. Clin. Psych., *42*(2):60, 1981.
14. Rees, J.M., and Worthington-Roberts, B.S.: Establishing a nutritional environment supportive of reproduction: Nutrition education issues. In Worthington-Roberts, B.S., Vermeersch, J., and Williams, S.R.: Nutrition in pregnancy and lactation. St. Louis, C.V. Mosby Company, 1981.
15. Rosso, P., and Lederman, S.A.: Nutrition in the pregnant adolescent. In Winick, M. (ed.): Adolescent Nutrition. New York, John Wiley & Sons, 1982.
16. Tanner, J.M.: Foetus into Man. Cambridge, Mass., Harvard University Press, 1978.
17. Thomas, J.A., and Call, D.L.: Eating between meals—a nutrition problem among teenagers? Nutr. Rev., *31*: 137, 1973.
18. Thompson, A.M.: Pregnancy in adolescence. In McKigney, J.I., and Munro, H.N. (eds.): Nutrient requirements in adolescence. Cambridge, Mass., M.I.T. Press, 1976.
19. U.S. Department of Health, Education and Welfare: Ten state nutrition survey, 1968–1970. Publ. No. (HSM) 73–8133. Health Services and Mental Health Administration, Center for Disease Control, Atlanta, 1973.
20. Wurtman, R.: Nutrients that modify brain function. Sci. Am., *246*(4):50, 1982.
21. Zlatnik, F.J., and Burmeister, L.F.: Low "gynecologic age"—an obstetric risk factor. Am. J. Ob. Gyn., *128*: 183, 1977.

Additional References

Baldwin, W., and Cain, V.S.: The children of teenage parents. Fam. P. Perspec., *12*:34, 1980.

Clancy, K.L., et al.: Snack food intake of adolescents and caries development. J. Dent. Res., *56*:568, 1977.

Coates, T., and Thoresen, C.: Treating obesity in children and adolescents: a review. Am. J. Public Health, *68*:143, 1978.

Coddington, R.D.: Life events associated with adolescent pregnancies. J. Clin. Psych., *40*:180, 1979.

DeLissovoy, V.: Child care by adolescent parents. Children Today, *2*:22, 1973.

Dwyer, J.: Nutritional requirements of adolescence. Nutr. Reviews, *39*:56, 1981.

Dwyer, J., et al.: Adolescent dieters: who are they? Physical characteristics, attitudes and dieting practices of adolescent girls. Am. J. Clin. Nutr., *20*:1045, 1976.

Erikson, E.H.: Identity, Youth and Crisis. New York, W.W. Norton, 1968.

Felice, M.E., et al.: The young pregnant teenager: impact of comprehensive prenatal care. J. Adol. Health Care, *1*:193, 1981.

Fried, R.I., and Smith, E.E.: Postmenarcheal growth patterns. J. Pediatrics, *61*:562, 1962.

Frisch, R.E.: Fatness of girls from menarche to age 18 years, with a nomogram. Human Biology, *48*:353, 1976.

Frisch, R.E.: Menarche and fatness: reexamination of the critical body composition hypothesis. Science, *200*:1506, 1978.

Greenwood, C.T., and Richardson, D.P.: Nutrition during adolescence. Wld. Rev. Nutr. Diet., *33*:1, 1979.

Hammar, S.L.: The role of the nutritionist in an adolescent clinic. Children, *13*:217, November-December, 1966.

Hammar, S.L., et al.: Treating adolescent obesity. Long range evaluation of previous therapy. Clin. Pediat., *10*:46, 1971.

Hertzler, A.A., et al.: Iron status and family structure of teenage girls in a low income area. Home Econ. Res. J., *5*: 92, 1976.

Hollingsworth, D.R., and Kreutner, A.K.: Teenage pregnancy: Solutions are evolving. N. Engl. J. Med., *303*:516, 1980.

Hurwitz, S.: Acne vulgaris. Am. J. Dis. Child., *133*:536, 1979.

Igoe, J.B.: Health Counseling and Teaching. In Howe, J.: Nursing Care of Adolescents. New York, McGraw-Hill Book Co., 1980.

King, J.C., et al.: Assessment of nutritional status of teenage pregnant girls. 1. Nutrient intake and pregnancy. Am. J. Clin. Nutr., *25*:916, 1972.

Klerman, L.V.: Adolescent pregnancy: a new look at a continuing problem. Am. J. Public Health, *70*:776, 1980.

Kreutner, A.K., and Hollingsworth, D.R.: Adolescent obstetrics and gynecology. Chicago, Year Book Medical Publishers, Inc., 1978.

Lucas, B.: Nutrition and the adolescent. In Pipes, P.: Nutrition in Infancy and Childhood. 2nd ed. St. Louis, C.V. Mosby Company, 1981.

Maier, H.W.: Three Theories of Child Development. New York, Harper & Row, 1978.

Marino, D.D., and King, J.C.: Nutritional concerns during adolescence. Ped. Clin. N. Am., *27*:125, 1980.

McKigney, J., and Munro, H.: Nutrient Requirements in Adolescence. Cambridge, Mass., M.I.T. Press, 1976.

Monello, L.F., and Mayer, J.: Obese adolescent girls, an unrecognized "minority" group? Am. J. Clin. Nutr., *13*:35, 1963.

Naeye, R.L.: Teenaged and pre-teenaged pregnancies: Consequences of the fetal-maternal competition for nutrients. Pediatrics, *67*:146, 1981.

Roche, A.F., and Davila, G.H.: Late adolescent growth in stature. Pediatrics, *50*:874, 1972.

Siantz, M.: The Nurse and the Developmentally Disabled Adolescent. Baltimore, University Park Press, 1977.

Slover, H.T., et al.: Lipids in fast foods. J. Food Sci., *45*:1583, 1980.

Stunkard, A., and Prestka, J.: The physical activity of obese girls. Am. J. Dis. Child., *103*:812, 1962.

Teen Pregnancy: The Problem That Hasn't Gone Away. New York, The Alan Guttmacher Institute, 1981.

Werkman, S.L., and Greenberg, E.S.: Personality and interest patterns in obese adolescent girls. Psychosom. Med., *29*: 72, 1967.

Winick, M., ed.: Adolescent Nutrition. New York, John Wiley & Sons, 1982.

Worthington-Roberts, B.S.: Nutritional needs of the pregnant adolescent. In Worthington-Roberts, B.S., Vermeersch, J., and Williams, S.R., Nutrition in Pregnancy and Lactation. St. Louis, C.V. Mosby Company, 1981.

Worthington-Roberts, B.S.: Suboptimal nutrition and behavior. In Worthington-Roberts, B.S.: Contemporary Developments in Nutrition. St. Louis, C.V. Mosby Company, 1981.

Yetley, E.A., and Roderuck, C.: Nutritional knowledge and health goals of young spouses. J. Am. Diet. Assoc., *77*:31, 1980.

Young, E.A., et al.: Perspectives on fast foods. Dietetic Currents, *5*:23, 1978.

Zifferblatt, S.M., and Wilbur, C.S.: Dietary counseling: Some realistic expectations and guidelines. J. Am. Diet. Assoc., *70*:591, 1977.

CHAPTER 15

Nutrition in Adulthood and the Later Years

Revised by
DEBORAH A. ROLAND, M.S., R.D.

The Process of Aging

Aging is a normal process. It begins with conception and ends only with death, but may progress at varying rates, depending upon several factors—among them nutrition. The best preparation for healthy later years begins in early childhood and possibly in utero.

From conception and during the period of growth, anabolic processes exceed catabolic or degenerative changes. When the body has reached physiological maturity, the rate of degenerative change becomes greater than the growth process. These changes impair the function of any organ to some degree. The decreased efficiency is caused by a loss of cells, leaving the functioning capacity of the organ to the remaining cells.

THEORIES OF AGING

PROGRAMMED CELL REPLICATION. Studies of cultures of human cells in vitro have shown that there is a limit to their proliferative capacities. The cells divide and produce new cells a specific number of times and then slow down to stop dividing. How the replication of cells is controlled or programmed in vivo is not understood,[6] but this process could be a reason for the aging of tissue.

CROSS-LINKAGE. The cross-linkage theory of aging states that the cells form defective RNA from the DNA. The defective RNA then designates the synthesis of defective proteins and defective enzymes. Cells are unable to function, so they die and are permanently lost. Tissues vary in their loss of functions. The percentages of remaining cells of some tissues are shown in Table 15–1.

During the aging process, the amount of soluble collagen decreases, probably because of an increase in cross-linkage in the collagen. Collagen becomes less elastic and stiffer, and it is likely that changes in collagen structure are involved in many of the diseases and disabilities associated with aging. The aging appearance of the skin, the slowness of wound healing and the reduction in vital capacity of the lungs may be due to the age-related structural changes of collagen.

IMMUNE SYSTEM. A deterioration of the body's immune system may cause the changes of aging. Antibody synthesis may become defective, so that antibodies against the body's own tissues are produced, with damaging results.

FREE RADICALS. Aging may be influenced by the duration and intensity of radiation. It is known that radiation can penetrate every cell and produce *free radicals*, which are intermediates with at least one unpaired electron. A free radical striking a polyunsaturated lipid may lead to peroxidation, which is destructive to the cell. The mitochondria and endoplasmic reticulum are vulnerable to peroxidation. The energy-generating process of electron transport and phosphorylation ceases. The cell then dies, and only a "clinker" remains. Cell age of tissue is determined by the ash or number of "clinkers" that remain.

Intracellular membranes that have a high content of polyunsaturated fatty acids are also susceptible to damage by free radicals. It is believed that *vitamin E*, which is an antioxidant, stabilizes the cell membranes and protects them from oxidation by free radicals.[21]

Ascorbic acid plays a role in the enzyme functions relating to the hydroxylation of proline in collagen biosynthesis. It reacts with glutathione, and through antioxidant synergism ascorbic acid increases its protective role. It has the ability to act as a synergist with vitamin E. Both vitamin E and ascorbic acid appear to be important in retarding the process of cellular aging.

Selenium also seems to have an important antioxidant role, although it is not defined in humans. *Glutathione peroxidase*, an enzyme that detoxifies harmful oxidation products, contains selenium. The function of glutathione seems to be enhanced by the presence of vitamin C, but further research in this area is needed. Although the causes of aging are not fully understood, it is agreed that the changes that occur are irreversible.

LONGEVITY AND NUTRITION

Since 1950 there has been no significant increase in the life expectancy of a person 20 years old, even though Americans spend several times more money on health care now than they did in 1950. Progress in medical care has resulted in a reduction of the death rate from infectious disease, and this is reflected in lower rates of infant and child mortality. However, as mortality from these diseases has declined, mortality from degenerative diseases such as atherosclerosis and diabetes mellitus has increased. It is known that the diseases of old age can be delayed somewhat by dietary changes, but the role of diet on the aging process still requires further study.

ENERGY. The hope of prolonging the period during which the characteristics of youth can be maintained is the impetus for a great deal of nutrition research. McCay and co-workers[11] contributed a series of studies on longevity, in which it was shown that restriction of energy, if started early in life, is the single most important factor for extending the life span. Ross, in experiments with rats, extended some life spans to 1800 days (normal life span is 700 to 1000 days) through severe underfeeding. This extended age corresponds to 180 years in human beings.[16] There is general agreement that lean rats live longest, and statistics for humans indicate that overweight in adults is associated with shortened life span. However, early energy restriction cannot be applied to humans at this point, because the division between beneficial and detrimental energy deprivation is not yet clear.

FAT. The amount of fat in the diet seems to be related to longevity. Results from a long-term study of women indicate that the greater the amount of fat in the diet at middle age, the shorter the life span. This was true even when the fat intake was not related to obesity.[18] This

Table 15–1. PERCENTAGE OF FUNCTIONS OF TISSUES REMAINING IN A 75-YEAR-OLD MALE

TISSUE	PER CENT REMAINING IN 75 YEAR OLD MALE
Body water content	82
Number of glomeruli in kidney	56
Number of nerve trunk fibers	63
Brain weight	56
Number of taste buds	36

(From Shock, N. W.: The physiology of aging. Scientific American, *206*:100, 1962. Copyright © 1962 by Scientific American, Inc. All rights reserved.)

same finding has been reported in rats fed high-fat diets early in life. We do not know how dietary intake affects growth and the life span, but the mechanism appears to be centered in the neuroendocrine and immunological systems of the body.

CARBOHYDRATE AND PROTEIN. Studies in animals in which protein alone is restricted show that there is little increase in life expectancy. There appears to be a slight increase in longevity when carbohydrate is restricted, but the greatest increase in longevity is demonstrated when all three variables of carbohydrate, protein and energy are restricted.[9]

Nutritional Needs in the Middle Years

Middle age is defined for the purposes of this text as the years from the late 20's to the early 60's—the largest portion of a person's life span. During this period human beings are usually most productive. It is a time of job achievement and recognition, child rearing and the establishment of lifestyle, values and attitudes that will be transmitted to one's children. Most people are in relatively good health at this age, but less than optimal habits can lead to poor health later. Cigarette smoking, stressful employment, little exercise, excessive alcohol intake and a diet high in saturated fat, cholesterol, sodium and sugar and low in fiber can be factors in the development of hypertension, overweight, atherosclerosis, diabetes mellitus and gastrointestinal problems. The middle years are an important time for education and medical care to preserve health and prevent or delay the onset of chronic disease. During these years, individuals are most able to afford the proper food and medical care necessary to maintain their health, but they may not necessarily have the motivation to take preventive measures for the maintenance of their health.

It is important when providing nutritional care for individuals in this age group to remind them of the importance of exercise and proper food habits. Attention to the improvement of exercise and eating habits can make a difference and make them feel their best now as well as later. The recommended dietary allowances for the majority of this group are defined as allowances for persons aged 23 to 50, as shown in Table 10–1.

Nutritional Needs in the Later Years

The physical, physiological and psychosocial factors of aging become more prominent and debilitating as the person gets older. For this rea-son the elderly person has particular nutrient needs related to his or her process of aging in a specific situation, just as the child has particular needs related to the individual process of growth. These needs are attracting more attention and research as the number of elderly in our population increases. At present, people aged 65 and over constitute nearly 12 per cent of the U.S. population, but if the U.S. birth rate continues to decline, the elderly are expected to constitute about 15 per cent of the population in the year 2000.

The elderly population is *not a homogeneous group*, and no general statements can be made about them. Each elderly person is an individual, and the health professional must be very conscientious to avoid the pitfall of stereotyping older people. The information presented in this chapter should function only as a flexible guideline for providing nutritional care for an elderly person.

The Effect of Aging on Nutritional Status

PHYSIOLOGICAL FACTORS

SENSORY. As a person ages, the senses of taste, smell, sight, hearing and touch diminish at individual and different rates. For example, the number of taste buds per papilla drops from 245 in children and young adults to 88 in people 74 to 85 years old.[1] Sensitivity to sweet and salt taste declines with age. It is also reported that the sense of smell declines more rapidly than the sense of taste. Schiffman has noted that the elderly have a reduced ability to detect odors compared with that of young persons.[17] Many of the medications taken by the elderly can change taste acuity, as shown in Table 21–3. As the sensory factors decline, it is not surprising that the enjoyment of eating is affected.

GASTROINTESTINAL. The following changes take place in the gastrointestinal system with age:

1. *Reduced salivary secretion* decreases the older person's ability to masticate and swallow food. This problem can be worsened by certain medications, such as antihypertensive drugs, which may make the mouth very dry. The decrease in saliva production can also result in rampant dental caries, because saliva produces a teeth-cleansing effect in the mouth.

2. About 50 per cent of persons over 65 years of age have lost all their teeth, and only 75 per cent of this group have satisfactory dentures. Those over 65 years of age who still have their teeth may be plagued by periodontal diseases and by dental caries resulting from years of *dental neglect*. Chewing and eating can become

painful and embarrassing. Persons with reduced mastication ability due to unreplaced tooth loss experience changes in food acceptability.[23] There is a tendency to eat softer, blander foods, which often have more calories in relation to their nutritive value than the fruits and vegetables that they tend to replace. These softer foods usually have less vitamin A, vitamin C, folic acid and fiber, and the change in eating pattern can lead to a deficient nutrient intake and to constipation.

3. *Decreased gastric secretion of hydrochloric acid* is suspected to be a cause of the decreased absorption of calcium and iron, although this has not been clearly demonstrated. There is also a decreased secretion of intrinsic factor, which is necessary for absorption of vitamin B_{12}, which over extended years can result in pernicious anemia in a small percentage of the elderly.

4. *Decreased secretion of pepsin* and the proteolytic enzymes appears to result in impaired digestion of protein.

5. *Decreased secretion of bile* makes digestion of food slower and less efficient. For this reason excessive fat can be a cause of indigestion. Absorption of fat and the fat-soluble vitamins may also be reduced.

6. *Decreased gastrointestinal motility* makes constipation a common problem in the elderly. There may be an increased amount of residue resulting from poor digestion and absorption, which leads to flatulence. These problems can be improved by increasing the amount of fiber and fluid in the diet and by encouraging increased exercise and regular bowel habits.

METABOLIC. *Glucose tolerance* appears to decrease with age. This decrease can be the result of two factors: (1) a diminished insulin secretion in response to a glucose challenge or (2) a decreased tissue response to the action of insulin. The latter may be due to an increased proportion of fat tissue in the elderly person regardless of whether he or she is overweight. Adipose tissue has a certain "insulin resistance." Whether diminished glucose tolerance is a natural process of aging or whether the person is truly a diabetic is difficult to determine. The use of glucose tolerance curves developed for younger adults to diagnose diabetes in an elderly person is now being debated. Some authorities believe that the declining glucose tolerance is a preliminary sign that true diabetes is emerging and may require treatment. Others feel that the changes in glucose tolerance are a non-pathological manifestation of the aging process and that the glucose tolerance test must be age-adjusted. How this adjustment should be made is still unclear.[8] Table 15–2 presents a system of treating diabetes in the elderly.

Basal metabolic rate decreases by 10 to 15 per cent or more after the age of 50, as shown in Figure 1–6, largely because of the decrease in lean body mass, since adiposity increases even in the presence of stable body weight.

The presence of *chronic disease* in the elderly can affect nutritional requirements by altering metabolic processes and by affecting digestion and the absorption, utilization and excretion of nutrients.

CARDIOVASCULAR. The capacity of the lungs and the amount of blood that the heart can pump diminish as total peripheral resistance increases with age. During the aging process blood vessels become less elastic and total peripheral resistance increases. Hypertension in the elderly, which is defined by systolic pressure above 160 mm. Hg and diastolic above 95 mm. Hg, is very common.[5] Maintaining the systolic pressure between 140 and 160 mm. Hg and diastolic between 90 and 100 mm. Hg is desirable when treating elderly persons who have hypertension.[4]

RENAL. The rate of blood flowing through the kidneys decreases and the number of nephrons diminishes. The composition of the blood may be modified, depending upon the functioning of the cells. The handling of excessive amounts of protein waste products or electrolytes becomes more difficult, and ample fluid intake is very important. The elderly individual is not able to respond as quickly to metabolic challenges in acid–base balance.

PSYCHOSOCIAL FACTORS

To promote optimal health and nutrition among the aging population several agencies, such as community home health care, chore worker services and community feeding centers, have been established. Use of these health-promoting services by the elderly can improve the quality of their lives. Because these services include a nutritional component, older persons are provided with an opportunity to improve their diets.

Special problems arise when the elderly lack variety in their diet or become uninterested in food. The primary causes of the failure to obtain an adequate diet are social isolation (separation) and retirement (reduced income). Because of a greater amount of leisure time, the person has time to think about his or her next meal and either may relish the idea of eating or may become critically despondent over its monotony. This is most likely to happen with persons who live alone or who have to do their own cooking. They find it easier to eat the same thing day after day and, unless watched carefully, may suffer from malnutrition even though overweight.

Table 15–2.   TREATMENT MODALITIES FOR OLDER PERSONS WITH DIABETES

A. Diet
1. Compliance is best if diet is planned after a careful history to determine patient's usual eating habits, and efforts are made to alter this by the least possible amount. In some patients, reduction of simple sugars may be the only change needed.
2. Often it is best to introduce changes gradually, rather than giving the patient a whole new diet all at once.
3. In most patients, priority should be given to weight reduction, while insuring adequate intake of protein, vitamins, and minerals.
4. In patients on insulin or oral agents, and some patients on diet alone, it may be important to establish regular meal times and consistent distribution of food among the meals.
5. It *may* be desirable to restrict fat consumption and emphasize polyunsaturated fats.
6. Diets high in fiber *may* assist in lowering the blood glucose and are probably indicated if patients have constipation or diverticulosis. Note that adding fiber to the diet of a person already well-controlled on insulin may lead to hypoglycemia, and a change in insulin dose may be needed.
7. Only rarely is the rigorously structured exchange-list type of diet ("ADA" diet) needed for older persons.

B. Exercise
1. Should usually be encouraged, to a degree consistent with cardiovascular fitness.
2. For patients who may be walking or running, instruction in foot care is mandatory.
3. In some patients, exercise may affect insulin absorption.

C. Insulin and oral agents
1. Older patients may be more prone to hypoglycemia when treated with insulin or long-acting oral agents such as chlorpropamide. In such patients, short-acting sulfonylureas, such as tolbutamide, may be preferable. All agents should be started in the lowest possible dose.
2. When prescribing insulin, first ascertain whether the patient has the agility and visual acuity needed to administer the intended dose accurately. Otherwise, use oral agents or arrange for another person to prepare the insulin injection.

D. Patient education
1. Because learning ability may be decreased, and attention span reduced, it may be necessary to modify the usual teaching program.
2. Priorities in patient education should be based on the intended modes of therapy and an appropriate *needs assessement*.
3. Because foot problems are a major cause of morbidity from diabetes in older patients, instruction in proper foot care should usually receive high priority.
4. All elements of the therapeutic plan must be periodically reviewed and knowledge reinforced, with both the patient, and, if appropriate, a responsible family member or friend.

(From Horwitz, D.L.: Diabetes and aging. Am. J. Clin. Nutr., *36*:803, 1982.)

SENSE OF LOSS. Depression may result from a sense of loss—loss of loved ones, productivity, a sense of worth, mobility, income and, finally, body image. The elderly person may avoid food in order to obtain attention that will overcome the sense of loss or may become a compulsive nibbler and overeat to compensate for the loss. Eating patterns may be erratic in some older persons. They may overeat one day and nibble on foods the next. Swanson found one case in which a woman's daily energy intake varied from 800 to 3700 kcal.[20]

REDUCED INCOME. Most people retire at age 60 to 65 and usually have several more years of life, during which they may be supported only by Social Security payments or by an employee pension plan. Frequently this income is inadequate and the elderly individual becomes poor. Unfortunately, food intake suffers. Although most poor elderly people are eligible for food stamp programs, they frequently do not use them. A survey of an urban population composed of low- to moderate-income elderly persons found that, while two thirds of the respondents were aware of the food stamp program, only 10 per cent said they used it, even though most of them would have been eligible.[19] Some reasons why an elderly person may not use food stamps are:

1. A feeling that food stamps are a form of charity.
2. The monthly trip to the food stamp office is inconvenient, dangerous or impossible.
3. The purchase of food stamps requires a large expenditure of money, leaving little for other necessities or emergencies.
4. The use of food stamps may stigmatize the person in the grocery store as poor and a recipient of charity.

ENVIRONMENTAL FACTORS

When plagued by decreased sight and physical handicaps, the elderly may be trapped by immobility. Food shopping is difficult. Some are confused by the variety of items in the stores. The distance from the stores and the inability to carry groceries are handicaps. The trend for small neighborhood grocery stores to close and be replaced by large supermarkets in shopping centers presents a great inconvenience to the urban dweller without a car. Walking long distances, having to cross busy highways and carting or carrying groceries can make the trip forbidding and hazardous, as shown in Figure 15–1. Using buses can be difficult when carrying groceries, assuming a bus system exists.

Because of reduced income the elderly person may be forced to live in poor, crime-ridden areas. This adds to the problem of isolation, making him or her fearful of leaving the home or apartment. A stroke, fracture or heart condition may decrease mobility even more. Moving to a smaller house, a first floor apartment or a house without stairs could help, but the poor elderly person is trapped financially; he or she cannot afford to pay for a move or to leave a house that is already paid for. Table 15–3 summarizes these and other factors that may lead to undernutrition in the elderly.

Nutritional Requirements of the Elderly

ENERGY

There is a decrease in energy requirements with age. In addition to a normal decline in metabolism of some 10 to 15 per cent after the age of 50, there is almost always a slackening of physical activity, which lowers the need for energy still further. It is difficult, however, to estimate the degree of reduction in physical activity of individuals in the later years of life. Both the reduction of physical activity and the decline in basal metabolic needs vary with indi-

Table 15–3. POSSIBLE CAUSE OF UNDERNUTRITION IN THE ELDERLY

Loss of income—poverty
Social isolation
Diseases that reduce appetite, decrease absorption or utilization of nutrients or increase requirements for nutrients
Drugs that affect food intake, or the absorption, utilization or excretion of nutrients
Ignorance about good nutrition or food preparation
Dental problems
Depression or mental problems
Decreased physical ability to buy food or prepare a meal
Alcoholism

viduals. The Food and Nutrition Board in the 1980 RDA proposed that energy allowances be reduced between 51 and 75 years of age to 90 per cent of the amount the person required as a young adult of age 23 or so, and for persons beyond age 75 years to about 75 to 80 per cent of that amount. If the person remains physically active after age 50, however, this reduction may not need to be as great.

The man and woman at age 23 need approximately 2700 and 2000 kcal. per day, respectively. Assuming that they maintain good health, normal activity and approximately the same weight, at age 51 to 75 they need approximately 2400 and 1800 kcal. per day, respectively. At age 76 and beyond they need approximately 2050 and 1600 kcal. per day, respectively. If their weight is greater at age 51 to 75 than it was at age 23, there has probably been addition of fat tissue.

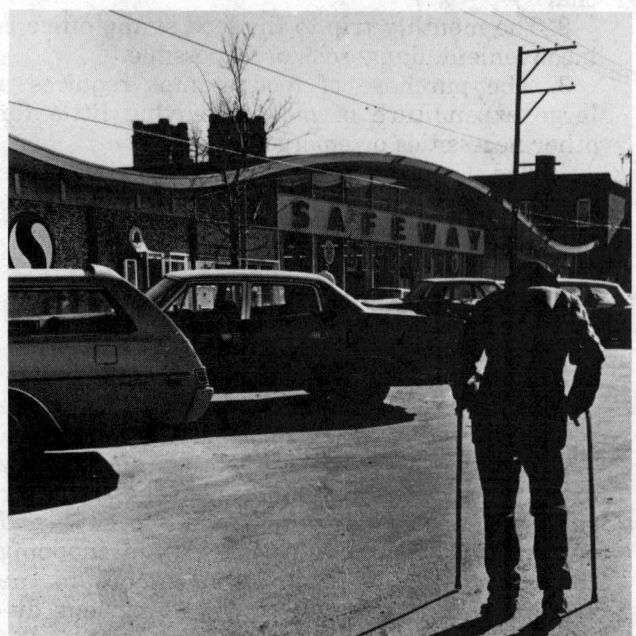

Figure 15–1. How will he carry groceries home? (From Sherman, E. M., and Brittan, M. R.: Contemporary food gatherers. Gerontologist, 13:358, 1973. Photo courtesy of Barbara Caley ACSW, St. Luke's Geriatric Clinic, Denver, Colorado.)

It seems advisable that most of the reduction in calories should come from a reduction in the carbohydrate and fat in the diet. Since aged persons require less energy but not less protein, vitamins or minerals, the foods eaten should obviously be good sources of these nutrients. Calories should not be wasted on low-nutrient foods such as candy, cola drinks, rich pastries and desserts. When kcalories are limited to less than 1800, careful planning is required to provide an adequate diet, as was clearly demonstrated by Swanson.[20] Food intakes falling below 1800 kcal. provided inadequate amounts of protein, calcium, iron and vitamins for nutritional safety.

PROTEIN

Body protein mass decreases with age. This is probably due in large part to a decrease in skeletal muscle mass. Visceral protein metabolism (for the internal organs) becomes more important. Total body protein increases from birth and reaches a maximum in the 20's, then slowly decreases throughout the middle and later years. The decrease seems to occur more rapidly in men than in women. In healthy elderly people body protein is 60 to 70 per cent of that of young adults. Although it seems that the protein needs of the old person would be less than those of a young adult, there is not enough information on the amino acid and protein needs of the elderly to make this statement. The requirements for certain amino acids (threonine, tryptophan and methionine) may be different from requirements for young adults, and the optimal pattern of essential amino acids may change with age.[24] In 1980 the Food and Nutrition Board concluded that the protein RDA of 0.8 gm./kg./day for younger adults is appropriate for the healthy elderly person.

Stressful physical and psychological stimuli can induce a negative nitrogen balance. Infection, altered gastrointestinal function and metabolic changes caused by chronic disease can reduce the efficiency of dietary nitrogen utilization. Even without disease the aging gastrointestinal tract has reduced protein digestion and absorption. For these reasons Young and Scrimshaw recommend a higher protein intake of 1 gm./kg./day.[25]

Dietary studies of older people frequently show low intakes of the foods that are good sources of protein. A low protein intake usually occurs with a low energy intake. Meat consumption decreases because of financial restraints, lack of cooking facilities, poor advice, lack of teeth and possibly other reasons. Negative nitrogen balances are often found when balance studies are made, and clinical protein deficiencies are also frequently observed. Such deficiencies contribute to edema, itching of the skin, chronic eczema, fatigue, muscle weakness and tissue wastage. Wounds heal slowly and body resistance is lowered. However, the question arises as to whether the protein deficiencies seen are caused solely by low intake or by a combination of low intake, incomplete digestion and assimilation and insufficient calories. A low intake of protein usually means a low vitamin and mineral intake, and vitamin deficiency could be present with protein deficiency.

CARBOHYDRATE

As mentioned, elderly people have a reduced glucose tolerance and therefore are more susceptible to temporary hypo- or hyperglycemia than a younger person is. When the blood sugar levels are increased by a load of sugar, the rate of return to lower values is significantly slower in an older person. The use of sugar and sweets should be reduced and the amount of complex carbohydrate and fiber should be increased. This change may improve insulin sensitivity.

FAT

Because of the relationship between serum cholesterol, saturated fatty acids and atherosclerosis, as discussed in Chapter 28, and because of the possible correlation between dietary fat and the level of serum cholesterol, it may be advisable to decrease the proportion of fat in the diet. From epidemiological evidence, serum cholesterol levels seem to peak in men between 50 and 59 years of age and in women between 60 and 69 years of age, and then to fall in the later years. Serum triglyceride levels rise with continuing age and probably reflect the decreased capacity of elderly persons to remove dietary fat from the blood. Restricting dietary fat, particularly saturated fat, may be helpful, but fat intake should still be about 30 per cent of the total energy intake.

Food sources of cholesterol include many protective foods (egg yolk, whole milk, liver and beef), and rigid restriction of these might lead to deficiencies of other nutrients. It does not seem advisable to restrict these foods rigidly in the daily diet of the person over 75 years of age, since the prevention of atherosclerosis in these people seems less significant than the risk of nutritional deficiencies.

The intake of the essential fatty acids should provide 2 per cent of the calorie intake. This is supplied by polyunsaturated fats (also a good source of vitamin E). Distributing the fat intake among all the meals also helps in the digestion and absorption.

MINERALS

Of the minerals, *calcium* and *iron* are probably of greatest importance in the nutrition of the aged. Fragility of bones may be attributed to low intake of calcium-rich foods such as milk. The 1971–1972 Health and Nutrition Examination Survey I (HANES) reported that one third of the white subjects 65 to 75 years of age with incomes above poverty level and one third of all black subjects regardless of income level did not meet the established standard for calcium—400 mg. for males, 600 mg. for females. Persons over 59 years of age are very likely to consume diets inadequate in calcium, and women have a lower intake than men.[10]

OSTEOPOROSIS. This is a condition of *reduced bone mass* that develops when more calcium is lost from bones than is taken in. It is more common in the later years of life. Although other factors are present in osteoporosis, one factor may be inadequate calcium intake over a period of years. A gradual decrease in bone mass takes place until finally there is pain and possibly fracture after a fall. From our present understanding of this disease it seems that the best protection against osteoporosis in old age is to include an adequate amount of calcium and vitamin D in the daily diet during adulthood and to remain physically active. Osteoporosis is discussed more fully in Chapters 7 and 33.

OSTEOMALACIA. This condition of *decreased bone mineralization*, commonly referred to as adult rickets, is caused by poor utilization of calcium induced by a severe lack of vitamin D. Elderly individuals who do not drink milk or who suffer from malabsorption, liver disease or kidney disease, who are taking anticonvulsant drugs or who do not get adequate exposure to sunlight can develop vitamin D deficiency and osteomalacia. Not enough calcium and vitamin D are available for normal bone maintenance, so the bones gradually weaken and fractures frequently result. Osteomalacia is further discussed more fully in Chapters 6 and 33.

NUTRITIONAL ANEMIA. This is frequently found in older persons and may be caused by deficiencies of iron, protein, vitamin B_{12}, folacin, ascorbic acid or, more likely, by a combination of factors including reduced gastric acidity. The Ten-State Nutrition Survey revealed that iron deficiency anemia is more prevalent in adults over 60 years of age than in younger people, regardless of income or race.[2] The HANES I data demonstrated that approximately 15 to 20 per cent of the elderly have lower than normal hemoglobin levels.[10]

PERIODONTAL DISEASE. Periodontal disease is characterized by demineralization of the alveolar bone of the mandible, which leads to loosening of the teeth, traumatization of the gingivae and hemorrhage and infection of the gums. It is thought that periodontal disease may be an early form of osteoporosis, in which case adequate calcium intake and the ratio of dietary phosphorus to calcium during the lifetime may be important. Periodontal disease is the most common cause of loss of teeth in Americans over the age of 35 and is discussed in Chapter 33.

VITAMINS

A number of studies have shown that increases in the vitamin intake of the aged give general health improvement. This could mean that the present allowances, which are the same as the allowances for younger adults, are not adequate for elderly people. More likely it reflects the fact that the elderly tend to have low intakes of vitamins. The HANES II preliminary data, which compare reported nutrient intakes of individuals over 65 with the RDA, are shown in Table 15–4. The data show that vitamin, mineral and other nutrient recommendations are not met. For example, 50 per cent of the men and 75 per cent of the women studied did not meet the RDA for vitamin A.

Some workers have shown that health is improved by giving B vitamins and vitamin C, while others have found that it takes large doses of the water-soluble vitamins to correct deficiencies of long standing in older people. Many of the so-called "normal" or "typical" characteristics of aging, such as slow adaptation of the eyes to darkness, follicular hyperkeratosis and certain conjunctival lesions, have been improved by prolonged and increased administration of vitamin A.

Mental and behavioral changes such as depression, anorexia and irritability can be partially caused by vitamin B deficiencies. To what extent latent or subclinical deficiencies of thiamin, niacin, folic acid or vitamin B_{12} affect behavior is still very unclear.

Also, to what extent are low serum levels of B vitamins "normal" in the aging person? For example, low serum B_{12} levels appear to be associated with the aging process and seem to be fairly common in a geriatric population. The low values are probably secondary to decreased absorption. Studies have shown that supplementing an older person's diet with vitamin B_{12} may not induce a change in serum B_{12} levels.[12] The elderly person should be assessed for the adequacy of vitamin B_{12} and treated accordingly.[3]

Folic acid deficiency, which can result in hyperchromic megaloblastic anemia, is frequently seen in an elderly population. This vitamin is not widely present in food, is easily destroyed during cooking, and may not be absorbed from the gastrointestinal tract, which may be the

Table 15–4.   REPORTED INTAKES OF INDIVIDUALS OVER 65 IN THE U.S. POPULATION: PRELIMINARY DATA FROM HANES II, 1977–1978

NUTRIENT	MEAN INTAKE AND STANDARD DEVIATION		RDA	PERCENTILE DISTRIBUTION OF INTAKES				
				5	25	50	75	95
MALES								
Kcalories	1828 ±	753	2000	948	1529	1966	2554	3481
Protein (gm.)	73.29 ±	34	56	29	50	67	89	135
Carbohydrate (gm.)	203.0 ±	92		72	140	193	253	366
Fat (gm.)	75.10 ±	40		27	49	68	93	141
Calcium (mg.)	698.0 ±	443	800	186	370	597	915	1564
Phosphorus (mg.)	1197 ±	541	800	483	813	1119	1468	2275
Iron (mg.)	14.09 ±	8.22	10	5.49	9.13	12.27	17.02	27.92
Sodium (mg.)	2892 ±	1620		1047	1843	2577	3593	5603
Vitamin A (I.U.)	6572 ±	12,535	5000	976	2229	3914	7062	17,161
Niacin (mg.)	19.93 ±	11.45	16	6.56	12.48	17.68	24.12	40.20
Thiamin (mg.)	1.33 ±	0.88	1.2	0.47	0.82	1.13	1.57	2.77
Riboflavin (mg.)	1.84 ±	1.35	1.4	0.57	1.07	1.56	2.25	3.95
Vitamin C (mg.)	100 ±	87	60	5	33	79	140	271
FEMALES								
Kcalories	1295 ±	503	1600	607	972	1221	1570	2173
Protein (gm.)	51.18 ±	23	44	21	36	48	63	92
Carbohydrate (gm.)	158.47 ±	69		64	111	151	194	285
Fat (gm.)	50.21 ±	26		16	33	46	62	99
Calcium (mg.)	541.9 ±	336	800	141	259	475	714	1156
Phosphorus (mg.)	880.0 ±	417	800	350	594	823	1078	1573
Iron (mg.)	10.23 ±	5.0	10	4.28	6.63	9.05	12.20	19.81
Sodium (mg.)	1990 ±	1086		678	1269	1818	2433	3891
Vitamin A (I.U.)	5486 ±	8090	4000	832	1990	3376	6255	15,500
Niacin (mg.)	14.44 ±	8.31	13	5.19	8.96	12.90	17.35	30.23
Thiamin (mg.)	0.99 ±	0.76	1.0	0.37	0.63	0.85	1.15	1.97
Riboflavin (mg.)	1.36 ±	1.12	1.2	0.42	0.79	1.13	1.60	2.88
Vitamin C (mg.)	105 ±	86	60	7	37	90	147	260

Values usually rounded to the nearest tenth.
(Abstracted from the preprint of HANES II Preliminary Statistics. Washington, D.C., Department of Health and Human Services, 1982, unpublished.)

problem for many elderly persons. Vitamin-dependent anemias are further discussed in Chapter 29.

Some individuals may need to supplement their diets with vitamin or mineral supplements. However, it is necessary to look at the diet before recommending a vitamin or mineral supplement. In many cases, a maintenance level multivitamin and mineral supplement may be well worth the expenditure and may cure latent nutritional deficiency states, which may be the basis for many chronic complaints. It is important to remember that foods containing vitamins provide calories, protein and fiber. Vitamin/mineral supplements do not. Individual vitamins are discussed in detail in Chapter 6.

Elderly people are often swayed by the claims made for health food and can spend money on organic vitamins, mineral supplements and special foods that are supposed to make them feel better. They may feel better, in fact, because of the improved nutrient intake. However, it would be better for them to spend their money on a general vitamin and mineral supplement than on health foods. The supplement would give the same results at a small fraction of the cost.

WATER

The importance of water in the diet increases with age. With diminished kidney function, water becomes increasingly important as a carrier and is reported to ease rather than burden the kidney. Drinking adequate amounts of fluids (five to eight glasses daily) also aids digestion and helps in the control of constipation, which so frequently plagues older people. Chapter 8 discusses the function of water in more detail.

REQUIREMENTS DURING CRITICAL ILLNESS

During the aging process, the cytoplasm of cells undergoes regressive and degenerative changes that lead to a depression of basic cellular mechanisms. The result is that the energy pathways that are crucial in times of stress do not function as efficiently in old cells. Second, the cellular potassium-sodium pump is not as efficient, which means that the aging body is less able to correct fluid and electrolyte imbalances quickly. Third, the aging cell does not have metabolic enzyme reserves that allow it to switch on new metabolic pathways and respond to challenges to homeostasis. Therefore, nutritional support for critically ill aged patients should include early and aggressive infusion of glucose, amino acids, electrolytes, vitamins and minerals.

NUTRIENT INTAKE AND NUTRITIONAL STATUS OF THE ELDERLY

The results of the 1968–1970 Ten-State Nutrition Survey of low-income people revealed that some of the elderly show evidence of general malnutrition.[2] The HANES I data revealed similar findings. For example, iron requirements were not met by the elderly in the low-income group. Calorie requirements were not met by any group regardless of socioeconomic background. Calcium, vitamin A and ascorbic acid intakes were below the standard for one third of the participants.[10]

However, it is a mistake to assume that the eating habits of all elderly are poor ones or that they all have poor nutritional status. Although the Ten-State Nutrition Survey revealed biochemical and clinical signs of nutritional deficiency, it was found that the nutrient quality of the diet of the elderly per 1000 kcal. was higher than that for adolescents. The problem seems to be not the quality of the diet but the *amount* of intake. In her study of 529 non-institutionalized elderly persons of all economic backgrounds aged 60 to 102 years,[22] Todhunter likewise found that the size of servings rather than the choice of foods was a major factor influencing nutrient intake. She also found that the adequacy of dietary intakes of those living alone did not differ significantly from that of those living with others.

From her study of elderly people, Todhunter concluded: "Their food habits and beliefs were free from faddism, they were willing to try new foods and to change at least some of their food habits, and they had a good appetite."[22]

Food for the Elderly

Helping older persons to provide an adequate diet for themselves often presents many problems. Education about a modified diet, usually as a valid part of medical care, frequently worsens the situation by further limiting the elderly person's food choices.

The nurse or dietitian should work *with* the aging person to plan a food pattern that the person can realistically follow. This is generally best accomplished by incorporating needed changes into the individual's already established patterns rather than planning a diet that would be completely new to the person. Helpful pamphlets, charts and booklets giving hints and simple information about food for the elderly are available from state health departments, offices of aging and Title IIIc Federal nutrition programs for the elderly.

Older people, just like people in other age groups, need a well-balanced diet that includes the protective foods, as discussed in Chapter 10. The protein from meat, fowl, fish, eggs, milk and milk products, or a combination of grains, legumes, nuts and vegetables, is essential, along with the vitamins and minerals from these foods. Fruits and vegetables are important protective foods. Dentures may limit consistency of food to the softened varieties, such as mashed, chopped or strained. Whole-grain breads and cereals are encouraged because they aid in maintaining normal bowel functions, as well as adding valuable food nutrients.

Milk is an important food in the diet of the aging. Yet too frequently it is omitted or replaced by tea or coffee. Some older people even resent being encouraged to drink milk, while others dislike it. It is frequently thought to cause gas, which may be true if lactase, the enzyme needed to digest milk, is absent, as is discussed in Chapter 23. As has been pointed out, milk is the chief source of calcium, a good source of protein, a rich source of riboflavin and, when fortified, an excellent source of vitamin D. If the elderly person does not tolerate milk or milk products, the nurse or nutritionist should look for other sources of vitamin D, calcium and riboflavin in the diet. If the diet still appears low in these nutrients, and ingestion of milk or milk products seems impossible, then dietary supplementation is recommended.

Foods that furnish few or no essential nutrients but many calories, such as rich sauces, gravies, pies, cakes, sugar, preserves, candies, oils, and fried and fatty foods, should be limited as necessary. However, such foods frequently offer a tremendous psychological boost and may be included for this reason.

For those with sensitive digestive systems the suggestions are to eat something hot at each meal, four or five light meals rather than three substantial ones, and the larger dinner meal at noon rather than in the evening.

The general principles governing the planning of a diet for the aging person are not fundamentally different from those for the mature younger adult. However, modifications may be necessary because of certain characteristics inherent in the process of aging and peculiar to the elderly, as already mentioned. Most important is that the food be nutritious, tasty and pleasant for the elderly person to eat.

FEEDING PROGRAMS

In Title IIIc, formerly Title VII of the 1973 Older Americans Act, the National Nutritional Program for the Elderly authorized funds for group feeding programs for the aging. These local programs are administered by health centers, church groups and senior citizen groups, and frequently are run by the elderly participants themselves. The daily meal provided is meant to be a pleasant social experience in addition to being nutritious. (It should provide one third of the RDA.) Outreach, transportation, nutrition education and social counseling are part of the program, in addition to the recreation and socialization surrounding the meal.

Participants who were interviewed gave equal importance to the food and the social aspects of the program. The group meals act as a catalyst for involving the elderly in social activities and in community responsibilities. It becomes very important to reach out *actively* to the elderly to participate, as illustrated by this excerpt:

The older American presents difficulties in outreach simply not found in other populations. He ordinarily pays his bills, lives within his means, obeys the laws, and is seldom found in the courts. He does not ordinarily march in the streets protesting his low pension, inadequate housing, or poor transportation. He gradually drops away from his social clubs and churches and stays within his own small circle of acquaintances and activities, calling no particular attention to his needs until he becomes ill enough to be hospitalized. In short, he is almost deliberately inconspicuous.[13]

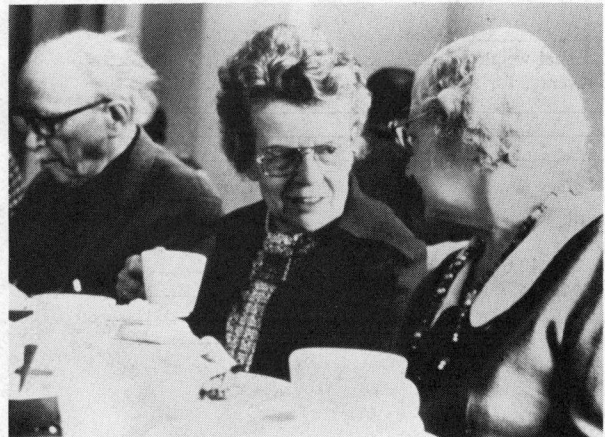

Figure 15–2. Community centers that offer meals often make eating more enjoyable for older people who live alone.

Nutrition education in these settings is more effective if presented by an informal group discussion approach than by the lecture approach. Nutrition education is also effective if utilized in the designing of program menus by a group of participants.[7]

FOOD STAMP PROGRAM

The present food stamp program has been modified so that it is useful to the elderly person who cannot get to the food stamp office. A proxy can be sent to enroll in the program and pick up the stamps. In some states food stamps can be purchased by mail and can be used to pay for Home Delivered Meals.

HOME DELIVERED MEALS

This feeding program, which is Federally funded through Title IIIc, provides home-delivered meals for persons who are homebound. To qualify for the program a person must be 60 years of age or older (or the spouse of an eligible client) and must be homebound. A small donation for the meals is suggested, but no one is denied meals because of an inability to pay. Chapter 17 provides further discussion of food programs.

NUTRITION EDUCATION

The 1981 Nutrition Education Conference for Older Americans was organized to address nutritional concerns of the elderly that could be ameliorated by educational programs.[15] One major goal of the conference was to identify strategies that would encourage the public and private sector to work together to remedy these problems. This meeting preceded the 1981 White House Conference on Aging, which also addressed nutrition-related concerns of the elderly and suggested the development of multipurpose senior centers that would provide nutrition and other services for the elderly. Another recommendation specified that registered dietitians be reimbursed by Medicare, Medicaid and private insurance for dietary counseling of the aging. A total of 600 recommendations were made during the conference to be used in the development of a national policy on aging.

For the elderly person to be motivated to change lifetime eating habits, the reason must be a good one and the approach humane. The traditional methods of presenting nutrition information in lecture or pamphlet form are not likely to be effective with this population. More appropriate are group discussions among elderly people who initiate questions or topics that they would like discussed.

During individual counseling, the counselor should try to understand *why* an elderly patient is or is not eating correctly or is not responsive to nutrition counseling. There may be a reason unrelated to food, cooking facilities, income or the ability to make a meal. The environment of an aged person is complex and changing as he or she accepts a new role in society. The ways in which each elderly person reacts to this change of life must be thoroughly understood before nutrition counseling or education can be meaningful and accepted.

Nutritional studies indicate that the elderly are relatively uninformed about nutrition compared with other age groups. When most of today's elderly people were in school, they received very little information about nutrition. The elderly may delude themselves into believing that nutrition does not matter for them. However, one important concern of elderly persons is their health. Once they accept the fact that proper nutrition is essential to good health, they are eager to learn how it can keep them healthy and living independently.[14]

NUTRITIONAL CARE IN NURSING HOMES AND OTHER CLINICAL SETTINGS

The nutritional care of the elderly in nursing homes and other clinical facilities must be directed toward meeting their physiological and psychological needs over a long period of time. These needs change depending upon the aging process, degenerative disease process and the emotional and mental status of the patient. It becomes very important to reassess the nutritional status and needs of the patient periodically in order to avoid continuing an unnecessary diet modification or missing an important unmet nutritional need. Table 15–5 presents a form for evaluating the nutritional status of an elderly person. Further discussion is found in Chapter 9.

Weight history is an important record of nutritional status. Each patient should be weighed weekly, and this should be recorded. Checking for other signs of malnutrition is especially important for the bedridden patient, who may be difficult to weigh. Table 15–6 gives the average weights for heights for persons aged 65 to 94 years of age.

The most important nutritional care activity performed by a nurse in a nursing home is noticing and recording the quantity and quality of fluid and food intake of the residents. Elderly people in a nursing home may not eat for various reasons, including the strangeness or unpalatability of the food. Improving the eating behavior of the elderly patient requires a special effort by the dietitian to make the foods he likes available in an attractive and palatable

Table 15–5. NUTRITIONAL STATUS EVALUATION OF THE ELDERLY

Name _____		Sex _____	Âge _____
Estimation of appetite:	Poor _____	Moderate _____	Good _____
Estimation of recent/past food intake:	Calories	Adequate	Inadequate
	Protein	Adequate	Inadequate
	Calcium	Adequate	Inadequate
	Folic acid	Adequate	Inadequate
	Iron	Adequate	Inadequate

Capability to consume food:
  Swallowing difficulties:
  Chewing problems:
  Physical handicaps:

ANTHROPOMETRIC DATA

Height _____ Usual weight _____ Recent losses _____
Current weight _____ % Usual weight _____
Body mass index (Table 27-1) _____ % Average for age (Table 15-6) _____
Triceps skinfold percentile (Appendix Table 31) _____
Midarm circumference percentile (Appendix Table 32) _____
Midarm muscle area percentile (Appendix Table 33) _____

LABORATORY DATA	*Normal Values*			*Current Value*
Serum albumin	3.5–5.5 gm./dl.			_____
Per cent expected creatinine/Ht.	72–80%			_____
Hemoglobin	14.0 gm./dl. M	12.0 gm./dl. F		_____
Hematocrit	44%	M	38% F	_____
Mean corpuscular volume	80 to 95			_____
Serum transferrin saturation	20%	M	15% F	_____

CLINICAL STATUS

History of chronic disease:
History of malabsorptive symptoms:
History of failure to care:

Prepared by Joan M. Karkeck, M.S., R.D., Assistant Professor, Department of Nutritional Sciences, University of Washington, Seattle, Washington.

Table 15-6. AVERAGE WEIGHT FOR HEIGHT: PERSONS AGED 65-94 YEARS

	MALES Age (yr.)						Height (in.)	FEMALES Age (yr.)					
Height (in.)	65-69	70-74	75-79	80-84	85-89	90-94		65-69	70-74	75-79	80-84	85-89	90-94
58							58	133	125	123		110	119
59							59	134	127	124	116	113	119
60							60	135	129	126	118	116	120
61	142	139	137				61	137	131	128	121	120	124
62	144	141	139	135			62	139	134	131	124	124	129
63	146	143	141	136	133		63	141	137	134	128	128	
64	149	146	143	138	135		64	144	140	137	132	133	
65	151	149	145	141	139	130	65	147	144	140	136	138	
66	154	152	148	144	142	133	66	151	147	143	140	142	
67	156	155	151	147	145	136	67	155	151	146	144		
68	159	158	154	150	148	140	68	159	155				
69	163	162	158	154	152	144	69	164	160				
70	167	165	162	159	156	149	70						
71	172	169	166	164	160	154	71						
72	177	173	171	170	165		72						
73	182	178	175				73						

(Adapted from Master, A.M., Lasser, R.P., and Beckman, G.: Tables of average weight and height of Americans aged 65 to 94 years. JAMA, *172*:659, 1960.)
Standards of height and weight for persons 65 to 94 years of age are calculated on the basis of data from 2925 males and 2694 females. The study notes that published figures are averages of actual measurements rather than optimal or ideal figures.

way, and an effort by the nurse to create a pleasant atmosphere, encourage independence in eating or, if necessary, help him eat. The attitudes of the nurse and the dietitian can be supportive or destructive and are reflected in the nutritional health of the elderly in the institution.

Problems and Suggested Topics for Discussion

1. List the ways in which the nutritional needs and food intake of an elderly person may differ from those of a normal younger mature adult.
2. What are the main nutritional problems of the elderly?
3. Interview an elderly man living alone. Identify the problems that he encounters in providing meals. Help him to plan an adequate diet.
4. Take a diet history from an elderly woman in the hospital or clinic. Assist her with improvements in her dietary program, taking into consideration any problems she may have connected with her diet. Check her diet for adequacy.

Cited References

1. Arey, L.B., Tremaine, M.J., and Monzingo, F.L.: The numerical and topographical relations of taste buds to human circumvallate papillae throughout the life span. Anat. Rec., 64:9, 1935.
2. Center for Disease Control: Ten-State Nutrition Survey, 1968–70. DHEW Publ. No. (HSM) 72–8134. Washington, D.C., U.S. Department of Health, Education and Welfare, 1972.
3. Elsborg, L., Lund, V., and Bastrup-Madsen, P.: Serum vitamin B$_{12}$ levels in the aged. Acta Med. Scand., 200:309, 1976.
4. Garvas, S., and Garvas, H.: Special considerations in treating hypertension in the elderly. Geriatrics, 35 (7):34, 1980.
5. Gordon, T.: Blood pressure of adults by race and area, United States, 1960–1962. Vital Health Statistics, Series 11, No. 5, 1964, pp. 1–20.
6. Hayflick, L.: The cell biology of human aging. N. Engl. J. Med., 295:1302, 1976.
7. Holmes, D.: Nutrition and health screening services for the elderly. J. Am. Diet. Assoc., 60:301, 1972.
8. Horwitz, D.L.: Diabetes and aging. Am. J. Clin. Nutr., 36:803, 1982.
9. Jakubczak, L.F.: Behavioral aspects of nutrition and longevity in animals, In Rockstein, M., and Sussman, M.L. (eds.): Nutrition, Longevity and Aging. New York, Academic Press, 1976.
10. Kerr, G., et al.: Relationships between dietary and biochemical measures of nutritional status in HANES I data. Am. J. Clin. Nutr., 35:294, 1982.
11. McCay, C.M., et al.: Nutrition requirements during the latter half of life. J. Nutr., 21:45, 1941.
12. Munro, H.: Nutrition and Ageing. Br. Med. Bull., 37:83, 1981.
13. Pelcovits, J.: Nutrition to meet the human needs of older Americans. J. Am. Diet. Assoc., 60:297, 1972.
14. Pelcovits, J.: Nutrition education in group meals programs for the aged. J. Nutr. Educ., 5:118, 1973.
15. Posner, B.: Nutrition education for older Americans: national policy recommendations. J. Am. Diet. Assoc., 80:455, 1982.
16. Ross, M.H.: Nutrition and longevity in experimental animals. In Winick, M. (ed.): Nutrition and Aging. New York, John Wiley & Sons, 1976, pp. 43–57.
17. Schiffman, S.: Food recognition by the elderly. J. Gerontol., 32:586, 1977.
18. Schlenker, E.D., et al.: Nutrition and health of older people. Am. J. Clin. Nutr., 26:1111, 1973.
19. Sherman, E.M., and Brittan, M.R.: Contemporary food gatherers. A study of food shopping habits of an elderly urban population. Gerontologist, 13:358, 1973.
20. Swanson, P.: Adequacy in old age. I. Role of nutrition. J. Home Econ., 56:651, 1964.
21. Tappel, A.L.: Where old age begins. Nutrition Today, 2:2, 1967.
22. Todhunter, E.N.: Life style and nutrient intake in the elderly. In Winick, M. (ed.): Nutrition and Aging. New York, John Wiley & Sons, 1976.
23. Wayler, A.H., et al.: Effects of age and dentition status on measures of food acceptability. J. Gerontol., 37:294, 1982.
24. Young, V.R., et al.: Protein and amino acid requirements of the elderly. In Winick, M. (ed.): Nutrition and Aging. New York, John Wiley & Sons, 1976.
25. Young, V.R., and Scrimshaw, N.S.: Protein needs of the elderly. Nutrition Notes, Dec., 1975, p. 6. (Published by the American Institute of Nutrition, Rockville, Md.)

Additional References

Booth, P., et al.: Taste acuity and aging: a review. Nutr. Res., 2:95, 1982.
Bortz, W.: Disuse and aging. JAMA, 248:1203, 1982.
Bowman, B., and Rosenberg, I.: Assessment of the nutritional status of the elderly. Am. J. Clin. Nutr., 35:1142, 1982.
Bozian, M.W.: Nutrition for the aged or aged nutrition. Nurs. Clin. North Am., 11:169, 1976.
Davies, L.: Nutrition education for the elderly. Proc. Nutr. Soc., 35:125, 1976.
Elwood, T.W.: Nutritional concern of the elderly. J. Nutr. Educ., 7:50, 1975.
Feldman, E.B.: Nutrition in the Middle and Later Years. Littleton, Mass., John Wright–PSG, Inc., 1983.
Gregor, J.L., and Sciscoe, B.S.: Zinc nutriture of elderly participants in an urban feeding program. J. Am. Diet. Assoc., 70:27, 1977.
Hutton, C.W., and Hayes-Davis, R.B.: Assessment of the zinc nutritional status of selected elderly subjects. J. Am. Diet. Assoc., 82:148, 1983.
Justice, C.L., Howe, J.M., and Clark, H.E.: Dietary intakes and nutritional status of elderly patients. J. Am. Diet. Assoc., 65:639, 1974.
Kent, S.: What nutritional deprivation experiments reveal about aging. Geriatrics, 31(10):141, 1976.
Kent, S.: Is diabetes a form of accelerated aging? Geriatrics, 31(11):140, 1976.
Limited food intake and longevity. Nutr. Rev., 40:314, 1982.
Lipolysis, aging and hormones. Nutr. Rev., 32:312, 1974.
Mitchell, C., and Lipschitz, D.: Detection of protein-calorie malnutrition in the elderly. Am. J. Clin. Nutr., 35:398, 1982.
Mitchell, C., and Lipschitz, D.: The effect of age and sex on the routinely used measurements to assess the nutritional status of hospitalized patients. Am. J. Clin. Nutr., 36:340, 1982.
Munro, H.N.: Major gaps in nutrient allowances. J. Am. Diet. Assoc., 76:137, 1980.
Nutrition and human needs. Part 14: Nutrition and the aged. Hearings before the Select Committee on Nutrition and Human Needs of the United States Senate, Ninetieth Congress (Second Session) and Ninety-first Congress (First Session), Sept. 9–11, 1969. Washington, D.C., U.S. Government Printing Office, 1968 and 1969.
O'Hanlon, P.: Dietary studies of older Americans. Am. J. Clin. Nutr., 31:1257, 1978.
Patten, S.: Nutrition and the elderly: a cultural perspective. Geriatrics, 37(5):141, 1982.

Rivlin, R.S., and Young, E.A. (eds.): Symposium on evidence relating selected vitamins and minerals to health and disease in the elderly population in the U.S. Am. J. Clin. Nutr., 36(5):Supplement, 1982.

Roe, D.A.: Geriatric Nutrition. Englewood Cliffs, N.J., Prentice-Hall, Inc., 1983.

Ross, M.H., Lustbader, E., and Bras, G.: Dietary practices and growth responses as predictors of longevity. Nature, 262:548, 1976.

Schaffer, J.: Getting elderly patients to eat properly. Geriatrics, 36(10):76, 1981.

Schumer, W.: The effect of aging on cellular and respiratory mechanisms—metabolic mechanisms of aging cells. In Siegel, J.H., and Chodoff, P. (eds.): The Aged and High Risk Surgical Patient: Medical, Surgical and Anesthetic Management. New York, Grune & Stratton, 1976, pp. 149–152.

Sempos, C., et al.: A dietary survey of 14 Wisconsin nursing homes. J. Am. Diet. Assoc., 81:35, 1982.

Shagan, B.P.: Diabetes in the elderly patient. Med. Clin. North Am., 60:1191, 1976.

Shaver, H., et al.: Nutritional status of nursing home patients. J. Parent. Ent. Nutr., 4:367, 1980.

Shock, N.W.: Physiologic aspects of aging. J. Am. Diet. Assoc. 56:491, 1970.

Sorenson, A., et al.: Appropriateness of vitamin and mineral prescription orders for residents of health related facilities. J. Am. Geriatr. Soc., 27:425, 1979.

Wallace, D.J.: The biology of aging: 1976, an overview. J. Am. Geriatr. Soc., 25:104, 1977.

Yearick, E., et al.: Nutritional status of the elderly: dietary and biochemical findings. J. Gerontol., 35:663, 1980.

Zanni, E., and Calloway, D.: Protein requirements of elderly men. J. Nutr., 109:513, 1979.

UNIT 4

NUTRITION, PEOPLE AND THE COMMUNITY

CHAPTER 16

Food Habits—Geographic and Cultural Dietary Variations

Food Patterns

Food patterns of a country are molded by its agricultural resources, technical progress, buying power and cultural patterns. In trying to understand the food habits of a people, one needs to learn about their country or, in the case of immigrants or refugees, the country from which they came.

GEOGRAPHICAL CHARACTERISTICS

The physical characteristics of a country are a strong influence on the eating habits of its people. For example, countries bordering an ocean are likely to have a variety of fish in the national diet, while in landlocked countries fish are eaten much less often.

Food patterns are based on the type of food production and service in a country. Distinct differences are apparent when the diets of areas where almost all food (plant and animal) is self-produced or gathered are compared with diets in those areas where the food is supplied from large-scale commercial agriculture (domestic and foreign). One of the differences is the ability of a people to *preserve* food, and this is reflected in the food pattern. Some cultures preserve food for future needs or for periods of scarcity. Other cultures do not preserve food and thereby experience a "feast or famine" way of life. The *distribution* of food (transportation, storage, and marketing facilities) affects the food pattern. In

some countries, the foods available in cities are different from those available in rural areas.

Urban food supply includes variety in food and variety in food service, while the characteristics of rural food supply are home-grown products that are home-processed, home-cooked, and home-served. In most Western industrialized countries, however, present shipping and shopping centers throughout the country give urban and rural dwellers equal opportunities of choice. Ready-to-eat foods are available and utilized in both the urban and rural areas, thus replacing many of the home-prepared foods.

CULTURE

Food patterns are interwoven with the culture of a people. They are the response of individuals or groups to social and cultural pressures in selecting, consuming and using portions of the available food supply.

Food patterns are based on *edible* materials one's culture considers to be food. For instance, while most Americans shy away from eating insects, fat crickets are sold at the market in Bangkok and sun-dried termites are a delicacy in Rhodesia.[10] Many foods may not be considered food by some cultures, but others eat them. In almost every culture, the people eat only a portion of the food supply available to them.

Different methods of *food preparation* influence food patterns as well as the nutritive value of foods (Fig. 16–1). One-pot dishes are used by

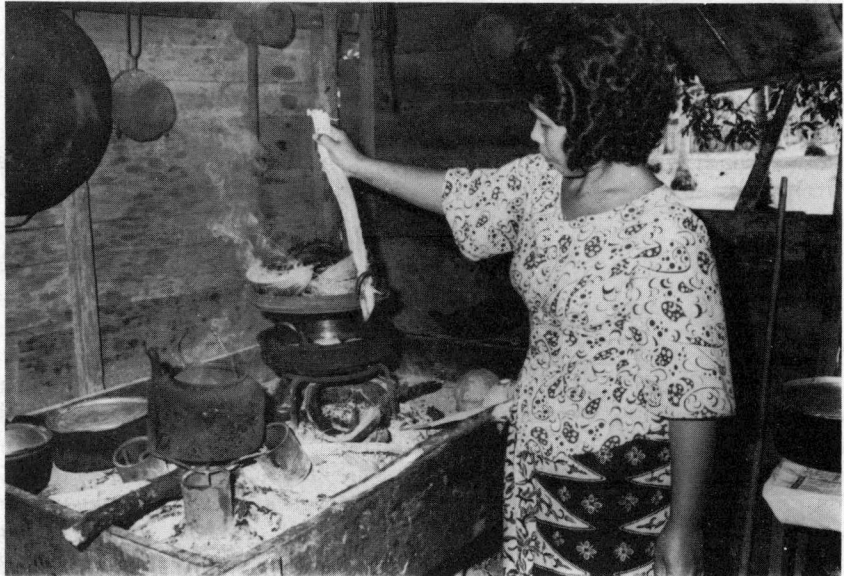

Figure 16–1. Food preparation in a Malay kitchen. (From Wilson, C. S.: J. Nutr. Educ., Winter 1971, p. 97.)

some cultures, while in other cultures baking and roasting in an oven are the familiar ways of preparing food.

Food habits are also influenced by *social organization*. Through the study of habits of primitive tribes, it was found that the role of food was related to the social status as well as to the physical status of the members of the tribe. During pregnancy women received favorite foods, the implication being that a prospective warrior might be born. However, in other cultures, pregnancy requires food restrictions, and often these are of foods that would be beneficial to the mother.

Food also has social and *ceremonial significance*. Many business transactions are conducted at the dining table in a club or restaurant. To maintain social position, women's clubs hold their meetings at a luncheon in a desirable hotel. Holidays are celebrated with special meals. Religious festivities are designated with feasts or banquets, and decisive moments in life, such as christenings, weddings, and funerals, are honored with serving of special food.

DEVELOPMENT OF FOOD HABITS

Food habits are largely established during childhood. The baby is taught to eat foods that the mother likes and that the mother had been taught to eat by her mother. If the mother likes sweetened cereal, the baby may establish a habit of eating sweetened cereal. The growing child is influenced by the environment and habits of the family group, the social group, the school group and, later, the work or professional

group. If there is an intercultural marriage, an adjustment or blending of the eating habits of the couple occurs. The offspring from this intermarriage are influenced by the food habits of each parent.

Changes in food habits are motivated by moral dictation, social desirability, scientific sanction or forced changes that are stimulated by physical circumstances, such as pressure for time, crop failures, or lowering of economic status of individuals, groups or nations. The most notable changes are those that have resulted from improvement in transportation.

With the present elaborate system of transportation, perishable foods are available the year round, as refrigeration, automated processing and packaging conspire to defy seasons and banish spoilage. Technological advancements have made it possible for innumerable new items to appear on grocery shelves and, ultimately, on the family table.

Dietary changes also occur when an individual, family or group immigrate into another country. Their food habits change to accommodate the new culture; and if the group is large enough, their food habits may influence the food habits of their new country. The taco is a good example of the Mexican-Americans' influence on U.S. eating habits.

Changes in food habits are also motivated by the bodily state of individuals during pregnancy, illness, aging and weight consciousness. An illness that imposes dietary restrictions or an unpleasant experience with food may result in a lifelong avoidance of some particular food or foods.

A full understanding of food habits and eating patterns requires the integration of various sciences: anthropology, psychology, biochemistry, agriculture, economics, genetics, physiology and sociology. The reader is encouraged to read the appropriate additional readings at the end of this chapter for further discussion of food habit development.

Dietary Patterns of Nationality Groups in North America

The dietary patterns of a number of countries are given in Tables 16–1 through 16–8. These should help the student obtain a better understanding of various foreign-born individuals and families who may need aid in meal planning, food budgeting and dietary instruction. Food composition tables for foods used by other than U.S. cultures are available.[8]

It is a very large undertaking to provide food and nutritional care for persons who immigrate to the United States under conditions of stress. The rapid influx of Cubans to Florida and Vietnamese, Laotians and Cambodians to California, for example, has led to crowded conditions, linguistic problems and unfamiliar foods for the newcomers.

Rapid change is taking place in all countries, and it should be kept in mind that, while the dietary patterns listed here consist of typical native foods and customs, what is typical today may not be in a few years. The best way to learn the eating patterns of a people is to talk

with them, eat with them and ask about their foods.

Because of the large number of Southeast Asians immigrating into North America and the fact that their culture is so different from ours, a detailed discussion of their food habits is included.

DIETARY PATTERNS OF SOUTHEAST ASIANS

by Andrea Carlson, M.S., R.D.

During the past few years the number of Southeast Asian refugees has increased dramatically worldwide. By the beginning of 1982, 567,000 refugees from Laos, Cambodia and Vietnam had entered the United States.[12] Among these refugees are numerous groups, each with a distinct language, culture and food habits. From Laos, Cambodia and Vietnam come the native ethnic groups, as well as Moslems and ethnic Chinese. From Laos, Thailand and Southern China come the nomadic hill people, the Hmong and the Mien. There are both urban and rural people, whose lifestyles differ considerably, even though they might come from the same country. In order to understand the refugees it is important to appreciate their tremendous diversity as well as recognize their common characteristics.

Southeast Asia is a humid and tropical area with a primarily agricultural economy. Outside of the cities, most people earn their living by fishing and/or raising crops and livestock.[14] A family raises enough food for its own consumption, with occasionally some left over to sell.

Table 16–1. THE SPANISH-AMERICAN–MEXICAN FOOD PLAN

FOODS	PREPARATION
Meats: Chicken, pork chops, weiners, cold cuts and hamburger.	Used only once or twice a week.
Other proteins: Eggs, beans.	Eggs used frequently and usually fried. In rural areas, chickens are kept for their eggs. Beans usually eaten mashed and refried with lard.
Vegetables: Potatoes, red and green chilies, fresh and canned tomatoes, pumpkin, corn, field greens, onions, carrots.	Potatoes are basic item, usually fried; may be used three times a day. Chilies are popular at each meal and are good source of vitamin A even when dried. Fresh tomatoes are very popular. Other vegetables used frequently.
Fruits: Bananas, melons, peaches, canned fruit cocktail, oranges, apples.	Oranges, apples used occasionally as snacks. Others are the more popular fruits.
Cereals and breads: Oatmeal, enriched white flour, packaged breakfast cereals, macaroni, white bread, tortillas, sweet rolls.	Sugar-coated packaged cereals are popular; oatmeal used occasionally. Macaroni is fried and served with beans and potatoes. Tortillas are homemade daily. Both purchased and homemade breads are used frequently. Purchased sandwich bread is a status symbol.
Milk: Limited availability, expensive. *Cheese:* Limited amounts used. *Fats:* Lard, salt pork, bacon fat. *Beverages:* Soft drinks; other sweets very popular.	Used liberally. Most foods are fried.

(Adapted from Cultural Food Patterns in the U.S.A. Chicago, American Dietetic Association, 1976.)

Table 16–2. THE CUBAN FOOD PLAN
(PRE-CASTRO REGIME)

FOODS	PREPARATION
Meats: Beef, pork, lamb, veal, poultry, sausages.	Pork is either roasted or fried. Beef and chicken are used in soups, stewed, roasted, broiled or barbecued. The sausages are used with beans.
Fish: All varieties of fish (fresh, salted, smoked and canned).	Fried, boiled, marinated, roasted or grilled.
Other proteins: Beans (black, red, kidney, navy, yellow, lima, green); split peas; eggs.	Black beans with rice and roast pork is a favorite dish and is eaten on Christmas day. Eggs are eaten daily: fried, scrambled or in dessert.
Vegetables: Native tubers such as *yuca, ñame, malanga* (white and yellow), *boniato* (white yams), *chayote, berenjena,* plantain, potatoes, lettuce, tomatoes, carrots.	The tubers are boiled and served with *mojo* (made with sour orange, crushed garlic, sliced onions and hot oil), or mashed with butter and milk. Fried ripe or green plantains are a favorite side dish.
Fruits: Anona, *mamey, guanábana, chirimoya,* papaya, banana, *zapote, marañón,* mangoes, grapefruit, oranges (sweet and sour), coconuts, *caimito.*	Eaten fresh, in juice, or in desserts such as pastes, jellies, puddings.
Cereals: Rice, cornmeal, cornstarch, imported breakfast cereals such as oatmeal, corn flakes.	The favorite is white (long grain) steamed rice; sometimes *bijol* is added to make it yellow as in *arroz con pollo* (yellow rice with chicken). White rice is eaten daily for dinner and supper.
Milk: Fresh cow's milk (whole, skimmed), condensed, evaporated, dry; sour cream; goat's milk for the sick, usually.	Adults use it in coffee; children use as beverage. Also used in cream sauces, gravies, desserts, etc.
Cheese: Gouda, cream, *queso de mano.*	The native cheese is *queso de mano* (hard cheese) made from milk, lactate of calcium and salt, which looks like compressed cottage cheese; usually eaten with guava paste.
Fats: Pork lard, olive oil, peanut oil, soy oil, butter, margarine and shortening.	Pork lard is most popular. Oil is used in salads and beans.
Desserts: Fruits, ice cream, cakes, pies, custards, puddings; guava, prune and mango pastes; *morón* cookies, *terrejas, boniatillo, buñuelos, cafiroleta.*	Eaten after each meal and also as snacks. *Raspadura* is very sweet and the most typical native dessert.
Seasonings: Oil, vinegar, cumin, oregano, *bijol,* salt, pepper, garlic, onion, green peppers.	
Beverages: Coffee, beer, wines, tea, carbonated beverages.	Dark strong coffee served demitasse, with or without sugar.

Foods are usually produced and consumed locally. In addition to cultivation, the rural and highland people also obtain food by hunting and gathering such foods as deer, rabbit, snake, monkeys, mushrooms, bamboo shoots, watercress and bananas.

Rice is the main crop and dietary staple, providing over 60 per cent of the calories in Southeast Asian diets.[2] In difficult times this percentage goes even higher. White, unenriched rice is very common. However, rice bran is sometimes added to fish pastes and pickled vegetables, thereby increasing the nutritive value of the diet.

In cities and villages, food shopping is done once or twice daily, since fresh foods are preferred. Canned or refrigerated foods are expensive and available only in the cities. Sometimes salt is the only food purchased by the Hmong and Mien. In rural areas there is no refrigeration, and cooking is done over open fires. Drying, salting, pickling and smoking are the most common methods of food preservation.

Lack of refrigeration prevents the widespread use of fresh cow's milk and other dairy products. Therefore, the calcium intake is generally low. Alternate native sources of calcium are tofu (soybean curd), fish pastes made from small whole fish, and soups or other dishes made from bones and vinegar. Unfortunately, these foods contain variable amounts of calcium and are not reliable sources. Soybean drinks do not contain significant amounts of calcium or protein.[7] Lactose intolerance has been reported to be a problem in many Southeast Asians.[1] However, most children accept milk readily, and many adults are able to drink it in small amounts without any discomfort.

Newly arriving refugees are at nutritional risk for a variety of reasons. They come from countries with limited food supplies caused by long histories of war and political strife. They may have spent as much as five years in refugee camps where food supplies were also limited. Poor sanitation has led to an increased incidence of parasites, and therefore an increase in anemia. General malnutrition, hypertension, dental caries and iron-deficiency anemia have been identified as problems among incoming refugees.[5]

Table 16–3. THE GREEK FOOD PLAN

FOODS	PREPARATION
Meats: Lamb is main meat. Some beef, goat, mutton, pork products; poultry is popular.	Meat is either cut into small pieces or ground. Poultry is cooked into broth. Lamb is cooked on skewers or cut up and browned in oil or fat with rice or flour and vegetables.
Fish: Salt-water fish (fresh, smoked or salted), shellfish, smoked roe, squid and octopus.	Fish is fried or steamed with vegetables. Used frequently.
Other proteins: Eggs, white beans and legumes.	Legumes are boiled, mashed or stewed and eaten either hot or cold. Soup made of dried beans, onions, celery and carrots is a national dish. Eggs are popular.
Vegetables: Cabbage, cauliflower, cucumbers, eggplant, greens, okra, onions, peppers, some potatoes, vine leaves, zucchini, tomatoes, salad greens, oranges and lemons.	Vegetables are boiled or fried in a small amount of olive oil and served hot or cold. Many vegetables are stuffed. Potatoes or vegetables are cooked with meat or fish. Lemon juice is used to dress salads and cold foods.
Fruits: Apricots, cherries, dates, figs, grapes, melons, nuts, plums, peaches, pears, quinces and raisins.	Fruits in season are eaten raw, grapes are pressed into wine or dried as raisins. Fruit for dessert.
Cereals and breads: Maize, rice and wheat.	Maize is used in polenta; rice is an ingredient for *pilawi* and stuffing for vegetables; wheat is made into bread. Bread used abundantly and white is preferred.
Milk: Cow's, goat's and sheep's milk.	Milk is boiled for children. Fermented milk or *yaourti* is eaten as dessert or with pastry.
Cheese: Soft and mild, hard and dry cheeses.	Cheese is popular.
Fats: Olive oil, seed oils, salted black olives and little butter.	Olive oil is used to dress salads and hot or cold vegetables and in cooking.
Seasonings: Caraway and pumpkin seeds, herbs, honey, nuts (hazel, pignolia and pistachio) and sesame.	Seeds are eaten between meals, and nuts are served as dessert.
Beverages: Coffee and wine.	Coffee (American) is the beverage served in the mornings. At other meals it is made and served Turkish style. Wine is served at meals.

Table 16–4. THE JAPANESE FOOD PLAN

FOODS	PREPARATION
Meats: The Buddhist tradition of not eating meat conforms with the physical necessities of agriculture. The Japanese consume very little meat, except beef. Since World War II, however, protein intake has increased; from 1950 to 1960 it increased 10 per cent and animal protein almost doubled.	Quantity is small. Usually cut into small pieces and served mixed with vegetables and cereal products.
Fish: Liked and one of the staple foods.	Prefer fish, shellfish and other marine life to meats of all types. Certain kinds of raw fish are considered great delicacies. Others cooked or dried.
Other proteins: Soybean preparations used freely. Eggs used when available.	Variety of soybean preparations.
Vegetables: Prefer plants such as seaweed, bamboo shoots, onions, large radishes, dried mushrooms (*shi-itake*) and beans. Potatoes and others when available.	Pickled is the favorite form. Others cooked with meat or fish.
Fruits: Principal fruit is *nasi* (tastes somewhat like pear, shaped like an apple; yellow, rough skin). Some persimmons and mulberries. Tangerines in mountain regions. Postwar increase in variety.	Dessert.
Cereals and breads: Rice is main food. Some barley, oats and rye.	Rice is mixed with barley by farmers and the poorer classes. Wheat bread, especially in urban communities.
Milk: Enjoy when available; mainly import evaporated or dry milk powder.	Mostly for children.
Cheese: Very little.	
Fats: Soy oil. Rice oil. Suet when available. Practically no butter and cream.	Used in cooking.
Seasonings: Salt, *sake* (liquor distilled from rice).	
Beverages: Tea, *sake*.	Tea freely used when afforded.

Table 16–5.   THE CHINESE FOOD PLAN

FOODS	PREPARATION
Meats: Pork (favorite), lamb, goat and poultry. Entire animal is eaten, including organs, brain, spinal cord, skin and coagulated blood.	Quantity is small and usually cut into small thin slices about 2 inches long and cooked in sesame or peanut oil with soy sauce, spices and a little water and served mixed with vegetables. Many methods for preserving and drying. Sweet and pungent pork or duck is a favorite (meat cubes rolled in batter and fried in oil, then simmered in sauce made of pineapple, green peppers, molasses, brown sugar, vinegar and seasonings.)
Fish: Fish and shellfish liked.	Fish is frequently baked with native spices or prepared in sweet-and-sour dishes. Many dried.
Other proteins: Hen, duck and pigeon eggs in abundance when afforded; soybean products; legumes.	Eggs are preserved and dried; also combined with chicken, mushrooms and bean sprouts and served with soy sauce (looks like vegetable omelet), termed *egg foo yong.* Egg roll served at beginning of meal is made of shrimp or meat and chopped vegetables rolled in thin dough and fried in deep fat. Soybeans used as sauce, as milk for infants in China and in many products. Legumes as substitute for meat.
Vegetables: Many plants such as carrots, onions, leeks, peas, cabbage, white turnips, corn, cucumbers, green and yellow beans, squash, shepherd's purse, radish leaves, sprouts (bean, bamboo, etc.), some white but more sweet potatoes.	Cut into uniform pieces and simmered or steamed with eggs or meat or added to meat and widely used in soups.
Fruits: Kumquat is favorite.	Preserved dessert.
Cereals and breads: Rice used freely. Some wheat, barley, corn and millet seed. Noodles are popular. Rice is main dish; others are side dishes.	Rice is used as main dish, plain or fried. Millet seed is made into cakes or used in a gruel. Noodles are small and fried. Steamed bread is eaten at breakfast.
Milk: Very little and generally not used. Given to children and invalids.	
Cheese: Little used.	
Fats: Chief oil is peanut oil. Some soy oil, rice oil, sesame oil or lard. Practically no butter or cream used.	Used in cooking.
Seasonings: Sesame seed, salt, ginger, garlic, fresh herbs, red pepper.	
Beverage: Tea is the national beverage.	Beverage at all meals, when afforded.

After refugees arrive in the United States, other factors contribute to their nutritional problems. They are thrust into a foreign country that has a completely new language, culture and society. They are faced with unfamiliar foods, food storage and food-buying habits. Many familiar foods are difficult or impossible to obtain. Low income limits their access to food, and they are susceptible to misleading food advertising.

Pregnant and lactating women, infants and children are at greatest risk because of their increased nutritional needs. Multiple pregnancies and extended periods of lactation are common in Southeast Asia. A pregnant woman is less concerned about her prenatal diet than her postpartum diet. However, in the third trimester of pregnancy weight gain is often restricted in order for the woman to have a small baby and easy delivery. Foods such as fruits, vegetables and certain meats are sometimes eliminated in the first postpartum month. A woman might lactate for as long as two years or until the next child is born. These practices, coupled with a low calcium intake, place great demands on a woman's nutritional stores.

Although in Southeast Asia most infants are breast-fed, in the United States infants of refugee women are usually fed formula. This alone does not constitute a problem, but it can lead to other problems. Improper dilution or unsanitary preparation and storage of formula are potential hazards. Misuse of the bottle, such as filling it with sweetened liquids, giving it to the infant at night, and using it as a frequent pacifier during the day can lead to nursing-bottle caries. This serious dental problem is frequently seen in refugee children.

Rice-and-water soup is a common first food for infants. The introduction of other solid foods is often limited, and weaning is delayed. At about one year of age formula is replaced with cow's milk. Iron-deficiency anemia easily develops in the refugee children who drink large amounts of milk and eat few iron-rich foods.

Southeast Asian refugees are often shorter and lighter than their Western counterparts.[9] Among children, weight for age, height for age

Table 16–6.   THE LAOTIAN FOOD PLAN

FOODS	PREPARATION
Meats: Pork, beef, chicken, rabbit, wild pig, buffalo, deer, snake, and elephant.	Eaten fresh, dried or salted. Prepared by frying, boiling, baking or broiling, mixed with vegetables and spices. Hmong and Mien might also eat monkey and bear.
Fish: Numerous varieties of freshwater fish and shellfish. Saltwater fish available in cities.	Eaten fresh, fermented, dried or salted. *Padek*, a fermented fish paste made from small whole fish, salt and rice bran is frequently eaten by lowland Lao, but not by the Hmong and the Mien.
Other proteins: Eggs, peanuts, black-eyed peas, kidney beans.	Soybean products not eaten by the Lao. Soybean curd (tofu) sometimes eaten by Hmong. Legumes often used in desserts.
Vegetables: Wide variety of vegetables, including pumpkin, squash, squash blossoms and young shoots, tomato, cabbage, spinach, green papaya, bamboo shoots, mushrooms, watercress, cucumber, and corn. See also Vietnamese vegetables.	Eaten raw, as juice or cooked with meat or fish. Preserved by drying or pickling.
Fruits: See Vietnamese fruits. Wide variety consumed.	Usually eaten fresh or as juice. Tamarinds sometimes salted and eaten as a snack.
Cereals and breads: Glutinous (sticky) rice, wheat, rice or bean thread noodles, French bread.	Sticky rice is rinsed several times and then soaked overnight. The soaking water is discarded and the rice is steamed. It is eaten with the fingers at meals or as a snack. The Hmong eat regular rice. Bread is eaten plain, with paté or coconut milk.
Milk: Sweetened condensed milk.	Sometimes diluted and used as infant formula. Also as a beverage for adults.
Fats: Lard.	
Seasonings: *Padek*, chili, lemon grass, coconut milk, coriander, tamarind, curry, monosodium glutamate, red and black pepper, salt, fish sauce, browned ground rice, mint.	*Padek* and chilies are characteristic seasonings of the lowland Lao.
Beverages: Soybean drink, sugar cane drink, tea, coconut juice, fruit or vegetable juice, beer, wine.	

(Developed by Andrea Carlson, M.S., R.D.)

and weight for height, when plotted on National Center for Health Statistics growth charts (Appendix Tables 15 to 22), are below the fifth percentile more frequently than for the reference population. The use of these measurements in nutritional assessment is discussed in Chapter 9. At present there are no reliable standards with which to evaluate the growth of refugee children. Both genetic and environmental factors affect growth. Chronic undernutrition, especially low protein, calcium and energy intakes, could contribute to poor growth in this population. In the countries of resettlement, improved diet and appropriate nutrition counseling to correct or prevent problems may improve the growth rates of refugee children and the health status of all refugees.

Dietary Restrictions and Patterns of Religious Groups

JEWISH FOOD CUSTOMS AND DIETARY LAWS[6]

The Jewish dietary laws are biblical ordinances codified and interpreted into rules regarding food. The rules pertain chiefly to the selection, slaughter and preparation of meat. Animals allowed to be eaten for food are the quadrupeds having a cloven hoof that chew a cud, specifically cattle, sheep, goats and deer; they are considered "clean." Permissible fowl are chicken, turkey, goose, pheasant and duck. All animals and fowl must be inspected for disease and killed by a ritual slaughterer according to specific rules. Only the forequarter of the quadruped may be used, except when the hip sinew of the thigh vein can be removed, in which case the hindquarter is also allowed.

Blood is forbidden as food, since blood is synonymous with life. Thus, the traditional process of "koshering" the meat and poultry removes all blood before cooking. Koshering involves soaking the meat in water, salting it thoroughly, allowing it to drain and then washing it three times to remove the salt.

Meat and milk cannot be combined in the same meal. Milk or milk foods may be eaten immediately before the meal, but not with it. After meat has been eaten, six hours must elapse before milk products may be used. Because of the rule of separating meat and milk products, traditional orthodox Jewish homes must keep two completely separate sets of dishes, silver and cooking equipment—one for meat meals and one for dairy meals.

Fish allowed are only those having fins and scales. This bars all shellfish and eels. Fish may be eaten with either dairy or meat meals.

Table 16–7.   THE VIETNAMESE FOOD PLAN

FOODS	PREPARATION
Meats: Pork, beef, chicken, sausage, chicken feet, ox tails, liver, stomach.	Pork is most common. Chicken is consumed only on special occasions. Meats are usually cut into small pieces and fried, boiled or steamed. (See also Chinese food plan for Chinese from Vietnam.)
Fish: Numerous types of freshwater and saltwater fish and shellfish.	Eaten fresh, dried, salted or fermented. Chinese like to steam fish, while Vietnamese like it fried and dipped in fish sauce.
Other proteins: Eggs, soybeans, peanuts, other legumes.	Soybeans eaten in processed forms such as soy sauce, soybean milk and soybean curd (tofu). Peanuts eaten in soups or as a snack. Legumes eaten in desserts (Chinese influence) or in soups.
Vegetables: Wide variety of vegetables, including bamboo shoots, bok choy, broccoli, carrots, cauliflower, napa cabbage, mustard greens, bittermelon, wintermelon, green beans, eggplant, corn, water chestnut, (see also Laotian vegetables).	Eaten fresh, dried or pickled. Usually eaten with meat or fish. Vietnamese eat raw vegetables more often than Chinese-Vietnamese.
Fruits: Wide variety of fruits, including bananas, mangoes, papayas, pineapples, melons, oranges, pears, grapefruit, longans, and tamarinds.	Usually eaten fresh. Sometimes cook pear or papaya to make a sweet soup for dessert.
Cereals and breads: Short-grain, long-grain and glutinous rice (See Laotian food plan), bean thread, wheat and rice noodles, French bread.	Rice is often eaten with every meal. It is rinsed several times before steaming. Bread eaten plain or with pork, paté, or sweetened condensed milk.
Milk: Sweetened condensed milk.	Served in coffee, with hot water or on bread. Also sometimes used as infant formula.
Fats: Lard, peanut oil.	
Seasonings: Oyster sauce, soy sauce, monosodium glutamate, black pepper, ginger, garlic, green onion, coriander, sesame oil (Chinese influence), curry (Indian influence), mint, dill, red pepper, lemon grass, vinegar, lemon, *nuoc mam* sauce.	Vietnamese food tends to be hotter than Chinese food. *Nuoc mam* sauce is a fish sauce, a thin extract made from fermented fish and salt.
Beverages: Tea, coffee, soft drinks, soybean milk, sugar-cane drink, beer and wine.	Tea is the most common beverage. Beer and wine are only for the men.

(Developed by Andrea Carlson, M.S., R.D.)

Table 16–8.   THE CAMBODIAN FOOD PLAN

FOODS	PREPARATION
Meats: Pork, beef, chicken, deer, wild pig, buffalo, rabbit.	Eaten fresh, dried or salted. Prepared by frying, boiling, baking, with spices. Not eaten as frequently as fish. Pork and chicken are expensive.
Fish: Numerous types of freshwater and saltwater fish and shellfish.	Very common food. *Prahoc*, a salted fermented fish paste, is a characteristic Cambodian food eaten with rice and raw vegetables. Fish also eaten fresh, smoked or dried.
Other proteins: Eggs, peanuts, soybeans, other legumes.	Eggs are expensive, so are not eaten often. Soybeans eaten only by Chinese Cambodians. Legumes eaten in desserts.
Vegetables: See Laotian and Vietnamese vegetables.	Eaten raw with *prahoc* or cut up small and cooked with other protein foods.
Fruits: See Vietnamese fruits.	Eaten raw as dessert or snack.
Cereals and breads: Long-grain, short-grain, glutinous (see Laotian food plan) and black sweet rice; rice and egg noodles, French bread.	Glutinous and black sweet rice used in desserts. French bread found mostly in cities.
Milk: Sweetened condensed milk.	Sometimes eaten on bread, or used as infant formula.
Fats: Lard.	
Seasonings: Prahoc, red pepper, vinegar, garlic, ginger, curry salt, monosodium glutamate, lemon, coconut milk, and coriander.	*Prahoc* is a characteristic seasoning. Food is generally not as hot as Laotian food.
Beverages: Tea, coffee, soft drink, beer, soybean drinks, sugar-cane drink.	

(Developed by Andrea Carlson, M.S., R.D.)

Eggs, too, may be used with either meat or milk. However, any egg yolk containing a drop of blood may not be used, since the blood is considered to be chick embryo or a sign of a new life.

Fruits, vegetables, cereal products and all of the other foods that make up a diet may be used without restriction. Bakery products and prepared food mixtures must be produced under acceptable kosher standards.

HOLIDAY OBSERVANCE. The most important of the holy days is the Sabbath, or day of rest, observed on Saturday. The meal on Friday night is the nicest of the week and usually includes both fish and chicken. No food is allowed to be cooked or heated on Saturday, so all food eaten on the Sabbath is cooked the previous day and either kept warm in the oven or eaten cold.

The festival holidays are Rosh Hashanah, the New Year, in September; Succoth, the fall harvest holiday; Chanukah, the feast of lights, in midwinter; and Purim, a joyous holiday in spring. Each holiday has delicacies associated with it.

Yom Kippur, or the Day of Atonement, occurs 10 days after Rosh Hashanah and is a day of fasting, with abstinence from all food and drink, including water, from sundown on the eve of the holiday to sundown on the holiday. Pregnant women and those who are ill do not fast.

Passover, a spring commemorative festival lasting eight days, requires special dietary consideration. During this period, leavened bread or cake is prohibited. Matzo, an unleavened bread, is eaten and all cake and baked products are made from flour of ground-up matzo or potato starch, leavened only with beaten egg whites. No salt is allowed in traditional Passover matzo. Variations of fried matzo or matzo meal pancakes are prepared with generous amounts of fat.

MUSLIM RELIGIOUS DIETARY CODE

The following dietary restrictions are followed by the Muslim:

1. Pork and pork products such as gelatin are prohibited.

2. Alcoholic beverages and alcohol products (such as vanilla extract) are prohibited.

3. All meat used for food must be slaughtered according to ritual letting of blood and while speaking the name of God. This may be done by anyone, since there is no special person designated for this function. Muslims use kosher meat products because they know they have been slaughtered in the proper manner.

4. Although all foods not specifically prohibited are allowed, certain foods are recommended: milk, dates, meat, seafood, sweets, honey and vegetable oil, especially olive oil.

5. Fasting is practiced during the month of Ramadan every year, which varies with the Islamic lunar calendar. Muslims will fast completely from dawn to sunset and will eat only twice a day—before dawn and after sunset. They are also encouraged to fast three days of every month. Menstruating, pregnant or lactating women are not required to fast, but must make up the fasting days at some other time.

6. Muslims are advised not to eat to capacity and always to share food.

ROMAN CATHOLIC DIETARY LAWS*

ON ABSTINENCE

1. Everyone, after the 7th birthday, is bound to observe the law of abstinence.

2. On days of complete abstinence, meat and soup or gravy made from meat may not be used at all. At the present time, these days are Ash Wednesday and the Fridays during Lent.

ON FAST

1. Everyone, from the 21st birthday to the 59th birthday inclusive, is also bound to observe the law of fast, except pregnant women and nursing mothers.

2. The days of fast vary because church laws have been changed.

3. On days of fast, only one full meal is allowed. Two other *light meatless* meals, sufficient to maintain strength, may be taken according to each one's needs. Meat may be taken at the principal meal on a day of fast, except on Ash Wednesday.

4. When health or ability to work would be seriously affected, the law of fast does not apply.

Vegetarianism

The cultural philosophies of so-called pure vegetarians are based mainly on Eastern religions and have many similarities; yet they are distinctly different.[4] Some regimens are nutritionally adequate and others are not.

The *lacto-ovo-vegetarian* diet consists of grains, fruits and vegetables supplemented with milk, cheese and eggs. Many legumes and nuts are included and used in a variety of ways. Meat of all kinds, fish and poultry are prohibited. The Seventh Day Adventists are advised by the church to follow this program but may elect not to.

Lacto-vegetarians eat all grains, fruits, legumes, seeds, nuts and vegetables supplemented with milk and cheese only. No other animal

---

*The dietary restrictions governing abstinence and fast have been liberalized. Customs vary in different localities and with individuals.

protein is permitted. Those who ingest vegetables only and prohibit the use of animal foods, dairy products and eggs are referred to as *vegans*. The *fruitarian* diet consists of only raw or dried fruits, nuts, honey and olive oil.

Pure vegetable and fruit diets without legumes, nuts and grains are nutritionally inadequate in protein, iron, calcium, riboflavin, vitamin B_{12} and possibly vitamin D. Mutual protein complementation using mixtures of vegetables, beans, grains and nuts can, if properly planned, supply a good balance of essential amino acids and adequate amounts of calcium, riboflavin, iron, vitamin A and vitamin D. Vitamin B_{12} would have to be given in supplement or obtained from a B_{12}-fortified soy milk. Further information on protein complementation can be found on pages 58 and 227, in Table 10–5 and in Cited Reference 11.

The Zen Buddhist believes that one's health and happiness depend on a proper balance between the "yin" and "yang" foods. This way of eating is known by some American groups as the Zen macrobiotic diet. The dietary pattern progresses through ten steps ranging from the lowest level diet, which includes 30 per cent vegetables, 30 per cent animal products, 15 per cent salad and fruits, 10 per cent soups, 10 per cent cereals and 5 per cent desserts, to the highest level, which contains 100 per cent cereals.[3] Several deaths and vitamin deficiencies have been reported in individuals who attempted the highest and most extreme levels of the diet.[13]

Problems and Suggested Topics for Discussion

1. What changes in food patterns have taken place in the United States? What caused these changes?
2. Interview someone with a different ethnic origin from your own and find out about his or her native food habits and social customs.
3. Evaluate one of the dietary patterns given in Tables 16–1 to 16–8 to make sure it contains the basic foods.
4. Plan field trips to restaurants and food shops offering foods of various nationalities.
5. Describe how the Laotian and the Vietnamese dietary patterns are similar. How are they different?
6. Select a family representing the most prevalent nationality in your neighborhood. Interview the homemaker of this family to determine the quality of the menus served for one week. How do they rate? What improvements in them are needed? How does the homemaker perceive the changes?
7. Design menus for two days for adequate diets for lacto-ovo-vegetarians, lacto-vegetarians, and vegans.

Cited References

1. Anh, N.T., et al.: Lactose malabsorption in adult Vietnamese. Am. J. Clin. Nutr., *30*:468, 1977.
2. Chang, K.C. (ed.): Food in Chinese Culture. New Haven, Yale University Press, 1977.
3. Council on Foods and Nutrition: Zen macrobiotic diets. JAMA, *218*:397, 1971.
4. Erhard, D.: The new vegetarians. Parts 1 and 2. Nutrition Today, *8(6)*:4, 1973, and *9(1)*:20, 1974.
5. Go, K., and Moore, I.: The food habits and practices of Southeast Asians. Public Health Service, Alameda County Health Care Services Agency, 1979.
6. Kaufman, M.: Adapting therapeutic diets to Jewish food customs. Am. J. Clin. Nutr., *5*:676, 1957.
7. Leung, W.T.W.: Some Native Foods in East and Southeast Asia—how nutritious are they? Bethesda, Md., Interdepartmental Committee on Nutrition for National Development, Office of International Research, Office of the Director, National Institutes of Health.
8. Nutrition Policy and Programmes Service: Food Composition Tables—Updated. Annotated bibliography. Rome, FAO, United Nations, 1975.
9. Peck, R.E., et al.: Nutritional status of Southeast Asian refugee children. Am. J. Pub. Health., *71*:1144, 1981.
10. Trager, J.: The Foodbook. New York, Grossman Publishers, 1970.
11. Trahms, C.M.: Vegetarianism as a way of life. In Worthington-Roberts, B.S.: Contemporary Developments in Nutrition, St. Louis, C.V. Mosby Company, 1981.
12. Tripp, R.E.: World refugee survey 1982. New York, U.S. Commmittee for Refugees, 1982.
13. White, P.L., and Mondeika, T.D.: Foods, fads and faddism. In Goodhart, R.S., and Shils, M.E. (eds.), Modern Nutrition in Health and Disease, 6th ed. Philadelphia, Lea & Febiger, 1980.
14. Whitmore, J.K. (ed.): An Introduction to Indochinese History, Culture, Language, and Life. Ann Arbor, Mich., Center for South and Southeast Asian Studies, 1979.

Additional References

Barer-Stein, T.: You Eat What You Are: A Study of Ethnic Food Traditions. London, Ontario, Canada, McClelland and Stewart, Ltd., 1979.
Cantoni, M.: Adapting therapeutic diets to the eating patterns of Italian-Americans. Am. J. Clin. Nutr., *6*:548, 1958.
Chang, B.: Some dietary beliefs in Chinese folk culture. J. Am. Diet. Assoc., *65*:436, 1974.
Committee on Nutrition, American Academy of Pediatrics: Nutritional aspects of vegetarianism, health foods and fad diets. Pediatrics, *59*:460, 1977.
Crane, N.T., and Green, N.R.: Food habits and food preferences of Vietnamese refugees living in Northern Florida. J. Am. Diet. Assoc., *76*:591, 1980.
Cronin, F.J.: Characterizing food usage by demographic variables. J. Am. Diet. Assoc., *81*:661, 1982.
Cultural Food Patterns in the U.S.A. Chicago, American Dietetic Association, 1976.
Drummond, J.C.: The Englishman's Food: A History of Five Centuries of English Diet. London, J. Cape, 1939.
Ellis, F.R., and Montegriffo, V.M.E.: Veganism, clinical findings and investigations. Am. J. Clin. Nutr., *23*:249, 1970.
Feitelson, M., and Fiedler, K.: Kosher dietary laws and children's food preferences: guide to a camp menu plan. J. Am. Diet. Assoc., *81*:453, 1982.
Gerhold, C.: Food habits of the valley people of Laos. J. Am. Diet. Assoc., *50*:493, 1967.
Gifft, H.H., Washbon, M.B., and Harrison, G.G.: Nutrition, Behavior and Change. Englewood Cliffs, N.J., Prentice-Hall, 1972.
Hardinge, M.G., et al.: Nutritional studies of vegetarians. J. Am. Diet. Assoc., *43*: 550, 1963, and *48*:25, 1966.
Hertzler, A., Wenkam, N., and Stardal, B.: Classifying cultural food habits and meanings. J. Am. Diet. Assoc., *80*: 421, 1982.

Jerome, N.W.: Northern urbanization and food consumption patterns of southern-born Negroes. Am. J. Clin. Nutr., *22*: 1667, 1969.

Joseph, S., et al.: Composition of Israeli mixed dishes. J. Am. Diet. Assoc., *40*:125, 1962.

Kaufman, M.: Vietnam, 1978: crisis in food, nutrition, and health. J. Am. Diet. Assoc., *74*:310, 1979.

Koroff, S.I.: The Jewish dietary code. Food Technology, *20*: 76, 1966.

Leung, W.W., et al.: Food composition table for use in East Asia. USDHEW Publication No. (NIH) 79–465, Washington, D.C., U.S. Department of Health, Education & Welfare, 1978.

Lowenberg, M.E., et al.: Food and People. 3rd ed. New York, John Wiley & Sons, 1979.

Molony, C.H.: Systematic valence coding of Mexican "hot"- "cold" food. Ecol. Food Nutr. *4*:67, 1975.

Natow, A.B., Heslin, J., and Raven, B.C.: Integrating the Jewish dietary laws into a dietetics program. J. Am. Diet. Assoc., *67*:13, 1975.

Pongborn, R.M., and Bruhn, C.M.: Concepts of food habits of other ethnic groups. J. Nutr. Educ., *2*:106, 1971.

Robson, J.K.R. (ed.): Food Ecology and Culture: Readings in the Anthropology of Dietary Practices. New York, Gordon and Breach, 1980.

Sakr, A.H.: Dietary regulations and food habits of Muslims. J. Am. Diet. Assoc., *58*:123, 1971.

Sakr, A.H.: Fasting in Islam. J. Am. Diet Assoc., *67*:17, 1975.

Sanjur, D.: Social and cultural perspectives in nutrition, Englewood Cliffs, N.J., Prentice-Hall, 1982.

Tannahill, R.: Food in History. New York, Stein and Day, Publishers, 1973.

Valassi, K.V.: Food habits of Greek-Americans. Am. J. Clin. Nutr., *11*:240, 1967.

Vy, T.: Nutritional value and composition of foodstuffs of the Vietnamese rural adult. Am. J. Clin. Nutr., *24*:38, 1971.

Wilson, C.S.: Food—custom and nurture: an annotated bibliography on sociocultural and biocultural aspects of nutrition. J. Nutr. Educ., *11*(4), Suppl. 1, 1979.

CHAPTER 17

Food and Nutrition in the Community

NATALIE GONZÁLEZ, M.S., R.D.

The nutrition of the individual reflects to some degree the nutrition of the community. The nutrition of the community is influenced by the safety, availability and economics of the food supply, the general health of the community, the availability of health care and education and the governmental policies supporting the nutrition programs necessary for the community. Efforts to monitor the food intake and the nutritional status of the members of the community are also an important activity.

National Food and Nutrition Surveys

Nutrition programs, whether federal, state or local, rely on national nutrition and health survey data for identifying their needs. This is due to the paucity of studies conducted at the state and county levels. National statistics are valid to use for planning nutrition programs on the local level in the United States because a mobile society and a nationwide system of marketing and transporting food have created a fairly homogeneous food supply. Food preparation methods across the United States may differ according to cultural background, but generally the groups of foods used do not.

FOOD SUPPLY DATA

The United States Department of Agriculture (USDA) keeps detailed information on "per capita consumption of all major food commodities," otherwise known as *food disappearance data*. Disappearance data are based upon total available food and not on actual consumption, and thus are difficult to interpret accurately, particularly because waste is not considered. Table 17–1 is an example of how disappearance data can be used to demonstrate trends over time as it gives the nutrient breakdown of the diet in the U.S. from 1910 to 1980. These data show that there has been a decrease in carbohydrate consumption, which is shown in more detail in Table 2–4. On the other hand, fat consumption has increased steadily, as shown in Table 3–4. Protein consumption has remained consistent at about 100 gm. per capita per day. The energy value of the diet dropped during the years from 1910 to 1957–1959 but has increased since then, so that in 1980 it is similar to that of 1910—about 3500 kcalories per day.

NATIONWIDE FOOD CONSUMPTION SURVEY (NFCS) 1977–78

To provide statistics that more closely reflect actual consumption, as opposed to the inflated

Table 17-1. NUTRITIVE VALUE OF DIETS PER PERSON IN THE UNITED STATES*

YEAR	KCALORIES	PROTEIN (gm.)	FAT (gm.)	CARBO-HYDRATE (gm.)	CALCIUM (gm.)	IRON (mg.)	VIT. A (I.U.)	THIAMIN (mg.)	RIBO-FLAVIN (mg.)	NIACIN (mg.)	ASCORBIC ACID (mg.)
1910	3500	101	123	498	0.84	15.3	7000	1.63	1.86	17.8	107
1920	3280	93	122	460	0.88	14.9	7400	1.53	1.86	16.2	107
1930	3450	92	134	477	0.90	14.3	7800	1.55	1.89	15.9	108
1940	3340	92	142	432	0.96	14.8	8200	1.55	1.95	16.5	122
1950	3250	95	144	401	1.03	17.1	8200	1.90	2.31	19.4	112
1955	3220	96	148	386	1.04	16.4	7400	1.85	2.34	19.7	108
1957–59[a]	3130	95	143	374	0.98	16.3	8100	1.85	2.31	21.1	105
1967	3240	99	152	373	0.95	16.4	7900	1.92	2.36	23.2	105
1974	3280	100	156	376	0.92	18.3	8200	1.99	2.37	23.9	117
1976	3290	102	157	376	0.93	18.6	8100	2.06	2.47	25.3	123
1980[b]	3520	103	168	406	0.89	17.6	8400	2.20	2.40	26.8	123

[a] Average

[b] Preliminary

* Sources: Trulson, M.F.: The American diet—Past and present. Am. J. Clin. Nutr., 7:93, 1959. Compiled from: Supplement for 1956, Consumption of Food in the United States, 1904–1952. Washington, D.C., U.S. Department of Agriculture, Agriculture Handbook No. 62, 1956.
"Dietary Levels of Households in the United States." Washington, D.C., U.S. Department of Agriculture, Agriculture Marketing Service and Agriculture Research Service Report No. 6.
Marston, R., and Friend, B.: Nutritional Review. National Food Situation, 158:25, November, 1976.
Marston, R., and Welsh, S.: Nutrient Content of the National Food Supply. National Food Review, Winter, 1981, p. 19.

Table 17–2. AVERAGE AMOUNTS OF FOOD EATEN IN ONE DAY
PER INDIVIDUAL*

FOOD (AS SERVED)	MEN	WOMEN
Milk and milk products (oz.)		
Milk, milk drinks	7.9	5.8
Yogurt	0.2	0.2
Cheese	0.8	0.6
Eggs (each) (medium)	3/4	1/2
Meat, poultry, fish (oz.)		
Beef	3.0	1.7
Pork	0.9	0.6
Other meat	1.2	0.6
Poultry	1.1	0.9
Fish, shellfish	0.5	0.6
Mixtures	3.3	2.3
Legumes, nuts, total (oz.)	1.1	0.7
Grain products		
Bread, rolls, biscuits (slices)	3 1/2	2
Other baked goods (oz.)	2.1	1.8
Cereals, pastas (oz.)	1.4	1.4
Mixtures (oz.)	2.6	1.5
Tomatoes, citrus fruit (cups)		
Tomatoes	1/8	1/8
Citrus fruit and juices	1/4	1/4
Dark green and deep yellow vegetables (tbsp.)	1	1
Potatoes (cups), white	1/3	1/4
Other vegetables and fruit (cups)		
Other vegetables	1/2	1/2
Other fruit	1/4	1/4
Sugars, sweets		
Sugar (gm.)	6	6
Candy (gm.)	2	3
Fats, oils (tbsp.)		
Table fats	1 1/4	1
Salad dressings	2/3	1/2
Beverages other than milk, juices and alcoholic drinks		
Tea (6 oz. cups)	1.0	1.0
Coffee (6 oz. cups)	1.7	1.6
Soft drinks (12 oz. bottles)	3/4	3/4

* Average amounts of food reported in one day (spring 1977) by men and women 23 to 34 years of age.

From NFCS 1977–78 Preliminary Report No. 2, Food and Nutrient Intakes of Individuals in 1 day, in the U.S., Spring 1977. USDA, SEA, Sept. 1980.

values provided by the disappearance data, the USDA also conducts national Food Consumption Surveys (FCS). The FCS are conducted approximately every ten years and provide yet another source of data on national food habits and trends. Table 17–2 shows the average daily consumption found in the NFCS* for two of the groups for which data were collected. While the FCS provide data of interest and use, caution is essential when comparing statistics over time,[39] as methodologies for measuring and collecting data are constantly changing. The most recent NFCS is a good example of a change in data collection from one decade to another. The most recent NFCS provides data similar to those collected by past FCS, but it also classifies members of various households and their dietary

information in ways never used before, such as: (1) dietary information for individuals including the kind and amount of each food eaten, (2) the time the food was eaten, (3) the type of food service, (4) the cost of the food eaten, (5) if the food eaten was typical for food usually consumed, (6) if the individual was on a special diet, (7) if the individual was a vegetarian and (8) if vitamins, minerals, or other supplements were consumed.[45]

However, even with the differences in data collection methods, enough similarities still exist to provide a basis for comparing one FCS with another. This type of a comparison provides interesting information on food consumption trends from one decade to another for particular food groups.

The average intake of milk and milk products decreased from 1965 to 1977, with the highest level of milk and milk products (butter not included) being consumed by children under one year of age and the next highest consumption

*The name has changed from Household Food Consumption Survey (through the 1965–66 survey) to the Nationwide Food Consumption Survey (1977–78).

level by boys aged 12 through 19 years.[9] Boys and men used more milk products than girls and women.[25] This kind of information is of use to educators, for example, those working with population groups who need to increase consumption of calcium-rich products.

Intakes of eggs, legumes, nuts and seeds decreased from the 1965 survey to the 1977 survey for those under the age of 35, while intakes for these same foods increased for individuals older than 35 years of age.

The heaviest consumers of grain products were teenage boys. Their average consumption of grain products was the equivalent of six slices of bread per day. Bread products (including rolls and biscuits) were preferred by more persons and in larger quantities than other items in this group of foods. Children 3 to 14 years of age were the largest consumers of cookies, crackers, doughnuts, pies, cakes and other pastries. Overall intakes of grain products declined from 1965 to 1977.

For all age groups, except adult women, intakes of fats and oils were less than half the amounts reported in 1965. The amount for adult women also declined, but not by as much.

Soft drink intake increased considerably from 1965, as shown in Figure 17–1. Still the overall

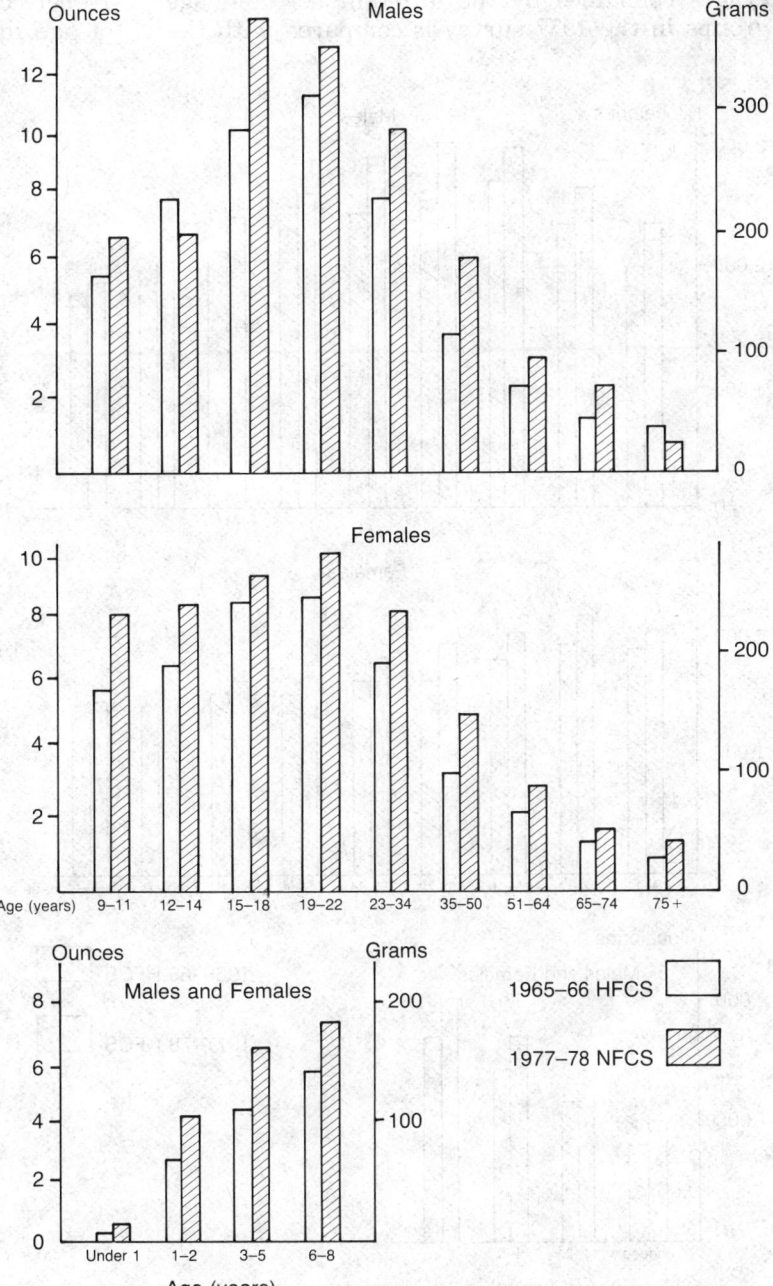

Figure 17–1. U.S. average intake of soft drinks per individual in a day, spring 1965 and 1977. (Adapted from USDA Household FCS 1965–66, Report No. 11, 1972, and USDA NFCS 48 States, Spring 1977, Preliminary.)

intake of sweets decreased from 1965. Teenage girls and adults over 35 years of age showed the largest decline in intakes of sugar and sweets.[45] This reduction in overall fat and sugar consumption is a good trend.

The average food energy intake for individuals in 1965 is compared with that of individuals in 1977 in Figure 17–2. For all age groups the average energy intake dropped in 1977 from the levels found in 1965. The distribution of the calories consumed is shown in Figure 17–3. Carbohydrate was the source of 42.8 per cent of the calories, and fat contributed 40.8 per cent in 1977.

The average nutritive content of food and beverages consumed by the different sex and age groups in the 1977 survey is compared with the 1980 Recommended Dietary Allowances (RDA) to examine the nutrient intake for the U.S. population. Table 17–3 shows that all 22 of the age-sex groups in the survey met the RDA for protein, riboflavin, niacin and vitamin C. Almost all age-sex groups met the RDA in full for phosphorus, vitamin A, thiamin and vitamin B_{12}. Calcium intakes for children under 3 years of age, children 6 to 8 years of age and males 19 to 34 years met the RDA, while females 12 years of age and older had the lowest intakes compared with the RDA (less than 79 per cent). Iron intakes averaged 100 per cent or more of the RDA for infants and men, while 1- to 2-year-olds and females 12 to 50 years of age met less than 70 per cent of the RDA. All groups over 2 years of age met less than 100 per cent of the RDA

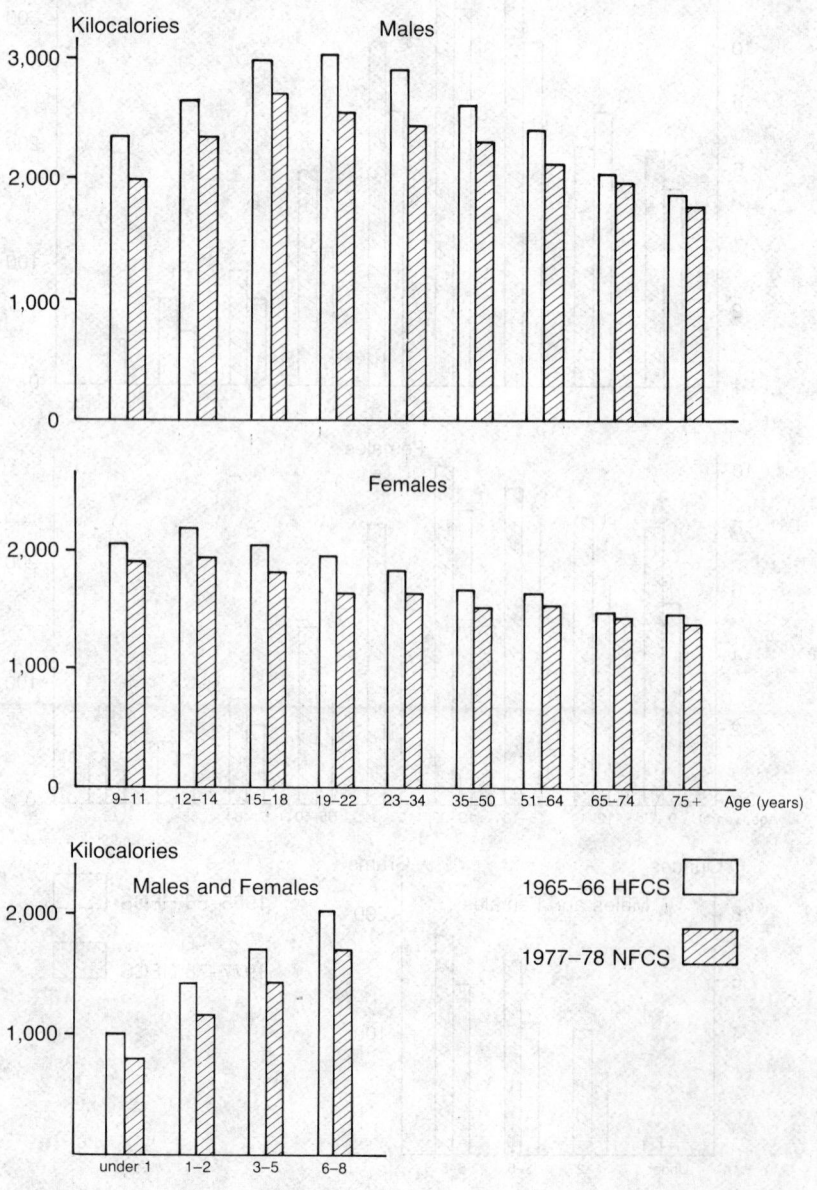

Figure 17–2. U.S. average food energy intake per individual in a day, spring 1965 and 1977. (Adapted from USDA Household FCS 1965–66, Report No. 11, 1972; and USDA NFCS 48 States, Spring 1977, Preliminary.)

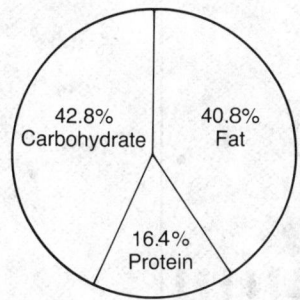

Figure 17–3. U.S. average intake of calories, by macronutrients in a day, spring 1977. (Redrawn from USDA NFCS 48 States, Spring 1977, Preliminary.)

for magnesium and vitamin B$_6$, with females over the age of 12 years meeting less than 79 per cent of the RDA.[45]

Information gathered by the NFCS is used by the USDA to update food plans, determine food stamp and other food program benefits, set requirements for regulatory programs, provide information on the adequacy of diets for the poor, and determine special needs of certain groups such as the elderly.[33] However, there are problems with the USDA using the NFCS data for determining requirements for food programs, particularly for low-income groups. Some of these problems are:

1. The survey's sample is too small to provide useful information in evaluating low-income families.

2. The methodology for obtaining this information has not been fully validated.

3. There are no assurances that the data obtained will represent the amount of food consumed.[46]

For decades the USDA food supply and consumption data were the only sources available on the nutrient and food intakes of the U.S. population. Although these are useful, the need for increased measures of surveillance on nutritional adequacy was recognized by many groups and individuals within and outside the government. This awareness and the White House Conference on Food, Nutrition and Health recommendations were motivating factors for conducting the nutrition surveys discussed later in this chapter.

WHITE HOUSE CONFERENCE ON FOOD, NUTRITION AND HEALTH

During the 1969 White House Conference on Food, Nutrition and Health[57] (WHC-FNH) the need for accurate nutrition data was recognized and several recommendations were made to that effect. Special emphasis was to be placed on those suffering from hunger and malnutrition. Many people, including policy-makers, did not want to admit that hunger and malnutrition existed in the United States. Fortunately, the President recognized the fact, and addressed the hunger issue in his remarks to Congress, opening the WHC-FNH on May 6, 1969; "We have awakened to the distressing fact that . . . many Americans suffer from malnutrition. . . . That hunger and malnutrition should persist in a land such as ours is embarrassing and intolerable." As a result of the WHC-FNH the government increased its participation in providing food programs for the needy and in conducting national nutrition surveys.

NATIONAL NUTRITION SURVEY 1968–70

The National Nutrition Survey or Ten-State Nutrition Survey[5] conducted by the U.S. Department of Health, Education and Welfare was designed to evaluate not only the dietary intake but also the nutritional status of the people. In addition to dietary intake information, data included socioeconomic information, anthropometric data, clinical findings and biochemical data. According to the findings of surveys conducted in ten states, many people in low-income areas were seriously malnourished. The trends in this survey suggested that economic status may be an important underlying factor in the families' nutritional patterns, along with the lack of concern, lack of knowledge of the right foods to eat or buy, and ignorance of health care. The clinical findings of anemia and reduced levels of serum albumin, vitamin A, ascorbic acid, and urinary thiamin and riboflavin clearly indicated the seriousness and magnitude of the problem. Obesity was a major problem, particularly among black women. Young children from poor families were smaller than young children from families with higher economic status, as shown for boys in Figure 17–4.

PRESCHOOL NUTRITION SURVEY 1968–70

In the Preschool Nutrition Survey,[48] 3400 children between one and six years of age from 36 states and the District of Columbia, representing whites, blacks, Spanish-Americans, and American Indians, were evaluated for nutritional status. Some of the findings from this survey were:

1. Low socioeconomic status was systematically associated with smaller size in white children.

2. Blacks tended to be smaller at birth than whites and remained smaller for the first two to three years of life. Thereafter, blacks tended to grow more rapidly.

3. As the socioeconomic status of the family

Table 17–3. NUTRIENT INTAKES BELOW 1980 RECOMMENDED DIETARY ALLOWANCES

Average Intake as Percentage of 1980 RDA, Spring 1977

SEX AND AGE (years)	PROTEIN	CALCIUM	IRON	MAGNE-SIUM	PHOS-PHORUS	VITA-MIN A	THIAMIN	RIBO-FLAVIN	NIACIN	VITA-MIN B6	VITA-MIN B12	VITA-MIN C
Males and females:												
Under 1												
1–2			•••									
3–5		••	•••	••						••		
6–8												
Males:												
9–11		•••		•••						•••		
12–14		•••	•	•••						•••		
15–18		•	•	•••						•••		
19–22				•••						•••		
23–34				••						•••		
35–50				••						•••		
51–64				••						••		
65–74		••		••						••		
75 and over		••		•						••		
Females:												
9–11		•••	•	•••						•••		
12–14		•••	•••	•••	••	•	••			•••		
15–18		•••	••••	•••						•••		
19–22		•••	••••	•••						•••		
23–34		•••	••••	•••						•••		
35–50		•••	••••	•••						•••		
51–64		•••	•••	•••						•••		
65–74		•••	•••	•••						•••		
75 and over		•••		•••						•••	•	

Blank indicates that intake meets 100% of the RDA.

• 90–99% RDA
•• 80–89% RDA
••• 70–79% RDA
•••• Below 70% RDA

From Nationwide Food Consumption Survey, 48 States. Spring 1977, preliminary.

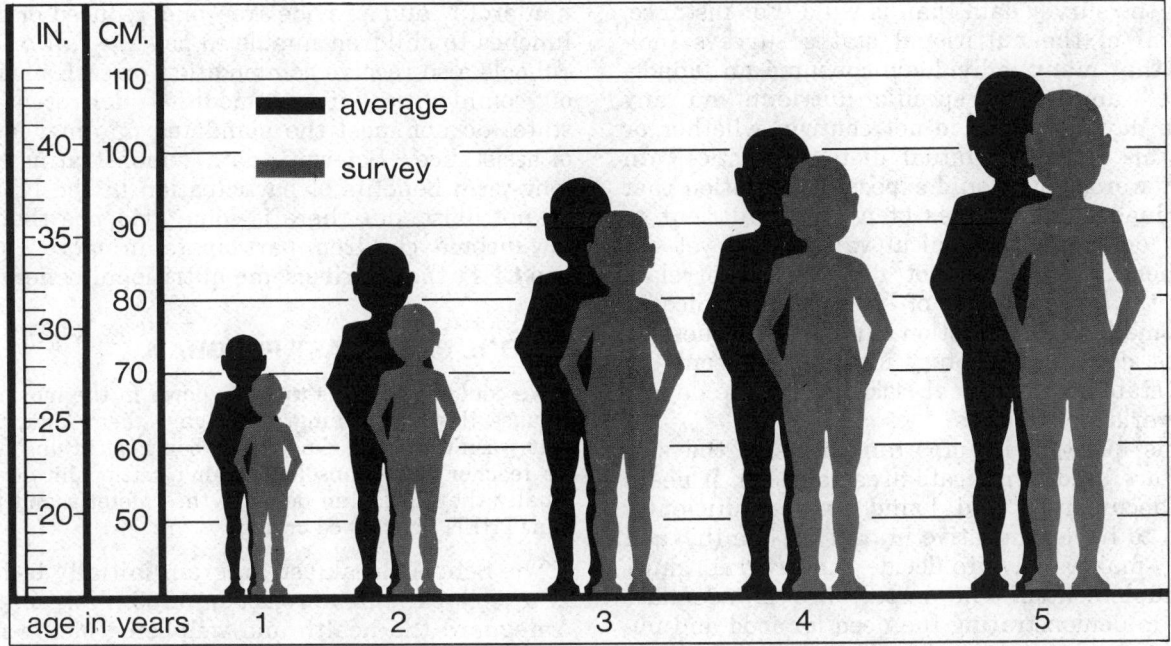

Figure 17–4. Relationship of height to age for boys five years of age and under, from low-income households included in the National Nutrition Survey, 1968, compared with average heights for boys. (From Nutrition Today, 4(1):10, 1969.)

improved, the nutrient intakes of the children improved. This was most evident for vitamin C.

4. Protein intakes of the subgroups averaged one and one half to two times the RDA. All children seemed to have adequate protein intakes.

5. Ten to 15 per cent of the children had borderline low intakes of ascorbic acid.

6. Twelve per cent of black, 10 per cent of Spanish-American and 7 per cent of white preschool children were classified as being anemic.

Most of these findings tended to confirm those related to children in the Ten-State Nutrition Survey.

HEALTH AND NUTRITION EXAMINATION SURVEY (HANES) 1971–74

The HANES survey of over 20,000 persons, representing the first health survey of the U.S. population with a nutritional component, was meant to assess and monitor the nutritional status of the American people over a period of time.[43] Population subgroups were defined according to sex, age, race and two levels of poverty.

Clinical data suggested that signs of nutritional deficiency such as tongue changes, bowed legs and knock knees, bleeding or swollen gums, goiter, and low urinary excretion of thiamin and riboflavin are more common in blacks than in whites. Obese black women were at the highest risk of suffering and dying from certain diseases, e.g., hypertension, heart disease and diabetes, and thus probably deserve special attention in both control and prevention programs.

Dietary intake data obtained by the 24-hour recall method showed:

1. Some population groups had mean intakes of protein, calcium, vitamin A and ascorbic acid that were lower than the RDA.

2. For the nutrients thiamin and riboflavin, adequate or more than adequate mean intakes were reported for all population groups.

3. For all population subgroups except adult white males, the mean intakes for iron were below the RDA.

However, without further biochemical and clinical evidence, it is impossible to say to what extent malnutrition exists in these populations.[32]

Because of the insufficient numbers of low-income or minority individuals in its sample, the HANES has been criticized as being inadequate. In recent years health data have been collected on Hispanics in national surveys, but Hispanics were sampled according to their proportion of the total population, which is relatively small. This has resulted in an insufficient number of Hispanics being included in the various surveys, so that the surveys have provided unreliable estimates on their health parameters. To remedy this, a Hispanic HANES is being conducted and data will be available in 1986.[44]

EVALUATING NUTRITION SURVEYS

When using the information from nutrition surveys, it is important not to interpret more from the survey data than is valid. For instance, several of the nutritional status surveys indicate that many individuals consume an "inadequate" amount of specific nutrients on any given day, but they do not confirm whether or not this reflects habitual dietary practice.[38] In other words, one would expect a population that had inadequate intakes of a given nutrient to show deficient biochemical values, and yet the biochemical data do not necessarily correlate with the large number of "poor" diets indicated by some food consumption surveys. The question arises, do the low dietary intakes represent the first state of nutritional risk or only the day-to-day variances in diets?

This question is important because the surveys are used to indicate areas of need. If needs are documented and found to be sufficiently large to have a negative impact on health, then policy-makers have to decide if a program must be implemented. The importance of adequate data in demonstrating the need for food and nutrition programs cannot be overstated. Another motivator for funding nutrition, as history has shown, has been the onset of a depression or a war.[28]

Food Assistance and Nutrition Programs

The feeding of children in the schools began in the early 1900's with the establishment of free, compulsory and universal education. Enlightened social scientists recognized that caring for the physical needs of children was essential if they were to learn. Philanthropic organizations, local school districts and private individuals took on the task of operating lunch programs in the early years. It took the great depression of the 1930's with its concomitant crop surpluses and depressed farm prices to involve the Federal government in school food programs.[19] This involvement was in the form of surplus commodities until World War II, when availability of surplus commodities dropped drastically and cash subsidies were given to schools in lieu of commodities. Table 17–4 provides a history of food and nutrition programs administered by the USDA.

NATIONAL SCHOOL LUNCH PROGRAM (NSLP)

The NSLP, permanently authorized in 1946, is the oldest and the largest of the Child Nutrition Programs (CNP). In fiscal year 1980 the Federal government spent more than 2.1 billion dollars on the NSLP. The NSLP must provide lunches meeting certain nutritional standards (the goal is to provide one third of the RDA), be non-profit, and provide free and reduced-priced lunches to children unable to pay the full price. Schools also receive commodities, or cash in lieu of commodities if commodities delivered to states do not meet the mandated minimal level of assistance.[19] Scientific data demonstrating the long-term benefits of participation in the NSLP do not exist, but there is some evidence that if low-income children participate in more than one CNP, they derive some nutritional benefit.[28]

SCHOOL BREAKFAST PROGRAM

We couldn't get kids to settle down in the morning because they were hungry. We gave them milk, but that wasn't enough. One day a boy kept crying and his teacher and counselor couldn't settle him down. Finally they took him down to the cafeteria and fed him. THEN he stopped crying.[28]

The School Breakfast Program initially began as a two-year pilot project in 1966, designed to "safeguard the health and well-being of the nation's children" and to provide a "coordinated comprehensive child food service in the schools."[28] Fortunately the program has continued beyond its infancy. Like the NSLP, this program provides free or reduced-priced meals to children who otherwise might go hungry. This program is also administered by the USDA.

CHILD CARE FOOD PROGRAM (CCFP)

In 1968 the CCFP began as a three-year pilot program and it has continued under the auspices of the USDA.[11] In 1975 amendments to the CNP legislation significantly expanded the scope and eligibility for this program. In 1980 the CCFP was the fastest growing of all of the CNP as non-profit, non-residential child care programs (day care centers and family day care homes) found they were eligible to feed children a lunch similar to that provided by schools in the NSLP, but cutbacks in Federal support have since curtailed growth of the program.

NUTRITION, EDUCATION, AND TRAINING (NET)

The NET section of the CNP bill passed in 1978 required the Secretary of Agriculture to formulate and carry out a nutrition information and education program by providing grants to state agencies to administer: (1) nutritional training of educational and food service personnel, (2) food service management training of food service personnel and (3) nutrition education activities in schools and child care institutions (including 24-hour child care residential facilities and day care programs for children).[10, 12]

The major goal of the program was to provide children with better learning opportunities re-

Table 17-4. FEDERAL FOOD AND NUTRITION PROGRAMS ADMINISTERED BY USDA

PROGRAM AND YEAR STARTED	ELIGIBLE INDIVIDUALS OR GROUPS	OBJECTIVES OF PROGRAM	COMPONENTS OF PROGRAM
Food Stamp Program 1964	Needy families and individuals in participating counties (almost all counties).	To supplement an individual's or a family's food-buying power.	Limited monthly allotment of food stamps at a reduced price, depending upon income. Stamps are used to pay for food.
Food Distribution Program (Donable Foods) 1930's	Supplemental food programs for mothers and infants. Elderly feeding programs. Schools and institutions.	To distribute surplus food to individuals and institutions to help agricultural support program.	Distribution of surplus food. Previously, to needy families. At present, only to eligible schools, institutions and persons in U.S. Trust Territories.
Supplemental Food Program for Women, Infants, and Children (WIC) 1974	Pregnant and lactating women and infants and children up to five years of age who live in an approved project area and who are judged to be at nutritional risk because of inadequate nutrition or income.	To improve the nutritional status of pregnant and lactating women and children up to five years of age in low-income areas.	Cash grants to state health departments and comparable agencies who make available supplemental foods through participating health clinics. Health clinics provide specified nutritious food supplements or vouchers for these foods. Regular health exam of mother and child required.
National School Lunch Program 1946	All children enrolled at participating schools, residential child care institutions, including homes for developmentally disabled up to 21 years of age, juvenile detention centers, and orphanages.	To provide a nutritious lunch (one that has as its objective to provide one third of the RDA for a child) at a reasonable cost to school children. To provide reduced-price or free lunches to needy eligible children.	Donated food to participating schools. Federal monetary support.
School Breakfast Program 1973	All children enrolled in participating schools.	To provide a nutritious breakfast at a low cost to children.	Donated food to participating schools. Federal monetary support.
Child Care Food Program 1968	Preschool children in non-profit facilities such as day care centers. Head Start centers and family day care homes.	To provide meal service for children in full-time day care centers and Head Start Programs and after-school care programs.	Federal monetary support. Cash in lieu of commodities available.
Special Milk Program* 1968	Schools, child care centers, summer camps, and institutions.	To reduce the cost of milk to children or provide it free to children who are also eligible for free meals.	Federal reimbursement to schools or centers for all or part of the cost of the milk served.
Summer Food Service Program for Children 1968	Public agency sponsored programs for preschool and school-age children in schools, recreation centers and summer camps and during vacations in areas with a continuous school calendar.	To provide free lunches to children in summer programs.	Federal monetary support.
Nutrition Education and Training 1978	All children enrolled in schools, residential child care institutions, child care food programs. Also teachers, and school-food service workers.	To provide nutrition education and training to children, teachers, and food service workers. To develop curriculum for teaching nutrition.	$0.50 available for every child enrolled in schools, institutions and child care food programs in the U.S. and Trust Territories.

*If a school is on the School Lunch Program, it cannot receive the Special Milk Program and vice versa.

garding food and nutrition so that they could learn about the relationship of nutrition to health and develop nutritional attitudes and practices necessary for health and well-being throughout life. However, full Federal funding of the program was discontinued in 1982.

SPECIAL SUPPLEMENTAL FOOD PROGRAM FOR WOMEN, INFANTS, AND CHILDREN (WIC)

In 1972, Congress created the WIC program as described in Table 17-4. The purpose of the program is to reduce the deleterious conse-

quences of poor nutrition for pregnant women during and after pregnancy and their infants and children during their formative years of development by providing them with supplemental nutritious foods. In 1978 substantive changes occurred in the program including the eligibility standards. Persons would not be eligible solely on the basis of low income but would also need to "exhibit evidence of nutritional risk, as determined by a competent professional authority, and that nutrition education was to be provided to all adult participants and that the State agency provide training to persons providing such nutrition education."[14]

The WIC program works because it combines all the factors necessary for a successful community health program. WIC meets an identified need through a very practical method—it provides food—insuring compliance by mothers and children certified to be at risk. It provides nutrition education and health services that recipients can also relate to. And, most importantly, documentation exists that WIC works. "Substantial evidence now exists to document the effectiveness of the WIC program in reducing the incidence of low birth weight in infants and averting subnormal infant development." At least one study has shown that the medical treatment of low-birth-weight infants is three times more expensive than the cost of prevention through the WIC program.[19]

FOOD STAMP PROGRAM

Through the Food Stamp Program (FSP) eligible low income households exchange an amount of money for an allotment of food stamps. Stamps may be used to purchase any foods except alcohol, pet food and certain imported items from retail stores. Their purpose is to assist low-income households to increase their food purchasing power and improve their diets. Changes in the FSP under the current political climate occur far too rapidly to report in any text. Up-to-date information can be obtained by contacting the Food Research Action Committee (see Table 17–12) and requesting the most current references and published literature. It is very important for a community health educa-tor to be knowledgeable and able to assist the poor, the disabled and handicapped, the elderly and children in obtaining adequate food stamp benefits. An educator can initiate nutrition education programs, but without sufficient *food* a recipient doesn't care much about the *nutrient* content of a diet.

The Cost of an Adequate Diet

Food requires the greatest share of the family budget at a low or moderate income level. This is particularly true of the large family, which may allot as much as half or even more of its income to food. In 1976, according to the Bureau of Labor Statistics, the urban working poor family spent almost 40 per cent of its disposable income on food,[17] and this is still true today. It costs more to feed a large family, but the average cost per person is less, because the small family generally cannot buy and prepare the meals as economically as the large one.

In the United States over 350 billion dollars a year is spent for food. This represents on the average slightly over 16 per cent of take-home pay.[23] The Economics and Statistics Service (ESS) of the USDA studied how the food dollar is spent in the average household with 2.95 persons and a before taxes income of $273.05. Figure 17–5 shows how the food dollar was spent based on the "money value of purchased food during the week preceding the 1977–78 NFCS" conducted by the USDA. These statistical values suggest behavioral patterns that may be used by

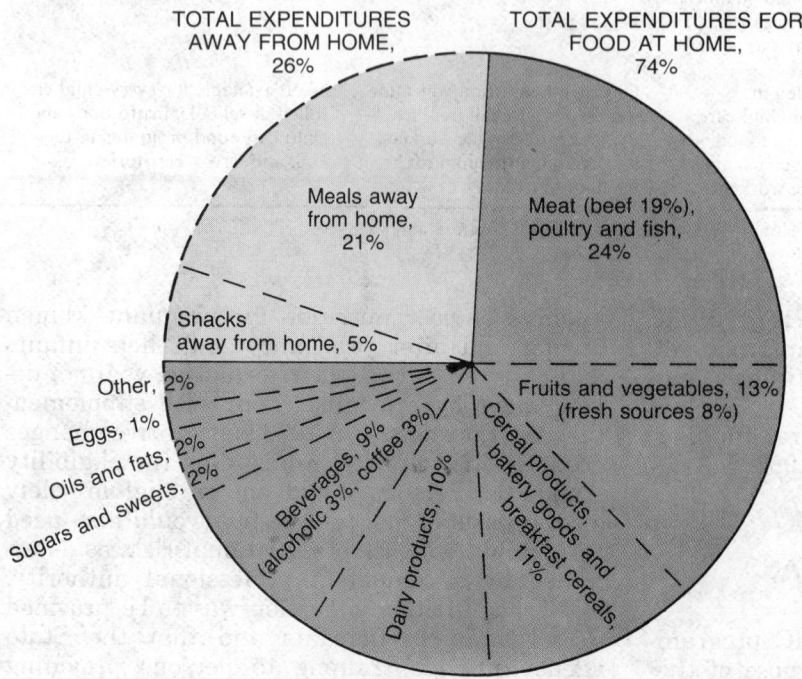

Figure 17–5. Average weekly household expenditures for food. Average number of people in a household was 2.95. Average household income before taxes was $273.05 per week. (Adapted from Impact of Household Size and Income on Food Spending Patterns. U.S. Department of Agriculture, Economics and Statistics Service. Technical Bulletin Number 1650, Washington, D.C., 1981.)

government policy-makers to anticipate the impact of government programs involving welfare payments for food purchases.[22]

USDA FOOD PLANS

Food plans are sets of nutritious diets, planned at four income levels, based on the latest information on food consumption and nutritional recommendations.[20] These four food plans —a thrifty, a low cost, a moderate cost and a liberal plan—are designed and published in booklet form by the Consumer and Food Economics Research Division, Agricultural Research Service, USDA. Each plan can be used as a guide for weekly budgeting, marketing, and individual or family food planning.

The USDA has updated the 1975 food plans to incorporate data collected in the 1977-78 NFCS, to reflect the 1980 RDA, the latest food prices and the most current nutrient composition data.[8a] The most significant change which deserves comment is the reduction of the 14 age-sex categories to 11. The food plans for children under one year of age and for pregnant and lactating women have been omitted. This is unfortunate considering the nutritional risk of these particular groups.[18]

CHARACTERISTICS OF DIETS AT DIFFERENT COST LEVELS

The *thrifty* plan (the least costly) is used as the basis for coupon allotment by the Food Stamp Program. The *low-cost* and especially the *thrifty* plans require skill in buying, storing and preserving food to insure that the family is well fed nutritionally. The *moderate-cost* plan is suitable for the average American family. It includes larger quantities of milk, eggs, meats, fruits and vegetables than the low-cost plan. It also has more variety and less home preparation. The *liberal* plan allows for more variety, more animal products, and more fruits and vegetables.

In general, the quantity of milk and milk products, leafy green and yellow vegetables, tomatoes and citrus fruits should not be changed very much, regardless of the amount spent for food. The greatest reduction in the cost of food can be made by reducing quantities of meat, fish, poultry and the group described as "other vegetables and fruits" and by increasing the intake of potatoes, cereals, dry beans and peas. Within any food group there are both expensive and less expensive sources of the essential nutrients. For example, evaporated or powdered milk can be used in place of fresh fluid milk; cereals cooked or made at home cost less than the ready-to-eat varieties; lower grades and cheaper cuts of meat can be used and fruits and vegetables can be grown at home, purchased in season or purchased in bulk from a food co-op. Knowing how to bake and cook can greatly lower the cost of meals. Ready-to-serve or partially prepared foods are proportionally expensive because the consumer is paying for the labor performed by the food manufacturer to save time for the consumer.

COST VERSUS ADEQUACY

Foods in the plans provide for a nutritionally adequate diet that meets the RDA for *most* individuals, even though the thrifty and low-cost plans contain less meat, poultry and fish than most families consume on the average. The 1975 plans do not meet the recommended dietary allowance for iron for young children, teenage girls and women of child-bearing age, when average selections are made. The 1975 plans provide about 6 mg. of iron per 1000 kcal. except if choices of particularly iron-rich food are made.[18, 20] Literature reviewing the nutritional content of the new 1983 food plans had not yet been published for inclusion in this text. Unlike the 1975 plans, the new plans also consider zinc, phosphorus, folacin, vitamin E, cholesterol, caloric sweeteners and sodium.[18, 20]

Studies have shown that there is a relationship between income and an adequate diet. This is demonstrated in Table 17-5, which shows the diet quality of households at four food cost levels. Education, or its lack, also is important in determining eating habits. In low-income groups, some diets were good, while in high-income groups some diets were poor. Education as to the foods that make up an adequate diet is essential. Studies of the food buying practices of urban low-income consumers indicate that they demonstrate considerable sophistication in grocery shopping. The majority of these consumers purchase groceries at supermarkets. They tend to stretch the food budget by buying canned and dried milk, canned fruits and vegetables, breads, potatoes, rice and other cereals to substitute in part for meat, fresh milk, fresh fruit and frozen foods.[16]

According to a Comptroller General's report to Congress, Americans want to select proper foods, but with the vast array of food products to choose from, consumers are finding it increasingly difficult to make the right food decisions. A report entitled "What Foods Should Americans Eat?" calls on the government to adopt a set of nutritional principles and provide authoritative guidance on safe levels of intake so that Federal agencies will be able to carry out their food programs and responsibilities for nutritional education more effectively.[56]

Table 17–5. DIET QUALITY OF HOUSEHOLDS AT FOUR FOOD COST LEVELS, 1977–78

FOOD COST LEVEL*	PERCENT OF HOUSEHOLDS USING FOOD THAT FURNISHED—	
	1974 RDA for 11 Nutrients†	*80 Percent of 1974 RDA for 11 Nutrients*
All households	50	71
Thrifty plan	9	33
Low-cost plan	31	64
Moderate-cost plan	52	81
Liberal plan	69	89

From Family Economics Review. Washington, D.C., U.S. Department of Agriculture, Agriculture Research Service, 1982

* Cost of food in the USDA food plans for a four-person household (man and woman 20–54 and children 6–8 and 9–11 years of age) adjusted for household size and economy of scale factors used in establishing the food stamp allotment.

† Protein, calcium, phosphorus, iron, magnesium, vitamin A value, thiamin, riboflavin, vitamin B_6, vitamin B_{12} and vitamin C.

National Nutrition Guidelines and Policies

NATIONAL NUTRITION POLICY (NNP)

The U.S. has a long history of policies and programs regarding agriculture, rural people, natural resources and, more recently, food aid and nutrition.[22] Some argue that these various programs form a U.S. food policy. Others argue that what the U.S. has are agricultural policies incidentally including nutrition and that this does not constitute a food policy. Fortunately, whatever the opinion, all seem to agree that the U.S. does need a coordinated approach to the various food, nutrition and agricultural issues that abound.[21] To form an effective food and nutrition policy new programs or policies do not necessarily have to be created, only existing ones coordinated. A NNP does not have to be complicated, as demonstrated in testimony given by the American Dietetic Association to Senator McGovern's Senate Select Committee on Nutrition and Human Needs. The ADA listed the following goals as important for the formation of a NNP:[1, 55] (1) maintenance and improvement of the health of the American people, (2) insuring adequate food production for domestic needs and global commitments, (3) maintenance of food quality, (4) guaranteed access to food supplies and (5) maintenance of freedom of choice as an essential feature of U.S. food distribution and allocation.

Unfortunately, the U.S. government is not any closer to a National Nutrition Policy in the 1980's than when the above suggestions were presented in 1975 or when the White House Conference on Food, Nutrition, and Health recommended similar goals in 1969.[57]

NATIONAL NUTRITION GUIDELINES AND GOALS

Food guides developed by government agencies for teaching consumers how to plan an adequate diet are not new, as shown in Table 17–6. The first formal recommendations were present-

Table 17–6. HISTORY OF ACTIONS BY PRIVATE AND PUBLIC HEALTH ORGANIZATIONS TOWARD DIETARY GUIDELINES FOR THE PUBLIC

1940	National Research Council appoints the first Food and Nutrition Board (FNB)
1943	Publication of the first *Recommended Dietary Allowances* by the FNB
	Publication of the first Basic Seven by USDA as part of the National Wartime Nutrition Program
1956	The USDA publishes the first Essentials of an Adequate Diet (*Basic 4*)
1961	The Ad Hoc Committee on Nutrition of the American Heart Association presents dietary advice
1968	The American Heart Association releases eight Dietary Guidelines
1969	The White House Conference on Food, Nutrition and Health makes numerous recommendations on a variety of food and nutrition issues
1977	*Dietary Goals for the United States*, 1st and 2nd Editions, are published by Senate Select Committee on Nutrition and Human Needs
1979	Surgeon General's report *Healthy People* is published
	Various agencies/organizations publish goals, guidelines, diet statements
1980	American Medical Association, American Heart Association update, American Society of Clinical Nutrition, National Cancer Institute, Food and Nutrition Board all publish various guidelines
	The Departments of Health and Human Services and Agriculture co-publish *Dietary Guidelines for the U.S.*
	The USDA publishes *Food 1* "The Hassle-Free Guide to A Better Diet," materials to assist Americans in following the Dietary Guidelines
1982	The USDA develops *Food 2* and *Food 3* booklets but does not publish them
	The American Dietetic Association agrees to publish the *Food 2* and *Food 3* booklets to enable the American consumer to have access to the information, at minimum cost
	The USDA and the DHHS form a task force to study the Dietary Guidelines for possible alternatives

ed simultaneously in 1943 with publication of the *Recommended Dietary Allowances (RDA)* by the Food and Nutrition Board and the Basic Seven by the USDA. While excellent for nutritionists and other scientists, the RDA has limited use for consumer education purposes. The RDA provides information on the amounts of nutrients needed but not on which foods to eat. To provide consumers with a guide for eating, the USDA developed the *Basic Seven*, later revised to become the *Basic Four*. The USDA became more involved with providing literature on nutrition when they published *Food I*, a booklet to help U.S. citizens consume a diet that would meet the Dietary Guidelines. See Additional Readings.

Except for revisions of the RDA every four to six years, the U.S. government had remained silent on nutrition recommendations, despite the proddings of the White House Conference on Food, Nutrition, and Health, until the legislative branch in 1977 published recommendations in the form of *"Dietary Goals for the United States, First Edition."* These goals were developed by Senator McGovern's Senate Select Committee on Nutrition and Human Needs. Controversy arose over both the content of the goals and the right of the government to publish dietary recommendations for the public.[3] Fortunately, the controversy over content was significantly reduced with publication of *"Dietary Goals for the United States, Second Edition."* Table 17–7 states the Goals from the second edition. While discussions continued on the validity and the applicability of the Goals, USDA home economists in the Agricultural Research Service (ARS) focused on the practicality of implementation. The USDA/ARS published *"The Dietary Goals and Food on the Table"* to interpret the goals in terms of the kinds and amounts of foods needed to be consumed to meet the Goals. Table 17–8 presents one option for altering the U.S. diet to meet the Goals.

Just as the nutrition community seemed to be reaching a consensus the USDA and the U.S. Department of Health and Human Services (DHHS) published *"Nutrition and Your Health, Dietary Guidelines for Americans"*[47] (Table 17–9) and the Food and Nutrition Board, National Academy of Sciences, published *"Toward Healthful Diets"*[27] (Table 17–10) which differed in one major aspect—the recommendation for fat. Table 17–11 summarizes the positions taken by various governments, U.S. agencies and voluntary health groups on this issue.

One of the most distressing aspects of the conflict (between those who supported the Goals and those who supported Healthful Diets) was that scientists seemed to be arguing from an emotional base, while purporting to protect the public from confusion.[31] The introduction of "To-

Table 17–7. DIETARY GOALS FOR THE UNITED STATES, SECOND EDITION

Goal 1.	To avoid overweight, consume only as much energy (calories) as is expended. If overweight, decrease energy intake and increase energy expenditure.
Goal 2.	Increase the consumption of complex carbohydrates and "naturally occurring" sugars from about 28% of energy intake to about 48% of energy intake.
Goal 3.	Reduce the consumption of refined and other processed sugars by about 45% to account for about 10% of total energy intake.
Goal 4.	Reduce overall fat consumption from approximately 40% to about 30% of energy intake.
Goal 5.	Reduce saturated fat consumption to account for about 10% of total energy intake; and balance that with poly-unsaturated and mono-unsaturated fats, which should account for about 10% of energy intake each.
Goal 6.	Reduce cholesterol consumption to about 300 mg. per day.
Goal 7.	Limit the intake of sodium by reducing the intake of salt (sodium chloride) to about 5 grams per day.

From Senate Select Committee on Nutrition and Human Needs: Dietary Goals for the United States. 2nd ed. Stock No. 052–070–04376–8. Washington, D.C., U.S. Government Printing Office, 1977.

ward Healthful Diets" stated that its publication was essential, "in an effort to reduce the confusion in the mind of the public that has resulted from these many conflicting recommendations" (from various agencies in government, voluntary health groups, etc.). During the period of strong disagreement no one "side" was worse than the other. Quite a few professionals raised the concern that the public would be confused by the plethora of recommendations. In confusion, or so the argument was made, the public would turn from health professionals due to lack of consensus or credibility. Others felt that this view was too simplistic,[32] as consumers are frequently faced with making health decisions rife with controversy.

When one examines the recommendations made by various governments, as well as agencies in the U.S., one can easily see that the areas of agreement far exceed those of disagreement, as summarized in Table 17–11. The major area of disagreement revolves around the issue of fat and cholesterol. The question should be asked, "If scientific consensus (if there is such a thing) does not exist over one issue, should guidelines, goals or recommendations not be issued?" It is recommended that one examine the original publications for all of the recommendations presented and determine for oneself if the data support acceptance or rejection on any one particular issue. "Problems related to the public and, to a large degree, professional understanding of nutrition issues today arise because we are depending too often on others to dig out facts, weigh various arguments, and make decisions for us regarding nutrition, diet, and health."[41]

Table 17–8. A DAY'S FOOD, AS SERVED, IN DIETS MODIFIED TO MEET THE GOALS BUT NOT NECESSARILY THE RDA,[1] AND FURTHER MODIFIED TO MEET THE RDA,[2] OPTION 1

FOOD[3] AND UNIT	MEET GOALS, NOT NECESSARILY RDA				MEET GOALS AND RDA
	Child, 6–8 Years[4]	Child, 9–11 Years[4]	Male, 20–54 Years[4]	Female, 20–54 Years	Female, 20–54 Years
Skim milk (cup)	2.9	3.3	1.7	1.3	1.2
Eggs (no. per *week*)	2.8	3.7	3.1	4.3	5.3
Mature beans or peas, cooked (tbsp.)	1.9	2.1	2.0	1.3	1.8
Meat, boned cooked lean (ounce)	1.3	1.8	2.7	2.2	1.6
Poultry and fish, cooked boned (ounce)	1.1	1.5	2.3	1.9	1.4
Vegetables and fruit (cup)	2.0	2.5	2.6	2.3	2.5
Cereal, pasta (ounce[5])	2.9	3.4	2.7	2.1	3.5
Bread or equivalent in bakery products (slices)	7.8	10.1	12.9	8.6	8.0
Margarine, oil (tbsp.)	3.4	4.1	3.6	2.5	2.9
Sugar, sweets (tsp.)	6.0	7.0	6.7	4.7	4.7

[1] Recommended Dietary Allowance (RDA) plus 5 percent for energy distributed as 30 percent or less from fat, 14 percent or less from protein, 56 percent or more from carbohydrate, and 10 percent or less from sugar other than that found naturally in foods such as milk and fresh fruit. Saturated fat provides 10 percent or less of energy intake and cholesterol intake is limited to no more than 300 milligrams per day plus 5 percent.

[2] RDA plus 5 percent for vitamin A value, thiamin, riboflavin, niacin, ascorbic acid, calcium, and iron.

[3] The assortment of meats, vegetables, and other groups of foods is based on food consumption of U.S. households in 1965–66.

[4] Diet modified to meet the Goals also meets the RDA for the 5 vitamins and 2 minerals studied.

[5] One serving is approximately 1 ounce of dry cereal.

From Peterkin, B.: "The Dietary Goals and Food on the Table." Outlook 78. Agricultural Research Service. Washington, D.C., U.S. Department of Agriculture, 1978.

Keeping current on nutritional issues, however, is not sufficient for an effective community nutrition educator. Knowing how to influence the processes that finance the programs and implement the regulations in the community is also essential.

Federal Funding and Legislation of Nutrition Programs

Since the majority of nutrition efforts and programs are funded on the federal level, knowledge of the federal legislative and rule-

making processes is important for the health professional interested in nutrition. This is especially true since the political climate in the early 1980's called for remanding responsibilities to states, in a process referred to as the "new federalism."

FEDERAL FUNDING OF NUTRITION PROGRAMS

The Federal government became involved in funding public health programs, because state governments generally were doing an inadequate job because of lack of either resources or recognition of the problem.[19] To be sure the funds appropriated were spent for the particular identified need, the Federal government instituted *categorical grants.* The USDA WIC program is an example of a categorical grant. Federal money is given to a state to administer the program according to specific rules and regulations set by the federal agencies responsible for the program. Government regulations are often cumbersome, but they also ensure that programs like nutrition are incorporated into health services. Some Federal grants require that a state also provide some money or a

Table 17–9. NUTRITION AND YOUR HEALTH

Dietary Guidelines for Americans

Guideline 1. Eat a variety of foods
Guideline 2. Maintain ideal weight
Guideline 3. Avoid too much fat, saturated fat and cholesterol
Guideline 4. Eat foods with adequate starch and fiber
Guideline 5. Avoid too much sugar
Guideline 6. Avoid too much sodium
Guideline 7. If you drink alcohol, do so in moderation

From Nutrition and Your Health. Dietary Guidelines for Americans. Home and Garden Bulletin No. 232. Washington, D.C., U.S. Department of Agriculture and Department of Health and Human Services, 1980.

Table 17–10. TOWARD HEALTHFUL DIETS

— Select a nutritionally adequate diet from the foods available, by consuming each day appropriate servings of dairy products, meats, legumes, vegetables and fruits, and cereal and breads.

— Select as wide a variety of foods in each of the major food groups as is practicable in order to ensure a high probability of consuming adequate quantities of all essential nutrients.

— Adjust dietary energy intake and energy expenditure so as to maintain appropriate weight for height; if overweight, achieve appropriate weight reduction by decreasing total food and fat intake and by increasing physical activity.

— If the requirement for energy is low (e.g., reducing diet), reduce consumption of foods such as alcohol, sugars, fats, and oils, which provide calories but few other essential nutrients.

— Use salt in moderation; adequate but safe intakes are considered to range between 3 and 8 grams of sodium chloride daily.

From Food and Nutrition Board, National Research Council: Toward Healthful Diets. Washington, D.C., National Academy of Sciences, 1980.

"match." Criticisms of categorical grants center on the fact that states are mandated to spend the money according to the dictates of the Federal government, not according to state's individual needs. Hence the initiation of "block" grants.

Block grants allow states more discretion as to how they choose to spend the allotted Federal funds. The problem with block grants, at least as instituted in the early 1980's, was that the total funding was less for each category placed into a "block" grant.

LEGISLATIVE AND RULE-MAKING PROCESSES

Figure 17–6 shows how a bill is introduced and becomes a law. Learning the system at the federal level assists in understanding how legislation is passed in all bicameral legislatures (those with two legislative bodies), as the mechanisms are similar.

The process does not end when a bill makes it through Congress and is signed into law by the President. Most laws enacted by Congress are too vague to be implemented immediately by the agencies responsible for regulating them, so rules and regulations must be promulgated. Regulations properly issued have the *force and effect of law*, just as if Congress had issued them. It is for this reason that one must become as familiar with the rule-making process as with the legislative process.

ADVOCACY AND LOBBYING

Advocacy and lobbying for an issue are essentially the same because, in both instances, an individual is seeking to influence the legislative and rule-making processes toward a particular end. One must be knowledgeable in all facets of the issue one is "lobbying" for, and be able to transmit that information to others in an intelligent manner. It is necessary to communicate with elected officials to let them know that a constituent of *theirs* is an expert in nutrition. It is important to let them know that one of their constituents would be glad to inform them of the impact of program changes in their district.

To be effective an advocate must know the pros and cons of each issue before contact is made with an elected official, a legislative staff member or an agency bureaucrat. To do that one must keep up with the abundance of reports, issues and legislation that affect programs for nutrition, and this is not easy. Table 17–12 provides various resources to assist the community health educator in understanding and staying current on relevant nutritional issues.

Agencies responsible for administering a program issue regulations and a whole host of reports, most of which are interesting, if not necessary, to read. The Federal Register can be extremely useful.[24] Not only do the administrating agencies issue documents but agencies with auditing responsibilities do also. Two major agencies responsible for auditing are the U.S. Government Accounting Office (GAO) and the Congressional Budget Office (CBO). These agencies also issue reports on a vast array of topics including food and nutrition programs. Reports from auditing agencies are read by members of Congress and their staffs as well as executive branch staff and officials, in order to evaluate a program's efficiency.

Laws and Rules Regulating Safety of Food

Since time immemorial humans have been developing methods of storing foods to insure against periods of famine. As humankind began to live in larger groups labor became increasingly divided, removing some individuals (i.e., skilled craft workers) from the chore of gathering, hunting, storing and growing food.[9] As human societies continued to grow in size and in areas of specialization the consumer began to lose more and more control over the direct production of foodstuffs, becoming vulnerable to the provider of the goods. At first guilds or fellow merchants regulated their own professions to insure protection for the consumer.[35] Soon most human societies had grown too large to allow the various professions to regulate themselves. Also food was being adulterated, contaminated and falsely advertised to the detriment of the public, forcing the government to

Table 17–11. COMPARISON OF DIETARY RECOMMENDATIONS TO PREVENT CHRONIC AND DEGENERATIVE DISEASES AS STATED BY VARIOUS AGENCIES/ORGANIZATIONS

TITLE OF PUBLICATION/ DATE AND SOURCE OF THE RECOMMENDATION	FATS/LIPIDS				MAINTAIN IDEAL WEIGHT	
	P:S Ratio	*Reduce Total Fat*	*Reduce Saturated Fat*	*Decrease Cholesterol*	*Through Exercise*	*Through Diet*
Dietary Goals for the United States, 2nd ed. 12/77. U.S. Senate, Select Committee on Nutrition and Human Needs.	—*	Yes	Yes	Yes	Yes	Yes
Healthy People. The Surgeon General's Report on Health Promotion and Disease Prevention. 7/79. Department of Health, Education and Welfare.†	—	Yes	—	Yes	Yes	Yes
Nutrition and Your Health— Dietary Guidelines for Americans. 2/80. USDA & DHHS.	—	Yes	Yes	Yes	Yes	Yes
Toward Healthful Diets. Food and Nutrition Board, National Research Council. National Academy of Sciences. 1980.	—	Yes	—	—	Yes	Yes
Concepts of Nutrition and Health, American Medical Association 11/79.	—	Yes‡	—	—	Yes‡	Yes‡
Am. J. Clin. Nutr. Symposium Report on Dietary Factors Relating to the Nation's Health. 1979. American Society of Clinical Nutrition.	—	Yes‡	Yes‡	Yes‡	—	Yes‡
Diet Heart Statement. Report of Nutrition Committee, American Heart Association 1982.	Yes	Yes	Yes	Yes	Yes	Yes
Diet, Nutrition, and Cancer. Committee on Diet, Nutrition and Cancer, National Research Council, National Academy of Sciences, 1982.	—	Yes	—	—	—	—
Recommendations for Prevention Programs in Relation to Nutrition and Cardiovascular Disease. Department of National Health and Welfare, Canada.	—	Yes	—	—	Yes	Yes
Nutrition and Health—on Norwegian Nutrition and Food Policy. National Nutrition Council, Norway, 1975.	Yes	Yes	Yes	—	Yes	Yes
Recommendations for Diet. Australia, 1979.	—	Yes	—	—	—	Yes

*Indicates no recommendation made or position stated.
†Currently called the Department of Health and Human Services (DHHS).
‡Specifies change only when a person is medically determined to be at risk.

Table 17–11. COMPARISON OF DIETARY RECOMMENDATIONS TO PREVENT CHRONIC AND DEGENER-ATIVE DISEASES AS STATED BY VARIOUS AGENCIES/ORGANIZATIONS (*Continued*)

CARBOHYDRATES		EAT A VARIETY OF FOODS	DRINK ALCOHOL IN MODERATION	REDUCE SODIUM/SALT INTAKE	SUPPORTED BY GOVERNMENT
Reduce Sugar	*Increase Complex Carbohydrate*				
Yes	Yes	—	—	Yes	No
Yes	—	—	Yes	Yes	Yes
Yes	Yes	Yes	Yes	Yes	Yes
Yes	—	Yes	Yes	Yes	No
Yes[‡]	—	Yes	Yes[‡]	Yes[‡]	No
Yes	—	—	Yes	Yes[‡]	No
—	Yes	—	—	Yes	No
—	Yes	—	Yes	—	No
Yes	Yes	Yes	Yes	Yes	Yes
Yes	Yes	Yes	—	—	Yes
Yes	Yes	Yes	Yes	Yes	Yes

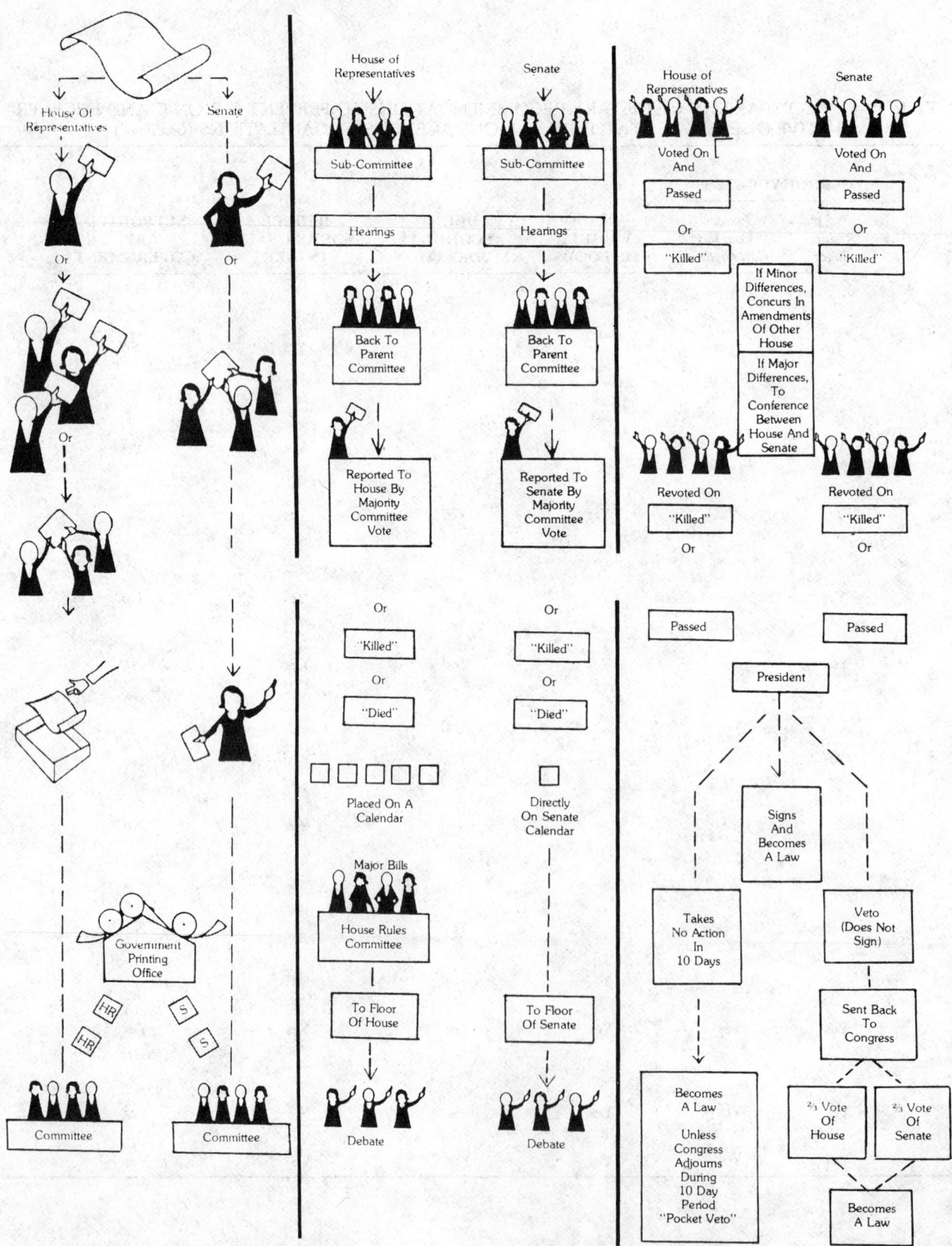

Figure 17–6. How a bill becomes law. The first column indicates the introduction of a bill or a group of similar bills by individual sponsors or cosponsors. (From League of Women Voters Education Fund.)

Table 17–12. PUBLICATIONS AND ORGANIZATIONS
USEFUL FOR PROVIDING INFORMATION ON NUTRITION
ADVOCACY

GROUP OR PUBLICATION	ADDRESS
Community Nutrition Institute A newsletter that informs of legislative and bureaucratic actions which affects all aspects of nutrition. An excellent resource.	1146 19th St. N.W. Washington, D.C. 20036 $35.00/year, published 50 weeks/year
Food Research Action Committee An organization that provides indepth up-to-date legislative analysis on federal food programs. Published books—"guides"—on understanding food-related issues.	1319 F St. N.W. Suite 500 Washington, D.C. 20004 $20.00/year for a newsletter and mailings on issues and guides to federal food programs
Family Economics Review Reports on research relating to economic aspects of family living, i.e., food stamps, NFCS analysis, nutrient/food dollar.	Family Economics Research Group Agricultural Research Service USDA, Federal Bldg. Hyattsville, Md 20782 $6.00/issue, Published quarterly
National Food Review Reports on a variety of research relating to economic, consumer, legislation, food situations, etc., that affect the USDA.	National Food Review Superintendent of Documents U.S. Government Printing Office Washington, D.C. 20402 $7.00/year, published quarterly
Consumer News Provides information on what the Federal government is doing for the consumer. Carries legislative and regulatory actions, and features stories of governmental and non-governmental programs affecting consumers. Covers more than food and nutrition issues.	U.S. Office of Consumer Affairs 621 Reporters Bldg. Washington, D.C. 20201 Was free but may be changed to include a minimum cost
A Brief Guide to Becoming a Nutrition Advocate A book describing actions to take for advocacy for food and nutrition programs.	Society for Nutrition Education 1736 Franklin Street Oakland, Calif. 94612 $3.75

regulate.[26] Table 17–13 summarizes the history of regulation of food in the U.S. in this century.

Some argue against any government regulations, but most responsible manufacturers recognize that in today's complex society, regulations are essential to protect the health, well-being and monetary investment of the consumer, particularly as our food system progresses toward more fabricated and formulated foodstuffs.[3, 54] Some manufacturers do not believe it is the responsibility of the food industry to replace nutrients lost during processing, even when unusual manufacturing techniques result in excess losses. The following expresses the attitude of some food processors and exemplifies why the consumer often distrusts manufacturers: "It is difficult to place full responsibility for the nutrition content of food products upon the manufacturer . . . a manufacturer justifiably may claim that his product makes so small a contribution that it is unimportant whether it contains nutrients." It is this kind of an attitude that motivates consumers to search for "unprocessed foods," "natural foods," or foods that still contain the nutrients originally present in the food.

Professionals need to assist the consumer in learning that the world is chemical whether the chemical is "natural" or "manufactured." For example, a good review has been written on the lack of benefits of "natural" versus "synthetic" vitamins.[37] The consumer must learn to differentiate between realistic caution and hypochondriacal fear, and that the food system is in equal danger from molds as from molecules. One of the first questions to ask is, "What are the greatest concerns regarding the food supply?" In 1978 the Food and Drug Administration (FDA) published a list of the greatest dangers to consumers from the U.S. food supply, and listed in the following order of importance: (1) foodborne toxigenic and pathogenic microorganisms, (2) malnutrition (diseases of under- and overnutrition), (3) environmental contaminants, (4) toxic natural constituents of food, (5) pesticide residues and (6) food additives.[30]

Table 17–13. HISTORY OF LAWS AND RULES REGULATING FOOD SAFETY AND QUALITY IN THE U.S.

NAME OF ACT AND DATE PASSED	CONTENT OF LEGISLATION
Wiley Act or "pure food and drug law." Passed 1906. The act itself was repealed 1938, but not some of amendments.	"An act for preventing the manufacture, sale or transportation of adulterated or misbranded or poisonous or deleterious foods, drugs, medicines and liquors, and for other purposes."
Meat Inspection Act, passed 1907.	Requires that "all meat and meat food products in interstate commerce be prepared under the supervision of the USDA."
Weight and Measure Amendment to Wiley Act, passed 1913.	Clarifies rules about stating the quantity of the contents of packaged foods.
Kenyon Amendment to Wiley Act, passed 1919.	Extends the weight and measure amendment to cover packaged meats.
McNary-Napes Amendment to Wiley Act, passed 1930.	Authorizes the USDA to establish minimum standards for the quality, condition and amounts of foods in containers, to be required of all canned foods except meat and milk.
Seafood Inspection Amendment to the Wiley Act, passed 1935.	Authorizes the USDA "to provide government inspection of the packaging of any seafood which might enter into interstate commerce" for those packers desiring such inspection service.
Food, Drug and Cosmetic Act, passed 1938.	Authorizes the Food and Drug Administration (FDA) to carry out the intent of Congress to ensure that foods are safe, pure, and wholesome; are made or processed under sanitary conditions; and are honestly labeled and packaged. To carry on research and public education. To set food standard regulations governing the definitions and standards of identity of foods, containers and labeling, to promote honesty and fair dealing in the interest of the consumer. Standards of identity to be obtained from the FDA free of charge. Minimum standards of quality were set for tenderness, color and freedom from defects. Standards for enrichment were set. Products labeled "enriched" or "fortified" must contain the exact specified amount of added nutrients.
Miller Pesticide Amendment, passed 1954.	Etablishes acceptable or relatively harmless levels for pesticide and chemical residues on raw agricultural commodities. The applicant must demonstrate the "usefulness" of a pesticide to the USDA's satisfaction and its "safety" to the FDA before its use.
Poultry Products Inspection Act, passed 1956.	Makes continuous inspection compulsory for fresh, frozen, ready-to-eat and canned poultry products. Labeling regulations were established for poultry products and enforcement powers were given to the USDA.
Food Additives Amendment to the Food, Drug and Cosmetic Act, passed 1958.	Requires that the safety of chemicals used in processing be proved by industry to be safe before being sold for use in foods. Previously the government was responsible for proving a chemical unsafe *after* it was on the market, often requiring court action for removal. Chemicals in use prior to 1959 were considered Generally Recognized as Safe (GRAS) and use was allowed to continue.
Delaney Clause to the Food, Drug and Cosmetic Act, passed 1958.	Requires that a food additive must be tested for safety on animals by the manufacturer or promoter and the results submitted to the FDA. If a food additive is found to produce cancer when ingested, in any amount by test animals of any species, the use of the additive is prohibited.
Color Additive Amendment to the Food, Drug and Cosmetic Act, passed 1960.	Requires manufacturers to prove that their color additives are safe, and authorizes the FDA to establish and enforce tolerances for the use of color additives in foods, drugs and cosmetics.
Fair Packaging and Labeling Act, passed 1967.	Requires prominent labels on packaged foods and the following information: (1) Statement of the food's identity must appear on the principal display panel in bold type. (2) Name and address of manufacturer, packer and distributor must be conspicuously stated. (3) Statement of the net contents must appear in concise standard measure. No qualifying terms such as "giant quart" may appear. (4) Statement listing ingredients, when required, must appear in type of legible size on a single panel of the label. The common names of the ingredients must appear in decreasing order of predominance. These regulations include proposals for special diet foods, with particular reference to vitamin and mineral supplementation and low-calorie foods.

FOOD-BORNE TOXIGENIC AND PATHOGENIC MICROORGANISMS

Over the past 20 years the few hundred food-borne outbreaks that have occurred in the U.S. have involved primarily pathogenic or toxigenic bacteria. Table 17–14 represents the typical distribution of cases in an outbreak. The vast majority of the food-borne outbreaks can be traced to poor sanitation practices in the home or food service establishments. Very few are attributable to commercial processing practices. Even honey, which is touted to be "organic" and "natural," can be highly toxic to infants under one year of age. The deadly bacterium *Clostridium botulinum* has been found to grow in honey, producing a type B toxin that has resulted in 43 documented cases of infant botulism in California since 1976.[7]

MALNUTRITION

Aspects of undernutrition are mentioned in Chapter 4, and overnutrition is discussed in Chapter 27 in detail. Malnutrition is discussed in this chapter as it pertains to food safety and consumer protection laws.

The consumer in 1980 is faced with over 10,000 food products, half of which did not exist 10 years ago. From this vast array of foods consumers are expected to make the proper food selections to meet their nutritional needs. To assist the consumer in making the correct food choices, informative labeling laws as discussed in Chapter 10 as well as consumer education programs are needed.

Enriched, Restored and Fortified Foods

The words *enriched, retored* and *fortified* are frequently confused. *Enriched* applies to flour, bread, degerminated corn meal and corn grits, for which standards have been established. Iron, niacin and thiamin are returned in about the same amounts as are lost in the milling of white flour from whole grain, while riboflavin is added in larger amounts than found in whole wheat. Calcium and vitamin D may also be added.

In *restored* foods the manufacturer may voluntarily replace the nutrients lost in the processing.

In *fortified* foods, the manufacturer adds nutrients not present in the food originally. For example, margarine is fortified with vitamin A and milk with vitamin D.

Definite limits had to be set for the addition of nutrients to food products in order to protect the public from combinations that are irritating or even harmful.

The 1953 joint report of the Food and Nutrition Board and the American Medical Association Council on Food and Nutrition approved the enrichment of flour, bread, degerminated corn meal and corn grits with thiamin, riboflavin and niacin.[2, 53] It also approved the nutritive improvement of whole grain corn meal and white rice, the retention or restoration of thiamin, niacin and iron in processed food cereals and the addition of vitamin D to milk (400 I.U. per qt.), vitamin A to margarine (15,000 I.U. per lb.), to bring it up to the average vitamin A content of butter, and iodine to table salt (1 part sodium or potassium iodide to 5000 parts salt). A well-controlled enrichment or fortification program can be an effective and inexpensive method of improving the intake of certain nutrients by a population.

ENVIRONMENTAL CONTAMINANTS

Safeguarding against environmental contaminants will become increasingly important as more solvents and byproducts of chemical reactions enter the food supply through increased processing and new packaging methods. Already it is evident that the mechanical deboning of meat (beef in particular) increases the amount of lead as well as calcium in the product. This happens as the process results in bone being pulverized and incorporated into the final product. Further discussion of lead can be found on page 798. Table 17–15 shows the chemical contaminants of concern in the U.S. for the last 10 years and probably for the next decade as well. An effective nutrition educator will need to stay current on issues such as these to ascertain

Table 17–14. CONFIRMED FOOD-BORNE DISEASES IN THE UNITED STATES IN 1978

MICROBIAL AGENTS	OUTBREAKS	CASES
Clostridium botulinum	12	58
Clostridium perfringens	9	617
Bacillus cereus	6	248
Salmonella spp.	45	1921
Shigella spp.	4	159
Staphylococcus aureus	23	1318
Vibrio parahaemolyticus	2	86
Other bacteria	4	59
Hepatitis A (virus)	5	300
Trichinella spiralis (parasite)	7	35
CHEMICAL AGENTS		
Naturally occurring seafood toxins	30	96
Toxic mushroom	1	7
Heavy metal	1	41
Other chemicals	5	19
Total	154	4964

From Foster, E.M.: How safe are our foods? Nutr. Rev., *40* (Suppl.):28, 1982.

Table 17–15. CHEMICAL CONTAMINANTS OF CONCERN IN FOODS, U.S., 1970–80

HEAVY METALS

1. Lead
2. Mercury
3. Cadmium
4. Selenium
5. Arsenic

HALOGENATED COMPOUNDS

6. Chlorine
7. Iodine
8. Vinyl chloride
9. Ethylene dichloride
10. Trichloroethylene
11. Polychlorinated biphenyls
12. Polybrominated biphenyls

OTHERS

13. Asbestos
14. Dioxins
15. Acrylonitrile
16. Lysinoalanine
17. Diethylstilbestrol
18. Heat induced mutagens
19. Antibiotics (in animal feed)

From Foster, E.M.: How safe are our foods? Nutr. Rev., *40* (Suppl.):28, 1982.

whether or not they pose a health problem for the public. Also, one must stay aware in order to be able to have an impact on the political process, answer questions by the consumer and alleviate fears if it is reasonable to do so.

TOXIC NATURAL CONSTITUENTS OF FOOD

Humans have learned through trial and error which foods contain naturally occurring toxicants. It did not take a lot of scientific knowledge for primitive humans to learn that eating a particular plant was unhealthy if a fellow tribal member died soon after eating it. In today's modern society loss of familiarity with wild foods has resulted in deadly problems, as in the case of persons in Arizona and Washington who mistakenly consumed foxglove instead of the expected herbal tea, comfrey.[8] Six other persons in New York and Pennsylvania were luckier in that the purchased herbal tea contained a "natural" cathartic that produced only severe diarrhea.[6]

Consumers must recognize that a toxin can produce death or disease whether it is found naturally in the food or is added to the food. In fact, some of the most potent carcinogens are naturally occurring.[36] Some foods naturally contain toxicants that would never be permitted by the FDA if they were potential food additives. *Safrole,* a "natural" flavoring agent found primarily in sassafras root, is not allowed as a food additive because research has found it to be

linked to liver cancer. But safrole is present in small amounts in a number of spices normally consumed, so it is impossible to avoid some contact with it.[40] Potatoes are another example. The potato contains *oxalic acid* (interferes with bodily absorption of calcium), *tannin* (poisonous and possibly cancer-producing), *nitrates* (can cause severe gastroenteritis), *solanine* (chemically related to nerve gas, and interferes with the transmission of nerve impulses) and *arsenic.*[40]

Certain molds are potent carcinogens. *Aflatoxins,* which grow on peanuts and have been found to cause cancer in rats, are an example.[50] Yet some people will consume molds when found on foods because they are natural and therefore perceived as good. Another very natural fungus that grows on poorly stored grain can cause a disease once known as St. Anthony's fire after a martyred saint who died by flame. This disease, now called ergotism, caused the hands and feet to turn charcoal black and eventually wither away.[40] This painful terminal disease was due to a naturally occurring substance. Table 17–16 lists some naturally occurring toxicants of concern.

It should not be assumed that merely citing these examples and other scientific facts will be enough to alter many people's deeply held beliefs that "natural is good." Food is something everyone is familiar with, so it should not be a surprise that some people regard "natural foods" as the answer to a myriad of real or imagined illnesses. Those diagnosed as having incurable illnesses are especially likely to turn to nutritional quackery or other alternatives that purport to offer hope.[4] Adherence to scientific principles is not of concern to the charlatan who peddles quackery for profit. Community health educators must be knowledgeable as to why people fall prey to quackery. One must be able to guide consumers toward information that will provide them with answers based on valid research in a way that they can comprehend.

PESTICIDE RESIDUES

Pesticides have played an important role in agriculture's phenomenal success and are expected to continue to be the chief deterrent against pests that menace food production. A disadvantage in their use is their poisonous nature, which gives rise to harmful residues. The effects of pesticides on other organisms in the environment and the amounts of residues on agricultural produce have been the subject of much debate and controversy. The current system for regulating residues on food is based on the "tolerance principle," which assumes that, while all pesticide chemicals can be poisonous

Table 17–16. COMPOUNDS OF TOXIC CAPABILITY FOUND IN NATURALLY OCCURRING SUBSTANCES

TOXIN	FOOD SOURCE	PRIMARY TOXIC EFFECT
Hemagglutinins	Several varieties of beans	Agglutination of red blood cells
Goitrogens[a]	Cabbage, kale, broccoli, other brassicae	Hypothyroidism (goiter)
Hydrogen cyanide[a]	Kernels of stone fruits, several varieties of beans, cassava	Cyanide poisoning
Pressor amines	Bananas, pineapple, aged cheeses, wine, chocolate	Increased blood pressure
Oxalates	Spinach, rhubarb, many others	Corrosive gastroenteritis, shock, death
Myristicin	Nutmeg, parsley, carrots	Hallucinations
Falcaranol	Carrots	Neurotoxicity
Aspergillus flavus (aflatoxin)	Corn, figs, grain, sorghum, cotton seed, certain tree nuts, peanuts	Liver carcinogen
Solanine	Skin of green potatoes, sprouts on "eyes" of potatoes	Interferes with transmission of nerve impulses
Ochratoxin	Barley, corn	Nephrotoxicity

[a]Not present in plants, but formed enzymatically from nontoxic precursors during processing or ingestion.

Sources: Rodricks, J.: Food hazards of natural origin. Fed. Proc. *37*:2587, 1978; Larkin, T.: Natural poisons in food. FDA Consumer. HEW Publ. No. (FDA) 76–2009, 1975.

at high levels, there are low levels at which injury does not occur.

The Food and Drug Administration sampled market baskets for residues of 20 chlorinated hydrocarbons, including DDT, and for organic phosphate–type insecticides. Most of the samples were reported to contain no residues or mere traces of chlorinated hydrocarbons; a few contained amounts measurable by extremely sensitive techniques; and only a few traces of organic phosphate residues were found. However, because of its lasting effects on the environment, DDT was banned in 1972 and can now be used only in very limited ways. The acceptable daily intakes of pesticide residues were established by the World Health Organization and the Food and Agricultural Organization of the United Nations and were revised in 1971.[49]

The system currently employed in regulating the agricultural use of pesticides focuses primarily on the problem of residues on agricultural products. It is well recognized that traces of pesticides retained on fruits, vegetables and forage material may be ingested either directly by humans or by animals that are in turn consumed by humans.

Pesticide residues left on foods as well as other aspects of conventional production (e.g., soil erosion and sedimentation, water pollution from runoff of fertilizers and pesticides) are a concern to a growing number of consumers. Some individuals and groups have blossomed this concern into the "organic" farming movement. To the majority of scientists and agriculturalists the use of the word organic to define a method of farming is inappropriate since organic only means the presence of carbon in a molecule. All food is organic since it all comes from plant and animal sources, which all contain carbon. To others *organic farming* is "a production system which avoids or largely excludes the use of synthetically compounded fertilizers, pesticides, growth regulators, and livestock feed additives. To the maximum extent feasible, organic farming systems rely upon crop rotations, crop residues, animal manures, legumes, green manures, off-farm organic wastes, mechanical cultivation, mineral bearing rocks, and aspects of biological pest control to maintain soil productivity and tilth, to supply plant nutrients, and to control insects, weeds, and other pests." One must be careful to differentiate between organic farmers and gardeners, just as is done with conventional growers, otherwise one will fall prey to the belief that organic farmers want to regress to agriculture as practiced in the 1930's. This is not true, since modern organic farmers use up-to-date machinery and methods.

The public connotation of organic involves the concept of soil as a living system and that food grown should be free of chemicals, pesticides and preservatives and not be overly processed. The problem is that only one Federal agency and three states define the term organic. There are no assurances in the vast number of cases that when one purchases "organically grown food" that it is indeed free of pesticide residues.

The concern community health educators should have regarding the use of organic foods is not with the process or the public's desire for locally grown, pesticide- and chemical-free food-stuffs, but with the lack of consistent legal definitions to protect the consumer. There are always opportunists present to take advantage of the consumer, and it is up to nutritionists to inform the purchasers of the lack of protection from fraudulently labeled products.

As of 1980 three states (Oregon, Maine and California) and the Federal Trade Commission (FTC) have developed legal definitions of organic agriculture. If a food is to be called "naturally grown," "wild," "ecologically grown," "biologically grown," "organically grown" or "organic" it must meet the following requirements:

1. It must be produced, harvested, distributed, stored, processed and packaged without application of synthetically compounded fertilizers, pesticides or growth regulators.

2. The area or field where perennial crops are to be grown must have been free from synthetically compounded fertilizers, pesticides or growth regulators for 12 months prior to planting and during the growing period.

3. Pesticide residues must not exceed 10 per cent of the level regarded as safe by the FDA.

4. Strict and clear labeling requirements must be met.[52]

It is the above information that must be transmitted to consumers to assist them in making an informed choice. It is not up to the nutrition educator to judge for the consumer by what method foods should be grown for consumption, particularly as eating organic foods is part of a belief system usually not open to scientific discussion.

FOOD ADDITIVES

While food additives receive the most publicity by the news media, they were viewed as the least hazardous issue by the FDA. Perhaps the public is so concerned about food additives because, of the six hazards listed by the FDA, they are the easiest to control through regulation. On the other hand toxins, bacteria, molds and insects will contaminate foodstuffs regardless of any law.

The Food Additives Amendment (Table 17–14) defines a *food additive* as:

. . . any substance the intended use of which results or may reasonably be expected to result, directly or indirectly, in its becoming a component or otherwise affecting the characteristics of any food (including any substance intended for use in producing, manufacturing, packing, processing, preparing, treating, packaging, transporting, or holding food; and including any source of radiation intended for such use . . .[13]

Simply put, a food additive is any substance that becomes part of a food product when added directly or indirectly to a food. In 1979 approximately 2800 substances were added to foods to produce a desired effect.[26] Perhaps if consumers were more familiar with the names, functions and uses of food additives (Table 17–17), they would not be so fearful of them. Perhaps if consumers knew whether or not food additives were used appropriately (Table 17–18), they would be more accepting of their use.[42] And perhaps if the consumer had a better understanding of how the government regulates the food industry, some measure of trust could be regained.[54]

In the U.S., regulations regarding food additives became more restrictive with the passage of the *1958 Food Additives Amendment*. Since 1958, if a petition for use is presented to the FDA then the petitioner must present evidence of the usefulness and harmlessness of the ingredients proposed to be used. Additives that were in use prior to passage of the amendment were "grandfathered" in by the amendment. In other words those particular substances were safe, based on the data available at the time, and were termed *"Generally Recognized as Safe"* *(GRAS)*. The FDA could not require a demonstration of safety for the continued use of the ingredients unless the FDA could demonstrate them to be unsafe. Then the FDA could remove them from use.[34]

The Food Additives Amendment requires exhaustive studies of proposed new additives while allowing continued use of the GRAS substances with little or no specific examination. The FDA initiated actions to alleviate this discrepancy by contracting with the Federation of American Societies for Experimental Biology (FASEB) to form a Select Committee to review the GRAS list.[51] By 1979 (the committee was formed in 1972) the FASEB Select Committee on GRAS Substances had 351 final or tentative evaluation reports of GRAS Substances. A majority (71 per cent) were found to be without hazard when used in food at current levels and at the future expected level of use; 15 per cent were found to be without hazard if use is limited to current levels of addition with no expected increase of use; 6 per cent were found to be without hazard when used in food at current levels, but due to uncertainties in the existing date, specific studies need to be conducted in the very near future; 4 per cent were found to exhibit adverse effects when used in food at the current level requiring safer usage conditions; and the final 4 per cent could not be evaluated owing to lack of available data.[34]

An example of a GRAS substance reviewed by the FASEB Committee on GRAS is caffeine. Caffeine was allowed for use as an additive in certain foods, and in cola-type beverages and as such was placed on the GRAS list. At its current level of use caffeine was found not to be

Table 17–17. FUNCTIONS AND USES OF COMMON FOOD ADDITIVES

FUNCTIONS	ADDITIVES USED	EXAMPLES OF FOODS IN WHICH ADDITIVES ARE USED
To improve nutritional value of certain foods.	Thiamin, riboflavin, niacin, iron, vitamin A, vitamin D, ascorbic acid, potassium iodide.	Wheat, flour, bread, rolls, biscuits, breakfast cereals, macaroni and noodle products, cornmeal, margarine, milk, iodized salt.
To maintain appearance, palatability and wholesomeness in certain foods (delaying undesirable changes in food caused by oxidation or microbial growth; preventing food spoilage caused by molds, bacteria, yeast).	Propionic acid, calcium and sodium salts of propionic acid, ascorbic acid, butylated hydroxyanisole (BHA), butylated hydroxytoluene (BHT), propylene glycol.	Bread, pie filling, cake mixes, potato chips, crackers, cheese, syrup, fruit juices, frozen and dried fruits, margarine, shortenings, lard.
To enhance flavor of certain foods.	Spices (cloves, ginger, cinnamon, etc.), citrus oils, amyl acetate, carvone, benzaldehyde, monosodium glutamate, vanilla.	Spice cake, gingerbread, ice cream, candy, carbonated beverages, fruit-flavored gelatins, toppings, sausage.
To give characteristic color to certain foods.	Annatto, carotene, cochineal, chlorophyll.	Baking goods, candy, carbonated beverages, cheese, margarine, ice cream, jams, jellies, oranges.
To maintain desired consistency in foods (emulsifiers and stabilizers).	Lecithin, mono- and diglycerides, gum arabic, carboxymethyl cellulose, carrageenan.	Bakery products, cake mixes, salad dressings, frozen desserts, ice cream, chocolate milk, candy, beer.
To control acidity or alkalinity in certain foods (leavening and neutralizing agents).	Potassium acid tartrate, tartaric acid, sodium bicarbonate, lactic acid, citric acid, adipic acid, fumaric acid.	Cakes, cookies, biscuits, crackers, waffles, muffins, butter, process cheese, cheese spreads, chocolates, carbonated beverages, confectionery.
To serve as maturing and bleaching agents.	Chlorine dioxide, chlorine, potassium bromate and iodate.	Wheat flour (to make it white), certain cheeses.
To help retain moisture (humectants), prevent caking or act as curing agents.	Glycerin, magnesium carbonate, sodium nitrate, calcium phosphate.	Coconut, marshmallows, table salt, garlic and onion powder, frankfurters, sausages, dietetic foods.

Adapted from: Food Additives—Every Day Facts. Manufacturing Chemists Association, 1825 Connecticut Ave. N.W., Washington, D.C., 20009.

hazardous, but uncertainties in the data led the FASEB committee to recommend caffeine's removal from the GRAS list. The primary reason for this seemingly contradictory recommendation was concern for children, especially very young children (one to five years) who are among the highest consumers of cola-type beverages. The uncertainties regarding the effect of chronic exposure to caffeine, during the period of brain growth and development, via cola-type beverages were sufficient that caffeine's removal from the list was recommended.[15]

Caffeine as a constituent of coffee, tea and chocolate was not reviewed by the FASEB committee, as the FDA cannot regulate naturally occurring caffeine under the food additive provisions of the law.[15] While this may seem capricious, remember that government regulatory agencies have the responsibility only to enforce the laws as Congress passes them.

In recent years the FDA has come under violent attack for enforcing the *Delaney Clause*, which is only one of the statements in the Food Additives Amendment to the Federal Food, Drug, and Cosmetic Act. The Delaney Clause states: "No additive shall be deemed to be safe if it is found to induce cancer when ingested by man or animal, or if it is found, after tests which are appropriate for the evaluation of the safety of food additives, to induce cancer in man or animal." It is the Delaney Clause that required the FDA to ban saccharin, nitrites and nitrates. The FDA did not decide on whether or

Table 17–18. APPROPRIATE AND INAPPROPRIATE USES OF FOOD ADDITIVES*

INAPPROPRIATE USES

1. To disguise faulty or inferior processes.
2. To conceal damaged, spoiled or inferior goods.
3. To deceive customers.
4. To gain some functional property at the expense of nutritional quality.
5. To substitute for economical, well-recognized good manufacturing processes and practices.
6. To use in amounts in excess of the minimum required to achieve the intended effect(s).

APPROPRIATE USES

1. To improve or maintain nutritional value.
2. To enhance quality.
3. To reduce waste.
4. To enhance consumer acceptance.
5. To improve keeping quality.
6. To make the food more readily available.
7. To facilitate food preparation.

From: Packard, V. S.: Processed Foods and the Consumer: Additives, Labeling, Standards and Nutrition. Minneapolis, University of Minnesota Press, 1976, p. 58.

* As compiled by the Food Protection Committee, National Academy of Sciences, 1970.

not the use of these additives was good or bad; the FDA only enforced the law as written. In the case of nitrites and nitrates the food industry lobbied Congress to exempt these two additives from the Delaney Clause. Consumers as well as industry decried the FDA's banning of saccharin as the banning of a "necessary" product. Congress responded to its constituency and allowed the continued use of saccharin.

Criticisms of the Delaney Clause abound, the most valid point being that only "food additives" as defined by the law that are found to be carcinogenic must be removed from the food supply.[36] The Delaney Clause does not in any way speak to the issue of naturally occurring carcinogens such as aflatoxin. At times it is found in amounts similar to those that produce cancer in rats. Another major problem with the Delaney Clause is that it is outdated, as scientific knowledge is far in advance of what it was in 1958.[26, 29] In 1958 scientists lacked the technology to assess adequately the risk presented by a particular chemical, whereas today chemicals can be identified and quantified at levels of one part per billion.[13] Currently the FDA is attempting to formulate new approaches to regulating the use of additives that more clearly reflect present knowledge.

The FDA has been monitoring the availability of foodstuffs for the consumer in the U.S. since the early 1900's and has done a very adequate job. Still the U.S. government must do more for the consumer than just monitor the availability of safe foods. The government must also insure that consumers can make informed choices.[56] Since food choices are influenced by attitudes and advertising as well as availability, the government must also regulate advertising, which shapes attitudes towards food.

Regulating Food Advertising

Within the federal government two agencies have the responsibility for regulating broadcast advertising, the Federal Trade Commission (FTC) and the Federal Communications Commission (FCC).

The FCC was given authority by the 1934 Communications Act to regulate advertising consistent with the public interest, convenience and necessity. The FTC was empowered in 1938 to protect the consumer as well as private competition by prohibiting false advertising and preventing unfair or deceptive acts or practices. In other words, the FCC regulates the amount and scheduling of advertising, while the FTC has jurisdiction over the content of the message.

Unlike the FDA, the FCC and FTC have allowed industry to regulate itself. This has led to the formation of the Children's Television Advertising Guidelines of the National Association of Broadcasters (NAB). Also, the Council of Better Business Bureaus monitors advertisements and acts on complaints by the public via their National Advertising Division (NAD). These voluntary guidelines are fairly permissive and really only restrict actual deceptive practices. Members of the public displeased with this lack of control by the government have formed consumer-interest groups such as the Action for Children's Television (ACT) and the Council on Children, Media and Merchandising (CCMM). These consumer-interest groups with concern for advertising, particularly as it pertains to children, file petitions with the regulatory commissions and the courts to force government action. Further discussion of the influence of the media on children's eating habits can be found in Chapter 13.

Consumers cannot expect a manufacturer to provide all the information regarding a product, particularly if some of the information is of a negative nature. The consumer who relies on advertising as the sole source of information will not be making informed choices. Marketing techniques used by advertising agencies on behalf of their clients have only one purpose—to sell a product. And that is fair, as long as the consumer is aware of that fact. Nutrition educators must communicate this point and inform consumers that it is their responsibility to become knowledgeable about the products and services they purchase. The government also must take some responsibility to protect the public from false and misleading advertising, but ultimately it is the individual who must make the decision.

Role of Community Health Educators

It is important to recognize that within everyone lies a dreamer who is willing to accept the impossible, to hope when all hope is gone. It is this very human part that makes all of us susceptible to those who would promise what is not realistically obtainable. The community nutrition educator's responsibility is to help others judge the facts, not to make judgments for them, and to educate people to recognize the difference between the promises and the reality. There are some questions that consumers need to ask of an expert or a product before they accept or purchase the idea or product. They are given in Table 17–19.

This is the type of rational questioning consumers must learn to ask if they are to sur-

Table 17–19. QUESTIONS TO CONSUMERS

1. Is the consumer being influenced to purchase something he or she would not ordinarily buy?
2. Are the credentials of the individual, company, etc. of a valid nature? How long has the product been on the market? Is the "expert" from a bona fide organization or university?
3. Does the product or individual purport to cure all the evils of humankind? Are statements made leading the consumer to believe that all diseases are due to a faulty diet?
4. Is the consumer led to believe that health can only be obtained through use of this particular product or via the wisdom of only this one individual?
5. Are promises of cures or long life or youth or a more active sex life made?
6. Does the product or individual use "case histories" or "taste tests" to stress the benefits of the product or idea?

vive in the complex world of today. It is the job of community nutrition educators to help the consumer differentiate between fact and fiction. To study the science of nutrition and to communicate these facts effectively to the consumer is indeed an art, the art of being an effective nutrition educator.

Problems and Suggested Topics for Discussion

1. Obtain and read the Final Report of the White House Conference on Food, Nutrition, and Health 1969. How many of the recommendations of Section 1 (Surveillance and Evaluation) and Section 4 (Nutrition Teaching and Education) have been met? By what agencies? By what programs?
2. Discuss the problems with comparing food consumption survey data (i.e., NFCS and disappearance data) from one decade to another? What are the problems with comparing these data with the RDA?
3. Review and discuss the new thrifty food plans designed by the USDA. Put together a menu meeting the monetary constraints of one on food stamps. Follow that diet for a week. Discuss the practicality of living on a food stamp budget.
4. Using Table 17–11, select a dietary guideline and research the original document. Set up panels to defend the assigned guidelines.
5. Contact one of your state legislators from each party to speak to your class on the legislative process. What are their stands on nutrition? How could you as a health professional influence them?
6. Discuss the purpose of and the legislation pertaining to food additives. List seven classes of food additives and give an example of each. Read the labels on ten canned or packaged foods and list the additives in each. What purpose does each of the listed additives serve?
7. From your local library obtain a copy of Federal Register Vol. 45, No. 20, Tuesday, January 29, 1980. Rules and legulations on "National School Lunch Program and School Breakfast Program: Competitive Foods." 7 CFR, Parts 210 and 220. Read this report with particular attention to page 6759, Section B, which discusses comments on the proposed rule regarding the sale of "junk food" in the schools. What is the importance of community nutritionists impact on the regulatory system? Can they have an impact?

Cited References

1. American Dietetic Association: Position paper on a national nutrition policy. J. Am. Diet. Assoc., *76*:596, 1980.
2. American Medical Association, Council on Foods and Nutrition: A statement of general policy concerning the addition of specific nutrients to foods. JAMA, *154*:145, 1954.
3. Beers, W.: The food industry and nutrition: challenge—responsibilities. Nutr. Rev., *40* (Suppl.):7, 1982.
4. Bruch, H.: The allure of food cults and nutrition quackery. Nutr. Rev., *32* (Suppl.):62, 1974.
5. Center for Disease Control: Ten-State Nutrition Survey, 1968–70. DHEW Publ. No. (HSM) 72–8130–34. Washington, D.C., U.S. Department of Health, Education and Welfare, 1972.
6. Center for Disease Control: Diarrhea from herbal tea. Morbidity and Mortality Weekly Report, *27*(29):248, 1978.
7. Center for Disease Control: Honey exposure and infant botulism. Morbidity and Mortality Weekly Report, *27*(29):249, 1978.
8. Center for Disease Control: Poisoning associated with herbal teas. Morbidity and Mortality Weekly Report, *26*(32):257, 1977.
8a. Cleveland, L. E., and Peterkin, B. B.: USDA 1983 Family Food Plans, Family Economics Review, No. 2, pp. 12–20, 1983.
9. Clydesdale, F.: Food Science and Nutrition: Current Issues and Answers. Englewood Cliffs, N.J., Prentice-Hall, 1979.
10. Code of Federal Regulations: Apportionment of funds for nutrition education and training. Final rule. 7 CFR, Part 227, 1979.
11. Code of Federal Regulations: Child care food program. Final rule. 7 CFR, Part 226, 1982.
12. Code of Federal Regulations: Nutrition education and training. 7 CFR, Part 227, 1979.
13. Code of Federal Regulations: Policy for regulating carcinogenic chemicals in food and color additives: advance notice of proposed rule making. 21 CFR, Chapter 1, 1982.
14. Code of Federal Regulations: Special supplemental food program for women, infants, and children. Final regulations. 7 CFR, Part 246, 1979.
15. Code of Federal Regulations: Soda water: standard of identity and caffeine deletion of GRAS status, proposed declaration that no prior sanction exists, and use on interim basis pending additional study, proposed regulations. 21 CFR, Part 165, 1980.
16. Coltrin, D.M., and Bradfield, R.B.: Food buying practices of urban low-income consumers. A review. J. Nutr. Educ., *1*:16, 1970.
17. Community Nutrition Institute: Food spending remains high for working poor. CNI Weekly Report, *7*(19):8, 1977.
18. Community Nutrition Institute: USDA ponders new food plans. Dietary guidelines review. CNI Weekly Report, *12*(48):4, 1982.
19. Congressional Budget Office: Feeding Children: Federal Child Nutrition Policies in the 1980's. Washington, D.C., U.S. Government Printing Office, 1978.
20. Consumer and Food Economics Institute: The Thrifty Food Plan. Hyattsville, Md., U.S. Department of Agriculture, Agricultural Research Service, 1975.
21. Economics and Statistics Cooperative Services: Structure Issues of American Agriculture. Agricultural Economics Report, No. 438. Washington, D.C., U.S. Department of Agriculture, 1979.
22. Economics and Statistics Service: Agricultural–food policy review: Perspectives for the 1980's. AFPR–4. Washington, D.C., U.S. Department of Agriculture, 1981.

23. Economics and Statistics Service: Impact of Household Size and Income on Food Spending Patterns. Tech. Bulletin No. 1650. Washington, D.C., U.S. Department of Agriculture, 1981.

24. Federal Register: What It Is and How to Use It. Publ. No. 022–003–00953–1. Washington, D.C., U.S. Government Printing Office, 1978.

25. Fincher, L.J., and Rauschert, M.E.: Diets of men, women and children in the United States. Nutrition Program News, Sept.-Oct., 1969.

26. Food and Drug Administration: More than You Ever Thought You Would Know About Food Additives. FDA Consumer. HEW Publ. No. (FDA) 79–2115. Washington, D.C., U.S. Government Printing Office, 1979.

27. Food and Nutrition Board, National Research Council: Toward Healthful Diets. Washington, D.C., National Academy of Sciences, 1980.

28. Food Research Action Committee: If We Had Ham, You Could Have Ham and Eggs . . . If We Had Eggs. A Study of the National School Breakfast Program. Washington, D.C., Food Research Action Committee, 1972.

29. Foster, E.M.: Food safety: problems of the past and perspectives of the future. Journal of Food Protection, 45:658, 1982.

30. Foster, E.M.: How safe are our foods? Nutr. Rev., 40 (Suppl.):28, 1982.

31. Harper, A.E.: Dietary goals—a skeptical view. Am. J. Clin. Nutr., 31:310, 1978.

32. Heyn, D.: The nutrition free-for-all, the facts behind the headlines. Family Health, Jan., 1980.

33. Highlights Fall 1978, Family Economics Review. Consumer Food Economics Institute. U.S. Department of Agriculture, Science and Education Administration, ARS–NE–36, 1978.

34. Irving, G.W.: Safety evaluation of the food ingredients called GRAS. Nutr. Rev., 36:351, 1978.

35. Janssen, W.F.: The U.S. Food and Drug Law: How It Came, How It Works. HEW Publ. No. (FDA) 79–1054. Washington, D.C., U.S. Department of Health, Education and Welfare, 1979.

36. Jukes, T.H.: Carcinogens in food and the Delaney Clause. JAMA, 241:617, 1979.

37. Kamil, A.: Commentary on how natural are those "natural" vitamins? J. Nutr. Educ., 4:92, 1972.

38. Kerr, G.R., et al.: Relationships between dietary and biochemical measures of nutritional status in HANES I data. Am. J. Clin. Nutr., 35:294, 1982.

39. Labuza, T.: The Nutrition Crisis: A Reader. San Francisco, West Publishing Company, 1975.

40. Larkin, T.: Natural Poisons in Food. FDA Consumer. HEW Publ. No. (FDA) 76–2009, 1975.

41. McNutt, K.: Dietary advice to the public: 1957–1980. Nutr. Rev., 38:353, 1980.

42. National Advisory Committee on Hyperkinesis and Food Additives: Final Report to the Nutrition Foundation. Washington, D.C., Nutrition Foundation, 1980.

43. National Center for Health Statistics: Health and Nutrition Examination Survey, 1971–74. Rockville, Md., Health Resources Administration, Public Health Service, 1977. Vital and Health Statistics; Series II; No. 202 (DHEW Publ. No. (HRA) 77–1647).

44. National Center for Health Statistics: Hispanic HANES Fact Sheet. Department of Health and Human Services, Public Health Service, 1981.

45. Nationwide Food Consumption Survey 1977–78: Preliminary Report No. 2, Food and Nutrient Intakes of Individuals in 1 Day in the U.S., Spring, 1977. Washington, D.C., U.S. Department of Agriculture, Science and Education Administration, 1980.

46. Nationwide Food Consumption Survey 1977–1978: Need for Improvement and Expansion. Report to the Select Committee on Nutrition and Human Needs by the Comptroller General of the U.S., CED 77–56, 1977.

47. Nutrition and Your Health. Dietary Guidelines for Americans. Home and Garden Bulletin No. 232. Washington, D.C., U.S. Department of Agriculture, U.S. Department of Health and Human Services, 1980.

48. Owen, G.M., et al.: A study of nutritional status of preschool children in the United States, 1968–70. Pediatrics, 53:597, 1974.

49. Pesticide Residues in Food. Report of the 1971 Joint FAO/WHO Meeting. WHO Technical Report No. 502. Geneva, World Health Organization, 1972.

50. Rodricks, J.: Food hazards of natural origin. Fed. Proc., 37:2587, 1978.

51. Siu, R.G.H., et al.: Evaluation of health aspects of GRAS food ingredients: lessons learned—questions unanswered. Fed. Proc., 36:2527, 1977.

52. Study Team on Organic Farming: Report and Recommendations on Organic Farming. Washington, D.C., U.S. Department of Agriculture, 1980.

53. The Addition of Specific Nutrients to Foods. Public Health Report No. 69, March, 1954, p. 275.

54. U.S. Senate. Hearings before the Subcommittee on Nutrition of the Committee on Agriculture, Nutrition and Forestry. Nutrition Labeling and Information, Part I. 95th Congress, August 9–10, 1978. Publ. No. 33–261–0. Washington, D.C., U.S. Government Printing Office, 1978.

55. U.S. Senate. Hearings before the Select Committee on Nutrition and Human Needs. Toward a National Nutrition Policy. 94th Congress. Washington, D.C., U.S. Government Printing Office, 1975.

56. What Foods Should Americans Eat? Better Information Needed on Nutritional Quality of Foods. Report to the Congress of the U.S. by the Comptroller General, General Accounting Office, CED 80–68, April 30, 1980.

57. White House Conference on Food, Nutrition and Health. Final Report. Washington, D.C., U.S. Government Printing Office, 1969.

Additional References

A Time to Choose: Summary Report on the Structure of Agriculture. Washington, D.C., U.S. Government Printing Office, 1981.

American Heart Association, Nutrition Committee; Rationale of the diet-heart statement of the American Heart Association. Arteriosclerosis, 4:177, 1982.

Bender, A.: Food manufacture and nutrition. Nutr. Rev., 40 (Suppl.):24, 1982.

Bureau of Nutritional Sciences, Health Protection Branch: Recommendations for Prevention Program in Relation to Nutrition and Cardiovascular Disease. Department of National Health and Welfare, Ottawa, Canada. JAMA, 242:2335, 1979.

Center for Science in the Public Interest: Battling junk food. How to get kids behind a better diet. Nutr. Action, 5(5):8, May, 1978.

Cleveland, L. E., et al.: Recommended Dietary Allowances as standards for family food plans. J. Nutr. Educ., 15:8, 1983.

Code of Federal Regulations: National school lunch program and school breakfast program: competitive foods. 7 CFR, Part 220, 1980.

Committee on Diet, Nutrition and Cancer, National Research Council: Diet, Nutrition and Cancer. Washington, D.C., National Academy of Sciences, 1982.

Committee on Food Protection, National Research Council: Toxicants Occurring Naturally in Foods. 2nd ed. Washington, D.C., National Academy of Sciences, 1973.

Dwyer, J.: Challenge of change—nutrition and policy. J. Nutr. Educ., 9:54, 1977.

Erdman, J., Jr.: Effect of preparation and service of food on nutrient value. Food Technology, 33:39, 1979.

Evaluation of Certain Food Additives. 25th Report of the Joint FAO/WHO Expert Committee on Food Additives. WHO Tech. Rep. Services, No. 669. Geneva, World Health Organization, 1981.

Feinstein, A.R., et al.: Commentary—coffee and pancreatic cancer. The problems of etiologic science and epidemiologic case-control research. JAMA, 246:957, 1981.

Food and Drug Administration: Animal Tests and Human Needs. HEW Publ. No. (FDA) 78–1036. Washington, D.C., U.S. Government Printing Office, 1977.

Gilchrist, A.: Food Borne Disease and Food Safety. Monroe, Wisconsin, American Medical Association, 1981.

Harper, A.E.: Dietary guidelines. Food and Nutrition News, 52(4), Mar.-Apr., 1981.

Healthy People. The Surgeon General's Report on Health Promotion and Disease Prevention. Public Health Service. Washington, D.C., U.S. Government Printing Office, 1979.

Herbert, V.: Laetrile: the cult of cyanide. Promoting poison for profit. Am. J. Clin. Nutr., 32:1121, 1979.

Herbert, V.: Nutrition Cultism. Philadelphia, George F. Stickley Company, 1980.

Kelsey, F.O.: Regulatory aspects of teratology. Role of the Food and Drug Administration. Teratology, 25:193, 1982.

King, J., et al.: Evaluation and modification of the basic four food guide. J. Nutr. Educ., 10:27, 1978.

Martinsen, C.S.: The American food supply. In Worthington-Roberts, B.S.: Contemporary Developments in Nutrition. St. Louis, C.V. Mosby Company, 1981.

Molitor, G.T.: The food system in the 1980's. J. Nutr. Educ., 12(Suppl.):103, 1980.

National Cancer Institute: Everything Doesn't Cause Cancer, but How Can We Tell Which Chemicals Cause Cancer and Which Ones Don't? NIH Publ. No. 80–2039. Bethesda, Md., National Institute of Health, 1980.

National Center for Health Statistics: Dietary Intake Source Data, 1971–74, United States. DHEW Publ. No. (PHS) 79–1221. Public Health Service, 1979.

Nutrition misinformation and food faddism. Nutr. Rev., 32 (Suppl.), July, 1974.

Office of Technology Assessment: Environmental Contaminants in Food. Summary. Washington, D.C., U.S. Government Printing Office, 1979.

Perspective on food legislation, special report. Nutr. Rev., 39: 413, 1981.

Peterkin, B.: Thrifty food plan (letter). J. Nutr. Educ., 12:44, 1980.

Research on the Effects of Television Advertising on Children. Report prepared for the National Science Foundation. Stock No. 038–000–00336–4. Washington, D.C., U.S. Government Printing Office, 1976.

Research on the Effects of Television Advertising on Children. A Review of Literature and Recommendations for Future Research. NSF/RA 770115. Washington, D.C., National Science Foundation, 1977.

Rodale, R.: The Cornucopia Papers. Emmaus, Pa., Rodale Press, 1981.

Royal Norwegian Ministry of Agriculture: On Norwegian Nutrition and Food Policy. Report No. 32 to the Storting, 1975–76.

Science and Education Administration: Food I. The Hassle-Free Guide to a Better Diet. Home and Garden Bulletin No. 228. Washington, D.C., U.S. Department of Agriculture, 1980.

Strange, M., and Hassebrook, C.: Take Hogs, for Example. The Transformation of Hog Farming in America. Walt Hill, Neb., Center for Rural Affairs, 1981.

Symposium. Report of the task force on the evidence relating six dietary factors to the nation's health sponsored by the American Society for Clinical Nutrition. Am. J. Clin. Nutr., 32(Suppl.):2621, 1979.

Tewksburg, J.G.: Measuring the societal benefits of innovation. Science, 209:658, 1980.

Thrifty Food Plan. Family Economics Review. Washington, D.C., U.S. Department of Agriculture, Agricultural Research Service, Fall, 1981.

Toward healthful diets. Nutrition News, 43(3), Oct., 1980.

U.S. Senate. Hearings before the Subcommittee on Nutrition of the Committee on Agriculture, Nutrition and Forestry. Nutrition Labeling and Information, Part III. 96th Congress, Feb. 9 and 23, 1979. Publ. No. 43–652–0. Washington, D.C., U.S. Government Printing Office, 1979.

U.S. Senate. Hearings before the Subcommittee on Nutrition of the Committee on Agriculture, Nutrition and Forestry. Nutrition Labeling and Information Amendments of 1979 to the Federal Food, Drug and Cosmetic Act. 96th Congress, Feb. 20 and Mar. 19, 1980. Publ. No. 61–331–0. Washington, D.C., U.S. Government Printing Office, 1980.

U.S. Senate. Hearings before the Subcommittee on Nutrition of the Committee on Agriculture, Nutrition and Forestry. Nutrition Labeling and Information, Part IV. 96th Congress, April, 1980. Publ. No. 62–339–0. Washington, D.C., U.S. Government Printing Office, 1980.

White, P.L., and Selvey, N.: Nutrition and the new health awareness. JAMA, 247:2914, 1982.

CHAPTER 18

Nutrition Education

HOLLY A. DIEKEN, M.S., R.D.

WHAT IS NUTRITION EDUCATION?

Many people view nutrition education as the process of teaching the science of nutrition to an individual or group. However, health professionals have a much different role in educating an individual in the clinic, community or long-term health care facility. In these settings the dietitian, nutritionist or nurse serves to assist or enable individuals to incorporate changes in eating patterns and behavior into their lives.

The major focus of this type of nutrition education is not knowledge and facts, but rather the development of permanent behavioral changes. This is the art of nutrition education—breaking down a large body of knowledge into small, individualized components that are presented to a patient or client at a rate and level at which he is able to absorb and use the information. Effective education is making nutrition information digestible and usable in an everyday setting.

WHO ARE THE LEARNERS?

Learners can be anyone—children in preschool and day-care facilities, older children in schools, pregnant women in community clinics and senior citizens living independently, to name a few. In the acute and long-term health care facilities the primary focus is on the patients or residents and teaching them how to change and modify their diets in order to meet their needs. The secondary focus for nutrition education is the professional staff—the doctor, medical student, nurse, nursing student, pharmacist and other allied health professionals. They need to know how to make or interpret appropriate dietary orders for patients and perhaps do some teaching related to the importance of dietary modifications in the maintenance or restoration of health.

WHEN TO TEACH

Teaching opportunities are always present; for the health professional the greatest problem is finding the time to teach. For the inpatient, dietary modifications should be taught during a patient's entire hospitalization rather than as the patient is packing to be discharged from the hospital. Professional staff inservices and hospital rounds provide an excellent opportunity to update clinicians or present new information. In the community, classes can be taught in health clinics, or private nutrition counseling appointments can be made with individuals. In elementary schools nutrition education can be integrated into all areas of the school curriculum, and in high school it can be a part of a health or biology class.

REASONS FOR TEACHING

By teaching individuals how to improve the quality of their diets or how to modify their diets to meet therapeutic prescriptions, the health professional attempts to improve the nutritional status and general health of individuals. Clients are made active partners in their health promotion. They learn to make appropriate decisions about food information and food selections at home, in the market place and in social gatherings.

WHERE TO TEACH

The hospital, nursing home, rehabilitation center, retirement center and neighborhood clinic are all examples of areas available for teaching nutrition. The public health nurse or dietitian frequently teaches clients in private homes, and professionals in private practice see clients in their offices.

HOW TO TEACH

There is no set style or format for teaching nutrition. The situation should set or determine the most appropriate style as will be discussed in this chapter. The needs and readiness of the individual should always be the major focus of the educational process. Assessment of needs, knowledge of the subject, and the ability to learn and use information should all be major considerations in preparing to teach the individual or group. Everyone has the potential to learn and incorporate changes into his or her diet. What needs to be remembered is that learning takes time, practice, feedback and a teacher who focuses on the needs of the learner.

Assessment of Educational Needs

THE INTERVIEWING PROCESS

Dietary interviews provide the foundation for the collection of information about individual food habits. Analysis of information collected provides the nutritionist or nurse with a basis from which to make recommendations for dietary modification, nutrition teaching and counseling. It is essential, then, that the information collected be as accurate and complete as possible. Skillful interviewing is an art requiring strong listening and verbal communication skills, combined with an empathetic and supportive attitude. It requires preparation and planning, objectives and the use of direct, open-ended questions.

The interviewing process contains four major steps or phases. The first is *preparation*. A dietary interview that is initiated without any preparation usually turns into a nonproductive or frustrating chat with little or inadequate information being collected. The purpose of the preparation phase is to collect background information on the client such as age, height, weight, medical history, medications, social history, educational level, occupation and family relationships. This information is usually obtained from a person's health record, a family member or a health professional. With this basic information the interviewer can establish objectives for collecting specific information during the interview. The second step is to *build rapport*. During this phase the interviewer introduces himself or herself, explains the purpose of the interview and begins to develop rapport with the client. This is a critical step in the interview, for without establishing a comfortable setting between health care professional and client, the flow of information between the client and interviewer may be hampered. Step three is *data collection*. During this step the interviewer questions the client about food habits based on the previously established objectives of the interview. Information is best obtained when open-ended, non-judgmental questions are used. Frequently clarification techniques will be used to explore vague responses or contradictory information. When the interviewer feels the objectives of the interview have been met, the fourth step, *closing*, is initiated. In the closing phase the interviewer summarizes the interview for the client to check completeness and accuracy. The interviewer then tells the client what will be done with the information and when the client will be contacted again for teaching or counseling or for evaluation of the data collected.

TOOLS FOR COLLECTING DATA ON DIETARY INTAKE

Dietary interviews are usually structured around three major types of data collection tools: the 24-hour recall, the diet history and the food record, all of which are discussed in detail in Chapter 9. The steps in the interview process remain the same regardless of the tool used or the type of information collected. However, the length of the interview will vary greatly, from 10 to 15 minutes for a 24-hour recall to one hour or more for a complete diet history.

An individual's food habits, as disclosed from a dietary interview, do not necessarily coincide with his or her knowledge of good nutrition. However, the dietary interview does provide a starting point from which the nutritionist or nurse can begin to assist the individual in modifying food selections toward more appropriate choices. Further, the dietary interview provides the interviewer with environmental information about the client. Such information is helpful in incorporating planned changes into a client's food pattern.

TOOLS FOR EVALUATING DIETARY INTAKE

There are a variety of evaluation tools that can be used to assess an individual's diet. The basic four food group system as discussed in Chapter 10, the diabetic exchange group system presented in Chapter 25, and the nutrient content of the diet as calculated by hand from food composition tables or with the aid of a computer all provide varying amounts of information about the adequacy of a diet. The basic four food group system identifies sources of major (sometimes referred to as leader) nutrients. Use of the diabetic exchange group system allows a rapid approximate analysis of the carbohydrate, protein, fat and energy content of the diet. Both the basic four food group and diabetic exchange group systems are relatively quick and easy to use once basic nutrients, portion sizes and group food values for carbohydrate, protein, fat and energy are committed to memory.

Calculation of the diet's nutrient content using food values is time-consuming. Although this provides a more exact picture of nutrient and energy adequacy, it is best suited for the research setting or special hospital cases that require very exact nutrient calculation. Computerized dietary evaluation will provide information similar to that from the hand-calculated method, assuming that the computer data base is developed from the standard food value handbooks currently in use, e.g., U.S. Department of Agriculture Handbooks No. 8 series, No. 456 or No. 72, as listed on page 12. The computer, however, will provide information quickly and with less possibility for error and is discussed further in Chapter 20. All of these methods are useful in establishing the quality of a client's diet. The method selected primarily depends on the individual situation and the time available.

Designing Instruction

Designing instruction is essentially the same, whether it be for a single diet modification or for a series of classes in a community clinic. The steps are outlined in Table 18–1.

Table 18–1. INSTRUCTION DESIGN

1. Identify learner's needs and learning goals
2. Assess knowledge of the learner
3. Establish behavioral objectives
4. Select an evaluation tool
5. Decide on instruction style
6. Prepare and organize information to be taught
7. Evaluate developed instruction
8. Revise
9. Teach
10. Evaluate learning

PREPARING TO TEACH

All planning begins with identifying the needs of the learner and goals for the instruction. The critical factor is differentiating between the needs of the learner and the needs of the instructor. Many health professionals leave teaching sessions feeling very self-satisfied with the knowledge they have conveyed while the client leaves essentially unfulfilled. The needs of the learners and their receptiveness to participate in the learning and change their behaviors are paramount in successful nutrition education. Once the needs of the learner and goals for instruction have been established, the teacher needs to assess the actual knowledge of the learner so that the teaching can be targeted at an appropriate level of understanding. This will also assist the teacher in determining the amount of time needed to teach and the suitability of educational materials for the learner.

At this point the teacher can outline specific behavioral objectives to be accomplished in the teaching session. These are based on the instructional goals and the assessment of the client's knowledge. It is important to establish objectives that are relatively simple to achieve so that the client may feel a sense of success in their accomplishment and be encouraged to maintain the new behavior. It is also important not to overwhelm the client with too many objectives at once, but to establish only as many objectives as can be achieved during each teaching session. Even these may not be met if the learning is slowed down for some reason; the teacher needs to remain flexible and open to change.

DEVELOPING AND USING BEHAVIORAL OBJECTIVES

Behavioral objectives, also termed performance or instructional objectives, are "statements of what students should be able to do when they complete a given set of instructional materials."[1] By identifying the important fact, principle or task to be learned, the health care professional targets the emphasis of instruction, provides a standard for measuring learning and identifies an area of concentrated learning for the student or client.

There are four components to an objective: (1) the learner or performer, (2) the behavior to be performed, (3) the conditions that exist during performance of the objective, and (4) the criteria for evaluating the performance of the objective. An example of an objective would be: "Given a list of foods, the learner will select, by circling foods on a list, those foods that are acceptable to eat routinely on a 2-gm. sodium diet." The components of this objective are the patient (the learner); "by circling foods on the list" (the behavior); "given a list of foods" (the condition); "which are acceptable to eat routinely on a 2-gm. sodium diet" (the criterion).

By using objectives in teaching clients, the health-care professional automatically establishes a means of evaluating learning. Asking a learner to perform an objective readily identifies whether further instruction or practice needs to be provided for the learner or whether a whole new teaching strategy needs to be developed to better teach the task or concept.

CHOOSING TOOLS TO EVALUATE LEARNING

Once the objectives are established, an evaluation tool can be developed to meet the learning situation. There are two major types of evaluation in learning—formal and informal. The objective test and performance evaluation are types of *formal evaluation*. *Objective tests*, though common in the academic setting, are not well suited for everyday use in an acute care setting, in a community clinic, with young children or with geriatric clients. Since nutrition education deals with food behaviors, performance evaluation can be used to evaluate learning in a practical setting. In *performance evaluation* a client is asked to complete a task based on the learning objectives. This would include such things as selecting appropriate menus for diabetics, identifying low-cholesterol foods from a local restaurant menu or planning a day's menu for a high-fiber diet. The important point is that the client is performing behaviors he is expected to perform when following his new dietary regime.

Informal evaluations are generally unstructured and include observation of food selection and eating behaviors as well as follow-up counseling. Observations may be made of patients in a hospital by making rounds at meal time to observe food selection. In a follow-up session a client may be asked to give a 24-hour recall in order to assess his compliance with his new dietary regimen. The significant factors to consider are whether the observed behaviors are consistent with the teaching objectives and whether the client can accomplish the objectives unassisted.

TYPES OF INSTRUCTION

The next step in planning instruction is to decide which of the many styles of instruction is most appropriate. This is based on the teaching situation, the client's ability to comprehend and use information, and the time available for instruction. Typically the most frequently used instructional formats are the lecture, the small group discussion, simulation, role playing, self-paced instruction and one-to-one counseling.

The university student is most familiar with the *lecture*, which has a predominance of one-way information flow, some use of audiovisuals and limited, if any, practice. The lecture format can be adapted with more client interaction and practice sessions, but is most suitable for a presentation to a large community group or other health professional.

The *small group discussion* employs some lecture but also a significant amount of interaction between the clients and teacher. Teaching small groups is especially beneficial in a clinical setting. Clients with similar diseases or problems can be brought together to learn new information and share common experiences, as shown in Figure 18–1. An example would be the use of a small group to teach people with diabetes how to follow their diabetic diets. Remember that the teacher needs to remain in control of the discussion so that it remains purposeful and objective-oriented.

Self-paced forms of instruction are well suited for use by a busy health care professional. Self-paced instructions are segments of information presented so that the client can read or view information, answer questions and receive feedback without the assistance of a teacher. Self-paced instruction, also called individual programmed instruction, comes in a variety of forms, the most common being a workbook format, but there are also slide-tape presentations and interactive computer programs.

PREPARING THE INFORMATION

Preparing the information for teaching is the next step. This includes evaluating the information available, matching the information to the objectives, preparing audiovisuals, deciding on appropriate practice sessions, and organizing the information and materials into a logical sequenced presentation. A detailed lesson plan is often needed for formal teaching presentations to groups, but for one-to-one or very small groups a simple outline will suffice. With these things the nurse or nutritionist should be ready to teach except for one last step.

PRE-TEACHING EVALUATION

Few professionals prepare and organize perfect instructions on the first attempt. Now is the time to evaluate what has been developed. Consider the questions listed in Table 18–2. If these questions are answered affirmatively the teacher is ready to begin teaching. If not, the instruction model needs to be revised until it conforms to these questions.

TEACHING AND EVALUATION OF LEARNING

During the actual teaching the teacher who is well prepared can focus on delivery of the material and the response of the learners. After the teaching is completed the evaluation tool is used to determine how well the client mastered the learning and what information needs to be retaught or practiced further.

Developing and Evaluating Educational Materials

One of the most beneficial teaching aids for the nutritionist or nurse is well-developed, field-tested, targeted material for nutrition education. Unfortunately, much of the volume of ma-

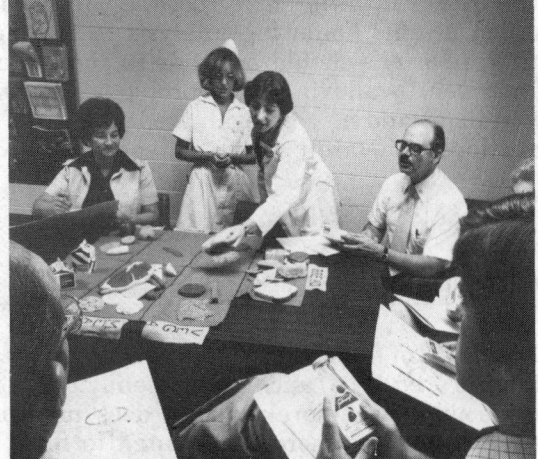

Figure 18–1. Dietitian and nurse teaching a group of patients about their diets. (Courtesy of Ms. Sheila Henderson, R. D. (deceased), and the nutrition staff of Lutheran General Hospital, Park Ridge, Ill.)

Table 18–2. EVALUATING PREPARED INSTRUCTION

Questions to Ask before Beginning Teaching

1. Are the objectives geared to the learner's needs?
2. Are the objectives obtainable in a single learning session?
3. Is the evaluation tool relevant to the client?
4. Is the instruction format relevant to the client?
5. Do the audiovisuals enhance the learning?
6. Does the information presented represent the established objectives?
7. Is the information presented in a logical sequence?
8. Is the learner given an opportunity to practice and receive feedback on the learning?

terials available is either developed haphazardly or used inappropriately. Few nutritionists or nurses are trained in development or evaluation of education materials, but they all are encouraged to use them to enhance learning and sometimes to substitute them for actual teaching.

Most of these materials fail because the reading level is too advanced for the client owing to the use of complex, scientific words and long sentences. Furthermore, users often select material that is not appropriately targeted for the education level, sociocultural background and interest of the client. Therefore one of the more useful tools for the teacher is a readability formula for determining the grade level of the material.[2] There are several references on readability cited at the end of the chapter, and directions for using the Gunning formula for determining grade level of printed material are presented in Table 18–3. If the nutritionist or nurse finds that available material is not appropriate for use with the client or that material is not available, then development of appropriate educational material is the next step.

Numerous types of materials may be created. Booklets, posters and flip charts represent the majority of commonly used educational materials, and overhead transparencies, slides and audio cassette tapes are also popular tools. Steps

Table 18–3. GUNNING FORMULA FOR DETERMINING GRADE LEVEL OF WRITTEN MATERIAL

1. Count a sample of about 100 words. Use more than 100 words if necessary to complete a sentence.
2. Count the number of sentences in the sample. Count each complete thought as a separate sentence. For example: "The diet must be individualized; a diet prescribed for one person is usually not suitable for another." (Two sentences.)
3. Divide the number of sentences into the total number of words. The result is the *average sentence length.*
4. Count the number of "difficult" words (more than two syllables).
   A. Count each repetition of the difficult word.
   B. Do not count capitalized words unless they begin a sentence.
   C. Do not count combinations of short easy words like "manpower," "insofar," and "however."
   D. Do not count verbs made into three syllables by adding "-ed" or "-es" like "restricted" and "reduces."
   E. Determine whether symbols, numbers and abbreviations have three syllables according to the way they are read aloud. For example: "e.g.—for example" contains a "difficult" word; "%—per cent" does not contain a "difficult" word.
5. Divide the number of "difficult" words by the total number of words in the passage and multiply by 100. The result is the *percentage of "difficult" words.*
6. Add the *average sentence length* and the *percentage of "difficult" words.* Multiply the resulting sum by the constant 0.4. The answer is the approximate grade level rating of the material.

in the development of such materials are essentially the same regardless of the type of material developed. The first step is to identify the needs of the target audience. Next, objectives need to be written for learning outcomes. Third, the content needs to be established based on the objectives, the total amount of information to be presented, the images to be drawn, and the level of language to be used. Fourth, attention needs to be given to layout and design.

Frequently educational materials appear as printed texts with little thought given to sectioning information to create white space, subtitling paragraphs, and using graphs, cartoons or illustrations instead of verbiage to present information. Concentration should be given to meeting the stated objectives clearly and avoiding presentation of too much information. There are many inexpensive tools that may be used to facilitate good layout and design, such as lettering guides, pressure-sensitive letters, and books of non-copyrighted art work that may be readily obtained at art supply stores. Having materials printed or photocopied on different color and weight paper also adds to the aesthetic quality of materials.

The most frequently omitted step in developing educational material is field testing the material. Field testing should simulate the actual conditions under which the material is to be used, in terms of learner population and teaching format. To field test the reliability and effectiveness of educational material a pre-test/post-test format is most helpful. Reliability can be checked by comparing the correctness of responses from one post-test to another. If a majority of clients miss the same question on the post-test, there is a problem with either the question or the material presented. All tests should be carefully analyzed to determine the significance of differences between pre- and post-test scores. Following analysis of the field testing, revisions should be made in the material in order to alleviate any problems. Revised materials should also be evaluated to ensure all corrections adequately meet the learners' needs.

Facilitation of Learning

The goal of nutrition education is to establish improved food and eating behaviors. Like all learning, behavioral change does not come easily, especially when it is related to food, because of the strong emotional, cultural and religious ties food holds for people. Several concepts that facilitate learning are important.

MOTIVATION

The use of motivation to ease the transition to new behaviors is an old tool. Many health professionals feel that clients either are motivated or have no motivation; this is an oversimplification of the issue. People are motivated in varying degrees, and all people can learn even if they have low levels of motivation. The key to motivation is success and support. A highly motivated individual can become discouraged through failure and lose interest in learning, while an individual with low motivation can increase his level of motivation and learning through small successful changes in behavior and encouragement and support from significant others.

To enhance motivation a teacher needs to concentrate the learning goals for teaching or counseling on the learner's needs. The nutritionist or nurse needs to be flexible and work within the client's lifestyle, striving for realistic and practical behavioral changes that the client can live with.

FOCUS ON THE INDIVIDUAL

Fleming[3] lists the following factors as being important in the process of teaching and learning.

1. Learning takes place more readily *when emphasis is placed on the individual.* Each individual is unique, with a different hereditary, social and home background. The aims and motivations of individuals differ and must be recognized. Individuals should participate in the planning of ways to accomplish their goals.

2. Learning tends to occur as *emphasis is placed on the learner's perception of the tasks to be accomplished.* The individual's perception of the task often differs from that of the teacher, and it is important that the teacher recognize this.

3. Learning is facilitated as *emphasis is placed on human factors.* As emphasis is given to the feelings, anxieties, concerns, questions and problems of the learner, a setting is created for growth. Feelings of belonging and of security are basic to maximum learning.

4. Learning is facilitated as *the learner is involved in an active way.* Learning is an active process and teachers should help students to clarify goals and plans and to experience, try out, manipulate and explore ideas. As learners assume responsibility, their growth is extended.

RESPONSIBILITY

The health professional needs to make the client responsible for his or her own behavior and not be so supportive or directive in teaching and counseling that the client puts the responsibility for success or failure on the teacher. It is rewarding for the professional to hear "you made my weight loss possible," but it is also untrue. It is the client who changed behavior and lost the weight.

ESTABLISHING A SUPPORTIVE ENVIRONMENT

As with interviewing, the establishment of rapport in the teaching process is very important. This facilitates the flow of information between client and practitioner and makes the client more receptive to learning. The practitioner, however, is but one resource; there are many people, places and things in the learner's environment that can, if carefully used, also contribute to the learning process. One or more support people to reinforce positive behavior can be identified by the client or learner.

Individual Counseling

DEFINING OBJECTIVES

Counseling involves aspects of interviewing and teaching. In an initial counseling session, such as that shown in Figure 18–2, a client will

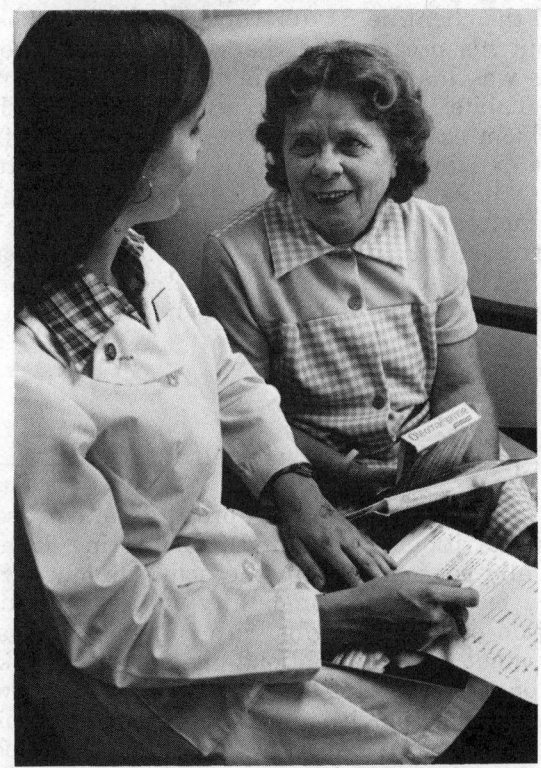

Figure 18–2. Dietitian and patient discussing dietary changes. (Photograph courtesy of Nutrition Department, Lutheran General Hospital, Park Ridge, Ill.)

be interviewed about food habits, medical history, physical activity and social history. The nutrition counselor will assess the food behavior for nutritional adequacy and, based on the client's problem, make some recommendations. The client and the counselor will then establish objectives based on the recommendations, and a plan to implement them. It is important throughout the counseling process that the counselor listen to what the client is saying and what may be implied. It is also important that goals be established with time frames for measuring behavioral change. As the client progresses toward a goal, the original plan may need to be modified to account for changes in progress or new goals.

FOLLOW-UP AND EVALUATION

Nutritional counseling follow-up, in order to evaluate learning, is an essential factor which needs to be included in the plan. After an initial interview, follow-up is usually planned for sometime during the next one to two weeks or perhaps at a later time in the same week. As clients progress toward a goal, follow-up visits are generally spaced further and further apart; in fact, follow-up may even be done over the phone. In a follow-up session the client's progress needs to be measured against the objectives and the client needs to receive positive feedback about his progress. In the event that no progress was made or the client slipped back into old habits, the counselor needs to pursue the problem assertively. Was the objective too difficult to achieve, e.g., was a 3-lb. weight loss too much to expect in one week? Were environmental factors too overwhelming, e.g., was having to restrict sodium while on a trip to Japan unrealistic? The problem needs to be identified and new goals or methods of achieving the goals established.

Summary

Nutrition education is a broad area; however, the nutritionists or nurses facilitating it are usually concentrated in the acute or long-term care facilities and community clinics. Most nutrition education begins with collection and assessment of information on dietary intake. Strong interviewing skills and a broad knowledge of food, nutrition, pathophysiology and biochemistry are important in analyzing food habits and making recommendations for improved or modified eating behaviors. In all aspects of teaching and counseling instructional objectives need to be established, the learner's

knowledge assessed, behavioral objectives written, evaluation tools devised, information needs screened and organized, education materials selected, and instruction critiqued and revised. It is also essential to keep the learner's needs in the forefront and work to maintain rapport with the client.

Education is not complete until the learning has been evaluated. Formal and informal tools may be used to measure learning against established objectives. Using evaluation helps identify if further teaching or clarification of information is needed. To some degree, demonstrating successful learning at evaluation reinforces continuance of new behaviors, which is the goal of nutrition education.

Problems and Suggested Topics for Discussion

1. Outline the steps in teaching a diabetic diet to a patient.
2. How would you deal with a client who does not seem to be learning?
3. How would you help the patient who needs follow-up after discharge from the hospital?
4. If you are not artistically talented, how could you make technical information interesting and easy to understand?
5. How would you handle sabotage behavior?
6. How do you know when you have given a patient enough information?

Cited References

1. Dick, W., and Carey, L.: The Systematic Design of Instruction. Glenview, Ill., Scott, Foresman and Company, 1978.
2. Alley-Crosby, M. L.: Selected Aspects of the Reading Difficulty of Diet Instruction Materials. Master's Thesis, University of Washington, 1975.
3. Fleming, R. S.: Principles of Learning. Proceedings of Nutrition Education Conference, April 1 to 3, 1957. USDA Publication No. 745. Washington, D.C., U.S. Department of Agriculture, 1957, p. 17.

Additional References

Anderson, M. L. F., Olson, C. M., and Rhodes, K.: Development and pilot testing of a tool for evaluating printed materials. J. Nutr. Educ. 12:50, 1980.
Andrew, B. J.: Interviewing and counseling skills. J. Am. Diet. Assoc. 66:576, 1975.
Burke, B. S.: The dietary history as a tool in research. J. Am. Diet. Assoc. 23:1041, 1947.
Engen, H. B., Iasiello-Vailas, L., and Smith, K. L.: Confrontation: a new dimension in nutrition counseling. J. Am. Diet. Assoc., 83:34, 1983.
Gagne, R. M., and Briggs, L. J.: The Principles of Instruction Design. 2nd ed. New York, Holt, Rinehart and Winston, 1979.
Gunning, R.: The Techniques of Clear Writing. New York, McGraw-Hill, 1968.
Mager, R. F., and Beach, K. M.: Developing Vocational Instruction. Palo Alto, Cal., Fearon Publishers, 1967.
Mager, R. F.: Developing Attitude Toward Learning. Palo Alto, Cal., Fearon Publishers, 1968.

Mason, M., Wenburg, B., and Welsh, P. K.: The Dynamics of Clinical Dietetics. 2nd ed. New York, John Wiley and Sons, 1982.

Office of Cancer Communications, National Cancer Institute: Pretesting in Health Communications. NIH Publication No. 81-1493. Washington, D.C., U.S. Department of Health and Human Services, 1981.

Purtillo, R.: Health Professional/Patient Interaction. 2nd ed. Philadelphia, W. B. Saunders Company, 1978.

Young, C. M.: The interview itself. J. Am. Diet. Assoc. *35*: 677, 1959.

Zifferblatt, S., and Wilbur, C. S.: Dietary counseling: Some realistic expectations and guidelines. J. Am. Diet. *70*:591, 1977.

Nutrition Education Resource Materials

American Diabetes Association, 18 E. 48th St., New York, NY 10020 (local affiliate also)

American Heart Association, 7320 Greenville Ave., Dallas, TX 75231 (local affiliate also)

Apple Press Newsletter, 1404 Sunnymede Ave., South Bend, IN 46615 (For K–6 audience to take home and share with their parents)

Currents in Food, Nutrition and Health, 1111 Plaza Dr., Schaumburg, IL 60195 (New quarterly newsletter from the Cereal Institute—free)

Department of Citrus, State of Florida, Florida Citrus Commission, Lakeland, FL 33802

General Mills, Inc., Nutrition Department, Dept. 45, PO Box 1112, Minneapolis, MN 55440 (Listing available–normal and therapeutic nutrition material)

Health Education Services, PO Box 802, 10000 Culver Boulevard, Dept. N2, Culver, CA 90230 (Food and nutrition catalogue available—filmstrips, books, charts, posters, transparencies, etc.) 800-421-4246 outside California, 213-839-2436 in California

Journal of Nutrition Education, Society of Nutrition Education (SNE), 2140 Shattuck Ave., Suite 1110, Berkeley, CA 94704 (Catalogue available)

Kellogg's Project Nutrition Unit, PO Box 9113, St Paul, MN 55191 (Nutrition education unit, grades 7–12)

McDonald's Action Packs, Box 14317, Dayton, OH 45414 (Nutrition action pack, grades 1–4; lesson plans and spirit masters)

Media People, 7117 East Camelback, Scottsdale, AZ 85251 (Hector Digestor program; filmstrips, teachers guide, spirit masters)

Nasco, Nutrition Teaching Aids, 901 Janesville Ave., Fort Atkinson, WI 53538, 414-563-2446 (Catalogue available—spirit masters, slides, games, films, food models and pamphlets)

National Dairy Council, 6300 N River Rd., Rosemont, IL 60018 (local affiliate also)(Catalogue available)

Nutrition for Everybody. Annotated list of resources—1981. From SNE—see Journal of Nutrition Education

Nutrition Graphics, P.O. Box 1527, Corvallis, OR 97330, 503-757-8820

Nutrition Information and Resource Center, Benedict House, The Pennsylvania State University, University Park, PA 16802 (Catalogue available)

Nutrition Today, Director of Circulation, Nutrition Today Society, Box 1829, Annapolis, MD 21404

Procter and Gamble Educational Services, PO Box 14009, Cincinnati, OH 45214 (Catalogue available)

Robert J. Brady Co., A Prentice-Hall Company, Bowie, MD 20715, 800-638-0220 outside Maryland, 301-262-6300 in Maryland (Audiovisual resource, catalogue available)

School Food Service Journal, American School Food Service Association, 4101 East Iliff Ave., Denver, CO 80222

Spectrum Films, 2785 Roosevelt St., Carlsbad, CA 92008, 714-729-3552

The Pennsylvania State University, Audio Visual Services, Special Services Bldg., University Park, PA 16802 (Nutrition education videocassettes, catalogue available)

The Pillsbury Company, Pillsbury Center, Minneapolis, MN 55402, 612-330-8732

The Polished Apple, 8881 Alma Real Dr., Pacific Palisades, CA 90272 (Catalogue available; produce A-V materials—films, filmstrips)

Tupperware Educational Services, Box 2353, Orlando, FL 32802 (Catalogue available-posters, etc.)

Walt Disney Educational Media Co., 500 S. Buena Vista St., Burbank, CA 91521 (Filmstrips with/audio cassettes and spirit masters, for a variety of primary and secondary classes)

This section of the book deals with the role of nutrition in the prevention and treatment of disease. All the therapeutic diets are modifications of the normal adequate diet pattern based on the Recommended Dietary Allowances as suggested by the Food and Nutrition Board of the National Research Council, with amounts of nutrients adjusted to cover the additional requirements created by disease or injury. Space does not permit the inclusion of all diets in use for each disease. Only those diets most generally accepted are outlined here.

Development of Diet Therapy

Nursing and medicine have always been concerned with the feeding of the sick. From the time of the Egyptian medical era, a relationship has been recognized between food and disease, and some form of diet therapy has been practiced. Celsus emphasized the role of foods in preventive medicine about 25 B.C., when he wrote: ". . . we come to those which nourish, namely food and drink. Now these are of general assistance not only in disease of all kinds but in preserving health as well." In 1671 Nicolai Venette recognized the efficacy of using vegetables and fresh fruits as antiscorbutics; and Bachstrom's writings in 1734 demonstrate that he recognized scurvy as a deficiency disease. As early as 1843, Jonathan Pereira, a member of the Royal College of Physicians in London, published a book in collaboration with Dr. Charles A. Lee of New York based on experimental work in the feeding of "paupers, lunatics, criminals, children and the sick in metropolitan institutions." In 1854, during the Crimean War, Florence Nightingale and her staff, located at Scutari, were as devoted to the problems of feeding the sick and wounded as they were to other phases of nursing. Florence Nightingale is historically recorded as the founder of dietetics as well as of nursing. In the early 1870's, Dr. F. W. Pacy, Fellow of the Royal College of Physicians, London, began a treatise on food and dietetics. It is recorded that in his lectures he emphasized that the correct feeding of the well and sick should be of deep concern. He stated, "Ill management of food kills off the weak and ruins the middling." Thus, the role of nutrient requirements in disease and the necessity of supplying certain essential nutrients as a preventive to disease were recognized by the earliest physicians.

Others became interested and approached and treated the subject from various angles. Cooking schools were founded in the East (New York, Boston and Philadelphia). In the 1880's, graduates from these schools began taking positions as instructors in foods and cookery in nurses' training schools, to teach the nurses how to prepare

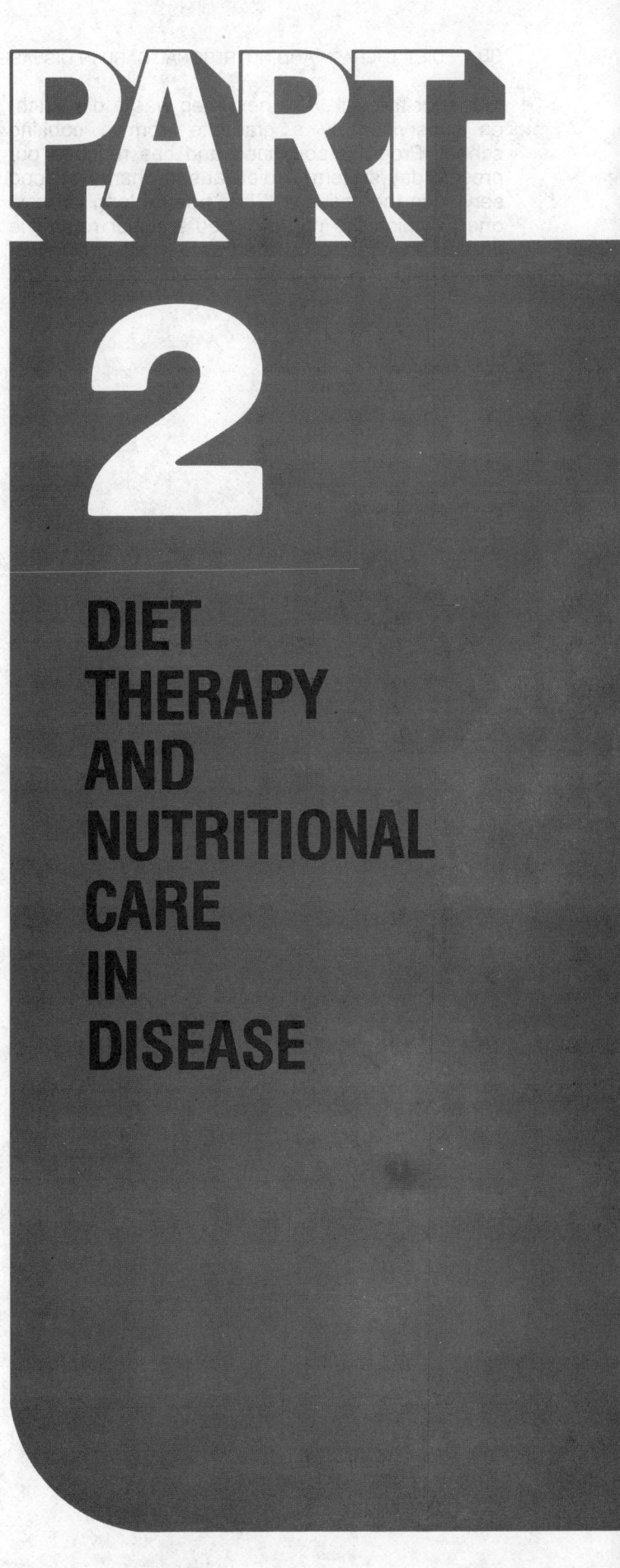

PART

2

DIET THERAPY AND NUTRITIONAL CARE IN DISEASE

foods for the sick. The next step was a diet kitchen supervised by a graduate from a cooking school. Progress continued and has reached our present-day system of dietitians in charge of food service in the hospital. It has been a long journey, one in which the nurse played a major role. The nurse continues to function as a vital and necessary member of the team in feeding the sick. She is with the patient more than anyone else, and when the food is served, she should be able to observe, encourage and guide the learning process intelligently. With the cooperation of everyone —nurse, doctor, dietitian and patient—effective management of the patient's dietary needs and provision of complete nutritional care will be achieved.

PRINCIPLES OF NUTRITIONAL CARE

The Nutritional Care Process

The Changing Picture of Nutritional Disease

Scientific progress is changing the picture of nutritional disease in America. In the early 1900's frank deficiency diseases—pellagra, beriberi, scurvy and rickets—were endemic. Today fully developed cases are rare or at least uncommon. In fact, in 1955 the United States Public Health Service discontinued reporting the occurrence of pellagra and other deficiency diseases. Today, the majority of cases of pellagra, beriberi, xerophthalmia and protein-energy malnutrition are the result of special conditioning circumstances, e.g., the existence of a primary disease that produces secondary nutritional deficiency disease. Nevertheless, sporadic cases do occur and could be diagnosed incorrectly if these diseases are not borne in mind.

Reasons for the changing face of nutritional disease include advances in research, steady improvement of general economic status, fortification and enrichment of foods, and education of the public. Along with these advancements there has been rapid and wide-reaching technological progress in the food industry itself.

However, while certain nutritional diseases are largely disappearing in America, there is a steady increase in the recognition of new nutrition-related disorders, most of which fall into one of four categories: (1) lack or imbalance of nutrients, (2) inborn errors of metabolism, (3) iatrogenic diseases (caused by medications and treatments affecting the intestinal flora, the appetite or the absorption, utilization and excretion of nutrients) and (4) overnutrition (obesity, diabetes mellitus, toxicity, atherosclerosis).

Definite relationships exist between diet and wound healing, stress, burns, gastrointestinal diseases, infectious diseases, diseases of the liver, diseases of the heart and circulatory system, diseases of the bone, cancer and possibly mental disorders. The relationship between nutrition and disease and the nutritional care needed with certain diseases will be described in subsequent chapters.

The Nutritional Care Process

In the course of a lifetime a person's nutritional status and nutritional needs will change. They will reflect the individual's environment and his or her phase in the life cycle. Because an individual is changing, the health care, including the nutritional care, must also be dynamic. Nutritional care is the *process* of meeting a person's changing nutritional needs. The type of care depends on the presence of disease or potential disease, on the environment and on the state of growth and development of the individual. The *nutritional care process* is the assessment of the individual's nutritional status, the identification of nutritional needs or problems, the planning of objectives of nutritional care to meet these needs, the implementation of nutritional activities, including education, necessary to meet the objectives, and the evaluation of the nutritional care.

For a healthy person, nutritional care may mean only assessment of nutritional status, identification of adequate nutritional health without problems and encouragement to continue the good work. A healthy person usually requires nutritional care in the form of education regarding eating habits that will help to prevent disease and maintain the present good health.

Nutritional care for the ill or hospitalized patient is more complex. It means far more than simply providing the hospitalized person with a tray of food three times each day. It should include the monitoring of food intake and, when intake is inadequate, should also include taking action through counseling the patient, providing emotional support and encouragement, or initiating a tube feeding, an elemental diet, parenteral nutrition, or protein, calorie or vitamin and mineral supplementation. It is obvious that thorough nutritional care requires the attention and contributions of many professionals, particularly those of the nurse, clinical dietitian, pharmacist and physician.

One of the reasons for the frequency of malnutrition in hospitals today (see page 398) is that no one health professional or group has taken complete responsibility for the nutritional care of the patient. This has happened in many phases of health care, and nutrition is no exception. Since nutritional care involves so many disciplines, several institutions have developed nutritional support teams composed of physicians, dietitians, nurses, surgeons, pharmacists and physical therapists, who can capitalize on each other's expertise and be responsible for the patient's nutritional care. They work with the primary care providers to ensure that the proper nutritional care is carried out.[7] For provision of effective nutritional care by all of these health professionals, a *nutritional care plan* or written documentation of the nutritional care process is a necessity. It allows for proper communication and the interaction necessary for complete nutritional care.

THE NUTRITIONAL CARE PLAN

The nutritional care plan consists of a nutritional assessment, the identification of nutritional problems, the setting of objectives of nutritional care, nutritional intervention activities (including education) and evaluation of the nutritional care.

Assessment

Collection of the data needed for assessment of nutritional status is discussed thoroughly in Chapter 9. This data base includes anthropometric, biochemical, clinical, dietary and psychosocial information that is pertinent to the nutritional status of the patient and is summarized in Table 19–1.

From the data base an assessment of nutritional status is made and any problems or needs are identified. The relative importance of these problems should also be evaluated so that they can be given levels of priority. Each problem is then numbered, and future notes are identified by the same number. This facilitates record keeping and allows a quick review of the care being provided for one nutritional problem. It is desirable that the nutritional problems, as the dietitian-nutritionist, nurse or physician perceives them, will be given the same priority by the patient, but frequently this is not the case.

The following is an example of a nutritional assessment and the identification of nutritional problems:

Patient: Ms. A.—20 years old, white, female. From the health record, laboratory data, anthropometric data and nutritional history, the following information serves as the data base:

Laboratory data:	Elevated fasting blood sugar. Ketosis. Hypoglycemia.
Anthropometric data:	Underweight; below-standard triceps skinfold thickness.
Dietary data:	Caloric intake below energy needs: 10-lb. weight loss in past year.
	Meals three times per day; coffee frequently.
Medical history:	Diagnosed one year ago as having insulin-dependent diabetes mellitus. Was given little instruction about diet and complains of hypoglycemia.

Nutritional Assessment: Ms. A., although diagnosed one year ago as having diabetes, is not in good control of her condition and does not completely understand her diet. She has been consuming fewer calories than she requires and does not follow a regular dietary pattern. Ms. A.'s *nutritional problem* can be stated as insulin-dependent diabetes mellitus in poor control. However, her nutritional problem could be stated more specifically as three problems: (1) hypoglycemic episodes related to poor control of diabetes mellitus, (2) weight loss and (3) little knowledge of proper dietary management.

The identification of nutritional problems, present and potential, evolves naturally from a thorough nutritional assessment. Identification of the potential problems brings attention to those that might be prevented by taking immediate action.

Objectives for Nutritional Care

After the identification of nutritional problems, the next step is to formulate a plan for dealing with each of them, with the greatest attention being paid to the problems of highest priority. If the nutrition information is not complete, the first objective would be to collect

Table 19–1. ASSESSMENT OF NUTRITIONAL STATUS—THE DATA BASE IN THE NUTRITIONAL CARE PROCESS

This data base includes all information—anthropometric, biochemical, clinical, nutritional-dietary and psychosocial—that is pertinent to the nutritional status, problems and care of the patient. It includes the following information:*

ANTHROPOMETRIC
  Weight, height and weight changes. Growth parameters (in infants, children, adolescents): chest circumference, head circumference; (in pregnant women): weight gain.
  Skinfold thickness: triceps, subscapular, abdominal, etc.
  Arm circumference and muscle circumference.
  Skeletal radiographic information.
BIOCHEMICAL
  Blood, serum, plasma measurements.
  Urinary measurements.
  Tissue assays or biopsies.
CLINICAL EXAMINATION
  Findings indicative of nutritional status.
  Findings indicative of disease that may affect nutritional status.
  Pertinent medical history—effect of disease, medications, recent surgery, radiation, chemotherapy or other treatments on nutritional intake, requirements and losses.
NUTRITIONAL HISTORY
  Dietary intake.
      24-hour recall.
      Food frequency questionnaire.
  Nutrition-related information.
      Use of vitamin and mineral supplementation.
      Allergies, food intolerances.
      Nutrition knowledge.
      Physical activity.
PSYCHOSOCIAL INFORMATION
  Cooking and eating atmosphere.
  Attitudes toward food and eating.
  Number of persons in household.
  Economic factors.
  Food buying and cooking facilities.
  Pertinent social history.
  Ethnic background.

*See Chapter 9 for a complete discussion.

more data. For example, one objective might be to find out when Ms. A.'s hypoglycemic attacks occur.

The objectives should be patient-centered, which means that they should be stated in terms that show what the patient will achieve if the objective is met. For example, the objective would be: "Ms. A. will be able to select a 2000-kcal. diet from the hospital menu after three days of instruction," rather than "I will teach Ms. A. how to select a 1500-kcal. diet from the hospital menu," which is not patient-centered. Stated in the latter way, the objective identifies what needs to be done but does not make the nurse, clinical dietitian or even Ms. A. responsible for Ms. A.'s learning. One session in which the dietitian does all the talking, and Ms. A does all the listening but learns little, would meet the objective but not the patient's needs. Patient-centered educational objectives are further discussed in Chapter 18.

In addition, the objectives should be realistic and should take into consideration the educational level of the patient and the economic and social resources of the patient and his family.

The objectives should be stated in *quantifiable* terms. In order to know if objectives have been met, they must be stated in measurable ways. The plan or objective of care for each problem should carry the same number in notations in the medical record as the problem it is designed to deal with. Returning to our example, the objectives for each of the three nutritional problems identified for Ms. A. might be the following:

Problem No. 1—Hypoglycemia episodes.

Objectives: (1) The nutrition counselor will find out when the hypoglycemic attacks occur, (2) Ms. A. will demonstrate an understanding of hypoglycemia through a verbal explanation of why it happens, what the body needs when it does happen and how to prevent it and (3) Ms. A. will modify her diet in order to avoid hypoglycemia.

Problem No. 2—Weight loss.

Objective: Ms. A. will stop losing weight and will demonstrate this by check-ups at three months, six months, nine months and one year.

Problem No. 3—Lack of knowledge about proper diet to control her diabetes.

Objective: Ms. A. will demonstrate understanding of the principles of her modified diet by being able to select the proper foods from the hospital menu to meet her dietary requirements.

Implementation of Nutritional Care

This part of the nutritional care process includes all of those activities or interventions that will enable the patient to meet the objectives already defined. Such activities include the diet prescription, nutritional counseling and education, provision of food and necessary nutritional supplements, vitamin and mineral medication, or activities such as public aid advice and food stamp counseling that will help the patient to meet his nutritional needs.

For each objective there are specific interventions or actions that are numbered to correlate with the objective they are designed to meet. The nutritional interventions should be complete and *specific* and should include the "what, where, when and how" of the activity. Nothing should be vague or left open to question. With complete and specific interventions outlined and documented, the entire health team (including the patient) will know what is being done, especially at those times when the primary care providers are not available. No one can be with a patient for 24 hours every day. Information about the treatment and progress of a patient should be accessible to the health team from a central record. Referring again to Ms. A., the nutritional interventions for each objective might be stated as follows:

Objective No. 1: Ms. A. will modify her diet in order to avoid afternoon hypoglycemia.

Intervention: No. 1–1. Carbohydrate will be distributed throughout the day as follows: breakfast (8:00 A.M.): 80 gm.; lunch (noon): 85 gm.; afternoon snack: 30 gm. and dinner (6:30 P.M.): 85 gm.

Objective No. 2: Ms. A. will stop losing weight.

Intervention: No. 2–1. Caloric intake will be increased to 2000 kcal. per day using the following diet: 280 gm. of carbohydrate, 43 gm. of protein and 80 gm. of fat.

Objective No. 3: Ms. A. will understand the principles of her modified diet and will be able to select the proper foods from the hospital menu.

Intervention: No. 3–1. Teach Ms. A. how to select a 2000-kcal. diet from the hospital menu by giving her the opportunity on February 7, 8 and 9 at 10:30 A.M. to select (with supervision and discussion) a 2000-kcal. diet from the hospital menu.

Evaluation of Nutritional Care

The last step is evaluation of the nutritional care provided. This step makes the nutritional care plan dynamic and responsive to the patient's needs. If the objectives have been written in measurable behavioral terms, the evaluation becomes very easy, since present behavior is being measured against behavior already defined. For example: "Ms. A. was not able to select a 2000-kcal. diet after three days of instruction because she does not understand the food exchange system." A revision in the care plan at this point might include the following: "Ms. A. will attend classes for diabetics during the week of February 14 to 18 in order to learn the concept of a food exchange."

Another aspect of this last step is the evaluation of the extent to which the patient's nutritional requirements are being met. This can be done by using the *nutritional index.*[4] The nutritional index quantifies the extent to which the patient's *actual intake* of a nutrient meets the recommended or *desirable intake* defined for that patient. The nutritional index (NI) can be used to evaluate the adequacy of the calorie, protein, vitamin or mineral intake of the patient. Nutrients of special importance in the patient's diet should be evaluated by using this method. To calculate the nutritional index:

$$\text{Nutritional Index (NI)} = \frac{\text{Actual Intake of Nutrient} - \text{Desirable Intake}}{\text{Desirable Intake}} \times 100$$

If the actual daily intake exceeds the desirable intake, the nutritional index is stated as a positive percentage. If actual intake equals desirable intake, the index is stated as $+1$ per cent to avoid an index of zero. If the actual intake is less than the desirable intake, then the nutritional index is stated as a negative percentage. Obviously, the goal of nutritional care is to meet the nutritional requirements of the patient and thus to have as many days as possible with a positive nutritional index. Having several days with a negative nutritional index means that the objectives of the nutritional care are not being met and that the care should be evaluated and changed.

Example: Mr. M., who was burned in a fire, requires 60 kcal. per kg. of body weight per day. His daily intake per kg. for one week was: Monday, 30 kcal.; Tuesday, 20 kcal.; Wednesday, 30 kcal.; Thursday, 36 kcal.; Friday, 40 kcal.; Saturday, 45 kcal. and Sunday, 60 kcal. The nutritional index for Monday would be calculated as follows:

$$NI = \frac{30 \text{ kcal./kg.} - 60 \text{ kcal./kg.}}{60 \text{ kcal./kg}} \times 100$$

$$NI = \frac{-30 \text{ kcal./kg.}}{60 \text{ kcal./kg.}} \times 100$$

$$NI = -0.5 \times 100 = -50\%$$

For the entire week the nutritional indexes are: Monday, -50 per cent; Tuesday, -66 per cent; Wednesday, -50 per cent; Thursday, -40 per cent; Friday, -33 per cent; Saturday, -25 per cent and Sunday $+1$ per cent. The average nutritional index for the week is -37.7 per cent.

On the seventh day Mr. M. finally achieved a positive nutritional index. During the week, Mr. M's average was 38 per cent below his desirable intake. The goal now would be to achieve equally high positive nutritional indexes to offset the days with negative indexes. At the least, the indexes should remain positive. If they do not, nutritional care should be modified, and parenteral nutrition, which is described in Chapter 35, may be necessary. The same kind of evaluation can be made for protein intake, vitamin C intake or the intake of any other nutrient. The NI for each nutrient can be plotted on a graph to provide a visual as well as a percentage evaluation of the patient's actual nutrient intake compared with the desirable intake.

As the evaluation reveals that objectives are not being met or that new needs have arisen, the process begins again with reassessment, identification of new needs, setting of objectives and so on. Table 19–2 summarizes the nutritional care process, including the criteria necessary for each step.

Table 19–2.   THE NUTRITIONAL CARE PROCESS

STEPS	COMPONENTS	FACTORS TO CONSIDER

1. *Assessment of Nutritional Status*
   Collect information (data base).
   Identify problems.
	Dietary history.
	Biochemical data.
	Clinical examination findings.
	Medical history.
	Anthropometric data.
	Psychosocial data.
		The information should be accurate, pertinent to the patient and appropriately interpreted.
		The problems should be numbered the same as those in the medical record, given priority ratings in the order of their importance, related to assessment data and should include present and potential problems.

2. *Planning of Nutritional Care* Set objectives.	Additional information needed. Available resources. Educational level of patient and family. Modification of dietary intake. Supplementation of nutrient intake. Measures to enable patient to meet nutritional requirements. Treatment of medical problems affecting nutritional status.	Objectives should be patient-centered, stated in behavioral terms, realistic, measurable, designated as short- or long-term and numbered according to problem that they are designed to deal with.
3. *Implementation of Nutritional Care* Determine nutritional interventions.	Modification of intake as required to make it acceptable to the patient. Teaching patient and family about the nutritional care plan. Provision of necessary nutritional supplements in acceptable form. Resolution of health problems. Enrollment of the patient in food assistance programs if necessary.	Interventions should be numbered according to the problem and objective, individualized for each patient and specific in describing what, how, why, when and where.
4. *Evaluation of Nutritional Care*	Monitoring of food and fluid intake; evaluation of intake for adequacy in meeting patient's nutritional needs. Assessment of nutritional knowledge as reflected in behavioral change. Monitoring of biochemical data related to nutritional status. Monitoring of anthropometric data. Monitoring of clinical condition.	Evaluation should include a comparison between observed behavior and expected behavior, a determination of the effectiveness of intervention in meeting objectives, an explanation of the effectiveness or ineffectiveness of intervention and suggestions for revision of the care plan based on evaluation.

THE NUTRITIONAL CARE RECORD

The nutritional care process, as applied to a patient in either a hospital or an outpatient setting, must be documented in the health record. Documentation of the nutritional care plan has the following advantages:

1. It helps the patient to understand his nutritional care and to know that he will have to be an active participant.

2. It helps ensure that nutritional care will be relevant, complete and effective by providing a record that identifies the problems and sets criteria for evaluating the care.

3. It allows the entire health team to understand the rationale for nutritional care and the means by which it will be provided.

4. It allows the entire health team to participate in the nutritional care and to reinforce the patient's education whenever there is an opportunity.

Fortunately, much of the information needed for nutritional care is already collected by various health professionals: dietitians, physicians, nurses and social workers. For example, a physician will ask about gastrointestinal disturbances and a nurse usually will weigh and measure the patient and ask about any food allergies. Social workers frequently ask about the amount of money available for food and about the patient's living conditions. But this information needs to be organized and recorded in one place as part of the nutritional care record, so that it can be used to make a nutritional assessment and formulate a picture of nutritional needs. The nutritional care record ensures that all aspects of nutritional care are noted in one place as part of the total health record.

A detailed nutritional care record may be kept by the clinical dietitian, but if this is the case, the information it contains should be summarized periodically in the permanent health record as shown in Figure 19–1. This detailed information is especially important for hospital care audits, professional standards reviews and other efforts to maintain quality health care. Figure 19–2 is an example of a nutritional care record.

Parts of the nutritional care record may be incorporated into the nursing care plan, which is a detailed record kept by the nurse and periodically summarized for inclusion in the medical record.

Nutritional Intervention—Diet Modification

ADEQUATE NORMAL DIET AS A BASIS FOR THERAPEUTIC DIETS

All therapeutic diets are modifications of the normal or adequate diet pattern. The hospital's general diet and the individual's normal diet are the basis for therapeutic diets. Regardless of the type prescribed, the aim or purpose of the diet is to supply needed nutrients to the body in a form the body can handle. Before any therapeutic diets, either general or specific, are discussed, the description of the adequate normal diet in Chapter 10 should be reviewed.

There are many ways to plan a diet that will be nutritious and adequate. The most legitimate way to determine if the diet is adequate for the individual, either sick or well, is through nutritional assessment of the patient as discussed in Chapter 9. However, this is not always possible, so the Recommended Dietary Allowances (RDA) (Table 10–1) are used to design diets for diseased persons. The RDA is not an ideal tool for this purpose, but at the moment there is nothing better.

For the normal healthy adult the foundation of an adequate diet or Daily Food Guide (Table 10–8) provides approximately 63 gm. of protein and 1200 kcal. To provide additional energy to achieve or maintain normal weight, more of the foods listed or other foods are added. Eating these additional foods will also raise the amounts of required nutrients taken in.

For the ill person the RDA and Daily Food Guide can be the basis of the diet, but there

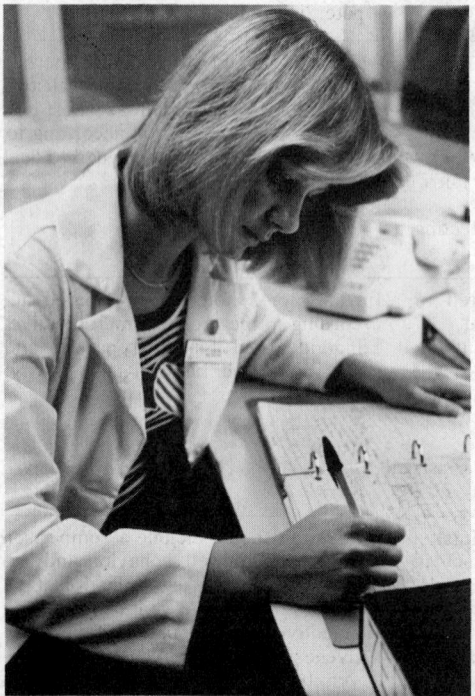

Figure 19–1. Dietitian documenting nutritional care. (Courtesy of Ms. Sheila Henderson, R. D. (deceased), and the nutrition staff of Lutheran General Hospital, Park Ridge, Ill.)

NUTRITIONAL CARE RECORD

	Rm. No._____	Nutritional Care Flow Sheet: Weights, Lab Values, I&O& Dates

Name_____
Address_____
and
Phone No._____

Age_____ Sex_____

Problem List

	Date									
Serum transferrin or serum pre-albumin or serum retinol-binding protein										
Wgt.										
Cal:N ratio										
Intake–tray pro./kcal.										
Intake–Supps. pro./kcal.										
Intake–P. Vein pro./kcal.										
Intake–C. Vein pro./kcal.										
Urine cc./24 hr.										
Stools Avg./24 hr.										

NUTRITIONAL CARE PLAN

Basal Energy Expenditure:_____ kcal.
Anabolic Req.: _____ kcal. _____ gm. pro. _____ gm. N
Maintenance Req.: _____ kcal. _____ gm. pro. _____ gm. N

Diet Calculation _____ kcal.
CHO =   Pro =   Fat =   Na$^+$ =

	P	F	C	PFC	PFC	PFC	PFC
Time							
Milk							
Meat							
Bread							
Fruit							
Fat							
Veg.							
Misc. CHO							
Total P F C							

EVALUATION OF NUTRITIONAL CARE— PROGRESS NOTES

Date

RECOMMENDATIONS FOR FOLLOW-UP

Figure 19–2. Nutritional care record shows assessment data, the nutritional care plan, intervention strategies and monitoring and evaluation data.

Illustration continued on following page

NUTRITIONAL CARE RECORD (*Continued*)

ASSESSMENT— Data Base

Diet HX _____ Date 24 Hr. Recall	Medications/Vits. & Mins./Supplements
	Date _____ Date _____
	Medical HX and Clinical Findings
	Biochemical findings
Allergies: Use of sugar: _____ salt: _____ Use of alcohol: _____ none _____ occas. _____ oz. _____ often Fluid intake _____	Social HX

Feeding and G.I. Habits
  Consistency of food:
  Appetite:
  Bowel habits:
  Recent chngs. in eating habits:
  Recent wgt. chngs.:
  Dental condition:
	Activities
	  Occup.: _____ hr./wk.
	  Exercise _____
	Anthropometry
	  Triceps skinfold thickness: Arm circumf.: % Body fat:
	  Arm muscle circumf.:
	Frame type: S M L IBW: Surface area:

Evaluation of Intake
  P _____ Cal. _____ _____ _____ _____
  F _____ _____ _____ _____
  C _____ _____ _____
	Patient's
	Hgt: Wgt: Wgt. goal: Usual wgt: % Usual wgt.:

Figure 19-2. *Continued*

must also be attention to nutrient needs affected by disease.

THE DIET PRESCRIPTION

Modifications of the normal diet pattern are indicated for a number of diseases. The following are some general principles of dietary management and nutritional care for a specific disease:

1. The therapeutic diet should vary from the individual's normal diet as little as possible, unless the normal diet is inadequate.

2. The diet should meet the body's requirements for essential nutrients as generously as the disease condition permits.

3. The diet regimen should recognize and take into account the patient's food intake habits and food preferences, his economic status and religious practices (Fig. 19–3), and any environmental factors that have bearing on the diet, such as where the meals are eaten and who prepares them.

The diet prescription in nutrition serves the same purpose as the drug prescription in medicine. It designates the type, amount, frequency weight and normal activity plus the amounts and forms of needed protein, fat, carbohydrate, minerals, vitamins and other substances such as fluid and fiber. The Recommended Dietary Allowances for different age groups may be used as a *guide* only, since variations or deviations from the average are not considered in the RDA. In the food prescription the individual variations are taken into account. The construction of the diet prescription will be discussed in detail.

Energy Allowance

It is possible to estimate the energy required by a normal person. Nature supplies a very good checking device, the appetite, and in most normally active people it regulates the weight with surprising accuracy. However, the appetite cannot be depended upon in disease. It is frequently necessary to calculate energy needs. In

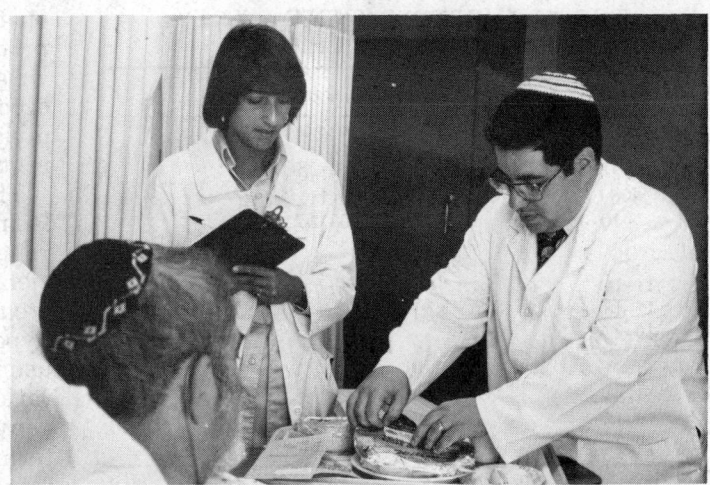

Figure 19–3. Rabbi blessing a meal. (Courtesy of Ms. Sheila Henderson, R. D. (deceased), and the nutrition staff of Lutheran General Hospital, Park Ridge, Ill.)

some instances, when it is possible, actual measurement of the basal or resting metabolic rate can be most useful. Some hospitals have mobile bedside carts that are able to measure a patient's oxygen consumption and resting metabolic rate.

The energy requirement of an individual may be calculated by either (1) calculating the number of kcal. per kilogram per day or (2) calculating the per cent increase over basal metabolic demands. To make the determinations, the desirable weight based on sex, age, height and body build (frame) is used (Appendix Table 27). Desirable or usual weight is used instead of actual weight in determining a patient's requirements because the present weight of the individual may be abnormal as a result of undernutrition or obesity.

The resting energy expenditure (REE) is calculated by using one of the methods described in Chapter 1. An additional factor is added depending upon the health and activity of the patient. This factor can be determined by measuring the daily urinary urea nitrogen loss as shown in Table 35–5, or the stress index as explained in Chapter 35. This will indicate whether the stress is mild, moderate or severe.

Patients with mild stress, such as those with uncomplicated surgery, require 0 to 20 per cent over their REE. Patients with multiple fractures or trauma are in moderate stress and may need up to 50 per cent over REE. A patient with acute major infection or burns may need up to 100 per cent over REE. Even the most hypermetabolic patients usually do not require more than 50 kcal./kg. ideal body weight for anabolism. Tables 19–3 and 19–4 present some guidelines, but the energy requirement should be determined from assessment of the individual.

Situations requiring energy intakes greater than 100 per cent over REE are usually those of excessive physical activity, as shown in Table 19–

Table 19–3. RECOMMENDED ENERGY ALLOWANCES FOR ADULTS*

CATEGORY	KCAL./ KG./DAY	PER CENT INCREASE OVER RESTING ENERGY EXPENDITURES
Activity		
Basal or standard	25	
Minimal (bed rest)	27.5	10
Very light (typist)	30–35	20–40
Light (student, teacher, nurse)	35–40	40–60
Moderate (homemaker, metal worker)	40–45	60–80
Hard (carpenter, housemaid at hard work)	45–50	80–100
Severe (farmer, dancer)	50–70	100–180
Very severe (miner, lumberman, athlete in hard training)	75	200
Illness and Disease		
Mild stress	30	0–20
Moderate stress	30–37	20–50
Severe stress	37–50	50–100

* Based on desirable weight.

Table 19–4. RECOMMENDED ENERGY REQUIREMENTS FOR CHILDREN*

AGE (yrs)	Kcal./kg./day
Both Sexes:	
3	70–140
4–6	65–115
7–10	60–120
Girls:	
11–14	30–65
15–18	20–55
19–22	30–45
Boys:	
11–14	45–80
15–18	30–60
19–22	35–50

* Data from Food and Nutrition Board, National Research Council: Recommended Dietary Allowances. 9th ed. Washington, D.C., National Academy of Sciences, 1980.

3. Athletes training for endurance events frequently need 100 to 200 per cent over REE for their energy intakes. This should be kept in mind when planning nutritional care for the athlete or any patient who is physically very active.

The determination of the energy requirement of an individual is illustrated in the following example.

Example: Suppose that the patient referred to earlier in this chapter (Ms. A.) is a 20-year-old student who has a height of 165 cm. (5 ft., 5 in.) and medium body build. According to Appendix Table 27 she has a desirable weight of 53.6 kg. (118 lb.). Her activity level is light, which, according to Table 19–3, shows that she requires 35 to 40 kcal. per kg. per day. Thus, her average calorie allowance would be 53.6 multiplied by 35 to 40 or 1876 to 2144 (average 2010) kcal. per day.

The energy requirement could also be calculated by determining the percentage increase over the REE. By consulting the third column in Table 19–3, one finds that there would be a 40 to 60 per cent increase over the student's basal demands. Energy requirements calculated for the same student by using this method would be as follows:

$$53.6 \text{ kg.} \times 25 \text{ kcal./kg./day} = 1340 \text{ kcal.} = \text{REE}$$

To this add 40 to 60 per cent for activity:

$$1340 + 536 \text{ to } 804 = 1876 \text{ to } 2144 \text{ kcal./day}$$

Protein Allowance

After the daily energy requirement is calculated, the protein fraction of the diet is determined. The recommended daily allowance based on the utilization value of 70 per cent for food proteins is 0.8 gm. of protein per kg. of body weight for adults. The RDA is usually considered adequate for previously well-nourished individuals who are ambulatory patients or who require only brief periods of hospitalization.

The patient with malabsorption, the patient losing protein (from burns, exudates, ascites or renal disease) and the patient not forming sufficient protein (hepatic disease) will require an increase in protein intake. For these patients in hypermetabolic states the protein allowance is usually determined based on a calorie:nitrogen ratio. Ratios of 100 to 200 kcal. per gm. of nitrogen intake are recommended and should be determined from nutritional evaluation of the patient as discussed in Chapter 9 and 35.

Severe depletion of body protein can lead to prolonged convalescence, poor wound healing, an increase in complications after surgery, anemia and increased susceptibility to infections, as well as other complications.

The determination of the protein fraction of an individual's diet is illustrated in the following example.

Example: Using the same 20-year-old female student previously mentioned, the protein allowance would be:

$$53.6 \times 0.8 = 43 \text{ gm. of protein per day}$$

Since her energy requirement is 1876 to 2144 kcal. per day, the calorie:nitrogen (Cal:N) ratio is determined by dividing these numbers by the grams of nitrogen in the diet. This comes to 272 to 311 calories per gm. of nitrogen. If Ms. A. were stressed or hypermetabolic it should be closer to 100 to 200 kcal. per gm. N as already mentioned. The lower the Cal.:N ratio, the greater the amount of protein in the diet.

Fat and Carbohydrate Allowances

Following the calculation of the protein fraction, the remainder of the calories in the diet are determined and are assigned to fat and carbohydrate. The correct or optimum proportion of fat to carbohydrate to meet the requirements of the body under various conditions is not completely understood and is discussed in each chapter dealing with a specific disease state. The present recommendations for Americans in order to decrease the risk of heart disease and cancer (Table 17–7) are to increase the carbohydrate content of the diet so that it provides 50 to 60 per cent of the calories and to reduce the fat content to 30 to 35 per cent of calories.[6] A suggested distribution of proteins, fats and carbohydrates in the diet is shown in Table 19–5.

The average daily food intake of a healthy or

Table 19–5.   SUGGESTED PROTEIN, FAT AND CARBOHYDRATE INTAKES

AGE OR CONDITION	PROTEINS (Gm./Kg.)	FATS (Gm./Kg.)	CARBOHYDRATES (Gm./Kg.)
Under 1 year	2.0–2.2	2–3	6–10
1–3	1.8	2–3	6–10
4–6	1.5	2–3	6–10
7–10	1.2	2–3	6–10
11–18	0.8–1.0	2–3	6–10
Adult	0.8	1–2	4–6
Pregnancy	+30 gm.*	1–2	4–6
Lactation	+20gm.*	1–2	4–6

*Indicates total additional protein needed, not gm./kg.

mildly stressed individual without dietary restrictions amounts to about 50 to 90 gm. of protein, 90 to 120 gm. of fat and 150 to 300 gm. of carbohydrate. This proportion may have to be varied to meet the needs caused by certain diseases or physical activity.

A rapid, satisfactory clinical method for calculating the constituents of a food prescription consists of dividing the total energy allowance into approximately 10 to 15 per cent protein, 25 to 35 per cent fat and 50 to 65 per cent carbohydrate.

Example: Continuing with the same 20-year-old female student used in the examples for calorie and protein allowances, the fat and carbohydrate needs are calculated.

Protein intake already determined: 43 gm.

$$4 \text{ kcal./gm.} \times 43 \text{ gm. protein} = 172 \text{ kcal. or } 8$$
per cent of kcal. from protein.

Fats make up 25 to 35 per cent of kcal., in this case 35 per cent. Total kcal. requirement (2010) × 0.35 = 703 kcal. from fat.

$$\frac{703 \text{ kcal.}}{9 \text{ kcal./gm. fat}} = 78 \text{ gm. of fat}$$

$$= 1.5 \text{ gm. fat/kg.}$$

Carbohydrates make up remainder of kcal.: 57 per cent in this case. Total kcal. requirement (2010) × 0.57 = 1146 kcal. from carbohydrate (CHO).

$$\frac{1146 \text{ kcal.}}{4 \text{ kcal./gm. CHO}} = 286 \text{ gm. CHO}$$

$$= 5.3 \text{ gm. CHO/kg.}$$

Minerals and Vitamins

In addition to total energy, protein, fat and carbohydrate allowances, the diet must satisfy the requirements for minerals and vitamins.

MINERALS. In acute conditions sodium, chloride, magnesium and potassium are of special concern. Zinc is important for wound healing. Iron is important in chronic illness or situations of poor gastrointestinal absorption. Chapter 7 discusses mineral requirements in detail, and the reader should also refer to the chapters discussing nutritional care for various diseases.

VITAMINS. Vitamin requirements under stress situations have not been completely determined, although understanding about them is increasing rapidly. Vitamin requirements during specific disease states or when using particular medications will be discussed in subsequent chapters.

Sometimes up to ten times the normal Recommended Dietary Allowances will be necessary. However, in many instances these large intakes are probably not indicated, and in the case of vitamins A and D they may be harmful. In arriving at the appropriate vitamin intake, the following should be considered: (1) requirements for normal individuals, (2) the nature of the disease or injury, (3) the known capacity of the body to store certain vitamins, (4) known losses through the skin, urine or intestinal tract produced by various phenomena, (5) interactions between drugs and vitamins and (6) the interrelations of nutrient requirements. Vitamins are discussed in detail in Chapter 6, and again the reader is referred to the various chapters dealing with nutritional care in disease states.

Fluids

Water, although not considered a food, is an indispensable nutrient and plays an important role in the proper functioning of the human body. Optimum convalescence demands normal tissue hydration. A normal healthy adult at rest and not perspiring needs 1800 to 2500 ml. of water daily to provide for urinary secretion and to replace losses from insensible perspiration. Additional fluids must be added to replace water lost by excessive sweating, vomiting, diarrhea,

Table 19–6.   CONSTRUCTION OF DAILY DIET PRESCRIPTION FOR A NORMAL ADULT BY TWO METHODS

STANDARD ALLOWANCES		DIET PRESCRIPTION
Desirable Weight for:		53.6 kg. (118 lb.)
Sex		Female
Age		20 yr.
Height		162.5 cm. (5 ft., 5 in.)
Protein Allowance		
0.8 gm./kg. ideal body weight (IBW) or approximately 10 to 20% of total calories.		53.6 × 0.8 = 43 gm. protein.
Fat and Carbohydrate Allowances		
Fats average 1 to 2 gm./kg. IBW or approximately 25 to 35% of total calories.		53.6 × 1.5 = 80 gm. fat.
Carbohydrates average 4 to 6 gm./kg. IBW or approximately 50% of total calories.		53.6 × 5.2 = 280 gm. carbohydrate.
Energy or Calorie Allowance		
Activity: light.		
Calories required per kg. IBW per day: 35 to 40 kcal.		53.6 × 35 to 40 = 1876 to 2144 kcal. (2010 avg.)
Calories from Food Constituents		
Protein = 4 kcal./gm.		43 × 4 = 172 kcal.
Fat = 9 kcal./gm.		80 × 9 = 720 kcal.
Carbohydrate = 4 kcal./gm.		280 × 4 = 1120 kcal.
		2012 kcal.
Mineral Allowances		
Calcium:	0.8 gm./day.	Calcium: 0.8 gm./day.
Iodine:	150 μg./day.	Iodine: 150 μg./day.
Iron:	18 mg./day.	Iron: 18 mg./day.
Phosphorus:	0.8 gm./day.	Phosphorus: 0.8 gm./day.
Magnesium:	300 mg./day.	Magnesium: 300 mg./day.
Zinc:	15 mg./day.	Zinc: 15 mg./day.
Vitamin Allowances		
Vitamin A:	4000 I.U. (800 R.E.)/day.	Vitamin A: 4000 I.U. (800 R.E.)/day.
Thiamin:	0.5 mg./1000 kcal./day.	Thiamin: 1.1 mg./day.
Riboflavin:	0.6 mg./1000 kcal./day.	Riboflavin: 1.3 mg./day.
Niacin equiv.:	6.6 mg./1000 kcal./day.	Niacin equiv.: 14.0 mg./day.
Folacin:	400 μg./day.	Folacin: 400 μg./day.
Vitamin B_6:	2.0 mg./day.	Vitamin B_6: 2.0 mg./day.
Vitamin B_{12}:	3.0 μg./day.	Vitamin B_{12}: 3.0 μg./day.
Ascorbic acid:	60 mg./day.	Ascorbic acid: 60 mg./day.
Vitamin D:	7.5 μg./day.	Vitamin D: 7.5 μg./day.
Vitamin E:	8 mg α-T.E.	Vitamin E: 8 mg α-T.E.

tube drainage or other conditions in which there is increased water loss. (See Chapter 8, Water and Electrolytes.) If sufficient water is not obtained through fluid intake and food, it must be supplied parenterally.

The sample in Table 19–6 shows how a completed food prescription for a normal adult, as described in the preceding pages, looks when finally assembled.

MODIFICATIONS OF THE NORMAL DIET

The normal diet may be modified and thereby become a specific therapeutic diet. The substitutions and modifications are made to help compensate for the dysfunction of the affected body part, to meet the specific needs induced by a disease or hypermetabolism or to prevent a disease from developing or worsening.

Therapeutic diets may be classified as qualitative and quantitative modifications of the normal diet. The *qualitative* diet is an adequate diet adjusted according to the type of food allowed. The *quantitative* diet is calculated with an increase or decrease in the amount of the food constituents. To illustrate: diets for management of gastrointestinal diseases are usually qualitative, whereas diets used in managing diabetes are usually quantitative.

The adjustment in diet may take any of the following forms:

1. Change in consistency of foods. Examples: liquid diet, soft diet, low fiber diet, high fiber diet.

2. Increase or decrease in energy value of diet. Examples: weight reduction diet, high calorie diet during recovery from trauma.

3. Increase or decrease in type of foods. Examples: sodium-restricted diet, lactose-free diet.

4. Omission of specific foods. Example: allergy diet.

5. Adjustment in the ratio and balance of food constituents: proteins, fats and carbohydrates. Examples: diabetic diet, ketogenic diet, high protein diet, low fat diet.

6. Rearrangement of the number and frequency of meals. Example: gastric ulcer diet or diabetic diet.

Some of the modifications may overlap in individual diets. For example, a patient may be on a diabetic diet but because of acute indigestion or poor teeth he may also require a soft diet.

Diets must be flexible in order to be practical and usable. Therefore, it is impossible to divide diets into separate and distinct categories. The recommended dietary allowances for food constituents established for normal body requirements are considered, with amounts of nutrients adjusted to cover the needs created by disease or injury, when modifications in the diet are indicated.

The Principal Sources of Food Constituents

To be familiar with the various foods included in a diet, it is necessary to know their nutrient composition. For that reason, Table 19–7 was planned as an aid in learning the contents of various foods. Knowing the nutrients contained in different foods is essential for correctly evaluating therapeutic diets. Chapter 10, particularly Tables 10–6 and 10–7, may also be helpful. A more complete analysis of the nutrient content of foods can be found in Appendix Table 1.

Table 19–7. THE PRINCIPAL SOURCES OF THE VARIOUS FOOD CONSTITUENTS*

Daggers on the chart below give a rough idea of how servings from groups of familiar foods contribute toward dietary needs—the more daggers, the better the food as a source of the nutrient. The percentages given below the chart are based on the National Research Council's recommended dietary allowances for a young, moderately active man. Some foods within a group have more of a nutrient, some less; but in a varied diet, which is common in this country, a group is likely to average as shown.

KIND OF FOOD	SIZE OF SERVING (READY-TO-EAT)	PRO-TEIN	CAL-CIUM	IRON	VIT. A	B VITAMINS[a] THIA-MIN	B VITAMINS[a] RIBO-FLAVIN	B VITAMINS[a] NIACIN	VIT. C	KCAL.
Milk	1 cup	†	††††		†	†	††			165
Cheese, process Cheddar	1 oz.	†	†††		†		†			105
Meat, poultry, fish	4 oz.	††		††	†	†	†	††		195
Eggs	1 large	†		†	†		†			80
Dry beans and peas, nuts	¾ cup cooked	††	†	†††		†	†	†		170
Whole grain or enriched products	2 slices	†	†	†		†	†	†		120
Citrus fruits	½ cup								†††††	50
Other fruits	½ cup			†	†				†	60
Tomatoes, tomato juice	½ cup			†	†††			†	†††	25
Dark green and deep yellow vegetables (except sweet potatoes)	½ cup		†	†	†††††		†		††††	40
Sweet potatoes	1 medium	†	†	†††††	†	†	†	†††		170
Light green vegetables[b]	½ cup	†	†	†				††		35
Potatoes	1 medium	†		†			†	†††		90
Other vegetables	½ cup	†						†		40
Butter, margarine	1 tbsp.			†						100
Other fats	2 tbsp.									220
Sugar, all kinds	2 tsp.									35
Molasses, syrups	2 tbsp.		††							110

†††††More than 50 per cent of daily need.   †††About 30 per cent of daily need.
††††About 40 per cent of daily need.   ††About 20 per cent of daily need.
†About 10 per cent of daily need.

[a]Foods supplying thiamin, riboflavin and niacin are good sources of other members of the B vitamin group.

[b]Includes asparagus, green snap beans, peas, green lima beans, green cabbage, brussels sprouts, green lettuce.

*From: Family Fare: Food Management and Recipes. Home and Garden Bulletin No. 1. Washington, D.C., U.S. Department of Agriculture, 1960.

Nutritional Care for the Hospitalized Patient

In the early 1970's it was documented that many patients in U.S. hospitals are in poor nutritional status.[2] This is due to their disease or to their poor eating habits before hospitalization. An appalling additional observation was that the nutritional status of many patients deteriorated while they were in the hospital.[1, 3, 5] This can be due to unfamiliarity with the food served or to side effects of medications which may decrease appetite, cause nausea or increase the requirements for certain nutrients. It can be due to treatments, tests, surgery or inattention to nutritional needs on the part of the hospital staff. As a consequence of this startling documentation there is now much more attention to nutritional assessment of the hospitalized patient. Nutritional support of patients is more aggressive and there are many more specialized nutritional products available for clinicians to feed patients, as shown in Tables 35–7 and 35–8.

Food service is equally important in nutritional support. It requires imagination and ingenuity in planning for a variety of foods familiar to patients. The appearance of the food on the tray —its color, texture, composition and temperature—is very important to most people. Making food taste good is an important part of nutritional care.

FOOD INTAKE

An important observation for the nurse to make is that the food *served* does not necessarily represent the food *intake* of the patient.

One of the ways to prevent iatrogenic malnutrition in hospitals is to observe and record the patient's intake frequently and as accurately as possible. The nutrient content of each person's recorded food intake can be determined by using a specially programmed computer as described in Chapter 20, or the dietitian can manually calculate the composition of the food intake.

Regardless of the type of diet prescribed for a patient, it is important to check both the food served and the food left on the tray in order to obtain an accurate indication of the patient's energy and nutrient intake. This is very important and should not be overlooked.

NUTRITIONAL ADEQUACY OF STANDARD HOSPITAL DIETS

All hospitals and institutions engaged in feeding the sick have some specific, basic, routine diets designed for uniformity and convenience of service. These standard diets are based on the foundation of an adequate diet pattern such as that outlined in Table 10–8, which is formulated from the Recommended Dietary Allowances, as already discussed in this chapter. It is important that these diets be as flexible as possible in order to meet the often increased nutritional needs of hospitalized individuals.

The types of standard diets are usually referred to as *general, light, soft* and *liquid*. These diets are used routinely for patients with certain physical conditions. It is important for the nurse and dietitian to be familiar with the principles and contents of the various diets, since they serve as a foundation for the diversified therapeutic diets.

The General or Adequate Normal Diet

In some hospitals the general diet is also known as the "regular," "full" or "house" diet. The general diet is a basic adequate normal diet of approximately 1600 to 2200 kcal. and usually contains 60 to 80 gm. of protein, 80 to 100 gm. of fat and 180 to 300 gm. of carbohydrate. All the protective foods outlined in the foundation of an adequate diet pattern, Table 10–8, which includes the basic four food groups (meat, milk, eggs, citrus fruits, vegetables, whole grain or enriched breads and cereals) are included. Additional foods or more of the same food, such as butter or margarine, desserts, salad dressing, crackers and sugar, are added to increase calories and to make the diet more palatable. There are no particular food restrictions. However, foods that may cause digestive disturbances, such as gas-forming foods, are used with discretion. A few hospitals are instituting the prudent diet of the American Heart Association or the Dietary Goals listed in Table 17–7, which are low in saturated fat and cholesterol, as the general diet.

An example of an average general diet is shown in Table 19–8. In most hospitals the general diet may be selected by the patient from a menu of nutritious foods. This allows the patient to select foods that he or she likes, yet controls the adequacy of the diet to some extent.

The Soft or Light Diet

The soft or light diet such as the sample diet shown in Table 19–9 is used as a transition diet. It is an adequate diet that is moderately low in cellulose and connective tissue and fat. The soft diet is planned for conditions in which mechanical ease in eating or in digestion or both is desired. It is also a diet low in residue. It is good for patients who have few or no teeth or ill-fitting dental plates. It is most useful when the

Table 19–8. GENERAL OR ADEQUATE NORMAL DIET

MEAL PLAN	SAMPLE MENU	SERVINGS GRAMS	SERVINGS HOUSEHOLD MEASURE
Breakfast			
Fruit	Fresh grapefruit	100	1 half (no skin)
Cereal	Cooked oatmeal (cooked weight)	118	½ cup
Egg	Soft cooked egg	50	1
Bread	Whole wheat toast	23	1 slice
Butter	Butter or fortified margarine	7	1 pat
Milk	Milk	244	1 cup
Cream	Cream	60	2 oz.
Sugar	Sugar	15	3 tsp.
Coffee	Coffee	200	2 coffee cups
Lunch			
Soup	Beef broth with rice	125	½ cup
Crackers	Saltines	8	2
Entrée	Macaroni and cheese	110	½ cup
Vegetable	Cooked asparagus	96	6 spears
Salad	Tomato and watercress	100	1 serving
Salad dressing	French dressing	15	1 tbsp.
Bread	Whole wheat roll	30	1 average-size
Butter	Butter or fortified margarine	7	1 pat
Milk	Milk	244	1 glass
Fruit	Stewed royal Anne cherries	100	10 cherries with juice
Dinner			
Meat	London broil	85	3 oz.
Potato	Stuffed baked potato	150	1 medium
Vegetable	Savory green beans	75	½ cup
Bread	Rye bread	23	1 slice
Butter	Butter or fortified margarine	7	1 pat
Dessert	Strawberry ice cream	62	1 average scoop (3½ oz. or ½ cup)
Milk	Milk	244	1 glass

patient's tolerance is the guide for inclusion of foods in the diet.

The average composition of the soft diet is 1800 to 2000 kcal. However, the energy as well as the protein, fat and carbohydrate allowances are adjustable according to the individual's needs, based on activity, height, weight, sex, age and any specific demands caused by disease.

The trend in diet planning fosters liberal interpretation of the soft diet, particularly with regard to vegetables and whole grain breads and cereals. Table 19–12 lists the foods included in a soft diet.

Liquid Diets

Liquid diets are commonly ordered for patients with conditions requiring easily digested and easily consumed nourishment that is free from mechanical irritants and irritating condiments or that has minimal residue. Patients who have chewing or swallowing difficulties or dental wiring may also require a liquid diet.

The two varieties of liquid diets are the full liquid diet and the clear or restricted liquid diet.

FULL LIQUID DIET. The full liquid diet such as that shown in Table 19–10, uses all foods that are liquid at room or body temperature. For example, ice cream is considered a liquid.

The diet, if properly designed and *consumed*, may be considered adequate for maintenance requirements, except with regard to fiber. The average composition of the diet is approximately 1300 to 1500 kcal., 45 gm. of protein, 65 gm. of fat and 150 gm. of carbohydrate. By careful planning, the diet can be increased in protein and caloric value to approach the normal diet or even a high-calorie diet. Increasing the protein and energy in a liquid diet is necessary when a patient must remain on such a diet for an indefinite period. Protein and vitamin supplements as listed in Table 35–8 can be added to the liquids to increase the protein and vitamin intake.

Full liquid diets can be planned to meet the needs of a patient with diabetes, renal disease

Table 19-9. SOFT OR LIGHT DIET

		SERVINGS	
MEAL PLAN	SAMPLE MENU	GRAMS	HOUSEHOLD MEASURE
Breakfast			
Fruit	Orange juice	124	½ glass
Cereal	Cooked farina (cooked weight)	119	½ cup
Egg	Poached egg on toast	50	1
Bread	Toasted bread (enriched)	23	1 slice
Butter	Butter or fortified margarine	7	1 pat
Cream	Cream	60	2 oz.
Milk	Milk	244	1 cup
Sugar	Sugar	15	3 tsp.
Coffee	Coffee	200	2 coffee cups
Lunch			
Soup	Tomato consommé	120	½ cup
Entrée	Baked macaroni and cheese	110	½ cup
Vegetables	Cooked asparagus tips or purée	96	6 spears
Bread	Light rye bread	23	1 slice
Butter	Butter or fortified margarine	7	1 pat
Fruit	Applesauce	127	½ cup
Milk	Milk	244	1 glass
Dinner			
Meat	Sliced chicken	85	3 oz.
Potato	Mashed potato	98	½ cup
Vegetable	Buttered spinach purée	90	½ cup
Bread	Light rye bread	23	1 slice
Butter	Butter or fortified margarine	7	1 pat
Dessert	Chocolate ice cream	62	1 average scoop (3½ oz. or ½ cup)
Milk	Milk	244	1 glass

Table 19-10. FULL LIQUID DIET—SAMPLE MENU*

A.M.

1/2 cup orange juice
1 cup farina with 2 tsp. fortified margarine, 1 tsp. sugar, and milk
Coffee or tea with sugar
1 cup pasteurized eggnog[†]

Between Meals

1 cup pasteurized eggnog[†]

Noon

1/2 cup apricot nectar
1 cup cream of potato soup with fortified margarine or butter
1 cup milk
1/2 cup Bavarian cream
Coffee or tea with sugar

Between Meals

Blenderized milkshake with 4 oz. milk, 2 tsp. chocolate syrup, 2 oz. ice cream (plain), and 2 tsp. sugar

P.M.

1/2 cup pineapple juice
1 cup strained cream of vegetable soup with 1 tsp. fortified margarine or butter
1 cup milk or pasteurized eggnog[†]
1/2 cup caramel custard
Coffee or tea with sugar

Bedtime

1/2 cup lemon gelatin
1 cup pasteurized eggnog

* To increase the calories, sugar, cream, butter, margarine or high-calorie supplements should be added whenever possible.
† Eggnog that is prepared in powdered form and mixed with milk. This avoids the use of raw eggs, which is not recommended owing to possible *Salmonella* poisoning and avidin binding of biotin.
(From American Dietetic Association: Handbook of Clinical Dietetics. New Haven, Yale University Press, 1981.)

or any other disorder. For the lactose-intolerant patient this is more difficult because the diet is usually based on milk as the protein source. One of the lactose-free products should be used. A fluid restriction might also make the full liquid diet inadequate because only a limited amount of it will be consumed. In this situation the liquids used should be very nutritious and highly concentrated.

Because this diet is inadequate in fiber, constipation may result from its prolonged use.

CLEAR OR RESTRICTED LIQUID DIET. The clear or restricted liquid diet such as that listed in Table 19–11 is frequently ordered for postoperative patients to furnish fluids, some electrolytes and small amounts of energy prior to the return of gastrointestinal function. It is an *inadequate* diet composed chiefly of water and carbohydrates; therefore, it is used a *very short time*. The average clear or restricted liquid diet contains 400 to 500 kcal., 5 to 10 gm. of protein, no fat and 100 to 120 gm. of carbohydrate.

The clear liquid diet composed of gelatin and sweetened beverages cannot replace the electrolytes lost in vomitus and diarrheal fluid. However, one bouillon cube contains 424 mg. of sodium, so a serving of bouillon can be a significant replacement for sodium losses.

The liquid is served at frequent intervals to supply the tissues with fluid and to relieve thirst. As the name indicates, the diet consists of clear liquids such as tea, broth, carbonated beverages, strained fruit juice and gelatin (liquid at body temperature). Milk and liquids prepared with milk are omitted. Some patients' stomachs become distended and very uncomfortable if they are given fruit juice, especially orange juice. Fruit juices that do not agree with the patient are omitted from the diet. Carbonated beverages, especially ginger ale, seem to be tolerated by the majority of patients. As usual, the diet is planned with due consideration to the patient's food preferences.

When a *nutritious* clear liquid is needed, an appropriate liquid elemental diet can be selected from Table 35–7.

Table 19–12 provides a summary of the basic hospital diets.

Psychological Factors in Feeding the Sick Person

Throughout the text an effort is made to bring out the psychological factors in feeding the sick. The three daily meals and between-

Table 19–11. CLEAR OR RESTRICTED LIQUID DIET

| | | SERVINGS | |
MEAL PLAN	SAMPLE MENU	Grams	Household Measure
	Breakfast		
Fruit juice	Orange juice (strained)	124	½ cup
Beverage	Coffee (decaffeinated)	200	2 coffee cups
Sugar	Sugar	10	2 tsp.
	10:00 A.M.		
Fruitade	Lemonade	240	1 cup
	Lunch		
Soup	Consommé	120	½ cup
Fruit juice	Grapefruit juice (strained)	123	½ glass
Tea	Tea	200	2 teacups
Sugar	Sugar	10	2 tsp.
	3:00 P.M.		
Carbonated beverage	Ginger ale	230	1 cup
	Dinner		
Soup	Chicken broth	125	½ cup
Gelatin	Raspberry gelatin	60	¼ cup
Tea	Tea	200	2 teacups
Sugar	Sugar	10	2 tsp.
	8:00 P.M.		
Fruit juice	Orange juice (strained)	248	1 cup

Table 19–12. SUMMARY OF BASIC HOSPITAL DIETS

FOOD	GENERAL OR ADEQUATE NORMAL DIET	SOFT OR LIGHT DIET	FULL LIQUID DIET	CLEAR LIQUID DIET
Milk, cream, buttermilk	Included.	Included.	Included.	Not included.
Eggs	Raw and cooked.	Included.	In beverages.	Not included.
Cheese	All varieties.	Cottage, pot, cream, mild American, Cheddar.	Not allowed.	Not included.
Fats	All kinds.	Butter, fortified margarine, oil, mayonnaise and French dressing.	Butter, fortified margarine, oil.	Not included.
Meat, fish, poultry	All included.	Ground and tender beef, lamb, veal; liver, bacon, fish, poultry.	Not allowed.	Not included.
Vegetables	All included.	Cooked vegetables of low fiber; lettuce and tomato salad; potatoes boiled, mashed, baked, creamed, scalloped; vegetable juices.	Vegetable juices, vegetable purée used in soups.	Vegetable water.
Fruits	All included.	Fruit juices, ripe bananas, cooked fruit without skin or seeds.	Fruit juices, fruitades.	Strained fruit juices, fruitades.
Breads	All varieties.	Fine whole grain, rye without seeds, enriched white, refined crackers.	Not allowed.	Not included.
Cereals	All varieties.	Refined; finely ground.	Cooked gruel.	Not included.
Cereal products	All varieties.	Cooked macaroni, spaghetti, noodles, rice.	Not allowed.	Not included.
Soups	All varieties.	Clear broth, consommé, strained cream and vegetable soups.	Clear broth, consommé; strained vegetable and cream soups.	Clear broth and consommé.
Beverages	All kinds.	All kinds.	Tea, decaffeinated coffee; carbonated beverages; eggnog.	Tea, decaffeinated coffee; carbonated beverages.
Desserts	All kinds.	Plain puddings, simple cakes and cookies; frozen desserts without nuts; custard, gelatin, milk-rennet pudding.	Plain gelatin dessert, ice cream without nuts and seeds; ices, sherbets, milk-rennet pudding, soft custard.	Plain gelatin desserts and ices.
Other			Liquid supplements listed in Table 35–8.	Elemental liquids such as shown in Table 35–7.

meal nourishments are often highlights of the day and are looked forward to by the patient, so the nurse and dietitian should attempt to make mealtime a pleasant experience. A comfortable temperature in a room free of drafts, a comfortable eating position in bed or on a chair located away from unpleasant sights, and pleasant conversation or music encourage good food intake. Most patients prefer to wash their hands and faces before eating and to eat from a table that is free of other objects.

The arrangement of the tray should reflect thoughtfulness and consideration of the patient's needs and wishes. The china, glassware and silver on the tray should be in a convenient location and within the patient's reach. Independence should be encouraged in patients who require assistance in eating. The nurse can accomplish this by having patients specify the sequence of foods to be eaten and by having them participate in eating, even if only by holding their bread.

A *patient's attitude* toward his illness and hospitalization frequently is reflected in the rejection of meals or the prescribed diet. Other reasons for poor acceptance of hospital meals may be unfamiliar foods and eating schedule and improper food temperatures. By giving patients an opportunity to express themselves and by accepting their attitudes, the nurse can help patients overcome their feelings and improve their acceptance of the hospital food. Food acceptance is also improved when selection of menus by the patients themselves is encouraged and when patients are given an explanation of why a particular diet has been prescribed. Problems with food acceptance that the nurse cannot handle should be communicated to the clinical dietitian.

If the nurse will take the time to encourage patients and show interest in their food, the result will often be most rewarding. Patients' acceptance of their diet is closely related to the nurse's attitude toward it. It is no more necessary to convince patients that they *like* their diets than it is to convince them that they *like* unpalatable medication. There is every need, however, to approach the patients and win their confidence so that they will accept the diet. The nurse who is convinced that the diet contributes to the restoration of her patients' health will communicate this conviction to them by her actions, her facial expressions and her conversation. Patients who understand that the diet contributes to the success of their medical or surgical therapy will usually accept it more willingly. In this capacity the nurse serves as an interpreter of the therapeutic diet.

When patients must adhere to a therapeutic dietary program indefinitely, the nurse may need to confer with the dietitian, the social worker or the community health nurse. She may want to bring the members of the health team together to help patients resolve their nutritional problems. In this role the nurse is a coordinator.

During the course of nursing care the nurse comes in contact with many individuals who do not require a therapeutic dietary program. Informal opportunities for discussing nutrition principles with all patients are often available, especially with those individuals receiving regular diets. Frequently, and usually most effectively, the nurse and dietitian can combine their skills to teach groups of patients normal nutrition or dietary modification for a disorder. Classes on diets for coronary artery disease, diabetes and hypertension have been developed. Support groups for patients with cancer, renal disease, ileostomies or other debilitating diseases can make their total care including their nutritional care more acceptable and feasible.

Problems and Suggested Topics for Discussion

1. Describe the nutritional care process.
2. What is meant by routine house diets and what purpose do they serve? What are their (a) advantages and (b) disadvantages or limitations?
3. Compare diets served in the hospital where you are located with those outlined in this chapter. If there are any differences between the diets, justify the discrepancy.
4. Plan a full liquid diet for a 46-year-old female patient requiring 2000 kcalories. Check with recommended allowances for adequacy.
5. List the foods usually allowed on a clear liquid diet. How adequate is a clear liquid diet? Why is it not necessary that the diet meet requirements for nutritional adequacy?
6. Discuss the conditions (diagnosis of patient, hospital management) for which it is advantageous to use the soft diet.
7. Discuss the advantages and disadvantages of the current trend for more liberal treatment and management of various diet plans.
8. List the psychological factors to be considered when feeding the sick. How can the nurse and dietitian help?
9. Design a nutritional care plan for a patient, including assessment, objectives, nutritional interventions and evaluation. What criteria will you use to evaluate the nutritional care? Did the patient meet the objectives?

Cited References

1. Bistrian, B.R., et al.: Protein status of general surgical patients. JAMA, *230*:858, 1974.
2. Bollet, A.J., and Owens, S.: Evaluation of nutritional status of selected hospitalized patients. Am. J. Clin. Nutr., *26*:931, 1973.
3. Butterworth, C.E., Jr.: The skeleton in the hospital closet. Nutr. Today, *9*(2):4, 1974.
4. Ghadimi, H. (ed.): Total Parenteral Nutrition: Premises and Promises. New York, John Wiley and Sons, 1975, p. 190.
5. Hill, G.L., et al.: Malnutrition in surgical patients: an unrecognized problem. Lancet, *1*:689, 1977.
6. Select Committee on Nutrition and Human Needs, U.S. Senate: Dietary Goals for the United States. Washington, D.C., U.S. Government Printing Office, 1977.
7. Wade, J.E.: Role of a clinical dietitian specialist on a nutrition support service. J. Am. Diet. Assoc., *70*:185, 1977.

Additional References

American Dietetic Association: Handbook of Clinical Dietetics. New Haven, Yale University Press, 1981.

American Hospital Association: Recording Nutritional Information in Medical Records. Chicago, American Hospital Association, 1976.

Bistrian, B.R., et al.: Prevalence of malnutrition in general medical patients. JAMA, *235*:1567, 1976.

Chicago Dietetic Association and South Suburban Dietetic Association: Manual of Clinical Dietetics. 2nd ed. Philadelphia, W.B. Saunders Company, 1981.

Cooper, L.F.: Florence Nightingale's contribution to dietetics. J. Am. Diet. Assoc., *30*:121, 1954.

Cousins, N.: Anatomy of an illness (as perceived by the patient). N. Engl. J. Med., *295*:1458, 1976.

Davis, J., and Hodges, R.E.: A "new" approach to diet therapy. Dietetic Currents, *1*(5), 1974. (Published by Ross Laboratories, Columbus, Ohio.)

Food and Nutrition Board, National Research Council: Recommended Dietary Allowances, 9th ed. Washington, D.C., National Academy of Sciences, 1980.

Goodhart, R.S., and Shils, M.E. (eds.): Modern Nutrition in Health and Disease, 6th ed. Philadelphia, Lea & Febiger, 1980.

Goodhue, P.J., Collins, M.E., and Baumgarten, S.: Continuing nutritional care for the discharged patient. Dietetic Currents, *3*(1), 1976.

Hegsted, D.M.: Nutritional requirements in disease. J. Am. Diet. Assoc., *56*:303, 1970.

Kocher, R.E.: Monitoring nutritional care of the long-term patient. J. Am. Diet. Assoc., *67*:45, 1975.

Mason, M., Wenberg, B.G., and Welsh, P. K.: The Dynamics of Clinical Dietetics. 2nd ed. New York, John Wiley and Sons, 1982.

Mayo Clinic: Mayo Clinic Diet Manual. 5th ed. Philadelphia, W.B. Saunders Company, 1981.

Selye, H.: On just being sick. Nutr. Today, *5*:2, 1970.

Weinsier, R.L., et al.: Hospital malnutrition: a prospective evaluation of general medical patients during course of hospitalization. Am. J. Clin. Nutr., *32*:418, 1979.

CHAPTER 20

The Computer in Nutritional Care

CHEDWAH J. STEIN, M.S., R.D.

Technological Development

People have always used tools to enhance their skills. Some of these are communication tools, like paper, the printing press, the telegraph and telephone, radio and television. Other tools are used for calculation, like the abacus and calculator. The computer has added a new dimension to both these functions. It is able to store large amounts of data, modify and analyze these data and present the resulting information very rapidly.

Computers are now used in many ways and new uses are continually being developed. Health care institutions are among the many that are making use of the advantages offered by the use of computers.

Use of Computers in Nutrition Services

MASTER MENU AND RECIPE FILES. The general and special diet menu cycles and the recipes of a hospital, nursing home or health care facility can be stored in a computer. They can be adjusted for seasonal and price changes, analyzed for nutritional content, and printed out as needed, as shown in Figure 20–1. With a computer, menus, recipes and foods needed for meal production can be printed daily. Purchasing can be made easier by summarizing foods needed for menu production for a week or a month, and these summaries can be used to control the food inventory. Food specifications can also be stored in the computer.[2]

NUTRIENT DATA. Nutrient data can be stored in a data file and used to calculate the nutrient content of menus, recipes and patients' individual food intake.[3] Figure 20–2 shows a printout of such data.

NUTRITIONAL ASSESSMENT. Methods and formulas to determine individual patient needs can be stored. A list of drugs and their nutritional implications, a list of normal and abnormal laboratory values with implications, and tables to evaluate height, weight and skinfold data can all be stored in the computer. Computer programs can compare an individual patient's data with the stored information and produce a nutritional assessment. These data need to be reviewed and interpreted by a qualified health professional, however, as a check on the accuracy of the results.[1, 5]

PATIENT INFORMATION. Relevant patient information can be stored in a master computer file and protected by a code to ensure privacy. Patients' diet orders can be entered into the file, as can such other information as the nutritional assessment, dietary intake, lifestyle factors that affect the diet, the nutritional care plan, and follow-up data to use for future planning. When patient orders are received, revisions can be quickly made in diet tallies, and food production and inventory information can be adjusted immediately.

PATIENT SERVICES. Thus a patient's personalized menu can be made easily available for the nurse or dietitian working with the patient. These menus can be adjusted for individual needs and food preferences.

PATIENT EDUCATION. Material for patient education also can be stored in the computer, adjusted to an individual patient's needs, and

DEPARTMENT OF NUTRITION AND DIETETICS--UMMC
MASTER MENU
WEEK 1 / 1 / 1 / 1

MONDAY   BREAKFAST   HOT

RECIPE NO	RECIPE NAME	G	S	LC	NA	LCNA	CO	MR	REN	P	CL	FL	CA	MM	SIZE/ PT SVG
PASTRY															
840629	DONUT CAKE, CAFE	X	X	.	.	.	.	.	X	X	.	.	C	P	51
890758	HOT CAKES	.	.	.	.	.	.	.	.	.	.	.	C	.	52
890456	TOAST FRENCH	.	.	.	.	.	.	.	.	.	.	.	C	.	102
090280	BISCUIT BAKING POWDER	.	.	.	.	.	.	.	.	.	.	.	C	.	64
ENTREES															
110850	EGGS SCRAMBLED MIX	U	X	X	.	.	.	X	H	.	.	.	C	X	65
111503	EGGS SCRAMBLED MIX LS	.	.	.	X	X	X	.	X	.	.	.	.	X	65
110108	BACON	U	.	X	.	.	.	X	H	.	.	.	C	X	15
110302	EGGS FRIED	.	.	.	.	.	.	.	.	.	.	.	C	P	51
110353	EGGS HARD COOKED	.	.	.	.	.	.	.	.	.	.	.	C	.	60
110833	OMELET HAM AND CHEESE	.	.	.	.	.	.	.	.	.	.	.	C	.	113
CEREAL, STARCH, GRAVIES															
120341	FARINA	X	X	X	.	.	.	X	.	X	.	X	X	X	120
121100	FARINA LS	.	.	.	X	X	X	.	X	.	.	.	.	X	120
400360	POTATO HASH BROWN DEHY	.	.	.	.	.	.	.	.	.	.	.	C	.	80
CONDIMENTS															
980285	GRAPE JELLY	U	X	.	X	.	X	.	X	H	.	.	.	P	14
130109	HONEY	.	.	.	.	.	.	.	.	.	.	.	.	.	15
BREADS															
800406	TOAST PLAIN	U	X	X	.	.	.	X	H	.	.	.	.	P	24

Figure 20–1. Computers are used to process menu data to facilitate food service cost control and patient care. This master menu computer printout is generated from the master menu file which contains such data as day, meal, temperature, menu category (entrée, salad, etc.) and texture modification. Diet categories are: G= general; S= simple; LC= low calorie; NA= low sodium; LCNA= low calorie and sodium; CO= coronary; MR= Minimum residue; REN= Renal; P= Pediatric; CL= clear liquid; FL= Full liquid; CA= Cafeteria. (Courtesy of Loretta W. Hoover, Ph.D., Department of Nutrition and Dietetics, University of Missouri Medical Center, Columbia, Missouri. Discussed in Hoover, L.W. et al.: Development of on-line real-time menu management system. J. Am. Diet. Assoc., 80:46, 1982.)

printed with the patient's name. "Interactive" patient education packages exist for computer use in hospitals, outpatient clinics and doctors' or dietitians' offices, as shown in Figure 20–3. Patients can use these programs to learn about the effect of different food choices on their diet. They can learn the basic principles of their diet selection before seeing a counselor, and the counselor will then be able to focus on the patient's questions and specific needs and concerns as discussed in Chapter 18.

QUALITY ASSURANCE. The latest nutrition information for use by staff and patients can be stored in the computer and updated as needed. Nutrition protocols can be stored in the computer and viewed by dietitians and nurses as needed. If the members of the health team all have access to the same protocols, patient care will be integrated and cohesive. Patient care plans can be entered in the patient's file, as can follow-up notes. Good, permanent, readily accessi-

ble records will enhance patient care and its evaluation.[4]

Skills Needed to Use the Computer Effectively

Computer analysts and programmers use a special language, and communication is easier if the professional is familiar with the terms defined in Table 20–1. The additional readings at the end of this chapter will help with learning this terminology. While it is not necessary to be able to program to use the computer, it is important to be able to outline the tasks required of the computer. Any task that involves manipulation of large amounts of data can best be handled by a computer. On the other hand, computer use is too costly for a task that will only occur once. Listing and ranking tasks will

```
                  NUTRITION & DIET SERVICES - CHEDWAH STEIN
JENNIFER LAUGHLIN: 3-DAY FOOD RECORD ANALYSIS:MAY 1983
FOOD GROUP TOTALS
NUTRIENT          UNITS CONTRIBUTED       AVERAGE   %        UNITS/KG    UNITS/CM
DESCRIPTION      DAY 1   DAY 2   DAY 3    UNITS    RDA       BDY WGHT    BDY WGHT

WATER       GM   1476    1584    812      1291               83.1        16.2
ENERGY      CAL  1386    852     788      1009     78        64.9        12.6
PROTEIN     GM   93      59      43       65       283       4.2         0.8
FAT         GM   59      25      27       37                 2.4         0.5
CARBOHYDRT  GM   122     101     101      108                6.9         1.4
FIBER       GM   13      10      6        10                 0.6         0.1
CALCIUM     MG   1229    1002    654      962      120       61.9        12.1
PHOSPHORUS  MG   1596    960     774      1110     139       71.5        13.9
IRON        MG   17      15      15       16       104       1.0         0.2
SODIUM      MG   3362    1162    725      1749               112.6       21.9
POTASSIUM   MG   3417    2467    1754     2546               163.9       31.9
MAGNSM      MG   182     88      69       113      75        7.3         1.4
COPPER      MG   0       0       0        0                  0.0         0.0
ZINC        MG   8       4       3        5        49        0.3         0.1
VIT A       IU   10676   9348    9647     9890     495       636.6       123.9
VIT D       IU   212     180     124      172      43        11.1        2.2
THIAMIN     MCG  954     761     559      758      108       48.8        9.5
RIBOFLAVIN  MCG  1868    1625    1152     1548     194       99.7        19.4
NIACIN      MG   16      12      9        12       137       0.8         0.2
ASC.ACID    MG   159     138     84       127      282       8.2         1.6
PANT.ACID   MG   1715    1747    928      1463               94.2        18.3
VIT B6      MCG  395     280     57       244      27        15.7        3.1
VIT B12     MCG  3       3       2        3        130       0.2         0.0
FOLIC ACID  MCG  267     237     120      208      208       13.4        2.6
HISTIDINE   MG   1616    1025    550      1064               68.5        13.3
ISOLEUCINE  MG   4146    3167    2233     3182               204.8       39.9
LEUCINE     MG   6275    4743    3320     4780               307.7       59.9
LYSINE      MG   5809    2978    1504     3431               220.8       43.0
TYROSINE    MG   3218    2293    1656     2389               153.8       29.9
PHENYLANAL  MG   3457    2713    2108     2759               177.6       34.6
THREONINE   MG   3339    1723    970      2011               129.4       25.2
TRYPTOPHNE  MG   1303    583     312      732                47.1        9.2
VALINE      MG   4453    3552    2554     3520               226.6       44.1
CYSTINE     MG   892     467     308      555                35.7        7.0
METHIONINE  MG   2040    1359    844      1414               91.0        17.7
SAT.F.ACID  GM   16      6       5        9                  0.6         0.1
MONO UN FA  GM   14      6       7        9                  0.6         0.1
LINOLEIC    GM   15      2       4        7                  0.4         0.1
POLY UN FA  GM   16      2       4        7                  0.5         0.1
CHOLESTERL  MG   492     334     286      371                23.9        4.6
LACTOSE     GM   26      24      15       22                 1.4         0.3
SUCROSE     GM   0       0       4        1                  0.1         0.0
SUGAR,TOTL  GM   26      24      19       23                 1.5         0.3

TOTAL COST       2.050   1.980   1.730

% CALORIES FROM PROTEIN: 25.4
% CALORIES FROM FAT: 32.6
% CALORIES FROM CARBOHYDRATES: 42.0
% CALORIES FROM ALCOHOL  0.0
RATIO U.F.A./ S.F.A. :   0.779
```

Figure 20–2. Computerized nutritional analysis of a three-day food record. Note that the daily average is determined for each nutrient and is stated based on the person's height and weight and as a percentage of the Recommended Dietary Allowances (RDA).

assist in making cost-effective decisions about their computerization.

In addition, health care professionals need to communicate the final form they wish the data

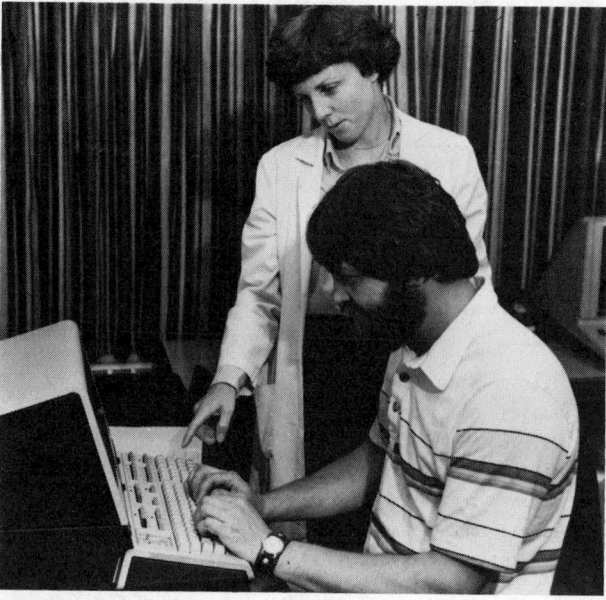

Figure 20–3. A nutritionist showing a patient how he can analyze his diet for its nutritional composition using a computer.

to take. Designing a form or "printout" is often the joint task of the user and the programmer.

The computer offers many advantages to the health professional, and as more is learned about how to use it effectively, more improvements in provision of care and greater time savings will be realized.

Table 20–1. COMPUTER TERMINOLOGY

Address	The number that defines a location in computer memory.
Algorithm	A set of instructions that directs the computer to accomplish a task.
Bit	The smallest unit of memory in the computer.
Bug	An error in a computer program.
Byte	A unit of memory consisting of 8 bits.
Compiler	Translates a more understandable set of instructions written in a higher level language such as Basic or Fortran into machine language that the computer understands.
CPU	The central processor unit. That part of the computer that controls the execution of machine language statements and performs all calculations.
CRT	A Cathode Ray Tube, similar to TV screen, that displays data per program instructions.
Data base	Set of information for a specific purpose, stored in the computer memory from which the computer can extract data and use it to solve a specific problem.
Debugging	Locating and removing errors from a computer program.
Disk	A type of magnetic recording medium used for storing data.
Hardware	Physical components of a computer complex.
Input	Data entered into the computer.
I/O devices	Computer components involved with input and output of data.
Memory	A device which accepts, stores and remits data values.
Menu	A list of programs.
Modem	A device that enables a computer to communicate with other computers via ordinary telephone lines.
Output	The transfer of data from the computer to various peripheral devices for display.
Program	A set of instructions written in a programming language which tells the computer how to perform a task.
Programming language	A language used to express an algorithm in a set of instructions.
Software	A program or collection of programs, user guides, and program documentation.
Storage devices	Memory devices that are not in the main computer, e.g., magnetic tape, disks.
Word processing	Using the computer to input, edit, store, output and transmit textual data.

Cited References

1. Danford, D.E.: Computer applications to medical nutrition problems. JPEN, 5:441, 1981.
2. Ford, M.G., and Wesley, N.W.: Dietitians improve patient care with computerized selective menus. Hospitals, 53:76, 1979.
3. Hoover, L., and Perloff, B.: Models for Review of Nutrient Data Base System Capabilities. Columbia, University of Missouri, 1981.
4. Lakness, J.A., and Doyle, M.K.: Computer assisted revision of a community diet manual. J. Am. Diet. Assoc., 76:477, 1980.
5. Rich, J.A.: A Programmable calculator system for the estimation of nutritional intake of hospital patients. Am. J. Clin. Nutr., 34:2276, 1981.

Additional References

Caldwell, R.: The computer as a teaching tool. Journal of Home Economics, 74:45, 1982.
Freiberger, S., and Chew, P.: A Consumer's Guide to Personal Computing and Microcomputers. Rochelle Park, N. J., Hayden Book Company, 1978.
Graham, N.: The Mind Tool. St. Paul, West Publishing Company, 1980.
Guley, H.M., and Stimson, J.P.: Computer simulation for production scheduling in a ready food system. J. Am. Diet. Assoc., 76:482, 1980.
Hoover, L.: Computer in Nutrition, Dietetics & Food Service Management. Columbia, University of Missouri, 1981.
Lambert, C.U., and Beach, B.L.: Computerized scheduling for cook/freeze food production plans. J. Am. Diet. Assoc., 77:174, 1980.
Maloff, C., and Zears, R.: Computers in Nutrition. Dedham, Mass., Artech, 1980.
Miller, J.W.: Computers for Everybody. 2nd ed. Beaverton, Ore., Dilithium Press, 1983.
Science, Vol. 215, No. 4534 Special Issue on Computers, Feb. 12, 1982.
Toong, H.D., and Gupta, A.: Personal computers. Sci. Am., 476(6):87, 1982.
Tuthill, B.H.: Dietitians use computer assistance to contain costs. J. Am. Diet. Assoc., 76:479, 1980.
Willard, R.: Computers in Dietetics. Dietetic Currents, 9(3), May-June, 1982.

CHAPTER 21

The Interactions Between Drugs, Nutrients and Nutritional Status

The management of many diseases today requires long-term care and drug therapy. In this situation, one of the factors that deserves attention is the interactions between drugs and the nutrient intake and nutritional status of the individual taking those drugs. Previously this was little appreciated, and it is still poorly understood. Both the side effects and the therapeutic effects of a drug can affect a person's nutrient intake, metabolism and requirements and ultimately, his nutritional status. Just as important, food and the nutrients in it can affect the action of a drug by altering its absorption, metabolism and excretion. When administering a drug, it is important to note its action and side effects in terms of nutritional implications. Some drugs have been reported as inducing actual clinical deficiency states in humans; others have caused decreased serum levels of certain nutrients; while still others have caused nutritional changes in animals only, and there is no evidence about their nutritional effects in humans.

Drug-induced malnutrition is most likely to develop in those patients receiving long-term drug therapy who take medication for the control of a chronic disease for many years. Children, the elderly and the chronically ill are most vulnerable. Clinical nutritional deficiency states related to drug ingestion are usually the result of a *combination of factors*. A nutritional deficiency is more likely to occur in those patients who have a marginal nutritional status before the drug is prescribed. If the nutritional status and the present intake are good, the patient is not as likely to become nutritionally deficient. Patients who have a catabolic disease, weight losses of 10 per cent or more of their ideal body weight, poor dietary intakes (alcoholics, for example), chronic disease of the gastrointestinal tract or increased nutritional requirements as a result of recent major surgery or infection, are more likely to be put into nutritional jeopardy by the use of certain drugs. If patients in these categories are then placed on long-term drug therapy, it becomes especially important to assess their dietary intakes and nutritional status and, if necessary, to institute preventive or rehabilitative measures such as providing additional food or vitamin and mineral supplements along with the drug therapy. An increased requirement for nutrients can usually be met by supplementation. Table 21–1 presents the effects of selected drugs on the major nutrients.

It is useful to categorize the interactions of drugs and nutrients into (1) those by which drugs affect the body's intake, absorption, metabolism and requirements for nutrients and (2) those in which nutrients, foods or poor nutritional status affects the absorption, metabolism, action and excretion of drugs.

The Effects of Drugs on Nutrient Intake, Absorption, Metabolism and Requirements

The effects of drugs on nutritional status can also be classified into various types of actions: (1) alteration of food intake, (2) alteration of nutrient absorption, (3) alteration of nutrient metabolism and utilization and (4) alteration of nutrient excretion, as summarized in Table 21–2.

DRUGS THAT AFFECT THE INTAKE OF FOOD AND NUTRIENTS

Drugs can affect the intake of food and nutrients either through a side effect accompanying their required action, or as the reason for their administration. An example that immediately comes to mind is the anorectic agents used to *diminish appetite* and thus the quantity of food consumed. These are used most often to aid in weight reduction. Because most of these agents are amphetamines and act on the central nervous system (CNS) to depress the appetite, they have several side effects, one of which is hyperactivity. The individual usually develops a tolerance to the drug's appetite-depressive effect after about 10 days, and consequently the use of such drugs for weight reduction should be only for a short time.

These same drugs are used to control behavioral difficulties in hyperactive children. Paradoxically, in hyperactive children the amphetamine dextroamphetamine and the structurally related compound methylphenidate have a calming effect. However, their use has been shown to cause growth retardation in children who take them for several months or longer.[28] When the medication is discontinued during the summer, a child grows faster than normal and experiences some "catch-up" growth.[29] Dextroamphetamine (Dexedrine) seems to have a greater growth-retarding effect than methylphenidate (Ritalin). Possibly this growth retardation is a result of the decreased food intake associated with the drug-induced appetite depression. Lucas and Sells studied two hyperactive boys and found reduced nutritional intakes on those days when the boys were taking drugs.[19] These reductions were enough to have caused the depressed growth in these children, and their findings suggest that some children may never develop a tolerance to the appetite-depressing effects of amphetamines. Ways to plan meals around the drug therapy and thus to increase the energy intake of these children are given in the article by Lucas and Sells.[19]

Some of the tranquilizing drugs such as chlorpromazine and lithium carbonate can lead to an increase in body weight. It is thought that these agents cause an increase in appetite secondary to their alteration of mental status or effect on the CNS. This effect is non-specific, but patients taking these drugs who have a weight gain should be evaluated and possibly the drug dosage should be reduced. Numerous other drugs decrease the appetite as a side effect of their action, and this should always be appreciated when they are administered. Information on the side effects of a particular drug usually states whether the appetite is affected.

Another side effect of drugs that affects the

Table 21–1. NUTRIENTS SIGNIFICANTLY AFFECTED BY SELECTED DRUGS

NUTRIENT	DRUG ACTION	DRUGS
Vitamin B_6	Function as vitamin B_6 antagonists or increase the turnover of B_6 in the body.	Isoniazid, cycloserine and other antituberculous drugs. Hydralazine. Penicillamine. L-Dopa. Oral contraceptives. Alcohol.

Table 21–1.   NUTRIENTS SIGNIFICANTLY AFFECTED BY SELECTED DRUGS (*Continued*)

NUTRIENT	DRUG ACTION	DRUGS
Folic Acid	Function as folic acid antagonists; affect the absorption of folic acid or increase the turn-over or loss of folate from the body.	Para-aminosalicylic acid. Methotrexate. Pyrimethamine. Isoniazid. Anticonvulsants. Triamterene. Trimethoprim. Oral contraceptives. Cycloserine. Salicylazosulfapyridine Acetylsalicylic acid. Pentamidine. Alcohol.
Vitamin B_{12}	Affect the absorption of vitamin B_{12}.	Neomycin. Biguanides. Para-aminosalicylic acid. Cholestyramine. Potassium chloride. Alcohol.
Niacin	By antagonizing Vitamin B_6, cause depletion, because vitamin B_6 is a necessary coenzyme in the synthesis of niacin from tryptophan.	Isoniazid.
Riboflavin	Decreases riboflavin absorption by increasing G.I. motility.	Thyroxine.
	Displaces riboflavin from plasma binding site and causes hyperexcretion of riboflavin.	Boric acid.
Thiamin	Impairs absorption of thiamin or impairs the formation of the coenzyme form of the vitamin.	Alcohol.
	Increase requirements.	Digitalis alkaloids.
Ascorbic Acid	Decrease the absorption or stimulate the metabolism of the vitamin.	Oral contraceptives.
	Deplete the tissues of the vitamin.	Acetylsalicylic acid. Alcohol. Anorectic agents. Anticonvulsants. Tetracycline.
	Depletes adrenal ascorbic acid.	Adrenal corticosteroids.
Vitamin A	Acts as a solvent for carotene and vitamin A and thus prevents absorption.	Mineral oil.
	Decrease absorption by damage to mucosa; inhibition of pancreatic lipase and inactivation of bile salts.	Cholestyramine. Neomycin. Alcohol. Colchicine (affects carotene).
Vitamin D	Affect absorption or metabolism of vitamin D.	Cholestyramine. Laxatives. Antacids. Mineral oil. Phenolphthalein.
	Accelerate the degradation of $25\text{-}OHD_3$.	Anticonvulsants. Glutethimide.
	Block the production of $1,25\text{-}OH_2D_3$ in the kidney.	Diphosphonates. Corticosteroids.
Vitamin E	Diminishes the carrier lipoprotein for vitamin E. Decreases absorption.	Clofibrate. Mineral oil. Isoniazid.

Table continued on the following page

Table 21–1. NUTRIENTS SIGNIFICANTLY AFFECTED BY SELECTED DRUGS (*Continued*)

NUTRIENT	DRUG ACTION	DRUGS
Vitamin K	Decrease synthesis of vitamin K_2 by intestinal bacteria, but no effect on vitamin status unless vitamin K intake is inadequate.	Tetracyclines and other broad-spectrum antibiotics.
	Decrease absorption of vitamin K.	Mineral oil. Neomycin. Cholestyramine.
	Cause vitamin K deficiency.	Coumarin anticoagulants. Aspirin and other salicylates.
Iron	Depresses iron absorption.	Bicarbonate.
	Increases iron absorption.	Isoniazide
	Impairs the uptake of iron into protoporphyrin; capable of causing sideroblastic anemia.	Cholestyramine.
Zinc	Cause excessive urinary excretion of zinc.	Alcohol. D-Penicillamine. Corticosteroids. Estrogen component of oral contraceptives. Chlorthalidone. Thiazides. Furosemide.
Magnesium	Increase urinary excretion of magnesium.	Chlorothiazide. Hydrochlorothiazide. Ethacrynic acid. Ammonium chloride. Mercurial diuretics. Alcohol.
	Drug-induced steatorrhea cuases formation of magnesium soaps and excessive fecal excretion of magnesium.	
Calcium	Cause malabsorption of calcium.	Prednisone and other glucocorticoids. Phenobarbital. Phenytoin. Primidone. Glutethimide. Diphosphonates. Phenolphthalein. Neomycin.
	Cause excessive urinary excretion of calcium.	Furosemide. Ethacrynic acid. Triamterene. Alcohol.
	Increase intestinal absorption of calcium.	Combination oral contraceptives.
Protein	Cause malabsorption of protein.	Neomycin.
	Inhibit protein synthesis.	Actinomycin D. Corticosteroids.
Fat	Cause malabsorption of fat.	Neomycin. Colchicine. Cholestyramine. Para-aminosalicylic acid.
Carbohydrate	Cause malabsorption of lactose.	Neomycin. Colchicine.
	Causes malabsorption of sucrose.	Neomycin.
Sodium and Potassium	Increase fecal excretion.	Neomycin. Colchicine.
Phosphate	Increase fecal excretion.	Aluminum hydroxide antacids.

Table 21–2. EFFECTS OF DRUG ACTION ON NUTRITIONAL STATUS

Alteration of food intake.
    Changes in appetite.
    Changes in sense of taste and smell.
    Decrease in salivary secretion.
    Gastric irritation.
    Nausea and vomiting.
Alteration of nutrient absorption.
    Luminal Effects
        Changes in gastrointestinal pH.
    Changes in gastrointestinal motility.
    Changes in bile acid activity.
    Formation of drug–nutrient complexes.
    Mucosal Effects
        Inactivation of absorptive enzyme systems.
        Damage to gastrointestinal mucosal cells.
Alteration of nutrient metabolism and utilization.
Alteration of nutrient excretion.

intake of food is *taste alteration*. Drugs can cause abnormal taste sensation (dysgeusia) or reduced acuity of the taste sensation (hypogeusia) or may leave an unpleasant aftertaste. Griseofulvin (an antifungal agent), D-penicillamine (a copper-chelating agent), clofibrate (an agent used to bind cholesterol in the gastrointestinal tract), 5-fluorouracil (a cancer chemotherapeutic agent) and some tranquilizers decrease or alter taste. Furthermore, they seem to have a systemic effect not related to the concomitant ingestion of food. Table 21–3 lists some drugs and their effects on the taste sensation.

Radiotherapy given to treat carcinoma of the tongue, tonsils or nasopharynx also reduces taste acuity by damaging the salivary glands and taste organs. When taking these drugs or receiving radiotherapy, patients should be informed of the possible alteration of taste, and every effort should be made to season their food well. Patients should be encouraged to eat well during periods when they are not receiving drugs or radiation therapy, as discussed in Chapter 36.

Zinc deficiency also causes hypogeusia and dysgeusia. Because of extended periods of inadequate nutritional intake or inadequate mineral supplementation, patients may become zinc-deficient and complain of taste changes. In this case, zinc supplements, usually in the form of zinc sulfate, are recommended.

Other drugs that affect food intake are those that cause nausea and vomiting as a side effect of their action. Still others are those that cause a dry mouth, which is a strong deterrent to eating. Many of the drugs used in the chemotherapy of cancer have this effect, as summarized in Table 36–2.

Some drugs may cause a craving or unusual desire for certain foods. For instance, patients taking diuretics may crave salt in their food because of the increased excretion of sodium, and will increase their sodium intake unless counseled about ways to avoid it.[17]

DRUGS THAT AFFECT THE ABSORPTION OF NUTRIENTS

Because most drugs and most nutrients are absorbed in the small intestine, it is not surprising that drugs affect nutrient absorption and vice versa. The interaction of food and drugs

Table 21–3. EFFECTS OF SOME MEDICATIONS ON TASTE SENSITIVITY*

DRUG	EFFECT
Acetyl sulfosalicylic acid	Decreased sensitivity.
Amphetamines	Decreased sweet sensitivity in some; differs with individuals. Increased bitter sensitivity.
Anesthetics	
Cocaine	Decreased sensitivity, especially sweet and bitter.
Eucaine	Decreased bitter and sweet sensitivity.
Amydricaine	Decreased bitter and sweet sensitivity.
Amylocaine	With high intake, loss of salt detection, decreased bitter sensitivity.
Isococaine and tropacocaine	Decreased sweet sensitivity.
Benzocaine	Increased sour sensitivity.
Amethocaine	Increased bitter sensitivity. Decreased sweet sensitivity.
Lidocaine	Decreased salt and sweet sensitivity.
Anti-thyroid agents	
Methimazole	Decreased sensitivity.
Methylthiouracil	Decreased sensitivity.
Bentyl	Decreased sensitivity.
Choloxin	Alterations in taste perception.
Clindamycin HCl hydrate	Bitter aftertaste.
Clofibrate	Decreased sensitivity; unpleasant aftertaste.
Dinitrophenol	Loss of salt taste; general hypogeusia.
5-Fluorouracil	Some alterations in bitter and sour sensitivity. Increased sweet sensitivity.
Griseofulvin	Decreased sensitivity.
Insulin	With prolonged use, decreased sweet and salt sensitivity.
Lithium carbonate	Strange, unpleasant taste.
Meprobamate	Decreased sensitivity.
Methicillin sodium	Aftertaste.
Oxyfedrine	Decreased sensitivity.
D-Penicillamine	General decrease in sensitivity.
Phenindione	Decreased sensitivity.
Phenytoin	Decreased sensitivity.
Probucol	Decreased sensitivity.
Propantheline bromide	Decreased sensitivity.

* Adapted from: Carson, J. A. S., and Gormican, A.: Disease-medication relationships in altered taste sensitivity. J. Am. Diet. Assoc., 68:550, 1976.

with the mechanical, secretory, digestive, absorptive and excretory functions of the gastrointestinal tract is complicated and depends on the drug dosage, type and amount of food, timing and the presence of disease or malnutrition.

In general, drugs can cause malabsorption by (1) exerting an effect in the intestinal lumen or (2) impairing the absorptive ability of the gastrointestinal mucosa. These effects can be limited and specific for a particular nutrient, or they can be general, resulting in a more severe malabsorption.

Luminal Effects

Drugs can *affect the transit time* of food and nutrients in the gut and reduce nutrient absorption. Cathartic agents such as podophyllin, jalap and colocynth may reduce gastrointestinal transit time. Calcium and potassium losses along with steatorrhea have been reported after use of these agents. Bisacodyl, oxyphenisatin, mannitol and phenolphthalein, commonly used as laxatives, can decrease the absorption of glucose.

A number of drugs *affect bile acid activity* and thus the absorption of fat, fat-soluble vitamins (A, D, E and K), carotene and other micellar components such as cholesterol. By sequestering bile acids through a binding effect, these drugs inhibit the intraluminal phase of fat digestion and absorption, and steatorrhea results. Drugs that have this action are cholestyramine, clofibrate, colestipol and neomycin. Cholestyramine, clofibrate and colestipol are usually given for the purpose of reducing cholesterol absorption and thus blood cholesterol, while neomycin is an antibiotic used to reduce the gut flora. Malabsorption has been reported in the form of vitamin K deficiency and hypoprothrombinemia.[9] Osteomalacia that responded to vitamin D therapy has also been reported;[13] however, the osteomalacia in this case was in a woman who also had a bile salt diarrhea, so that a deficiency of bile salts may have also contributed to the vitamin deficiency. Fat-soluble vitamins and possibly calcium should be given to patients taking cholestyramine.[18]

The status of fat-soluble vitamins in patients receiving these drugs should be monitored with periodic determinations of serum carotene for vitamin A status, of serum calcium, serum $25(OH)D_3$ and serum alkaline phosphatase for vitamin D evaluation, of serum alpha-tocopherol for vitamin E status and of prothrombin time to assess vitamin K status. Night blindness, osteomalacia, hemolysis of red blood cells when exposed to H_2O_2, and easy bruising are clinical signs that may reflect a deficiency of one or more of these fat-soluble vitamins, as discussed in Chapter 9.

Another drug that *prevents the absorption* of the fat-soluble vitamins is mineral oil, frequently used as a laxative. Of course, excessive use of this oil is more likely to cause a deficiency than occasional use. The vitamins become dispersed in oil, with the result that they are not absorbed but excreted in the feces. Mineral oil may also impair micelle formation in the gastrointestinal lumen.

Finally, a drug may *affect the environment of the gastrointestinal lumen* and prevent the absorption of a nutrient. Antacids change the pH of the stomach and if used extensively and frequently can significantly reduce the absorption of iron, which requires an acidic gastric environment in order to be changed from the ferric to the absorbable ferrous form. The absorption of iron is reduced in an alkaline environment.

Mucosal Effects

The drugs with the greatest effect on nutrient absorption are those that *damage the intestinal mucosa*. Such drugs destroy the structure of the villi and microvilli, which results in an inhibition of the brush border enzymes and intestinal transport systems needed for optimal nutrient absorption. The result is general or specific malabsorption of varying degrees. The irritating cathartics already mentioned may have this effect and thus cause a mild steatorrhea. This often happens with chronic laxative abuse.

Neomycin is known to cause histological changes in the gut mucosa within six hours of administration and results in diminished absorption of sucrose and xylose.[16] This action of neomycin is in addition to its bile acid binding activity, which has already been discussed. Increased excretion of protein, sodium, potassium and calcium also occurs. Neomycin causes malabsorption by three mechanisms: (1) mucosal damage, (2) precipitation of bile salts and (3) inhibition of pancreatic lipase. Mucosal damage probably has the greatest effect on nutrient absorption.

One drug that *affects the intestinal transport mechanisms* of the mucosa is colchicine, an anti-inflammatory agent used in the treatment of gout. Patients taking colchicine have reduced serum cholesterol levels; increased fecal excretion of bile acids, sodium, potassium, fat and protein; and impaired absorption of vitamin B_{12}. Although the drug causes some change in the intestinal mucosa, this does not seem to be enough to account for the extensive reduction in absorption. The malabsorptive effect of colchicine may be a result of changes in the mucosal transport systems.[25]

Para-aminosalicylic acid (PAS) seems to reduce the absorption of vitamin B_{12} in a similar fashion. It does not appear to interfere with the production of intrinsic factor or with its binding to vitamin B_{12} but rather with the uptake and transport of the vitamin across the mucosal wall.[31]

It has also been postulated that the biguanides phenformin and metformin cause a malabsorption of sugars from the gastrointestinal tract by blocking a mucosal enzyme and thus the transport of sugar across the mucosa into the blood stream. This is the reason for their use in the treatment of hyperglycemia.

Sulfasalazine, a drug used in the treatment of ulcerative colitis, reduces absorption of folate by inhibiting the jejunal enzyme responsible for the hydrolysis of polyglutamyl folate to the monoglutamyl form. In addition, the intestinal transport of folate is reduced by this drug.[11]

DRUGS THAT AFFECT THE METABOLISM AND EXCRETION OF NUTRIENTS

Antivitamins

Drugs that *interfere with the action of a vitamin by affecting its enzymes* can be antimetabolites, antivitamins or enzyme inducers. Antivitamins and antimetabolites, with structures similar to those of the real vitamins and metabolites, can block enzymatic reactions. The enzymes take up the antivitamin or antimetabolite instead of the actual vitamin or metabolite. Cancer chemotherapeutic agents operate on this principle. The antivitamins are taken up by the most rapidly growing cells in the body, the cancer cells, which die or malfunction when the antivitamin does not function like the real vitamin. Common antivitamins are the folate antagonists methotrexate and pyrimethamine. Methotrexate is used to treat leukemia, choriocarcinoma and psoriasis that is resistant to other forms of therapy. Pyrimethamine is used in the treatment of chloroquine-resistant malaria and ocular toxoplasmosis. These drugs act as folic acid analogs and are bound to the dihydrofolate reductase enzyme instead of folic acid. Folic acid is then unable to bind with the enzyme and is put out of the metabolic system and excreted. Without the real folic acid, deoxyribonucleic acid (DNA) synthesis, which depends on the presence of folic acid, is inhibited, cell replication stops and the cell dies. In addition, the folic acid deficiency can cause macrocytic anemia, as discussed in chapter 29.

Clinical rickets and osteomalacia in patients receiving long-term anticonvulsant therapy (phenytoin, phenobarbital, carbamazepine) are due to increased induction of hepatic enzymes, which interfere with the metabolism of vitamin D_3 to $25\text{-}OHD_3$ so that there is a smaller amount of active vitamin D available.[21] It appears that the concentration of $24,25(OH)_2D_3$ is also diminished, especially by phenobarbital. $1,25(OH)_2D_3$ does not seem to be as affected.[34] It is usually recommended that patients taking anticonvulsants receive a vitamin D supplement and possibly a folate supplement, as discussed on page 418. From 8000 to 10,000 I.U. of vitamin D has been recommended weekly, especially for blacks, patients with limited sun exposure and patients with limited activity.[10]

A drug may also affect the metabolism of a nutrient by *forming a complex* with it, making it unavailable for use by the body. Isoniazid (isonicotinic acid hydrazide, INH) functions in this manner. This drug, used in the long-term treatment of tuberculosis, forms a complex with pyridoxine (vitamin B_6) with the result that the pyridoxine is excreted in the urine and is not used by the body. Urinary levels of vitamin B_6 breakdown products are then above normal and indicate a biochemical vitamin B_6 deficiency. Other drugs that function as vitamin B_6 antagonists are hydralazine, penicillamine, L-dopa and cycloserine. Clinical signs of vitamin B_6 deficiency are, in order of appearance, seborrheic dermatitis, glossitis, stomatitis, cheilosis, conjunctivitis and later, severe sensory neuritis. Cycloserine and pyrazinamide (other antituberculous drugs) when given in conjunction with isoniazid will cause a sideroblastic anemia that is not seen when isoniazid is given alone. A dose of 50 mg. of vitamin B_6 daily will protect against vitamin B_6 deficiency when the patient is taking one of these drugs.

Excretion of Nutrients

Drugs act to increase the excretion of a nutrient by *displacing the vitamin from its binding site on a plasma protein*. If unbound to a protein, the vitamin will be filtered through the kidneys and excreted.[25] Aspirin may alter the transport of folate by competing for sites on the serum proteins that transport folate, and thus folate is excreted.[2]

D-Penicillamine, used to treat heavy metal poisoning (such as lead poisoning), Wilson's disease, cystinuria or rheumatoid arthritis, besides chelating with the intended metal such as lead or copper, may also *chelate with other metals* and increase their excretion in the urine. D-Penicillamine increases the excretion of zinc through formation of a zinc-penicillamine chelate.[22] In the reported cases, the patient's absorption of zinc from food offset the excessive loss of that mineral, so that a balance was maintained. However, an ill patient who is not eating could not maintain that balance. EDTA (ethylenediaminotetraacetate) administered intravenously to treat lead poisoning may also cause excessive urinary excretion of zinc.[6]

Drugs can also increase the excretion of a nutrient by *decreasing its reabsorption by the kidneys.* Oral diuretics such as furosemide, etha-crynic acid and triamterene can produce significant hypercalciuria by reducing reabsorption of calcium from the convoluted tubule in the kidney. Because of this, furosemide has also been utilized as a temporary measure to control symptoms of hypercalcemia. Diuretics may also affect the status of magnesium and zinc in the body by increasing renal excretion of these minerals.[33] Table 21–4 gives a synopsis of the nutritional implications of the use of selected drugs. For more extensive lists of interactions see Cited References 7 and 26.

Table 21–4. EFFECTS OF SOME DRUGS ON NUTRITIONAL STATUS

DRUG	POSSIBLE MECHANISM	NUTRITIONAL IMPLICATION
Amphetamines		
Dextroamphetamine	CNS effect on appetite	Weight loss
Methylphenidate	CNS effect on appetite	Decreased rate of growth in children due to decreased intake
Analgesics		
Alcohol	Toxic effect on intestinal mucosa	Decreased absorption of thiamin, folic acid, vitamin B_{12}
	Impairs pancreatic enzyme secretion	Increased urinary excretion of magnesium and zinc
		Decreased serum vitamin B_{12}
Aspirin (salicylates)	Decreases leukocyte uptake of ascorbic acid and alters ascorbic acid distribution	Decreased plasma and platelet ascorbic acid levels
	May uncouple energy source necessary for renal tubular resorption of amino acids	Increased urinary loss of ascorbic acid, potassium and amino acids
		Decreased absorption of tryptophan, possibly other amino acids and glucose
Colchicine	Decreases activity of intestinal disaccharidases	Decreased absorption of vitamin B_{12}, fat, carotene, sodium, potassium, lactose, xylose, protein
	Damages G.I. mucosa by blocking mucosal cell replication	Decreased serum cholesterol, carotene and vitamin B_{12}
Indomethacin	Increases rate of gastric emptying	Decreased plasma and platelet ascorbic acid levels
	May uncouple energy source for mucosal active transport of amino acids	Dyspepsia
		Decreased absorption of amino acids and xylose
		May cause anemia
Antacids		
Aluminum hydroxide	Decreases absorption of phosphate	Phosphate depletion
		Decreased vitamin A absorption
Others	Basic environment inactivates thiamin and prevents formation of ferrous from ferric iron	Inadequate amount of thiamin
		Decreased absorption of iron
Anticoagulants		
Coumarins	Antagonize vitamin K and vice versa	Increased prothrombin time
	Drug effect antagonized by high doses of vitamin E	
Anticonvulsants		
Phenobarbital	Increase turnover of vitamin D, may block hydroxylation of vitamin D	Decreased serum levels of 25-hydroxy-vitamin D_3 and calcium and magnesium
Phenytoin		Possible osteomalacia or rickets
Primidone	May increase biliary excretion of vitamin D	Decreased serum levels of folate, vitamin B_{12}, pyridoxine
		Can cause megaloblastic anemia
Barbiturates	Accelerate inactivation of vitamin D	Increased need for vitamin D and folic acid with long-term use
		Decreased absorption of thiamin
		Increased urinary excretion of vitamin C

Table 21–4.   EFFECTS OF SOME DRUGS ON NUTRITIONAL STATUS (*Continued*)

DRUG	POSSIBLE MECHANISM	NUTRITIONAL IMPLICATION
Barbiturates (*Continued*)		Decreased serum vitamin B_{12} Can cause megaloblastic anemia
Antidepressants		
Amitriptyline Imipramine		Interfere with riboflavin metabolism
Lithium carbonate	May increase appetite May inhibit magnesium-dependent enzymes or alter magnesium distribution	Possible weight gain Altered blood glucose Increased plasma magnesium Increased calcium excretion Decreased calcium uptake by bone
Antifungals		
Amphotericin B	Nephrotoxicity	Increased urinary excretion of potassium and nitrogen Decreased serum magnesium and potassium Increased blood urea nitrogen (BUN)
Antimicrobials		
Chloramphenicol	Decreases protein synthesis by blocking mRNA-ribosome bond	Possibly increased need for riboflavin, pyridoxine and vitamin B_{12} Possible peripheral neuritis, optic neuropathy Can antagonize response to folate, iron and vitamin B_{12} therapy
Penicillins	Carry potassium with them into urine Possibly induce hyperaldosteronism	Hypokalemia
Tetracyclines	Chelate divalent ions May decrease synthesis of mucosal iron-carrier protein	Decreased absorption of calcium, iron, magnesium, zinc, xylose, amino acids and fat. Net effect with minerals not clinically significant Increased urinary excretion of vitamin C, riboflavin, nitrogen, folic acid and niacin Decreased synthesis of vitamin K by intestinal bacteria
Neomycin (Some of these changes also seen with kanamycin and paromomycin)	Decreases activity of disaccharidases Causes mucosal injury Precipitates bile acids and disrupts micelle formation	Decreased absorption of fat, MCT, carbohydrate, protein, fat-soluble vitamins A, D and K, vitamin B_{12}, calcium and iron
Gentamicin	Nephrotoxicity	Increased urinary excretion of magnesium and potassium
Viomycin	Induces hyperaldosteronism	May cause hypomagnesemia, hypokalemia, hypocalcemia, alkalosis
Cephalosporins	Nephrotoxicity Damages gastrointestinal mucosa	May cause hypokalemia May cause vitamin K deficiency with prolongation of prothrombin time
Antineoplastics	Cytotoxic	Extensive effects discussed in Chapter 36
Antitubercular Agents		
Paraaminosalicyclic acid	Affects mucosal transport mechanism Decreases intestinal mucosal disaccharidases	Decreased absorption of vitamin B_{12}, iron, folate, fat and xylose Possible peripheral neuritis
Isoniazid	Structurally related to pyridoxine and niacin	Increased urinary excretion of pyridoxine Causes pyridoxine depletion Can cause polyneuropathy, megaloblastic anemia Causes niacin depletion, pigmented rash, cheilosis, and diarrhea Decreased serum folate
Cycloserine	Acts as a pyridoxine antagonist	Decreased protein synthesis May decrease absorption of calcium and magnesium May decrease serum folate, vitamin B_{12} and pyridoxine
Antivitamins		
Methotrexate	Inhibits dihydrofolate reductase; decreased formation of active folate	Malabsorption of vitamin B_{12}, folate, fat and xylose

Table continued on the following page

Table 21–4. EFFECTS OF SOME DRUGS ON NUTRITIONAL STATUS (*Continued*)

DRUG	POSSIBLE MECHANISM	NUTRITIONAL IMPLICATION
Methotrexate (*Continued*)	Causes gastrointestinal mucosal injury	Weight loss, diarrhea, nausea, anorexia, vomiting, gingivitis and stomatitis
Biguanides Metformin	Decreases activity of maltase, isomaltase and sucrase in jejunum	Decreased absorption of glucose, xylose, vitamin B_{12} Decreased serum folate, vitamin B_{12}
Phenformin	May affect active transport mechanisms	Decreased rate of glucose absorption in human ileum Decreased absorption of vitamin B_{12}, fat, calcium and amino acids
Cardiac Drugs Propranolol		Decreased carbohydrate tolerance Increased BUN
Digitalis glycosides	Inhibit glucose absorption	Diarrhea; cachexia Increased urinary excretion of magnesium, calcium and potassium
Cathartics	Can cause intestinal hyperperistalsis May irritate intestine	Can cause steatorrhea Can increase intestinal calcium and potassium loss Decreased glucose absorption
Phenolphthalein		Decreased absorption of vitamin D
Chelating Agents Penicillamine	Chelates with pyridoxine Chelates with zinc and copper	Increased urinary excretion of pyridoxine, zinc and copper Can cause pyridoxine depletion Decreased taste acuity; unpleasant taste
Corticosteroids	Stimulate protein catabolism Depress protein synthesis	Decreased absorption of calcium and phosphorus Increased urinary excretion of ascorbic acid, calcium, potassium, zinc and nitrogen Decreased serum zinc Increased blood glucose, serum triglycerides and serum cholesterol Increased need for vitamin B_6, ascorbic acid, folate and vitamin D Decreased bone formation Decreased wound healing
Diuretics Ethacrynic acid	May interfere with glucose-carrier complex	Decreased carbohydrate tolerance Increased urinary excretion of calcium, magnesium, potassium. Possible hypokalemia and hypomagnesemia
Furosemide		Increased urinary excretion of calcium, magnesium, potassium and zinc Decreased serum and muscle magnesium and potassium Decreased carbohydrate tolerance
Mercurials	Renal tubule damage	Increased urinary excretion of thiamin, magnesium, calcium and potassium Possibly induced magnesium depletion and bone resorption
Spironolactone		Increased urinary excretion of calcium and magnesium
Thiazides	May increase intestinal calcium absorption or increase bone resorption	Increased urinary excretion of potassium, magnesium, zinc and riboflavin Decreased carbohydrate tolerance Possible potassium and magnesium depletion
Triamterene	Competitive inhibition of dihydrofolate reductase; reduces activation of folic acid	Decreased serum folate Possibly increased calcium excretion
Hypocholesterolemics Cholestyramine	Binds bile salts and disrupts micelles Binds intrinsic factor at ileal pH	Decreased absorption of cholesterol, vitamins A, D, K and B_{12}, folate, fat, medi-

Table 21–4. EFFECTS OF SOME DRUGS ON NUTRITIONAL STATUS (*Continued*)

DRUG	POSSIBLE MECHANISM	NUTRITIONAL IMPLICATION
Cholestyramine (*Continued*)	Binds iron	um-chain triglycerides (MCT), glucose, xylose, carotene and iron Decreased calcium absorption Decreased serum calcium and vitamin B_{12} Increased urinary excretion of calcium
Clofibrate	May decrease activity of intestinal disaccharidases	Decreased taste acuity, unpleasant aftertaste Decreased absorption of carotene, glucose, iron, MCT, vitamin B_{12} and electrolytes
Colestipol	Bile acid sequestrant	Reduced serum cholesterol Lowered plasma and serum levels of vitamins A and E
Hypotensive Agents		
Hydralazine	Inactivates pyridoxine May chelate trace metals	Increased excretion of pyridoxine; pyridoxine depletion Possible peripheral neuritis
Diazoxide	May cause pancreatic damage	Hyperglycemia Decreased tubular excretion of uric acid
Reserpine		Increased G.I. motility and secretion May cause weight gain
Sodium nitroprusside	Binds vitamin B_{12}	Increased urinary B_{12} excretion Decreased plasma B_{12}
Laxatives		
Mineral oil (Petrolatum, liquid)	Dissolves fat-soluble vitamins Increases intestinal motility	Decreased absorption of carotene, vitamins A, D, E and K, calcium and phosphate
L-Dopa (levodopa)	Pyridoxine involved in metabolism of L-dopa Antagonizes pyridoxine	Possible polyneuropathy related to pyridoxine depletion Increased need for ascorbic acid and pyridoxine Decreased absorption of tryptophan and other amino acids Increased urinary excretion of sodium and potassium
Oral Contraceptives	May increase catabolism, decrease absorption or alter tissue uptake of vitamin C May inhibit folate conjugase May increase transport proteins for vitamin A Estrogens increase the rate of conversion of tryptophan to niacin	Altered tryptophan metabolism Decreased serum vitamin C levels Possibly decreased serum vitamin B_{12}, folate, pyridoxine, riboflavin, magnesium and zinc Increased hemoglobin, hematocrit, serum levels of vitamins A and E, total lipids, triglycerides, iron, total iron-binding capacity (TIBC) and plasma copper Possible polyneuropathy, peripheral neuritis and megaloblastic anemia
Parasympatholytic Agents		
Atropine	Decreases gastric acidity	May decrease iron absorption
Potassium Supplements	Slow release of potassium chloride causes decrease of ileal pH (acidification)	Decreased absorption of vitamin B_{12}
Sedative-Hypnotics		
Glutethimide	Possibly increases inactivation of 25-hydroxy vitamin D_3	Increased vitamin D turnover Increased bone resorption Polyneuropathy
Sulfonamides		
Salicylazosulfapyridine (Sulfasalazine)	Inhibits intestinal transport of folate Inhibits action of polyglutamyl folate conjugase	Decreased absorption of folate Decreased serum folate and serum iron Decreased response to folate supplement
Other sulfonamides		Peripheral neuritis Increased urinary excretion of ascorbic acid
Tranquilizers		
Chlorpromazine	Hepatotoxic May interfere with riboflavin metabolism	Can reduce physical activity Possible weight gain Increased serum cholesterol

Table continued on the following page

Table 21–4.   EFFECTS OF SOME DRUGS ON NUTRITIONAL STATUS (*Continued*)

DRUG	POSSIBLE MECHANISM	NUTRITIONAL IMPLICATION
Uricosuric Agents		
Probenecid	Action on renal tubule	Increased urinary excretion of riboflavin, calcium, magnesium, sodium, potassium, phosphate and chloride
		Decreased urinary excretion of pantothenic acid
		Decreased absorption of riboflavin and amino acids
Urinary Germicides		
Nitrofurantoin	May inhibit intestinal folate conjugase	Decreased serum folate
		Possible megaloblastic anemia and peripheral neuritis

Data from Roe, D. A.: Handbook, Interactions of Selected Drugs and Nutrients in Patients. 3rd ed., Chicago, American Dietetic Association, 1982.

SUMMARY OF SOME OF THE ACTIONS OF SOME COMMON DRUGS

Anticonvulsants

In addition to the vitamin D deficiency state already discussed, the anticonvulsants phenytoin, phenobarbital and primidone are also capable of inducing a biochemical or clinical folate deficiency state. The prevalence of megaloblastic anemia in people who take anticonvulsants ranges from 0.15 to 0.75 per cent.[25] It is thought by some that these drugs interfere with the conversion of folic acid to 5-methyltetrahydrofolate, the active form of folic acid. Others feel that these drugs, particularly phenytoin, impair the absorption of folate from food by inhibiting intestinal conjugase, which is necessary for breaking down the polyglutamates of folic acid in food to the monoglutamate form that can be absorbed. Vitamin B_{12} levels, although usually unaffected by the use of anticonvulsants, may fall if folic acid is given to remedy low serum folate levels. The increased hematopoiesis increases the body's need for vitamin B_{12}. Serum B_{12} should always be watched when the patient taking anticonvulsant therapy is also being given folate treatment.[25] Folate supplementation can also cause a decrease in the effectiveness of the anticonvulsants.

Oral Contraceptives

Oral contraceptives have many effects on nutrition, some of which are clinically important. Women using estrogen-containing oral contraceptives showed increased plasma cholesterol, triglyceride, low density lipoprotein and very low density lipoprotein levels, but high density lipoprotein levels were similar to those in controls. The increases were positively correlated with the amount of estrogen in the agent. The effects were not so pronounced when estrogen was taken for menopausal reasons.[32] These metabolic changes due to oral contraceptive use seem to be clinically relevant because there is an increased risk of cardiovascular disease in women taking oral contraceptives.[20]

Oral contraceptives also cause alterations in carbohydrate metabolism that lead to hyperglycemia and reduced glucose tolerance. However, it appears that the alteration in carbohydrate metabolism is due more to the progestogens contained in oral contraceptives than to the estrogens. It appears at this point that products with 50 μg. or less of estrogen and a weak progestogen such as norethindrone are the most appropriate for avoiding these lipid and carbohydrate metabolism changes mentioned.[30]

Oral contraceptives also increase serum vitamin A, vitamin E, iron and total iron-binding capacity. Plasma copper also is increased.[27] The high estrogen preparations alter tryptophan metabolism and carbohydrate metabolism and decrease serum and leukocyte ascorbic acid levels and red blood cell (RBC) folate, as well as serum levels of vitamin B_{12} and B_6.[26] These nutritional effects appear to be determined by the amount of estrogen in the contraceptive agent and the interaction of the two hormones.

The fact that these changes are not found in all women illustrates that some women are more sensitive to the effects of oral contraceptive agents (OCAs) than others. Dietary intake probably influences the development of a biochemical deficiency.

Vitamin B_6 metabolism is affected so that there is an increased excretion of tryptophan metabolites after a tryptophan loading test. Thus, the requirement for vitamin B_6 is increased. Another result is a decrease in the brain amine serotonin and its metabolite 5-hydroxyindoleacetic acid (5-HIAA). This decrease could cause the depression sometimes seen in women who have biochemical signs of vitamin B_6 deficiency. In these women, depression was relieved when vitamin B_6 was given. Such women should probably take a vitamin B_6 supplement of 20 to 40 mg. daily.[1] Vitamin B_6 is probably not routinely necessary for all women taking contraceptives.

Some women who take oral contraceptives develop biochemical signs of folate deficiency; that is, lowered serum folate and lowered red cell folate with increased excretion of formiminoglutamic acid (FIGLU), a urinary metabolite of folic acid. Whether folate deficiency develops while a woman is taking oral contraceptives depends largely on her intake of folate and use of folate supplements. One theory postulates that oral contraceptives interfere with the deconjugation of polyglutamic acid to the monoglutamate form that is necessary for folic acid absorption from the gastrointestinal tract.

Changes in plasma levels of minerals are likely a result of the redistribution of the minerals within the body rather than of excessive excretion or impaired absorption of the minerals.

Antihypertensives

Diuretics can cause increases in serum lipid and lipoprotein concentrations and they can impair glucose tolerance. In addition the beta-adrenoceptor blocking agents (beta-blocking drugs), often used in conjunction with diuretics to lower blood pressure, increase serum triglyceride and decrease concentrations of high density lipoproteins. It is suggested that these changes are due to an insulin resistance caused by the drug.[3] However another study showed that only propranolol and not metoprolol impaired glucose tolerance and that the mechanism remains uncertain.[8]

The Effect of Nutrients and Nutritional Status on the Absorption and Metabolism of Drugs

Effect on Absorption

The absorption of many drugs from the gastrointestinal tract is affected by the presence of food and nutrients in the lumen as summarized in Table 21–5. Generally, drugs are absorbed more slowly when they are taken with food, and thus the total absorption may be reduced, usually because of delayed gastric emptying and dilution. By reducing the absorption of a drug, food reduces its therapeutic dosage. The drug may never reach effective levels in the blood, or the slow absorption may act as a sustained release, prolonging the effects of the drug.

Table 21–5.   EFFECT OF FOOD ON SERUM LEVELS OF SOME DRUGS

DRUG	EFFECT OF FOOD
Antihypertensives	
Canrenone (metabolite of spironolactone)	Increases absorption, increases drug levels
Hydralazine	Increases serum drug levels
Bronchodilators	
Theophylline	Decreases absorption, decreases serum drug levels with high-protein diet
Cardioactives	
Digoxin	Decreases absorption, decreases serum drug levels
Propranolol	Increases absorption, increases serum drug levels
Metoprolol	Increases absorption
Antibiotics	
Ampicillin	Decreases absorption
Isoniazid (antitubercular)	Decreases absorption, decreases serum drug levels
Oxacillin	Decreases absorption
Penicillin	Decreases absorption
Rifampin (antitubercular)	Decreases serum drug levels
Tetracycline	Decreases absorption with calcium-containing foods.
Amoxicillin (analogue of ampicillin)	No effect
Metronidazole	No effect
Antifungal Agents	
Griseofulvin	Increases absorption with fatty foods
Antiepileptics	
Carbamazepine	Increases serum drug levels

Adapted from Decker, E.L.: Drug and food interactions. R.D., *2*(3):2, 1982.

These actions can be clinically significant. *Changes in gastrointestinal acidity* generally affect the rate of absorption of a drug rather than the total amount of drug absorbed.

The *rate of gastric emptying*, influenced by the type of meal or food ingested, can influence the absorption of a drug. For example, drugs such as L-dopa and penicillin G are metabolized or degraded in the stomach, so that situations of delayed gastric emptying would cause increased destruction of these drugs and a smaller effective dosage. On the other hand, delayed gastric emptying in the case of nitrofurantoin, a broad-spectrum antibacterial agent, would increase the time the product is in the stomach, allowing a greater portion of the drug to be dissolved by the gastric juice before it entered the duodenum where the absorption would be maximal. Food in this case would increase the effective dosage of a drug. Hydralazine, an antihypertensive, is another drug that is more completely absorbed when given with food.

Certain *nutrients can affect the absorption* of drugs. Foods of dairy origin, which contain large amounts of calcium, inhibit the absorption of tetracycline because calcium forms a complex with the drug that prevents its absorption from the gastrointestinal tract. Tetracycline derivatives should be taken without milk or milk products at the time that they are administered.

Another example of a nutrient affecting the absorption of a drug is the effect of a high-fat meal on the absorption of griseofulvin. A large intake of fats increases the absorption of griseofulvin, which is highly lipid-soluble. It may be that the fat stimulates the secretion of bile, which makes the drug more water-soluble. Table 21–6 lists the effects of food on the absorption and serum levels of some drugs.

EFFECT ON METABOLISM

Drug metabolism may be altered in states of nutritional deficiency or nutritional manipulation, since the activity of the hepatic microsomal enzyme drug-metabolizing system (mainly the cytochrome P_{450}-dependent "mixed function oxidase" system) is influenced by the intake of protein, carbohydrate and lipid. For example, manipulation of the diet from a normal one to a high-protein, low-carbohydrate diet resulted in a 35 to 40 per cent reduction in the plasma half-lives of antipyrine and theophylline.[15] These drugs were metabolized more rapidly by the liver during the period when subjects were ingesting the high-protein diet. This effect was seen even when carbohydrate or protein was given as a supplement to the diet.[4] Asthmatic children treated with the bronchodilator theophylline had fewer wheezing episodes on the high-carbohydrate, low-protein diet than those on the high-protein, low-carbohydrate diet.[5]

Table 21–6. MECHANISMS BY WHICH FOOD INTERFERES WITH DRUG THERAPY*

Alteration of absorption of orally administered drugs by affecting:

    gastrointestinal transit time and motility.
    gastrointestinal secretions and pH.
    osmolality of gastrointestinal tract.
    ionization of drug.
    stability of drug.
    solubility of drug.
    complexation of drug with a dietary component.
Alteration of drug's distribution.
Alteration of drug's metabolism.
Alteration of drug's excretion.
Exertion of antagonistic pharmacological response by active substance in food.

*Adapted from Hethcox, J. M., and Stanaszek, W. F.: Interactions of drugs and diet. Hospital Pharmacy, 9(10): 373, 1974.

Whether the diet was high in carbohydrate or fat as opposed to protein did not appear to make a difference.[4] Manipulation of major components of the diet could be of particular clinical significance in some situations, such as a protein increase for weight reduction or postoperative therapy using only intravenous glucose.

Vitamin C status may be important in drug metabolism in the liver. Vitamin C deficiency in animals impairs drug oxidation, but there has been no documented enhanced effect of vitamin C administration on drug metabolism in humans.[4]

Polycyclic aromatic hydrocarbons in the environment are known to accelerate the metabolism of a number of drugs, including antipyrine, theophylline, phenacetin and caffeine. Broiling of meats over charcoal results in the formation of these polycyclic aromatic hydrocarbons, and it has been shown that with the ingestion of charcoal-broiled beef, there are enhanced oxidation rates of a variety of drugs in humans.[14]

Brussels sprouts, cabbage and cauliflower contain substances that are powerful inducers of the "mixed function oxidase" activities in the liver and intestine. In one study, clearance of phenacetin by the liver was enhanced when these vegetables were present in the diet.[23]

Other factors that influence the metabolism of drugs are the rate of intestinal absorption and delivery of the drug to the liver; the presence of other disease, including malnutrition; liver function; and the concomitant administration of other drugs that can either increase or decrease the metabolism of the first drug.

An example of an interaction between a drug and a food constituent is seen with the monoamine oxidase (MAO) inhibitors (used to treat depression) and the tyramine and dopamine content of food. These drugs, which include phenelzine sulfate and tranylcypromine sulfate, block MAO activity, and thus tyramine and dopamine are not deaminated in the liver but are allowed to reach the circulation. These monoamines are powerful pressor substances, which cause constriction of blood vessels and elevation of blood pressure. The patient gets an occipital headache and a severe increase in blood pressure that may result in intracranial hemorrhage. Normally these monoamines are metabolized to their harmless metabolites by MAO systems. However, in the presence of MAO inhibitors the body's defense against their activity is removed. For example, the pressor effect of tyrosine may be enhanced 100-fold in the presence of MAO inhibitors.[12] Foods such as cheeses and wine, which contain tyramine, should be avoided by patients taking MAO inhibitors. Other foods that have been fermented or aged or in which protein breakdown is used to increase flavor are not permitted, since they contain bacteria capable of forming amines from amino acid precursors. See Table 21–7 for a complete list.

Table 21–7. TYRAMINE- AND DOPAMINE-RESTRICTED DIET*

FOODS ALLOWED	FOODS EXCLUDED
Beverages	
All except those specifically to be avoided; decaffeinated coffee, coffee, tea	Alcoholic beverages, wines, ale, beer
Breads and Bread Substitutes	
All not specifically excluded, including commercial bread	Homemade yeast breads with substantial quantities of yeast, breads or crackers containing cheese
Fats	
All except those excluded	Soured cream
Fruits	
Orange (limit to 1 small orange daily, 2 1/2 in. diameter, which provides 1 mg. of tyramine); any other fruits not specifically excluded	Bananas (contain dopamine), red plums, avocados (contain dopamine), figs, raisins (permitted on diets not restricted in dopamine)
Meats and Meat Substitutes	
Cottage cheese and meats not specifically to be avoided, eggs	Aged game, liver, and canned meats; yeast extracts; commercial meat extracts; stored beef liver; chicken livers; salami; sausage; aged cheese: blue, Boursault, brick, Brie, Camembert, cheddar, colby, Emmentaler, Gouda, mozzarella, Parmesan, provolone, Romano, Roquefort, Stilton; salted dried fish such as herring, cod, or camlin; pickled herring
Vegetables	
Tomato (limit to 1/2 cup daily), all other vegetables not specifically excluded	Italian broad beans (pods contain tyramine), green bean pods, eggplant
Miscellaneous	
Fresh homemade gravies; all not specifically excluded	Yeast concentrates, marmite, soup cubes, products made with concentrated yeasts, commercial gravies or meat extracts, soups containing items that must be avoided, soy sauce,† any protein-containing food that has been stored improperly or that may have been spoiled or is putrid, i.e., all except those that have been freshly prepared

* This diet eliminates all known major sources of tyramine and dopamine including those foods containing bacteria with enzymes capable of decarboxylating the amino acid tyrosine to tyramine. This diet provides less than 2 mg. of tyramine daily.

† Contains 1.7 mEq./gm. of tyramine.

Adapted from American Dietetic Association: Handbook of Clinical Dietetics. New Haven, Yale University Press, 1981.

EFFECT ON EXCRETION

Food and nutrients can affect the excretion of drugs. By changing the pH of the urine, food and nutrient intake can affect drug excretion. For example, acidic drugs are excreted faster in an alkaline urine. Drug excretion can be affected by body levels of minerals. Such is the case with the drug lithium carbonate. With sodium depletion there is increased reabsorption of both sodium and lithium. With a low sodium intake, serum lithium rises more rapidly and peaks at a higher level. With sodium supplementation or increased fluid intake there is an increase in lithium excretion.[24]

Problems and Suggested Topics for Discussion

1. Evaluate one of your patients for possible nutritional problems resulting from his or her drug therapy. What are your recommendations for nutritional care?
2. Why are drugs more likely to induce nutritional deficiency in chronically ill, debilitated patients? What can be done to prevent this?
3. Evaluate a patient with a malabsorption syndrome (sprue, regional enteritis or small bowel resection, for example). Is he or she taking any medication? How is the absorption of medication changed? Evaluate the patient's nutritional status. What nutritional care would you recommend?
4. Evaluate a patient receiving a cancer chemotherapeutic agent. Chapter 36 may be helpful.
   a. Is he or she suffering from oral or gastrointestinal side effects of the therapy? What are these side effects?
   b. Is the nutritional intake adequate? Is there any weight loss? If so, why?
   c. What would you recommend for nutritional care?
   d. How would you help the patient make any necessary changes in his or her diet?

Cited References

1. Adams, P.W., et al: Effect of pyridoxine hydrochloride (vitamin B_6) upon depression associated with oral contraceptives. Lancet, *1*:897, 1973.
2. Alter, H.J., Zvaifler, M.J., and Rath, C.E.: Interrelationship of rheumatoid arthritis, folic acid and aspirin. Blood, *38*:405, 1971.
3. Ames, R.P., and Hill, P.: Improvement of glucose tolerance and lowering of glycohemoglobin and serum lipid concentrations after discontinuation of antihypertensive drug therapy. Circulation, *65*:899, 1982.
4. Anderson, K.E., Conney, A.H., and Kappas, A.: Nutritional influences on chemical biotransformations in humans. Nutr. Rev., *40*:161, 1982.
5. Feldman, C.H., et al.: Effect of dietary protein and carbohydrate on theophylline metabolism in children. Pediatrics, *66*:956, 1980.
6. Fell, G.S., et al.: Urinary zinc levels as an indication of muscle catabolism. Lancet, *1*:280, 1973.
7. Grant, A.: Nutritional Assessment Guidelines. 2nd ed. 1979, pp. 63–103. Available from Box 25057, Northgate Station, Seattle, Wash. 98125.
8. Groop, L., et al.: Influence of beta-blocking drugs on glucose metabolism in patients with non–insulin de-

pendent diabetes mellitus. Acta Med. Scand., 211:7, 1982.

9. Gross, L., and Brotman, M.: Hypoprothrombinemia and hemorrhage associated with cholestyramine therapy. Ann. Intern. Med., 72:95, 1970.

10. Hahn, T.J., et al.: Serum 25-hydroxycalciferol levels and bone mass in children on chronic anticonvulsant therapy. N. Engl. J. Med., 292:550, 1975.

11. Halstead, C.H., Gandhi, G., and Tamura, T.: Sulfasalazine inhibits the absorption of folates in ulcerative colitis. N. Engl. J. Med., 305:1513, 1981.

12. Headache, tyramine, serotonin and migraine. Nutr. Rev., 26:40, 1968.

13. Heaton, K.W., Lever, J.V., and Barnard, D.: Osteomalacia associated with cholestyramine therapy for postileectomy diarrhea. Gastroenterology, 62:642, 1972.

14. Kappas, A., et al.: Effect of charcoal-broiled beef on antipyrine and theophylline metabolism. Clin. Pharmacol. Ther., 23:445, 1978.

15. Kappas, A., et al.: Influence of dietary protein and carbohydrate on antipyrine and theophylline metabolism in man. Clin. Pharmacol. Ther., 20:643, 1976.

16. Keusch, G.T., Troncale, E.J., and Plant, A.G.: Neomycin-induced malabsorption in a tropical population. Gastroenterology, 58:197, 1970.

17. Langford, H.G.: Rationale for diets modified in sodium and potassium. Paper presented at the 57th Annual Meeting of the American Dietetic Association, Philadelphia, 1974.

18. Longstreth, G.F., and Newcomer, A.D.: Drug-induced malabsorption. Mayo.Clin. Proc., 50:284, 1975.

19. Lucas, B., and Sells, C.J.: Nutrient intake and stimulant drugs in hyperactive children. J. Am. Diet. Assoc., 70:373, 1977.

20. Mann, J.I., and Vessey, M.P.: Trends in cardiovascular disease mortality and oral contraceptives. Br. J. Fam. Plan., 6:99, 1981.

21. Matheson, R.T., et al.: Absorption and biotransformation of cholecalciferol in drug-induced osteomalacia. J. Clin. Pharmacol., 16:426, 1976.

22. McCall, J.T., et al.: Comparative metabolism of copper and zinc in patients with Wilson's disease (hepatolenticular degeneration). Am. J. Med. Sci., 254:13, 1967.

23. Pantuck, E.J., et al.: Effect of dietary Brussels sprouts and cabbage on human drug metabolism. Clin. Pharmacol. Ther., 25:88, 1979.

24. Platman, S.R., and Fieve, R.R.: Lithium retention and excretion. The effects of Na^+ and fluid intake. Arch. Gen. Psych., 20:285, 1969.

25. Roe, D.A.: Drug-induced nutritional deficiencies. Westport, Conn., Avi Publishing Co., 1976, p. 135.

26. Roe, D.A.: Handbook: Interactions of Selected Drugs and Nutrients in Patients. 3rd ed. Chicago, American Dietetic Association, 1982.

27. Rubinfeld, Y., et al.: A progressive rise in serum copper levels in women taking oral contraceptives: a potential hazard? Fertility and Sterility, 32:599, 1979.

28. Safer, D.J., Allan, R.P., and Barr, E.: Depression of growth in hyperactive children on stimulant drugs. N. Engl. J. Med., 287:217, 1972.

29. Safer, D., Allan, R.P., and Barr, E.: Growth rebound after termination of stimulant drugs. J. Pediatr., 86:113, 1975.

30. Spellacy, W.N.: Carbohydrate metabolism during treatment with estrogen, progestogen and low-dose oral contraceptives. Am. J. Obstet. Gynecol., 142:732, 1982.

31. Toskes, P.P., and Deren, J.J.: Selective inhibition of vitamin B_{12} absorption by para-aminosalicylic acid. Gastroenterology, 62:1232, 1972.

32. Wallace, R.B., et al.: Altered plasma lipid and lipoprotein levels associated with oral contraceptive and estrogen use. Lancet, 2:111, 1979.

33. Wester, P.O.: Zinc during diuretic treatment. Lancet, 1:578, 1975.

34. Zerwekh, J.E., et al.: Decreased serum 24, 25 dihydroxyvitamin D concentration during long-term anticonvulsant therapy in adult epileptics. Ann. Neurol., 12:184, 1982.

Additional References

American Dietetic Association: Handbook of Clinical Dietetics. New Haven, Yale University Press, 1981.

Briggs, M.H., and Briggs, M.: Randomized prospective studies on metabolic effects of oral contraceptives. Acta Obstet. Gynecol. Scand. (Suppl.), 105:25, 1982.

Carson, J.A.S., and Gormican, A.: Disease-medication relationships in altered taste sensitivity. J. Am. Diet. Assoc., 68:550, 1976.

Carson, J.A.S., and Gormican, A.: Taste acuity and food attitudes of selected patients with cancer. J. Am. Diet. Assoc., 70:361, 1977.

Clinical nutrition: Folic acid absorption, anticonvulsant and contraceptive therapy. Nutr. Rev., 32:39, 1974.

Cummings, J.H., et al.: Laxative-induced diarrhea: A continuing clinical problem. Br. Med. J., 1:537, 1974.

Faloon, W.W. (ed.): Symposium: Drug-nutrient relationships. Am. J. Clin. Nutr., 26:103, 1973.

Goodman, L.S., and Gilman, A. (eds.): The Pharmacological Basis of Therapeutics, 6th ed. New York, Macmillan Publishing Company, 1980.

Hahn, T.J.: Bone complications of anticonvulsants. Drugs, 12:201, 1976.

Hartshorn, E.A.: Food and drug interactions. J. Am. Diet. Assoc., 70:15, 1977.

Leary, W.P., and Reyes, A.J.: Diuretics, magnesium, potassium and sodium. S. Afr. Med. J., 61:279, 1982.

Malnutrition and drug metabolism in man. Nutr. Rev., 34:237, 1976.

Moore, A.O., and Powers, D.E.: Food-Medication Interactions. Tempe, Ariz., Food-Drug Interactions, 1981.

Symposium: Oral contraceptives and nutrients. Am. J. Clin. Nutr., 28:371, 1975.

Varda, V.A., Bartak, B.R., and Slowie, L.A.: Nutritional therapy of patients receiving lithium carbonate. J. Am. Diet. Assoc., 74:149, 1979.

Visconti, J.A.: Drug-food interaction. In Nutrition in Disease. Columbus, Ohio, Ross Laboratories, 1977.

Wynn, V.: Vitamins and oral contraceptive use. Lancet, 1:561, 1975.

DISEASES OF THE GASTROINTESTINAL SYSTEM

Nutritional Care in Esophageal or Gastric Disease

Gastrointestinal diseases can be classified as (1) organic or (2) functional. The latter are the more common. An *organic* disease of the gastrointestinal tract is one in which a definite pathological change has taken place in the structural tissues. Peptic ulcer and cancer are examples. A *functional* disorder is a disturbance, either sensory, motor, absorptive or secretory in origin, for which no structural, infective or biochemical cause can be found. One fifth of the patients who consult a gastroenterologist have symptoms that cannot be explained.[17] Functional disorders have, in addition, a hard-to-define emotional and psychological component. Some disorders have both organic and functional components. For example, a "functional" disorder such as ulcerative colitis has characteristic pathological manifestations; and an "organic" disorder such as peptic ulcer is caused by excessive gastric acidity, a functional aspect.

A gastrointestinal disorder, whether it is the patient's primary disease or the gastrointestinal manifestation of a systemic disease, is a potential threat to the individual's nutritional status. The objectives of the nutritional care are not only to alleviate the gastrointestinal symptoms but also to maintain good nutritional status.

The first objective requires application of knowledge about how various foods may affect the gastrointestinal tract and aggravate the present pathological condition. The second objective, maintenance of good nutritional status, requires an understanding of the way in which the gastrointestinal disorder impairs the individual's ability to consume, absorb and utilize nutrients. It is important to recognize the *nutrient limitations* of the therapeutic diet modifications, especially when the patient must change usual dietary intake patterns and is suffering from anorexia, nausea and vomiting, constipation or diarrhea.

GASTROINTESTINAL REACTIONS TO MEDICATIONS. Many medications taken for gastrointestinal disease or other disease can cause gastrointestinal side effects. These can aggravate or cause gastrointestinal problems and affect nutritional status. This should always be kept in mind when assessing the patient with a gastrointestinal complaint. See Chapter 21.

Nutritional Assessment

The assessment of nutritional status, especially the dietary history, is crucial in the nutritional care of a patient with a gastrointestinal disorder. Besides being the basis for setting the nutritional care objectives, as discussed in Chapter 19, the assessment has special significance in gastrointestinal disease. First the dietary history can reveal eating patterns or changes that reflect symptoms characteristic of a disorder. For example, the patient who complains of pain four to five hours after a fatty meal gives a clue of possible gallbladder disease. Esophageal dis-

Table 22–1. DIETARY HISTORY INFORMATION THAT CAN GIVE CLUES TO
GASTROINTESTINAL DISEASE

SYMPTOM	POSSIBLE DISORDER
Ingestion of solid food causes distress but liquids do not.	Esophageal stricture or tumor.
Difficulty in swallowing; food sticks in throat.	Esophageal spasm; achalasia.
Epigastric pain when eating.	Gastric ulcer.
Pain 2–5 hours after a meal, relieved upon eating.	Duodenal ulcer.
Abdominal pain several hours after a fatty meal.	Pancreatic or biliary tract disease.
Cramps, distention and flatulence several hours after drinking milk.	Lactose intolerance probably due to lactase deficiency.
Heartburn after a fatty meal.	Hiatal hernia; achalasia; esophageal motility problem.

ease should be considered when the patient gives a history of difficulty in swallowing dry foods such as bread or toast. Table 22–1 presents more clues to be gained from the dietary history.

Second, the nutritional status assessment can forewarn the nurse and nutritionist about potential nutritional problems. Gastrointestinal disease will probably worsen borderline nutritional status, and measures should be taken to prevent this.

Third, a nutritional assessment performed after the patient has started a therapeutic regimen can reveal how the patient is coping with the disease and its treatment, especially when he is at home. Because eating problems are individual, because eating can be painful and because food and the gastrointestinal reactions related to it are fraught with mystery and misconception, patients may follow very restricted and inadequate diets that are different from what was prescribed.

Diseases of the Esophagus

In normal swallowing, the muscles of the pharynx, upper esophagus and upper esophageal sphincter are smoothly coordinated with the muscles of the lower esophagus and lower esophageal sphincter.* The entire esophagus functions as one tissue during swallowing. The bolus of food is voluntarily moved from the mouth to the pharynx. The upper sphincter relaxes, the food moves into the esophagus, and the lower esophageal sphincter (LES) relaxes to receive the food bolus. Peristaltic waves move the bolus down the esophagus and into the stomach, as shown in Figure 22–1. For a more complete discussion of the physiology of the esophagus the reader is referred to other texts.[12, 13]

---

*Although these muscles are referred to as "sphincters" they are really no different from the rest of the esophagus; however, physiologically they remain constricted and closed.

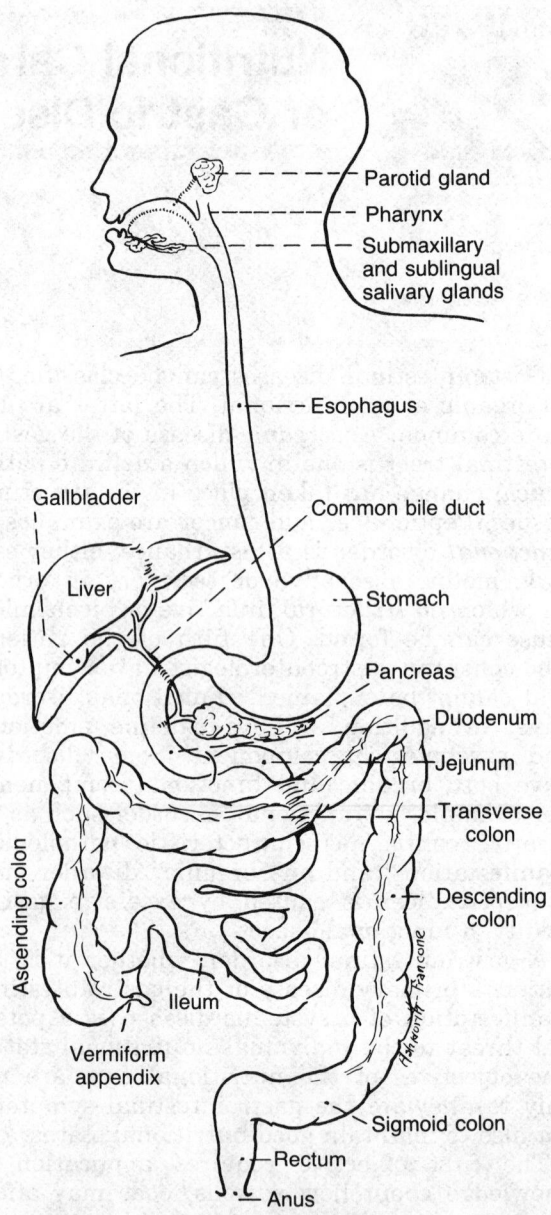

Figure 22–1. The digestive system and its associated structures. (From: Jacob, S. W., and Francone, C. A.: Structure and Function in Man, 5th ed. Philadelphia, W. B. Saunders Co., 1982.)

Disorders of the esophagus are due to obstruction, inflammation or derangement of the swallowing mechanism. Although all esophageal disorders are potential deterrents to the person's ability to consume food, only those common disorders for which nutritional care is indicated will be discussed here.

ACHALASIA (ESOPHAGEAL DYSSYNERGIA)

Achalasia, also called *esophageal dyssynergia,* is a disorder of lower esophageal motility. Because of impaired cholinergic innervation of the esophageal musculature there is failure of the LES to relax and open during swallowing. Consequently, patients complain of *dysphagia,* or difficulty in swallowing, and describe the sensation of food sticking in the esophagus under the sternum. Dysphagia, which can be mild and infrequent, becomes severe and painful as the achalasia worsens. During eating, the esophagus fills with food and fluid until either the pressure forces the esophageal sphincter to open and allow small amounts of food to enter the stomach, or the person is forced to vomit up the food. Extreme dilatation of the esophagus develops, while the LES opening narrows. When the patient finally seeks help, he or she is usually eating very little because of the physical and social discomfort involved and has usually lost weight.

Treatment

Achalasia is treated by *pneumatic dilatation,* the forceful dilatation of the LES with small inflatable bags. In this way, dysphagia can be relieved for years and perhaps permanently; however, esophageal motility is not restored. Surgery is often required, although pneumatic dilatation may be performed first in order to rehabilitate the patient nutritionally prior to surgery. After dilatation or surgery the esophagus, now permanently open, functions by means of gravity and oropharyngeal pressure.

Until the LES can be opened, the use of antacids along with liquid foods and fluids with meals will facilitate swallowing and maintain the patient's nutritional intake. If this method does not result in adequate nutritional intake, feeding by means of a nasogastric tube, jejunostomy or gastrostomy, as described in Chapter 35, may be necessary.

Permanent opening of the LES through dilatation or surgery alleviates dysphagia, but it also allows reflux of the gastric contents into the esophagus. The gastroesophageal reflux is highly acidic and can cause inflammation of the esophagus or *esophagitis.*

ESOPHAGITIS

Esophagitis usually occurs in the lower esophagus as a result of the irritating effect of acidic gastric reflux on the esophageal mucosa. The common symptom is *heartburn,* a burning epigastric substernal pain. In the rare situation when esophagitis appears in the upper esophagus, it is usually a consequence of iron deficiency (Plummer-Vinson syndrome.) Iron deficiency causes atrophic changes in the esophageal mucosa that make it vulnerable to the minor trauma from food.

Esophagitis can be either acute or chronic. *Acute* esophagitis is caused by ingestion of an irritating agent, viral inflammation or intubation. *Chronic* esophagitis is a result of recurrent gastroesophageal reflux due to a hiatal hernia, reduced LES pressure, recurrent vomiting or other factors. When lower esophagitis is chronic, an inflammatory stricture and eventually dysphagia can develop. Gastroesophageal reflux esophagitis is due to several factors. The content of the gastric reflux, the esophageal mucosal resistance, the esophageal clearing rate and gastric emptying are important in addition to the competency of the LES. It is known that LES tone is important in preventing gastroesophageal reflux, but there is poor correlation between the basal LES pressure and clinical evidence of reflux disease.[24] It appears that there can be transient relaxations of the LES with subsequent reflux in normal persons, but it may be more frequent in those with esophagitis.[6] Gastroesophageal reflux also commonly occurs owing to transient increased abdominal pressure.[8]

The LES pressure is controlled by many factors, one of which is hormonal control. Many gastrointestinal hormones and peptides have been proposed as possible physiological regulators of LES pressure, but they remain controversial. Gastrin, once thought to be important, does not seem to affect LES pressure significantly at present. The most clinically relevant hormone now seems to be progesterone. LES pressures decrease during pregnancy, in women taking progesterone-containing oral contraceptives, and even in normal women in the late stage of a normal menstrual cycle.[7, 32] This may explain the frequent occurrence of heartburn during pregnancy.

Nutritional Care

The objectives of nutritional care for esophagitis are (1) to prevent irritation of the inflamed esophageal mucosa in the acute phase, (2) to prevent esophageal reflux and (3) to decrease the irritating capacity or acidity of the gastric juice.

In the acute phase, the patient may want a liquid diet, which is less abrasive to the esophagus. Orange juice and other citrus and tomato products can be irritating because of their acidity, and omission of these from the diet can be helpful.

Certain foods affect LES pressure:

1. Fatty meals *decrease* LES pressure.

2. Chocolate, which contains caffeine and theobromine, *decreases* LES pressure.

3. Coffee, which contains caffeine, *decreases* esophageal pressure and stimulates gastric acid secretion.

4. Alcohol *decreases* LES pressure.

5. Cigarette smoking (nicotine) *decreases* LES pressure.

6. Peppermint and spearmint oils, such as might be found in liqueurs, *decrease* LES pressure.

Those foods and other factors that decrease LES pressure should be restricted or omitted from the diet. Practically speaking, this means a diet low in fat that excludes alcohol, carminatives (peppermint and spearmint), chocolate and caffeine-containing beverages.

To decrease the irritating capacity or acidity of the gastric juice, the patient is advised to take antacids and Gaviscon. Gaviscon is a mixture of aluminum hydroxide and alginic acid that floats on top of the gastric acid pool. It prevents the movement of gastric acid into the esophagus. However, it is probably no more effective than antacids. Antacids, besides lowering gastric acidity, also raise LES pressure.

Other helpful suggestions are for the patient to sleep on a bed that has its upper portion raised 4 to 6 inches and to lose weight if overweight. Table 22–2 summarizes the nutritional care for esophagitis.

Bethanechol, a cholinergic drug, increases

LES pressure and may be prescribed if the esophagitis does not respond to other measures. Metoclopramide, a dopamine antagonist, also shows promise in treating gastroesophageal reflux. However, its neurological and psychotropic side effects are disturbing. Lastly, the histamine H_2 receptor blocking agent cimetidine has been used to decrease gastric acid production. It decreases symptoms, but has not consistently been shown to aid in healing esophagitis. It has no effect on LES pressure. Esophagitis that does not respond after three to six months of medical therapy should be treated surgically. This is the case in 5 to 10 per cent of patients with gastroesophageal reflux.[24]

HIATAL HERNIA

Hiatal hernia is an outpouching of a portion of the stomach into the chest through the esophageal hiatus of the diaphragm. Depending on the form of the outpouching, a hiatal hernia may be *paraesophageal* or *sliding*, in which part of the stomach but not the esophagus herniates through the diaphragm into the thorax, or it can be *gastroesophageal*, in which the lower esophagus and part of the stomach protrude through the diaphragm into the thorax as shown in Figure 22–2. The major symptoms of either type of hernia are reflux of gastric contents into the esophagus and esophagitis.

Treatment

Treatment aims to reduce gastroesophageal reflux, so the nutritional care is similar to that for esophagitis. Especially important is weight reduction if obesity is a problem. Decreased weight will result in decreased abdominal pressure. Again, surgical repair is indicated if the esophageal distress is resistant to medical therapy.

Diseases of the Stomach

INDIGESTION

Indigestion or dyspepsia is an indefinite term frequently used to describe any discomfort occurring from a disorder of the digestive tract. The core of the trouble may be in the stomach, or it may be a symptom of the derangement of some other organ, such as the colon, or of gallbladder disease, chronic appendicitis or diabetes. Indigestion as a manifestation of psychoneurosis is frequently encountered. The association between emotional and gastrointestinal disturbances is so frequent that the relationship cannot be denied. Many people complain of

Table 22–2. NUTRITIONAL CARE FOR PATIENTS WITH ESOPHAGITIS

The patient with esophagitis should:

1. Avoid those foods that he knows will cause heartburn.
2. Eat small, frequent meals to prevent stomach distention and resulting gastric acid secretion.
3. Avoid high-fat meals and decrease fat in the diet. Fat decreases lower esophageal sphincter pressure.
4. Avoid chocolate, alcohol and caffeine-containing beverages such as coffee, tea and cola drinks, which decrease lower esophageal sphincter pressure.
5. Avoid lying down, bending over or straining immediately after eating.
6. Avoid eating within two to three hours of going to bed.
7. Avoid tight-fitting clothing, especially after a meal.
8. Lose weight if overweight.

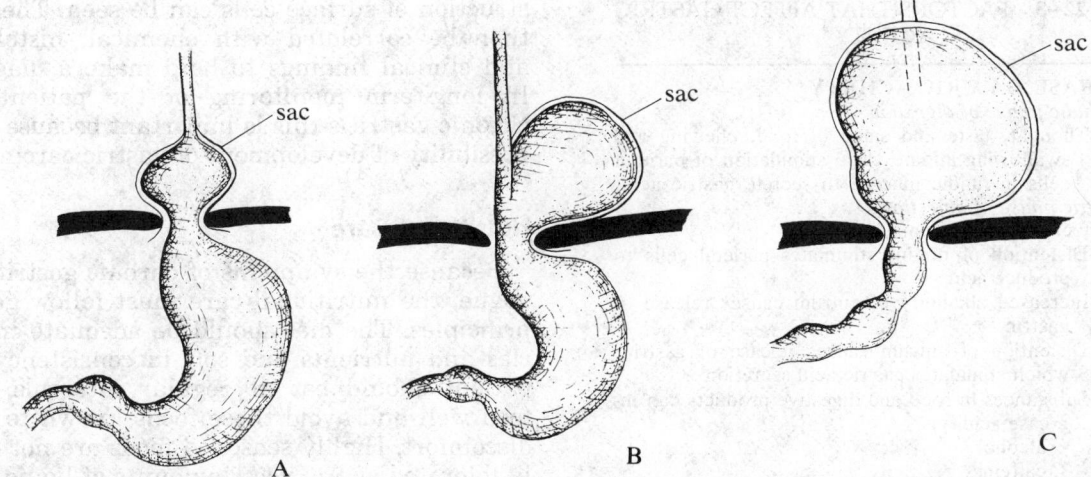

Figure 22–2. Sketches of various types of hernias. *A,* Bell (or sliding) hernia; *B,* paraesophageal hernia; *C,* massive (or gastro-esophageal) hernia. (From: Hagarty, G.: A classification of esophageal hiatus hernia with special reference to sliding hernia. *Am. J. Roentgenol., 84*:1056, 1960.)

a "nervous stomach," which they attribute to the eating of certain foods. Besides psychic disturbance, other avoidable causes of indigestion are rapid eating, poor mastication, overindulgence in rich foods and a poor diet.

Nutritional Care

Before dietary treatment begins, the cause of indigestion must be determined. The symptoms may be a warning of a more serious illness. A therapeutic diet for simple indigestion is seldom necessary, since a well-balanced diet plus correct eating habits is usually sufficient. Treating the cause, whether it is a mental or a physical one, is the important factor. Emphasis should be placed on the improvement of the patient's customary dietary and eating habits.

ACUTE GASTRITIS

Acute gastritis is an inflammation of the gastric mucosa, sudden and sometimes violent in onset, but the term is often applied to any stomach discomfort. True gastritis is usually manifested by nausea and vomiting, hemorrhage, pain, malaise, anorexia or headache. Attacks very often follow the eating of specific foods to which the individual is sensitive, eating too fast or eating when overtired or emotionally upset. Too much alcohol, tobacco and highly seasoned foods may also be contributing factors. Food poisoning or ingestion of a corrosive substance can also cause acute gastritis. Drugs such as salicylates, reserpine, indomethacin and phenylbutazone can cause gastritis. Occasionally acute gastritis will follow radiation therapy, trauma, burns, surgery, hypoxia, shock, fever,

jaundice, or renal failure. Rarely, it can complicate a bacterial infection.

The initial treatment is to remove the cause or get rid of the offending substance as soon as possible. It may be necessary to empty the stomach by induced vomiting, lavage or both. Irrigation of the colon and the administration of a laxative may also be of value in hastening the cleansing process.

Nutritional Care

To allow the stomach to rest and heal, food is usually withheld for 24 to 48 hours or longer, depending upon whether there is bleeding or pain. If there is bleeding, nasogastric lavage with ice water brings hemostasis in most patients. Fluids are given intravenously.

Following the fasting period, liquids are added as tolerated. The amount of food and the number of feedings are increased according to the patient's tolerance until he or she is eating a full regular diet. Highly seasoned foods as well as foods listed in Table 22–3 that increase gastric acidity may need to be avoided for a while. The nurse or dietitian should discuss the patient's customary dietary pattern, eating habits and any changes needed.

CHRONIC GASTRITIS

The cause of chronic gastritis is not known. Chronic gastritis often precedes the development of organic gastric lesions such as cancer or ulcer. It may be due to an antral defect that closely resembles these diseases. It may also be related indirectly to diseases such as tuberculosis, myocardial failure and nephritis. The same

Table 22–3. FACTORS THAT AFFECT GASTRIC ACIDITY

INCREASE GASTRIC ACIDITY
  Cephalic phase of digestion
      Thought, taste and smell of food, chewing and swallowing initiate vagal stimulation of parietal cells in fundic mucosa to secrete gastric acid.
  Gastric phase of digestion
    Effect of food in stomach:
      Distention of fundus stimulates parietal cells to produce acid.
      Increased alkalinity of antrum causes release of gastrin.
      Distention of antrum causes release of gastrin, which stimulates gastric acid secretion.
      Substances in food and digestive products can increase acidity:
          alcohol
          caffeine
          decaffeinated coffee
          red pepper
          cola beverages
          polypeptides and amino acids (products of protein digestion).

DECREASE GASTRIC ACIDITY
  Gastric phase of digestion
      Acidification of antrum reduces gastrin release and thus gastric acid secretion.
      Food, especially protein, has an initial buffering effect.
  Intestinal phase of digestion
      Fat, acid and hyperosmolarity in the small intestine stimulate release of one or more gastrointestinal hormones which inhibit gastric acid secretion.

dietary indiscretions listed for acute gastritis seem to be frequent causes of chronic gastritis. Although symptoms may be vague or absent, the most usual ones are similar to symptoms of indigestion—loss of appetite, a feeling of fullness, belching, vague epigastric pain, and nausea and vomiting.

There are three types of chronic gastritis: *superficial,* which causes an inflamed mucosa with hemorrhages and small erosions; *atrophic,* which occurs in all layers of the stomach, results in a decreased number of parietal and chief cells (see Chapter 5), is frequently associated with gastric ulcer and cancer and is invariably present in pernicious anemia; and *hypertrophic,* which causes the mucosa to be dull, nodular and irregular with frequent hemorrhages.

Endoscopy

An endoscope, a flexible tube with a light at one end and an eye piece, can be passed down the esophagus into the stomach, and the appearance of the stomach mucosa can be viewed, studied and even photographed. Erosions, ulcerations, changes in the blood vessels, and de-

struction of surface cells can be seen. These can then be correlated with chemical, histological and clinical findings to help make a diagnosis. In long-term monitoring of the patient with chronic gastritis this is important because of the possibility of development of gastric carcinoma.

Nutritional Care

Because the symptoms of chronic gastritis are vague, the nutritional care must follow general principles. The diet should be adequate in calories and nutrients and soft in consistency. The patient should eat at regular intervals, chew food well and avoid those foods known to cause discomfort. Highly seasoned foods are not usually tolerated well. Excess amounts of liquids with meals tend to cause discomfort because of stomach distention. The principles followed in care of ulcers, which are summarized in Table 22–4, are also followed in the treatment of gastritis. Most important is to determine foods and situations that cause discomfort and then to prescribe individualized treatment.

In atrophic gastritis, which results in atrophy and loss of stomach oxyntic cells, there is achlorhydria (a loss of gastric secretion) and possible vitamin B_{12} malabsorption. This is due to a lack of intrinsic factor. Vitamin B_{12} status should always be assessed in these patients.

GASTRIC AND DUODENAL ULCERS

An eroded lesion in the gastric mucosa or intestinal mucosa (duodenum) is termed an *ulcer.* The location of the ulcer determines its nomenclature. That is, if the ulcer is located in the stomach, it is a *gastric ulcer;* if it is located in the duodenum, as shown in Figure 22–3, it is called a *duodenal ulcer.* Often both types are grouped together under the general term *peptic ulcer.* Since the treatment for both types is essentially the same, the nutritional care for

Table 22–4. PRINCIPLES OF NUTRITIONAL CARE FOR PEPTIC ULCER DISEASE

The patient with peptic ulcer disease should:
  1. Eat three regular meals daily.
  2. Eat small meals to avoid stomach distention.
  3. Avoid drinking coffee, tea, cola and other caffeine-containing beverages and alcohol.
  4. Cut down on or quit smoking cigarettes.
  5. Avoid using large amounts of aspirin or other drugs known to damage the stomach lining.
  6. Avoid using excessive amounts of pepper in cooking or on food.
  7. Avoid those foods or drinks that cause discomfort.
  8. Eat meals in as relaxed an atmosphere as possible.
  9. Take antacids 1–3 hours after meals and prior to bedtime.

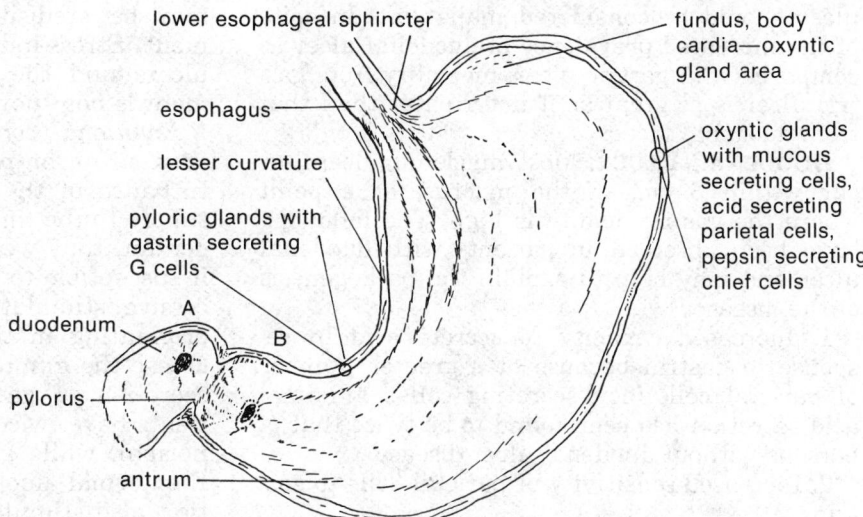

Figure 22–3. Diagram showing stomach and duodenum with eroded lesions. *A,* Duodenal ulcer; *B,* gastric ulcer.

them will be considered together. Duodenal ulcers are much more common than gastric ulcers, and both kinds occur in the male (80 to 85 per cent of duodenal ulcer patients and 60 per cent of gastric ulcer patients) more frequently than in the female, usually in people who are naturally tense, hard-working and hard-worrying. Duodenal ulcer tends to occur initially in younger people, the peak age of initial appearance in males being about 20 to 30 years of age and in females 40 to 50 years. Gastric ulcers tend to have their initial appearance between ages 50 and 60 years.

It is reported that approximately 10 per cent of the population is or has been afflicted with gastric or duodenal ulcers. Sometimes during routine x-ray examination ulcer scars are found, although the individual never knew that the disorder existed. This would seem to indicate that healing sometimes takes place spontaneously. Ulcers tend to recur in 75 to 80 per cent of patients. The disease appears to run a course that lasts about 15 years.[10]

Presently there is a decline in the incidence of duodenal ulcer that cannot be explained until more is known about the pathogenesis of peptic ulcer disease.[23] However, the frequency of duodenal ulcer seems to be increasing among U.S. females, possibly as a result of the fact that more American women are now pursuing aggressive careers.

Pathogenesis of Ulcer Disease

An acidic gastrointestinal environment is believed to be the principal cause of peptic ulcer disease. Normally, the mucosa of the stomach is protected from the strongly acidic digestive juices by the mucus secreted by glands located in the gastrointestinal walls from the lower esophagus to the upper duodenum. The duodenum is also protected by the pancreatic secretions, which contain large quantities of sodium bicarbonate that neutralize the hydrochloric acid in the gastric juice. In the alkaline environment, pepsin is inactivated and cannot digest the duodenal mucosa.

The reasons why the gastric or duodenal acidity gets too high and why the mucosa loses its resistance to normal gastric acidity are not clear, but many theories have been suggested.

GASTRIC ULCER. Most gastric ulcers are found in the antrum of the stomach. Their pathogenesis seems to be different from that of duodenal ulcers in that there usually is not gastric acid hypersecretion in gastric ulcer patients as is seen in most duodenal ulcer patients. Impaired gastric mucosal resistance is the major factor in gastric ulcer, whereas gastric acid hypersecretion is the major factor in pathogenesis of duodenal ulcer. The following are possible pathological processes of gastric ulcers:

1. Gastritis or inflammation of the antrum or pyloric gland area tends to occur with gastric ulcer and may be a "pre-ulcer" condition.

2. Chronic backward diffusion of H^+ ions after the normal gastric mucosal barrier is disrupted results in gross mucosal damage. The mucosal damage leads to release of pepsin in large quantities, which contributes to further mucosal damage.

3. A disturbance in antroduodenal motility can cause bile acids from the duodenum to reflux back into the stomach, where they break the mucosal barrier and cause gastritis. The damaged mucosa then becomes susceptible to peptic ulceration. Other agents that break the barrier are salicylates and alcohol.

In the instance when there is no detectable gastric acid secretion (achlorhydria), the gastric ulcer should be considered malignant. In spite of the increased prevalence of duodenal ulcer as compared with gastric ulcer, mortality from gastric ulcer is as great as if not greater than that from duodenal ulcer.

DUODENAL ULCER. Most duodenal ulcers occur within 3 cm. of the pylorus, at a point where the gastric acidity is high. The following have been observed in patients with duodenal ulcer and may help to explain the pathogenesis of the disease:[15, 33]

1. Increased capacity to secrete acid in response to gastrin because of a greater number of parietal cells (acid-secreting cells). Maximal acid secretion has been found to be twice that of persons without duodenal ulcer disease.

2. Increased sensitivity of parietal cells to gastrin.

3. Hypersecretion of gastrin in response to meals.

4. Decreased ability to inhibit gastrin release when the acidity of the gastric contents drops too low.

5. Abnormally long gastric secretory response to a meal that continues into a latent postprandial period.[19]

6. Increased nocturnal gastric acid secretion.

7. Rapid entry of acidified chyme into the duodenum and it cannot be neutralized rapidly enough.

All of these abnormal functions result in an increased acid load to the duodenum and the development of a duodenal ulcer.

Although chronic ulcer usually follows a typical course and produces characteristic symptoms, occasionally the symptoms may be either non-existent or indefinite, and hemorrhage or perforation may be the first sign of the illness. Ulcers can perforate into the peritoneal cavity or penetrate into an adjacent organ (usually the pancreas), and they may erode an artery and result in massive hemorrhage.

Predisposing Factors

Faulty dietary habits, excessive smoking, excessive aspirin ingestion and *excessive drinking of coffee and cola drinks* are associated with an increased risk of developing an ulcer.[11] Rushing through meals, improper selection of food and irregular mealtimes are poor habits that seem to set the stage for ulcer development.

Heredity has been mentioned as a possible factor in the development of ulcers. The capacity of the stomach to secrete hydrochloric acid is a function of the number of parietal cells in the gastric mucosa, and this is thought by some to be genetically determined.[26]

Physical stress can cause ulcers. Therefore, inadequate sleep and rest, disease and trauma may be predisposing factors in their development. Stress-induced ulcers usually are gastric ulcers and the mechanism for their development is not known.

Emotional conflicts, psychological stress, nervous strain or *psychic trauma* can cause a disturbance of the nerves that control the blood supply to the lining of the stomach and the duodenum, thus weakening the lining and making it susceptible to attack by the gastric juices. Excessive stimulation of the vagus by impulses originating in the cerebrum is thought to increase the number of parietal cells and thus the secretion of gastric acid. Duodenal ulcer patients have twice the number of parietal cells as normal, while gastric ulcer patients have half the normal amount.[21] In addition, vagal stimulation also stimulates gastrin release, lowers the threshold of the parietal cell to circulating gastrin, and directly stimulates gastric acid secretion by the parietal cells.

Protective factors in unrefined foods may help to prevent ulcer disease. Based on epidemiological studies in populations that eat unrefined diets, some investigators feel that factors present in fiber can protect the gastrointestinal epithelium from ulcer disease through a buffering activity.[31]

Treatment

The objectives of treatment are relief of pain, healing of the ulcer, reduction of the tendency to recurrence and maintenance of good nutritional status. Unfortunately, there is no cure for peptic ulcer disease, and the ulcers do tend to recur.

MEDICAL THERAPY. The accepted medical treatment at present for peptic ulcer is based on the fact that these ulcers do not exist in the absence of hydrochloric acid. Accordingly, therapy is directed toward the neutralization of acids and the reduction of acid secretion by the stomach. By elevating the pH of the gastric contents, the proteolytic activity of pepsin and the damaging effect of acid are reduced. In addition, therapy aims to preserve the resistance of the epithelium to the destructive action of gastric juice. With these objectives, therapy consists of taking antacids and medications, modifying the diet and avoiding stressful situations.

Rest. Because resistance must be kept at a high level, physical and mental rest are important. If the ulcer is moderately advanced, bed rest either at home or in the hospital may be advocated for a period of one to three weeks. An equal period of convalescence is prescribed, particularly for the working person, who should stay away from disturbing office situations. In mild cases the patient can usually continue his regular routine work activities while following the diet and taking medication. If the atmosphere and surroundings at home or at work are unpleasant and cause emotional upsets, the patient may be advised to consider a complete change.

Antacids. Antacids have long been clinically effective in reducing the pain from duodenal ulcer, and it was always thought that relief was due to a reduction in gastric acidity. This is questionable now in the light of evidence showing that pain relief in duodenal ulcer patients was the same whether they were given an antacid or a placebo that looked and tasted like chalky white antacid but had no buffering capacity.[29] This does not exclude the use of antacids but suggests that factors other than acid neutralization are important in the relief of ulcer pain. The degree to which a patient responds to antacids depends on the individual, the extent of the parietal cell mass, the rate at which the antacid is emptied from the stomach and the gastric acid response to eating. Antacids vary in their ability to neutralize acid, and this should be considered when prescribing the amount to be used. For most effectiveness antacids should be taken between meals and before bed.

The preferred antacid contains aluminum hydroxide, which has good acid-neutralizing ability and is not absorbed by the body. However, aluminum hydroxide binds phosphorus in the gut and prevents its absorption, which could result in a lowered serum phosphate level. Antacids containing calcium, such as calcium carbonate preparations, are less desirable. Calcium stimulates gastrin secretion, which increases gastric acid secretion. Magnesium frequently is added to antacid mixtures to prevent constipation.

Antacids should be taken one to three hours after eating. Taken this way they have a longer buffering effect, about three to four hours. More antacid is usually required for the patient with duodenal ulcer than for the patient with gastric ulcer, because the duodenal ulcer patient usually has hypersecretion of acid.

Other Drugs. Although anticholinergics decrease gastric acid secretion and gastric motility, their regular use in treatment of peptic ulcer disease has been a disappointment and they have no value in treatment of duodenal ulcer.[21] They inhibit vagal stimulation of acid-secreting parietal cells, vagal-stimulated release of gastrin and gastric motility. They may be given during the active phase of ulcer disease. During inactive phases they may be taken only at night, since during sleep basal gastric acid secretion increases. Unfortunately, they have side effects such as mouth dryness, blurred vision and retention of urine.

Cimetidine (Tagamet), which blocks the stimulatory action of histamine on acid-secreting parietal cells, is widely used and effective in treatment of peptic ulcer disease. One cautionary note is that antacids inhibit the absorption of cimetidine, probably due to the binding of the drug by aluminum hydroxide. For this reason antacids and cimetidine should not be taken simultaneously.[27]

Prostaglandins (PGE_1 and PGE_2) inhibit the secretion of gastric acid and may also increase the resistance of mucosal cells to injury. The synthetic analogues of these, when given to ulcer patients, have been shown to be effective in inhibiting gastric secretions and hastening healing.

Mucosal barrier fortifiers such as carbenoxolone have been shown to be effective in preventing hydrogen ion back-diffusion into the mucosa and in stimulating mucus production that enhances healing of gastric ulcer. However, this treatment may lead to severe side effects, including salt and water retention and occasionally hypokalemia and hypertension.[2]

Several gastrointestinal hormones lead to decreased gastric acid secretion, including secretin, cholecystokinin-pancreozymin, gastric inhibitory peptide and others (see Table 5–1).

NUTRITIONAL CARE. Like the other measures, nutritional care aims to reduce the secretion of stomach acid, to neutralize it, to maintain the resistance of gastrointestinal epithelial tissue to the acid and to restore the patient's nutritional status. There is little disagreement about these objectives of nutritional care, but controversy does exist regarding the dietary modifications needed to meet these objectives. As is usually the case, the controversy exists because of the ignorance regarding what happens to an individual food item in the gut, its effect on the alimentary tube and the explanation of symptoms that might follow its ingestion. Many of the diets used are a result of deep-rooted practice, without true scientific justification.

It is known that sight, smell and taste, water and practically anything else taken into the stomach stimulate gastric secretions to some degree. Neither those foods that are chemically, mechanically or thermally irritating to the mucosa nor those that are soothing have been determined. Although the chemical composition and physical properties of foods before ingestion are available, correlations between the nature of a food and its gastrointestinal effects in most cases are unknown.

When trying to reduce gastric acidity, it is important to consider both the immediate and delayed effects of foods and even of antacids. Antacids and food act as buffers, so their immediate effect is a lowering of gastric acidity. However, when the acidity gets too low, a feedback mechanism in the stomach stimulates it to begin secreting acid again.

Food Acidity. The effect of acidic foods on gastric acidity must be evaluated. The pH of foods ranges from about 2 in lime juice to 8 in egg whites. Most foods have a pH of between 5 and 7. The pH of both orange juice and grapefruit juice is 3.2 to 3.6, which is considerably less acidic than the normal gastric pH of about 1.6. Theoretically (on the basis of their immediate acidity), acid fruit juices are contraindicated only for patients who have oral or esophageal lesions and possibly for patients with gastric lesions, particularly if the stomach is achlorhydric (atrophic gastritis). Otherwise, the pH of a food before it is ingested has little therapeutic importance.

Foods That Cause Gas. In thinking about foods that give them distress, many ulcer patients will mention several foods that cause them to belch and have gas. The many factors that influence its production are discussed on page 439.

Factors That Damage Gastrointestinal Mucosa. Usually the stomach is protected by its epithelium, and the duodenum is protected by the thick alkaline mucoid secretions of Brunner's glands. There is only limited knowledge about the dietary and environmental factors that cause epithelial irritation and possible breakdown. Alcohol is known to damage the gastric mucosa, however. Black pepper, chili powder, cloves, nutmeg and mustard seed have been thought to cause a slight reddening of the mucosa. Black pepper has been shown to be an irritant causing a specific and localized hyperemia, whereas other spices are apparently innocuous in this respect.[25] Salicylates and some other drugs can cause damage to gastric mucosa.

Foods That Stimulate Gastric Acid Secretion. Caffeine is known to stimulate secretion of gastric juices when consumed by itself and should be avoided by ulcer patients. Decaffeinated coffee also increases gastric acid secretion.[20,31] A recent study showed that the acid responses to Sanka, regular coffee and Kava were similar.[20]

Cigarette smoking may increase gastric acid secretion and gastric motility or may impair neutralization of gastric acid by inhibiting pancreatic bicarbonate secretion, but this has not been proved.[3,28] Garlic, paprika, horseradish, mustard and other spices have been shown to increase gastric secretion, but only when they were used alone and in fairly large amounts.[5] Many more studies show that nonspicy diets are no more effective in reducing ulcer pain or in aiding ulcer healing than are regular diets.

Factors that increase or decrease gastric acidity are listed in Table 22–3. Pepsin secretion in response to the intake of different foods tends to parallel gastric acid secretion. The production of mucus in response to various foods is not known.

Diet and Eating Pattern Recommendations

Frequent and regular meals and antacid therapy are more important than the type of food ingested. It is important to eat small meals frequently (every three hours or so) so that the buffering action of food will be present in the stomach and yet the stomach will not be distended with a large meal, which enhances gastric acid secretion.

Protein foods have a dual role related to gastric content and secretions. They act as a buffer, but their buffering action is only temporary. As the protein digestion products (amino acids and polypeptides) reach the antrum, they stimulate the secretion of gastrin and thus the secretion of gastric acid.

Fat inhibits gastric secretion. However, there are no experimental observations to verify that the dairy fats traditionally recommended to the ulcer patient are any more effective in depressing gastric secretions than are other animal fats, vegetable oils or foods fried in vegetable oil.

Whether or not a food will be tolerated by an ulcer patient is best determined by trial. Intelligent individuals will probably avoid any food that they know from experience causes indigestion, pain or other digestive symptoms. Doll and associates[9] observed 121 patients with peptic ulcer who received a controlled dietary regimen and reported that a conventional bland diet does not increase the healing rate. Lennard-Jones and Babouris reported no difference in the gastric acidity of 12 duodenal ulcer patients whether they received a "free choice" diet or a traditional ulcer diet.[18] In fact, gastric acidity frequently was lower when a free-choice diet was taken. Todd[30] found no proof that the avoidance of certain foods customarily considered irritating is beneficial, unless these foods cause immediate distress. In summary, then, *there is no proof that a bland diet increases the healing rate or prevents the recurrence of peptic ulcer.*

THE LIBERAL APPROACH. In 1971, the American Dietetic Association stated that nutritional care for the patient with ulcer disease should be liberalized considerably, based on information showing that the bland diet has had no significant effect on the healing of ulcers.[1] The liberal approach as outlined in Table 22–4 is recommended. There is no necessity to eat six small feedings since there has been found to be little difference in gastric acid secretion between a three meal per day pattern and that of six small feedings per day.[16]

Counseling the Patient. The application of the liberal concept centers on the person rather than the diet and on normal nutritional needs rather than a special regimen. Regularity and frequency of meals and moderation in eating habits are important in the long-term care. An understanding, common-sense approach to the dietary treatment, which considers the patient as a whole person and not just the ulcer, will provide the essential nutritional needs and acid-reducing features that are therapeutic to the individual (Fig. 22–4). Some anxious, worrisome patients may need a strict diet plan for emotional and psychological reasons, while others are comfortable with less rigidity and more freedom of choice. Using such an approach, the nurse or dietitian might ask, for example, what changes should the patient make in the present dietary pattern to provide the necessary calories and nutrients? What changes can be made in eating habits? How will the patient implement the changes? What changes must he or she make in lifestyle? Who can help in making these changes?

TRADITIONAL ULCER DIET. Although it is not recommended in this text, the traditional treatment remains widely used and for that reason is presented here. A survey of 240 gastroenterologists revealed that 48 per cent still prescribed a bland or restricted diet to their ulcer patients notwithstanding the ADA guidelines.[22]

Unlike the foods used in the liberal approach, foods included in the conventional ulcer diet are soft in consistency, with a minimum amount of fiber. All foods *believed* to stimulate gastric secretion and gastric motility are omitted.

Milk. In 1915 Sippy introduced a progressive regimen. Milk (or milk and cream) was the basis of the diet and was conventionally used for its acid-buffering capacity. It is now questionable whether milk should be used to such a large extent in the diet for the ulcer patient. In a study of five patients with duodenal ulcer and five patients without gastrointestinal disease, it was shown that milk (whole, low-fat or skim) significantly increased gastric acid secretion in all patients, and that this stimulatory effect lasted for at least three hours. Its initial buffering and pain-relieving ability is not long-lasting.[14] Second, in other patients who received hourly drinks of milk and cream, gastric contents were more acidic (pH 1.3) than in patients who received only three meals per day.[16] Third, calcium, of which milk is a rich source, is known to increase gastric acid secretion by stimulating gastrin release. It may be that ulcer pain that occurs two to four hours after a meal is due to milk ingestion with that meal. Fourth, whole

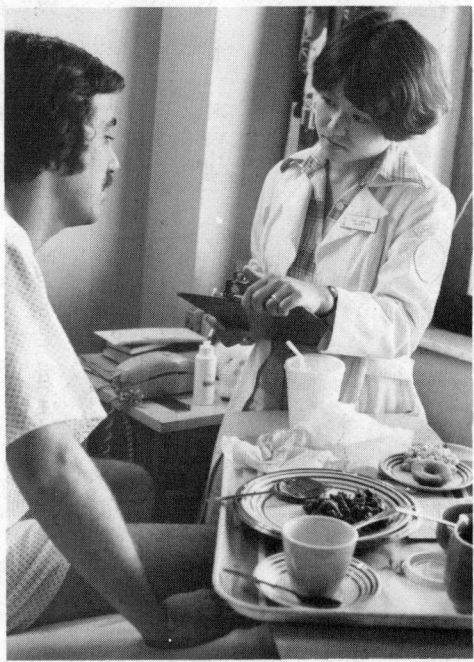

Figure 22–4. Clinical dietitian and peptic ulcer patient discussing problem foods and individualizing a diet plan. (Courtesy of Ms. Sheila Henderson, R.D.(deceased), and the nutrition staff of Lutheran General Hospital, Park Ridge, Ill.)

milk and whole milk products contribute saturated fat to the diet. The milk-based diet predisposes patients who follow it to atherosclerosis and myocardial infarction because of the high content of saturated fat. The neutralizing effects of cream, whole milk and skim milk are identical. Fifth, the excessive use of milk, especially combined with absorbable antacids (sodium bicarbonate or calcium carbonate), can lead to the rare instance of *milk-alkali syndrome* and resulting hypercalcemia and calcium deposition.

Stages of Traditional Peptic Ulcer Diet Therapy. The acute phase dietary management is given in Table 22–5. When used, this is prescribed for a short time for the patient with bleeding or acute pain. As pain disappears, small feedings of soft-fiber foods are added to or replace some of the milk or milk and cream feedings.

Many physicians who still follow traditional dietary management would then prescribe the six-feeding restricted bland diet given in Table 22–6. Small feedings (12 to 20 oz.) are given six times a day. Fried foods, most raw fruits and vegetables, caffeine, alcohol, coarse breads and cereals, highly seasoned foods and any other foods known to cause the patient discomfort are omitted. Table 22–7 gives a sample menu. The diet contains approximately 100 gm. of protein, 90 gm. of fat, 280 gm. of carbohydrate and 2300 kcal. If fewer calories or a reduction of serum

Table 22–5. ACUTE PHASE OF TRADITIONAL DIETARY MANAGEMENT FOR PEPTIC ULCER

	8 A.M.	10 A.M.	12 NOON	3 P.M.	6 P.M.
First Stage 3 to 4 oz. milk or milk and cream (half-and-half) served every 1 to 2 hours on the hour, 7 A.M. through 9 P.M. and during the night if necessary.					
Second Stage					
Supplementary feedings added as tolerated (6 to 8 oz.)					
1 feeding	Farina with cream and sugar				Baked custard
2 feedings	Boiled rice with cream and sugar				Gelatin and cream
3 feedings	Farina with cream and sugar	Milk toast			Vanilla ice cream with sugar cookies
4 feedings	Oatmeal with cream and sugar	Poached egg on toast	Cream soup with soda crackers		Cream soup with croutons
5 feedings	Cream of Wheat with cream and sugar	Soft-cooked egg with 1 slice toast	Boiled rice with cream and sugar	Bread pudding with cream	

434

Table 22–6.   SIX FEEDING RESTRICTED BLAND DIET

FOOD GROUPS	FOODS RECOMMENDED	FOODS WHICH MAY CAUSE DISTRESS
Milk and Milk Products (2 or more cups daily)	All milk and milk drinks	None
Vegetables (2 or more servings daily)	All vegetable juices Cooked vegetables as tolerated Salads made from allowed foods	Raw vegetables, dried peas and beans, corn Gas-forming vegetables such as broccoli, Brussels sprouts, cabbage, onions, cauliflower, cucumber, green pepper, rutabagas, turnips and sauerkraut
Fruits (2 or more servings daily)	All fruit juices Cooked or canned fruit Avocado and banana Grapefruit and orange sections without membrane	All other fresh and dried fruit Berries and figs
Breads and Cereals (4 or more servings daily)	Enriched breads and cereals	Very coarse cereals such as bran Seeds in or on breads, rolls and crackers Bread and bread products made with nuts or dried fruit Any fried breads
Potatoes or Substitutes	Potatoes Enriched rice, barley, noodles, spaghetti, macaroni and other pastas	Potato chips, fried potatoes, fried rice, wild rice
Meats or Substitutes (6 or more ounces daily)	All lean, tender meats, poultry, fish and shellfish Eggs; crisp bacon; lean ham Mild cheeses Smooth peanut butter Soybean and other meat substitutes	Highly seasoned, cured or smoked meats, poultry or fish, such as corned beef, luncheon meats, frankfurters and other sausages, sardines, anchovies and strong-flavored cheeses Chunky peanut butter
Fats	Butter or fortified margarine Mayonnaise All fats and oils	Salad dressings
Soups	Mildly seasoned meat stock and cream soups made with allowed foods	All other soups
Sweets and Desserts	Sugar, syrup, honey, jelly, seedless jam, hard candies, plain chocolate candies, molasses, marshmallows Cakes, cookies, pies, puddings, custard, ice cream, sherbet and Jello made from allowed foods	All sweets and desserts containing nuts, coconut or fruit that is not allowed Fried pastries such as doughnuts
Beverages	Decaffeinated coffee, cocoa, fruit drinks, 99% caffeine-free cola and other carbonated beverages, except other cola drinks.	Coffee, tea, alcohol and all cola drinks
Miscellaneous	Iodized salt, flavorings Mildly flavored gravies and sauces Mild herbs and spices	Strongly flavored seasonings and condiments such as ketchup, pepper, barbeque sauce, chili sauce, chili pepper, horseradish, garlic, mustard, vinegar Olives, pickles, popcorn, nuts and coconut

From Manual of Clinical Dietetics. 2nd ed. Researched and approved by Chicago Dietetic Association and South Suburban Dietetic Association of Cook and Will Counties. Philadelphia, W. B. Saunders Company, 1981.

lipids is desired, skim milk and milk products should be used along with less added fat and smaller portions.

Possible Nutritional Inadequacies. Energy and protein deficiencies can accompany ulcers, especially during the initial treatment, and in-terfere with the healing of the lesions. Avitaminosis, particularly of vitamin C, may develop unless vitamin supplements or specific vitamin-rich foods are added to the diet.

Secondary anemia may develop in the ulcer patient during treatment with antacids. Iron ab-

Table 22–7. SAMPLE MENU FROM THE SIX FEEDING RESTRICTED BLAND DIET

BREAKFAST	LUNCH	DINNER
½ cup orange juice	2 oz. beef patty	2 oz. broiled chicken
1 poached egg or egg substitute	½ cup rice	½ cup mashed potatoes
1 slice toast	½ cup spinach	½ cup peas
1 tsp. butter or margarine	1 slice bread	1 tsp. butter or margarine
1 cup decaffeinated coffee	1 tsp. butter or margarine	1 cup decaffeinated coffee
1 oz. cream or non-dairy creamer	4 oz. milk (whole or low-fat)	1 oz. cream or non-dairy creamer
2 tsp. sugar		2 tsp. sugar

MIDMORNING SNACK	MIDAFTERNOON SNACK	BEDTIME SNACK
½ cup oatmeal	6 oz. vegetable soup	½ cup cottage cheese
8 oz. milk (whole or low-fat)	½ cup sherbet	½ cup apricots
2 tsp. sugar	2 sugar cookies	2 saltine crackers
½ cup peaches	1 cup decaffeinated coffee	4 oz. milk (whole or low-fat)
	1 oz. cream or non-dairy creamer	
	2 tsp. sugar	

APPROXIMATE NUTRITIVE VALUE OF SAMPLE MENU

Protein	95 gm.	Riboflavin	1.985 mg.
Fat	85 gm.	Thiamin	1.467 mg.
Carbohydrate	280 gm.	Calcium	1028 mg.
Calories	2265	Phosphorus	1466 mg.
Vitamin A	16,354 I.U.	Iron	14.3 mg.
Vitamin C	124 mg.	Sodium	3047 mg.
Niacin	20 mg.eq.	Potassium	3015 mg.

From Manual of Clinical Dietetics. 2nd ed. Researched and approved by Chicago Dietetic Association and South Suburban Dietetic Association of Cook and Will Counties. Philadelphia, W. B. Saunders Company, 1981.

sorption depends upon an acid medium; thus, neutralization of gastric acids interferes with iron absorption. Possible blood loss from an unhealed ulcer can result in an iron deficiency.

Patients receiving restricted ulcer diets need careful supervision. Whenever there is doubt about the adequacy of the diet, protein, vitamin and iron supplements should be added. Radiographs show that complete healing takes from 14 to 100 days, with an average of 40. This is why medical treatment is sometimes continued for six to seven weeks.

Surgery

Peptic ulcer is primarily a medical disease, but surgery is advised when the ulcer is complicated by hemorrhage, perforation, obstruction or intractability or when the patient is unable to follow the medical regimen. Surgical procedures for peptic ulcer have been summarized in the review by Cooperman.[4] The nutritional implications of vagotomy, antrectomy and gastric resection are covered in Chapter 34. After the ulcer has been removed, the patient should be informed that permanent lifestyle changes are essential, since an operation is not a cure-all. Recurrences of ulcers are common following both medical and surgical treatment.

CARCINOMA OF THE STOMACH

The etiology of carcinoma of the stomach is unknown and is believed by some authorities to include a number of causes rather than a single cause, as discussed in Chapter 36. Symptoms are so slow to manifest themselves and the growth of the tumor is so rapid that frequently carcinoma of the stomach is overlooked until it is too late for an effective cure. Because it is a disease of middle age, any unusually prolonged gastric discomfort appearing at this stage in life should be investigated, even though it seems slight. Loss of appetite, loss of strength and loss of weight frequently precede other symptoms. Achylia gastrica or achlorhydria has been shown to exist for years preceding the onset of gastric carcinoma.

Periodic physical examinations or check-ups are encouraged for middle-aged people. X-ray examinations and gastroscopy aid in making a very early diagnosis, so that surgical treatment is more likely to be successful. Speculation as to the role of diet in the etiology of cancer of the stomach has been growing, and Chapter 36 deals with this subject more fully.

Nutritional Care

The dietary regimen for carcinoma of the stomach is determined somewhat by the location of the cancer, the nature of the functional disturbance and the stage of the development of the disease. The patient with advanced, non-operable cancer should receive a diet adjusted to provide comfort. Any food preferences, unless definitely harmful, are granted, and living should be made as bearable as possible. In the later stages of the disease the patient may tolerate only a liquid diet, and it may be necessary to resort to parenteral nutrition. As long as other therapeutic procedures such as surgery, radiation therapy or chemotherapy are being performed, the nutritional support for the patient should be equally aggressive, as described in Chapter 36.

Anorexia is almost always present in patients who have stomach cancer, from the early stages throughout the entire course of the disease. Patients who are encouraged to select their own menus and who suggest foods that are appealing to them usually ingest more than when they are not involved in the selection or when they are forced to eat.

Chemotherapy and radiation therapy affect gastric function, and the necessary nutritional care for patients receiving these treatments is discussed in Chapter 36.

Surgery is often necessary in cases of carcinoma of the stomach. The nutritional care outlined for gastric surgery is discussed in Chapter 34.

Problems and Suggested Topics for Discussion

1. Interview a patient with dysphagia due to achalasia. Obtain a dietary history and assess his or her nutritional intake. With the patient, plan the nutritional care.
2. What are the principles of dietary treatment for peptic ulcer? Give the rationale for each principle.
3. Compare the medical dietary treatment for ulcers used in your hospital with the dietary treatment outlined in this chapter.
4. Study the eating habits of three ulcer patients of different nationalities who are in the hospital. Check for adequacy.
5. Obtain the diet history of a patient with duodenal ulcer admitted to the hospital. What were the symptoms? What was involved in the diagnosis? If possible, follow the patient's progress in the outpatient clinic.
6. Obtain a dietary history from a patient who complains of indigestion. How adequate is his or her dietary pattern? Indicate where improvement is needed. How will he or she implement the changes?

Cited References

1. American Dietetic Association: Position paper on bland diet in the treatment of chronic duodenal ulcer disease. J. Am. Diet. Assoc., 59:244, 1971.
2. Baron, J.H.: Effect of carbenoxolone sodium on human gastric acid secretion. Gut, 18:721, 1977.
3. Boden, G., et al.: Effect of nicotine on serum secretin and exocrine pancreatic secretion. Am. J. Dig. Dis., 21: 974, 1976.
4. Cooperman, A.M. (ed.): Peptic ulcer disease. Surg. Clin. N. Am., 56(6):1976.
5. Demling, L., and Koch, H.: Condiments. Acta Hepatogastroenterol., 21:377, 1974.
6. Dent, J., et al.: Mechanism of gastroesophageal reflux in recumbent asymptomatic human subjects. J. Clin. Invest., 65:256, 1980.
7. Dodds, W.J., Dent, J., and Hogan, W.J.: Pregnancy and the lower esophageal sphincter (editorial). Gastroenterology, 74:1334, 1978.
8. Dodds, W.J., et al.: Mechanisms of gastroesophageal reflux in patients with reflux esophagitis. N. Engl. J. Med., 307:1547, 1982.
9. Doll, R., Friedlander, P., and Pygott, F.: Dietetic treatment of peptic ulcer. Lancet, 1:5, 1956.
10. Fry, J.: Peptic ulcer: A profile. Br. Med. J., 2:809, 1964.
11. Grossman, M.I., et al.: A new look at peptic ulcer. Ann. Intern. Med., 84:57, 1976.
12. Guyton, A.C.: Textbook of Medical Physiology, 6th ed. Philadelphia, W.B. Saunders Company, 1981, pp. 784–815.
13. Hightower, N.C.: Applied anatomy and physiology of the esophagus. In Bockus, H.L.: Gastroenterology. Vol. 1. 3rd ed. Philadelphia, W.B. Saunders Co., 1974.
14. Ippoliti, A.F., Maxwell, V., and Isenberg, J.I.: The effect of various forms of milk on gastric acid secretion. Ann. Intern. Med., 84:286, 1976.
15. Isenberg, J.I., et al.: Increased sensitivity to stimulation of acid secretion by pentagastrin in duodenal ulcer. J. Clin. Invest., 55:330, 1975.
16. Kirsner, J.B., and Palmer, W.L.: Effect of various antacids on the hydrogen ion concentration of the gastric contents. Am. J. Dig. Dis., 7:85, 1940.
17. Lennard-Jones, J.E.: Functional gastrointestinal disorders. N. Engl. J. Med., 308:431, 1983.
18. Lennard-Jones, J.E., and Babouris, N.: Effect of different foods on the acidity of the gastric contents in patients with duodenal ulcer. Gut, 6:113, 1965.
19. Malagelada, J.R., et al.: Gastric secretion and emptying after ordinary meals in duodenal ulcer. Gastroenterology, 73:989, 1977.
20. McArthur, K., Hogan, D., and Isenberg, J.I.: Relative stimulatory effects of commonly ingested beverages on gastric acid secretion in humans. Gastroenterology, 83: 199, 1982.
21. McGuigan, J.E.: Peptic ulcer disease. In Dietschy, J.M. (ed.): Disorders of the Gastrointestinal Tract. Disorders of the Liver. Nutritional Disorders. Vol. 1, The Science and Practice of Clinical Medicine. New York, Grune & Stratton, 1976.
22. McHardy, G.G.: Diet therapy: perspective and current practice in peptic ulcer disease: an update. New York, Biomedical Information Company, 1979.
23. Mendeloff, A.I.: What has been happening to duodenal ulcer? Gastroenterology, 67:1020, 1974.
24. Richter, J.E., and Castell, D.O.: Gastroesophageal reflux. Pathogenesis, diagnosis and therapy. Ann. Intern. Med., 97:93, 1982.
25. Schneider, M.A., De Luca, V., Jr., and Gray, S.J.: Effect of spice ingestion on stomach. Am. J. Gastroenterol., 26:722, 1956.
26. Sleisenger, M.H., and Fordtran, J.S.: Gastrointestinal Disease. 2nd ed. Philadelphia, W.B. Saunders Company, 1978.
27. Steinberg, W.M., Lewis J.H., and Katz, D.M.: Antacids inhibit absorption of cimetidine. N. Engl. J. Med., 307: 400, 1982.
28. Solomon, T.E., and Jacobson, D.E.: Cigarette smoking

and duodenal ulcer disease. N. Engl. J. Med., *286*: 1212, 1972.

29. Sturdevant, R.A.L., et al.: Antacid and placebo produced similar pain relief in duodenal ulcer patients. Gastroenterology, *72*:1, 1977.

30. Todd, J.W.: Treatment of peptic ulcer. Lancet, *1*:113, 1952.

31. Tovey, F.: Duodenal ulcer and diet. In Burkitt, D.P., and Trowell, H.C. (eds.): Refined Carbohydrate Foods and Disease: Some Implications of Dietary Fiber. London, Academic Press, 1975.

32. Van Thiel, D.H., Gavaler, J.S., and Stremple, J.F.: Lower esophageal sphincter pressure during normal menstrual cycle. Am. J. Obstet. Gynecol., *134*:64, 1979.

33. Walsh, J.H., Richardson, C.T., and Fordtran, J.S.: pH dependence of acid secretion and gastrin release in normal and ulcer subjects. J. Clin. Invest., *55*:462, 1975.

Additional References

Arachidonic acid stimulates prostaglandin synthesis in cytoprotection of gastric mucosa. Nutr. Rev., *41*:90, 1983.

Atkinson, M.: Dysphagia. Br. Med. J., *1*:91, 1977.

Brown, M., et al.: Personality factors in duodenal ulcer. Psychosom. Med., *12*:1, Jan.-Feb., 1950.

Brunner, L.S.: What to do (and what to teach your patient) about peptic ulcer. Nursing '76, *6*:27, 1976.

Buchman, E., et al.: Unrestricted diet in the treatment of duodenal ulcer. Gastroenterology, *56*:1016, 1969.

Burkitt, D.P.: Hiatus hernia: is it preventable? Am. J. Clin. Nutr., *34*:428, 1981.

Castell, D.O.: Diet and the lower esophageal sphincter. Am. J. Clin. Nutr., *28*:1296, 1975.

Cohen, S., and Booth, G.H.: Gastric acid secretion and lower esophageal sphincter pressure in response to coffee and caffeine. N. Engl. J. Med., *293*:897, 1975.

Friedman, G.D., Siegelaub, A.B., and Seltzer, C.C.: Cigarettes, alcohol, coffee and peptic ulcer. N. Engl. J. Med., *290*:469, 1974.

Hartroft, W.S.: The incidence of coronary artery disease in patients treated with the Sippy diet. Am. J. Clin. Nutr., *15*:205, 1964.

Isenberg, J.I.: Peptic ulcer, epidemiology, nutritional aspects, drugs, smoking, alcohol and diet. In Winick, M. (ed.): Nutrition and Gastroenterology. Vol. 9, Current Concepts in Nutrition. New York, John Wiley & Sons, 1980.

Isselbacher, K.J., et al. (eds.): Harrison's Principles of Internal Medicine. 9th ed. New York, McGraw-Hill, 1980.

Laureta, H.C., et al.: An appraisal of the management of peptic ulcer including comparative studies of the value of a polyunsaturated fat nutritional preparation in the management of gastric hypersecretion. Am. J. Clin. Nutr., *15*:211, 1964.

McMillan, D.E., and Freeman, R.B.: The milk alkali syndrome. A study of the acute disorder with comments on the development of the chronic condition. Medicine, *44*: 485, 1965.

Moeller, H.C.: Conventional dietary treatment of peptic ulcer. Am. J. Clin. Nutr., *15*:194, 1964.

Morson, B.C.: Precancerous lesions of upper gastrointestinal tract. JAMA, *179*:311, 1962.

Odell, A.C.: Ulcer dietotherapy: Past and present. J. Am. Diet. Assoc., *58*:447, 1971.

Price, S.F., Smithson, K.W., and Castell, D.O.: Food sensitivity in reflux esophagitis. Gastroenterology, *75*:240, 1978.

Sanchez, P.E.: Concept of the mucous barrier and its significance, changes in the gastric mucosa produced by the local actions of spices and other irritative agents. Gastroenterology, *18*:269, 1951.

Sandweiss, D.J.: The Sippy treatment for peptic ulcer: fifty years later. Am. J. Dig. Dis., *6*:929, 1961.

Schneider, M.A., DeLuca, V., and Gray, S.J.: The effect of spice ingestion upon the stomach. Am. J. Gastroenterol., *26*:722, 1956.

Sippy, B.W.: Gastric and duodenal ulcers: medical cure by an efficient removal of gastric juice erosion. JAMA, *64*: 1625, 1915.

Snorf, L.D.: Emotional factors in gastrointestinal disorders. JAMA, *162*:857, 1956.

Solanke, T.: The effect of red pepper on gastric acid secretion. J. Surg. Res., *15*:385, 1973.

Wright, L.E., and Castell, D.O.: The adverse effect of chocolate on lower esophageal sphincter pressure. Dig. Dis. Sci., *20*:703, 1975.

CHAPTER 23

Nutritional Care in Intestinal Disease

Physiology and Functions of the Intestines

The absorption of food is practically completed in the small bowel. Food is emptied from the stomach into the duodenum where the breaking-down process continues. Secretions from the intestine, the pancreas and the liver have prepared the gastric contents for absorption, which for the most part takes place in the upper half of the small intestine. The only substances that are absorbed in the distal small intestine (the terminal ileum) are fats, bile salts and vitamin B_{12}.

The large intestine or colon takes up considerable space in the abdomen. It is about 1.5 meters long and starts with the cecum, the segment from which the appendix projects. From the lower right side of the abdomen, the colon extends upward (ascending), crosses (transverse) underneath the liver and stomach to the spleen and turns downward (descending)

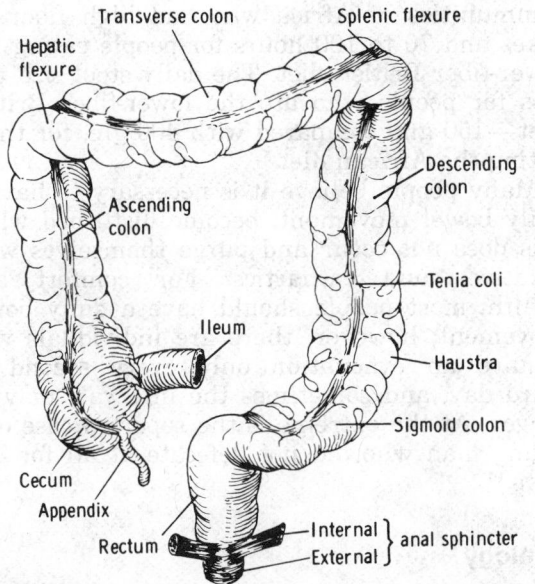

Figure 23–1. The human colon (From: Ganong, W. F.: Medical Physiology, 11th ed. Los Altos, California, Lange Medical Publications, 1983.)

on the left side, as shown in Figure 23–1. It is connected with the rectum by a small section called the sigmoid.

The main functions of the colon are (1) the absorption of water and (2) the transfer of feces from the ascending colon to the descending colon, then via the rectum to the exterior. This latter function is accomplished mainly by periodic, relatively frequent intervals of progressive mass peristalsis. The sigmoid sphincter prevents the passage of fecal material into the rectum until the urge to defecate is felt. Normal rectal sensibility is needed for the desire for evacuation, and regularity of habit and ample roughage are prime requisites for proper functioning of the colon.

The mechanism of the entire alimentary tract is controlled by the nervous and endocrine systems. When an individual becomes tense or overfatigued, the colon may go into a single spasm or series of spasms. The constriction may be associated with alternating constipation and diarrhea.

This brief review has been presented as a guide to better understanding of the various diseases in the intestinal region and their dietary treatment. A review of Chapter 5 is recommended. Figure 5–8, illustrating the sites of normal absorption of nutrients from the small bowel, will be helpful when studying intestinal disease and the necessary nutritional care.

Since many intestinal disorders appear to be functional ones, that is, involving motility, absorption and secretion problems in the absence of recognizable pathological conditions, it seems probable that diet is related to both the exacerbation and remission of these diseases. However, this area of study is largely unexplored, and there is only limited evidence to incriminate certain foods in some individuals. In these cases, elimination of individual foods may be beneficial. Distress after ingestion would seem to incriminate that particular food. Although there are some general principles to follow, *nutritional care for all patients with diseases of the intestines must be individualized.* The principles presented here are only *guidelines.*

Flatulence

Because human gas production has not been studied extensively, it is not well understood. Almost all intestinal gas is composed of five gases: N_2, O_2, CO_2, H_2 and CH_4 (methane). The normal individual usually excretes less than 100 ml. of gas per hour. If this amount is exceeded, he or she usually complains of "excessive gas."

The causes of excessive gas are (1) *aerophagia* (the swallowing of air while eating or drinking), (2) increased intestinal motility (decreased intestinal transit time) and (3) excessive bacterial fermentation of bowel contents.

An analysis of rectal gas can give a clue to the reason for excessive flatulence. Excessive amounts of H_2 and CO_2, which are not present in the atmosphere in large quantities, indicate excessive bacterial fermentation and point to malabsorption of a fermentable substrate such as lactose. High N_2 and O_2 concentrations in the flatus result from aerophagia. Methane is produced by only one third of the population. However, a person's flatus is rarely analyzed for its composition. If it were, suggestions and methods for nutritional care to minimize gas production would be more effective.

Patients with "too much gas" frequently do not have more gas than other people, but may have problems with gastrointestinal motility. Normally, gas is reabsorbed through the colonic wall as the feces move down to the rectum. If colonic motility is increased for any reason, less gas can be reabsorbed. If colonic motility is disordered so that gas cannot pass through to the rectum, the result is eructation, pain and distention.

Nutritional Care

Nutritional care begins with cautioning the patient to eat slowly, chew with the mouth closed and avoid gulping food. The patient can also be counseled about the effects of certain foods. The following fruits and vegetables could *possibly* be gas-forming. Trial periods of omitting them and observing the results can determine which of them affect individual patients.

VEGETABLES

Beans, kidney	Onions
Beans, lima	Peas, split or black-eyed
Beans, navy	Peppers, green
Broccoli	Pimentos
Brussels sprouts	Radishes
Cabbage	Rutabagas
Cauliflower	Sauerkraut
Corn	Scallions
Cucumbers	Shallots
Kohlrabi	Soybeans
Leeks	Turnips
Lentils	

FRUIT

Apples (raw)	Cantaloupe
Avocados	Honeydew melon
	Watermelon

Last, it should be determined whether the patient has lactase deficiency or some other intestinal enzyme inadequacy. Lactase intolerance (due to lactase deficiency) is the most common, and if it is suspected, a trial of omission of all milk and lactose-containing products (ice cream, puddings, custards) from the diet should be tried. See page 458 for a lactose-free diet and further discussion.

Constipation

Definition

The definition of constipation is very subjective. In the minds of individuals it may mean that their stools are too hard, too small, too infrequent or too difficult to expel or that they have a feeling of incomplete evacuation. All of these complaints are difficult to quantify. Devroede has given constipation an objective definition—constipation exists if a person passes fewer than three stools (fewer than five in men) per week while eating a high residue diet, or if he or she skips more than three days without a stool, and if the stools weigh less than 35 gm. per day.[7]

Under normal conditions, the residue of food eaten one morning will reach the large bowel (but not the rectum) the following morning. Defecation takes place normally 24 to 72 hours or longer after the intake of food. The type of diet eaten is believed to influence to some degree the length of time before defecation takes place. A diet high in fiber content resists enzymatic digestion or absorbs liquids in its passage along the intestinal tract and thereby produces bulk, a stimulant to defecation. The opposite is true of a diet low in fiber. Burkitt found that the transit time for food through the gut was approximately 30 to 40 hours for people in rural

communities of Africa who had high fiber intakes and 70 to 100 hours for people eating the lower-fiber British diet. The daily stool size was less for people who ate the lower-fiber British diet—150 gm. compared with 400 gm. for those eating the African diet.[5]

Many people believe it is necessary to have a daily bowel movement, become disturbed when this does not occur and purge themselves with laxatives and cathartics. For comfort and health, most people should have a daily bowel movement; however, there are individuals who require an evacuation only every second or third day, and sometimes the intervals may be longer. At the extreme is the reported case of a young man who did not defecate at all for 368 days.[10]

Etiology

Constipation is not a disease but a symptom of various diseases. The diseases that cause constipation are either systemic or gastrointestinal, as shown in Table 23–1.

Repeated lack of response to the urge for defecation, failure to establish a regular time for defecation, lack of exercise (which causes a loss of tone in the intestinal musculature), the use of cathartics for long periods of time, nervous strain and worry are the most common causes. Hypothyroidism, dehydration and certain medications such as those containing iron, aluminum or calcium compounds can cause constipation. Insufficient fiber in the diet may cause constipa-

Table 23–1. CAUSES OF CONSTIPATION

SYSTEMIC
  Side effect of drug
  Metabolic and endocrine abnormalities, such as hypothyroidism, uremia and hypercalcemia
  Lack of exercise
  Social habits
  Vascular disease of the large bowel
  Systemic neuromuscular disease leading to deficiency of voluntary muscles
  Nutrient deficiencies

GASTROINTESTINAL
  Diseases of upper gastrointestinal tract
    Celiac sprue
    Duodenal ulcer
    Gastric cancer
    Cystic fibrosis
  Diseases of the large bowel that result in:
    Failure of propulsion along the colon (colonic inertia)
    Failure of passage through anorectal structures (outlet obstruction)
  Excessive mucosal absorption capacity in the large bowel due to:
    Disorders of innervation, such as Hirschsprung's disease, multiple sclerosis, Parkinson's disease or paraplegia
    Disorders of the other bowel structures, such as tumors, hernias, strictures, diverticular disease, irritable colon and anal fissure

tion because there is little residue reaching the colon, and stool bulk is needed to promote normal peristalsis. Lack of thiamin can also cause constipation.

Chronic constipation may result from an organic disorder such as a physical defect, obstruction or constriction associated with a debilitating disease.

Treatment

The treatment is to develop regularity of habit through a bowel training program and the establishment of good health habits: regular meals, adequate diet providing ample fiber, regular time for elimination, rest, relaxation, adequate intake of fluids and exercise. In the case of constipation due to bowel obstruction, the treatment is removal of the obstruction, which usually involves surgery.

Nutritional Care

The adequate normal diet is used for patients with constipation, except that it is high in fiber —at least 14 gm. of crude fiber. Fiber is defined on page 30. Table 23–2 gives a high-fiber diet. The diet includes enough bulk (vegetables, fruit

Table 23–2.   HIGH-FIBER DIET

FRUIT 3–5 servings daily		VEGETABLES 4 servings daily		CEREAL 1 serving daily
[a]Apples	Grapefruit	Asparagus	Okra	Oatmeal
[a]Apricots	[a]Peaches	Broccoli	Onions	Shredded wheat
Bananas	[a]Pears	Brussels sprouts	Parsnips	Whole-wheat cereal
Berries	Pineapple	Carrots	Peas (all varieties)	Bran cereal
Cherries	[a]Plums	Cabbage	Peppers	Puffed wheat
Figs	Prunes	Cauliflower	Potatoes (white,	Brown rice
Oranges	Dried fruit	Celery	sweet)	Bran (include 2 tblsp. daily)
		Corn	Radishes	
		Eggplant	Rhubarb	
		Endive	Sauerkraut	
		Kohlrabi	Spinach	
		Lettuce	Squash	
		Greens (all varieties)	Tomatoes	
		Green beans	Turnips	
		Lima beans	Watercress	
		All other beans		
		Mushrooms		

SOUPS As desired	PROTEIN 3 servings daily		BREAD 3–5 servings daily
Hearty varieties such as vegetable, minestrone, chowder, bean, chili	Beef	Pork	100% whole-wheat bread
	Veal	Bacon	Cracked wheat bread
	Lamb	Eggs	Rye bread
	Fish	Chicken	Buckwheat bread
	Ham	Peanut butter	Corn bread made with
	Turkey	(crunchy)	coarse-ground meal

DESSERTS As desired	MISCELLANEOUS	FATS As desired
Ices and sherbets	Sunflower seeds	Butter
Fruit (fresh, frozen, canned)	Pumpkin seeds	Margarine
Fruit whips	Popcorn	Cream
	Nuts	Salad oil
		Salad dressing

BEVERAGES 6–8 glasses daily	AVOID
Water	Highly refined cereals:
Milk (2–3 cups)	white rice
Fruit juice	cream of wheat
Cocoa	farina
Tea	white bread
Coffee	pastries
	pies
	cakes
	macaroni
	spaghetti
	noodles
	Ice cream

From Department of Food and Nutrition Services, Shands Teaching Hospital and Clinics, University of Florida, Gainesville, Florida, 1975.
[a]Unpeeled.

and whole-grain cereal products) so that the fiber residue left in the bowel after digestion will encourage the movement of the intestinal contents and stimulate periodic evacuation. Appendix Table 4 gives the fiber content of foods.

Prunes and prune juice have been found to stimulate intestinal motility by pharmacological means. The laxative substance found in prunes is *dihydroxyphenyl isatin*. Other foods may have this same ability; but data on pharmacological laxative properties of food are very limited.

Because water is absorbed by the colon, the habitual intake of eight to ten glasses of fluid daily is necessary. If the fluid intake is less than this, constipation is likely to result. Some people believe milk to be constipating. Usually the cause for the constipation will be found in other factors.

Bran, the most concentrated source of food fiber, should be used in moderation. Excessive amounts given right away may irritate a sensitive alimentary tract, and large quantities may cause flatulence, loose stools or intestinal blockage. Patients should start with 1 tbsp. per day and gradually increase the amount to 5 to 6 tbsp. per day. The large amount of phytates in bran may reduce absorption of calcium, magnesium, iron and zinc. However, bran should be included gradually in the diet in breakfast cereals and bran muffins or added to stews and baked goods.

Laxatives

There are several types of laxatives: bulk-increasing agents, stool softeners, chemical stimulants and saline cathartics. Cellulose and hemicellulose derivatives and psyllium are common bulk-increasing agents. Magnesium hydroxide is another osmotic laxative. The excessive use of mineral oil can affect nutritional status by interfering with the absorption of the fat-soluble vitamins A, D and K and carotene, as discussed in Chapter 21. The regular use of laxatives that stimulate peristaltic activity should be discouraged because it tends to cause dependence and may lead to a spastic constipation.

Irritable Bowel Syndrome or Spastic Colon

The irritable bowel syndrome (also known as *spastic colitis, spastic colon* or *mucous colitis*) is a common disorder of unknown cause that does not appear to be characterized by any organic abnormality. The syndrome probably includes numerous other as yet unidentified diseases. At present there are three areas of investigation into the cause of this disorder: (1) motility disturbances, (2) psychiatric disorders and (3) dietary deficiencies or intolerance. It appears that patients with irritable bowel syndrome (IBS) have a lower threshold for pain and feel pain at lower levels of intestinal distention.[21]

IBS is the result of overstimulation of the intestinal nerve endings that causes irregular contractions of the bowel. There is excessive or uncoordinated sigmoidal motility and loss of rectal sensibility, which can cause either rapid transit through the bowel or constipation. It is accompanied by abdominal pain and sometimes by nausea, constipation or diarrhea, which may alternate. Mucus may be found in the stool. Because of the spasms, the fecal mass moves irregularly along the intestinal tract. Attacks are frequently associated with an emotional upset or a prolonged period of stress. Contributing causes vary and include the excessive use of laxatives and tobacco, drinking too much caffeine or alcohol, previous gastrointestinal illness, antibiotic therapy, enteric infections and lack of regularity in sleep, rest, fluid intake and bowel movements. Patients complain of heartburn, distention, flatulence, a full feeling and mild or severe cramping pain.

Treatment

A therapeutic regimen must include helping the patient to cope with stressful situations and to relieve pent-up emotions. Good habits of personal hygiene must be established, with adequate time allowed for a bowel movement.

Nutritional Care

Persons suffering from IBS are frequently underweight, tense and upset. Because of past experience they are afraid to eat and fearful of additional pain. The aim of the nutritional care is to relieve the condition, nourish the patient and bring the patient's weight back to normal.

The normal diet is recommended, with emphasis on high-fiber foods that will add bulk to the stool and relieve the constricting pressure and promote normal bowel motility. An increase in dietary fiber is not the cure-all for irritable bowel syndrome that many people believe it to be. A study of patients who were given either high-bran or regular biscuits daily found no difference in the relief of their symptoms.[23] The beneficial effect of bran for some people may be a placebo effect.

If the high-fiber diet fails to control the diarrhea, then the use of anticholinergic or antidiarrheal agents may be necessary. If there is any suggestion that psychological factors are involved, then psychiatric help is recommended. Biofeedback and learning techniques of relaxation and stress reduction may also be helpful to the patient.

Hemorrhoids

Hemorrhoids are ruptured blood vessels located around the anal sphincter. They may be either external or internal and may or may not cause pain and discomfort (Fig. 23–2). It is important for the patient with hemorrhoids not to become constipated, because the pressure from the dry, hard feces often causes bleeding and severe pain. Surgery usually is advised if the hemorrhoids become progressively worse. Some of the causes of hemorrhoids are constipation, pregnancy and the prolonged and continued use of cathartics or enemas. Sometimes they appear without any identifiable cause.

Nutritional Care

Diet can be a treatment for the condition but is primarily to provide comfort for the patient and possibly to prevent the development of more hemorrhoids. The high-fiber diet shown in Table 23–2 plus 8 to 10 glasses of water or liquids per day is recommended to avoid constipation and reduce straining at defecation. In addition, bulking agents to soften and increase the size of the stools may also be recommended. A discussion with the patient of a normal diet and regular eating and elimination habits is indicated. In the acute phase of hemorrhoid flare-up, the patient may require a low residue, low-fiber diet as described in Table 23–3. Gradual return to the high-fiber diet should be the objective.

Diarrhea

Diarrhea, which is a symptom and not a disease, is the occurrence of frequent liquid stools. The passage of food through the intestines is abnormally rapid and impairs complete digestion and absorption. The fecal matter passes through the colon so quickly that there is no chance for the fluid to be absorbed. Because of this, fluid replacements are necessary. The symptoms of diarrhea and constipation are direct opposites. However, the physiological mechanisms are not. Diarrhea results from luminal or mucosal changes, while constipation is believed to result almost entirely from motility disorders in the colon.

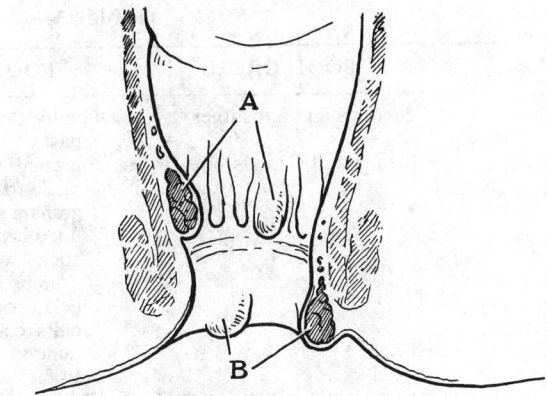

Figure 23–2. Hemorrhoids. *A*, Internal hemorrhoids; *B*, external hemorrhoids.

Classification and Etiology

Diarrhea should be distinguished from dysentery. *Diarrhea* refers to the character of the stools alone, while *dysentery* refers both to symptoms of intestinal dysfunction, such as abdominal cramps, and stool characteristics, chiefly the presence of blood and mucus.

Diarrheal disorders may be acute or chronic and of one or more general types: osmotic, secretory, exudative or limited mucosal contact. *Osmotic diarrheas* are caused by the presence in the intestinal tract of osmotically active solutes that are poorly absorbed. Diarrhea occurring in dumping syndrome and after lactose ingestion by the lactase-deficient person is osmotic diarrhea. *Secretory diarrheas* are the result of active secretion by the intestinal epithelium of electrolytes and water. Acute secretory diarrheas are caused by bacterial exotoxins, certain laxatives such as castor oil, viruses and increased intestinal hormone secretion. Unlike osmotic diarrheas, secretory diarrheas are generally not relieved by fasting. *Exudative diarrheas* are always associated with mucosal damage, which leads to an outpouring of mucus, blood and plasma proteins and to a net accumulation of electrolytes and water. The diarrheas of chronic ulcerative colitis and radiation enteritis are exudative. Prostaglandin release may be involved. *Limited mucosal contact diarrheas* are those resulting from situations of inadequate mixing of chyme and inadequate exposure of chyme to intestinal epithelium. The diarrhea of Crohn's disease and that following extensive bowel resection are from limited mucosal contact. This type of diarrhea is usually also complicated by steatorrhea resulting from bacterial overgrowth and reduced luminal concentrations of conjugated bile acids.

Caffeine consumption in amounts of 75 to 300 mg. per day (the amount in one to two cups of

Table 23–3. MINIMAL-FIBER DIET

FOOD GROUP	FOODS ALLOWED	FOODS NOT ALLOWED
Potatoes and Substitues	Potatoes without skin; rice, pasta	Kasha
Breads and Cereals	Enriched white bread or rolls made from finely milled flour; graham crackers, saltines, refined cereals, croutons; bread sticks without seeds; bread crumbs, rusks, matzoth, bagels, pancakes, waffles, biscuits, cornbread, French toast	All-Bran, cracked wheat bread and rolls, bran flakes, shredded wheat, Wheat Chex, Grape Nuts Flakes, Pettijohns, barley
Fruit	Strained fruit juices	All fruits
Fats	Any fat	None
Combination Dishes	Those made with rice or pasta and meat, cheese or fish	Any made with vegetables, fruits or other foods not allowed
Snacks	Plain crackers without seeds or cracked grain, potato chips, pretzels, corn chips (note: because of the nature of these foods, patients may not want them)	Any made from foods not allowed.
Beverages		
Milk	Any	None
Milk-free Beverages	Any	None
Available Supplements	Any	None
Soups	Any creamed or broth-based soups without vegetables	Soups with vegetables
Animal Protein		
Meat	Any	None
Poultry	Any	None
Fish	Any	None
Non-meat Protein		
Dairy Products	Any cheese	None
	Yogurt made without fruit or seeds	Yogurt with seeds or fruit
	Any eggs	
Other Sources	Meat extenders	Dried beans, peas, nuts, seeds, lentils, chunky peanut butter
Vegetables	None	All vegetables
Desserts and sweets	Any without seeds or fruit	Any made with cracked wheat, seeds or fruit
Miscellaneous	Salt, spices, herbs, sugar substitute, meat tenderizers, MSG, mustard, catsup, soy sauce, Worcestershire sauce, brewer's yeast, extracts, flavorings, food coloring, vinegar, Tabasco sauce, baking powder, baking soda, cornstarch, horseradish, gravy without vegetables	Pickles, relishes, olives, gravy with vegetables such as onions

From Handbook of Nutrition Care, 6th ed. St. Louis, Mo., Barnes Hospital, 1982.

coffee) may cause diarrhea in some people. In these doses, caffeine increases intestinal secretion, which may account for the diarrhea.[25] Patients should be questioned about their caffeine consumption, and a trial period of decreased intake may be effective. Table 23–4 gives the caffeine content of some beverages.

Nutritional Care

For all types of diarrhea the nutritional care is similar. The aim of the medical treatment is to remove the cause. The diet generally adopted is one that will leave very little residue in the intestinal tract. The low-fiber diet presented in Table 23–3 is used.

In the beginning of the dietary treatment for severe diarrhea, a fast of 24 to 48 hours is often prescribed to provide rest for the gastrointestinal tract. The nature and severity of the diarrhea determine the duration of the rest.

Besides bowel rest, the nutritional care for adults includes replacement of lost fluids and electrolytes by increasing the oral intake of liq-

Table 23–4. CAFFEINE CONTENT
OF BEVERAGES

BEVERAGE	CAFFEINE[a] (mg./200 ml.)
Prepared coffee[b]	66–150
Tea	70–150
Cola drinks	20–26
Decaffeinated coffee	1.8–6
Cocoa	0.25–345

From Handbook of Nutrition Care, 5th ed. St. Louis, Mo., Barnes Hospital, 1975.

[a] It is obvious that there is a wide range of figures represented in the literature. Part of this variance is due to the fact that the caffeine content of beverages is based on the amount of water, the method of brewing, and the blend of coffee or tea used. Since caffeine is water soluble, the longer the exposure to hot water, the greater will be the extraction of caffeine.

[b] Coffee prepared by the drip or vacuum method has less caffeine than percolated coffee.

uids, sodium and potassium. Fruit juices and bouillon are examples of fluids high in potassium and sodium, respectively. (See Appendix Table 10 for more foods high in sodium and potassium.) Losses of electrolytes, especially of potassium and sodium, should be corrected early with saline solutions that have potassium added. If the parenteral feeding must be continued for longer than 72 hours, amino acids in a 3 per cent solution may be added to prevent further protein catabolism. In the event that the diarrhea continues and cannot be diagnosed or treated, total intravenous hyperalimentation as described in Chapter 35 may be necessary, especially if exploratory surgery is anticipated.

Acute diarrhea is most dangerous in infants and small children, who can easily become dehydrated from the large fluid losses. In these cases parenteral administration of fluids and electrolytes is usually necessary as discussed in Chapter 38.

Pectin has value in the treatment of diarrhea. Scraped raw apple or liberal amounts of applesauce may be given every two to four hours, as tolerated, for their pectin content. When the diarrhea stops and the patient begins to tolerate food, the amounts given should be increased gradually as the patient can accept them. The foods given should be low in fiber and concentrated in protein and calories. Because the activity of the enzyme lactase may be decreased in a period of gastroenteritis, it is wise to avoid lactose at first. Lactase deficiency is discussed on page 458. Diet changes are always guided by the patient's condition and toleration for foods. The return to the normal diet is gradual. High calorie and protein intakes may be required for several months to correct protein deficiencies.

If the diarrhea becomes chronic, it may be associated with a number of nutritional deficiencies. Besides possible impaired absorption there is a heavy loss of electrolytes, vitamins, minerals and protein, which will have to be replaced. Potassium is probably the most important electrolyte lost, reflecting tissue depletion rather than specific changes in the circulating plasma levels. The loss of potassium alters bowel motility, encourages anorexia and can introduce a cycle of bowel distress. Loss of iron from gastrointestinal bleeding may be severe enough to cause anemia. Protein may be poorly digested and absorbed. If antibiotic therapy is used, intestinal synthesis of some of the B vitamins is impaired. Deficiencies of folic acid and vitamin B_{12} can occur.

In diseases associated with chronic diarrhea, low-fiber diets may have to be used initially. In some cases, enteral feeding will not be tolerated, and parenteral nutrition, which is discussed in Chapter 35, will be necessary. When enteral feeding is tolerated, it should begin with an easily digested nutritious formula; some of these formulas are described in Table 35–7.

After the diarrhea begins to lessen, adding more fiber to the diet may be effective. A larger stool bulk helps to restore normal bowel motility. Large quantities of fluid (2 to 3 qt. daily) are required in an attempt to replace body fluids lost in the stools.

STEATORRHEA

Steatorrhea, characterized by an excess of fat in the stool, is a symptom of malabsorption. It is generally indicative of serious organic disease. The excessive amount of exogenous fat in the stool may result from (1) failure of proper digestion, as in pancreatitis (Chapter 24), and following gastric resection (Chapter 34); (2) bile salt deficiency, as in diseases of the liver and biliary tract system, blind loop syndrome or ileal resection (Chapter 34); (3) failure of normal absorption due to mucosal damage, as occurs in sprue and regional enteritis, and after gastrointestinal radiation therapy; and (4) decreased fat re-esterification and decreased chylomicron formation and transport, as seen in abetalipoproteinemia and intestinal lymphangiectasia. Table 23–5 gives examples of diseases that can lead to steatorrhea.

Normally, the fecal fat amounts to about 4 per cent of ingested fat or 2 to 5 gm. daily, but when there are defects in absorption or digestion, fat from food appears in the stool in amounts as high as 60 gm. daily. Occasionally, the fecal fat level may be high in a normal person after ingestion of large amounts of dietary fat.

Table 23–5. EXAMPLES OF DISEASES MANIFESTING STEATORRHEA FROM POSSIBLE DEFECTS IN FAT ABSORPTION

POSSIBLE DEFECT	REPRESENTATIVE DISEASE	DEGREE OF STEATORRHEA
Decreased lipolysis	Chronic pancreatitis	Severe
	Pancreatic carcinoma	Severe
	Cystic fibrosis	Moderate
Decreased micellar solubilization	Extrahepatic or intrahepatic biliary obstruction	Mild
	Intestinal stasis (blind-loop syndrome)	Mild
	Ileal resection	Mild to moderate
	Drugs, e.g., cholestyramine	Mild
Decreased mucosal uptake	Gluten enteropathy	Moderate
	Tropical sprue	Mild
	Nongranulomatous jejunitis	Moderate
	Whipple's disease	Moderate
	Amyloidosis	Mild
	Extensive intestinal resection	Severe
	Lymphoma	Moderate
Decreased re-esterification	Small bowel ischemia (?)	Mild to moderate
Decreased chylomicron formation	Abetalipoproteinemia	Mild
Decreased chylomicron transport in lymph	Intestinal lymphangiectasia	Moderate
	Retroperitoneal fibrosis or malignancy	Moderate

Adapted from Westergaard, H., and Dietschy, J. M.: Normal mechanisms of fat absorption and derangements induced by various gastrointestinal diseases. Med. Clin. North Am., *58*:1413, 1974.

Nutritional Care

Since steatorrhea is a symptom and not a disease, the underlying disorder must be determined and treated. Weight loss is always present; so patients require an increased energy intake. Dietary protein should be high, with carbohydrates and fats added as tolerated to meet individual needs. Multiple vitamin and mineral deficiencies are common, making supplemental vitamin-mineral therapy necessary, with special emphasis on fat-soluble vitamins, calcium, zinc, magnesium and iron. Foods high in these vitamins and minerals are recommended, plus medication as necessary. Hematopoietic factors, such as vitamin B_{12} and folic acid, should be included when macrocytic anemia is present, as discussed in Chapter 29. Potassium should be increased in the diet and, in some cases, is required as medication.

MEDIUM-CHAIN TRIGLYCERIDES. Inadequate energy intake resulting from faulty digestion and absorption of fat may be alleviated by the use of medium-chain triglycerides (MCT) in the diet. MCT are hydrolyzed more rapidly than the longer-chain fats for a given lipase concentration and can rely on the small amount of intestinal lipase rather than on pancreatic lipase. The products of MCT hydrolysis are easily dispersed and absorbed without the presence of bile acids. Resynthesis of free fatty acids into triglycerides within the mucosal cell is not necessary with these fatty acids. Following absorp-

tion, the short- and medium-chain fatty acids enter the portal venous blood and are transported to the liver directly, without being resynthesized into triglycerides. Besides being more easily absorbed, MCT have also been found to be more rapidly absorbed, approximately as fast as glucose. MCT are available in oil and dry powder preparations, which also supply protein, carbohydrate, minerals and vitamins. The infant formula Pregestimil and the elemental diet Flexical (both by Mead Johnson) and others listed in Table 35–7 contain MCT oil. MCT are used as a source of calories for the patient with steatorrhea and not as a primary form of therapy, unless the steatorrhea cannot be treated in any other way.

Because these triglycerides are not very palatable, most patients cannot tolerate more than 50 gm. per day, which supplies about 400 kcal. MCT are discussed further on page 41.

Diverticular Disease

Diverticula are herniations of the colonic wall that are either congenital (or "true") diverticula or acquired (or "false") diverticula. *Diverticulosis* of the colon is a collection of acquired false diverticula and is considered to be abnormal.

While some patients with diverticulosis experience no symptoms, most complain of abdominal distention, cramping pain, tenesmus, diarrhea or constipation, symptoms similar to those of irritable bowel syndrome. It is thought that the outpouchings result from segmentation of the colon and the resulting high intracolonic pressures,[19] as shown in Figure 23–3. In addition, there is probably decreased strength of the musculature of the colon. With aging, normal tensile strength of intestinal mucosa is decreased, probably accounting for the fact that the incidence of diverticulosis increases with aging.

The diverticula may occur anywhere along the intestinal tract but are most frequently observed in the colon. The accumulation of fecal matter in these pockets often results in infection and inflammation and sometimes causes ulceration or even perforation. This is *diverticulitis*. Surgery is sometimes advised, especially if perforation occurs. Approximately 10 to 15 per cent of patients with diverticulosis develop diverticulitis.

Nutritional Care

The reason why segmentation and high intracolonic pressures occur has not been definitely elucidated, but a most plausible theory is that of Burkitt, Painter and their colleagues.[5, 19] They theorize that the decreased stool size resulting from decreased fiber intake leads to increased intracolonic pressure, which is responsible for the development of diverticular disease. This argues against old diet therapy. Because undigested fragments of fiber were frequently found near perforated diverticula that required surgery, physicians and surgeons felt that roughage aggravated the condition and prescribed low-roughage diets. Now it appears that a fiber-deficient diet favors the development of diverticulosis.

Painter reported that his patients who had diverticulosis defecated easier, had less pain and less distention when the dietary fiber was increased. The swiftly passed soft stool subjects the sigmoid to less strain and does not favor the development of diverticula. After treating 70 patients who had diverticulosis by giving them unprocessed bran, all-bran cereal and whole-meal bread, Painter found that 2 tsp. of bran three times per day (the equivalent of 2 to 3 gm. of fiber) relieved the symptoms of the disease for most patients.[20] Table 23–2 lists a variety of foods that provide a high-fiber diet.

Patients with diverticular disease who are taught about the high-fiber diet may require extensive encouragement, because the high-fiber approach is probably the complete opposite of all previous advice the patient has received. Some patients following a high-fiber diet complain initially of bloating or gas, but these side

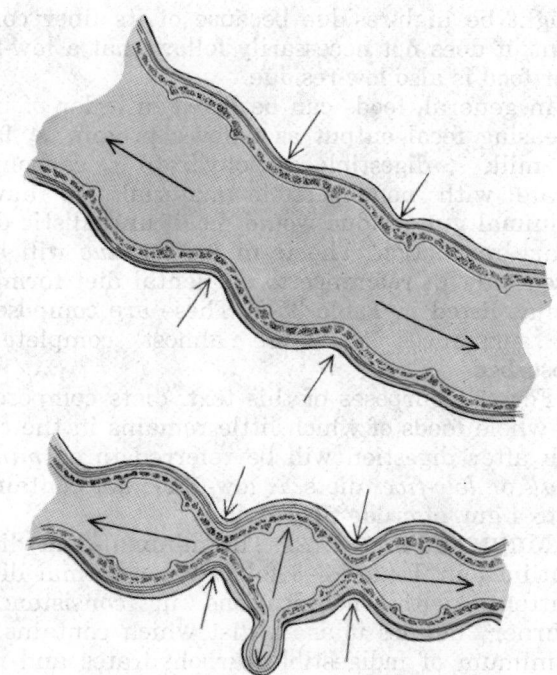

Figure 23–3. Mechanism by which low-fiber, low-bulk diets might generate diverticula is shown schematically. Where colon contents are bulky (top) muscular contractions exert pressure longitudinally. If lumen is smaller (bottom), contractions can produce occlusion and exert pressure against colon wall, which may produce a diverticular "blowout."

effects usually disappear shortly. In cases in which patients cannot consume the necessary amount of bran, the bulking agents methylcellulose and psyllium have been used with good results.

Surgery may be necessary in situations of recurrent diverticular hemorrhage, recurrent diverticulitis, acute perforations or fistula development.

"**FIBER,**" "**ROUGHAGE**" AND "**RESIDUE**" **DIETS.** Because they are still referred to occasionally, an explanation of the difference between the terms low residue and low fiber is necessary. The word *residue* is mistakenly used to describe two different characteristics: (1) the indigestible content of a food, i.e., the dietary fiber, and (2) the increased fecal output from a food, regardless of whether any portion of the food would remain after laboratory chemical digestion.

All foods leave some residue. In fact, even if no food is eaten, there is residue in the intestinal tract from the normal body metabolism and intestinal secretions. Milk and fats seem to increase the bulk of stools, although they are actually low in fiber content. Milk, while reported and considered by many to be a high-residue food, should be classified as medium-residue on the basis of fecal studies. Thus, while a food might be high-residue because of its fiber content, it does not necessarily follow that a low-fiber food is also low-residue.

In general, foods can be listed in order of increasing fecal output as follows: protein < fat < milk < digestible carbohydrate < carbohydrate with non-digestible material. To have minimal gut residue would mean unrealistic dietary restriction. The term *low residue* will be used only in reference to elemental diet formulas as listed in Table 35–7. These are composed of substances that are almost completely absorbed.

For the purposes of this text, diets composed of whole foods of which little remains in the colon after digestion will be referred to as *minimal-* or *low-fiber* diets. A low-fiber diet contains 0 to 4 gm. of crude fiber daily.

MINIMAL-FIBER DIET. The minimal-fiber diet outlined in Table 23–3 follows the normal diet pattern, with modifications in consistency. Turner[24] defines it as "a diet which contains a minimum of indigestible carbohydrates and no tough connective tissue."

HIGH-FIBER DIET. The high-fiber diet contains foods providing 13 to 20 gm. of crude fiber or 30 to 60 gm. of dietary fiber. This diet presented in Table 23–2 provides large amounts of foods that resist digestion.

Inflammatory Bowel Disease

Crohn's disease (regional enteritis) and ulcerative colitis are two diseases that usually are distinct but occasionally are indistinguishable. Simply stated, when an inflammatory process involves one or more lengthy segments of small intestine, whether or not the right colon is involved, the disease is *Crohn's disease*. When the inflammation is in the rectum with extension into the colon without affecting the right colon or small intestine, the disease is clearly *ulcerative colitis*. However, in 10 to 15 per cent of all inflammatory disease patients, the entire colon and rectum are involved or there is distal colonic disease without rectal involvement. In these patients the distinction is blurred and correct clinical diagnosis is difficult. Rectal biopsy is used to make the diagnosis. The incidence of Crohn's disease in the United States and Western Europe seems to be increasing, while the incidence of ulcerative colitis is remaining the same or declining slightly. Various viruses, cell-wall defective bacteria and autoimmunity have all been implicated in the pathogenesis of inflammatory bowel disease, but no single agent has been found to be responsible for either Crohn's disease or ulcerative colitis.[14]

CROHN'S DISEASE (REGIONAL ENTERITIS)

Crohn's disease is a chronic, progressive granulomatous disorder. It affects the submucosa rather than the mucosa of the intestine and usually the submucosa in the ileum and colon. There may be secondary lesions in the regional lymph nodes, liver, skin, eyes and joints. The number of macrophages (a cell involved in the immune system) in the mucosa is increased, but what this means in the disease process is not clear.

Crohn's disease may take a benign course and eventually disappear, or it may become severe, with complications such as intestinal obstruction or fistula formation. When confined to the colon, Crohn's disease has a patchy distribution and thus is more likely to be successfully managed through surgical removal of the diseased sections. However, when found in the small intestine Crohn's disease is diffuse and continues to spread and damage the intestine even after surgical resection. The patient who has Crohn's disease in the small intestine will probably have many problems and require a number of surgical resections in attempts to control the disease.

The disease occurs most often in patients between the ages of 10 and 40 years; both sexes are equally affected; and it is two to three times more common among Jews of European extraction than among non-Jews or Jews of African or Oriental descent. The cause of the disease is unknown, but current theories include genetic, infectious and immunological factors. Psychological factors are probably not primary but may be involved in flare-ups of the disease.

Patients typically complain of fatigue, anorexia, variable weight loss, right lower quadrant pain or cramping, diarrhea and fever. They may also have eye problems, arthritis and skin changes. This is frequently the case with adolescents. In children one of the first symptoms of Crohn's disease may be a decrease in growth. Failure of growth and development of children is a serious complication of inflammatory bowel disease (IBD), especially in those with Crohn's disease. The possible causes are inadequate food intake, loss of protein into the gut lumen, fever, low-grade but chronic intestinal obstruction, malabsorption of fat and protein and possibly secondary zinc deficiency.[2, 22]

Anemia is also common, usually as iron deficiency anemia due to blood loss. However, iron absorption is also decreased in both patients with Crohn's disease and patients with ulcerative colitis.[26] Megaloblastic anemia is less common in IBD and is usually due to folate deficiency, although it may be due to a vitamin B_{12} deficiency.

Treatment

Emotional support is especially important, since the disease is chronic with unknown etiology and variable prognosis. The patient, usually a young person, frequently is resentful about this physical weakness in the most productive period of his or her life.

Most important during acute periods, are maintenance of fluid and electrolyte balances and administration of an antidiarrheal agent. Salicylazosulfapyridine (sulfasalzine) may be given to suppress bowel activity. Corticosteroids are given in severe cases that do not respond to other measures. Immunosuppressive agents such as 6-mercaptopurine may also be used. Surgical removal of the diseased portion of the ileum or colon is indicated in cases of recurrent, complicated Crohn's disease. However, following any type of surgery for Crohn's disease there is a recurrence rate of about 15 per cent per year. It is not clear why this happens, but it may be that the disease already exists in normal-appearing tissue and that surgery merely provokes further activity.[4]

The result of surgery may be an ileostomy. The nutritional care for patients with ileostomies is discussed on page 698.

Nutritional Care

The diet should be high in caloric value, liberal in animal proteins and rich in vitamins and minerals. It should not be restricted but individualized to the patient's tolerance.

In Crohn's disease with steatorrhea, there usually is improvement when fats are restricted to 25 per cent of calories (about 50 gm.) per day; sometimes severe restriction (to 10 per cent of calories) is necessary. Table 24–4 describes a fat-restricted diet. Improvement may result from the use of medium-chain triglycerides. Ideally, fat in the patient's stool should be less than 10 gm. daily.

If there is growth failure, special attention should be given to nutritional support. One study showed that aggressive protein and energy supplementation, through a nocturnal nasogastric tube in order to bypass the anorexia that plagues these patients, resulted in diminished gastrointestinal protein loss, a weight gain and lean body mass deposition in adolescents with Crohn's disease. The intake was increased by 40 per cent so that the supplemented average intake was 96 kcal./kg./day.[17] The results suggested that dietary insufficiency rather than chronic inflammation or corticosteroid therapy is a major factor associated with the growth failure.

If a lactase deficiency is present, secondary to the intestinal damage, a lactose-free or limited diet can be prescribed. With drug therapy and improvement of the patient, the diet should be quickly liberalized and the patient should be allowed to eat anything tolerated. There are no foods known to provoke flare-ups of the disease.

If iron is indicated to correct anemia, it should be given intramuscularly to avoid irritation of the mucosa and the poor iron absorption in the active stage of the disease.

If megaloblastic anemia is present, it should be determined whether the anemia is due to folate or vitamin B_{12} deficiency, and the appropriate supplementation should be provided. Vitamin B_{12} deficiency occurs in Crohn's disease patients who have disease of the ileum, resection of the ileum, or overgrowth of gastrointestinal bacteria that compete for vitamin B_{12}.

Drug therapy may cause nutritional status changes in the patient. See Table 21–4 for the nutritional implications of sulfasalazine. One of these is decreased absorption of folate.

Elemental diet formulas (see Chapter 35) or total parenteral nutrition may be necessary if the patient cannot absorb nutrients or if food exacerbates the diarrhea. This kind of nutritional support allows the bowel to be put at rest, and in cases of small-bowel involvement, symptomatic relief in terms of reduced pain and diarrhea and closing of fistulae can be seen in five to ten days. Total parenteral nutrition (TPN) is the treatment of choice for IBD patients with acute symptoms. However, enteral feeding is still the preferred route, provided the gastrointestinal tract can be used safely. When enteral feeding is to be attempted, the patient should be given a 3-day trial with oral feeding that is carefully monitored. If the patient is unable to ingest 1000 to 1500 kcal. per day, then tube feeding should be started. Even when intubated, the patient can continue to eat orally, with the objective of having the oral intake meet his nutritional requirements. Tube feeding is further discussed in Chapter 35. Frequently IBD patients will need a chemically defined diet because of malabsorption.

Patients with Crohn's disease seem to have lower serum and leukocyte vitamin C levels than do normal individuals.[11] This could be a result of the low-fiber diets that these patients usually follow, which are low in vitamin C, or it could be due to an increased need for vitamin C as a result of this disease. Since it has also been found that patients who developed fistulas also had ileal tissue and blood ascorbate levels lower than patients without fistulas, it has been postulated that fistulas might form more easily in patients who have a depressed vitamin C content. Possibly the defect occurs in the collagen formation process which requires vitamin C.[11] Increased intake of vitamin C (at least 500 mg. per day) is indicated until the levels of the vitamin improve.

Ureteral calculi are seen in patients with Crohn's disease because of the *hyperoxaluria* that can accompany the disease. The hyperoxaluria is caused by increased colonic absorption of oxalate due to colonic mucosa damage and decreased luminal calcium, which normally binds with oxalate and prevents its absorption. With steatorrhea there is an increase in the free fatty acids in the intestines. They combine with calcium to make calcium soaps, leaving little calcium available to bind with oxalate. In the situation of ureteral calculi in Crohn's disease, a low-fat diet as listed in Table 24–4 supplemented with calcium is often beneficial. Dietary oxalates should also be restricted. Table 30–13 explains how this can be done.

ULCERATIVE COLITIS

Ulcerative colitis is a chronic inflammation and ulceration of the mucosa of the large intestine as shown in Figure 23–4. It most commonly also involves the rectum, rectosigmoid and left colon. The etiology is unknown, although a number of theories have been offered by medical authorities. The two most common theories are: (1) it is of infectious origin, and (2) it is an autoimmune disorder. That individuals who develop the disease are frequently depressed, irritable and emotionally unstable is a common observation. In addition, there is a genetic factor. A combination of causal factors probably is involved.

The general characteristics of severe ulcerative colitis are rectal bleeding, diarrhea accompanied by pain and spasm, fever, ulcerative

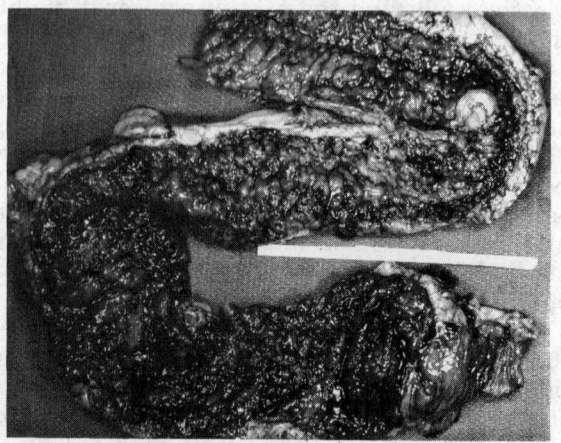

Figure 23–4. The mucosal lining of the colon in ulcerative colitis is greatly disturbed. (From: Sabiston, D.C. (ed.): Davis-Christopher Textbook of Surgery, 12th ed. Philadelphia, W. B. Saunders Co., 1981.)

lesions in the mucosa of the large intestine, nutritional edema, negative nitrogen balance, avitaminosis, dehydration, electrolyte imbalance, anorexia and malnutrition. Anemia may be present as a result of blood loss. However, some patients can have no symptoms, and it may be the systemic manifestations that bring them in for health care. They may have chronic debilitating polyarthritis or polyarthralgia. Uveitis, a feature of this disease, may bring the patient to the ophthalmologist. Skin changes also accompany the disease.

The disease usually occurs in young people (under age 40 to 50), though no age is exempt. Chronic ulcerative colitis has a striking tendency to exacerbation and remission.

If medical treatment fails to produce results, surgery may be advised. Surgery is required for 20 to 30 per cent of patients with chronic ulcerative colitis. Because this disease is so nutritionally debilitating, the patient should always receive nutritional support and rehabilitation prior to surgery.

Nutritional Care

As with Crohn's disease, nutritional care is an important part of the therapy. If it does not receive attention, multiple nutritional deficiencies will develop. The diet should consist of adequate nutrients that are not disturbing to the patient's physiological condition. Severe dietary restrictions not only cause nutritional deficiencies but also add to the problems most individuals with this ailment exhibit.

The importance of restoring normal nutrition in patients with ulcerative colitis cannot be overemphasized; in some cases this alone may initiate improvement. A daily intake of 2500 to 3500 kcal., including 1.0 to 1.5 gm./kg./day of protein, is recommended. High-protein, high-calorie diets are discussed in Chapters 34 and 35 and Table 27-9. There should also be assessment for folate deficiency, since folate absorption is decreased in ulcerative colitis.[26] If the patient has a folate deficiency, there should be supplementation with folate.

The foods included in the diet should provide large amounts of vitamins and minerals. Vitamin and mineral supplements are recommended. The recommendation with regard to iron in Crohn's disease applies to ulcerative colitis as well.

Frequent small feedings are advised and are usually more acceptable to the individual than the customary three meals a day. The frequent small feedings are more beneficial, permitting better absorption of the nutrients in the diet.

The nurse can be of great help by giving encouragement and understanding to these patients, who are frequently described as dependent, immature, obsessive and hostile. These individuals are often highly vulnerable to the ordinary events of life. An understanding of their emotional difficulties is indispensable to the effective treatment of ulcerative colitis. Attention to the attractive service of food, cheerful surroundings, efforts to inspire confidence and encouragement to eat the diet prescribed, are of primary importance to effective total therapy. The nurse has an opportunity to study the patient's eating habits and to assist in making the changes or improvements that are indicated in his or her customary diet. As with all patients who have intestinal diseases, the dietary regimen should be individualized.

During acute flare-ups, the nutritional care described for the patient with Crohn's disease is also appropriate for the patient with ulcerative colitis.

Gastrointestinal Allergy

Although there are many claims for the existence of gastrointestinal allergy, only two clinical situations have been established as disease entities due to food hypersensitivity: celiac sprue, which is discussed on page 452, and cow's milk intolerance, which will be considered in Chapter 31. A hypersensitivity reaction in the gastrointestinal tract may cause nausea, vomiting, diarrhea, pain, bleeding, anorexia or weight loss. Treatment consists of identifying the problematic food or foods and eliminating them, as discussed in Chapter 31.

EOSINOPHILIC GASTROENTERITIS

Eosinophilic gastroenteritis is a chronic relapsing condition that often exists for long periods without symptoms. It occurs in the stomach or small bowel and is characterized by clinical symptoms of abdominal pain, belching, bloating, distention, flatus and diarrhea. Pathologically, there is tissue edema and infiltration of the intestinal wall with eosinophils and protein-losing enteropathy. This disorder is thought to be an allergic reaction, but no definite relationship to food hypersensitivity has been defined. The patient often will respond dramatically to corticosteroid therapy, and the treatment can be short.

Nutritional care consists of eliminating those foods known to cause exacerbation.

Malabsorption Syndromes

A number of disorders interfere with adequate intestinal absorption of essential food elements, or cause *malabsorption*. Many will be

Table 23–6. SOME DISEASES AND CONDITIONS ASSOCIATED WITH MALABSORPTION

Inadequate Digestion
    Pancreatic insufficiency
    Gastric acid hypersecretion
    Gastric resection
Altered Bile Salt Metabolism with Impaired Micelle Formation
    Hepatobiliary disease
    Interrupted enterohepatic circulation of bile salts
    Bacterial overgrowth
    Drugs that precipitate bile salts
Abnormalities of Mucosal Cell Transport
    Biochemical or genetic abnormalities
      Disaccharidase deficiency
      Monosaccharide malabsorption
      Specific disorders of amino acid malabsorption
      Abetalipoproteinemia
      Vitamin B_{12} malabsorption
      Non-tropical sprue (gluten-sensitive enteropathy)
    Inflammatory or infiltrative disorders
      Regional enteritis
      Ulcerative colitis
      Amyloidosis
      Scleroderma
      Tropical sprue
      Gastrointestinal allergy
      Infectious enteritis
      Whipple's disease
      Intestinal lymphoma
      Radiation enteritis
      Drug-induced enteritis
    Endocrine and metabolic disorders
    Inadequate absorptive surface after surgery
Abnormalities of Intestinal Lymphatics and Vascular System
    Intestinal lymphangiectasia
    Mesenteric vascular insufficiency
    Chronic congestive heart failure

described in this chapter. Causes of malabsorption discussed in other chapters include the toxic influences of some drugs (Chapter 21), pancreatitis (Chapter 24) and the short bowel syndrome (Chapter 34). Table 23–6 lists some disorders associated with malabsorption. Abnormal laboratory findings in malabsorption are listed in Table 23–7.

Table 23–7. LABORATORY ABNORMALITIES FOUND IN THE MALABSORPTION SYNDROME

Macrocytic, hyperchromic, hypochromic or normochromic anemia (B_{12} and folic acid deficiency)
Microcytic, hypochromic anemia (iron and protein deficiency)
Hypocholesterolemia
Low prothrombin
Low serum calcium
Low serum phosphorus
Low serum potassium
Low serum albumin
Elevated alkaline phosphatase

From Ross, J. R., and Moore, V. A.: Axioms of malabsorption. Hospital Medicine, *11*:98, 1975.

CELIAC SPRUE

Celiac sprue is a disease in which there is (1) actual or potential intestinal malabsorption of virtually all nutrients, (2) a characteristic lesion of the small intestinal mucosa and (3) prompt clinical improvement following withdrawal of gluten from the diet. It is estimated that one in 2500 people in the United States has celiac sprue, but there may be more since the typical celiac sprue lesion and the potential for developing overt disease may be present in asymptomatic individuals. The highest incidence is in West Ireland, where it is 1:300. Celiac sprue is often called *celiac disease, non-tropical sprue, adult celiac disease,* or *gluten-sensitive enteropathy.*

In 1954 the intestinal lesion was accurately described from study of surgical biopsy material, and through this technique it was shown that celiac disease in children and non-tropical sprue in adults are identical. The intestinal biopsy has become the method of diagnosis of the disease. The typical diagnostic procedure is biopsy, institution of a gluten-free diet, rebiopsy to note intestinal villi improvement, and then gluten challenge followed by another biopsy six weeks later. One-hour blood xylose or five-hour urinary xylose tests are also used to assess absorption after a xylose load.

The disease affects primarily the mucosa of the small intestine. The villi of the intestinal mucosa become atrophied and flattened, so that the absorptive surface is decreased and the cells of the villi become deficient in disaccharidases and peptidases needed for digestion and in the carriers needed for the transport of nutrients into the blood stream. Figure 23–5 shows the effect of the disease on the villi. The result is a malabsorption of lipid, carbohydrate, protein, iron, magnesium, zinc and vitamins, especially the fat-soluble ones. The length of small intestine involved varies with the patient. The disease is sometimes limited to the proximal bowel. In other cases additional parts of the intestine are involved, but the proximal bowel has the most severe involvement.

Two other diseases that may present like celiac sprue but that do not resolve with removal of gluten from the diet are *collagenous sprue* and *refractory sprue.* The outlook for patients with these diseases is grim.

It has been found that almost all patients with *dermatitis herpetiformis* have at least a mild mucosal lesion consistent with celiac sprue. Recent evidence suggests that dermatitis herpetiformis is gluten-dependent and improves with gluten withdrawal.[16] Only a few patients with celiac sprue have dermatitis herpetiformis. Much remains to be learned regarding the interesting relationship between these two diseases.

There is a genetic factor in the etiology of celiac sprue. However, many relatives with the disease confirmed after biopsy had either no symptoms or mild symptoms so that they were unaware that they had the disease. The genetic marker HLA-B8 is present in 80 per cent of persons with celiac sprue. The mode of inheritance is not clear but is thought to be autosomal dominant with incomplete penetrance.

The intestinal mucosa reverts toward normal after institution of a gluten-free diet; however, some patients may require months or even years before there is maximal return to normal. Complete reversion to normal is relatively uncommon. Gluten intake is positively related to the degree of mucosal damage. As gluten intake increases, severity of mucosal damage increases.[6]

One possible explanation is that the disease is due to an abnormal (either defective or deficient) enzyme in the mucosal cell that fails to digest a toxic peptide contained in the *gliadin* fraction of gluten (the protein in wheat and other grains). Another possibility is that the reaction to gluten is an immune reaction in the mucosal cell membrane that allows gluten to act as a cytotoxic agent.

Apparently, the intestinal epithelium of patients who have this disease cannot tolerate the *glutamine*-rich polypeptide contained in gluten, and so this polypeptide acts as a cytotoxin. It interferes with the normal maturation of the intestinal epithelium, thus injuring the mucosa and causing the pathological changes.[1]

Symptoms

Depending on the extent of small-intestine involvement, symptoms can range from devastating and life-threatening malabsorption to refractory iron deficiency anemia or evidence of osteomalacia due to malabsorption, as listed in Table 23–8. Naturally, untreated celiac sprue will have exacerbations and remissions. The disease may first become apparent when the infant begins eating gluten-containing cereals, or it may not appear until middle age. Then it may be unmasked by gastrointestinal surgery, stress, pregnancy or viral infection.

The most common symptoms in children six months to three years of age are diarrhea, growth failure, projectile vomiting and a bloated abdomen. The frequency and nature of the stools vary but can be in excess of ten stools per day. Severe dehydration, electrolyte depletion and even acidosis may develop, especially in infants and children. The stools usually are watery or semiformed, light tan or gray, oily and frothy with a foul, rancid odor.

In adults the typical picture is variable. Increased appetite, weight loss, weakness and fatigue are common complaints. Diarrhea may or may not be present, and some patients may even have constipation. Their infrequent bowel movements uually are large and putty colored; the stools tend to float because of the high fat content.

The amount of weight that the patient might lose depends upon the extent of the disease and the ability of the patient to compensate with increased food intake. Many patients have large appetites and lose little weight. However, there is frequently anorexia and weight loss. In some patients there may be severe hypokalemia resulting from loss of potassium in the stool and severe muscle weakness. Although there is frequently abdominal distention and flatus, only rarely is there abdominal pain.

There is evidence that cholecystokinin release

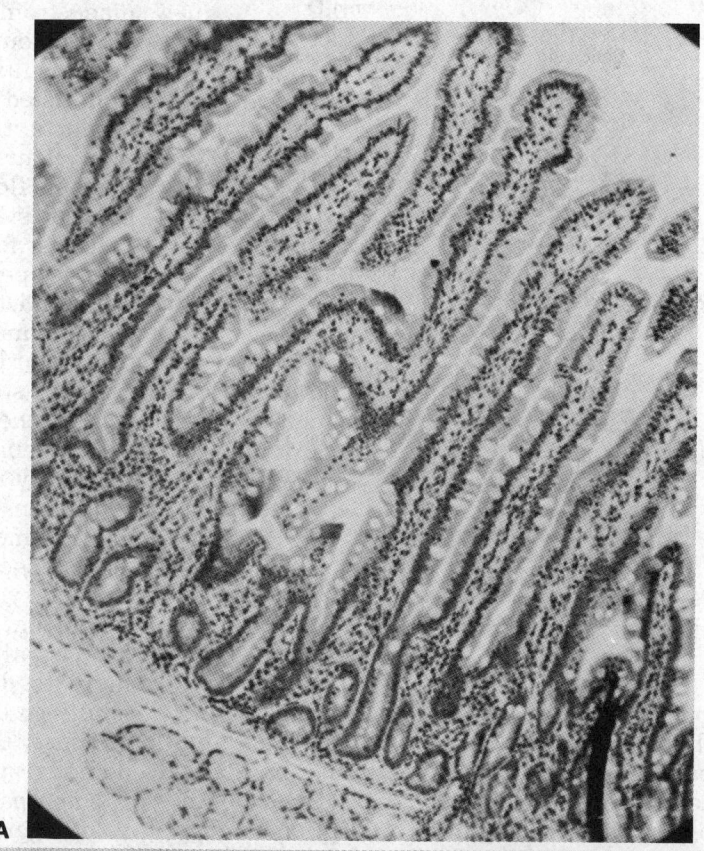

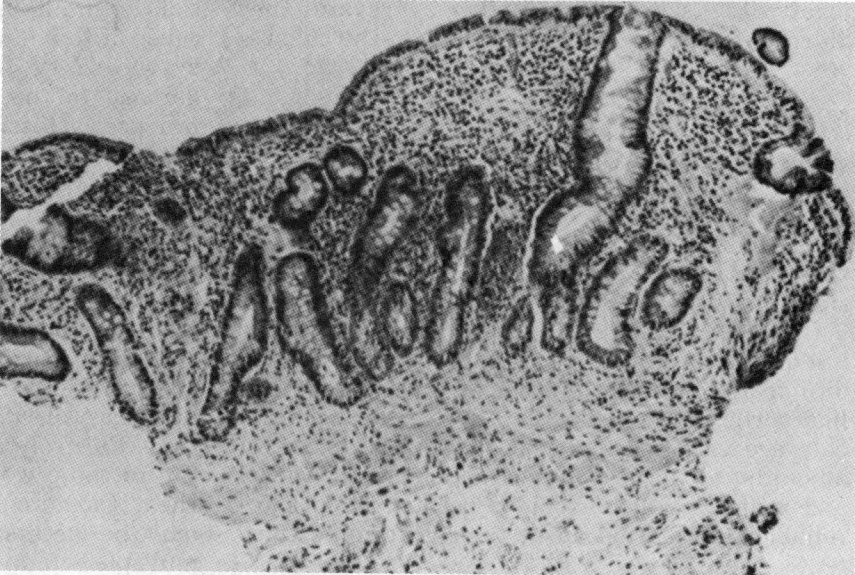

Figure 23–5. *A*, Low-power photomicrograph (X 100) of a normal human duodenal mucosa. Note the long, thin villi. *B*, Low-power photomicrograph (X 100) of a peroral small-bowel biopsy specimen from a patient with gluten enteropathy. Note the complete loss of villi and the heavy infiltrate of white blood cells in the lamina propria. (From Floch, M. H.: Nutrition and Diet Therapy in Gastrointestinal Disease. New York, Plenum Medical Book Co., 1981.)

Table 23–8. EXTRAINTESTINAL MANIFESTATIONS OF CELIAC SPRUE

ORGAN SYSTEM	MANIFESTATION	PROBABLE CAUSE
Hematopoietic	Anemia	Iron, folate, vitamin B_{12} or B_6 deficiency
	Hemorrhage Purpura	Hypoprothrombinemia usually due to impaired intestinal absorption of vitamin K
Skeletal	Osteomalacia	Impaired absorption of vitamin D
	Osteoporosis Bone pain	Formation of insoluble calcium soaps by fatty acids in intestinal lumen and thus defective calcium transport and absorption
Muscular	Paresthesias Muscle cramps Tetany	Calcium depletion and/or magnesium depletion due to poor absorption
	Weakness	Hypokalemia due to potassium loss
Neurological	Peripheral neuropathy	Vitamin deficiencies such as thiamin and vitamin B_{12}
Endocrine	Secondary hyperparathyroidism	Calcium and vitamin D malabsorption causing hypocalcemia
	Secondary hypopituitarism	Malnutrition due to malabsorption
	Adrenocortical insufficiency	Hypopituitarism
Integumentary	Follicular hyperkeratosis	Vitamin A deficiency
	Petechiae and ecchymoses	Hypoprothrombinemia

in response to a meal is impaired, which means that there is diminished delivery of bile and pancreatic enzymes into the gut lumen and that digestion is compromised. Further, if the ileum is involved, there is impaired absorption of conjugated bile salts, which further aggravates the diarrhea by direct cathartic action on the colon.

Nutritional Care

The treatment includes correcting the nutritional malfunction of the small bowel and thus the deficiency states. Removal of gluten from the diet results in the histological appearance of the intestinal mucosa returning to the normal state illustrated in Figure 23–5A.

GLUTEN-FREE DIET. A specific diet that omits the glutamine-bound fraction (glutenin and gliadin) of protein is the treatment of choice for celiac sprue. In this diet wheat, rye, barley and oats are excluded, since they all contain large amounts of this protein fraction. Buckwheat and millet are also excluded because of lack of reliable information about their glutamine content.

The gluten-free diet means that all bakery products and packaged foods must be scrutinized before they are used. Labels must be read carefully because, besides being a basic ingredient, gliadin-containing grains may be added as a derivative when the food is processed or prepared. For example, hydrolyzed vegetable protein may be made from soya or corn, or it may be made from mixtures of wheat, corn and soya. Table 23–9 shows the recommended diet. Table 23–10 contains a list of ingredients that may be made from wheat and that require information on the source. Additional recipes may be found by consulting the resources for patient education listed at the end of this chapter. Cereal products that can be used as substitutes are corn flour, cornmeal, potato flour, rice flour, soybean flour, tapioca flour and starch, and arrowroot starch. Table 23–11 provides some suggestions for incorporating these substitutions into recipes. During the first few weeks of gluten restriction, the diet should be supplemented with vitamins and minerals and be high in protein in order to cure deficiencies and replenish nutrient stores.

Both the immediate and prolonged effects of the gluten-free diet have been clinically satisfactory. Any relapses are usually due to dietary indiscretions and promptly subside when gluten is again removed from the diet.

Just because the person with celiac sprue is free of symptoms after eating gluten does not mean that there is not villi damage. There usually is, although it may take eight weeks or more to develop. It has been observed that if adults go on and off a gluten-free diet a number of times, they may reach a stage at which they do not respond to a gluten-free diet.

Some patients with untreated celiac sprue develop aggravation of their symptoms after ingestion of milk or milk products. The probable cause of this milk intolerance is lactase deficiency secondary to the reduced number of and damage to the intestinal absorptive cells that produce lactase. Milk and milk products should be removed initially (see Table 23–11), but most patients develop milk tolerance as intestinal structure and function approach normal after gluten withdrawal.

If the disease has been severe, patients may need supplements in addition to the gluten-free diet. Anemic patients should receive iron, folate and/or vitamin B_{12}, depending upon the type of anemia. Vitamin K should be given if there is purpura, bleeding or prolonged prothrombin time. Electrolyte and fluid replacement is essential in those with dehydration from severe diarrhea. Calcium and vitamin D administration may be necessary to correct osteomalacia. A multiple vitamin-mineral supplement should be

Table 23–9. GLUTEN-FREE DIET

(Wheat, Rye, Oat, and Barley Free) *

This diet is designed to provide adequate nutrition while eliminating wheat, rye, oats, and barley from the diet.

Gluten may be present in foods either as a basic ingredient (that is, listed as wheat, rye, oats or barley), or added as a derivative when a food is processed or prepared. Thus, *reading labels carefully is very important.*

Since flour and cereal products are quite often used in the preparation of foods, it is important to be aware of the methods of preparation used as well as the foods themselves. This is especially true when dining out.

FOOD GROUP WITH RECOMMENDED DAILY INTAKE	FOODS ALLOWED	FOODS TO AVOID
Milk: 2 or more cups	Fresh, dry, evaporated or condensed milk; cream; sour cream,[†] whipping cream; yogurt[†]	Malted milk; some commercial chocolate drinks; some non-dairy creamers[‡]
Meat, fish, poultry: 2 or more servings	All kinds of fresh meats, fish, other seafood, poultry; fish canned in oil or brine; some prepared meat products, such as hot dogs[‡] and lunch meats[‡]	Prepared meats that contain wheat, rye, oats or barley, such as some sausages,[‡] hot dogs,[‡] bologna,[‡] luncheon meats,[‡] chili con carne,[‡] sandwich spreads[‡]; bread-containing products, such as: Swiss steak, croquettes; meat loaf; tuna canned in vegetable broth,[‡] and turkey with hydrolyzed vegetable protein injected as part of the basting solution
Cheeses (can be used for meat and milk groups)	All aged cheeses, such as cheddar, swiss, edam, parmesan; cottage cheese,[†] cream cheese,[†] pasteurized processed cheese[†‡]	Any cheese product containing oat gum as an ingredient
Eggs	Plain or in cooking	Eggs in sauce made from gluten-containing ingredients (such as a regular, wheat-based white sauce)
Potato or other starch: 1 or more servings	White and sweet potatoes, yams; hominy; rice; wild rice; special gluten-free noodles (Aprotein) made by Henkel Corp.; some oriental rice and bean noodles	Regular noodles; spaghetti; macaroni; most packaged rice mixes[‡]
Vegetables: 2 or more servings	Use all plain, fresh, frozen or canned vegetables; dried peas and beans; lentils; some commercially prepared vegetables[‡]	Creamed vegetables[‡]; vegetables canned in sauce[‡]; some canned baked beans[‡]; commerically prepared vegetables and salads[‡]
Fruits: 2 or more servings	All fresh, frozen, canned or dried fruits; all fruit juices; some canned pie fillings	Thickened or prepared fruits; some pie fillings[‡]
Breads: 3 or more servings	Specially prepared breads using only allowed flours; examples of commercially available brands: Ener-G Foods Brown Rice Bread and White Rice Bread	All others containing wheat, rye, oat or barley flour
Cereals: 1 or more servings of enriched cereal	Hot cereals made from cornmeal, cream of rice, hominy, rice; cold cereals as follows: Puffed Rice, Kellogg's Sugar Pops; Post's Fruity and Chocolate Pebbles, special cereals	All others containing wheat, rye, oats or barley; bran, graham; wheat germ; malt; kaska; bulgar; buckwheat[§]; millet[§]
Flours and thickening agents		Wheat starch (mfr. states it contains gluten); all flours containing wheat, rye, oats, or barley
Good thickening agents	Arrowroot starch, cornstarch, tapioca starch	
Good when combined with other flours	Corn flour, cornmeal, potato flour, potato starch flour, rice bran, rice flours (plain, brown, sweet), rice polish, soy flour	
Best combined with milk and eggs in baked product	Corn flour, cornmeal, potato flour, potato starch flour, rice flours (plain, brown, sweet), rice polish, soy flour	
Grainy-textured products	Corn flour, cornmeal, sweet rice flour	
Drier product than with other flours	Potato flour, potato starch flour, plain and brown rice flours	
Moister product than with other flours	Sweet rice flour	
Adds distinct flavor to product: use with moderation	Rice polish, soy flour	
Crackers and snack foods	Rice wafers[‡]; pure cornmeal tortillas; popcorn, some crackers[‡] and chips[‡]	All others containing wheat, rye, oats or barley
Fats	Butter; margarine; vegetable oil; nuts; peanut butters; hydrogenated vegetable oils; some salad dressings[‡]; mayonnaise[‡]	Some commercial salad dressings[‡]
Soups	Homemade broth and soups made with allowed ingredients; some commercially canned soups[‡]	Most canned soups[‡] and soup mixes[‡]; bouillon

Table continued on the following page

Table 23–9. GLUTEN-FREE DIET (*Continued*)

FOOD GROUP WITH RECOMMENDED DAILY INTAKE	FOODS ALLOWED	FOODS TO AVOID
Desserts	Cakes, quick breads, pastries, puddings prepared with allowed ingredients; corn-starch, tapioca, and rice puddings; gela-tin desserts; custard; vanilla-flavored ice cream from: Arden, Carnation, Darigold, Foremost, Lucerne‡; some pudding mixes‡	Commercial cakes, cookies, pies, etc., made with wheat, rye, oats or barley; prepared mixes‡; ice cream cones; pudding‡
Beverages	Instant and ground coffee; instant tea; tea; carbonated beverages‡; pure cocoa pow-der; unfortified wines; rums; some root beers‡; vodka distilled from grapes	Ovaltine; malted milk; ale; beer; gin; whiskies‖; vodka distilled from grain
Sweets	Jelly; jam; honey; brown and white sugar; molasses; most syrups‡; some candy‡; chocolate; pure cocoa; coconut	Some commercial candies‡
Miscellaneous	Salt; pepper; herbs; extracts; food coloring; cloves; ginger; nutmeg; cinnamon; chili powder; tomato puree and paste; olives; pickles; cider and wine vinegar; yeast; bircarbonate of soda; baking powder; cream of tartar; dry mustard; some other condiments‡; monosodium glutamate (MSG)	Some curry powder‡; some dry seasoning mixes‡; some gravy extracts‡; some meat sauces‡; some catsup‡; some mustard‡; horseradish‡; some soy sauce‡; chip dips‡; some chewing gum‡; distilled white vinegar‖

* Diet developed by Elaine I. Hartsook, M. Ed., R.D., Member, National Digestive Disease Advisory Board, National Institutes of Health, Public Health Service, U.S. Department of Health and Human Services.

† Check vegetable gum used.

‡ Product ingredients should be investigated.

§ Although botanically different from other gluten-containing grains, additional information is needed before this can be cleared.

‖ Distilled white vinegar uses grain as a starting material. Whiskies, including "corn whisky," use wheat, rye, oats, or barley in their mash. Gluten-intolerant persons are advised to use the cider and wine vinegar in food preparations such as making salad dressings, pickles, and in cooking. Avoid all whiskies.

Commercially prepared pickles, ketchup, mustard, mayonnaise, steak sauce, and other condiments are usually made with distilled grain vinegar; however, the maximum amount of gluten that would be present in such products via the vinegar would be insignificant. Thus, moderate use of the above commercial condiments is recommended.

Table 23–10. GLIADIN-CONTAINING DERIVATIVES*

Always check the source of the following nebulous ingredients before eating any product containing them.

INGREDIENT (as appears on label)	INCLUDE	AVOID
"Hydrolyzed vegetable protein" (HVP)	Soy, corn	Mixtures of wheat, corn and soya (soy)
"Flour" or "cereal products"	Rice flour, corn flour, cornmeal, potato flour, soy flour	Wheat, rye, oats or barley
"Vegetable protein"	Soy, corn	Wheat, rye, oats or barley
"Malt" or "malt flavoring"	Those derived from corn	Those derived from barley or barley malt syrup
"Starch"	When listed as such on a U.S. manu-facturer's ingredient list, it is *cornstarch*	
"Modified starch" or "modified food starch"	Arrowroot, corn, potato, tapioca, waxy maize, maize	Wheat starch
"Vegetable Gum"	Carob bean, locust bean, cellulose gum, guar gum, gum arabic, gum acacia, gum tragacanth, xanthan gum	Oat gum
"Soy sauce" or "soy sauce solids"	Those that *do not* contain wheat, such as Chun King	Those that *contain* wheat

* Developed by Elaine I. Hartsook, M. Ed., R.D., Member, National Digestive Disease Advisory Board, National Institutes of Health, Public Health Service, U.S. Department of Health and Human Services.

These questionable ingredients must be cleared with the manufacturer before they are eaten. When writing the manufacturer, request in-formation on the specific starting material(s) used in their nebulous ingredient. For example, when "modified food starch" appears as a la-beling ingredient, ask for the specific type of starch used, i.e., potato starch, tapioca starch, etc.

A combination of wheat, corn and soya is primarily used as starting material for hydrolyzed vegetable protein, and thus is not allowed on a gluten-free diet. When wheat protein is "hydrolyzed," its large amino acid chains are broken down into smaller chains. Some protein researchers believe the sequence of amino acids found in these smaller chains contain the same toxicity as the intact gliadin sub-fraction of the gluten protein. Thus, HVP made from wheat is not recommended for use on a gluten-free diet.

Table 23–11. SUGGESTIONS FOR SUBSTITUTIONS FOR WHEAT FLOUR IN RECIPES

One cup of wheat flour may be substituted in standard recipes by the following:

  1 cup corn flour
  ¾ cup coarse cornmeal
  1 scant cup fine cornmeal
  ⅝ cup potato flour
  ⅞ cup rice flour

There are some problems in the use of substitutes for wheat flour. The following suggestions will improve the eating quality of the final product:

1. Rice flour and cornmeal tend to have a grainy texture. A smoother texture may be obtained by mixing the rice flour or cornmeal with the liquid called for in the recipe, bringing this mixture to a boil and then cooling before adding to the other ingredients.
2. Soy flour must always be used in combination with another flour, not as the only flour in a recipe.
3. When using other than wheat flour in baking, longer and slower baking is required. This is particularly necessary when the product is made without milk and eggs.
4. When using coarse meals and flours in place of wheat flour, the amount of leavening must be increased. For each cup of coarse flour, use 2½ tsp. of baking powder.
5. Substitutes for wheat flour do not make a satisfactory yeast bread.
6. Muffins or biscuits, when made with other than wheat flour, are of better texture if baked in small sizes.
7. Dryness is a common characteristic of cakes made with flours other than wheat. Moisture may be preserved by (a) frosting or (b) storing in closed containers.

From Ohlson, M. A.: Experimental and Therapeutic Dietetics, 2nd ed. Minneapolis, Burgess Publishing Co., 1972, pp. 142–143.

taken regularly by those with celiac sprue who continue to have malabsorption.

Drugs

Corticosteroids are given only if there is evidence of secondary adrenal insufficiency. Steroids are rarely used in the treatment because a gluten-free diet is safer and more specific.

Prognosis

In children a gluten-free diet always results in a return to normal absorption; however, this is not always so in adults. Even though they gain relief with a gluten-free diet, some adults still have intestinal abnormalities, as revealed by biopsy. Likewise, persons with celiac sprue who eat gluten but do not have clinical symptoms still show damage to intestinal villi. One does not outgrow celiac disease. There is still destruction of villi upon gluten ingestion, even though clinical symptoms may abate.

Several reports suggest an increased incidence of malignant disease in adults with celiac sprue than in the general population. Gastrointestinal carcinomas and lymphomas seem to be the most common.[13] The true increase in this incidence is open to speculation. It is not known whether strict adherence to a gluten-free diet reduces the incidence of intestinal lymphoma or other malignancies in celiac sprue patients.

TROPICAL SPRUE

Tropical sprue is a syndrome of unknown etiology. It has a peculiar geographic distribution and is found in tropical areas except in Africa, south of the Sahara. Although the cause is not known, it is suggested that an infectious agent is involved. Nutritional deficiency, which is frequently present, may increase the patient's susceptibility to an infectious agent. The nutrients thought to be lacking are folic acid and vitamin B_{12}.

As in celiac sprue the intestinal villi are shortened, but the surface cell alterations are much less severe than those seen in patients with untreated celiac sprue. The gastric mucosa may be atrophied and inflamed, and the patient may have hypochlorhydria and diminished secretion of intrinsic factor.

Symptoms include diarrhea, anorexia, and abdominal distention and symptoms of nutritional deficiency, such as night blindness, glossitis, stomatitis, cheilosis, pallor and edema. Anemia may result from iron, folic acid and vitamin B_{12} deficiencies.

Nutritional Care

The first goal of care is to control the diarrhea through medication. Severe fluid and electrolyte imbalances and deficiencies are corrected by parenteral supplementation. Mortality can be significantly reduced by management of the dehydration and electrolyte imbalances. A high-energy, high-protein diet is appropriate. Specific nutritional deficiency states, such as megaloblastic anemia and iron deficiency, should be treated. Oral supplementation of folate and iron is possible, since iron and folate appear to be adequately absorbed. Vitamin B_{12} should be given parenterally because it frequently is poorly absorbed.

Intestinal Brush Border Enzyme Deficiencies

Intestinal enzyme deficiency states involve deficiencies of the brush border disaccharidases, which hydrolyze disaccharides at the mucosal cell membrane and allow the absorption of monosaccharides (see Table 2–1). Deficiencies or low levels of these enzymes can result in malabsorption of the carbohydrates, causing diarrhea, flatulence, abdominal distention and pain.

There are three types of disaccharidase deficiencies: (1) rare congenital defects, such as sucrase-isomaltase or lactase deficiencies seen in the newborn, (2) generalized forms that are secondary to diseases such as Crohn's disease or celiac sprue, which damage the intestinal epithelium, and (3) an acquired form of lactase deficiency, which usually appears after childhood but can appear as early as two years of age.

ACQUIRED LACTASE DEFICIENCY

Intolerance to lactose, the sugar in milk, is very prevalent in the world population, especially among blacks, Asians, Orientals and South Americans. In fact, most populations except for Northern European Caucasians and white American ethnic groups have high incidences of adult lactose intolerance. The majority of human adults in the world are non-digesters of lactose. Kretchmer proposes that lactose intolerance is the normal state; lactose tolerance is the abnormal condition.[15] It has been estimated that there are 30 million people in the United States, including 2 million elementary school children, who cannot absorb lactose.[3]

It is not known why acquired lactase deficiency develops with age in some people, but there are several hypotheses: (1) two lactases may exist, one "infantile" and one adult, and the adult lactose non-digester does not have the adult form; (2) the condition may be a genetic phenomenon with a delayed expression; (3) a lactase enzyme inhibitor may develop with age; and (4) the deficiency may be a permanent result of transient small-bowel disease. There is no evidence to support the notion that lactase activity is adaptively regulated by the concentration of dietary lactose and that the persistence of lactase is induced by continuation of milk in the diet after weaning.

Figure 23–6 summarizes the effects of lactose intolerance. Unable to be hydrolyzed into galactose and glucose, lactose is not absorbed but remains in the gut and acts osmotically to draw water into the intestines. In addition, bacteria ferment the undigested lactose and generate lactic acid and other organic acids, carbon dioxide and hydrogen gas. The result is bloating, flatulence, cramps and diarrhea. In neonates with congenital lactase deficiency this physiological process begins as soon as breast milk or cow's milk formula is taken. In these patients failure to thrive, fluid and electrolyte imbalances and protuberant abdomen are usually the presenting symptoms. It is presumed that the

person with lactase deficiency can utilize the protein, fat, vitamins and minerals in milk.

Lactase deficiency is diagnosed from a history of gastrointestinal symptoms that occur after milk ingestion, from a breath or hydrogen test, an abnormal lactose tolerance test or biopsy of the intestinal mucosa. For a *lactose tolerance test*, the patient takes an oral dose of lactose (1.5 to 2 gm. per kg. of body weight or up to 50 gm. in an adult—the equivalent of the amount of lactose in 1 qt. of milk) after an overnight fast. Measurements are made of the blood glucose at specified times afterward. For the *breath test*, the amount of H_2 produced by the bacteria acting on lactose and then released into the gut is measured in the breath. In the lactose-intolerant person, gastrointestinal symptoms will appear after administration of the lactose, and blood glucose will increase less than 25 mg. per 100 ml. of serum above the fasting level. Although some patients will appear abnormal when tested, they will have no history of intolerance to milk. This raises the question of whether the blood glucose level is truly an indicator of lactose intolerance. Such patients appear able to tolerate the small amount of milk in their diets but cannot accommodate the large test load of 50 gm. when it is given undiluted and on an empty stomach. Other diagnostic tests are stool examination for reducing sugars, a low stool pH, increased stool lactic acid level and a mucosal enzyme assay of biopsy material, which is the most definitive. For further reading on lactose intolerance the reader is referred to the work by Paige and Bayless.[18]

Nutritional Care

With the reduction or omission of milk and lactose-containing foods, the symptoms of lactose intolerance are alleviated. Cheese contains very minute amounts of lactose, but most patients can tolerate it. The amount of lactose in creamed cottage cheese varies widely, since lactose is an optional ingredient added to the creaming mixture.[8] Yogurt contains lactose but for some unknown reason is tolerated by some patients.[9] It may be that enough of the lactose has been degraded by the culture so that it is lower in lactose content.

Dietary lactose has no significant effect on the absorption of protein, ascorbic acid and vitamin A in lactose-intolerant adults. Most lactose-intolerant adults can consume some lactose without symptoms. Lactose in milk with a meal is better tolerated than alone. There do not appear to be any great nutritional consequences in healthy lactose-intolerant adults who consume milk and milk products in small amounts.

For others lactose may have to be omitted. Ice

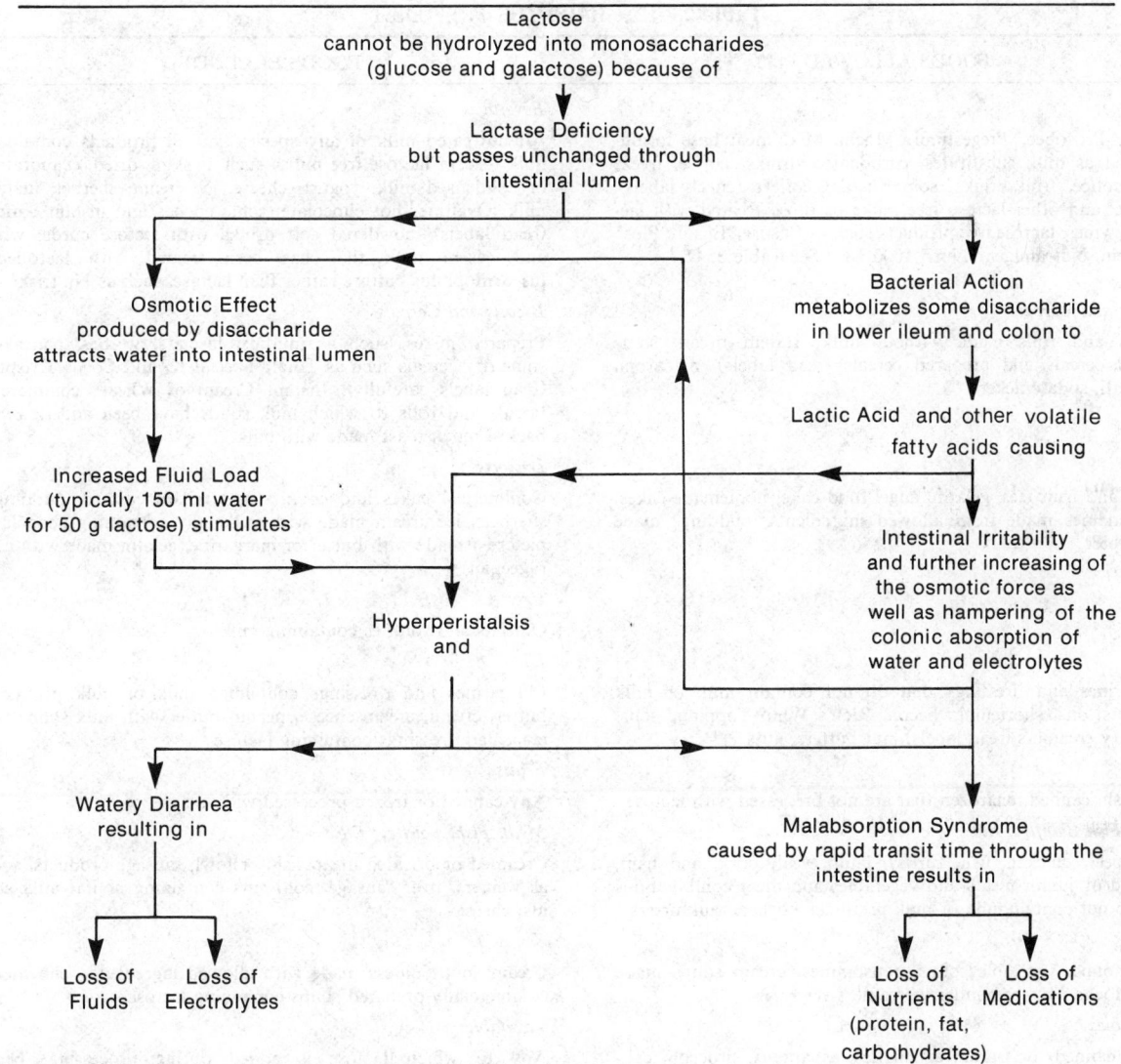

Figure 23–6. Pathogenesis and clinical implications of lactose intolerance. (From: Ensure Plus. Columbus, Ohio, Ross Laboratories, 1977, p. 11.)

cream and other milk dishes, cooked or uncooked, contain lactose and should be avoided or restricted. See Table 23–12 for a lactose-free diet. The diet should be evaluated for calcium and vitamin D adequacy and supplemented if necessary.

If after strict adherence to a lactose-free diet the symptoms do not disappear, then lactose intolerance is probably not the reason for the gastrointestinal symptoms, and another cause should be sought.

SUCRASE DEFICIENCY

Sucrose intolerance exists when there is a deficiency of the enzyme sucrase. The symptoms that develop are the same as those of lactose intolerance and result from bacterial fermentation of the undigested sugar. Much less

commonly than lactose intolerance, sucrose intolerance may develop temporarily as a result of severe gastroenteritis. See Table 39–11 for a sucrose-free diet. Fructose, sorbitol and artificial sugar substitutes can be used as sweeteners.

Blind Loop Syndrome

Blind loop syndrome is a disorder characterized by intestinal stasis and bacterial overgrowth that results from obstructive disease, stricture, fistula formation or surgical repair of the intestine (see Chapter 34). Because stasis favors their growth, the bacteria undergo a population explosion. Bacteria unconjugate bile salts, which besides being cytotoxic in the unconjugated form are also less effective as micelle

Table 23–12.   LACTOSE-FREE DIET

FOODS ALLOWED	FOODS EXCLUDED
Beverages	*Beverages*
Isomil,[a] Prosobee,[b] Pregestimil,[b] Mocha Mix,[c] meat base formulas used as milk substitutes, carbonated drinks, coffee, freeze dried coffee, fruit drinks, some instant coffees (check labels), Lidalac[d] and other lactose free milks or those treated with lactase enzymes; lactose free products such as Ensure,[a] Ensure Plus[a] Citrotein, Nutramigen,[b] Nutri 1000 LF.[e] See Table 35–7	All untreated milk of any species and all products containing milk (except lactose free milk), such as skim, dried, evaporated, or condensed milk; yogurt; cheese; ice cream; sherbet; malted milk; Ovaltine;[f] hot chocolate; some cocoas and instant coffees (read labels); powdered soft drinks with lactose curds; whey and casein milk that has been treated with lactobacillus/acidophilus culture rather than lactase, such as Nu-trish[g]
Breads and Cereals	*Breads and Cereals*
Breads and rolls made without milk, Italian bread, some cooked cereals and prepared cereals (read labels), macaroni, spaghetti, soda crackers	Prepared mixes, such as muffins, biscuits, waffles, pancakes; some dry cereals such as Total,[h] Special K,[i] and Cocoa Krispies[i] (read labels carefully); Instant Cream of Wheat[j]; commercial breads and rolls to which milk solids have been added; zwieback; French toast made with milk
Desserts	*Desserts*
Water and fruit ices; gelatin; angel food cake; homemade cakes, pies, cookies made from allowed ingredients; puddings made with water	Commercial cakes and cookies and mixes, custard, puddings, sherbets, ice cream made with milk; any containing chocolate, pie crust made with butter or margarine, gelatin made with carrageenan
Eggs	*Eggs*
All	Omelets and soufflés containing milk
Fats	*Fats*
Margarines and dressings that do not contain milk or milk products, oils, shortening, bacon, Rich's Whip Topping,[k] some nondairy creamers (read labels), nut butters, nuts	Margarines and dressings containing milk or milk products, butter, cream, cream cheese, peanut butter with milk solids fillers, salad dressings containing lactose
Fruits	*Fruits*
All fresh, canned, or frozen that are not processed with lactose	Any canned or frozen processed with lactose
Meat, Fish, Poultry, Etc.	*Meat, Fish, Poultry, Etc.*
Plain beef, chicken, fish, turkey, lamb, veal, pork, and ham; strained or junior meats and vegetables and meat combinations that do not contain milk or milk products; kosher frankfurters	Creamed or breaded meat, fish, or fowl; sausage products, such as weiners, liver sausage, cold cuts containing nonfat milk solids; cheese
Soups	*Soups*
Clear soups, vegetable soups, consommés, cream soups made with Mocha Mix[c] or nondairy creamers	Cream soups unless made with allowed ingredients, chowders, commercially prepared soups containing lactose
Vegetables	*Vegetables*
Fresh, canned, or frozen: artichokes, asparagus, broccoli, cabbage, carrots, cauliflower, celery, chard, corn, cucumber, eggplant, green beans, kale, lettuce, mustard, okra, onions, parsley, parsnips, pumpkin, rutabagas, spinach, squash, tomatoes, white and sweet potatoes, yams, lima beans, beets	Any to which lactose is added during processing; peas; creamed, breaded, or buttered vegetables; instant potatoes, corn curls, and frozen French fries if processed with lactose
Miscellaneous	*Miscellaneous*
Soy sauce, carob powder, popcorn, olives, pure sugar candy, jelly or marmalade, sugar, corn syrup, carbonated beverages, gravy made with water, baker's cocoa, pickles, pure seasonings and spices, wine, molasses (beet sugar), pure monosodium glutamate, instant coffees that do not contain lactose	Chewing gum; chocolate; some cocoas; toffee; peppermint; butterscotch; caramels; some instant coffees, dietetic preparations (read labels); certain antibiotics and vitamin and mineral preparations; spice blends if they contain milk products; monosodium glutamate extender; artificial sweeteners containing lactose, such as Equal,[l] Sweet n' Low,[m] Wee Cal;[n] some nondairy creamers (read labels)

From The American Dietetic Association: Handbook of Clinical Dietetics, New Haven, Yale University Press, 1981, pp. D–15–16.
[a] Ross Laboratories, Columbus, OH 43216.
[b] Mead Johnson and Co., Evansville, IN 47721.
[c] Presto Food Products, Los Angeles, CA 90021.
[d] Lidano Co., Kalunborg, Denmark.
[e] Cutter Laboratories, Berkeley, CA 94710.
[f] Ovaltine Products, Villa Park, IL 60181.
[g] Knudsen Bros., North Haven, CT 06473.
[h] General Mills, Minneapolis, MN 55435.
[i] Kellogg Co., Battle Creek, MI 49016.
[j] Nabisco, Inc., East Hanover, NJ 07936.
[k] Rich Products Corp., Buffalo, NY 14212.
[l] G.D. Searle and Co., Skokie, IL 60076.
[m] NIFDA (National Institutional Food Distributor Associates, Inc.), Atlanta, GA 30325.
[n] Domino Amstar Corporation, New York, NY 10020.

formers. With reduced micelle formation, steatorrhea secondary to the bowel stasis results. There is also malabsorption of vitamin B_{12} because the bacteria use the vitamin for their own growth. Treatment is directed toward removal of the blind loop or control of the bacterial growth with antibiotics.

Protein-Losing Enteropathy

Protein-losing enteropathy, a disorder secondary to many diseases, is a condition of excessive gastrointestinal loss of protein and can occur anywhere along the G.I. tract. Four mechanisms have been proposed to explain this abnormal loss of protein into the gut:[12]

1. Because of an inflamed or ulcerated mucosa, plasma proteins may pass into the G.I. lumen (regional enteritis, ulcerative colitis).

2. Disordered mucosal cell structure may permit plasma protein loss (non-tropical sprue).

3. Increased lymphatic pressure causes increased movement of plasma proteins into the lumen through spaces between mucosal cells in the epithelium.

4. Dilated lymph vessels in the intestinal mucosa rupture and discharge their protein-rich contents into the lumen (idiopathic intestinal lymphangiectasia).

A normal person will catabolize 5 to 10 per cent of the intravascular albumin pool daily, but the person with protein-losing enteropathy will catabolize 50 to 60 per cent.

Nutritional Care

Treatment aims to relieve the underlying disorder and to supply large amounts of calories and protein (150 gm. or more daily) to offset the protein loss. This is done with a high-protein diet and protein supplements, with a defined-formula diet that is high in protein (see Table 35–7) or with total parenteral nutrition. It is very important to maintain nutritional status in these patients so that they will respond to the medical treatment.

Problems and Suggested Topics for Discussion

1. Describe the physiology and functions of the intestines.
2. Classify foods into low- and high-fiber types.
3. Research the "fiber hypothesis" and explain how fiber is related to many intestinal diseases.
4. Interview an adolescent with Crohn's disease. Find out about his lifestyle and eating patterns. Analyze his diet for nutrient content. Is he taking any supplements? Is the intake adequate? Evaluate his growth.

5. Perform a nutritional assessment of a patient hospitalized for an acute attack of ulcerative colitis. Plan her nutritional care. Is she able to take food orally? Can she meet her needs by this route? If not, what would you recommend for enteral feeding?
6. What are the principles of a diet for chronic diarrhea? Differentiate between diarrhea and steatorrhea.
7. Interview a patient with lactose intolerance and find out which foods bother him or her. Is the patient afraid to eat certain foods? Is his or her diet adequate? What changes would you recommend?
8. What are the general principles of nutritional care for a patient with a malabsorption syndrome?
9. Do a nutritional assessment of a patient with gluten-sensitive enteropathy.
10. Plan a "convenience-food" menu for one day for a young single person with celiac sprue who does not like to cook.

Resources for Patient Education

Gluten Intolerance Group of North America
P.O. Box 23053
Seattle, Washington 98102

American Celiac Society
45 Gifford Avenue
Jersey City, New Jersey 07304

American Digestive Disease Society
7720 Wisconsin Avenue
Bethesda, Maryland 20014

National Foundation for Ileitis and Colitis
295 Madison Avenue
New York, New York 10017

National Digestive Disease Education and Information Clearinghouse
1555 Wilson Boulevard, Suite 600
Rosslyn, Virginia 22209

Cookbooks

GIG Cookbook
Gluten Intolerance Group of North America
P.O. Box 23053
Seattle, Washington 98102

Weiss, M., Davis, J., and Smith, A.: Pointers for Parents Coping with Celiac Sprue, 1982.
Clinical Dietetics
The Children's Memorial Hospital
2300 Children's Plaza
Chicago, Illinois 60614

Cited References

1. Baker, H., Frank, O., and Sobotka, H.: Mechanisms of folic acid deficiency in nontropical sprue. JAMA, *187*: 119, 1964.
2. Bayless, T.M.: Special problems of adolescents with inflammatory bowel disease. In Korelitz, B.I. (ed): Inflammatory Bowel Disease: Experience and Controversy. London, John Wright, PSG Inc., 1982.
3. Bedine, M.S., and Bayless, T.M.: Intolerance of small amounts of lactose by individuals with low lactase levels. Gastroenterology, *65*:735, 1973.
4. Bruno, M.S.: An internist's view of inflammatory bowel disease. In Korelitz, B.I. (ed.): Inflammatory Bowel Disease: Experience and Controversy. London, John Wright, PSG Inc., 1982.
5. Burkitt, D.P., Walker, A.R.P., and Painter, N.S.: Effect

of dietary fiber on stools and transit-times and its role in causation of disease. Lancet, 2:1408, 1972.

6. Congdon, P., et al.: Small-bowel mucosa in asymptomatic children with celiac disease. Am. J. Dis. Child., 135:118, 1981.

7. Devroede, G.: Constipation: mechanisms and management. In Sleisenger, M.H., and Fordtran, J.S. (eds.): Gastrointestinal Disease: Pathophysiology, Diagnosis, Management. 2nd ed. Philadelphia, W.B. Saunders Company, 1978.

8. Feeley, R.M., Criner, P.E., and Slover, H.T.: Major fatty acids and proximate composition of dairy products. J. Am. Diet. Assoc., 66:140, 1975.

9. Gallagher, C.R., Molleson, A.L., and Caldwell, J.H.: Lactose intolerance and fermented dairy products. J. Am. Diet. Assoc., 65:418, 1974.

10. Geib, D., and Jones, J.D.: Unprecedented case of constipation. JAMA, 38:1304, 1902.

11. Gerson, C.D.: Ascorbic acid deficiency in clinical disease including regional enteritis. Ann. N.Y. Acad. Sci., 258:483, 1975.

12. Greenberger, N.J., and Isselbacher, K.H.: Disorders of absorption. In Thorn, G.W., et al. (eds.): Harrison's Principles of Internal Medicine. 8th ed. New York, McGraw-Hill Book Co., 1977, p. 1535.

13. Harris, O.D., et al.: Malignancy in adult coeliac disease and idiopathic steatorrhea. Am. J. Med., 42:899, 1967.

14. Korelitz, B.I.: Evidence for Crohn's disease as an extensive process. In Korelitz, B.I. (ed.): Inflammatory Bowel Disease: Experience and Controversy. London, John Wright, PSG Inc., 1982.

15. Kretchmer, N.: The significance of lactose intolerance. In Paige, D.M., and Bayless, T.M. (eds.): Lactose Digestion: Clinical and Nutritional Implications. Baltimore, The Johns Hopkins University Press, 1981.

16. Leonard, J., et al.: Gluten challenge in dermatitis herpetiformis. N. Engl. J. Med., 308:816, 1983.

17. Motil, K.J., et al.: Whole body leucine metabolism in adolescents with Crohn's disease and growth failure during nutritional supplementation. Gastroenterology, 82:1359, 1982.

18. Paige, D.M., and Bayless, T.M. (eds.): Lactose Digestion: Clinical Nutritional Implications. Baltimore, Johns Hopkins University Press, 1981.

19. Painter, N.S.: Diverticular disease of the colon: a disease caused by fiber deficiency. Plant Foods for Man, 1(1):67, 1973.

20. Painter, N.S., Alameida, A.Z., and Colebourne, K.W.: Unprocessed bran in treatment of diverticular disease of the colon. Br. Med. J., 1:137, 1972.

21. Ritchie, J.: The irritable bowel syndrome. II. Manometric and cineradiographic studies. Clin. Gastroenterol. 6:622, 1977.

22. Sandstead, H.H.: Zinc as an unrecognized limiting nutrient. Am. J. Clin. Nutr., 26:790, 1973.

23. Søltoft, J., et al.: A double-blind trial of the effect of wheat bran on symptoms of irritable bowel syndrome. Lancet, 1:270, 1976.

24. Turner, D.: Handbook of Diet Therapy. 5th ed. Chicago, University of Chicago Press, 1970.

25. Wald, A., Back, C., and Bayless, T.M.: Effect of caffeine on the human small intestine. Gastroenterology, 71:738, 1976.

26. Wisch, N.: Hematologic complications of inflammatory bowel disease and its drug therapy. In Korelitz, B.I. (ed.): Inflammatory Bowel Disease: Experience and Controversy. London, John Wright, PSG Inc., 1982.

Additional References

Ament, M.E.: Inflammatory disease of the colon: ulcerative colitis and Crohn's colitis. J. Pediatr., 86:322, 1975.

Bayless, T.M., Yardley, J.H., and Hendrix, T.R.: Adult celiac disease: treatment with gluten-free diet. Arch. Intern. Med., 111:83, 1963.

Burkitt, D.P., and Trowell, H.C. (eds.): Refined Carbohydrate Foods and Disease: Some implications of Dietary Fiber. New York, Academic Press, 1975.

Debry, G., and Drouin, P.: Diet in functional disorders of the colon. Prog. Food Nutr. Sci., 2:1, 1976.

Dworken, H.J.: Gastroenterology: Pathophysiology and Clinical Applications. Boston, Butterworth Inc., 1982.

Elsborg, L., and Bastrup-Madsen, P.: Folic acid absorption in various gastrointestinal disorders. Scand. J. Gastroenterol., 11:333, 1976.

Farmer, R.G.: The protein manifestations of Crohn's disease. Postgrad. Med., 57:129, 1975.

Floch, M.H.: Nutrition and Diet Therapy in Gastrointestinal Disease. New York, Plenum Medical Book Company, 1981.

Goldstein, F.: Diet and colonic disease. J. Am. Diet. Assoc., 60:499, 1972.

Idea Exchange: Fiber in the diet. J. Am. Diet. Assoc., 66:50, 1975.

Kaufmann, M.: Answers to questions on gastrointestinal allergy. Hospital Medicine, 11:61, 1975.

Kirsner, J.S., and Shorter, R.G.: Recent developments in "nonspecific" inflammatory bowel disease. Pt. 1 and 2. N. Engl. J. Med., 306:775 and 837, 1982.

The lactose tolerance test and milk consumption. Nutr. Rev., 34:302, 1976.

Levine, G.M.: Nutritional support in gastrointestinal disease. Surg. Clin. North Am., 61:701, 1981.

Levitt, M.D., et al.: Studies of a flatulent patient. N. Engl. J. Med., 295:260, 1976.

McCarthy, C.F.: Nutritional defects in patients with malabsorption. Proc. Nutr. Soc., 35:37, 1976.

Matthan, V.I.: Tropical sprue. In Sleisenger, M.H., and Fordtran, J.S. (eds.): Gastrointestinal Disease: Pathophysiology, Diagnosis, Management. 2nd ed. Philadelphia, W.B. Saunders Company, 1978.

Mendeloff, A.I.: Dietary fiber. Nutr. Rev., 33:321, 1975. The role of lactose in the diet. Dairy Council Digest, 45(5), 1975 (Published by the National Dairy Council, Chicago).

Moesgaard, F., et al.: High-fiber diet reduces bleeding and pain in patients with hemorrhoids. Dis. Col. Rect., 25:454, 1982.

Rombeau, J.L.: Enteral nutrition therapy in inflammatory bowel disease. Clin. Consult. Nutr. Support, 1(3):1, 1981.

Ruffin, J.M., et al.: Gluten-free diet for nontropical sprue: immediate and prolonged effects. JAMA, 188:42, 1964.

Simoons, F.T., Johnson, J.D., and Kretchmer, N.: Perspective on milk during drinking and malabsorption of lactose. Pediatrics, 59:98, 1977.

Sleisenger, M.H., and Fordtran, J.S. (eds.): Gastrointestinal Disease: Pathophysiology, Diagnosis, Mangagement. 2nd ed. Philadelphia, W.B. Saunders Company, 1978.

Tasman-Jones, C.: Constipation. N.Z. Med. J., 90:204, 1979.

Thompson, W.G.: Constipation and catharsis. Can. Med. Assoc. J., 114:927, 1976.

Trier, J.S.: Celiac sprue disease. In Sleisenger, M.H., and Fordtran, J.S. (eds.): Gastrointestinal Disease: Pathophysiology, Diagnosis, Management. 2nd ed. Philadelphia, W.B. Saunders Company, 1978.

Trowell, H.: Definition of dietary fiber and hypotheses that it is a protective factor in certain diseases. Am. J. Clin. Nutr., 29:417, 1976.

Nutritional Care in Disease of the Liver, Exocrine Pancreas and Biliary System

Physiology and Functions of the Liver

In the metabolism of food, the liver is one of the most important of the body organs. It is the largest glandular organ of the body, contributing between 2.5 and 3 per cent of the body weight. Figure 24–1 shows the location of the liver and other organs of the upper abdomen.

The liver also has the greatest number of and most varied functions of any organ in the body. Most of the end products of the digestion of food are transported directly to the liver. Compounds that it manufactures or stores are sent to other parts of the body as needed. Poisons that enter the body through food or that are produced in other parts of the body are detoxified in the liver. Drugs are metabolized in the liver. Since the liver has many functions in the metabolism of all major nutrients, a brief summary of its role in the metabolic process follows.

CARBOHYDRATE METABOLISM

The hepatic cells serve as a storehouse for glycogen, which is formed in the liver from the glucose, fructose and galactose received from the portal circulation (glycogenesis). When glucose is needed by the body, glycogen is converted to glucose (glycogenolysis) and returned to the blood stream. When glucose concentration in the blood begins to fall below normal, conversion of protein and fat to glucose (gluconeogenesis) occurs in the liver, after which it is sent to the blood stream to maintain normal blood glucose level.

FAT METABOLISM

The liver synthesizes fat from fatty acids, deaminized amino acids (keto acids) and carbohydrates. It synthesizes cholesterol and converts about 80 per cent of it into bile salts; the remainder is transported in the form of lipoproteins in the blood. Triglycerides are synthesized from fatty acids, as are phospholipids. Both are incorporated into lipoproteins for transport to the adipose tissue, where they are stored. Oxidation of fatty acids to acetoacetic acid and then to acetyl-CoA occurs in the liver. Acetyl-CoA in turn can enter the Krebs cycle and be oxidized to liberate energy. About 60 per cent of all initial oxidation of fatty acids in the body takes place in the liver.

PROTEIN METABOLISM

In the metabolism of proteins, deamination of the amino acids must take place in the liver cells before they can be used for energy or converted to carbohydrate and fats. Keto acids and ammonia are also formed from this deamination process. Conversion of amino acids into other amino acids (non-essential) occurs in the liver through several stages of *transamination*. They are released from the liver to maintain normal blood levels of each amino acid. Other important chemical compounds (such as purines and pyrimidines) are synthesized from amino acids through transamination. The formation of urea by the liver removes ammonia, which is excreted. The carbon residues are converted into fatty acids or glucose for energy or eventual storage. Most of the plasma proteins (albumin, globulin, fibrinogen, prothrombin and heparin) are synthesized by the hepatic cells. A reserve of these proteins is maintained in the liver to replenish serum proteins as needed.

MINERALS AND VITAMINS

The greatest portion of the body's iron is stored in the liver in the form of *ferritin* until needed by the body. Copper is also stored in the liver and is necessary for the production of hemoglobin. Iron is an integral part of hemoglobin, and vitamin B_{12} (also stored in the liver) brings about the maturation and release of red blood cells in the bone marrow. The iron from discarded red blood cells is recovered and stored by the liver.

All the fat-soluble vitamins are present in the liver. Considerable amounts of vitamins A, D and K are stored there, as are small amounts of vitamin E. The liver converts carotene into vitamin A, vitamin K into prothrombin and vitamin D into an active form ($25\text{-}OHD_3$). It also stores appreciable amounts of ascorbic acid and the B-complex vitamins.

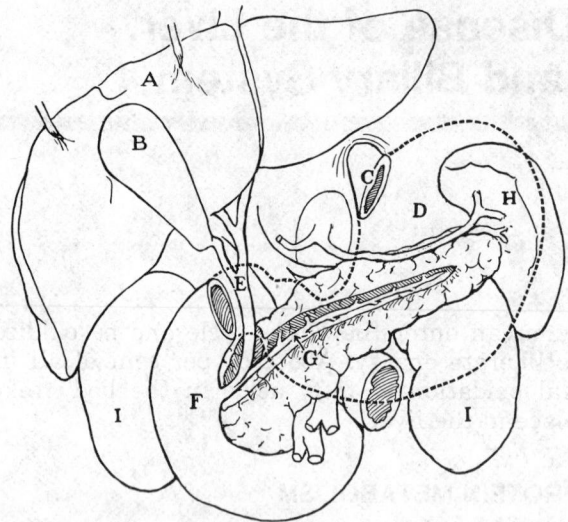

Figure 24–1. Schematic drawing showing relationship of organs of the upper abdomen. *A*, Liver (retracted upward); *B*, gallbladder; *C*, esophageal opening of stomach; *D*, stomach (shown in dotted outline); *E*, common bile duct; *F*, duodenum; *G*, pancreas and pancreatic duct; *H*, spleen; *I*, kidneys.

Diseases of the Liver

VIRAL HEPATITIS

Hepatitis is an inflammation of the liver caused by a virus, toxin, obstruction, parasite or drug (chloroform, carbon tetrachloride). Viral hepatitis is caused by three major agents and several minor ones. The vast majority of cases are caused by hepatitis viruses A and B, and the so-called non-A, non-B agents.

Hepatitis caused by the type A virus is also referred to as *hepatitis A* or *infectious hepatitis*. This disease, common among children and young adults, is mildly contagious and readily transmitted through contaminated drinking water, food or sewage. In the acute phase there are symptoms of nausea, vomiting, anorexia, fever, headache, weight loss, fatigue and abdominal discomfort.

While most attacks are not serious, they may be severe in older people. If liver damage is extensive in older patients, fatty infiltration of the liver may occur, and hepatic encephalopathy and coma may develop.

In contrast to hepatitis A, *hepatitis B* (caused by the type B virus and formerly known as *serum hepatitis*) may cause a wide variety of acute or chronic hepatic and extrahepatic diseases. The clinical course of hepatitis B is more variable and usually more prolonged than that of hepatitis A. This disease can be transmitted through transfusions of blood or serum from a person who is a carrier of the virus or through improperly sterilized medical instruments, den-

tal drills, tattooing needles or any other skin-puncturing instrument that has come in contact with contaminated blood. Less commonly, it can also be transmitted by other than the parenteral route, which makes its specific cause more obscure. In 5 to 10 per cent of cases, hepatitis B patients develop chronic active hepatitis and some become asymptomatic carriers of the hepatitis B antigen (HB_sAg). These people are the most dangerous to the health of the community.

CIRRHOSIS

Cirrhosis is the most serious or final stage of liver injury and degeneration. The normal liver tissue is gradually destroyed and inactive fibrous connective tissue replaces the liver cells, following fatty degeneration of long standing, as shown in Figure 24–2. An intermediate stage called *alcoholic hepatitis* may develop, in which some liver cells die and cause necrotic inflammation. In contrast to the enlarged fatty liver, the cirrhotic liver is contracted and has lost most of its function. Once the dense vascular and fibrous bands have formed, scarring is reported to be permanent.

Etiology

ALCOHOL. Chronic alcoholism is the most common cause of cirrhosis. The alcohol-induced liver injury is due to the constant presence of alcohol itself and the metabolic derangements it causes, rather than to the malnutrition commonly associated with alcoholism.[12] However, in most cases malnutrition is also involved. Alcohol causes disordered liver metabolism because of its conversion to acetaldehyde and the excessive production of hydrogen that results from this reaction. The metabolic and toxic effects of alcohol are diagrammed in Figure 24–3. Fatty liver commonly occurs even after acute alcohol ingestion.

Not all alcoholics go on to develop alcoholic hepatitis and cirrhosis. Whether they do depends on the duration and amount of their alcohol intake and on undefined genetic and possibly immunological factors. An adequate diet does not protect against the development of fatty liver, alcoholic hepatitis or cirrhosis in the alcoholic.

Studies by Lieber[11] indicate that an intake of 11 to 12 oz. of 86 proof whiskey per day can lead to the development of fatty liver in humans, regardless of the maintenance of an adequate diet. When rats were fed this amount of alcohol, a fatty liver could be produced within two to six weeks, even though a well-balanced and controlled dietary intake was maintained.

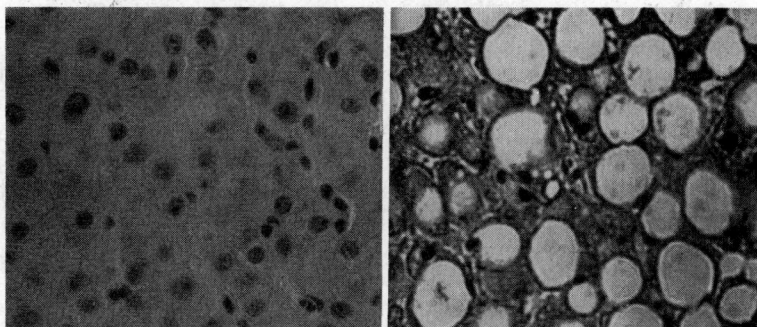

Figure 24–2. Fatty changes in the liver. (From: Halpern, S.L.: Nutrition and chronic disease. Reprinted from Health News, monthly publication of the New York State Department of Health, September, 1955.)

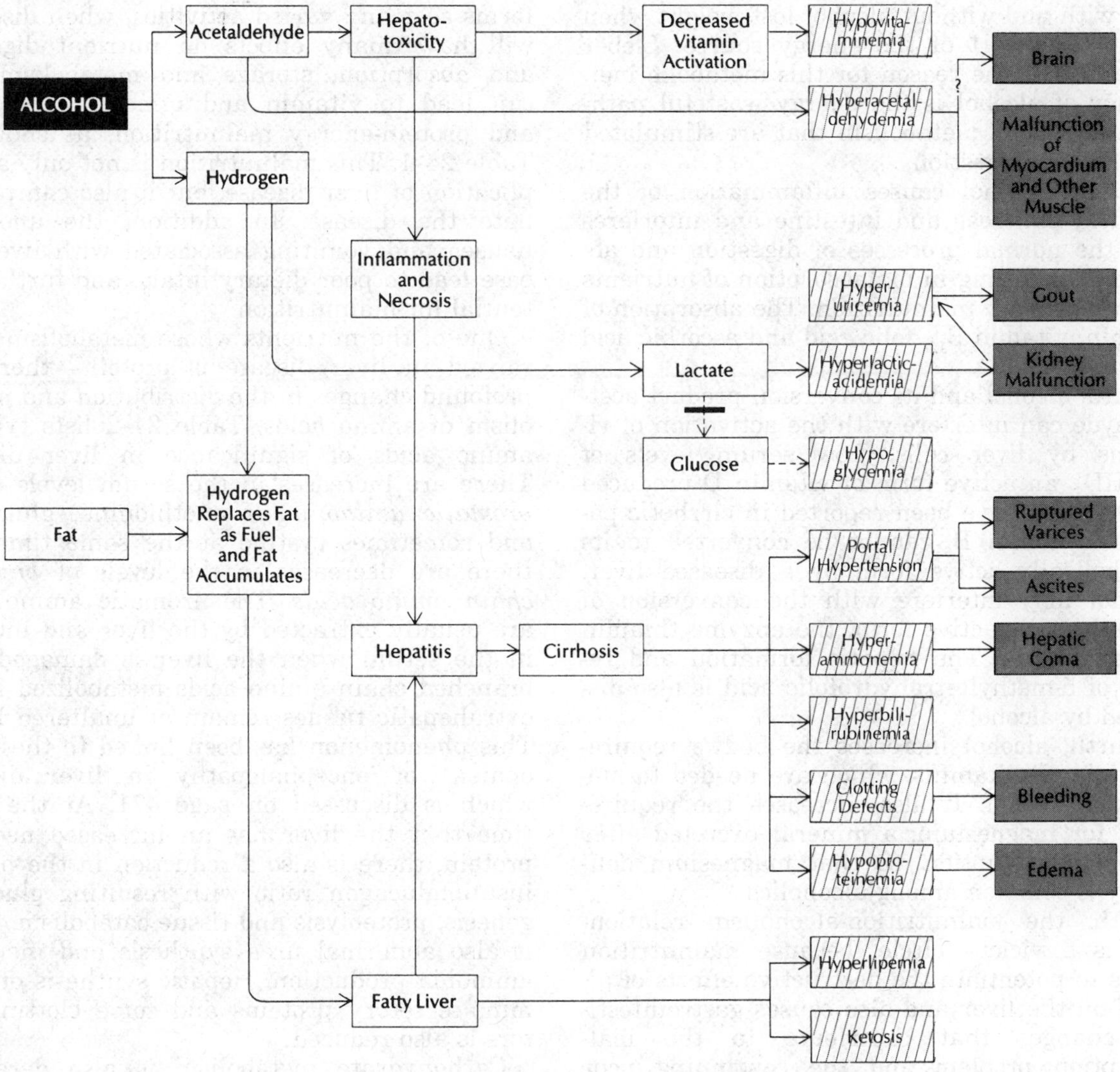

Normal liver   Fatty infiltration of liver

Figure 24–3. Complications of excessive alcohol consumption stem largely from excess hydrogen and from acetaldehyde. Hydrogen produces fatty liver and hyperlipemia, high blood lactic acid and low blood sugar. The accumulation of fat, the effect of acetaldehyde on liver cells and other factors as yet unknown lead to alcoholic hepatitis. The next step is cirrhosis. The consequent impairment of liver function disturbs blood chemistry, notably causing a high ammonia level which can lead to coma and death. Cirrhosis also distorts liver structure, inhibiting blood flow. High pressure in vessels supplying the liver may cause ruptured varices and accumulation of fluid in the abdominal cavity. There are individual differences in response to alcohol; in particular, not all heavy drinkers develop hepatitis and cirrhosis. (From: Lieber, C.S.: The metabolism of alcohol. Sci. Am., *234*:33, 1976. Copyright © 1976 by Scientific American, Inc. All rights reserved.)

MALNUTRITION. The chronic alcoholic with liver disease is usually also malnourished for several reasons. First, alcohol replaces food in the diet. It is possible for humans to obtain some of their maintenance energy needs from the calories in the alcohol consumed, but they will be malnourished because of an inadequate intake of nutrients. Alcohol is a notable source of empty calories, since 20 oz. of 86 proof liquor provides 1500 kcal., or about one half to two thirds of the daily caloric requirement, but it contains no protein, vitamins or minerals. However, even though alcohol provides 7 kcal./gm., its energy efficiency is not comparable to that of other nutrients. Humans consuming isocaloric diets with and without alcohol lost weight when alcohol was part of the energy source. Lieber suggests that the reason for this metabolic inefficiency of alcohol is the energy wasteful pathways of ethanol metabolism that are stimulated with alcohol ingestion.

Second, alcohol causes inflammation of the stomach, pancreas and intestine and interferes with the normal processes of digestion and absorption, resulting in malabsorption of nutrients and a secondary malnutrition. The absorption of thiamin, vitamin B_{12}, folic acid and ascorbic acid is depressed.

Third, alcohol and its conversion product acetaldehyde can interfere with the activation of vitamins by liver cells. Low serum levels of $25\text{-}OHD_3$, an active form of vitamin D produced by the liver, have been reported in cirrhotic patients. Vitamin B_6 cannot be converted to its metabolically active form by a diseased liver. Alcohol may interfere with the conversion of thiamin to its active form, the enzyme thiamin pyrophosphate. The hepatic formation and release of 5-methyltetrahydrofolic acid is also disturbed by alcohol.

Fourth, alcohol increases the body's requirements for B vitamins, which are needed to metabolize alcohol. It also increases the requirement for magnesium, a mineral excreted after alcohol consumption, so that magnesium deficiency is common among alcoholics.

Fifth, the malnutrition-alcoholism relationship is a vicious circle, because malnutrition seems to potentiate the destructive effects of alcohol on the liver and also causes gastrointestinal changes that contribute to the malabsorption problem and the continuing poor nutritional status already provoked by the alcohol. Folate deficiency and, to a lesser extent, protein deficiency seem to be most responsible for the malabsorption caused by malnutrition.[1]

These reasons combined with social and economic factors usually lead to a malnourished chronic alcoholic. He or she will frequently exhibit signs of clinical deficiency, such as cardiac changes from thiamin deficiency or macrocytic anemia from folate deficiency.

OTHER CAUSES. Cirrhosis may also be caused by various toxic and infectious agents that cause destruction of the liver cells, as is seen in viral hepatitis, which ultimately leads to fibrosis of the liver.

NUTRITIONAL CARE IN LIVER DISEASE

Because the type of nutritional care is directly related to the liver's functions, an understanding of its role in the metabolic process is necessary to determine the character of the diet for any hepatic disturbance. An organ that performs so many varied activities, when diseased, will have many effects on nutrient digestion and absorption, storage and metabolism that can lead to vitamin and mineral deficiencies and protein-energy malnutrition, as shown in Table 24-1. This malnutrition is not only a complication of liver disease, but it also can perpetuate the disease. In addition, the anorexia, nausea and vomiting associated with liver disease lead to poor dietary intake and further potential for malnutrition.

One of the nutrients whose metabolism is deranged in liver disease is protein—there are profound changes in the distribution and metabolism of amino acids. Table 24-2 lists types of amino acids of significance in liver disease. There are increases in the serum levels of the *aromatic amino acids*, methionine, glutamine and sometimes cystine at the same time that there are decreases in the levels of *branched chain amino acids*. The aromatic amino acids are usually extracted by the liver and increase in the serum when the liver is damaged. The branched chain amino acids metabolized in the extrahepatic tissues remain at unaltered levels. This phenomenon has been linked to the development of encephalopathy in liver disease, which is discussed on page 471. At the same time that the liver has an increased need for protein, there is also a reduction in the plasma insulin:glucagon ratio with resulting gluconeogenesis, proteolysis and tissue catabolism. There is also abnormal urea synthesis and increased ammonia production. Hepatic synthesis of albumin, secretory proteins and some clotting factors is also reduced.

Carbohydrate metabolism is also deranged. Hepatitis patients may experience fasting hypoglycemia due to decreased glycogen stores and serum insulin elevations. In cirrhosis there may be glucose intolerance due to elevated serum insulin, insulin resistance and growth hormone and glucagon elevation which lead to mobilization and utilization of endogenous protein for energy.

Table 24-1. NUTRITIONAL CONSEQUENCES OF LIVER DISEASE

NUTRIENT	ABERRATION	CONSEQUENCE
Protein and amino acids	↑ Serum levels of tyrosine, methionine, phenylalanine, glutamine and sometimes cystine	Theory: ↑ aromatic amino acids in brain lead to formation of false neurotransmitters and encephalopathy
	↓ Serum levels of branched chain amino acids—valine, leucine and isoleucine	
	Reduction in plasma insulin:glucagon ratio	Gluconeogenesis, proteolysis of protein and catabolism of tissue
Carbohydrate	Glucose intolerance due to elevated serum insulin, insulin resistance and growth hormone and glucagon elevation	Mobilization and utilization of endogenous protein for energy
Lipid	Decreased synthesis of lipid-transport proteins	Decreased high density lipoprotein
	Decreased absorption of long chain fatty acids	Steatorrhea
Vitamins	↓ Formation of 25-OHD$_3$ in the liver	↓ Serum 25-OHD$_3$ Osteoporosis
	↓ Degradation of pyridoxal phosphate	Possible vitamin B$_6$ deficiency
	↓ Formation of vitamin A transport protein	↓ Serum vitamin A Night blindness
	Inadequate retention of folate in the liver	Possible folate deficiency
Minerals	Steatorrhea resulting in calcium soaps and decreased absorption of calcium	↓ Serum levels of zinc, magnesium and calcium
	Magnesium excreted after alcohol consumption	Possible zinc deficiency
	Zinc excretion increased in cirrhosis	

There are also alterations in lipid metabolism. Low levels of high density lipoproteins (HDL) are characteristic as are low levels of beta-lipoproteins, the principal transport protein for vitamin E.

OBJECTIVES. The objectives of nutritional care are: (1) to maintain or improve the patient's nutritional status through the provision of adequate energy and nutrients, (2) to prevent or ameliorate hepatic encephalopathy and (3) to prevent further degeneration of the liver and to enable the liver to regenerate new tissue to the maximum extent possible. These three principles of nutritional care apply for all hepatic disturbances.

LIVER FUNCTION TESTS. During the course of liver disease, liver function can change drastically, and the nutritional care must be adjusted according to the deteriorating or improving liver function. For example, a serum albumin level reflects protein nutriture. A decreased serum albumin level shows that the liver is unable to synthesize protein. An elevated level of serum ammonia indicates that the liver is unable to synthesize urea from ammonia in the blood and that too much ammonia is entering the bloodstream from the action of colonic bacteria on protein in the gut. The tests listed in Table 24-3 provide clues to changing liver function.

ENERGY. Since there is often extreme weight loss, a high-calorie diet with at least 45 to 50 kcal. per kg. desired body weight per day is indicated to rehabilitate the patient with liver disease.

CARBOHYDRATE. Increased carbohydrate in the diet for patients with liver disease is well tolerated and seems to have a definite therapeutic value. The carbohydrate content of the diet protects and supports hepatic function. Three hundred to 400 gm. per day is recommended to spare the available protein and to aid in recovery.

Table 24-2. AMINO ACIDS OF APPARENT IMPORTANCE IN LIVER DISEASE AND ENCEPHALOPATHY

AROMATIC AMINO ACIDS—AAA

   tyrosine
   phenylalanine*
   tryptophan*

Branched chain amino acids—BCAA

   valine*
   leucine*
   isoleucine*

Ammoniogenic amino acids

   glycine
   serine
   threonine*
   glutamine
   histidine*
   lysine*
   asparagine

*Denotes essential amino acids.

Table 24–3. COMMON LIVER FUNCTION TESTS

DIAGNOSTIC TEST	FUNCTION EVALUATED
Van den Bergh Icterus index Urine bilirubin Urobilinogen Fecal urobilinogen	Formation and excretion of bile
Total protein Albumin Globulin Fibrinogen Thymol turbidity Cephalin flocculation	Protein metabolism and formation of albumin, globulin, fibrinogen
Prothrombin time	Production of prothrombin
Urea Uric acid Ammonia	Formation of urea and uric acids and removal of ammonia

Glucose tolerance
Galactose tolerance
	Carbohydrate metabolism
	  Gluconeogenesis
	  Glycogenesis
	  Glycogenolysis

Serum phospholipids, triglycerides Cholesterol (total or ester) Ketone	Lipid metabolism Synthesis of cholesterol Formation of ketone bodies
Bromsulphalein (BSP) Hippuric acid	Detoxification Excretion of substances withdrawn from the blood Conjugation, oxidation or reduction
Serum glutamic-oxaloacetic transaminase (SGOT) Serum glutamic-pyruvic transaminase (SGPT) Lactic dehydrogenase (LDH) Alkaline phosphatase Leucine aminopeptidase (LAP) 5′-Nucleotidase Cholinesterase	Enzyme production

From Given, B. A., and Simmons, S. J.: Gastroenterology in Clinical Nursing, 2nd ed. St. Louis, C. V. Mosby Co., 1975, p. 273.

Table 24–4. FAT-RESTRICTED DIET

FOODS ALLOWED	FOODS EXCLUDED
Beverages	*Beverages*
Skim milk or buttermilk made with skim milk; coffee, tea, Postum, fruit juice, soft drinks, cocoa made with cocoa powder and skim milk	Whole milk, buttermilk made with whole milk, chocolate milk, cream in excess of amounts allowed under fats
Bread and Cereal Products	*Bread and Cereal Products*
Plain, nonfat cereals, spaghetti, noodles, rice, macaroni; plain whole grain or enriched bread	Biscuits, breads, egg or cheese bread, sweet rolls made with fat, pancakes, doughnuts, waffles, fritters, popcorn prepared with fat, muffins, natural cereals and breads to which extra fat is added
Cheese	*Cheese*
Cottage, 1/4 cup to be used as substitute for an ounce of cheese, or specially processed American cheese containing less than 5% butterfat	Whole milk cheeses

Table continued on the opposite page

Table 24-4.   FAT-RESTRICTED DIET (*Continued*)

FOODS ALLOWED	FOODS EXCLUDED
Desserts	*Desserts*
Sherbet made with skim milk; fruit ice; gelatin; rice, bread, cornstarch, tapioca, or Junket pudding made with skim milk; fruit whips with gelatin, sugar, and egg white; fruit; angel food cake; meringues	Cake, pie, pastry, ice cream, or any dessert containing shortening, chocolate, or fats of any kind, unless especially prepared using part of fat allowance
Eggs	*Eggs*
3 per week prepared only with fat from fat allowance; egg whites as desired; low fat egg substitutes	More than 1/day unless substituted for part of the meat allowed
Fats	*Fats*
Choose up to the limit allowed on diet among the following (1 serving in the amount listed equals 1 fat choice): 1 tsp. butter or fortified margarine 1 tsp. shortening or oil 1 tsp. mayonnaise 1 tbsp. Italian or French dressing 1 strip crisp bacon 1/8 avocado (4″ diameter) 2 tbsp. light cream 1 tbsp. heavy cream 6 small nuts 5 small olives	Any in excess of amount prescribed on diet; all others
Fruits	*Fruits*
As desired	Avocado in excess of amount allowed on fat list
Lean Meat, Fish, Poultry	*Meat, Fish, Poultry*
Choose up to the limit allowed on diet among the following: poultry without skin, fish, veal (all cuts), liver, lean beef, pork, and lamb, with all visible fat removed—1 oz. cooked weight equals 1 equivalent; 1/4 cup water packed tuna or salmon equals 1 equivalent	Fried or fatty meats, sausage, scrapple, frankfurters, poultry skins, stewing hens, spareribs, salt pork, beef unless lean, duck, goose, ham hocks, pig's feet, luncheon meats, gravies unless fat free, tuna and salmon packed in oil, peanut butter
Milk	*Milk*
Skim, buttermilk or yogurt made from skim milk	Whole, chocolate, buttermilk made with whole milk
Seasonings	*Seasonings*
As desired	None
Soups	*Soups*
Bouillon, clear broth, fat free vegetable soup, cream soup made with skimmed milk, packaged dehydrated soups	All others
Sweets	*Sweets*
Jelly, jam, marmalade, honey, syrup, molasses, sugar, hard sugar candies, fondant, gumdrops, jelly beans, marshmallows	Any candy made with chocolate, nuts, butter, cream, or fat of any kind
Vegetables	*Vegetables*
All plainly prepared vegetables	Potato chips; buttered, au gratin, creamed, or fried vegetables unless made with allowed fat; commercially frozen vegetables; casseroles, or frozen vegetables in butter sauce.

DAILY FOOD ALLOWANCES FOR 50 GM. FAT DIET

Food	Amount	Approximate fat content (gm.)
Skim milk	2 cups or more	0
Lean meat, fish, poultry	6 oz. or 6 equivalents	18
Whole egg or egg yolks	3 per week	3
Vegetables	3 servings or more, at least 1 or more dark green or deep yellow	0
Fruits	3 or more servings, at least 1 citrus	0
Breads, cereals	As desired	0
Fat exchanges*	5–6 exchanges daily	25–30
Desserts and sweets	As desired from permitted list	0
	Total fat	46–51

* Additional fat servings are listed in Table 25–8. Fat content can be reduced further by reducing the fat exchanges. 1 fat exchange = 5 gm. fat.

From American Dietetic Association: Handbook of Clinical Dietetics. New Haven, Yale University Press, 1981, p. E-4

PROTEIN. A liberal protein intake is essential for the repair of hepatic cells. A daily intake of 1.0 to 1.5 gm. per kg. of desired body weight per day is usually adequate. *A cause for exception to the high protein intake is hepatic coma,* which is discussed on page 471. Both the quality and quantity of protein are important. Patients seem to tolerate vegetable and dairy proteins better than most other forms of protein, perhaps because of their low aromatic and ammoniogenic amino acid content.[8, 15] Tables 27–9 and 35–3 give high-calorie, high-protein diets. In addition, several resources at the end of Chapter 36 give recipes for high-calorie, high-protein foods.

CONCENTRATED ORAL AND PARENTERAL PROTEIN. If a patient is too ill to eat or has a poor appetite and cannot consume the large quantity of protein food he or she needs, concentrated protein may be included, such as calcium caseinate, dried milk, soybean flour, dried yeast or other products can be added to the diet. Table 35–8 identifies high-calorie and high-protein nutritional supplements. Tube feeding may be necessary. Parenteral nutrition may be prescribed if the oral consumption is inadequate. Discussion of branched chain amino acid (BCAA) supplementation is on page 472.

VITAMINS. A therapeutic vitamin preparation that is a good source of the vitamin B complex, especially folic acid, should be given. All of the vitamins should be supplied in abundance to fortify the liver against stress and to repair damage already done. If beri-beri, Wernicke-Korsakoff syndrome or polyneuritis is present, then thiamin should be given. Since the liver is responsible for synthesizing the active forms of several B vitamins and would be unable to do so in disease, ideally B vitamin supplements should be given in their active forms.

If there is steatorrhea, water-soluble forms of vitamins A, D and E may be necessary. In severe cirrhosis with problems of vitamin storage, metabolism and transport, intramuscular injections of A, D and K may be necessary. Vitamin K should be prescribed if evidence of hypoprothrombinemia exists.

FAT. The lowering of dietary fat to 25 per cent of total calories has been shown to reduce the amount of fatty deposition in the liver when alcohol is being consumed. Substitution of medium-chain triglycerides (MCT) for normal longer-chain dietary fats also resulted in a reduced accumulation of fat in the liver. Whether these measures hasten the recovery from alcoholic fatty liver after the patient has stopped drinking is not known.

Steatorrhea is found in about 50 per cent of cirrhotic patients, whether they are alcoholics or not. This malabsorption of fat appears to have several causes, which vary among patients: cirrhosis-associated pancreatic insufficiency, decreased amounts of bile salts, administration of neomycin, administration of cholestyramine, and, possibly, lymphatic or portal congestion. Use of MCT oil or liquid feedings containing some MCT rather than all long-chain triglycerides might be useful. The absorption and function of MCT is discussed on page 446.

In situations where MCT use is not effective as a substitute for dietary fat, it may be necessary to reduce the total fat in the diet. Food is more palatable (which is important with the anorexic patient) and easier to prepare when moderate amounts of fat are allowed especially in light of the high protein requirements. In addition, the inclusion of fats increases the energy content of the diet. Thus 70 to 100 gm. of fat, or about 25 to 30 per cent of total calories, is recommended. Table 24–4 outlines such a diet. Occasionally a patient will tolerate dairy fats when not able to tolerate those contained in fried foods.[15]

FLUIDS AND SODIUM. One of the complications of advanced cirrhosis is the development of edema and *ascites* (the accumulation of fluid in the abdominal cavity). It is thought that the ascites is due to (1) hypoalbuminemia, (2) high portal pressure from obstruction by the damaged liver and (3) renal sodium retention from secondary hyperaldosteronism. Abnormalities in the sympathetic nervous system and prostaglandin concentrations may also be factors.

To reduce the fluid accumulation, sodium and fluids are restricted according to the individual's needs (100 to 1500 ml. of fluid per day). Sodium is restricted to between 500 mg. and 1500 mg. per day (20 to 65 mEq.), depending upon the rate of diuresis and the tolerance of the patient. Sodium-restricted diets are discussed in Chapter 28. Diuretics are also given. Since potassium is also lost by the cirrhotic patient, a potassium-sparing diuretic is used.

Patients should be weighed and their abdomens palpated daily to check for fluid retention. As diuresis progresses there will be weight loss, until the patient is "dry." Then if the patient was underweight there should be a steady, slow gain in weight as the nutritional status improves.

PROBLEMS IN FEEDING. Great care should be taken to serve the patient food that is attractive. This cannot be overemphasized, since the appetite is almost always poor, and much difficulty is frequently encountered in maintaining nutritional intake. Dividing the day's intake into six to eight small feedings per day is usually more inviting than three large meals. Patients tend to experience nausea at the end of the day, so the major part of the intake should be given in the morning. The patient's understanding of the importance of the nutritional therapy helps him to eat the necessary food. Guidance from the nurse or dietitian in assisting the person to make the right choices is helpful. Appetite tends to improve as the patient eats more, and establishing a regular eating pattern often helps.

PRECAUTIONS AGAINST CONTAMINATION. When serving the patient with hepatitis the additional factor of contamination must be considered. Disposable dishes, utensils, cups and trays should be used when serving food to the patient who has viral hepatitis of *either the A or B type.* The paper or plastic service and all uneaten food should be disposed of in the patient's room, not in the central dishwashing area of the hospital. Nurses or family members who feed the patient should take all precautions to avoid contracting the disease or spreading it to other patients or staff.

HEPATIC ENCEPHALOPATHY OR COMA

In patients having severely impaired liver function, particularly those having advanced cirrhosis or vascular shunts between the portal and caval venous systems, hepatic encephalopathy is a common occurrence. Signs of encephalopathy or impending hepatic coma include confusion, apathy, personality changes, muscle contractions ("flapping"—tremor of the hands when extended in front of the chest) and spasticity.

HYPERAMMONEMIA. An elevated level of serum ammonia is one cause of portal-systemic encephalopathy but not the only one. Ammonia gains access to the general circulation, raising the blood ammonia and causing intoxication of the central nervous system. Following ingestion of protein or an episode of bleeding into the gastrointestinal tract, intestinal bacteria act on the protein to produce ammonia, which passes through the intestinal wall into the blood stream. The diseased liver is unable to convert ammonia to non-toxic urea, and ammonia accumulates in the blood stream. The accumulation of blood in the gastrointestinal tract has the same effect as the ingestion of a high-protein meal because of the very high protein content of blood.

NEUROTRANSMITTERS. Another approach in exploring the etiology of hepatic encephalopathy involves the neurotransmitters in the brain, which are described on page 665, and those amino acids that are their precursors. It is proposed that abnormally high levels of aromatic amino acids lead to the formation of false neurotransmitters that produce encephalopathy.[4] If the protein given orally or by infusion to pa-tients with impaired liver function could be low in the aromatic amino acids that are precursors of false neurotransmitters, then encephalopathy could be avoided. When such amino acid mixtures were given intravenously to patients who had hepatic dysfunction, there was a reduction in encephalopathy.[6] This treatment has also been shown to have a similar effect when given enterally.[7]

Nutritional Care

While generous quantities of protein are essential in the treatment of liver diseases, they must be avoided in impending hepatic coma. This results in a frustrating problem in nutritional care. The amount of protein that the patient requires for good nutritional support may aggravate the encephalopathy. When signs and symptoms of ammonia intoxication are manifested (such as "flapping"), the dietary intake of protein must be markedly reduced to about 30 to 40 gm. (0.5 gm. per kg. body weight) per day or even eliminated completely. With improvement, the dietary protein is gradually increased until a normal or high protein intake is tolerated, but the patient must always be watched for signs of impending coma, and serum ammonia should be monitored. Protein intakes as low as 30 to 40 gm. daily (using protein of high biological value) will usually permit nitrogen balance in an otherwise adequate diet supplying adequate calories. Table 24–5 outlines a protein-restricted diet.

In the case that nitrogen balance is not achieved with restricted protein intake, the clinician is left with a frustrating nutritional problem. The amount of protein that the patient requires for nitrogen balance, or even positive nitrogen balance to allow rehabilitation, induces encephalopathy. Added to this is the possibility that the negative nitrogen balance and malnutrition may lead to further hepatic deterioration. Further restrictions may be necessary.

AMMONIA CONTENT OF FOODS. Some foods are more potent in causing hyperammonemia

Table 24–5. PROTEIN-RESTRICTED DIET

FOOD	GM. PROTEIN
Meat, fish or poultry (2 to 3 oz.)	14–21
Milk (8 oz.)	8
Bread and cereals (3 servings)	6
Vegetables (2 to 3 servings)	4
Non-protein foods: enough to supply calories needed (sugar, jelly, fruit, oil, salt-free butter)	0
Vitamin and mineral supplements	0
Total	32–39

than others because they contain substantial amounts of pre-formed ammonia along with protein. Eliminating these foods could help patients with hyperammonemia. Table 24–6 gives the ammonia content of some foods as well as their nitrogen or protein content (gm. of nitrogen $\times$ 6.25 = gm. of protein). Those foods that raise the serum ammonia the most in cirrhotic patients are: several varieties of cheese, chicken, buttermilk, gelatin, hamburger, ham, potatoes, onions, peanut butter and salami.[14]

Other foods have an ammoniogenic effect because they contain large amounts of certain amino acids* that are deaminated in the patient's tissues and produce ammonia, which then enters the blood stream. One can speculate that, if amino acid precursors (alpha ketoacids) were given to the patient, perhaps they would combine with the excess ammonia to make amino acids and thus use up the excess ammonia.[3]

---

*Glycine, serine, threonine, glutamine, histidine, lysine and asparagine.

These newly formed amino acids would also improve the nutritional status of the patient.

Other methods which are commonly used to reduce blood ammonia are the oral administration of neomycin to destroy gut flora and the use of lactulose, a non-digestible carbohydrate that induces diarrhea and so removes the intestinal contents. Lactulose may also reduce colonic absorption of ammonia by lowering the luminal pH.

BRANCHED CHAIN AMINO ACIDS. Another protocol for nutritional management of encephalopathy is administration either orally or enterally of solutions that have branched chain amino acids as 37, 42, or 50 per cent of the total amino acid content as opposed to 22 per cent in the usual amino acid mixtures. According to Fischer[5] this branched chain amino acid (BCAA) support improves encephalopathy by (1) promoting protein synthesis in the muscle, (2) enhancing the uptake and incorporation of aromatic amino acids by muscle, (3) reducing intracerebral aromatic amino acid levels by competing

Table 24–6. AMMONIA (NH_3) CONTENT OF SELECTED FOODS

FOOD	N (gm./100 gm. Wet Weight)	NH_3-N (% Total N)	FOOD	N (gm./100 gm. Wet Weight)	NH_3-N (% Total N)
American cheese[a]	3.712	2.19	Half milk/half cream	0.512	2.27
Apples	0.032	3.36	Ham[b]	2.704	0.58
Bacon	4.864	0.33	Hoap cheese[b]	3.520	1.75
Banana	0.176	0.00	Hot dog	2.000	0.32
Beer	0.048	1.62	Idaho potatoes[b]	0.416	2.33
Beer cheese[b]	3.760	2.44	Lemon juice (frozen)	0.080	2.90
Bread	0.320	0.94	Lettuce	0.144	0.55
Breakfast cereal (Rice Krispies)	0.944	0.00	Lima beans	1.344	0.21
			Margarine	0.096	21.96
Brewer's yeast	6.208	0.35	Mayonnaise	0.176	23.33
Broccoli	0.496	1.26	Milk	0.560	0.35
Brussels sprouts	0.512	2.15	Mushrooms	0.304	2.18
Buttermilk[a]	0.576	2.75	Mustard	0.352	1.00
Cabbage	0.208	0.82	Onions[b]	0.240	11.20
Carrots	0.176	0.81	Orange juice (frozen)	0.112	3.16
Catsup	0.320	11.00	Peaches	0.064	3.78
Cauliflower	0.302	1.41	Peanut butter[b]	4.448	1.10
Celery	0.144	0.00	Pears	0.112	2.67
Cheddar cheese[a]	4.000	2.76	Pecans	1.472	0.48
Chicken[b]	3.808	0.45	Pickle relish	0.080	10.84
Corn	0.560	0.25	Potato chips	0.848	2.83
Cucumbers	0.144	3.27	Radishes	0.160	2.77
Domestic blue cheese[a]	3.440	4.00	Raisins	0.400	2.37
Egg white	0.744	0.05	Rice	0.320	0.04
Egg yolk	2.560	0.16	Salami[a]	2.800	3.97
French dressing	0.096	14.00	Spanish olives	0.224	4.16
Grapefruit	0.800	2.07	Spinach	0.480	0.20
Grapes	0.208	4.20	Squash	0.192	4.28
Grape wine	0.016	11.20	String beans	0.160	0.46
Gelatin[a]	13.696	0.25	Sweet potatoes	0.288	0.61
Green peas	1.008	0.60	Tilsit cheese[b]	4.000	1.38
Grits (corn)	0.192	0.00	Tomatoes	0.176	2.09
Ground beef (hamburger)[a]	3.872	0.26	Turnip greens	0.400	0.73

[a] and [b] These foods are exceptionally high in NH_3-N or ammonia. Foods marked with a are higher than foods marked with b.

From Rudman, D., et al.: Ammonia content of food. Am. J. Clin. Nutr., 26:487, 1973.

for a common transport system across the blood brain barrier and (4) increasing hepatic protein synthesis. Figure 24–4 presents a diagram of these concepts. Defined formula diets containing high BCAA are presently commercially available (Hepatic-Aid, McGaw). Parenteral solutions are also available. Ornithine salts of the keto-analogues of the BCAA are also available and have been shown to be effective.[9]

If the patient remains neurologically clear after about a week on the low-protein diet (BCAA supplemented or not), protein intake should be increased by 10 to 15 gm. intervals each week until a level of 1 gm. per kg. of body weight per day (65 to 85 gm.) or higher is reached. If encephalopathy develops, the dietary protein must again be reduced or BCAA given or further ammonia-reducing treatments given.

WILSON'S DISEASE

Wilson's disease, hepatolenticular degeneration, is a disease characterized by accumulation

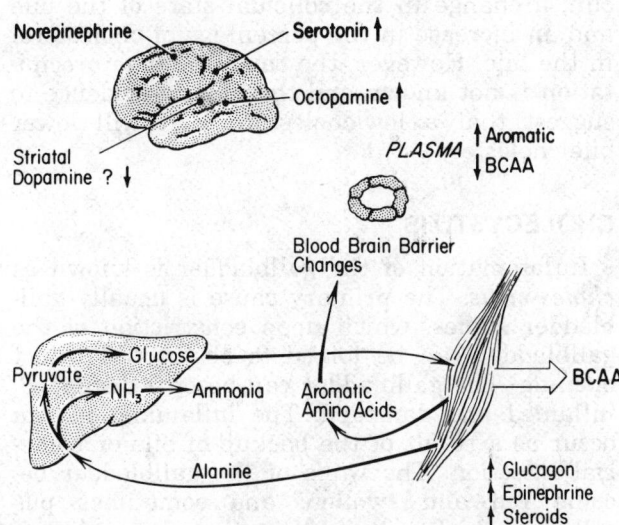

Figure 24–4. The overall metabolic scheme leading to hepatic coma is shown. A state of sustained gluconeogenesis is present in the periphery. Steroids are increased, as is epinephrine, secondary presumably to decreased catabolism in liver disease. Glucagon is increased because of release by the aromatic amino acids and perhaps a signal suggesting decreased glucose output by the liver. The result is sustained catabolism and breakdown of protein for gluconeogenesis. The aromatic amino acids, depending on the liver for their catabolism, are not metabolized and accumulate. The branched chain amino acids are oxodized by the periphery in muscle as well as in fat and therefore are decreased. Blood-brain barrier changes are also important in producing a deranged brain amino acid pattern. The result is a distorted aminergic central neurotransmitter balance with decreased putative neurotransmitters, norepinephrine and striatal dopamine, and increased beta-hydroxyphenylethanolanimes and serotonin. BCAA=valine, leucine and isoleucine. Aromatic amino acids=tyrosine, tryptophan and phenylalanine. (From Fischer, J. E., and Bower, R. H.: Nutritional support in liver disease. Surg. Clin. N. Am., *61*:653, 1981.)

of excessive copper in body tissues that most likely is due to a genetic absence of a liver enzyme. There is a deficiency in the liver's synthesis of serum copper-binding protein, ceruloplasmin. Treatment is a diet low in copper. Increasing the intake of zinc may also improve the management of this disease and necessitate less use of penicillamine, which, as discussed in Chapter 21, has serious side effects. For the copper content of foods the reader is referred to the Pennington and Calloway reference.

Physiology and Function of the Gallbladder

The gallbladder, shaped like a pear with the large end pointing upward as shown in Figure 24–1, is attached to the right side of the undersurface of the liver. Variations in shape and position are not unusual. Diseases of the biliary tract and gallbladder are closely associated with liver disorders.

The main task of the gallbladder is to store the bile secreted by the liver. The bile is composed of bile salts and acids, color pigments, lipids, mucin and water, and after secretion from the liver it passes through the hepatic ducts and is concentrated in the gallbladder. During the concentration process water and electrolytes are reabsorbed by the gallbladder mucosa. Other constituents, particularly the bile salts, and lipid substances such as cholesterol are not reabsorbed. They become highly concentrated in the gallbladder bile. Approximately one quart of bile is produced daily.

Bile assists in the digestion and absorption of fats and in the absorption of fat-soluble vitamins A, D, E and K and the minerals iron and calcium. It is necessary for the formation of *micelles*, the form in which fat, cholesterol and fat-soluble vitamins are absorbed. In addition it has a slightly laxative action and is believed to retard fermentation.

The rate of secretion of bile is directly related to the type of food digested. Fatty foods excite the secretory activity of the gallbladder. A high percentage of the bile salts that pass into the intestines is reabsorbed in the terminal ileum, enters the portal vein and returns to the liver to be secreted again into bile. This *enterohepatic circulation* of bile salts maintains the bile salt pool. The bile is a carrier of waste products such as bile pigments, which are finally excreted with the feces and account for the normal brown color of feces.

The gallbladder is ordinarily full and relaxed between meals, with the sphincter of Oddi closed. During the course of digestion, food fat

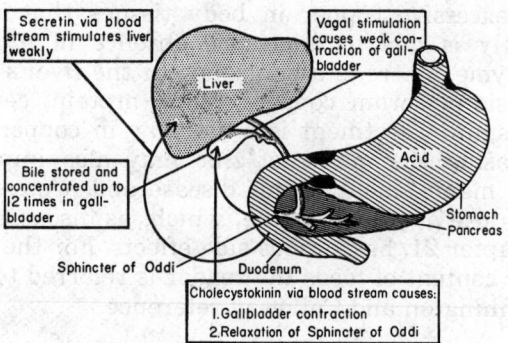

Figure 24–5. Mechanisms of liver secretions and gallbladder emptying. (From: Guyton, A.C.: Textbook of Medical Physiology. 6th ed. Philadelphia, W.B. Saunders Company, 1981.)

or fatty acids reach the duodenum and stimulate the production of the hormone *cholecystokinin* in the intestinal mucosa. When brought to the gallbladder by the blood stream, this hormone causes the gallbladder to contract and the sphincter of Oddi to relax, thus releasing the concentrated bile into the duodenum via the common duct at a site called the ampulla of Vater. This common duct also carries the digestive enzymes from the pancreas. It is because of this joining of hepatic, biliary and pancreatic ducts, which is illustrated in Figure 24–5, that diseases of these organs often affect one another.

Diseases of the Gallbladder

Women are victims of gallbladder disease more frequently than men are. It is a disease that occurs most often in obese women over 40 years of age. The common diseases of the biliary tract are biliary dyskinesia, cholecystitis (acute and chronic) and gallstones.

BILIARY DYSKINESIA

Biliary dyskinesia produces vague abdominal complaints. The sphincter of Oddi, which controls the opening and closing of the bile duct into the duodenum, does not open properly and can go into spasm. Bile then builds up in the gallbladder, causing increased pressure. This spasm of the sphincter of Oddi can exist even after cholecystectomy.

CHOLELITHIASIS

The formation of gallstones without infection of the gallbladder is called *cholelithiasis*. *Choledocholithiasis* develops when stones slip into the common bile duct, producing obstruc-

tion and cramps. The existence of stones may cause no symptoms and the patient may be unaware of their presence until this happens. In this situation the patient would probably complain of severe right upper quadrant pain. In choledocholithiasis, the passage of bile into the duodenum is interrupted and cholecystitis can develop. Without the presence of bile in the intestine, the absorption of fat and fat-soluble vitamins is impaired, and stools become light-colored because they contain no bile pigments. If not corrected, the backup of bile can cause liver damage, biliary cirrhosis or pancreatitis. In most cases, however, the stones remain stationary and the symptoms are similar to chronic inflammation. If the gallbladder and stones are removed by surgery, the majority of patients are cured completely. Most gallstones in the American population are composed of *cholesterol* crystals or of bile salt and pigment, or both, and some calcium. Most stones are found to contain a high percentage of cholesterol. Therefore, the stones are probably caused by stagnation of the bile, with the formation of calculi, a change in the colloidal state of the bile and an increase in the percentage of cholesterol in the bile. However, the cause of stone precipitation is not known and there is no evidence to suggest that a low-cholesterol diet will lower bile cholesterol.

CHOLECYSTITIS

Inflammation of the gallbladder is known as *cholecystitis*. The primary cause is usually gallbladder stones, which upon constriction of the gallbladder can be forced to obstruct the duct opening. The gallbladder can become distended, inflamed and damaged. The inflammation can occur as a result of the backup of bile or bacterial infection. The walls of the gallbladder become red and swollen, and sometimes pus collects, which causes distention. During such episodes, the patient is aware of pain in the region of the gallbladder, accompanied by nausea, vomiting, flatulence and soreness in the upper right side of the abdomen. Jaundice may appear.

Jaundice, a symptom of various diseases of the biliary tract, is a discoloration of tissues and body fluids by bile pigment. Much of the pigment that gives the bile its greenish color is derived from the breakdown of red corpuscles. Should the biliary tract become obstructed by a stone or by inflammation so that bile is no longer able to reach the intestine, the coloring matter undergoes changes and returns to the circulation as bilirubin. This overflow of bile into the general circulation as bilirubin causes the yellow pigmentation of the skin and discoloration of the eyes that are typical of jaundice. Jaundice may be either *obstructive,* the result of a complete or partial obstruction caused by stones, tumor or inflammation within the common bile duct or duodenum (see Fig. 24–1), or *hepatocellular,* which means it is caused by a liver disease or injury.

Nutritional Care

Because fats stimulate gallbladder secretion and sphincter of Oddi action, they should be moderately restricted by the patient with a gallbladder problem. The patient learns through experience that he is more comfortable if he eats plain, simple foods and avoids rich pastries, nuts, sauces, gravies, oil, chocolate and fatty, fried foods. Condiments and highly seasoned foods may cause distention and increase peristalsis, which ultimately results in irritation to the gallbladder. However, *the disturbance varies with the individual patient* and the dietary management should be individualized. The suggestion that cholecystitis is precipitated by the ingestion of fatty foods probably is invalid.

ACUTE ATTACK. An acute attack almost always occurs in connection with an obstruction. When it does occur, the gallbladder should be kept as inactive as possible. Sometimes, oral feedings are discontinued. However, when the patient does eat, all visible fat in the diet is omitted. An all-liquid diet of 2 to 3 liters per day and parenteral supplementation may be required. The protein (30 to 40 gm.) is supplied by skim milk, and carbohydrate (200 to 300 gm.) is obtained from sweetened fruit juices, fruit nectars and gelatin. As soon as tolerated, limited amounts of fat and solid food are added.

The patient is advised to adhere to a low-fat (about 50 gm. of fat) diet until it is known whether surgical removal of the gallbladder is indicated. A combination of foods to provide 50 gm. of fat is shown in Table 24–4. Skim milk, low-fat cottage cheese, cereals, breads, vegetables, fruits, ices, Jello and puddings made with skim milk are used. A regimen free of fat would restrict the protein foods to skim milk, cream-free cottage cheese and egg whites only, with no meat, margarine or butter. No fat of any kind would be allowed in cooking or otherwise added to food.

CHRONIC CONDITION. For the nutritional care of patients with chronic cholecystitis it is desirable to keep the diet *low in fat* (about 25 per cent of total calories). Too strict limitation, however, is undesirable, since fat in the intestines is important for some gallbladder stimulation and drainage of the biliary tract. Many patients with cholecystitis or gallstones are overweight and attention should be given to weight reduction.

The *protein* allowance is kept at the normal requirement and the carbohydrate allowance is normal, decreased or increased to maintain the patient's weight at the desired level. Increasing the amount of *carbohydrate* serves as a therapeutic measure in cases complicated by jaundice since it does not stimulate gallbladder contraction and potential bile backup.

Individuals differ considerably as to the foods that are "gas-forming" or cause them discomfort. It is best to discuss this with the patient, who can then eliminate those foods that bother him. See page 440 for a list of potentially gas-forming foods. A survey of patients hospitalized with gallbladder disease failed to show any greater incidence of specific food intolerances than among patients without gastrointestinal disorders.[10]

Vitamin Supplementation. Because fat and therefore the fat-soluble vitamins are poorly absorbed, administration of water-soluble forms of vitamins A, D, E and K may be necessary. Vitamin K plays an important role in controlling bleeding in individuals afflicted with certain types of jaundice. When given parenterally or orally with bile salts, vitamin K can be transported to the liver where it helps to produce prothrombin, which is necessary for blood clotting.

POSTOPERATIVE CHOLECYSTECTOMY DIET. If the patient has the gallbladder removed surgically, it is still advisable to continue the low-fat diet regimen for a few weeks following the operation to permit the inflammation to subside. When the gallbladder is removed, the bile is stored in the large common duct connecting the liver and small intestine. The tube stretches to perform its new function.

CHENODEOXYCHOLIC ACID AND LECITHIN. Although surgery is the treatment of choice for gallstones, conservative management is sometimes indicated. *Chenodeoxycholic acid (CDCA),* a normal constituent of human bile, will dissolve gallstones in most patients when given in a daily dose, but this therapy may be necessary for 6 to 30 months. It appears the CDCA reduces hepatic cholesterol synthesis and thus the biliary concentration of cholesterol. There are mild side effects such as abdominal discomfort and diarrhea that can be controlled by modification of dosage but, more importantly, the long-term effects of CDCA on hepatic function are not known.[2] *Lecithin,* another natural bile component, also dissolves gallstones and it too is being used with good results. Lecithin is discussed further on page 44.

Physiology and Function of the Pancreas

The pancreas is located deep in the upper abdomen, behind the stomach, as shown in Figure 24–1. Some of its cells manufacture insulin (endocrine function) and others secrete powerful enzymes that aid in the digestion of protein, fats and carbohydrates in the intestine (exocrine function). This *exocrine* function, known to be under the control of gastrointestinal hormones (see Table 5–1), may also be controlled by the endocrine function of the pancreas.[13] The duct leading from the pancreas joins a common tube through which both bile and pancreatic juices drain into the duodenum.

PANCREATITIS

Pancreatitis is an inflammation of the pancreas characterized by edema, cellular exudate and fat necrosis. It can be mild and self-limiting or severe, with necrosis of pancreatic tissue. It can be acute or chronic, with pancreatic destruction so extensive that exocrine or endocrine pancreatic function is lost and steatorrhea or diabetes results.

The symptoms of pancreatitis can range from those of a mild upset stomach to severe upper abdominal pain, nausea and vomiting, distention, steatorrhea, edema and shock, and death may result.

Etiology and Pathogenesis

The precise mechanisms that cause pancreatitis and pancreatic destruction are unknown, but the following are associated with and perhaps are causes of pancreatitis: chronic alcoholism, biliary tract disease, ingestion of certain drugs, trauma and hypercalcemia.

One theory states that an obstruction to the flow of pancreatic juice develops, either from a malfunctioning sphincter of Oddi, a stone in the common duct or a protein plug in a pancreatic ductule. The pancreatic juices then back up into the pancreas. Somehow, these pancreatic enzymes become activated, possibly by backed-up bile, and they move out of the ductules and into the pancreatic parenchyma, where they begin to digest the organ itself. In severe cases the enzymes move out of the pancreas and begin to digest surrounding fat tissue. When this happens, serum calcium falls to a dangerously low level, which is a bad prognostic sign. It may be that serum calcium falls because of "soap" formation by the calcium and the fatty acids created by fat necrosis. Serum amylase and lipase, two pancreatic enzymes, move from the inflamed pancreas into the lymphatic system and the blood stream, leading to elevated serum amylase and lipase levels, which are characteristic of pancreatic disease.

A common cause of pancreatitis is alcoholism. Presumably alcohol causes duodenitis and edema of the papilla of Vater, where the common bile duct opens into the duodenum. This condition obstructs pancreatic and bile flow, which back up into the pancreas. It is also possible that alcohol has a direct cytotoxic effect on the pancreas by causing excessive precipitation of protein in the pancreatic ductules, which blocks the release of pancreatic juice.

Some tests for monitoring pancreatic function are given in Table 24–7.

Nutritional Care

The liberation and activation of the potent pancreatic digestive enzymes are brought about by a strong stimulus such as food or alcohol. In addition, fatty foods excite the secretory activity of bile. Thus, the nutritional care for pancreatitis must be adjusted to provide foods that will not stimulate these systems into action.

During severe acute attacks of pancreatitis, all oral feeding is withheld, and a nasogastric tube frequently is used to remove all gastric acid. After 24 to 48 hours the patient may be given a clear liquid diet to see how he tolerates it. One of the biggest mistakes made in treating these patients is to start them eating again too soon. A nutritious clear liquid diet can be made by giving the patient a defined formula diet consisting of amino acids, glucose and a small amount of fat. This diet is "predigested" and will not stimulate pancreatic secretions. Total parenteral nutrition may be necessary in prolonged severe pancreatitis. Chapter 35 discusses these feedings in greater detail.

In less severe attacks, easily digested, nonstimulating foods that are very low in fat,

Table 24–7. SOME TESTS OF PANCREATIC FUNCTION

TEST	SIGNIFICANCE
Secretin Stimulation Test	Measures pancreatic secretion, particularly bicarbonate, in response to secretin stimulation
Glucose Tolerance Test	Assesses endocrine function of pancreas by measuring insulin response to a glucose load
72-Hour Stool Fat Test	Assesses exocrine function of pancreas by measuring fat absorption, which reflects pancreatic lipase secretion

with increased carbohydrate and protein, should be given. Foods are better tolerated if divided into six small meals rather than the usual three. The low-fat diet described in Table 24–3 can be used.

Chronic pancreatitis ensues when inflammation fails to subside or recurs at intervals. The patient almost always presents feeding problems because food provokes nausea and vomiting, which make it difficult to maintain good nutritional status. To complicate matters, the pancreas does not secrete a sufficient amount of enzymes, and maldigestion and malabsorption result.

Steatorrhea is a common occurrence and results in malabsorption of the fat-soluble vitamins. Water-soluble forms of the vitamins will be necessary. *Pancrease*, a pancreatic enzyme replacement, administered orally after each meal to facilitate digestion of carbohydrate, protein and fat, is the primary treatment for steatorrhea, but lowering the dietary fat intake may bring additional benefit. In order to promote weight gain the level of fat in the diet should be the maximum that the patient can tolerate without an increase in steatorrhea or pain. Use of MCT for dietary fat may bring further improvement in fat absorption and weight gain. Since pancreatic bicarbonate secretion will frequently be defective, antacids should also be given to maintain the optimum pH level for enzyme activity. Effort should be made to cater to the patient's tolerances and preferences insofar as the diet prescription permits. Alcohol is prohibited, since it acts as an intestinal irritant and encourages recurrences.

In chronic cases with extensive pancreatic destruction, the insulin-secreting capacity of the pancreas decreases and glucose intolerance develops. Treatment with insulin and nutritional care similar to that used for a patient with diabetes mellitus, as described in Chapter 25, is then required.

Malabsorption of vitamin B_{12} has been observed in some patients with pancreatic insufficiency, so for these patients vitamin B_{12} status should be assessed, and the vitamin should be given parenterally if needed.

ZOLLINGER-ELLISON SYNDROME

A gastrin-secreting tumor or gastrinoma of the pancreas is the cause of this disease. The high serum levels of gastrin cause hypersecretion of gastric acid and the development of duodenal ulcers in 95 per cent of cases. The nutritional care is the same as that for a duodenal ulcer as discussed in Chapter 22; however, the preferred treatment is surgical removal of the tumor.

Problems and Suggested Topics for Discussion

1. List the various functions of the liver and then determine the relationship of each function to the metabolism of food.
2. Take a dietary history of a patient with cirrhosis of the liver. Identify the areas of his diet that need improving. How will the patient implement the changes?
3. Under what conditions does hepatic coma appear? Why is a low-protein diet used?
4. Adjust the diet in problem 2 to limit sodium to 250 mg. When would such a diet be required in cirrhosis of the liver?
5. Plan a diet containing 30 gm. protein for a patient with hepatic coma. The patient is a 40-year-old male requiring 2600 kcal. Why is it important to maintain adequate energy intake?
6. Obtain the dietary history of a patient with gallbladder disease. What adjustments need to be made to restrict the diet to 40 gm. of fat? Adjust the protein and carbohydrate to meet the individual's caloric needs. Why does a patient with gallbladder disease experience pain on the ingestion of fat?
7. What is the rationale for using a high-protein diet in treating viral hepatitis?
8. What are the principles of diet for chronic pancreatitis? Plan a diet and meal pattern for a patient with chronic pancreatitis who is 50 years old and requires 2300 kcal.
9. Explain why a chemically defined diet or "predigested diet" is useful in the nutritional care of a patient with pancreatitis.

Cited References

1. Baraona, E., and Lindenbaum, J.: Metabolic effects of alcohol on the intestine. In: Lieber, C.S. (ed.): Metabolic Aspects of Alcoholism. Lancaster, England, MTP Press Ltd., 1977, p. 107.
2. Carey, M.C.: Editorial: Cheno and urso: What the goose and the bear have in common. N. Engl. J. Med., *293*:1255, 1975.
3. Close, J.H.: The use of amino acid precursors in nitrogen-accumulation diseases. N. Engl. J. Med., *290*:663, 1974.
4. Fischer, J.E., and Baldessarini, R.J.: False neurotransmitters and hepatic failure. Lancet, *2*:75, 1971.
5. Fischer, J.E., and Bower, R.H.: Nutritional support in liver disease. Surg. Clin. N. Am., *61*:653, 1981.
6. Fischer, J.E., et al.: The effect of normalization of plasma amino acids on hepatic encephalopathy in man. Surgery, *80*:77, 1976.
7. Freund, H., Yoshimura, N., and Fischer, J.E.: Chronic hepatic encephalopathy. Long-term therapy with a branched-chain amino-acid-enriched elemental diet. JAMA, *242*:347, 1979.
8. Greenberger, N.J., et al.: Effect of vegetable and animal protein diets in chronic hepatic encephalopathy, Am. J. Dig. Dis., *22*:845, 1977.
9. Herlong, H.F., Maddrey, W.C., and Walser, M.: The use of ornithine salts of branched-chain keto acids in portal systemic encephalopathy. Ann. Intern. Med., *93*:545, 1980.
10. Koch, J.F., and Donaldson, R.M.: A survey of food intolerances of hospitalized patients. N. Engl. J. Med., *271*:657, 1964.
11. Lieber, C.S.: The prolonged cocktail hour and liver disease. JAMA, *185*:419, 1963.
12. Lieber, C.S., and De Carli, L.M.: Metabolic effects of alcohol on the liver. In: Lieber, C.S. (ed.): Metabolic Aspects of Alcoholism. Lancaster, England, MTP Press Ltd., 1977, p. 45.

13. Malaisse-Lagae, F., et al.: Exocrine pancreas: Evidence for topographic partition of secretory function. Science, 190:795, 1975.
14. Rudman, D., et al.: Ammonia content of food. Am. J. Clin. Nutr., 26:487, 1973.
15. Spiro, A.H.: Nutritional therapy in liver disease. Clin. Consult. Nutr., 2(3)(Suppl.):1, 1982.

Additional References

American Dietetic Association: Handbook of Clinical Dietetics, New Haven, Yale University Press, 1981.

Baraona, E., et al.: Alcoholic hepatomegaly: Accumulation of protein in the liver. Science, 190:794, 1975.

Dworken, H.J.: Gastroenterology. Pathophysiology and Clinical Applications, Boston, Butterworth, 1982.

Freund, H., et al.: Infusion of branched chain enriched amino acid solution in patients with hepatic encephalopathy, Ann. Surg., 196:209, 1982.

Gracie, W.A., and Ransohoff, D.F.: The natural history of silent gallstones. The innocent gallstone is not a myth. N. Engl. J. Med., 307:798, 1982.

Guyton, A.C.: Textbook of Medical Physiology. 6th ed. Philadelphia, W.B. Saunders Company, 1981.

Hepner, G.W., Roginsky, M., and Moo, H.F.: Abnormal vitamin D metabolism in patients with cirrhosis. Am. J. Dig. Dis., 21:527, 1976.

Kater, R.M.H., et al.: Relationship of serum tocopherol to beta-lipoprotein concentrations in liver diseases. Am. J. Clin. Nutr., 23:913, 1970.

Leevy, C.M., Thompson, A., and Baker, H.: Vitamins and liver injury. Am. J. Clin. Nutr., 23:493, 1970.

Maddrey, W.C., et al.: Effects of keto analogues of essential amino acids in portal-systemic encephalopathy. Gastroenterology, 71:190, 1976.

Makhlouf, G.M.: Function of the gallbladder. Nutr. Today, 17(1):10, 1982.

Morrison, S.A., et al: Zinc deficiency: a cause of abnormal dark adaptation in cirrhotics. Am. J. Clin. Nutr., 31:276, 1978.

Muscle protein catabolism in cirrhotic patients reduced by branched-chain amino acids. Nutr. Rev., 41:146, 1983.

Panel report on nutritional support of patients with liver, renal and cardiopulmonary diseases. Am. J. Clin. Nutr., 34:1235, 1981.

Pennington, J.T., and Calloway, D.H.: Copper content of foods. J. Am. Diet. Assoc., 63:143, 1973.

Soeters P.B., and Fischer, J.E.: Insulin, glucagon, amino acid imbalance and hepatic encephalopathy. Lancet, 2:880, 1976.

Symposium on nutrition and liver injury. Pts. I and II. Am. J. Clin. Nutr., 23:445 and 579, 1970.

Toskes, P.P., et al.: Vitamin B_{12} malabsorption in chronic pancreatic insufficiency. N. Engl. J. Med., 284:627, 1971.

Tuzhilin, S.A., et al.: The treatment of patients with gallstones by lecithin. Am. J. Gastroenterol., 65:231, 1976.

NUTRITION AND ALCOHOLISM

Alcohol, gastritis, and nutrient absorption. Nutr. Rev., 35:8, 1977.

Isselbacher, K.J.: Metabolic hepatic effects of alcohol. N. Engl. J. Med., 296:612, 1977.

Lieber, C.S.: The metabolism of alcohol. Sci. Am., 234:25, 1976.

Morgan, M.Y.: Alcohol and nutrition. Br. Med. Bull., 38:21, 1982.

Pirola, R.C. and Lieber, C.S.: The energy cost of the metabolism of drugs, including ethanol. Pharmacol., 7:185, 1972.

Williamson, D., and Turl, M.: Nutrition in the treatment of the alcoholic. Dietetic Currents, 2(1), 1975. (Published by Ross Laboratories, Columbus, Ohio.)

DISEASES OF METABOLISM AND THE ENDOCRINE GLANDS

Nutritional Care in Disease of the Endocrine Pancreas: Diabetes Mellitus and Hypoglycemia

Diabetes Mellitus

Diabetes mellitus is an ancient disease. The name comes from the Greek words *diabetes*, meaning "to flow through a siphon," and *mellitus*, meaning "honeyed" which was added many centuries later to describe the sweet taste of the urine.

Classification

It is now apparent that diabetes is a heterogeneous disease, as Table 25–1 indicates. The two major forms of diabetes are Type I or *insulin-dependent diabetes* (IDDM), which appears in youth and may be called juvenile-onset diabetes, and Type II or *non–insulin-dependent diabetes* (NIDDM), which usually appears in middle-aged adults and is called maturity-onset diabetes. Type II is much more common; about 90 per cent of all diabetics have NIDDM.

The main differences between these two types of diabetes are that IDDM begins abruptly, manifests severe symptoms immediately and requires insulin to control, whereas NIDDM develops insidiously, has milder symptoms and can frequently be controlled by diet alone. Table 25–2 lists further differences that distinguish the two main types of diabetes.

As many as 10 million Americans or about 5 per cent of the population have diabetes mellitus and the incidence is increasing by about 6 per cent per year.[18] The cost in morbidity and mortality is tremendous. The long-term complications of the disease reduce life expectancy by one third. The mean life expectancy in patients with IDDM is about 40 years from the age of diagnosis. Compared with non-diabetics, diabetics show a rate of blindness 25 times higher, of kidney disease 17 times higher, of gangrene five times as high, and of heart disease twice as high. The clinical syndrome of diabetes is characterized by (1) an impaired ability to metabolize carbohydrates, (2) an increased concentration of glucose in the circulating blood (hyperglycemia) and (3) the excretion of varying amounts of glucose in the urine (glycosuria).

Etiology

The causes of both types of diabetes are unknown, but current evidence suggests that IDDM is a heterogeneous disorder that in most cases results from a virally initiated autoimmune destruction of beta cells of the pancreas. NIDDM is probably also heterogeneous, is genetically determined, and is expressed with age or the influence of other factors such as obesity, diet and inactivity. Impaired insulin secretion (beta cell defect), tissue insensitivity to insulin and abnormal hepatic glucose metabolism are probably all factors in the different types of NIDDM, as diagrammed in Figure 25–1.

GENETIC FACTOR. Although it is known that heredity is involved in the development of dia-

Table 25–1. CLASSIFICATION AND KEY DIAGNOSTIC FEATURES
OF DIABETES MELLITUS

TYPE	CHARACTERISTICS	DIAGNOSTIC CRITERIA
Insulin-dependent diabetes mellitus (IDDM) (formerly called juvenile-onset DM)	Ketosis-prone Insulin-deficient	1. Classic symptoms of diabetes such as polyuria, polydipsia, ketonuria and rapid weight loss together with random plasma glucose (PG) > 200 mg./dl. 2. Fasting plasma glucose (FPG) ≥ 140 mg./dl. 3. FPG < 140 mg./dl. but sustained elevated plasma glucose during the oral glucose tolerance test (OGTT) on more than one occasion: both the 2 hr. sample and some other sample taken between administration of the glucose and 2 hr. later must be ≥ 200 mg./dl.
Non-insulin dependent diabetes mellitus (NIDDM) (formerly called adult-onset DM)	Ketosis-resistant May develop ketosis during stress or infection Obesity may or may not be present Treatment involves diet and perhaps hypoglycemic agents and insulin Hyperinsulinemia and insulin resistance in some	1. Classic symptoms as described above 2. FPG ≥ 140 mg./dl. 3. FPG < 140 mg./dl. but sustained elevated plasma glucose on OGTT as described above
Impaired glucose tolerance (formerly called chemical, latent or subclinical DM)	Non-diagnostic fasting glucose levels Possible increased risk of atherosclerotic disease	1. FPG < 140 mg./dl. 2. PG 2 hr. after glucose administration in an OGTT must be between 140 and 200 mg./dl. 3. PG between ½ and 1½ hr. after the glucose administration in OGTT must be ≥ 200 mg./dl.
Gestational Diabetes	Glucose intolerance has its onset or recognition during pregnancy Associated with increased perinatal complications	1. Two or more of the following values during the OGTT must be met or exceeded: FPG = 105 mg./dl. 1 hr. PG = 190 mg./dl. 2 hr. PG = 165 mg./dl. 3 hr. PG = 145 mg./dl.
Diabetes mellitus associated with certain conditions or syndromes (formerly called secondary diabetes mellitus)	Associated with certain conditions and syndromes: pancreatic disease; hormonal; drug- or chemical-induced; insulin receptor abnormalities; certain genetic syndromes; other types	1. Diagnosis of diabetes (as described above) and the presence of the associated condition or syndrome

From National Diabetes Data Group: Classification and diagnosis of diabetes mellitus and other categories of glucose intolerance. Diabetes, *28*:1039, 1979.

betes, or its metabolic variations that lead to vascular complications, its role is poorly understood. Since the work of Pincus and White in 1933, the mode of transmission has been thought to be Mendelian autosomal recessive. Subsequent genetic studies, however, have brought this into question. It is now supposed that the diabetic predisposition is due to a number of genetic characteristics (upon which environment has an influence) that result in the final clinical presentation. The susceptibility and not the disease is inherited. It has also been

clearly established that there is a genetic difference between childhood diabetes and that which develops in an adult. From studies in twins, it is now apparent that genetic factors are predominant in NIDDM but additonal factors, presumably environmental, are needed for the development of IDDM.

Studies have shown that for pairs of identical twins in which one twin has NIDDM, the other one will have it almost 100 per cent of the time. However, if one twin has IDDM the other will have it only 50 per cent of the time.[40]

Table 25–2. DIFFERENCES BETWEEN TYPE I (IDDM) AND TYPE II (NIDDM) DIABETES

FEATURES	TYPE I INSULIN-DEPENDENT	TYPE II NON–INSULIN-DEPENDENT
Age at onset	Usually under 40	Usually over 40
Proportion of all diabetics	Less than 10%	Greater than 90%
Seasonal trend	Fall and winter	None
Family history of diabetes	Uncommon	Common
Appearance of symptoms	Acute or subacute	Slow
Metabolic ketoacidosis	Frequent	Rare
Obesity at onset	Uncommon	Common
Beta cells	Decreased	Variable
Insulin	Decreased	Variable
Insulin receptors	Normal	Low or normal
Inflammatory cells in islets	Present initially	Absent
HLA association	Yes	No
Antibody to islet cells	Yes	No
Clinical remission	Short-lived after treatment started	May be prolonged (if weight loss successful)
Primary immediate objective of dietary management	Synchronization of food intake and insulin injections	Weight reduction

Much attention is now directed toward the histocompatibility antigens or the human leukocyte antigens (HLA). These antigens are proteins on the surface of all body cells with nuclei that allow the body to recognize itself and reject foreign tissue. The genes that code the histocompatibility complex, located on chromosome 6, are receiving attention because it seems that certain histocompatibility complex genes (particularly HLA-B8) are associated with IDDM. It may be that genetically controlled differences in the immune response influence the development of diabetes. In fact, researchers have identified islet cell antibodies in the serum of newly diagnosed diabetics that react with the alpha, beta and delta cells in the islets of Langerhans.[19] It might be that there is an inherited deficient immune response to agents that preferentially attack beta cells; this would allow beta cell damage and diabetes to result.[28] This seems to fit with the observation that in patients with IDDM there is a decrease in the number of insulin-containing beta cells, and early in the course of the disease inflammatory cells are also found in the islets of Langerhans. In patients with NIDDM it appears that other hereditary mechanisms confer genetic susceptibility.

VIRAL FACTOR. Because it is known that some viruses replicate in the pancreas and cause beta cell damage, viral infection is strongly suspected as a possible factor in the etiology of IDDM. Several viruses, including mumps, rubella and coxsackie are being investigated. It is thought that the susceptibility to pancreatic damage (and thus

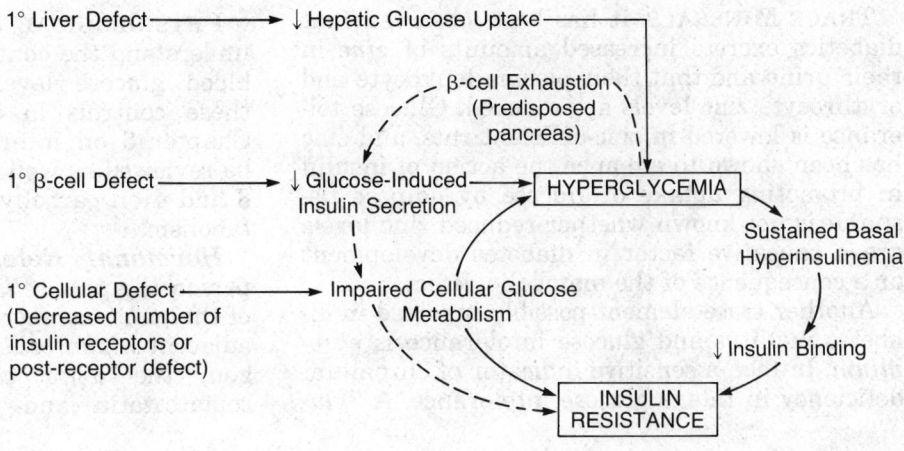

Figure 25–1. Schematic representation of the potential pathogenetic mechanisms contributing to the insulin resistance observed in non-insulin-dependent diabetes mellitus (NIDDM). Adapted from DeFronzo, R. A., and Ferrannini, E.: The pathogenesis of non-insulin-dependent diabetes. Medicine, *61*:125, 1982.)

deficient insulin production) resulting from viral infection has a genetic link.[12]

OBESITY. The onset of NIDDM in adulthood is usually associated with obesity. With every 20 per cent increase in body weight, the chance of becoming diabetic doubles. Hyperinsulinism is also seen, and it is thought that insulin resistance develops from an increase in adipose tissue mass. The number of insulin receptors located on the surface of the cells is decreased in the obese person. The insulin is not able to attach to the receptor and so cannot exert its effect.

It is hypothesized that the increased food intake associated with obesity initially leads to the secretion of excessive amounts of insulin into the circulation. The hyperinsulinemia acts through a negative feedback process to reduce the number of insulin receptors on the cells. This decrease in receptors makes the cells less responsive to insulin and an "insulin resistance" develops. The cell is less capable of utilizing glucose. The number of receptors increases as body fat decreases, which makes weight reduction and maintenance of appropriate body weight the cornerstone of treatment in NIDDM. In the obese with more severe hyperinsulinemia there is not only a decrease in the number of receptors but probably also a postreceptor (within the cell) defect. In either case the effective treatment is weight reduction.

STRESS. The ramifications of stress in the development of diabetes are poorly understood. Infectious diseases such as influenza, pneumonia and scarlet fever, accidents or trauma or the physiological stress of pregnancy may precipitate symptoms of diabetes. These situations decrease glucose tolerance in the diabetic. Diseases of the liver, gallbladder, thyroid, pituitary and pancreas are frequently associated with diabetes. Mental stress may aggravate the disease by causing the release of catecholamines, which decrease glucose tolerance and promote mobilization of fatty acids and possible ketoacidosis.

TRACE MINERALS. It has been observed that diabetics excrete increased amounts of *zinc* in their urine and that their plasma leukocyte and erythrocyte zinc levels are reduced. Glucose tolerance is lowered in zinc-deficient rats, and zinc has been shown to enhance the action of insulin in promoting uptake of glucose by adipose tissue. It is not known whether reduced zinc levels are a causative factor in diabetes development or a consequence of the metabolic defect.

Another trace element possibly involved in diabetes mellitus and glucose intolerance is *chromium*. In fact, a sensitive indicator of chromium deficiency in rats is glucose intolerance. A "*glucose tolerance factor*" (GTF) has been identified as a natural form of chromium. This factor seems to potentiate the action of insulin by facilitating its binding with receptors. Chromium deficiency, often seen with advancing age, may account for impaired glucose tolerance in some elderly persons. Supplementation with chromium-rich brewer's yeast also has been found to reduce the serum glucose and insulin levels in older people, but the effect does not appear to be predictable.[30] Long-term oral supplementation with chromium was found to improve glucose tolerance in some diabetic persons, probably in those with a chronic low-chromium state.[27] Chromium may also have a role in controlling blood lipids in those with impaired glucose tolerance.[41]

Progression of the Disease

Diabetes can be thought of as beginning at conception with a genetic tendency. The time between conception and the development of overt diabetes varies from months to years, depending upon environmental factors.

In the case of NIDDM the first stage is impaired glucose tolerance. Fasting blood glucose levels are normal, but the glucose tolerance test or two hour postprandial blood glucose test indicates a reduced clearance of glucose. These patients seem to have a decreased insulin sensitivity. If adequate hyperinsulinemia cannot be generated to overcome this defect in insulin action, then carbohydrate intolerance develops.

The next stage is insulin resistance severe enough that a fasting hyperglycemia and overt diabetes exist. Besides having fewer insulin receptors, there is also probably a post-receptor defect. It is proposed that the greater is the postreceptor defect, the more severe is the fasting hyperglycemia.[31]

Physiological Disturbances and Symptoms

PHYSIOLOGICAL DISTURBANCES. In order to understand the controls for maintaining normal blood glucose levels and the impairment of these controls in diabetes, the discussion in Chapter 5 on intermediary metabolism should be reviewed as well as the sections in Chapter 2, 3 and 4 on carbohydrate, lipid and protein metabolism.

Hormonal Relationships. In the healthy person the *beta cells* in the islets of Langerhans of the pancreas secrete the hormone insulin, the adjacent *alpha cells* secrete the hormone glucagon, the *delta cells* secrete the hormone somatostatin and the pancreatic *polypeptide cells* secrete pancreatic polypeptide. All four are important in controlling the blood glucose level. Insulin lowers and glucagon raises blood glucose. Somatostatin inhibits the secretion of both insulin and glucagon and it also inhibits the release of growth hormone, increased levels of which have been seen in uncontrolled diabetes. The complete function of pancreatic polypeptide is not yet clear. Other hormones such as cortisol and epinephrine are also involved in blood glucose control. In diabetes mellitus insulin is absent, deficient or ineffective, and this accounts for the metabolic derangements which will be discussed.

Glucose from dietary carbohydrate, protein and fat and from liver glycogen (glycogenolysis) maintains blood glucose levels. Normally glucose combines with a carrier substance in the cell membrane and is transported through the membrane, where it is released to the interior of the cell in most tissues of the body. This movement is dependent upon the presence of insulin attached to the insulin receptor sites on the cells. An exception to this is in the brain, where glucose transport is more dependent on diffusion through the blood-brain barrier than through the cell membrane.

As glucose enters the bloodstream it is normally handled by the body in several ways: (1) it may be utilized for energy at once (cell oxidation), (2) it may be converted to glycogen for storage in the liver (glycogenesis), (3) it may be converted to fat for storage in adipose tissue (lipogenesis) or (4) it may be converted to muscle glycogen. All depend on the movement of glucose into cells and the action of insulin. This rapid disposition prevents the concentration of blood glucose from rising above the threshold established by the kidneys. The diabetic, however, with little or no insulin or reduced insulin effectiveness, has lost the ability to perform these functions completely, because the glucose cannot cross the cell membrane and be oxidized through the glycolytic pathway in the cell to supply energy, and it cannot be converted or stored. Hyperglycemia and glycosuria follow.

The normal renal threshold for glucose averages 160 to 180 mg. per 100 ml. of blood. The non-diabetic may, however, have a normally low threshold. If so, glucose may be excreted from the kidneys, but this does not mean that he has diabetes. Whether the person has a low or high renal threshold is determined by the glucose tolerance test, which also includes measurement of urine glucose.

Fatty acid synthesis decreases and fatty oxidation increases in untreated IDDM. When the glycogen stores are depleted, fatty acids are used for energy through acetyl-CoA and the citric acid cycle. When the acetyl-CoA cannot be used fast enough it is converted into the *ketone bodies* beta-hydroxybutyric acid and acetoacetic acid, which accumulate rapidly in the blood. They combine with basic ions and are excreted in the urine. Acetone is excreted by the lungs and gives a "fruity" odor to the breath. *Ketonuria,* the presence of ketone bodies in the urine, is a serious condition in IDDM and requires immediate adjustment of diet or insulin. Acidosis develops when the basic ions are depleted; diabetic coma then ensues and, if not treated, results in death.

In the absence of insulin or effective insulin activity, free fatty acids, triglycerides, cholesterol and phospholipids increase in the blood. These high concentrations have been suggested as factors in the development of atherosclerosis in people with diabetes.

Protein synthesis is affected by insulin, since it promotes the transport of amino acids through the cell membrane in a similar carrier transport system that transports glucose. Normally the total quantity of protein stored in the tissues of the body is increased by insulin. In diabetes protein catabolism increases, particularly in IDDM. Amino acids are deaminized, and the non-nitrogenous part of the molecule is used to synthesize glucose and fatty acids. This leads to an increase of glucose and incompletely oxidized fatty acids in the blood and an increased excretion of nitrogen and potassium in the urine.

SYMPTOMS. Because of the previously described physiological changes in untreated or uncontrolled diabetes, symptoms of the disease usually include *increased thirst (polydipsia), increased urination (polyuria), increased appetite (polyphagia),* failing strength and loss of weight. Pruritus vulvae, skin infection or irritation and visual disturbances are frequently present. Excessive urinary output and the failure to balance it by fluid intake causes dehydration and electrolyte imbalance. Inability of tissues to heal and degenerative changes occur, especially in advanced cases. Acidosis or ketosis is a symptom of the accumulation of ketones in the blood and is often seen in IDDM. The failing strength and loss of weight result from starvation, because the body is unable to utilize food. However, in NIDDM there is usually obesity and only in severe untreated cases will weight loss be apparent.

Glucose is usually present in the urine, although glycosuria is not necessarily diagnostic of diabetes because it may have another cause such as emotional upset, overeating, hyperthyroidism or renal malfunction. There are four other carbohydrates that may appear in the urine without creating any suspicion of the disease: pentose, galactose, fructose and lactose. Glucose is the specific sign in the urine of the diabetic.

Diagnosis

Diagnosis of diabetes mellitus is usually made by measuring a fasting plasma glucose (FPG), sometimes combined with an oral glucose tolerance test (OGTT) or a postprandial plasma glucose. FPG is elevated in all but the mildest cases of diabetes (usually called "impaired glucose tolerance"); the normal plasma glucose level is 70 to 115 mg./dl. Diabetes exists if on two separate occasions the FPG is greater than 140 mg./dl. The two hour postprandial plasma glucose indicates how well the person handles the glucose from a meal. It will be elevated in the person with diabetes.

The OGTT indicates the ability of the patient to utilize a specific amount of glucose (75 gm. in adults or 1.75 gm./kg. in children).

A plasma glucose estimate is made before the glucose preparation is given and again one-half hour, 1 hour, 2 hours, and 3 hours and possibly 4 and 5 hours after the glucose preparation has been taken. Urine glucose is also frequently measured at the same time.

The OGTT is not well accepted for diagnostic purposes because it is difficult to do correctly and if done incorrectly can be abnormal owing to factors other than the presence of diabetes. For example, it should not be used to diagnose the elderly, a person under stress or an ill person. If it is done it should always be preceded by three days of carbohydrate intake of at least 150 gm. per day. For the OGTT to be diagnostic of diabetes the two hour plasma glucose must be greater than 200 mg./dl. and any measurement between the administration of glucose and two hours must be greater than 200 mg./dl. See Table 25-1.

MANAGEMENT OF DIABETES

Clinical Versus Chemical Control

CLINICAL CONTROL. The methods by which adequate control of diabetes may be accomplished have been the subject of much study and debate. On the one hand, the patient may be treated by permitting him to eat what he likes so long as he is free from clinical symptoms, maintains or gains weight (as necessary) and is free from ketosis and hypoglycemia. Continuous glycosuria and hyperglycemia are permitted as long as the patient maintains his normal weight and shows no ketone bodies in the urine. This is known as clinical control.

CHEMICAL CONTROL. In contrast is chemical control in which diet, exercise and insulin, when indicated, are regulated in order to maintain plasma glucose within normal limits and to keep the urine free or nearly free of glucose. This is now more easily achieved with the continuous subcutaneous insulin infusion (page 486), home glucose monitoring (page 487) and "intensified" conventional therapy.

The question arises as to whether the meticulous glycemia control gained by using the regulated diet with nearly perfect insulin balance will minimize the incidence of complications throughout the years. The group advocating a liberal diet feels that glycosuria is not incompatible with well-being and intimates that vascular damage is perhaps inevitable and not delayed by strict control. However, the weight of evidence suggests that the microvascular complications of diabetes (retinopathy, nephropathy and possibly neuropathy) are decreased by reduction and control of blood glucose concentration.[10, 13, 37] Whether the macrovascular complications (coronary artery disease, cerebrovascular accidents and peripheral vascular disease) can be influenced is still unknown. Many years of study and observation are needed for the complete answer.

On the other hand, with the trend toward meticulous control and the use of continuous subcutaneous insulin infusion, there must be attention to the risk of brain damage from hypoglycemia. Maybe "near normalization" of the glycemic profile (plasma glucose < 130 mg./dl. after fasting and < 180 mg./dl. postprandially) is a therapeutic target preferable to "normalization."[46]

Hormonal Therapy

INSULIN. Since their introduction in 1922, commercial insulin preparations have been the cornerstone of treatment of IDDM. Because he does not make insulin or enough insulin, the IDDM patient must provide his body with insulin daily. This can be supplied either as injections or as a continuous subcutaneous insulin infusion (CSII). A balance must be maintained between the insulin and the glucose received from food and metabolized in activity.

The NIDDM patient produces insulin, and in fact may have hyperinsulinemia, but the insulin is not effective because of aberrations or a decrease in the number of insulin receptor sites. Weight reduction is most important; however, insulin is used in those Type II patients who do not respond to weight reduction and dietary control. In some of these patients insulin administration is effective in controlling hyperglycemia most frequently because the Type II patient may have a decreased number of receptors, which can be overcome with more insulin, or he may have a beta cell problem in which insufficient insulin is released in response to a glucose load.

Commercial Insulin. Insulin is a protein extracted from the pancreas of animals and is packaged in crystalline form. A *standardized unit of insulin* provides for the use of 1.5 to 3.0 gm. of glucose. Regardless of its source, insulin is sold in a standard potency, U-100 (100 units per ml.).

There are three general types of commercial insulin: (1) the quick-acting regular crystalline or unmodified insulin, (2) the slow-acting protamine zinc insulin and (3) the intermediate insulin. The types and characteristics of the insulins available in the United States are summarized in Table 25–3. The diabetic's response to the insulin determines the kind and amount that the physician will prescribe.

Administration of Insulin. The insulin preparations currently available require subcutaneous administration because the digestive juices would digest insulin, which is a protein.

The type, dosage and frequency of insulin administration is individualized for the patient, depending upon his stage of growth, physical state, activity and psychological stability. It may be a single dose or a mixture of insulins in one injection or a regimen of two or three injections during a 24-hour period. It may be given as a CSII with small additional amounts before meals and snacks.

Insulin administration must be continued during the period when the pancreas is unable to function adequately. Very often improvement occurs for a short period of time after insulin has been started in the IDDM patient. This clinical remission may last for a period of weeks or up to a year but is only temporary. During the remission insulin is either reduced or omitted, as discussed on page 791. The NIDDM patient who requires insulin at first may, after sufficient weight loss, be able to control his or her diabetes by diet alone or by diet plus one of the oral hypoglycemic agents and no longer require insulin. The *severity* and the *nature* of the diabetes determine whether insulin must be continued.

In contrast is the *Somogyi phenomenon,* in which there is deterioration of diabetic control in the face of increasing dosages of insulin. The person becomes overinsulinized, as is frequently seen in children when attempts are made to eliminate glycosuria completely. This should be suspected in a child receiving more than 1.5 units of insulin per kg. body weight per day. The insulin dosage should be slowly reduced or split into two injections.

Table 25–3. TYPES AND CHARACTERISTICS OF INSULIN

TYPE OF INSULIN	APPEAR-ANCE	ACTION	DURATION (*Hours*)
Regular Crystalline	Clear	Rapid	5–7
Semilente®	Turbid	Rapid	12–16
Globin	Clear	Intermediate	18–24
NPH	Turbid	Intermediate	24–28
Lente®	Turbid	Intermediate	24–28
Protamine Zinc	Turbid	Prolonged	36+
Ultralente®	Turbid	Prolonged	36+

Adapted from Waife, S. O. (ed.): Diabetes Mellitus. 8th ed. Indianapolis, Lilly Research Laboratories, Eli Lilly & Company, 1980, p. 46.

Insulin is best injected where the skin is loose, in a pocket between the fat and muscle. The sites of injection should be frequently changed or rotated (see Figure 25–2). Because the nurse most often has the responsibility of teaching the use and administration of the insulin to a patient, she should become very familiar with the various techniques.

Frequently, there will be atrophy or hypertrophy of the adipose tissue in the areas where insulin is injected. The cause of this phenomenon is immunologic injury in response to impurities in the insulin (usually protamine zinc insulin). Fortunately newer insulins are purer and re-

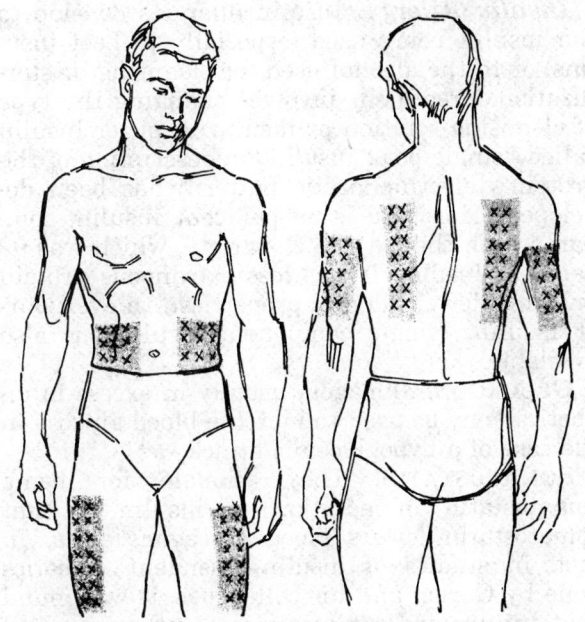

Figure 25–2. Sites for insulin injection. (From Luckman, J., and Sorensen, K. C.: Medical-Surgical Nursing. Philadelphia, W. B. Saunders Co., 1974, p. 1329.)

duce these effects. Rotating injection sites will also help to prevent this problem.

CONTINUOUS SUBCUTANEOUS INSULIN INFUSION. Continuous subcutaneous insulin infusion (CSII) pumps are becoming more widely available and are being used by a greater number of diabetic patients, particularly those with IDDM. These are insulin pumps worn outside the body that are programmed to give an approximation of basal insulin levels with additional increments of insulin just before meals or snacks. The patient must monitor the blood glucose with glucose-oxidase reagent strips and use this information to adjust the insulin infusion. Data show that there is improved metabolic control and possible reduction in metabolic complications. There is already some evidence of a decrease in complications such as neuropathy.[36]

Research continues for a device capable of monitoring blood glucose and delivering insulin into the blood stream when necessary—a "closed loop" system. There would be enough insulin within the device to keep the person supplied for an extended period. Problems of miniaturization of a reliable glucose sensor remain.

Insulin Resistance. In some cases antibodies to injected insulin can develop. An immune reaction occurs, and the insulin becomes ineffective. Depending on the degree of resistance, insulin dosages are greatly increased, sometimes up to several hundred units per day. It is then necessary to switch to another type of insulin (from pork to beef, for instance). More common causes of insulin resistance are physiological stresses such as pregnancy, infection, an endocrine disorder or obesity.

Insulin Allergy. Insulin allergies develop to the insulin being used (especially to beef insulins) or to the alcohol used for cleansing or sterilization. Treatment involves changing the type of cleansing solution or insulin. A purer insulin called "single peak insulin" (a description of the protein's electrophoretic pattern) has been developed. This type is 99 per cent insulin, compared with the old U.S.P. variety, which was 92 per cent insulin. It has less extraneous protein and thus fewer allergic properties. An even purer insulin, "single component insulin," is also available.

GLUCAGON. Glucagon, usually in excess in diabetics, may be used to increase blood glucose in the case of a hypoglycemic attack.

SOMATOSTATIN. The rationale for using somatostatin in addition to insulin is that somatostatin lowers blood glucagon levels. In fact, in studies of insulin-dependent diabetics done by Gerich and his colleagues, it was found that insulin and somatostatin together resulted in lower blood glucagon levels after a meal and lower blood glucose levels than when insulin alone was used.[20]

Because glucagon seems to be a key in the development of ketoacidosis, it is postulated by Gerich that somatostatin may be more effective than insulin in the treatment of ketoacidosis, since it can reduce the level of blood glucagon more effectively.

At present, there are several problems with the use of somatostatin: (1) it can be given only by infusion rather than injection because of its short half-life, (2) it may be inappropriate for children because it also inhibits the release of growth hormone and (3) it has been shown by some researchers to exert a transient effect on the aggregation of platelets.

Oral Hypoglycemic Agents

The hypoglycemic agents presently in use for treatment of NIDDM in the U.S. are the sulfonylureas, some of which are listed in Table 25–4. They lower the blood sugar level and reduce glycosuria in certain diabetic patients by *stimulating the pancreatic beta cells to secrete endogenous insulin.* These compounds are effective only in diabetics who have beta cells that can respond to the stimulus. However, they also enhance insulin sensitivity apparently by increasing insulin receptor binding.[33] They are considered a second line of therapy after weight reduction in NIDDM.

The *biguanides,* although no longer in use in the U.S., are still in use in other countries. They function differently from the sulfonylureas since they seem to *stimulate glucose utilization by the tissues,* possibly through affecting the insulin receptor sites on cells.[21] They also reduce hepatic glucose production. However, these drugs have unpleasant side effects and dangerous physiological consequences such as lactic acidosis.

Table 25–4. AVAILABLE ORAL HYPOGLYCEMIC COMPOUNDS

Sulfonylureas
  Tolbutamide
    (Orinase)
  Acetohexamide
    (Dymelor)
  Chlorpropamide
    (Diabinase)
  Tolazamide
    (Tolinase)
  Glyburide
  Glipizide
  Glibornuride
  Gliclazide
  Gliquidone

Reports of the University Group Diabetes Program in 1970 linked sulfonylurea use to subsequent cardiovascular complications. However, subsequent evaluation has shown the data to be weak. There was no greater incidence of cardiovascular complications in patients taking the sulfonylurea tested (tolbutamide).

DRUG-NUTRIENT INTERACTION. Alcohol may dangerously potentiate the hypoglycemic effect of hypoglycemic agents. It may cause facial burning and flushing. Aspirin, phenylbutazone, sulfonamides and monoamine oxidase inhibitors may enhance hypoglycemic effects of sulfonylureas but are not the hazard of alcohol. Corticosteroids have a hyperglycemic effect, as do oral contraceptives and thiazide diuretics.

Home Glucose Monitoring

Self-monitoring of glycemia using glucose-oxidase reagent strips (i.e. Dextrostix, Chemstrip) read visually or with a reflectance meter (glucometer) has greatly helped patients improve their glycemia control. Both can be done at home with a finger prick sample of blood. Read visually the glucose-oxidase reagent strips give a general evaluation of blood glucose level, while a reflectance meter can give the individual the exact blood glucose level.* It allows patients to adjust daily insulin dosages and diet in accordance with the observed effect on blood glucose. This leads to better control of glycemia and potential reduction in the complications of diabetes. As long as glycosuria is consistently present, home glucose monitoring is not needed, because virtually all plasma glucose values will exceed 180 mg./dl. An obvious exception is patients with lowered maximal tubular reabsorption of glucose, of which the commonest example is pregnant women.

Glycosylated Hemoglobin (Hemoglobin A_{1c})

Glycosylated hemoglobin or hemoglobin A_{1c} level is an integrated measure of long-term (past 60 to 90 days) blood glucose level. Because high concentrations of glucose in the serum form chemical bonds with the hemoglobin, it gives a picture of long-term blood glucose control. The longer the blood glucose is high, the higher the hemoglobin A_{1c}. The level of glycosylated hemoglobin is a measure of long-term

---

*Any of the visual or electronically read tests, when carefully done, will give results within 10 to 15 per cent of glucose concentrations measured by standard laboratory methods.

blood glucose control and is not helpful in adjusting daily insulin doses.

Urine Testing

Urine glucose and acetone concentrations are very crude measurements of the adequacy of diabetes management. If they are used, urine specimens should be checked four times daily: before breakfast, lunch, dinner and bedtime. Ideally, the specimens should be *double-voided*, which means emptying the bladder and then testing the urine voided half an hour later. The insulin dosage or food intake is then adjusted depending upon the presence or absence of glycosuria or ketonuria.

Exercise

Physical exercise reduces the insulin requirement and improves glucose tolerance in patients with IDDM.[47] Even normal trained athletes have normal or supernormal glucose tolerance despite plasma insulin responses that are lower than those of untrained individuals. In patients with NIDDM insulin sensitivity improved with regular physical training and the improvement correlated with rise in maximal aerobic capacity.[43]

Nutritional Care

The diet of a diabetic is a normal diet which consists of sufficient energy for activity and the maintenance of ideal weight and is adequate in carbohydrate, protein, fat, minerals and vitamins. At present much controversy, research and change exist regarding the principles of nutritional care for the person with diabetes. However, authorities do agree on the following goals:[2]

1. To improve the overall health of the individual by achieving and maintaining optimal nutritional status.

2. To achieve and/or maintain ideal level of body fat or ideal body weight.

3. To provide for normal physical and psychosocial development of the child or adolescent with diabetes mellitus.

4. For the pregnant woman with diabetes, to provide for optimal health during pregnancy and growth and development of the fetus. For the nursing mother with diabetes, to provide for adequate nutrition for successful lactation and nourishment of her infant.

5. To maintain plasma glucose as near the normal physiological range as possible.

6. To prevent or delay the development and/or progression of cardiovascular, renal, reti-

nal, neurological and other complications of diabetes, insofar as these are related to metabolic control.

7. To modify the diet as necessary for nutritional care for complications of diabetes or associated diseases.

8. To make the dietary plan as attractive and realistic as possible and to provide each patient with an individualized educational and follow-up program.

To achieve these goals in the insulin-dependent diabetic it is important to consider the timing of meals, the composition of the diet, the energy content of the diet and the physical activity. In the NIDDM patient timing of meals is not as important (unless insulin or oral hypoglycemic agents are used), but the energy content is perhaps more important since weight reduction is the most effective treatment.

ENERGY. The same procedure used to plan the normal diet is followed when computing a diet prescription for a diabetic patient. First, a guide to the energy requirement is determined, based on the patient's height, weight, age, sex and occupation or activity. Details are given in Chapter 1. However, this is just a guide; the most effective way to determine the appropriate energy intake is through monitoring of weight and adjusting energy intake depending upon the weight change. Energy requirements can be generally calculated in the following way:

1. To determine the basal energy expended for 24 hours, the patient's ideal weight in pounds is multiplied by 10 or in kilograms by 4.5.

2. If the person is young, tall, or male, 100 to 200 calories are added to the basal energy requirement.

3. If the person is elderly, short or female, 100 to 200 calories are subtracted from the basal energy requirement.

4. Light activity requires 30 per cent added to the calculated basal energy need. Greater activity requires an addition of 50 to 75 per cent of the calculated basal energy need.

5. If the person is obese, subtract 500 to 750 kcal. from the calculated daily energy requirement to promote weight loss. However, this is only a guide, and some obese people may need to take in even less energy in order to lose weight, as discussed in Chapter 27.

PROTEIN. Next, the amount of protein is determined, which is essentially the same as that listed for the normal individual in Table 10–1 and may vary from 0.8 to 1.7 gm./kg. of desirable body weight or 0.4 to 0.7 gm./lb depending on age.

Untreated or poorly regulated diabetics excrete large quantities of nitrogen in the urine, the result of the increase in the conversion of protein to glucose to meet the need for glucose. Because of this a large protein deficit may occur. It is advisable to allow 1.5 gm. of protein during the beginning few weeks of the treatment to correct this deficit. Later in the course of management, 0.8 gm./kg. of desirable body weight of protein daily will be sufficient for an adult. Children need between 0.9 and 1.7 gm./kg. Protein should account for 12 to 20 per cent of the total energy intake.

CARBOHYDRATE. The amount and type of carbohydrate in the diet is the next consideration. The estimation is guided by the patient's blood sugar, urinalysis and available insulin. Carbohydrates provide 45 to 50 per cent of the total energy in the diet of most Americans. In diabetics this percentage should be higher.

According to current evidence it appears that the insulin-dependent person can ingest diets varying in carbohydrate content without a serious impact on blood glucose control. A high-carbohydrate diet also seems to lower blood glucose and enhance glycemia control in Type II diabetes also. Some studies have shown that high-carbohydrate diets will not lead to hypertriglyceridemia in the long term.[48] It is recommended that carbohydrate make up 50 to 60 per cent of total energy, although the diet should be individualized to fit the patient's lifestyle and present eating habits as much as possible.

It had always been assumed that the majority of the carbohydrate in the diet for the diabetic should be of the complex type due to slower digestion and absorption, and that simple sugars should be avoided because of potential rapid rises in plasma glucose. These recommendations were based on chemical analysis of foods rather than the in vitro response of plasma glucose to the ingestion of the carbohydrate.

From recent studies of the actual physiological response to food ingestion, there is now considerable evidence that different carbohydrate-containing foods, even though they contain similar amounts of carbohydrate by chemical analysis, cause widely different blood glucose response curves after ingestion.[15, 16, 23, 25] The rate of digestion of the food and the glycemic response correlate well for both diabetic and non-diabetic individuals. It is becoming apparent that the rate of carbohydrate digestion and absorption may be more important than the actual amount of carbohydrate consumed.

Other components in some carbohydrate foods that have been identified as having an important influence on the glycemic response to a food are the enzyme inhibitors. Enzyme inhibitors are substances that can occur naturally in foods and affect the intraluminal digestion and absorption of a food. An example is alpha-amylase inhibitor in wheat, which inhibits amylase which digests starch. Most enzyme inhibitors in foods are broken down in the small intestine. The pharmaceutical industry is already developing forms of enzyme inhibitors that may be able to be taken with food in order to slow down the digestion and absorption of food. Acarbose is one such example that has been tested in man.

Jenkins has coined the term "lente" carbohydrate in referring to those foods that are rich in viscous unabsorbable plant gums, pectins and storage polysaccharides such as guar and tragacanth, and natural enzyme inhibitors. Legumes are the richest source of the gel-forming fibers and enzyme inhibitors and seem to produce the flattest glycemic response. They even flatten the glycemic response to the meal taken after their ingestion.[24] Pectins and polysaccharides such as gums and mucilages (see page 30), which can form gels in the small intestine and result in slower carbohydrate absorption, are more effective than structural fibers such as wheat bran in lowering a glycemic response.[23] In addition there may be other components, such as phytates, sugars, fats, proteins, starches, protein-starch interactions and the structure of food, which influence the rate of digestion and absorption of a food and thus the glycemic response to that food.

Jenkins and colleagues have tested some 62 foods and given them a *glycemic index,* which is the blood glucose response for two hours after the food is ingested as a percentage of the two-hour response to ingestion of an equivalent amount of glucose.[25] The lower the glycemic index, the smaller the glycemic response to the ingestion of that food. Table 25–5 gives the glycemic range for some commonly eaten foods.

The same foods that have low glycemic indexes also act to reduce blood cholesterol and triglyceride levels and should make up the major portion of the carbohydrate in the diet for diabetics.

It is now obvious that the rate of absorption of food and the blood glucose response can be manipulated by dietary means. The principles established will probably have considerable impact both on the diet recommended to diabetic patients and the development of pharmacological approaches. Perhaps purified viscous fiber supplements and enzyme inhibitors will be used regularly in the dietetic management of diabetes.

An individual's glycemic response to an ingested food is unpredictable at this point in light of these new observations. For example, consumption of potato starch yields postprandial glucose and insulin levels indistinguishable from those after the ingestion of a comparable amount of dextrose, while rice yields a relatively flat curve as shown in Figure 25–3. Further-

Table 25–5. THE GLYCEMIC INDEX FOR SELECTED FOODS*

100%	60–69%	40–49%	20–29%
Glucose	Bread (white)	Spaghetti (wholemeal)	Kidney beans
	Rice (brown)	Porridge oats	Lentils
80–90%	Muesli	Potato (sweet)	Fructose
Cornflakes	Shredded Wheat	Beans (canned navy)	
Carrots[†]	"Ryvita"	Peas (dried)	**10–19%**
Parsnips[†]	Water biscuits	Oranges	
Potatoes (instant mashed)	Beetroot[†]	Orange juice	Soya beans
Maltose	Bananas		Soya beans (canned)
Honey	Raisins	**30–39%**	Peanuts
	Mars bar	Butter beans	
70–79%		Haricot beans	
	50–59%	Blackeye peas	
Bread (wholemeal)		Chick peas	
Millet	Buckwheat	Apples (Golden Delicious)	
Rice (white)	Spaghetti (white)	Ice cream	
Weetabix	Sweet corn	Milk (skim)	
Broad beans (fresh)[†]	All-bran	Milk (whole)	
Potato (new)	Digestive biscuits	Yoghurt	
Swede[†]	Oatmeal biscuits	Tomato soup	
	"Rich Tea" biscuits		
	Peas (frozen)		
	Yam		
	Sucrose		
	Potato chips		

*The glycemic index is the area under the two-hour blood glucose response curve for each food expressed as a percentage of the area under the curve after taking the same amount of carbohydrate as glucose. 50 gm. carbohydrate portions were used in most cases except where specified. Results are the means of 5 to 10 normal, nondiabetic individuals.

[†]25 gm. carbohydrate portions tested.

From Jenkins, D.J.A.: Lente carbohydrate: A newer approach to the dietary management of diabetes. Diabetes Care, 5:634, 1982.

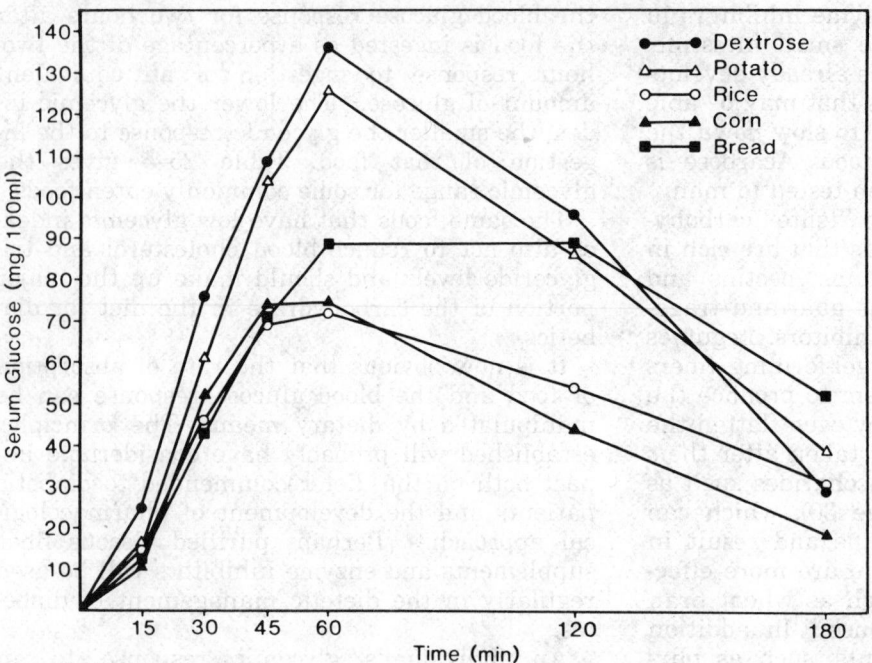

Figure 25–3. Mean change in serum glucose in response to dextrose, potato, rice, corn, and bread in inidividuals with NIDDM. Fifty-gm. carbohydrate portions of the foods were given, and results are the mean of the responses of 20 non-insulin-dependent diabetic patients. (From Crapo, P. A., et al: Comparison of serum glucose, insulin, and glucagon responses to different types of complex carbohydrate in noninsulin-dependent diabetic patients. Am. J. Clin. Nutr., *34*:184, 1981.)

more, within the range of normal subjects, the magnitude of the differences in postprandial responses to various starches is related to each individual's degree of glucose intolerance. Thus, the most glucose-tolerant patients exhibited the smallest differences in postprandial responses, whereas the least glucose-tolerant normal subjects exhibited the greatest differences.[16] There have even been reported variable responses to the administration of simple sugars. The ingestion of sucrose leads to lower blood glucose concentrations than does dextrose, and fructose ingestion has resulted in relatively flat blood glucose response curves compared with either sucrose or dextrose.[9]

FIBER. It is now being generally recommended that the diet for the patient with diabetes, either Type I or II, contain a high level of fiber. Dr. James Anderson and several others have shown that high-carbohydrate (70 per cent of calories), high-fiber (65 gm. of dietary fiber) diets containing sustained-release carbohydrate improved diabetic control in IDDM and NIDDM patients. Many patients on high-fiber, high-carbohydrate (HCF) diets are able to reduce the amount of insulin required daily and some on lower doses can eventually eliminate it.[4] The high-fiber diets seem to enhance tissue sensitivity to insulin by some unknown mechanism, as evidenced by an increase in insulin receptors on monocytes.[6, 34]

When patients are started on HCF diets insulin requirements and blood glucose should be closely monitored and insulin dosage reduced as

necessary. It now seems reasonable to estimate the amount of dietary, not crude, fiber in the diabetic diet, and a realistic amount seems to be about 30 to 50 gm. of dietary fiber. See Chapter 2 for a definition of fiber. High-fiber diets are accompanied by lower fasting and postprandial plasma glucose values as well as lower insulin requirements than are low-fiber diets. High-fiber diets composed of commonly available natural foods have been accompanied by improved glucose metabolism, which has been sustained for up to four years without discernible adverse side effects.[3] Anderson and colleagues recommend a diet in which 70 per cent of the calories are from carbohydrate and which provides 65 gm. of dietary fiber (40 gm./1000 kcal.). Besides finding better glucose control, they have also been able to lower the serum triglycerides by 18 per cent and serum cholesterol by 25 per cent in patients.[3] The effects of fiber on lipid metabolism are further discussed in Chapter 28. On intakes of only 55 to 60 per cent of the energy as carbohydrate and 50 gm. daily of dietary fiber, they have also seen a response, but it is slower and not nearly as dramatic. This is what is recommended for long-term home maintenance. Anderson has also shown that in his patients following the HCF diet there was no development of a vitamin or mineral deficiency.[8] A typical HCF diet as proposed by Anderson and the nutritional analysis of the exchange system used to calculate the HCF diet are given in Table 25–6. Notice that fiber is considered in food groupings. For additional information see the

Anderson reference under Resources for Patients at the end of this chapter.

Other researchers have used fiber supplements in the diets of diabetic patients in order to provide increased fiber. Jenkins used guar gum baked into a very acceptable bread and was able to lower glycemic response. In general the viscous fibers (guar, tragacanth, konjac mannan and pectin) have been most effective in flattening postprandial glycemia in normal and diabetic individuals and reducing urinary glucose loss. Part of this action may stem from the ability of these fibers to slow gastric emptying and reduce the rate of small intestinal absorption. The action of fiber naturally occurring in foods may be to reduce the rate of small intestinal digestion by impeding the penetration of the food by digestive enzymes.

However, there is now question as to whether it is the fiber or some other aspect of the food form that is responsible for the apparent success of long-term, high-fiber diets in diabetes. The reason for this questioning is the finding of Jenkins and coworkers that the glycemic response to pasta was much lower than to wheat bread and the fiber content was not that different.[22, 26] It seems that the form of the food may be an important factor in determining the glycemic response. From this finding these researchers recommend increased use of pasta in the diet of diabetics.

In order to be most effective, fiber supplements must be intimately mixed with carbohydrate portion of the foods as is the case with natural whole foods. Fiber supplements taken separately or sprinkled on top of food have not been found to be as effective.

An analysis including fiber of the present ADA exchange lists is given in cited Reference 7 and the fiber content of foods can be found in Appendix Table 4. Table 25–6 gives an example of a 2000 kcal. high-carbohydrate (55 to 60 per cent of total calories), high-fiber (50 gm.) maintenance diet.

FAT ALLOWANCE. To balance the energy requirement, the remaining energy in the diet is supplied by fats. It is recommended that fat be restricted to between 30 and 35 per cent of calories and contain mostly polyunsaturated fatty acids as a preventive measure against atherosclerosis. Others recommend even further reduction to 20 to 25 per cent of total energy intake from fat.[3] It will need to be this low if carbohydrate intake reaches 70 per cent of total energy intake.

ALCOHOL. Even though the metabolism of alcohol does not require insulin, alcohol in the diet still has several disadvantages for the person with diabetes. First, it is rather concentrated energy providing 7 kcal./gm. yet very low in nutrients. This is a disadvantage for the diabetic who needs to lose weight. Second, it causes an increase in serum triglycerides that aggravates a bad situation in the uncontrolled diabetic who may already have hypertriglyceridemia. Third, in some patients taking sulfonylureas, alcohol can produce hypoglycemia.

However, there will be times when the diabetic will want some alcohol. One way to work the occasional drink into the diet is to exchange the kcalories from alcohol for the kcalories in fat. Therefore one average drink (1.5 oz. of alcohol) would be equal to three fat exchanges. Patients should be encouraged to mix liquor with non-caloric, non-sugar-containing mixers whenever possible. Twelve oz. of regular beer would be the equivalent of three fat exchanges, while 12 oz. of light beer or 4 oz. of wine would be the equivalent of two fat exchanges.

MINERALS AND VITAMINS. Vitamin and mineral requirements of patients with well-controlled diabetes do not differ significantly from those of normal people. There is no necessity for mineral and vitamin supplements when the diet is adequate and the glycosuria is controlled. The possible exception is in the case of chromium or GTF. A supplement of 150 to 200 µg. of chromium per day as a chromium salt or 4 gm. per day of brewer's yeast (a rich source of GTF) has been shown to be effective in improving glucose tolerance. It takes three months before an improvement will be observed.

MEAL PLANNING WITH EXCHANGE LISTS. In 1950 the American Diabetes Association, working jointly with the U.S. Public Health Service and the American Dietetic Association, published a simplified, widely used method of calculating a diabetic diet and planning the diabetic's meals. An effort was made to reclassify and standardize food values and reduce the complexity of diabetic diets by classifying foods into six groups according to their protein, fat and carbohydrate content. In 1971 this system was updated and now takes into consideration the recommendations for a reduced fat, especially saturated fat, intake. The present booklet, "Exchange Lists for Meal Planning," is available at small cost for use in planning menus. See reference under Patient Resources at the end of this chapter. See Table 25–7 for a summary of the ADA exchange lists. Exchange lists merely list the serving sizes of various foods.

The weaknesses of the present ADA exchange list system have been alluded to and are:

1. The foods in the lists are grouped according to their nutritional analysis, not by the glycemic response to their ingestion. For example, 1/2 cup portions of rice, noodles or mashed potatoes are treated as equal and exchangeable although their glycemic indexes are different.

Table 25–6. ANDERSON EXCHANGE SYSTEM FOR HIGH-CARBOHYDRATE, HIGH-FIBER DIETS

Average Compositions *

EXCHANGE[†]	CARBOHYDRATE gm.	PROTEIN gm.	FAT gm.	FIBER gm.	ENERGY kcal.
Milk	11	8	0.5	0	80
A Vegetable	2	1	0	2	13
B Vegetable	4	2	0	2	24
C Vegetable	15	2	0.5	3	75
Beans	12.5	6.6	0.5	8	80
Cereal	13	2.5	0.5	3	70
Bread	11	2	0.5	2	60
Fruit	9.5	0.5	0	2	40
Meat	0	8	2	0	50
Fat	1.5	0	4	0	40

HIGH-CARBOHYDRATE, HIGH-FIBER MAINTENANCE DIET.
2000 KCAL., 55% CARBOHYDRATE.

		EXCHANGE
Breakfast	Skim milk, 8 oz.	1 milk
	Whole oats, ¼ cup	1 cereal
	Whole wheat toast, 2 slices	2 bread
	Grapefruit, ½	1 fruit
	Margarine, 2 pats	2 fat
Noon Meal	Kidney bean & rice casserole, 1 cup	1 bean
		1 A vegetable
		1 B vegetable
		1 C vegetable
	Cooked kale, 1 cup	2 A vegetable
	Cucumber & onion salad	1 A vegetable
	Boiled potatoes, ½ cup	1 C vegetable
	Cantaloupe, 1 cup	1 fruit
	Whole wheat bread, 2 slices	2 bread
	Margarine, 4 pats	4 fat
Snack	Yogurt, 5 oz.	1 milk
	Fresh strawberries, 1 cup	1 fruit
Evening Meal	Roast beef, 4 oz.	4 meat
	Lima beans, ½ cup	1 bean
	Sliced tomato, 1 small	1 B vegetable
	Steamed asparagus, ½ cup	1 B vegetable
	Winter squash, 1 cup	1 C vegetable
	Blackberries, ¾ cup	1 fruit
	Whole wheat bread, 2 slices	2 bread
	Margarine, 4 pats	4 fat
Snack	Fresh apple, 1 small	1 fruit
	Rye wafers, 6	2 bread

*The nutrient, fiber and energy values are average values for the foods in a given exchange
Adapted from Anderson, J. W., Sieling, B., and Chen, W.-J.: Professional Guide to HCF Diets.
HCF Diabetes Research Foundation, Inc., 1872 Blairmore Road, Lexington, Kentucky 40502.
†Foods included in each exchange group are given in the above reference.

Table 25–7. COMPOSITION OF FOOD EXCHANGE GROUPS

EXCHANGE GROUP	WEIGHT (gm.)	APPROX. MEASURE	COMPOSITION FOR 1 EXCHANGE OR 1 SERVING[a]	CALORIES
List 1	240	1 cup	Milk (C, 12 gm.; P, 8 gm.; F, trace)	80
List 2	100	½ cup	Vegetables (C, 5 gm.; P, 2 gm.)	25
List 3	varies	varies	Fruit (C, 10 gm.)	40
List 4	25 (varies)	1 slice ⎫ Other	Bread exchanges (C, 15 gm.; P, 2 gm.)	70
List 5	30 (varies)	1 oz. ⎬ items	Meat exchanges (P, 7 gm.; F, 3 gm.)	55
List 6	5 (varies)	1 tsp. ⎭ vary	Fat exchanges (F, 5 gm.)	45

[a]C = carbohydrate, P = protein, F = fat.

2. The foods are grouped without taking into account their fiber content, which will affect the levels of serum triglycerides and cholesterol as well as the blood glucose as has been discussed. For example, 1/3 cup of apple juice and one very small apple are considered exchangeable, but their fiber content is significantly different.

At present, however, this is the most widely used system of diabetic education. *Patients using the ADA exchange lists should be instructed to eat their food in as whole a form as possible and to choose foods with glycemic indexes of 50 per cent or lower, as listed in Table 25–5.*

THE DIET PLAN. Keeping in mind the total energy intake and the recommended composition for protein, fat and carbohydrate which has already been discussed, the nutrition counselor evaluates the patient's present dietary pattern and uses it as a foundation for planning necessary diet changes.

The foods to meet the carbohydrate allowance are reviewed first. The analysis of some carbohydrate-containing foods shows that they also contain fat and protein. For example, using the exchange list, 8 oz. of skim milk contains 12 gm. of carbohydrate, 8 gm. of protein and a trace of fat. A slice of bread from list 4 contains 15 gm. of carbohydrate and 2 gm. of protein. There should be special attention to including the vegetable, bread and fruit exchanges, which are high in dietary fiber as indicated in Appendix Table 4, and foods with low glycemic indexes such as beans, pasta and apples.

Most of the protein foods contain a percentage of fat. For example, 3 oz. of a lean meat such as boiled ham contains 21 gm. of protein and 9 gm. of fat. The patient should be encouraged to select protein foods that are lower in fat.

The fat allowance is the last adjustment made in the diet. Because butter, fortified margarine, oil and mayonnaise are considered pure fats, their inclusion or exclusion from the diet can be easily and simply adjusted to meet the fat requirement. The ADA exchange lists are given in Table 25–8.

See Table 25–9 for the method of planning a diabetic diet. Table 25–10 shows how this is translated into an eating pattern and sample menu.

Meal Planning

The type and amount of insulin, the time of insulin administration and the timing, type and amount of daily activity and exercise determine the optimal amount and timing of food intake throughout the day. Since good control of glycemia is thought now to be very important in preventing diabetic complications, it is impor-

tant to match insulin activity, food intake and exercise as much as possible. Now that patients are able to monitor their blood glucose at home they can also match their insulin administration and food intake more closely. Self-management is based on trial and error and the correlation of blood glucose measurements with food intake, insulin administration and exercise. Consistency in food intake makes the regulation easier, but more flexibility for the patient who wants it is now possible with good education in diabetes management and conscientious use of home glucose monitoring.[35] The following recommendations for nutrient distribution, particularly carbohydrate, throughout the day are merely guidelines from which to adjust the diet and tailor it to the patient's needs and lifestyle.

USING NO INSULIN. When no insulin is prescribed, the daily carbohydrate allowance usually is spread evenly throughout the day. Patients should monitor their blood glucose to see if this is appropriate, and if not, should adjust food intake accordingly with the advice of the nutrition counselor. Protein and fat are distributed at meals or snacks according to the patient's preference, activity and control.

USING REGULAR (CRYSTALLINE) INSULIN. When regular, quick-acting (crystalline) insulin before each meal is employed, the carbohydrate allowance is divided equally into three meals, following the same proportions suggested when using no insulin. Regular insulin is used in CSII pumps and in patients receiving multiple daily injections. Frequently, it is used in children in conjunction with a slower-acting insulin to give better control of blood sugar.

USING PROLONGED-ACTING INSULINS. Protamine zinc insulin, for example, has a prolonged activity of approximately 36 hours. The maximum availability of glucose from foods should coincide with the maximum availability of insulin. Thus, when protamine zinc insulin is administered, an evening feeding (bedtime) is usually required to prevent hypoglycemia during the night or early morning. Some protein is also given in the bedtime feeding to provide for long-term plasma glucose maintenance (58 per cent of protein is metabolized to glucose) and prevention of hypoglycemia during sleep.

USING INTERMEDIATE-ACTING INSULINS. The intermediate-acting insulins have an action that is intermediate in duration and intensity. When an insulin of intermediate action (NPH or Lente) is given before breakfast, a late afternoon nourishment (3:30 to 4:00 P.M.) is frequently required to counteract any hypoglycemic tendency at this time. A bedtime feeding often is unnecessary when intermediate insulin preparations are used.

CONTINUOUS SUBCUTANEOUS INSULIN IN-

Text continued on page 498

Table 25–8.   DIABETIC EXCHANGE LISTS

*List 1—Milk Exchanges (Includes **Non-fat**, Low-fat and Whole Milk)*

This list shows the kinds and amounts of milk or milk products to use for one Milk Exchange. Those that appear in **bold type** are **non-fat.** Low-fat and whole milk contain saturated fat. One Exchange of milk contains 12 grams of carbohydrate, 8 grams of protein, a trace of fat and 80 calories.

TYPE	AMOUNT
Non-Fat Fortified Milk	
Skim or non-fat milk	1 cup
Powdered (non-fat dry, before adding liquid)	⅓ cup
Canned, evaporated skim milk	½ cup
Buttermilk made from skim milk	1 cup
Yogurt made from skim milk (plain, unflavored)	1 cup
Low-Fat Fortified Milk	
1% fat fortified milk	1 cup
(omit ½ Fat Exchange)	
2% fat fortified milk	1 cup
(omit 1 Fat Exchange)	
Yogurt made from 2% fortified milk (plain, unflavored)	1 cup
(omit 1 Fat Exchange)	
Whole Milk (omit 2 Fat Exchanges)	
Whole milk	1 cup
Canned, evaporated whole milk	½ cup
Buttermilk made from whole milk	1 cup
Yogurt made from whole milk (plain, unflavored)	1 cup

List 2—Vegetable Exchanges

This list shows the kinds of vegetables to use for one Vegetable Exchange. One Exchange is ½ cup. One Exchange of vegetables contains about 5 grams of carbohydrate, 2 grams of protein and 25 calories. All vegetables listed are non-fat.

Asparagus	Greens:
Bean sprouts	Mustard
Beets	Spinach
Broccoli	Turnip
Brussels sprouts	Mushrooms
Cabbage	Okra
Carrots	Onions
Cauliflower	Rhubarb
Celery	Rutabaga
Cucumbers	Sauerkraut
Eggplant	String beans, green or yellow
Green pepper	Summer squash
Greens:	Tomatoes
Beet	Tomato juice
Chard	Turnips
Collards	Vegetable juice cocktail
Dandelion	Zucchini
Kale	

The following raw vegetables may be used as desired:

Chicory	Lettuce
Chinese cabbage	Parsley
Endive	Radishes
Escarole	Watercress

Starchy vegetables are found in the Bread Exchange list.

From Exchange Lists for Meal Planning. American Diabetes Association, Inc., 1 West 48th Street, New York, New York 10020; and American Dietetic Association, 430 N. Michigan Avenue, Chicago, Illinois 60611, 1976.

Table 25–8.   DIABETIC EXCHANGE LISTS (*Continued*)

List 3—Fruit Exchanges

This list shows the kinds and amounts of fruits to use for one Fruit Exchange. One Exchange of fruit contains 10 grams of carbohydrate and 40 calories. All fruits listed are non-fat.

FRUIT	AMOUNT	FRUIT	AMOUNT
Apple	1 small	Mango	½ small
Apple juice	⅓ cup	Melon	
Applesauce (unsweetened)	½ cup	Cantaloupe	¼ small
Apricots, fresh	2 medium	Honeydew	⅛ medium
Apricots, dried	4 halves	Watermelon	1 cup
Banana	½ small	Nectarine	1 small
Berries		Orange	1 small
Blackberries	½ cup	Orange juice	½ cup
Blueberries	½ cup	Papaya	¾ cup
Raspberries	½ cup	Peach	1 medium
Strawberries	¾ cup	Pear	1 small
Cherries	10 large	Persimmon, native	1 medium
Cider	⅓ cup	Pineapple	½ cup
Dates	2	Pineapple juice	⅓ cup
Figs, fresh	1	Plums	2 medium
Figs, dried	1	Prunes	2 medium
Grapefruit	½	Prune juice	¼ cup
Grapefruit juice	½ cup	Raisins	2 tablespoons
Grapes	12	Tangerine	1 medium
Grape juice	¼ cup		

Cranberries may be used as desired if no sugar is added.

List 4—Bread Exchanges (Includes Bread, Cereal and Starchy Vegetables)

This list shows the kinds and amounts of breads, cereals, starchy vegetables and prepared foods to use for one Bread Exchange. Those that appear in **bold type** are **low-fat**. One Exchange of bread contains 15 grams of carbohydrate, 2 grams of protein and 70 calories.

FOOD	AMOUNT	FOOD	AMOUNT
Bread		**Starchy Vegetables**	
White (including French and Italian)	1 slice	**Corn**	⅓ cup
Whole wheat	1 slice	**Corn on cob**	1 small
Rye or pumpernickel	1 slice	**Lima beans**	½ cup
Raisin	1 slice	**Parsnips**	⅔ cup
Bagel, small	½	**Peas, green (canned or frozen)**	½ cup
English muffin, small	½	**Potato, white**	1 small
Plain roll, bread	1	**Potato (mashed)**	½ cup
Frankfurter roll	½	**Pumpkin**	¾ cup
Hamburger bun	½	**Winter squash, acorn or butternut**	½ cup
Dried bread crumbs	3 tbsp.	**Yam or sweet potato**	¼ cup
Tortilla, 6″	1		
		Prepared Foods	
Cereal		Biscuit, 2″ dia.	1
Bran flakes	½ cup	(omit 1 Fat Exchange)	
Other ready-to-eat unsweetened		Corn bread, 2″ × 2″ × 1″	1
cereal	¾ cup	(omit 1 Fat Exchange)	
Puffed cereal (unfrosted)	1 cup	Corn muffin, 2″ dia.	1
Cereal (cooked)	½ cup	(omit 1 Fat Exchange)	
Grits (cooked)	½ cup	Crackers, round butter type	5
Rice or barley (cooked)	½ cup	(omit 1 Fat Exchange)	
Pasta (cooked)		Muffin, plain small	1
Spaghetti, noodles, macaroni	½ cup	(omit 1 Fat Exchange)	
Popcorn (popped, no fat added)	3 cups	Potatoes, french fried, length 2″ to 3½″	8
Cornmeal (dry)	2 tbsp.	(omit 1 Fat Exchange)	
Flour	2½ tbsp.	Potato or corn chips	15
Wheat germ	¼ cup	(omit 2 Fat Exchanges)	

Table continued on the following page

Table 25–8.   DIABETIC EXCHANGE LISTS (*Continued*)

List 4—Bread Exchanges (Includes Bread, Cereal and Starchy Vegetables) (Continued)

This list shows the kinds and amounts of breads, cereals, starchy vegetables and prepared foods to use for one Bread Exchange. Those that appear in **bold type** are low-fat. One Exchange of bread contains 15 grams of carbohydrate, 2 grams of protein and 70 calories.

FOOD	AMOUNT	FOOD	AMOUNT
		Pancake, 5″ × ½″	1
Crackers		(omit 1 Fat Exchange)	
Arrowroot	3	Waffle, 5″ × ½″	1
Graham, 2½″ sq.	2	(omit 1 Fat Exchange)	
Matzoth, 4″ × 6″	½		
Oyster	20		
Pretzels, 3⅛″ long × ⅛″ dia.	25		
Rye wafers, 2″ × 3½″	3		
Saltines	6		
Soda, 2½″ sq.	4		
Dried Beans, Peas and Lentils			
Beans, peas, lentils (dried and cooked)	½ cup		
Baked beans, no pork (canned)	¼ cup		

List 5—Meat Exchanges (a) Lean Meat

This list shows the kinds and amounts of lean meat and other protein-rich foods to use for one low-fat meat exchange. One Exchange of lean meat (1 oz.) contains 7 grams of protein, 3 grams of fat and 55 calories. To plan a diet low in saturated fat, select only those exchanges that appear in **bold type**.

TYPE		AMOUNT
Beef:	**Baby beef (very lean), chipped beef, chuck, flank steak, tenderloin, plate ribs, plate skirt steak, round (bottom, top), all cuts rump, spare ribs, tripe**	1 oz.
Lamb:	**Leg, rib, sirloin, loin (roast and chops), shank, shoulder**	1 oz.
Pork:	**Leg (whole rump, center shank), ham, smoked (center slices)**	1 oz.
Veal:	**Leg, loin, rib, shank, shoulder, cutlets**	1 oz.
Poultry:	**Meat without skin of chicken, turkey, cornish hen, guinea hen, pheasant**	1 oz.
Fish:	**Any fresh or frozen**	1 oz.
	Canned salmon, tuna, mackerel, crab and lobster	¼ cup
	Clams, oysters, scallops, shrimp	5 or 1 oz.
	Sardines (drained)	3
Cheeses containing less than 5% butterfat		1 oz.
Cottage cheese, dry and 2% butterfat		¼ cup
Dried beans and peas (omit 1 Bread Exchange)		½ cup

List 5—Meat Exchanges (b) Medium-Fat Meat

This list shows the kinds and amounts of medium-fat meat and other protein-rich foods to use for one medium-fat meat exchange. For each Exchange of medium-fat meat omit ½ Fat Exchange.

TYPE		AMOUNT
Beef:	Ground (15% fat), corned beef (canned), rib eye, round (ground commercial)	1 oz.
Pork:	Loin (all cuts tenderloin), shoulder arm (picnic), shoulder blade, Boston butt, Canadian bacon, boiled ham	
Liver, heart, kidney and sweetbreads (these are high in cholesterol)		1 oz.
Cottage cheese, creamed		¼ cup
Cheese:	Mozzarella, ricotta, farmer's cheese, Neufchatel,	1 oz.
	Parmesan	3 tbsp.
Egg (high in cholesterol)		1
Peanut butter (omit 2 additional Fat Exchanges)		2 tbsp.

Table 25–8.   DIABETIC EXCHANGE LISTS (*Continued*)

List 5—Meat Exchanges (c) High-Fat Meat

This list shows the kinds and amounts of high-fat meat and other protein-rich foods to use for one high-fat meat exchange. For each Exchange of high-fat meat omit 1 Fat Exchange.

TYPE		AMOUNT
Beef:	Brisket, corned beef (brisket), ground beef (more than 20% fat), hamburger (commercial), chuck (ground commercial), roasts (rib), steaks (club and rib)	1 oz.
Lamb:	Breast	1 oz.
Pork:	Spare ribs, loin (back ribs), pork (ground), country style ham, deviled ham	1 oz.
Veal:	Breast	1 oz.
Poultry:	Capon, duck (domestic), goose	1 oz.
Cheese:	Cheddar types	1 oz.
Cold cuts		4½″ × ⅛″ slice
Frankfurter		1 small

List 6—Fat Exchanges

This list shows the kinds and amounts of fat-containing foods to use for one Fat Exchange. To plan a diet low in saturated fat select only those Exchanges that appear in **bold type.** They are **polyunsaturated.** One Exchange of fat contains 5 grams of fat and 45 calories.

FOOD	AMOUNT
Margarine, soft, tub or stick†	1 tsp.
Avocado (4″ in diameter)††	⅛
Oil: corn, cottonseed, safflower, soy, sunflower	1 tsp.
Oil, olive††	1 tsp.
Oil, peanut††	1 tsp.
Olives††	5 small
Almonds††	10 whole
Pecans††	2 large whole
Peanuts††	
Spanish	20 whole
Virginia	10 whole
Walnuts	6 small
Nuts, other††	6 small
Margarine, regular stick	1 tsp.
Butter	1 tsp.
Bacon fat	1 tsp.
Bacon, crisp	1 strip
Cream, light	2 tbsp.
Cream, sour	2 tbsp.
Cream, heavy	1 tbsp.
Cream cheese	1 tbsp.
French dressing†††	1 tbsp.
Italian dressing†††	1 tbsp.
Lard	1 tsp.
Mayonnaise†††	1 tsp.
Salad dressing, mayonnaise type†††	2 tsp.
Salt pork	¾ inch cube

† Made with corn, cottonseed, safflower, soy or sunflower oil only
†† Fat content is primarily monounsaturated
††† If made with corn, cottonseed, safflower, soy or sunflower oil can be used on fat modified diet

Table continued on the following page

Table 25–8. DIABETIC EXCHANGE LISTS (*Continued*)

List 7—Beverages, Seasonings, Condiments and Foods Allowed as Desired

The following may be used as desired, unless the physician finds a special reason to limit them. The foods listed have no appreciable carbohydrate, protein or fat content if used in ordinary amounts.

Coffee	Rennet tablets	Garlic	Parsley seasoning
Tea	Celery seasoning	Lemon	Pepper
Clear broth	Cinnamon	Mint	Saccharin, Sucaryl and other non-caloric sweeteners
Bouillon, without fat		Mustard	Vinegar
Gelatin, unsweetened		Nutmeg	Pickles (sour or unsweetened dill)
		Onion seasoning	

FUSION. For patients using the CSII pump, meal timing can be more flexible because the person can administer an additional bolus prior to a meal or a snack to cover the increased insulin needs at that time. The amount of insulin administered continuously throughout the day and the amount administered before a meal is determined based on trial and error and the observations of patients frequently testing their blood glucose and correlating it with their food intake and exercise. Studies have shown that the diet can be liberalized without loss of glycemia control. However, it was also noticed that when patients using CSII liberalized their diet they tended to take a rather high fat intake (about 51 per cent of total calories). Despite this, serum lipids and body weight remained normal.[14] In a study of 12 pump users, all 12 reported eating larger meals and adjusting the insulin bolus. Over half experimented with foods and adjusted their insulin. Ten of the 12 reported weight gains of 5 to 15 lb., probably due to better utilization of food energy through tight control of blood glucose along with occasionally increased food consumption.[38] This necessitates follow-up nutritional care of pump users in order to educate them to prevent weight gains and to learn how to work new foods into their diets.

SPECIAL DIABETIC FOODS AND SWEETENERS. Contrary to popular belief, the purchase or

Table 25–9. EXAMPLE OF A METHOD FOR PLANNING A DIABETIC DIET

Diet Prescription: Calories 1800; carbohydrate, 252 gm.; protein, 68 gm.; fat, 57 gm. Approximate % of calories: C = 55%, P = 15%, F = 30%

	TOTAL DAY'S FOOD				
FOOD	AMOUNT	LIST	C (gm.)	P (gm.)	F (gm.)
Milk, skim exchanges	1	1	12	8	
Vegetable exchanges	5	2	25	10	
Fruit exchanges	5	3	50		
			87 (total)		
Bread exchanges	11	4	165	22	
				40 (total)	
Meat exchanges	2	5a		14	6
	2	5b		14	11
					17 (total)
Fat exchanges	8	6			40
		Totals:	252	68	57

The number of servings of bread, meat and fat exchanges required to complete the diet prescription were determined in the following way:

1. Subtract the carbohydrate grams (87) furnished by the milk, vegetables and fruit from the grams of carbohydrate prescribed (252); divide the result by 15, which is the amount of grams of carbohydrate in one bread exchange (List 4).

   252 − 87 = 165; 165 ÷ 15 = 11 bread exchanges

2. The protein grams in a diet are adjusted by the addition of one or more meat exchanges (List 5). Subtract the amount of protein in milk, vegetable, fruit and bread exchanges (40) from the amount prescribed (68). Divide the result by 7, the grams of protein in 1 meat exchange.

   68 − 40 = 28; 28 ÷ 7 = 4 meat exchanges

3. The fat grams in a diet are adjusted by the addition of one or more fat exchanges (List 6). Subtract the amount of fat in meat exchanges (17) from the amount prescribed (57). Divide the result by 5, the grams of fat in 1 fat exchange.

   57 − 17 = 40; 40 ÷ 5 = 8 fat exchanges

Table 25–10. AN EXAMPLE OF AN EATING PATTERN FOR AN ADULT WITH NIDDM USING NO INSULIN OR USING ORAL HYPOGLYCEMIC AGENTS

Diet Prescription: Calories 1793; protein, 68 gm.; fat, 57 gm.; carbohydrate, 252 gm. The carbohydrates are divided approximately as follows: breakfast, 61 gm.; lunch, 71 gm.; dinner, 70 gm.; afternoon snack, 35 gm.; and evening snack, 15 gm.

TOTAL DAY'S FOOD

FOOD	AMOUNT*	LIST	C gm.	P gm.	F gm.
Milk, skim exchanges	1 serving	1	12	8	
Vegetable exchanges	5 servings	2	25	10	
Fruit exchanges	5 servings	3	50		
Bread exchanges	11	4	165	22	
Meat exchanges					
lean	2 servings	5a		14	6
medium-fat	2 servings	5b		14	11
Fat exchanges	8 servings	6			40
		(total)	252	68	57

EXCHANGES		SAMPLE MENU
Breakfast:	1 fruit exchange:	½ grapefruit
	3 bread exchanges:	¾ cup dry cereal
		2 slices whole wheat toast
	½ milk exchange:	½ cup skim milk
	1 fat exchange:	1 tsp. margarine
Lunch:	2 meat exchanges:	Sandwich: Sliced chicken, 2 oz.
	3 bread exchanges:	Bread, 2 slices
	1 fat exhange:	Mayonnaise, 1 tsp.
		Tomato, sliced
		¼ cup baked beans
	1 fat exchange:	1 tbsp. Italian dressing
	2 vegetable exchanges:	Lettuce and carrot salad
	1 fruit exchange:	1 small orange
	½ milk exchange:	½ cup skim milk
Mid-Afternoon:	2 fruit exchanges:	1 banana
	1 bread exchange:	3 Rye-krisp crackers
Dinner:	2 meat exchanges:	Hamburger, lean, 2 oz.
	3 vegetables exchange:	Broccoli, ckd ½ cup
		Eggplant, ckd ½ cup
		Lettuce and tomato salad
	3 bread exchanges:	Corn, ckd. ²⁄₃ cup
		Whole wheat roll, 1 small
	5 fat exchanges:	3 tbsp. French dressing
		Margarine, 2 tsp.
	1 fruit exchange:	1 very small apple
	Tea or coffee, as desired	
Evening:	1 bread exchange:	Whole wheat roll, 1
	1 fat exchange:	Margarine, 1 tsp.

*For foods included and serving size consult Table 25–8.

preparation of special diabetic foods is not necessary. The diabetic patient can and should eat the same variety of foods as the rest of the family, with the exception of glucose and foods prepared with glucose, dextrose or sucrose. These should be limited. Canned and frozen fruits present the greatest problem because of the syrup in which they are prepared. However, water-packed fruits, and fruits packed in their own juices, are quite widely available and are becoming more equitable in price.

It now appears that *fructose* elicits a lower glucose and insulin response after ingestion than either glucose or sucrose either when consumed alone or in a sweetened product.[1, 17] However, as glucose tolerance worsens in individuals, there is an increasingly greater glycemic response to fructose. Fructose appears to be an acceptable nutritive sweetener for moderately controlled or well-controlled diabetic patients. It is a nutritive sweetener, however, so its caloric contribution to the diet must be considered.[17]

Xylitol, the alcohol of xylose, is as sweet as sucrose and is also used as a sweetener in the diets of diabetics. Like sorbitol and mannitol (see Chapter 2), this sugar can be taken by diabetics because it is absorbed less quickly than sucrose. However, these sugars are eventually absorbed and metabolized to glucose and therefore must be considered in the diet calculation. In summary, the use of fructose, sorbitol or xylitol in amounts of 50 to 60 gm. per day is acceptable.[32]

Sugar Substitutes. To replace sugar and sweetness in the diet for the diabetic, non-nutritive sweeteners have been developed. The oldest of these sweeteners is *saccharin*. In early 1977 the FDA proposed banning the use of this sweetener in foods because Canadian studies reported the development of bladder tumors in rats that were fed large doses of saccharin. However, it is still available as a non-prescription drug. The Joint FAO/WHO Expert Committee on Food Additives and the British Diabetic Association recommend that *the acceptable daily intake of saccharin be 2.5 mg. per kg. of body weight.*[29]

Cyclamate, a popular, good-tasting sweetener, was banned in 1971. Because of the controversy about saccharin and cyclamates, new sweeteners are being used or being developed.

One such product is *aspartame*, which was approved for use by the FDA in 1981. It is made from the amino acid phenylalanine, has been rigorously tested and is very acceptable as a sweetener in cold items that do not require cooking or baking. However, it is not to be used by those individuals with phenylketonuria. An acceptable daily dosage is 40 mg./kg. body weight. One 12 oz. can of diet drink contains 150 mg. of aspartame.[49]

FOOD VALUE SYSTEM. The composition of the most frequently served foods can be found in Appendix Tables 1 and 4. The classifications of fruits and vegetables according to their carbohydrate content are given in Appendix Table 3. These tables along with food composition information on food labels may be useful in the education of well-motivated, intelligent patients who desire maximum flexibility in food choice. The patient learns the actual protein, fat, carbohydrate and, perhaps, fiber content of foods and the amount of each nutrient to consume throughout the day.

The total value of the ingredients makes up the nutrient value of any prepared dish. For example, when a custard is analyzed for its nutrient value, the ingredients of the custard are listed, namely milk or cream, sweetening, egg, and flavoring. The nutrient value of the custard is the total of its component nutrients.

Other Exchange Systems. Other exchange systems have certain merits that probably warrant their continued use. For example, some clinicians and educators use fewer groupings of food, combining fruits and some vegetables into one group, including milk with the meat group and other vegetables on the free food list, or other simplifications.

DIABETES IN PREGNANCY AND CHILDHOOD

The diet of the pregnant diabetic woman is discussed in Chapter 11. Aspects of diabetes that particularly relate to children are discussed in Chapter 38.

DIABETES IN THE ELDERLY

Glucose tolerance declines with age, so that a large number of elderly patients seem to have diabetes. For this reason several authorities argue that different glucose tolerance standards should be used in diagnosing true cases of maturity-onset diabetes in the elderly. Since the relationship between blood glucose control and the development of the debilitating vascular complications of diabetes is still unclear, how best to care for the elderly patient has not been definitely established. Table 15–2 presents one approach.

The long-term effects of oral hypoglycemic agents have already been discussed, and the use of insulin can mark the end of independence for an elderly patient and force him or her into accepting outside supervision or chronic institutionalization. Insulin injections can often be hazardous for the nearly blind, forgetful, frightened and unconfident elderly patient. Hypoglycemia is always a danger because the elderly patient may neglect to eat or may give himself a second injection, forgetting that he had already injected himself.

Before treating diabetes, it should be clear to what extent the person is afflicted by it. Dietary control of blood glucose levels should be tried first, before other measures. This change itself may be difficult for the patient and will require a great deal of time and empathy on the part of the clinician.

DIABETES AND SURGERY

If the diabetic patient's condition has been kept under control, he may undergo needed surgery without any unusual risk. When the surgery is an emergency, preoperative preparation is impossible. In emergency surgery cases, the regulation of insulin, intravenous fluids and blood glucose is begun during the actual operation and carried on after its completion.

In elective surgery, it is advisable to plan a preoperative program for the patient, following the same principles suggested for the non-diabetic. To prevent dehydration, large amounts of fluids are administered by mouth or parenterally, especially the day preceding the operation. The degree of severity of the surgery will help to guide the preoperative and postoperative nutritional care.

To maintain fluid and electrolyte balance, abundant amounts of saline fluids are administered parenterally immediately after the operation. Glucose is usually given in the fluid, with adequate injections of insulin to metabolize the glucose.

There is some recent evidence that insulin-requiring diabetic patients undergoing elective surgery may have better blood glucose control after surgery if they receive 3.5 per cent crystalline amino acid solutions without dextrose.[42] However, patients need to be monitored very carefully.

Food in liquid form is usually the first type of food permitted orally. After minor surgery, the patient may be given his usual diet immediately. The diet advances in a procedure similar to that described for the non-diabetic. The blood glucose determinations govern the amount and type of insulin injections.

DIABETIC DIETS IN EMERGENCIES

Illness

During an illness insulin should still be taken, although caloric intake should be decreased by about 20 per cent, because insulin requirements usually increase during febrile illness. Glucagon levels also increase, which puts the diabetes out of control. The person should be watched for the development of ketoacidosis and treated with insulin accordingly.

Sometimes a diabetic patient may become too ill to eat. Even in this situation it is important that the IDDM patient still take some insulin. If possible, carbohydrate should still be given at the rate of 50 to 75 gm. every six to eight hours to prevent ketosis of starvation. The intake may be in the form of more simple carbohydrate such as juices and even sugar-containing drinks as listed in Table 25–11. A soft or liquid diet may be tried. If necessary, the protein and fat allowances may be sacrificed and the amounts limited to provide maximum comfort for the patient.

Here are some suggested adjustments that may be made to the prescribed diabetic diet:

1. Fruit juices and ginger ale may be served instead of whole fruits.
2. Cooked cereal may be diluted with the milk allowance in the diet to make a soft gruel, which is usually tolerated by a sick person.

Table 25–11. CARBOHYDRATE CONTENT OF SOME FOODS USED DURING ILLNESS

FOOD	CARBOHYDRATE CONTENT (gm./240 c.c.)
Whole milk	12
Orange juice	24
Coke	20
Ginger ale	21
Other soft drinks	25
Sugar	5/tsp.
Candy bar	22/oz.
Honey	16/tbsp.

3. Soft cooked cereal may be substituted for the potato or bread included in the diet.
4. Some of the bread and milk allowance can be served as milk toast.
5. Eggs or cottage cheese or both may be substituted for the meat allowed in the diet. Use the eggs for an eggnog or custard and blend with the milk allowed in the diet.
6. The cooked vegetables may be puréed and then diluted with some of the milk allowance in the diet to make a vegetable-milk soup.

Diabetic Coma

Uncontrolled diabetes can lead to ketosis followed by ketoacidosis and coma. This *ketoacidosis* occurs in IDDM when there is an *insulin lack* through either deliberate or unavoidable omission of prescribed insulin injections, an infection, surgical operation or other stress. In an attempt to maintain blood glucose the body metabolizes fatty acids with the result that ketones may accumulate in the blood when fatty acids cannot be metabolized fast enough. The patient requires more insulin, and if this urgent need is not recognized and the insulin supplied immediately, the patient may go into a diabetic coma.

Ketoacidosis does not usually appear in maturity-onset diabetics because, even though there is not enough effective insulin for proper glucose uptake by the tissues, enough still exists to inhibit excessive fat mobilization and development of ketonemia. For this reason, another less common diabetic coma is seen in adults with NIDDM—the *non-ketotic hyperosmolar coma*. It has an insidious onset and is frequently seen in adults with undiagnosed or mild diabetes who experience a precipitating stress, such as acute pancreatitis, myocardial infarction, septicemia or gastroenteritis. The resulting hyperglycemia, 600 to 3000 mg. per dl., leads to a hyperosmolarity and osmotic diuresis. The inevitable consequence is severe dehydration and hypovolemia, leading to compromised renal blood flow and thromboembolic complications and eventually to cerebral dehydration and coma.

A last form of diabetic coma occurs from *lactic acidosis*, but the reason for its association with diabetes is obscure. It is characterized by even greater acidosis and compensatory deep breathing than that seen in ketoacidosis. Both hyperosmolar coma and lactic acidosis are variants of ketoacidosis from the point of view of therapy as well as pathophysiology.

The *warning symptoms of coma* are: thirst and dry mouth, flushed face, progressive drowsiness, nausea, vomiting, abdominal pain, cold and dry skin, characteristic acid breath (ketoacidosis), difficult breathing, headache, dizziness, pain in back and legs and extreme weakness. When one of the symptoms occurs, it may not indicate anything seriously wrong, but when several or all of the symptoms appear, it is cause for alarm. The urine will contain large amounts of sugar.

TREATMENT. Coma caused by ketoacidosis, hyperglycemic hyperosmolarity or lactic acidosis may prove fatal if not treated promptly and efficiently. Speed in treatment is essential.

The treatment consists of (1) insulin, (2) electrolytes and (3) fluids. Regular insulin is given intravenously as a low dose constant infusion or as an hourly intramuscular injection. In severe ketoacidosis, fluid and electrolyte replacement requires the intravenous route and consists of normal saline solution and sometimes bicarbonate. As hyperglycemia and glycosuria diminish, 5 per cent glucose is added. However, the patient should not be fed orally for 24 hours, since a flare-up of autonomic neuropathy could lead to emesis and aspiration. Intravenous administration should be maintained until oral intake is possible. Potassium is also given, preferably monitored by electrocardiogram, and urinary output must be adequate.

Insulin Reaction (Hypoglycemia)

Insulin reactions occasionally experienced by diabetics result from the sudden decline of the percentage of glucose in the blood—*hypoglycemia*. The early symptoms are usually sweating, impatience, double vision, hunger, pallor, trembling, palpitation, headache, faintness and an "all gone" feeling. Although fleeting, these reactions can be relieved by the immediate consumption of an easily digested carbohydrate such as fruit juice, candy or sugar.

An insulin reaction from regular insulin is rapid and requires immediate recognition and treatment; with a slow-acting insulin the onset is more gradual. When the reaction occurs from a slow-acting insulin, it may be necessary to repeat for several hours the administration of a rapidly absorbed carbohydrate plus a more slowly absorbed food such as crackers and milk. When severe reactions result in unconsciousness, the patient usually receives glucose intravenously. Assuming that the insulin is given before breakfast, reactions from regular unmodified insulin often occur before lunch (between three and six hours after injection); reactions from intermediate-acting insulins (NPH, Lente) are apt to occur in the afternoon before the evening meal; and reactions from protamine zinc insulin occur later. Reactions may be caused by an unusual amount of exercise, a delay in eating, the omission of a meal or of the prescribed amount of food, by an error resulting in the administration of an excessive amount of insulin or by a decreased need for insulin such as with the switch to a diet containing a high fiber content.

A more serious type of insulin reaction is one that develops slowly and results from an excessive and continuous overdosage of insulin. The result is not only a lowering of blood sugar but also a depletion of glycogen reserves. Central nervous system involvement finally results, and gastric stasis often is present. In this case the use of oral glucose is futile, and the patient should be given intravenous glucose or glucagon immediately, followed by oral glucose after the person responds to intravenous treatment.

If reactions occur too frequently, the insulin dose should be adjusted to prevent permanent brain damage. Patients taking insulin are advised to carry lump sugar or hard candy for such emergencies, and to avoid dangerous delays, diabetics should carry cards of identification. More than one staggering diabetic afflicted with an insulin reaction has been shunned as being intoxicated.

Glucagon produced in the alpha cells of the islets of Langerhans may be used in the treatment of hypoglycemic reactions. Subcutaneous injection of 1 or 2 mg. is used. Glucagon stimulates glycogenolysis in the liver, and glucose is released rapidly into the blood stream.

COMPLICATIONS OF DIABETES MELLITUS

Diets for control of diabetes should be designed not merely to maintain blood glucose control but also to minimize the development of complications. The modern treatment of the diabetic patient has as its primary goal the prevention of vascular degenerative complications. Evidence is accumulating that early control of diabetes can postpone and minimize the onset of such complications as retinopathy, neuropathy, severe atherosclerosis and renal vascular disease.

DEGENERATIVE VASCULAR COMPLICATIONS. The increased life span of the diabetic made possible by improved control of the disease has brought a steady increase in the incidence of vascular complications in these patients. The vascular disease is of two types: atherosclerosis and microangiopathy. The relationship between diabetes and the vascular diseases is not clear, but it is known that they frequently appear together. *Atherosclerosis* is not specific to diabetes, but it generally develops at an earlier age in diabetics than in non-diabetics and is the major cause of death in patients with maturity-onset diabetes. The atherosclerosis may be due to elevated lipid levels. In a study of IDDM patients poor diabetic control was associated with statistically significant increases in total serum cholesterol and total serum triglyceride.[44]

Microangiopathy, unique to diabetes, is characterized by a thickening of the capillary basement membrane and accounts for most of the deaths in IDDM patients. It has been stated that microangiopathy is seen before clinical symptoms of diabetes and thus is independent of the hyperglycemia and metabolic changes of that disease. This has been the rationale for liberal control of the diabetic patient. Evidence is accumulating, however, that refutes this idea and supports the hypothesis of R. G. Spiro:

The metabolic hypothesis holds that diabetic microangiopathy is a true consequence or "complication" of insulin deficiency. Either the lack of insulin itself or secondary phenomena such as hyperglycemia and/or somatotropin elevation would be responsible for capillary alterations.[45]

In 1982 the National Institute of Arthritis, Diabetes and Digestive and Kidney diseases initiated a multicenter clinical trial, the Diabetes Control and Complications Trial (DCCT), to address the issue of whether good metabolic control as assessed by blood glucose will affect the development of complications of diabetes mellitus.[39] There is still no agreed-upon answer to the question of which comes first: the small vessel disease or the metabolic disorder. At present the evidence suggests that the metabolic disorder comes first and that the small vessel disease is a result of constant hyperglycemia and lipoprotein abnormalities due to the lack of insulin.

To explain the vascular changes and the relationship to hyperglycemia, some diabetologists refer to the *polyol pathway* of glucose metabolism. This insulin-dependent pathway functions in the lens of the eye, in some nerve cells, in the aorta and in capillary tissue of the diabetic with hyperglycemia. Via this pathway, sorbitol and fructose accumulate within the cell, causing an increase in osmotic pressure. In the eye this results in a movement of water into the lens and a disruption of the lens fibers, allowing cataracts to form. A similar process takes place in the aorta and capillaries. Areas of disruption become necrotic and fill with cholesterol, and atherosclerotic plaques develop.

Another hypothesis to explain the thickening of the capillary basement membrane is that the diabetic is merely experiencing *premature aging* of cells. A third hypothesis contends that high concentrations of glucose in the blood cause glucose molecules to form chemical bonds with the amino groups of cellular proteins, a reaction known as *glycosylation*. For example, it has been shown that in the blood of diabetics, glycosylated forms of hemoglobin are unusually common (see page 487). Many researchers believe that this same process is going on in other tissues as well, but the question still remains about whether it is responsible for the basement membrane thickening.

Besides involving the eyes, the vascular complications can affect the kidneys (*nephropathy, Kimmelstiel-Wilson syndrome*) and lead to renal failure; the heart and coronary arteries, causing impairment of physical activites; and the limbs (*dermopathy*), which are frequently the site of mild to extreme degeneration of the arteries, resulting in gangrene of one or both legs. Wounds heal slowly, especially in the feet, so the diabetic should take reasonable precautions. *Neuropathy*, or deterioration of nervous tissue, can also develop in the diabetic.

For the diabetic patient with atherosclerosis, a reduction of total fat to between 25 and 30 per cent of total calories, with a polyunsaturated to saturated fat ratio of 2:1, and a high fiber intake, especially from oats and beans, are recommended. Atherosclerosis is discussed in Chapter 28.

INFECTIONS. The diabetic is highly susceptible to infection. Uncontrolled diabetes favors uncontrollable infections. The nurse must be aware of this and be alert to any signs. Usually an infection will destroy the glucose-insulin homeostasis and put the diabetes "out of control."

BODY WEIGHT IMBALANCE. The diabetic should determine his ideal weight, and try to reach it or maintain it. Overzealous insulin therapy will result in a weight gain as the resulting hypoglycemia triggers an appetite response and increased food consumption. In addition, the diabetic under treatment is not losing as much energy through glycosuria.

Uncontrolled diabetics will often lose weight, especially during the onset of the disease, because of the body's inability to utilize glucose. The underweight condition is more prevalent in diabetic children than in adults. Children have the additional physiological stress of body growth and development. See Chapter 38 for discussion of diabetes mellitus in children.

EDUCATION OF THE PATIENT

Every person with diabetes should know how to calculate and plan his own diet, adjust his exercise, adjust his insulin when necessary, and monitor his serum glucose. If for any reason this is not possible; he should be involved in the planning of a program that he can reasonably follow. Changes in eating habits and dietary pattern are not easily attained, particularly when weight reduction is necessary as is so often the case, and frequent adjustments are necessary until an acceptable pattern evolves. It is important that the nurse and dietitian recognize when the patient is *ready to learn* about his disease and the management of it. Frequently, when a person realizes that he has diabetes, learning about appropriate diet is the least important focus of his attention. He is likely to be much more concerned about giving himself an insulin injection, and the education regarding his diet may have to wait until a more appropriate time.

The first step in the teaching-learning process, as discussed in Chapter 18, is to begin with the patient's customary dietary patterns and eating habits and retain as many of them as possible. The more familiar he becomes with food values the better he is able to meet changing situations. Timing and spacing of meals, so important in the treatment of IDDM, should be planned with the person to conform to his lifestyle. The diet and the insulin dosage should be adjusted to the person and not vice versa.

At each follow-up visit to the clinic, hospital or doctor's office, the interview should begin with a determination of the dietary pattern the patient is now following. If there has been a change in weight or abnormal blood and urine tests, or both, the well-informed diabetic usually knows the reason. Many times he needs assistance in adjusting to changing conditions in his life.

Standardized diet sheets are seldom applicable to the person's educational needs. Distributing the sheets and going over them with the person requires little preparation and could be done by a clerk. It is the role of the professional interviewer (dietitian, nurse, physician) to involve the diabetic person in planning and monitoring his own program. The time thus spent will be rewarding to all concerned.

Most people resist changes in diet. Furthermore, they resist being different from other people. The nurse can help to develop a healthy mental attitude in the patient. Her daily association with the patient at mealtime, during the administering of insulin and at other times offers an opportunity to help him accept his disease. Teaching aids to demonstrate the importance of substituting foods equal in energy, protein, carbohydrate, fat, fiber, mineral and vitamin content should be used. An understanding of the function of foods, the relationship of the diet to health and the purpose of insulin administration, body care and the testing of urine or blood for glucose content will alleviate fear.

The diabetic patient requires skillful care and thoughtful guidance to help him gain confidence. The cooperation of the physician, dietitian, nurse and patient is important. If there is failure in the control of the diabetic condition, it may be attributed to the patient's ignorance of the complications and consequences. To the diabetic patient, "knowledge is freedom."

Programs for patients with diabetes are available throughout the United States, sponsored by various health agencies, diabetic associations, hospitals and clinics. The aim is to give practical and continuing education, guidance and support to the diabetic and his family.

The bimonthly magazine *Forecast* published for diabetics by the American Diabetes Association and the paper published by the American Association of Diabetic Educators contain helpful information about the disease, diets and recipes based on the Exchange Lists, plus interesting and pertinent stories.

Hypoglycemia

Hypoglycemia is not a disease but a symptom of a derangement in carbohydrate metabolism. As mentioned, hypoglycemia may occur in the diabetic person (from not eating or from too much insulin) but may also be caused by other disorders. It is usually defined as a plasma glucose level below 50 mg./dl. (blood glucose of 40 mg./dl. or less) after a meal or glucose load *combined with symptoms*. A person may have recurring symptoms after meals that are compatible with hypoglycemia yet not have the documented plasma glucose of 50 mg./dl. Because of the problems with the oral glucose tolerance test, it is now accepted by most that hypoglycemia exists if the blood sugar falls to a low point after a meal and not if it is only elicited after the large glucose load of the OGTT. Symptoms must also be present at the nadir of the blood glucose. The mixed meal tolerance test (MMTT) entails measuring the plasma or blood glucose at specified times after consumption of a meal that contains 75 gm. carbohydrate combined with fat and protein as would exist in a normal meal.[11]

The symptoms of sweating, weakness, hunger, tachycardia and "inward trembling" are produced by a compensatory increase in epinephrine secretion as the body attempts to increase hepatic glycogenolysis to offset the falling blood glucose level. Other non-specific symptoms are headache, blurred vision, mental confusion, incoherent speech, bizarre behavior or convulsions, which usually result from a slow and severe decline in blood sugar.

Basically, hypoglycemia is of two types: that which is present in the fasting state (*organic hypoglycemia*) and that which is present in the "fed" state. *Fasting hypoglycemia* is characterized by the development of hypoglycemic symptoms eight or more hours after a meal. Although fasting hypoglycemia is rare in occurrence, there are several possible causes, some of which are: hypersecretion of insulin due to an insulinoma (tumor of the pancreatic islet beta cells), other endocrine tumors, an endocrine deficiency, overadministration of insulin or sulfonylureas, liver damage, starvation or cancer. The treatment for this type of hypoglycemia is to remove the tumor, correct the underlying medical problem or treat the symptoms with diazoxide, which decreases secretion of insulin and elevates blood glucose.

Hypoglycemia in the "fed" state, or *reactive hypoglycemia*, is caused by intake of food, especially of carbohydrates, in sensitive individuals. Such individuals are those with certain inherited metabolic disorders, alimentary hypoglycemia resulting from gastrojejunostomy dumping syndrome as discussed in Chapter 34, or *functional hypoglycemia*, a poorly understood disorder that has also been called *diabetic type hypoglycemia*.[5] In the opinion of some authorities this represents one of the earliest manifestations of the diabetic state and is characterized by a delay in insulin secretion with the peak insulin response occurring between 90 and 180 minutes after a meal as opposed to a normal peak occurring between 30 and 60 minutes postprandially. The liver has already started taking up glucose at this time, so that serum glucose is not maximal at the same time as serum insulin. Thus the late-arriving insulin causes an excessively large drop in serum glucose between 180 and 270 minutes after food intake, and hypoglycemia and symptoms result. The symptoms are relieved with carbohydrate intake.

The work-up for the patient complaining of hypoglycemic symptoms should include a dietary history to determine the content of the diet and timing of symptoms. In addition, there should be questioning about what relieves the symptoms. Symptoms of true hypoglycemia should be relieved by carbohydrate intake.

NUTRITIONAL CARE

Surgery to remove the pancreatic tumor is the preferred treatment when a tumor is established definitely as the cause. Some patients refuse to have an operation, and others, with mild symptoms, may prefer to try medical regimens, including diet. The basic principles of the dietary treatment for hypoglycemia focus upon slowing the quick absorption and utilization of carbohydrates, which stimulate the islet cells of the pancreas to secrete insulin and draw glucose from the blood. Because the glucose available after the absorption and metabolism of complex carbohydrate, fiber and protein is released into the blood stream evenly and more slowly, causing less stimulation of insulin secretion, a diet rich in these components is recommended.

The diet for hypoglycemia is calculated in a procedure similar to that used to plan the diabetic diet, and the Exchange Lists given in Table 25–8 can be used. A diet divided into five or six meals, with some protein and fiber in each meal in order to provide a less rapidly available source of glucose and slow down glucose absorption, helps maintain blood glucose at a normal level.

The energy content of the diet is based upon the patient's normal requirements, and this procedure has been discussed previously. After the energy requirement is determined, the amounts of protein and carbohydrate are determined. A moderate protein content of 70 to 130 gm. (15 to 20 per cent of calories) is average; and a moderate carbohydrate content of 40 to 55 per cent of calories is the usual range. After deducting these two requirements, the balance of the calories is allotted to fats. Caution must be exercised to prevent the development of any dietary inadequacies.

Since most concentrated sweets are still assumed to be rapidly absorbed and stimulate insulin production, sugar, sweetened desserts, jelly, jams, honey, syrups, candy, sweetened fruits, fruits high in carbohydrates and soft drinks are omitted. Fruits, vegetables, breads, cereals and potatoes should make up the carbohydrate in the diet.

Alcohol should be omitted or restricted to one drink per day, since alcohol can potentiate hypoglycemia by blocking gluconeogenesis. Caffeine should also be omitted because it affects blood glucose levels through epinephrine stimulation.

Problems and Suggested Topics for Discussion

1. What is diabetes mellitus? Describe some theories about its causation. What tests are used to diagnose the disease?

2. List the symptoms of an untreated diabetic. How can they be controlled?
3. What is the purpose of insulin? Describe the different kinds and point out how they differ.
4. Describe the oral hypoglycemic agents and explain their use in the treatment of diabetes mellitus.
5. Describe diabetic acidosis or ketosis. What is the cause and treatment?
6. What is an insulin reaction? How is it treated?
7. What percentages of carbohydrate, protein and fat are metabolized to glucose in the body?
8. Interview a patient who has just learned that he has diabetes and show how his present dietary pattern can be modified for diabetic management.
9. Plan a menu guide with the patient, using the Exchange Lists, that is 60 per cent carbohydrate and high in fiber.
10. Check the planned menus for nutritional adequacy.
11. Research further the new information regarding the glycemic response to food ingestion. What factors seem to affect it?
12. Study several different diabetic diet educational systems and evaluate them for ease of learning, practicality and effectiveness in blood sugar control.
13. (a) Calculate a diet for a patient with reactive hypoglycemia. Does he or she have any lifestyle factors that will need changing? What would you suggest as alternatives?
    (b) Determine the total calories.
    (c) Plan a meal pattern.

Resources for Patients

A.D.A. Exchange Lists for Meal Planning and A.D.A. Forecast (published bimonthly). Available from American Diabetes Association, Inc., 1 West 48th Street, New York, N.Y., 10020.

Anderson, J.W.: Diabetes. A Practical Guide to Daily Living. New York, Arco Press, 1981.

Anderson, J.W., Sieling, B., and Chen, W.-J.: User's Guide to HCF diets, Lexington, Ky., HCF Diabetes Research Foundation, Inc., 1980. Available from University of Kentucky Diabetes Fund, P.O. Box 811, University of Kentucky Medical Center, 800 Rose Street, Lexington, Ky. 40536.

Donahoe, V.: Diabetic Cooking Made Easy. Minneapolis, Burgess Publishing Co., 1976.

Fischer, A.E., and Horstmann, D.L.: A Handbook for the Young Diabetic. 4th ed. New York, Intercontinental Medical Book Corp., 1972.

Gormican, A.: Controlling Diabetes with Diet. Springfield, Illinois, Charles C Thomas, 1971.

MacRae, N.: How to Have Your Cake and Eat It Too! 2nd ed. Anchorage, Alaska Northwest Publishing Co., 1982.

Middleton, K., and Hess, M.A.: The Art of Cooking for the Diabetic. Chicago, Contemporary Books, Inc., 1979.

Cited References

1. Akgun, S., and Ertel, N.H.: A comparison of carbohydrate metabolism after sucrose, sorbitol and fructose meals in normal and diabetic subjects. Diabetes Care, 3:583, 1980.
2. American Diabetes Association: Principles of nutrition and dietary recommendations for individuals with diabetes mellitus. Diabetes, 28:1027, 1979.
3. Anderson, J.W.: Dietary fiber and diabetes. In Spiller, G.A., and Kay, R.M. (eds.): Medical Aspects of Dietary Fiber. New York, Plenum Medical Book Company, 1980.
4. Anderson, J.W., and Ward, K.: High carbohydrate, high fiber diets for insulin-treated men with diabetes mellitus. Am. J. Clin. Nutr., 32:2312, 1979.
5. Anderson, J.W.: Reactive hypoglycemia. In Conn, H.F. (ed.): Current Therapy. Philadelphia, W.B. Saunders Company, 1979.
6. Anderson, J.W.: High carbohydrate, high fiber diets for patients with diabetes, In Camerini-Davalos, R.A. and Hanover, B. (eds.): Treatment of Early Diabetes. New York, Plenum Medical Book Company, 1979.
7. Anderson, J.W., Lin, W.-J., and Ward, K.: Composition of foods commonly used in diets for persons with diabetes. Diabetes Care, 1:293, 1978.
8. Anderson, J.W., et al.: Mineral and vitamin status on high-fiber diets: long term studies of diabetic patients. Diabetes Care, 3:38, 1980.
9. Arvidsson-Lenner, R.: Studies of glycemia and glycosuria in diabetics after breakfast meals of different compositions. Am. J. Clin. Nutr., 29:716, 1976.
10. Brownlee, M. and Cahill, G.F., Jr.: Diabetic control and vascular complications. In Paoletti, R., and Gotto, A.M., Jr. (eds.): Atherosclerosis Reviews. New York, Raven Press, 1979.
11. Buss, R.W., et al.: Mixed meal tolerance test and reactive hypoglycemia. Horm. Metab. Res., 14:281, 1982.
12. Cahill, G.F., Jr., and McDevitt, H.O.: Insulin-dependent diabetes mellitus: The initial lesion. N. Engl. J. Med., 304:1454, 1981.
13. Cahill, G.F., Jr., Etzwiler, D.D., and Freinkel, N.: Control and diabetes. N. Engl. J. Med., 294:1004, 1976.
14. Chantelau, E., et al.: Diet liberalization and metabolic control in Type I diabetic outpatients treated by continuous subcutaneous insulin infusion. Diabetes Care, 5:612, 1982.
15. Crapo, P.A., et al.: Comparison of serum glucose, insulin and glucagon responses to different types of complex carbohydrate in noninsulin-dependent diabetic patients. Am. J. Clin. Nutr., 34:184, 1981.
16. Crapo, P.A., et al.: Postprandial hormonal responses to different types of complex carbohydrate in individuals with impaired glucose tolerance. Am. J. Clin. Nutr., 33:1723, 1980.
17. Crapo, P.A., Kolterman, O.G., and Olefsky, J.M.: Effects of oral fructose in normal, diabetic and impaired glucose tolerance subjects. Diabetes Care, 3:575, 1980.
18. Crofford, O.: Report of the National Commission on Diabetes to the Congress of the United States (DHEW Publication No. NIH 76-1018). Washington, D.C., U.S. Government Printing Office, 1975.
19. Dobersen, M., et al.: Cytotoxic autoantibodies to beta cells in the serum of patients with insulin-dependent diabetes mellitus. N. Engl. J. Med., 303:1493, 1982.
20. Gerich, J.E., et al.: Prevention of human diabetic ketoacidosis by somatostatin: evidence for an essential role of glucagon. N. Engl. J. Med., 292:985, 1975.
21. Holle, A., et al.: Biguanide treatment increases the number of insulin-receptor sites on human erythrocytes. N. Engl. J. Med., 305:563, 1981.
22. Jenkins, D.J.A., et al.: Glycemic response to wheat products: reduced response to pasta but no effect of fiber. Diabetes Care, 6:155, 1983.
23. Jenkins, D.J.A.: Lente carbohydrate: A newer approach to the dietary management of diabetes. Diabetes Care, 5:634, 1982.
24. Jenkins, D.J.A., et al.: Slow release dietary carbohydrate improves second meal tolerance. Am. J. Clin. Nutr., 35:1339, 1982.
25. Jenkins, D.J.A., et al.: Glycemic index of foods: a physiological basis for carbohydrate exchange. Am. J. Clin. Nutr., 34:362, 1981.
26. Jenkins, D.J.A., et al.: Lack of effect of refining on the glycemic response to cereals. Diabetes Care, 4:509, 1981.
27. Levine, R.A., Streeten, D.H.P., and Doisy, R.J.: Effects of oral chromium supplementation on glucose tolerance of elderly human subjects. Metabolism, 17:114, 1968.

28. Notkins, A.L.: The causes of diabetes. Sci. Am., *241*:62, 1979.
29. Nutrition Subcommittee of the British Diabetic Association's Medical Advisory Committee: Dietary recommendations for diabetics for the 1980's—a policy statement by the British Diabetic Association. Human Nutrition: Applied Nutrition, *36A*:378, 1982.
30. Offenbacher, E.G., and Pi-Sunyer, F.X.: Beneficial effect of chromium rich brewer's yeast on glucose tolerance and blood lipids in elderly subjects. Diabetes, *29*: 919, 1980.
31. Olefsky, J.M., Koltermann, O.G., and Scarlett, J.A.: Insulin action and resistance in obesity and noninsulin-dependent type II diabetes mellitus. Am. J. Physiol., *243*:E15, 1982.
32. Olefsky, J.M., and Crapo, P.A.: Fructose, xylitol and sorbitol. Diabetes Care, *3*:390, 1980.
33. Olefsky, J.M., and Reaven, G.M.: Effects of sulfonylurea therapy on insulin binding to mononuclear leukocytes of diabetic patients. Am. J. Med., *60*:89, 1976.
34. Pedersen, O., et al.: Increased insulin receptors on monocytes from insulin-dependent diabetes after a high starch, high fiber diet. Diabetologia, *19*:306, 1980.
35. Peterson, C.M., Forhan, S.E., and Jones, R.L.: Self-management: an approach to patients with insulin-dependent diabetes mellitus. Diabetes, *3*:82, 1980.
36. Pietri, A., Ehle, A.L., and Raskin, P.: Changes in nerve conduction velocity after six weeks of glucoregulation with portable insulin infusion pumps. Diabetes, *29*:668, 1980.
37. Pirart, J.: Diabetes mellitus and its degenerative complications: a prospective study of 4400 patients observed between 1947 and 1973. Diabetes Care, *1*:168, 1978.
38. Powers, M.: Pump users and diet behavior. Infusion, *2* (1):6, 1983.
39. Protocol for Diabetes Control and Complications Trial (DCCT). Diabetes Care, *5*:XXIX, 1982.
40. Pyke, D.A., and Nelson, P.G.: Diabetes mellitus in identical twins, In Creutzfeldt, W., Koberling, J., and Neel, J.V. (eds.): The Genetics of Diabetes Mellitus. New York, Springer Verlag, 1976.
41. Riales, R., and Albrink, M.J.: Effect of chromium chloride supplementation on glucose tolerance and serum lipids including high-density lipoprotein of adult men. Am. J. Clin. Nutr., *34*:2670, 1981.
42. Sizemore, D.A.: Peripheral vein feeding in the diabetic patient. Clin. Consult. Nutr. Support, *1*(2):9, 1981.
43. Soman, V.R., et al.: Increased insulin sensitivity and insulin binding to monocytes after physical training. N. Engl. J. Med., *301*:1200, 1979.
44. Sosenko, J.M., et al.: Hyperglycemia and plasma lipid levels. A prospective study of young insulin-dependent diabetic patients. N. Engl. J. Med., *302*:650, 1980.
45. Spiro, R.G.: Search for a biochemical basis of diabetic microangiopathy. Diabetologia, *12*:1, 1976.
46. Unger, R.H.: Meticulous control of diabetes: benefits, risks and precautions. Diabetes, *31*:479, 1982.
47. Vranic, M., and Berger, M.: Exercise and diabetes mellitus. Diabetes, *28*:147, 1979.
48. West, K.M.: Diabetes mellitus. In Schneider, H.A., Anderson, C.E., and Coursin, D.B.: Nutritional Support of Medical Practice. Hagerstown, Md., Harper & Row, 1977.
49. Wong, G.S.: Position statement (Canadian Diabetes Assoc.): Aspartame and its safe use. Diabetes Dialogue, *29*(Spring):3, 1982.

Additional References

American Diabetes Association: Statement on hypoglycemia. Diabetes Care, *5*:72, 1982.
Anderson, J.W., Sieling, B., and Chen, W.J.: Professional Guide to HCF Diets, Lexington, Kentucky, HCF Diabetes Research Foundation, Inc., 1981. Available from University of Kentucky Diabetes Fund, P.O. Box 811, University of Kentucky Medical Center, 800 Rose St., Lexington, Kentucky, 40536.
Anderson, J.W., Midgley, W.R., and Wedman, B.: Fiber and Diabetes. Diabetes Care, *2*:369, 1979.
Bantle, J.P., et al.: Postprandial glucose and insulin responses to meals containing different carbohydrates in normal and diabetic subjects. N. Engl. J. Med., *309*:7, 1983.
Bar, R.S., et al.: Regulation of insulin receptors in normal and abnormal physiology in humans. Adv. Intern. Med., *24*:23, 1979.
Blood glucose response to various foods. Nutr. Rev., *41*:8, 1983.
Craighead, J.E.: Current views on the etiology of insulin-dependent diabetes mellitus, N. Engl. J. Med., *299*:1439, 1978.
Cryer, P.E., and Gerich, J.E.: Relevance of glucose counterregulatory systems to patients with diabetes: critical roles of glucagon and epinephrine. Diabetes Care, *6*: 95, 1983.
DeFronzo, R.A., and Ferrannini, E.: The pathogenesis of non-insulin dependent diabetes. Medicine, *61*:125, 1982.
El-Beheri Burgess, B.R.B.: Rationale for changes in the dietary management of diabetes. J. Am. Diet. Assoc., *81*: 258, 1982.
Felig, P.: Disorders of Carbohydrate Metabolism. In Bondy, P.K., and Rosenberg, L.E.: Metabolic Control and Disease. 8th ed. Philadelphia, W.B. Saunders Company, 1980, pp. 276–392.
Hofeldt, F.D., et al.: Are abnormalities in insulin secretion responsible for reactive hypoglycemia? Diabetes, *23*:589, 1974.
Kaplan, S.A., et al.: Diabetes mellitus, UCLA conference. Ann. Intern. Med., *96*:635, 1982.
Kolata, G.: Dietary dogma disproved. Science, *220*:487, 1983.
Miranda, P.M., and Horwitz, D.L.: High fiber diets in the treatment of diabetes mellitus. Ann. Intern. Med., *88*:482, 1978.
National Diabetes Data Group: Classification and diagnosis of diabetes mellitus and other categories of glucose intolerance. Diabetes, *28*:1039, 1979.
Nuttall, F.Q.: Diet and the diabetic patient. Diabetes Care, *6*: 197, 1983.
Pincus, G., and White, P.: On the inheritance of diabetes mellitus. Am. J. Med. Sci., *186*:1, 1933.
Shagan, B.P.: Diabetes in the elderly patient. Med. Clin. North Am., *60*:1191, 1976.
Whitehouse, F.W.: Classification and pathogenesis of the diabetes syndrome: a historical perspective. J. Am. Diet. Assoc., *81*:243, 1982.

Nutritional Care in Disease of the Adrenal Cortex, Thyroid Gland or Parathyroid Glands

The adrenal cortex, thyroid gland and parathyroid glands are very potent endocrine glands, and the consequences of their functioning abnormally are extensive. This malfunctioning can affect metabolism and cause nutritional imbalances, body weight changes and much discomfort. Fortunately, hormonal replacement therapy is very effective and usually restores the patient to productive and comfortable living. Nutritional care is important to help maintain metabolic balance during the acute phase of the disease and to rehabilitate the patient nutritionally after the hormonal treatment has started.

Adrenal Cortex

FUNCTION. The adrenals, two small glands of vital importance, are deeply imbedded in the back tissues near the kidneys. They consist chiefly of two parts. The central portion (medulla) contains cells originating from nerve structures that secrete *epinephrine* and *norepinephrine*. The outer shell (cortex) secretes *aldosterone,* a *mineralocorticoid* that controls water and electrolyte balance; the *glucocorticoids* cortisol (hydrocortisone) and cortisone, which function in gluconeogenesis; and the *androgens,* which stimulate protein synthesis and the formation of sex hormones.

ADRENAL CORTEX INSUFFICIENCY

Addison's disease is a rare metabolic disorder in which there is an insufficiency of the hormones of the adrenal cortex, either because of the failure of the adrenal glands or because the pituitary for some reason does not secrete *adrenocorticotropic hormone (ACTH),* which stimulates the adrenal glands. Most cases of Addison's disease are probably due to an autoimmune disorder, while some are the result of an infection such as tuberculosis or histoplasmosis.

MINERALOCORTICOID DEFICIENCY. In Addison's disease the lack of aldosterone decreases sodium reabsorption and allows the excretion of sodium ions, chloride ions and water in the urine in excessive quantities. A greatly decreased extracellular fluid volume results; acidosis develops because of the failure of hydrogen ions to be excreted in exchange for sodium reabsorption; potassium retention is increased and serum potassium rises sharply; blood volume falls and cardiac output decreases. A crisis develops in a few days.

GLUCOCORTICOID DEFICIENCY. Because of the lack of cortisol secretion, it is impossible for the person to maintain normal blood glucose levels between meals, since he cannot synthesize sufficient amounts of glucose by gluconeogenesis. Rapid glycogen depletion occurs and *hypoglycemia* follows. Severe hypoglycemia may be experienced by a person without food for several hours or after a high-carbohydrate meal. Mobilization of fats and protein from tissues is reduced, and many other metabolic functions are depressed. These patients frequently experience abdominal discomfort, diarrhea, nausea, vomiting, anorexia and weight loss. The prognosis for Addison's disease was grave, but hormonal therapy has improved the outlook considerably.

Treatment

HORMONAL. Supplying the missing adrenal cortex hormones to the patient is the main therapy. Cortisone, cortisol, prednisone or hydroxycortisone is given to meet glucocorticoid needs, and fluorocortisol or desoxycorticosterone is given to meet mineralocorticoid needs. Hormone therapy has enabled the person with adrenocortical insufficiency to lead a normal life, provided the proper medication is taken faithfully.

NUTRITIONAL. Hormone replacement therapy causes the release of serum potassium and the retention of salt and water, with the sodium and potassium reaching or approaching a normal concentration. However, 4 to 6 gm. of additional salt daily is often advised to spare the need for hormones and thus reduce the expense of the treatment. In a few cases, sodium chloride therapy alone is sufficient to relieve the symptoms for years. If electrolyte balance is not thus achieved, then active cortical extracts or aldosterone is given.

Because of the tendency to hypoglycemia and

the extreme weakness experienced by patients with Addison's disease, frequent feedings of an adequate diet, moderate to high in protein and moderate in carbohydrate—similar to that described for hypoglycemia in Chapter 25—may be necessary. The individual with Addison's disease must understand the symptoms of hypoglycemia, and carry food with him to control attacks if they occur frequently. He should have a fairly substantial meal at bedtime in order to prevent an early morning hypoglycemic reaction.

Because the sufferer is frequently dehydrated, a generous intake of fluids is required. Vitamins, particularly ascorbic acid and those of the B complex that function as components of metabolic enzymes, should be given in liberal amounts to provide for the increased metabolism. A vitamin supplement may be prescribed. Foods listed in Appendix Table 10 which are rich in potassium should be included, along with a potassium supplement, since hormonal therapy tends to cause potassium depletion.

Anorexia is often a symptom of untreated chronic adrenocortical insufficiency, and many such patients will have lost weight. A return to normal weight through dietary management as described in Chapter 27 may need to be included in the treatment.

ADRENOCORTICOTROPIC HORMONE THERAPY

The *glucocorticoids* (e.g., cortisone, prednisone, dexamethasone) and the *adrenocorticotropic hormone* (ACTH) of the anterior pituitary gland, which stimulates the adrenal cortex, are used for the treatment of a variety of disorders. The effect of their long-term usage on metabolism is important to note.

MINERALS. Therapeutic doses of cortisone may produce a mineralocorticoid effect evidenced by hypokalemia, and hypochloremic alkalosis. Potassium is provided by an adequate intake of fruits, fruit juices, vegetables, vegetable juices, whole-grain cereals, meat and broth.

Sodium retention along with edema may develop, so some sodium restriction is recommended.

PROTEIN METABOLISM. The administration of a large amount of cortisone may result in a negative nitrogen balance and wasting of muscle tissue, thinning of skin, dissolution of vertebral bone, poor wound healing and growth retardation in children. A diet sufficient in energy, high in protein (at least 1 gm./kg./day) and liberal in carbohydrate to exert the maximum protein-sparing effect against the protein catabolizing effect of the glucocorticoids will help to maintain nitrogen balance.

LIPID METABOLISM. Glucocorticoids increase total body fat, but the mechanisms by which the lipid metabolic changes take place are still unclear. Fat deposition occurs in the face ("moon face"), supraclavicular areas ("buffalo hump") and over the lower cervical vertebrae of the trunk. This can be disconcerting to patients and must be explained to them. Little can be done to prevent this other than regulating the hormonal medication.

CARBOHYDRATE METABOLISM. Cortisone therapy stimulates gluconeogenesis. Insensitivity to insulin is manifested, so diabetics taking cortisone require additional insulin. Previously unrecognized latent diabetes often is unmasked in these patients and may become clinical diabetes requiring insulin.

ASCORBIC ACID. Considerable amounts of ascorbic acid are present in adrenal tissue. ACTH depletes the adrenal tissue of this vitamin. A supplement of ascorbic acid may be necessary with ACTH therapy.

VITAMIN D. Glucocorticoids have an antagonistic effect on vitamin D metabolism so that a negative calcium balance is the result. Osteoporosis may develop, but small doses of 25-OHD$_3$ daily may prevent this effect.[4]

OTHER MANIFESTATIONS. Adrenocortical steroid therapy increases hydrochloric acid secretion. Peptic ulceration may develop and if not treated may result in hemorrhage. Frequent feedings are indicated, along with the use of antacids.

Thyroid Gland

Normal Thyroid Function

The thyroid gland secretes the hormones *thyroxine (T$_4$), triiodothyronine (T$_3$), reverse triiodothyronine (rT$_3$),* and *calcitonin.* Their release by the thyroid is regulated by *thyrotropin (thyroid-stimulating hormone, or TSH)* secreted by the anterior pituitary. Only 20 to 30 per cent of the T$_3$ is secreted by the thyroid; about 70 to 80 per cent of the circulating T$_3$ is derived from the peripheral conversion of T$_4$ to T$_3$. T$_3$ is about four times more metabolically potent than T$_4$. However, since the serum concentration of T$_3$ is only one fifth that of T$_4$ and since it binds to the thyroxine transport protein with much less affinity than T$_4$, it is estimated that these hormones contribute equally to biologic activity. T$_4$ is not just a "precursor" for T$_3$ but has its own important function in metabolism. rT$_3$ is also present in the circulation at much lower levels and is metabolically inactive.

Thyroid hormones are made from iodine, a dietary nutrient for which no other function is known in humans; hence the interest of nutritionists in this particular hormone's function. See Chapter 7 for further discussion of iodine.

Dietary Influences on Thyroid Metabolism

Low-energy diets, starvation, catabolic illness and stress decrease the activity of the enzymes responsible for deiodinating T_4 to T_3 with the result that there is a lowering of the serum T_3 levels and thus the metabolic rate. This situation exists in dieting patients and may explain the plateau that dieters reach in weight loss after dieting for several weeks. In the catabolic patient, low serum T_3 levels reflect the body's attempt to protect nutritional reserves.

The amount of carbohydrate in the diet has also been shown to affect the level of T_3, especially when the energy intake is low. The greater the amount of carbohydrate in the diet, the greater the level of T_3. Fat has the opposite effect. See Chapter 27 for further discussion of the thyroid in weight control.

HYPERTHYROIDISM (GRAVES' DISEASE)

Hyperthyroidism is a condition in which the thyroid gland is overactive, with a consequent increase in the rate of metabolism. The condition is also referred to as exophthalmic goiter, thyrotoxicosis or Graves' disease. Figure 26–1 shows a patient with hyperthyroidism. It is thought to be an autoimmune disorder and is much more common in women than in men. It can develop postpartum; one study showed a prevalence of thyroid dysfunction of 5.5 per cent, the majority being hyperthyroidism. Thyroid dysfunction was also four times more prevalent in women giving birth to girls than in those giving birth to boys. It was usually transient and had resolved by six months postpartum.[1]

Disorders of carbohydrate metabolism (with abnormal blood glucose curves and glucose intolerance), increased protein metabolism, calcium imbalance, and bone turnover due to altered vitamin D metabolism, disordered creatine metabolism and depressed serum cholesterol and triglyceride levels are frequently present. Vitamin requirements are increased because of enhanced cellular metabolism and accelerated degradation of vitamins.

The patient may complain of perspiration and heat intolerance. There may be slightly elevated basal body temperature. In children, a first sign of hyperthyroidism is acceleration of linear growth and bone maturation. But if the hypermetabolic state continues, decreased nutrition, weight loss and retarded growth may be present.

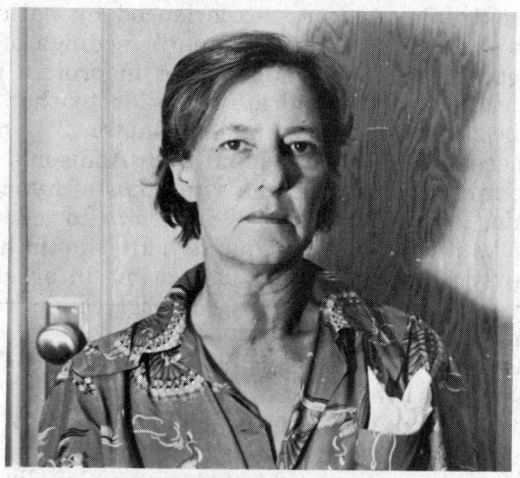

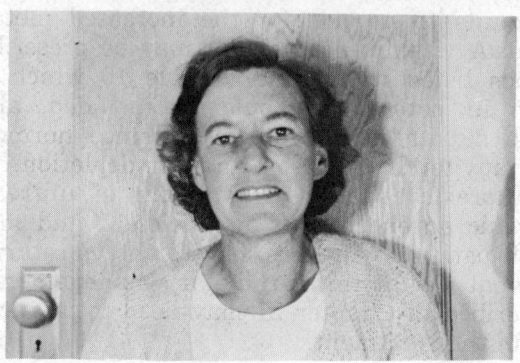

Figure 26–1. Before and after ½ months of treatment for severe hyperthyrodism (without exophthalmos). An antithyroid drug was administered. Patient was later treated with I^{131} and made a complete recovery despite a stormy course. Note weight loss, enlarged thyroid (goiter) and tense expression before treatment. (Courtesy of Dr. R. H. Hoffman.)

Treatment

MEDICAL. Treatment for hyperthyroidism includes one of the following therapies, with the choice depending on the patient's age and the extent of the disease: (1) administration of antithyroid drugs such as propylthiouracil or methimazole, (2) radioiodine therapy or (3) surgery. In many cases, a partial thyroidectomy is performed. However, even following a successful operation, many symptoms remain. Therefore, the medical treatment is of paramount importance.

NUTRITIONAL CARE. Since in hyperthyroidism all the metabolic processes in the body are accelerated, a high-energy diet is indicated to prevent the destruction of body tissue and a rapid loss of weight.

Energy. The increase of energy over normal allowances should be in accordance with the elevation of the metabolic rate. In mild cases the increase may be from 15 to 25 per cent above the normal allowance, while in severe cases an increase of 50 to 75 per cent is required. A diet containing 4500 to 5000 kcal. or more is frequently prescribed and consumed, since these patients exhibit a ravenous appetite. The dietary additions given in Table 27–9 can be used to increase the energy content of the diet.

Protein. Hyperthyroidism is characterized by *negative nitrogen balance* and a decrease in muscle mass. Therefore, the protein allowance should be liberal—sufficient to meet the increased need for nitrogen. If sufficient energy is supplied through carbohydrates and fats, an allowance of 100 gm. of protein will usually be adequate to maintain nitrogen balance.

Carbohydrate. Carbohydrate intake should be liberal in order to spare the proteins in the diet. If there is glucose intolerance, the carbohydrate should be of the complex type with limitation of simple sugars.

Minerals and Vitamins. The diet should be abundant in all essential food nutrients. Supplements, especially B vitamins, should be a regular part of any diet program to meet the greatly increased demand.

Iodine. Iodine administration plays a significant role in the treatment of Graves' disease. Iodine is an essential component of the thyroid hormone *thyroxine*, the active principle of the thyroid gland. In hyperthyroidism, administration of iodine in large doses (as potassium iodide) will increase the storage of thyroid hormone and prevent its release. Consequently its effects on hyperthyroidism are striking, even if only temporary. It is normally used only for a short period of time in conjunction with antithyroid drugs and before surgery or other therapy.

Many people in developed countries, and especially the U.S., have excessive dietary intakes of iodine due to the use of iodized salt and the use of iodate as a conditioner in bread. This excess iodine in the diet may be reponsible for the decreased effectiveness of antithyroid drugs as a form of treatment for hyperthyroidism.[2]

Stimulants. The stimulating effect of tea, coffee, tobacco and alcohol is limited or avoided, as indicated or ordered by the physician.

Psychology of Feeding. The psychological aspect of hyperthyroidism is important and should be considered seriously in nutritional care. When the person is *involved in planning* the dietary regimen, successful adoption of the prescribed diet is apt to occur. Physical rest and peace of mind are essential in the successful treatment of these patients.

HYPOTHYROIDISM

Hypothyroidism is characterized by the deficient activity and reduced secretion of T_4 or T_3 or both. In adults, the medical term for the advanced stage of this difficulty is *myxedema*. In women it is frequently caused by *Hashimoto's thyroiditis*. Often, it develops after treatment for hyperthyroidism.

A similar disorder in children, termed *cretinism* or infantile myxedema, develops in fetal life or early infancy if the mother has severe hypothyroidism. It will be discussed in Chapter 38.

In myxedema the thyroid undergoes a slow, progressive, specific type of atrophy. The cause is unknown. Symptoms may develop slowly and proceed unrecognized.

Because of the lowered basal metabolic rate (ranging from 15 per cent to 30 per cent, or more), there is rapid increase in weight despite decreased appetite, elevated blood cholesterol and triglyceride levels, cold intolerance, dry skin, constipation and lethargy. There also is a flattened oral glucose tolerance curve due to slowed absorption of glucose from the intestine. There is also a decrease in the conversion of carotene to vitamin A and serum carotene levels are often increased. Falling off of growth may be a first sign of hypothyroidism in children. See Table 26–1 for a list of symptoms. Myxedema is more frequent in the female than the male. A patient with myxedema is shown in Figure 26–2.

Treatment

Treatment consists of the administration of *thyroid extract*, preferably by mouth, and regulation of the diet. Because most of the patients suffering with hypothyroidism are overweight, a low-energy diet is indicated. The energy content of the diet should be reduced in accordance with the low metabolic rate and the degree of overweight. This, combined with the administration of thyroid hormone, should result in a return to normal weight. Principles of energy reduction are described in Chapter 27.

Table 26–1. CLINICAL FEATURES OF HYPOTHYROIDISM

Physical and mental slowness; drowsiness
Dry skin and hair
Decreased hearing acuity
Slow thick speech
Decreased appetite
Intolerance to cold
Constipation
Menorrhagia and sterility in menstruating women
Paresthesia of hands and feet
Muscular aching and cramping

All or most of these symptoms and signs may be present in patients with severe hypothyroidism, but only a few are noted in patients with early or mild hypothyroidism.

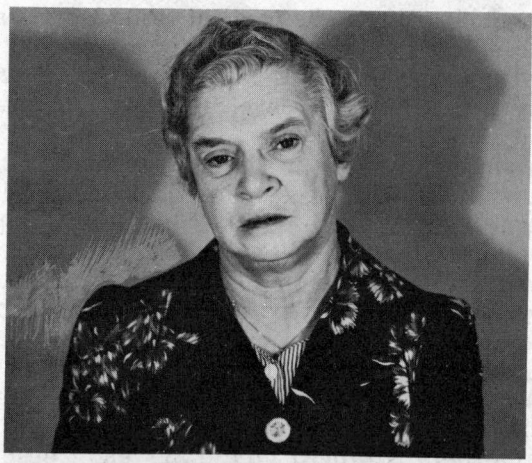

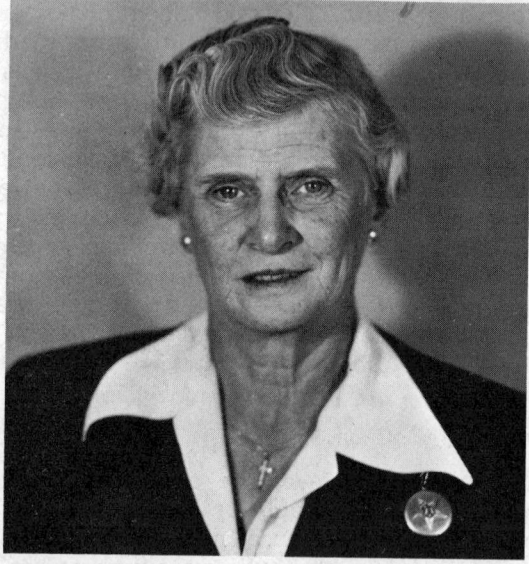

Figure 26-2. Above, severe case of myxedema prior to therapy. Below, same case following adequate thyroid therapy. (Courtesy of Arnold S. Jackson, M.D., Jackson Clinic, Madison, Wisconsin, and JAMA, *165*:122, 1957.)

Because hypothyroidism causes decreased peristalsis, which results in constipation, nutritional care during rehabilitation should include serving high-fiber, natural laxative foods such as bran, prunes or apples and encouraging the patient to drink six to eight glasses of water per day. See Table 23-2 for a high-fiber diet.

Parathyroid Glands

HYPOCALCEMIA

Hypocalcemia is a condition of low serum calcium. In adults it occurs most commonly as a result of injury to the parathyroids during a thyroidectomy. However, other etiologies are idiopathic failure of the parathyroid glands, magnesium deficiency, a defect in the receptor mechanism for parathyroid hormone (pseudohypoparathyroidism), and a defect in the hormone molecule itself. In children the cause of hypocalcemia may be neonatal immaturity or congenital absence of the parathyroid glands. Severe gastrointestinal disease, pancreatitis, osteomalacia or kidney disease may also lead to parathyroid abnormality and hypocalcemia.

If allowed to progress, hypocalcemia can lead to tetany, which is manifested by convulsions, cramps and muscle twitching.

Nutritional Care

If hypocalcemia is due to parathyroid hormone abnormality, that should be corrected if possible with parathyroid hormone (Paroidin). If the cause of the hypocalcemia cannot be treated, then a normal adequate diet, emphasizing the foods rich in calcium and vitamin D, is prescribed. (See Table 7-2 and Appendix Table 9 for foods high in calcium content.) Milk and cheese are excellent sources of calcium and should be included in the daily diet. In addition to foods rich in calcium, supplemental calcium is also given, because it is difficult to get the large doses of calcium required (1 to 2 gm. per day) through food alone. Vitamin D is given to promote the absorption and utilization of calcium. Usually large amounts of vitamin D are necessary to treat hypocalcemia because it is usually a metabolic problem and not a dietary inadequacy. A daily dosage of 25,000 to 200,000 I.U. of vitamin D may be necessary. It is more effective to determine at what step the vitamin D is not being hydroxylated properly and to give the metabolically active form or an analogue. This is discussed on page 621. In patients with hypocalcemia due to hypoparathyroidism, supplementation with magnesium may improve the response to vitamin D and calcium.[3]

HYPERCALCEMIA

Like hypocalcemia, hypercalcemia is a symptom of many disorders. In addition to hyperparathyroidism, it is often caused by malignancies. Various other bone diseases, including carcinoma of the bone, hyperthyroidism, overconsumption of antacids and milk in ulcer therapy (milk-alkali syndrome), vitamin D intoxication and rarely vitamin A intoxication, are also known causes. Hypercalcemia (defined as serum calcium levels higher than 5.8 mEq. per liter) is usually found in combination with hypophosphatemia; as serum calcium levels increase, serum phosphorus levels decrease. Some of the symptoms of this combined disorder are osteoporosis, kidney stones, nausea, anorexia, constipation, lethargy and irritability.

Treatment

Hypercalcemia is treated by caring for the underlying disorder. However, in the event that this must be delayed, the following medical therapy is usual.

FLUIDS. A high fluid intake is encouraged to prevent formation of calcium-containing renal stones.

DIURETICS. Thiazide diuretics promote renal clearance and excretion of calcium.

ACID-ASH DIET. This diet acidifies urine and prevents calcium stone formation, as discussed in Chapter 30. Prune juice and cranberry juice, for example, result in an acidic urine.

PHOSPHATE. Phosphate promotes deposition of calcium into the skeleton and is used as intravenous therapy in hypercalcemia. Complications of intravenous therapy are metastatic calcification and acute renal failure. They appear less commonly with oral phosphate therapy; however, diarrhea is a common problem with oral therapy.

Problems and Suggested Topics for Discussion

1. (a) Interview a patient with Addison's disease and obtain a diet history.
   (b) Plan with the patient a menu pattern that meets his requirements.
   (c) Check the menu for adequacy of calcium, protein, iron, vitamins and calories.
2. Interview a patient receiving steroid therapy.
   (a) Note the fat distribution of the person.
   (b) Note whether the person requires insulin.
   (c) Ask if his appetite or diet has changed since beginning ACTH therapy.
3. (a) Interview a patient suffering with Graves' disease and obtain a list of her average daily food intake.
   (b) Has she had any weight changes?
   (c) Estimate the amount of protein and energy in her daily intake.
   (d) Estimate the *normal* daily calorie and protein requirements for the patient and compare with the estimated intake.
   (e) With the patient, plan a diet that will meet her psychological and physiological needs.
   (f) Check the nutritional adequacy of the menus, particularly for minerals and vitamins.
4. (a) Obtain the diet history of a patient suffering with myxedema.

(b) Determine the patient's *normal* calorie requirements per day.
(c) Estimate her average calorie intake for the day and compare with her normal requirement.
5. Describe the many processes involved in the maintenance of serum calcium homeostasis.
6. Read the chart of a patient with hypercalcemia.
(a) Note the cause of the hypercalcemia.
(b) What kind of therapy is the patient receiving?

Cited References

1. Amino, N., et al.: High prevalence of transient postpartum thyrotoxicosis and hypothyroidism. N. Engl. J. Med. *306*:849, 1982.
2. Molith, M.E., Dahms, W.T., and Bray, G.A.: Endocrinology. In Schneider, H.A., Anderson, C.E., and Coursin, D.B. (eds.): Nutritional Support of Medical Practice. Hagerstown, Md., Harper & Row, 1977.
3. Potts, J.T., and Deftos, L.J.: Parathyroid hormone, calcitonin, vitamin D, bone and bone mineral metabolism. In Bondy, P.K., and Rosenberg, L.E. (eds.): Duncan's Diseases of Metabolism. 8th ed. Philadelphia, W.B. Saunders Company, 1980.
4. Vitamin D in health and disease. Symposium. Ann. Intern. Med., *96*:674, 1982.

Additional References

Astwood, E.B.: Management of thyroid disorders. JAMA, *286*:585, 1963.
Bondy, P.K.: The adrenal cortex. In Bondy, P.K., and Rosenberg, L.E. (eds.): Duncan's Diseases of Metabolism. 8th ed. Philadelphia, W.B. Saunders Company, 1980.
Eisenstein, A.B., and Singh, S.: Hormonal control of nutrient metabolism. In Goodhart, R.S., and Shils, M.E. (eds.): Modern Nutrition in Health and Disease. 6th ed. Philadelphia, Lea & Febiger, 1980.
Jastrup, B., et al.: Serum levels of vitamin D metabolites and bone remodelling in hyperthyroidism. Metabolism, *31*:126, 1982.
Kutsky, R.J.: Handbook of Vitamins, Minerals and Hormones. 2nd ed. New York, Van Nostrand Reinhold Company, 1981.
Larsen, P.R.: Thyroid-pituitary interaction. N. Engl. J. Med., *306*:23, 1982.
MacFarlane, I.A., et al.: Vitamin D metabolism in hyperthyroidism, Clin. Endocrinol., *17*:51, 1982.
Maxon, H.R., Apple, D.J. and Goldsmith, R.E.: Hypercalcemia in thyrotoxicosis. Surg. Gynecol. Obstet., *147*:694, 1978.
McConahey, W.M.: Hypothyroidism. Hosp. Med. *11*:98, 1975.
Sterling, K.: Thyroid hormone action at the cell level. N. Engl. J. Med., *300*:117, 1979.

UNIT 8

IMBALANCE OF BODY WEIGHT

CHAPTER 27

Nutritional Care for Weight Management*

KARON J. SANDE, M.S., R.D. ● L. KATHLEEN MAHAN, M.S., R.D.

The Regulation of Energy Intake and Balance of Body Weight

The balance between energy intake and energy expenditure is very precise, as evidenced by the observation that most people maintain a constant body weight throughout adulthood. This is illustrated by several studies as shown in Figure 27–1. Individuals tend to fluctuate in weight around a "setpoint" body weight. When this weight is disturbed by either underfeeding or overfeeding, physiological and psychological changes occur such that an individual's normal weight is defended. This is frustrating to individuals who wish to lose weight, maintain a reduced weight or gain weight; however, it also serves as a clear indicator that body weight is under regulatory controls. Thus, research is focusing more intensely upon identifying regulators of body weight and food intake and dismissing the simplistic notion that obesity is only a direct result of gluttony and lethargy.

Because an energy supply is important to an animal for the maintenance of its life, it is not surprising that energy balance is under physiological regulation. The control of energy intake and expenditure is the result of many neural, chemical and hormonal influences. An imbalance between energy intake and expenditure leads to weight gain or loss. If weight is regulated, why does an imbalance occur? It is clear

that social and environmental influences can have an effect on weight regulation. An individual may gain or lose weight in a new environmental situation; however, within a given environment, body weight settles at a new weight and this weight is defended. Thus, to assess an individual's body weight, one must take into account environmental stimuli, but also realize that genetics and physiological controls may be important variables regulating the individual's body weight.

NEURAL CONTROL

Traditionally, the hypothalamus has been considered to be the neural center for the control of food intake. The hypothalamus is a portion of the brain that composes less than 1 per cent of the total volume of the brain. Two areas of the hypothalamus have been regarded as important in the control of food intake: the *ventromedial hypothalamus (VMH)* and the *lateral hypothalamus (LH)*, as shown in Figure 27–2.

The VMH has been labeled the "satiety center" for the following reasons. Electrical stimulation of the VMH leads to cessation of eating. Even if an animal is starving, it stops eating (as if satiated) when the VMH is stimulated. Destruction of the VMH causes the animal to become hyperphagic (to overeat), eventually leading to extreme obesity. The animal overeats by increasing the size of individual meals as if it cannot detect when it is satiated.

The LH has been labeled the "feeding center" for similar reasons. Electrical stimulation of the LH causes animals to begin eating. A lesion in the LH area causes animals to undereat by de-

---

*Sections of this chapter are from Mahan, L.K.: Obesity: New knowledge and current treatments. In Worthington-Roberts, B.S.: Contemporary Developments in Nutrition. St. Louis, C.V. Mosby Co., 1981. With permission.

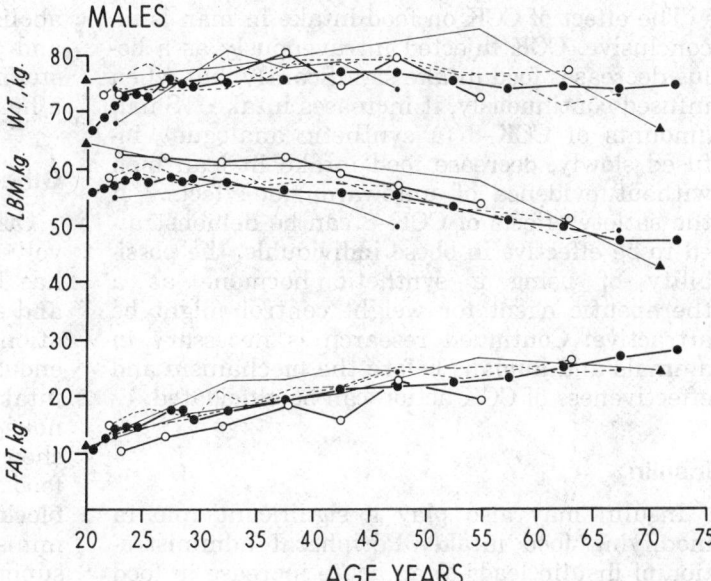

MALES

Figure 27–1. The relative stability of body weight with increasing age in males (cross-sectional measurement from several studies) and changes in body composition are shown. Note the rise in percentage of body fat and decline in percentage of lean body mass (LBM). (From Forbes, G. B., and Reina, J. C.: Adult lean body mass declines with age: some longitudinal observations. Metabolism, 19:653, 1970.)

creasing the size of individual meals, as if they are satiated earlier or cannot detect hunger. These animals become aphagic, lose a significant amount of weight and may die if not force-fed.

Such animal studies have led to the practice of dividing the brain into a "satiety center" (VMH) and a "feeding center" (LH). This subdivision of the hypothalamus into these two distinct centers is an attractive concept; however, it is probably far too simplistic. It is clear that the brain is not organized into discrete centers that control specific functions. The observed results of the VMH and LH lesion studies are now considered to be due to a number of factors, including damage to fiber tracts within the nervous system, alteration of "setpoint" and alteration of hormonal balance.[51] Investigators have begun to question whether the hypothalamus itself has any role in feeding behavior. It is doubtful that the hypothalamus directly affects feeding behavior; the regulation of food intake is more complex than originally proposed. It is becoming apparent that food intake is controlled by neural and neuroendocrine influences that remain to be defined. When this is accomplished, there will be a clearer picture of the role the hypothalamus plays in regulating feeding behavior.

HORMONAL CONTROL

Gut Peptides

A promising area of investigation related to food intake is that polypeptide hormones secreted during digestion may also function as satiety signals. This theory is based upon two facts: (1) feeding often stops before significant quantities of ingested food have been absorbed; and (2) food stimulates the release of gut peptides by contacting the mucosal surface of the gut (i.e., prior to absorption).[83] Thus, it has been hypothesized that one or more gut peptides released by pre-absorptive food stimuli act as peripheral negative feedback signals to stop feeding behavior.[20]

For example, the gastrointestinal hormone *cholecystokinin-pancreozymin* (CCK-PZ or CCK) may serve as a satiety factor in addition to its known function as a stimulator of the gallbladder and exocrine pancreas. Injection of this hormone into animals[21, 22, 35] induces cessation of eating.

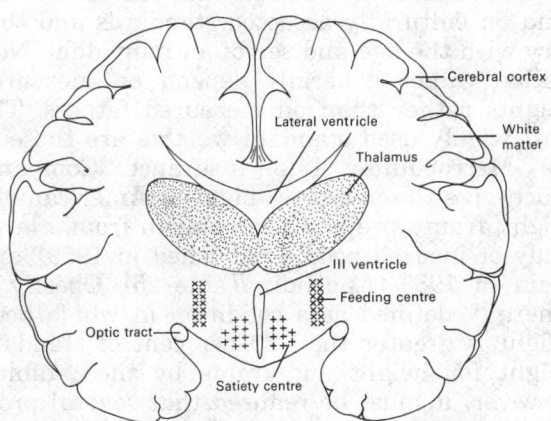

Figure 27–2. Cross-section of the brain indicating the feeding centers below the thalamus (hypothalamic area). (From Davidson, S., Passmore, R., and Brock, J. F.: Human Nutrition and Dietetics, 6th ed. Baltimore, Williams & Wilkins Co., 1976.)

The effect of CCK on food intake in man is inconclusive. CCK injected intravenously as a bolus decreases food intake significantly, but when infused continuously, it increases intake.[90] Small amounts of CCK–8 (a synthetic analogue), infused slowly, decrease food intake in lean men without evidence of untoward side-effects.[48] If the satiety effects of CCK–8 can be demonstrated to be effective in obese individuals, the possibility of using a synthetic hormone as a therapeutic agent for weight control might be attractive. Continued research is necessary in animals and humans before the mechanism and effectiveness of CCK action can be elucidated.

Insulin

Insulin may also play a significant role in modifying food intake. Peripheral administration of insulin leads to an acute increase in food intake. This response is attributed to peripheral hypoglycemia, which is a potent stimulus for eating. If hypoglycemia is prevented at the time insulin is peripherally administered, a decrease in food intake is observed in animals.

Insulin has been found in the cerebrospinal fluid, where its concentration is increased by systemic infusions of glucose or insulin and is proportional to its concentration in plasma.[65] Binding sites characteristic of insulin receptors are found in areas of the brain that are influential in feeding behavior. When insulin was infused into the lateral cerebral ventricles (i.e., into the cerebrospinal fluid) of free-feeding baboons, a dose-dependent suppression of food intake and body weight was observed as shown in Figure 27–3A. Suppression of body weight and food intake ceased when insulin infusions were stopped. These studies suggest that insulin may be capable of acting to influence food intake. Note that body weight and food intake returned to baseline levels; but body weight recovered sooner than food intake as shown in Figure 27–3B.[97] The reason for this is not understood, but it suggests that changes in energy efficiency may have occurred to defend normal body weight.

Estrogen

Estrogen has been shown to influence food intake in experimental animals. When given estrogen and estrogenlike compounds, animals eat less. It has also been noted that in female rats there is a cyclic pattern of food intake. On the day of estrus (phase characterized by high estrogen levels, LH surge and ovulation) there is a decrease in food intake, whereas in the nonestrus phase of the cycle, food intake rises. This cyclic pattern of food intake can be abolished by castration, resulting in weight gain and an increase in body fat. These and other studies support the speculation that estrogen is a hormone involved in regulation of food intake.

Other Peptides and Hormones

Other peptides and hormones may be involved in food intake regulation. Much evidence has been generated indicating that exogenous and endogenous opiates have a role in the initiation of food intake. Morphine, the classic exogenous opiate, has been reported to increase food intake. *Endorphins* and *enkephalins* (endogenous morphinelike compounds) have been shown to initiate feeding in rats and to increase food intake. Naloxone, an opiate antagonist, blocks opiate receptors. When naloxone is administered to animals or humans, food intake is suppressed.

A series of very potent endogenous compounds similar in structure to endorphins has recently been discovered. These have been named *dynorphins* (*dynas* = powerful; *orphins* = morphine). They initiate feeding when injected into the brain. These and other recently discovered or yet-to-be discovered compounds may play a major role in energy regulation and food intake. With a more thorough understanding of gastrointestinal peptides and neuroendocrinology, the mystery surrounding appetite regulation may be solved in the near future.

Identifying the Obese

Obesity is a condition of excess adipose tissue relative to lean body mass. It reflects a long-term imbalance between energy intake and energy expenditure. Overweight and obesity may be defined in relation to normal values that depend on culturally accepted standards and that vary with the age and sex of an individual. Normative values generally depend on measured weights rather than on measured fatness. The most widely used standard weights are those of the Metropolitan Life Insurance Company, which give the average weight of Americans by height, frame size and sex as taken from a large study of insured people published in 1959[57] and again in 1983 (Appendix Table 25). Obesity is generally defined as a condition in which body weight is greater than 20 per cent of standard weight for height and frame by these tables. However, it must be realized that several problems arise with the use of these tables for the determination of obesity.

The first problem is that these weight norms may not represent an accurate cross-section of the U.S. population. Second, the proper use of

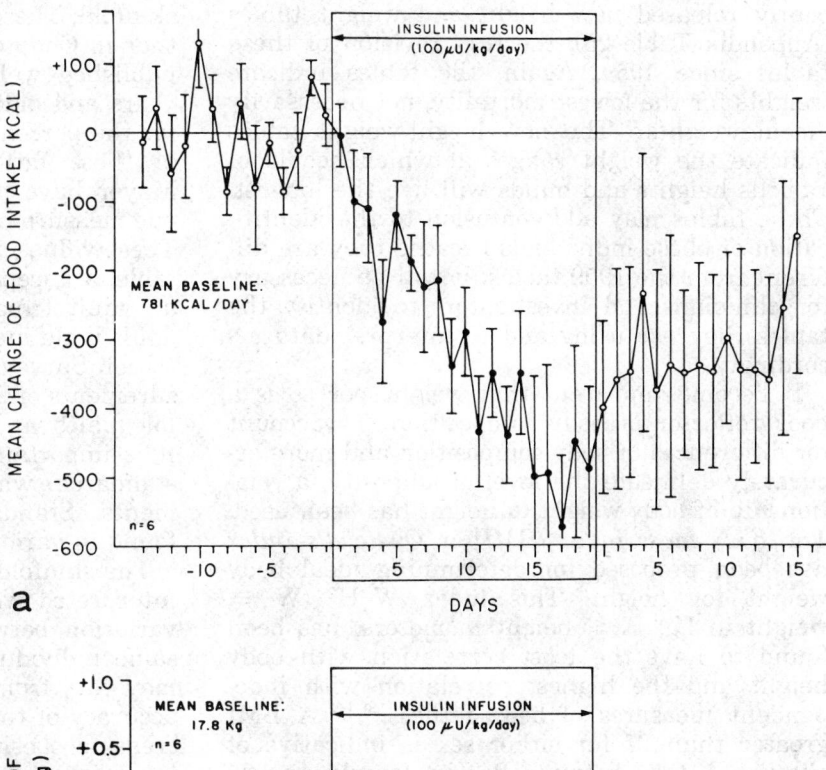

Figure 27-3. *a*, The effect of intraventricular insulin (100 μU./kg./day) on food intake in free-feeding baboons. Note the progressive effect of a constant infusion and the delayed recovery time. *b*, The effect of intraventricular insulin (100 μU./kg./day) on body weight. Note that body weight recovers sooner than food intake. (From Porte, D., Jr., and Woods, S. C.: Insulin and food intake, regulation of food intake and body weight by insulin. *Diabetologia*, 20:274, 1981.)

the tables requires the assessment of frame size. When the tables were first developed, *frame size* was arbitrarily defined and no standard method was designated by which to assess it. In the 1983 edition frame size is determined using elbow breadth as described in Appendix 26.

To deal with this problem, an adaptation of this table may be used in which the mean weight for the medium frame size is used as a reference point, with acceptable body weight ranging between the lowest level for the small frame and the highest level for the large frame. Appendix Table 27 gives these norms. Individuals above the upper limits of this top weight for height may be classified as overweight. These upper limits are approximately 15 per cent above median weight for medium frame size.

Third, use of these standards makes it difficult to distinguish if an individual who is "overweight" according to these standards is, in fact, "overfat." Differences in skeletal size and

weight can contribute to variations in body weight among individuals of similar height, as can lean body mass. Increased muscular development can increase body weight above the standard weight without the individual being obese. Athletes (e.g., football players) may be classified as overweight secondary to excess muscle mass rather than adipose mass. However, in most cases, people who are overweight according to the tables are obese, and the excess weight is fat relative to lean body mass.

Fourth, a person within the proper weight range may have excess body fat and lower than optimal lean body mass, and in fact be obese despite a normal body weight.

Fifth, the standards merely indicate the weight ranges at which people of various heights and builds will have the lowest mortality and do not necessarily represent "ideal" weights.

The Metropolitan Life Insurance Company recently released new height and weight tables (Appendix Table 25), the first revision of these tables since 1959. Again, the tables indicate weights for the lowest mortality, not necessarily "ideal weights." The new height-weight tables indicate the weight ranges at which people of various heights and builds will live the longest. These tables may add confusion to the identification of obese individuals because they are different from the 1959 tables. It will be necessary for clinicians and investigators to identify the tables they are using and to interpret data accordingly.

It becomes apparent that weight per se is a poor reflector of body composition. To account for differences in body composition and more accurately delineate the level of adiposity, a relationship of body weight to height has been used. The *body mass index (BMI)* or *Quetelet's index* has been proposed for determining ideal body weight for height. This index W/H^2 (W = weight in kg; H = height in meters) has been found to have the least correlation with body height and the highest correlation with independent measures of body fatness.[46, 47] A BMI greater than 27 for either sex is indicative of obesity. A BMI between 24 (for females) or 25 (for males) and 27 is defined as overweight, not obesity.[16] Table 27–1 gives the body mass indexes for several heights and weights.[17]

Thus, one may compare the body weights of individuals by using standard weight tables or a body mass index such as W/H^2. As stated earlier, individuals have been arbitrarily classified as obese if they are 20 per cent above "ideal" weight or have a BMI greater than 30. Clearly, there is no single definition of obesity and it is difficult to assess adiposity accurately on the basis of height and weight. Since obesity is defined as an excess of body fat, this parameter should be assessed as accurately as possible.

Methods are available by which body fat can be accurately determined. Two methods that are quite accurate but clinically impractical are underwater weighing and measurement of total body potassium. These methods are utilized primarily for research purposes. In addition there are many other less well known methods that are used for research purposes.

A method that is practical in a clinical setting is measurement of the subcutaneous fat. From measurement of fat just under the skin, called the fatfold or skinfold, the amount of total body fat can be estimated, assuming that 50 per cent of body fat is subcutaneous. To improve the accuracy of the assessment of body fat, it is recommended that the fatfold be measured at several sites on the body. The most common measurements are the triceps skinfold, biceps skinfold, subscapular skinfold and suprailiac

skinfold. These measurements are discussed further in Chapter 9. Durnin and Womersley have published well-accepted standards for men 17 years and older and women 16 years and older for the percentage of body fat based on the sum of these fatfold measurements.[29] Seltzer and Mayer have published standards based on just one measurement, that of the triceps skinfold.[78,79] These values are given in Table 27–2. Using this table, a triceps skinfold of 28 mm. or greater in an adult female and 16 mm. or greater in an adult male indicates obesity. The Ten State Nutrition Survey, 1968–1970, used the triceps measurements of 25.1 mm. for females and 18.6 mm. for males as indicative of obesity in adults.[91] It is important to use sex- and age-appropriate standards when evaluating fatfold measurements. Standards for use with children are found in various references.[28, 33, 61]

The skinfold thickness measurements must be interpreted with caution because there can be variation between measurements done on the same individual, and methods of measurement may vary from those used in the standards. The accuracy of the measurement decreases with increasing obesity secondary to the compressibility of fat and difficulty in getting an accurate measurement of subcutaneous fat.

At present there is no simple, precise and clinically useful method by which to assess body composition. To assess obesity, one must rely on as many parameters as possible. As technology becomes more advanced, it is projected that new methods will be developed by which body composition can be accurately and simply determined.

Types of Obesity

Obesity might be classified as either "exogenous," meaning that it is caused by excessive energy intake, or "endogenous," meaning there is an inherent metabolic problem that promoted the obesity. Examples of endogenous obesity are certain clinical conditions in which the appetite is abnormally elevated or the energy intake for weight maintenance is much lower than normal. Syndromes in this category of obesity include the Prader-Willi syndrome, Laurence-Moon-Biedl syndrome, Cushing's syndrome, or hyperphagia resulting from a tumor affecting the hypothalamus. However, it has recently been questioned whether "exogenous" obesity truly exists because all obesity may be "endogenous" and explained by metabolic differences in otherwise normal people.

Physiologically, obesity can be categorized on the basis of adipose cellularity. Fat cells may increase in number (hyperplasia) or size (hypertro-

Table 27-1. BODY MASS INDEX*†

Height (Inches)	Height (Meters)	45.3 (100)	49.90 (110)	54.43 (120)	58.97 (130)	63.50 (140)	68.04 (150)	72.57 (160)	77.11 (170)	81.65 (180)	86.18 (190)	90.72 (200)	95.25 (210)	99.79 (220)	104.33 (230)	108.86 (240)	113.40 (250)	117.93 (260)	122.47 (270)	127.01 (280)	131.54 (290)	136.08 (300)
55	1.397	23.24	25.56	27.89	30.21	32.54	34.86	37.19	39.51	41.84												
56	1.422	22.43	24.67	26.92	29.16	31.40	33.65	35.89	38.13	40.37	42.62											
57	1.448	21.64	23.80	25.96	28.13	30.29	32.46	34.62	36.79	38.95	41.12	43.28										
58	1.473	20.90	22.99	25.08	27.17	29.26	31.35	33.44	35.53	37.62	39.71	41.80	43.89									
59	1.498	20.20	22.22	24.24	26.26	28.28	30.29	32.32	34.33	36.35	38.37	40.39	42.41	44.43								
60	1.524	19.53	21.48	23.43	25.39	27.34	29.29	31.25	33.20	35.15	37.11	39.06	41.01	42.96	44.92	46.87	48.82	50.78	52.73	54.68	56.64	58.59
61	1.549	18.89	20.78	22.67	24.56	26.45	28.34	30.23	32.12	34.01	35.90	37.79	39.68	41.57	43.46	45.35	47.24	49.13	51.02	52.90	54.79	56.68
62	1.575	18.29	20.12	21.95	23.78	25.61	27.44	29.26	31.09	32.92	34.75	36.58	38.41	40.24	42.07	43.90	45.72	47.55	49.38	51.21	53.04	54.87
63	1.600	17.71	19.48	21.26	23.03	24.80	26.57	28.34	30.11	31.88	33.66	35.43	37.20	38.97	40.74	42.51	44.28	46.06	47.83	49.60	51.37	53.14
64	1.626	17.16	18.88	20.60	22.31	24.03	25.75	27.46	29.18	30.90	32.61	34.33	36.05	37.76	39.48	41.20	42.91	44.63	46.34	48.06	49.78	51.49
65	1.651	16.64	18.30	19.97	21.63	23.30	24.96	26.62	28.29	29.95	31.62	33.28	34.94	36.61	38.27	39.94	41.60	43.26	44.93	46.59	48.26	49.92
66	1.676	16.14	17.75	19.37	20.98	22.60	24.21	25.82	27.44	29.05	30.67	32.28	33.89	35.51	37.12	38.74	40.35	41.96	43.58	45.19	46.81	48.42
67	1.702	15.66	17.23	18.79	20.36	21.93	23.49	25.06	26.62	28.19	29.76	31.32	32.89	34.46	36.02	37.59	39.15	40.72	42.29	43.85	45.42	46.99
68	1.727	15.20	16.72	18.24	19.77	21.29	22.81	24.33	25.85	27.37	28.89	30.41	31.93	33.45	34.97	36.49	38.01	39.53	41.05	42.57	44.09	45.61
69	1.753	14.77	16.24	17.72	19.20	20.67	22.15	23.63	25.10	26.58	28.06	29.53	31.01	32.49	33.96	35.44	36.92	38.39	39.87	41.35	42.82	44.30
70	1.778	14.35	15.78	17.22	18.65	20.09	21.52	22.96	24.39	25.83	27.26	28.70	30.13	31.57	33.00	34.44	35.87	37.30	38.74	40.17	41.61	43.04
71	1.803		15.34	16.74	18.13	19.52	20.92	22.32	23.71	25.10	26.50	27.89	29.29	30.68	32.08	33.47	34.87	36.26	37.66	39.05	40.45	41.84
72	1.829		14.92	16.27	17.63	18.99	20.34	21.70	23.05	24.41	25.77	27.12	28.48	29.84	31.19	32.55	33.90	35.26	36.62	37.97	39.33	40.69
73	1.854		14.51	15.83	17.15	18.47	19.79	21.11	22.43	23.75	25.07	26.39	27.71	29.02	30.34	31.66	32.98	34.30	35.62	36.94	38.26	39.58
74	1.879		14.12	15.41	16.69	17.97	19.26	20.54	21.83	23.11	24.39	25.68	26.96	28.25	29.53	30.81	32.10	33.38	34.66	35.95	37.23	38.52
75	1.905			14.99	16.25	17.50	18.75	20.00	21.25	22.50	23.75	25.00	26.25	27.49	28.75	30.00	31.25	32.50	33.75	35.00	36.25	37.50
76	1.930			14.61	15.82	17.04	18.26	19.47	20.69	21.91	23.13	24.34	25.56	26.78	27.99	29.21	30.43	31.65	32.86	34.08	35.30	36.52

WEIGHT, kg. (lb.)

* From Bray, G.A., et al.: Evaluation of the obese patient. 1. An algorithm. JAMA, 235:1487, 1976.
† Expressed as weight (kg.)/height (meters)².

Table 27–2. OBESITY STANDARDS
FOR CAUCASIAN AMERICANS
(MINIMUM TRICEPS SKINFOLD
THICKNESS IN MILLIMETERS
INDICATING OBESITY)*†

AGE (YEARS)	SKINFOLD MEASURE-MENTS	
	Males	*Females*
5	12	14
6	12	15
7	13	16
8	14	17
9	15	18
10	16	20
11	17	21
12	18	22
13	18	23
14	17	23
15	16	24
16	15	25
17	14	26
18	15	27
19	15	27
20	16	28
21	17	28
22	18	28
23	18	28
24	19	28
25	20	29
26	20	29
27	21	29
28	22	29
29	23	29
30–50	23	30

*From Seltzer, C. C., and Mayer, J.: A simple criterion of obesity. Postgrad. Med., *38*: 101A, 1965. © McGraw-Hill, Inc.

†Figures represent the logarithmic means of the frequency distributions plus one standard deviation.

phy), as indicated in Table 27–3. In some forms of obesity there is a greater number of fat cells than there would be at normal weight *(hyperplastic)*. There may also be a combination of enlarged fat cells with an increased number of fat cells, which is classified *hyperplastic-hypertrophic* obesity. This type of obesity usually begins in childhood, and the fat tends to be distributed over the entire body. This obesity tends to be associated with fewer metabolic aberrations than later onset or adult-onset obesity. *Hypertrophic*

Table 27–3. MORPHOLOGICAL TYPES OF OBESITY

	HYPERTROPHIC	HYPERPLASTIC-HYPERTROPHIC
Cell size	↑	↑ ↑
Cell number	Normal	↑ ↑
Severity	Moderate	Marked
Age of onset	As adult	As child
Fat distribution	Central	Central and peripheral

obesity is associated with an enlargement of existing fat cells, and the number of fat cells is not significantly greater than the number of fat cells seen in the normal weight person. This form of obesity is characterized by a fat distribution that is more central over the body, and it is commonly associated with metabolic disorders such as hyperinsulinemia, non-insulin-dependent diabetes mellitus, hyperlipidemia, abnormal glucose tolerance or hypertension.

It is difficult to make a specific diagnosis of obesity type in a clinical setting. However, a presumptive diagnosis may be made based on age of obesity onset, the presence of metabolic findings such as abnormal glucose tolerance, elevated serum cholesterol and triglycerides, hypertension, and distribution of body fat.[15]

Diagnosis of the type of obesity may influence the goal and therapy for weight reduction. Weight reduction to the point where the adipose cells have a normal lipid content is a possible goal for all obese people. In those individuals with adult-onset obesity, this goal may mean achievement of ideal body weight as determined by the standards of weight for height or skinfold thicknesses. The same goal in the person with an increased number of fat cells may not result in ideal weight as defined by traditional standards. Perhaps the realistic therapy goal should be weight reduction to the point where fat cells are down to normal size and the metabolic abnormalities associated with obesity are corrected, even though this may not be ideal body weight.

Health Risks of Obesity

Obesity is associated with the presence of several diseases: hypertension, coronary heart disease, thrombophlebitis, diabetes mellitus, hyperlipidemia, respiratory disease, gallbladder disease and intestinal disorders. Obesity may increase mortality secondary to diseases associated with obesity. Obese individuals are also at greater risk for accidents, emotional disorders and social discrimination. However, obesity is not necessarily accompanied by these disorders and the disorders are not always accompanied by obesity.

As an individual gains weight, the following metabolic abnormalities associated with atherosclerosis often develop: hyperinsulinemia, impaired glucose tolerance, hyperlipidemia and hypertension. In the female, obesity also leads to the predisposition of toxemia of pregnancy, osteoarthritis, malignancy of the endometrium, menstrual abnormalities, ovarian dysfunction and breast cancer.

The Framingham study showed that each 10

per cent gain in weight in the males studied resulted in an average 6.6 mm. rise in blood pressure, an average 2 mg./dl. rise in blood glucose and an average 11 mg./dl. rise in blood cholesterol. In females, these changes were about half those in the males.[36] The mechanism by which excess storage of calories in the adipose tissue raises blood lipids, elevates blood pressure, impairs glucose tolerance and promotes hyperuricemia is not clear. Karam proposed that the enlargement of the fat cell and the resulting insulin resistance cause these changes.[44] However, with weight reduction, these metabolic abnormalities are reversed. Thus, some individuals with hypertension or adult-onset diabetes might be advised to lose weight before more aggressive therapies are employed in treatment.

Not all authorities are convinced that obesity is the medical health hazard it is thought to be.[56] Is obesity the cause of various disease states, or is it that individuals with a genetic propensity toward a specific disease also have a tendency to become obese? The confusion may exist due to the fact that obesity as a disease entity is not fully defined. Various types of obesity may be associated with different complications and problems.

In summary, obesity is associated with a number of health disorders and is considered to be a risk factor in a number of diseases as shown in Figure 27–4. Thus it can be concluded that obesity is harmful to health if it exacerbates other health problems (e.g., hypertension, glucose intolerance). If this is the case, weight loss is strongly advised.

Causes of Obesity

The cause of obesity is multifactorial and this issue is further complicated by the fact that there are, most likely, multiple forms of obesity.

NATURE VERSUS NURTURE

In humans, obesity appears to be more prevalent in some families and in some ethnic or social groups. The role genetics plays in the etiology of obesity is not clear; however, there is evidence supporting the fact that heredity is a contributor to the development of obesity.

It has been reported that a child has a 10 per cent chance of becoming obese if the parents are of normal weight, a 40 per cent chance if one parent is obese, and an 80 per cent chance if both parents are obese. Data from the Ten State Nutrition Survey demonstrated that children from two lean parents tended to be thin, whereas children from two obese parents tended to be fat.[34] Thus, there is substantial resemblance of body weight and fatness among family members.

Mono- and dizygotic twin studies have been conducted to distinguish between hereditary and environmental influences. Newman found larger average differences in body weight between identical twins raised apart as compared with those raised together. Greater differences in body weight were observed between fraternal versus identical twins.[59] This indicates that both environment and genetics play a role in body weight regulation. It has also been observed that fatfold thickness in dizygotic twins was three times more likely to differ when compared with that of monozygotic twins.[13]

The issue is clouded by environmental interactions, which may have a significant impact on the expression of obesity. Thus, genetics may provide an individual with a propensity toward obesity; the environment may act to suppress or express the genetic propensity.

ADIPOSE CELL SIZE AND NUMBER

Since obesity is characterized by an increase in adipose mass, it is necessary to achieve a

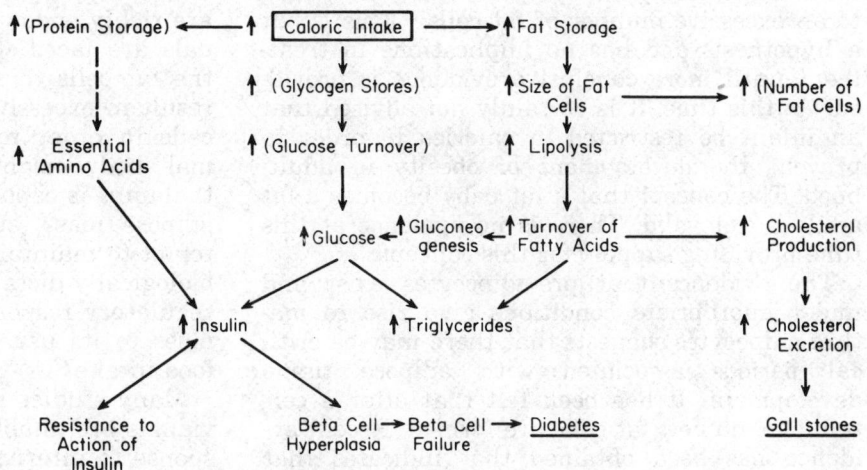

Figure 27–4. A schematic diagram for some of the metabolic consequences of ingesting excess calories. The parentheses and broken lines indicate uncertainty about the proposed metabolic changes. This diagram allows a formulation of the pathogenesis of gallstones and diabetes, two of the major diseases associated with obesity. (From Bray, G. A.: The Obese Patient. Philadelphia, W. B. Saunders Co., 1976, p. 265.)

more thorough understanding of the development of adipose tissue in order to distinguish between gene action and environmental impact. Such understanding may have future significance in obesity treatment.

As mentioned, adipose mass increases by either an increase in fat cell size or an increase in fat cell number, or both. In normal-weight children, fat cell size increases and fat cell number triples or quadruples between birth and two years of age.[40] In normal-weight children, fat cell number changes very little between two years of age and puberty. A further increase in fat cell number does not again occur until puberty.[50] Obese children, on the other hand, have a different pattern of adipose tissue development. An increase in fat cell number occurs during the period between two years of age and puberty. Additionally, obese children, older than two years of age, have increased fat cell size as compared with normal-weight children.[31,49]

Other observations in obese children suggest that two subpopulations exist: one in which obesity is evident by one year of age, and another in which it occurs later in childhood.[18] The earlier-onset group was characterized by elevated fat cell number. In this subpopulation, the obesity could not be controlled or reversed, fat cell number continued to increase, and postpubertal follow-up suggested that aggressive dietary restriction may have interfered with linear growth.[38, 53] Perhaps this type of obesity constitutes some form of inborn error characterized by resistant metabolic alterations.

The mechanisms involved in the development of excessive adiposity are not fully understood. There is evidence in animals and humans that pre-adipocytes, the precursors of adipocytes, exist and may be important in fat development.[92] One hypothesis states that these cells are formed early in infancy and become filled with fat. During this growth phase, if there is excessive energy intake, there is a greater deposition of fat into these pre-adipocytes, which may lead to an excessive number of fat cells.[71] This is but a hypothesis and has no implications in treatment until more conclusive evidence is provided. At this time, it is certainly not advised that an infant be restricted in calories in order to prevent the development of obesity in adulthood. The concept that a fat baby becomes a fat adult is not valid. There is no evidence at this time providing support for this concept.

The evidence that pre-adipocytes exist and under appropriate conditions give rise to mature adipocytes suggests that there may be critical periods associated with adipose tissue development. It has been felt that after a certain age, no new fat cells are formed. Recent evidence has been obtained that indicates that new fat cells can be formed at an adult age in animals provided conditions are suitable.[7] There is some evidence of this in humans; however, further research is required before this can be substantiated.

Psychology of Obesity

The psychological approach to obesity assumes that hyperphagia is the primary cause of obesity. Included in this approach are the following concepts. Obese people eat in response to external cues and there is no metabolic basis promoting continuous overeating. Obese people respond to external cues and stimuli and eat even if satiated. They should eat less and lose weight when provided with different sources of stimulation.

EXTERNALITY THEORY

Data from Stunkard and Koch and from Schachter and coworkers support this "externality theory" as a cause of overeating and obesity development.[74, 88] Researchers found that obese people are relatively insensitive to "internal" cues of hunger and satiety and are more sensitive to "external" cues such as the smell, taste or sight of food or food-related activities. The obese are more likely to eat, or eat more than normal-weight people, when food-relevant cues are present than when they are not.

The psychological portrayal of the obese individual as being overresponsive to external cues and underresponsive to internal cues has come under scrutiny and reassessment. An alternative concept that has been developed to account for feeding behaviors in the obese individual is that of restrained and non-restrained eating.

RESTRAINED AND NON–RESTRAINED EATING

Nisbett proposed that some obese individuals are richly endowed with fat cells. These individuals are faced with two alternatives: (1) allow the fat cells to achieve repletion, which would result in excessive obesity; or (2) deplete the fat cells in order to attain and maintain a "normal" body weight and appearance.[60] If the hypothalamus is capable of sensing or regulating the adipose mass, such obese individuals who attempt to maintain a weight below that which is biologically dictated will risk activating counterregulatory responses aimed at returning the fat mass to its usual level. How would this affect food intake?

Many studies have suggested that obese individuals are unable to regulate food intake in response to internal cues. Interestingly, the obese consumed somewhat *more* after consuming a snack than after consuming nothing. This was in contrast to normal-weight subjects who showed a significant decrease in intake following a snack.[74] However, one must consider that many obese individuals are ordinarily dieting in an attempt to lose weight or maintain a new low weight, and this may influence feeding behavior.

Perhaps any individual who is suppressing his or her weight should demonstrate "obese" eating patterns. This was assessed in normal-weight individuals who differed only in the degree to which they demonstrated evidence of dieting or weight suppression.[39] Food intake was measured after a preload drink. As expected, the *restrained eaters* (the dieters or weight suppressors) resembled Schachter's obese subjects— they failed to compensate for the preload in their total energy intake. Subjects forced to drink milkshakes ate more ad libitum than those who did not drink milkshakes. The *unrestrained eaters* (non-dieters) demonstrated a fair degree of caloric compensation after the preload. Thus, unrestrained subjects compensated, whereas restrained subjects, even though of normal weight, counterregulated. It appears that obese individuals fail to show compensatory responses to a preload only to the extent that they are dieters. Obese dieters differ little from dieters of normal weight. It is theorized that when given a preload, dieters become disinhibited and eat unrestrainedly.

The concept of restrained eating may be able to explain a number of "obese behaviors." There is increased evidence that restrained eaters are overly emotional and overreactive relative to non-restrained eaters. Such behaviors appear to be related to dieting, not to obesity per se. The obese individual tends to be continuously worrying about or attempting to diet, and thus is in a continual restrained eating pattern. This restraint continues to be necessary in order to maintain a new reduced body weight. This can be a stressor and, clearly, the turmoil that confronts the obese and reducing individual must be contemplated. It appears that dieting and stress are related; thus, awareness of this emotional state must be appreciated in the obese individual attempting to lose weight. Within this milieu of factors, feeding behavior and body weight regulation are interrelated physiologically and psychologically. It is this concept that researchers and clinicians must now contend with.

SOCIAL DISCRIMINATION

The obese are subject to severe discrimination. Ironically, they are the "afflicted" in a society that encourages eating so very much. Fashion trends, insurance programs, college placements, and employment opportunities all discriminate against the obese person. The obese person learns self-defeating and self-degrading social responses. The person may come to believe that fat is "bad," and this leads to a vicious cycle of low self-esteem, depression, overeating for consolation, increased fatness, social rejection and further lowering of self-esteem.[30]

Physiology of the Obese State

The adipose mass is in a continuous dynamic process of fat storage and fat release. The first process involves the uptake of triglyceride from the blood stream under the influence of the enzyme *adipose tissue lipoprotein lipase (AT–LPL)*. This enzyme is produced by the adipose cell and has its site of action on the surface of the blood capillary endothelium close to the adipose cell. It acts to hydrolyze triglycerides from chylomicrons and very low density lipoproteins into free fatty acids and free glycerol. Fatty acids pass into the fat cell to be re-esterified into triglyceride; glycerol proceeds to the liver.

Since lipoprotein lipase is associated with the transport of energy into the fat cell, it may be speculated whether it has any significance in obesity. Moderately elevated levels of AT–LPL per fat cell have been observed in obese adults.[67] This enzyme initially falls with fasting in obese subjects but begins to increase with prolonged dieting.[63] More important, it has been demonstrated that reduced obese individuals have AT–LPL levels severalfold greater than persons of normal weight[76] or greater than their non-reduced state levels.[77] It is postulated that this enzyme may be involved in a mechanism that accounts for the difficulty most previously obese persons have in maintaining a reduced weight. The high level of this enzyme, which promotes fat storage, works against maintenance of a reduced body weight and promotes the return of the fat cell to its original size.

Because the adipose mass is maintained at a relatively constant level over the long term, it is felt that the adipose mass is regulated by a sensitive feedback mechanism. What is the signal that is sensed, perhaps in the hypothalamus? Perhaps signals from the adipose mass or lean body mass are released when "normal" body composition is disturbed. The signal has not been identified, although several have been suggested: blood levels of free fatty acids or glycerol released from the adipose tissue during lipolysis, or serum insulin. Insulin may be a signal sensitive to fat mass that also has the potential of affecting food intake and thus body weight regulation.[65] At present, the mechanisms involved in regulation of adipose mass are far from understood.

There is a significant relationship between the degree of adiposity and fasting insulin levels. The more obese an animal or human, the higher the fasting insulin levels. However, many obese individuals appear to be insulin-resistant, as evidenced by an abnormal glucose tolerance curve. It seems that as fat cells enlarge, insulin sensitivity decreases.[72] This insulin resistance develops even in normal weight individuals who are forced to gain weight by excessive caloric intake. However, it is also known that administration of insulin to normal weight individuals can stimulate the appetite, leading to overeating and weight gain. Thus, it is not clear whether insulin levels determine adiposity or adiposity determines insulin levels, or if there is a more complex interaction. It is known, however, that insulin resistance, impaired glucose tolerance and associated hyperlipidemia can be corrected with weight loss.

A number of investigators suggest that total energy reserves are regulated. The *lipostatic theory* has been developed, which suggests that the hypothalamus is sensitive to the adipose mass and that there is a "lipostatic" regulation of food intake. Adipose reserves are "sensed" so that a constant body weight can be maintained by changes in physiological parameters, that is, absorption, metabolism or energy expenditure. Several types of evidence support this hypothesis. When human volunteers are force-fed to gain weight, they stop eating or reduce their daily intakes as soon as the force-feeding stops, and they return to their normal weight.[82] In animals with a lesion of the ventromedial hypothalamus that results in hyperphagia and weight gain, the animals overeat but the intake gradually tapers off and stabilizes. At a new elevated weight, food intake is just sufficient to maintain the new weight. More impressive is that the new weight is defended from deviations secondary to energy restriction or overfeeding. It appears as if the body has assumed a higher "set point," often termed the "ponderostat" for adipose reserves.

The lipostatic theory may have significance for formerly obese individuals who have difficulty maintaining a new reduced weight. Studies suggest that while the adipose cell size decreases with weight loss, the adipose cell number does not. When individuals lose weight, their fat cells may be "starving" and they may experience extreme hunger symptoms. Losing weight may not be normal for these people, and at the reduced weight they may be in a chronic, starvation-like state in which they are genuinely hungry.[60] It is theorized that their bodies are meant to have a certain amount of fat and their bodies constantly try to maintain or regain that "setpoint" of fat stores during periods of re-

duced energy intake. Thus, maintenance of a weight below that which the body metabolically prefers is difficult. Even though obese, an individual may be at his or her biologically normal weight.

THERMOGENESIS

Thermogenesis is the ability of the body to get rid of excess energy through heat production. It can be exercise-induced, cold-induced or diet-induced. In the normal person, there is an increase in metabolic rate after eating that is thought to be related to thermogenesis. This phenomenon was demonstrated in subjects who were force-fed in order to gain weight. Subjects consumed 7000 to 10,000 kcal. per day for periods of 200 days or more. Normal subjects who were forced to gain weight required more kcal. per kg. to maintain their new higher weight than their old baseline weight, implying that calories were being "wasted."[82]

Animal studies suggest that the mechanism of diet-induced thermogenesis is the same as that for non-shivering thermogenesis (NST), which occurs in brown adipose tissue (BAT) and allows animals and young infants to maintain body temperature.

Some investigators have shown that the obese have a reduced thermogenic response to eating while others have shown a normal response. Jung has shown that some obese humans show a blunted thermogenic response to the catecholamine norepinephrine, which stimulates thermogenesis.[43] It is not clear what relevance these observations have in energy balance; however, differences in thermogenic responses among individuals may explain why some can overeat and not gain weight while others cannot. The concept of thermogenesis gives rise to an important question: Is obesity secondary to an increase in food intake and/or more efficient utilization of energy?

Evidence has been obtained suggesting that a specific metabolic derangement underlies the "cause" of obesity. The enzyme sodium-potassium activated Mg^{2+}–dependent adenosine triphosphatase ($Na^+ + K^+ + Mg^{2+}$–ATPase) is the enzyme involved in the active transport of Na^+ out of and K^+ into cells. Because of this role, it is more commonly known as the Na^+K^+ *pump ATPase*. ATPase enzymes split ATP, thus they "burn" energy. If there were fewer Na^+K^+ pump units, it is possible that less energy would be burned; conversely, increased ATPase-mediated energy consumption would "waste" energy.

DeLuise and coworkers[23] measured the number of Na^+K^+ pumps or ATPase units in the red blood cells of 21 obese subjects and found that they had an average of 22 per cent fewer as compared with those of non-obese controls. The absolute number of pump sites was negatively correlated with the percentage of ideal body weight. This study suggested that fewer ATP-burning pump sites would lead to less energy consumption; this might be a metabolic abnormality leading to obesity.

It may be that thermogenic factors play a role in weight maintenance when individuals attempt to maintain a weight different from that normally maintained. Greater efficiency in energy metabolism has been shown to occur during weight loss[26] as illustrated in Figure 27–5. Does this reduction in metabolic rate persist in reduced obese individuals, and could this be responsible for the clinical observations that reduced obese individuals are more energy efficient than their lean counterparts who have not lost weight? One study concludes that there is a reduction in energy requirements for weight maintenance after weight loss relative to baseline weight. However, the resting metabolic rates of the reduced obese subjects are similar to those of subjects of comparable weight who have not reduced.[25] This suggests that there are no differences in energy efficiency between the two groups. However, is the resting metabolic rate an accurate indicator of energy efficiency? This study cannot conclude that the reduced obese individual is not more energy efficient; perhaps some other unmeasured parameter is responsible for the energy efficiency that appears to exist in the reduced obese individuals.

Do obese individuals require less energy for weight maintenance than do lean individuals? Some studies suggest that obese individuals require less energy for weight maintenance; however, it may be that lean individuals are more active than obese individuals are and consequently require more energy. More likely it is body composition that makes a difference. An inverse relationship does exist between kcal./kg. and degree of adiposity as determined by percentage of ideal body weight or relative body weight (RBW) as shown in Figure 27–6. Thus, on a per kilogram basis, an obese individual may require 20 kcal./kg., whereas a lean individual may require 30 to 35 kcal./kg. However, if obese and lean individuals are compared on the basis of lean body mass, they do not differ in energy efficiency. It is becoming evident that lean body mass is a major determinant of caloric requirements.

THYROID HORMONE

Thyroid hormone is a principal hormone regulating basal metabolism. Peripheral thyroid metabolism has been shown to be affected by energy restriction and energy excess.

In severe caloric restriction, metabolically active serum 3,3',5-triiodothyronine (T_3) decreases

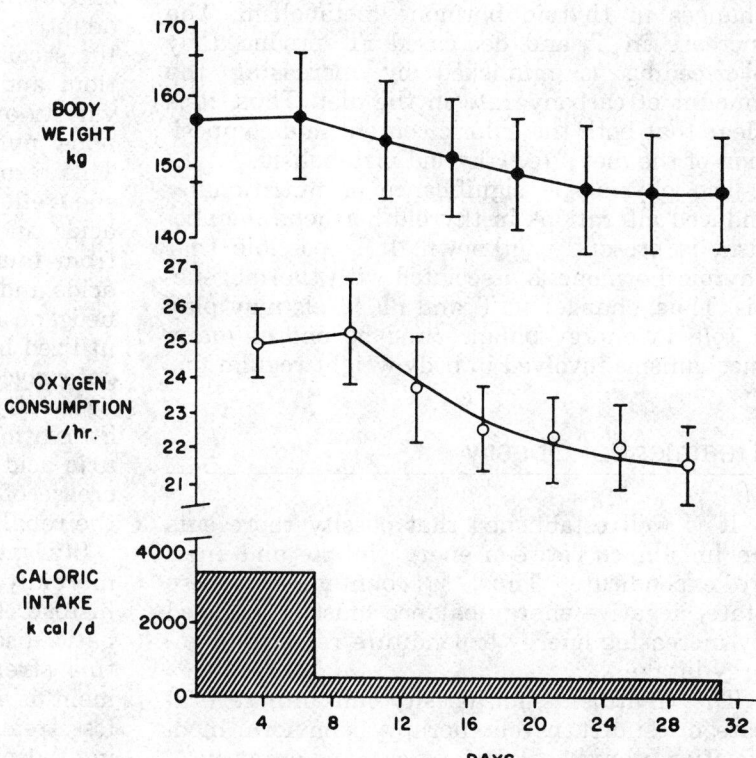

Figure 27–5. Oxygen consumption in six obese patients during caloric restriction. After 7 days on a 3500 calorie diet, intake was restricted to 450 calories and maintained for an additional 24 days. By the end of this period, the decline in oxygen consumption approximated 17 per cent of the prerestriction values, while body weight had declined less than 3 per cent. (From Bray, G. A.: Effect of caloric restriction on energy expenditure in obese patients. Lancet, 2:397, 1969.)

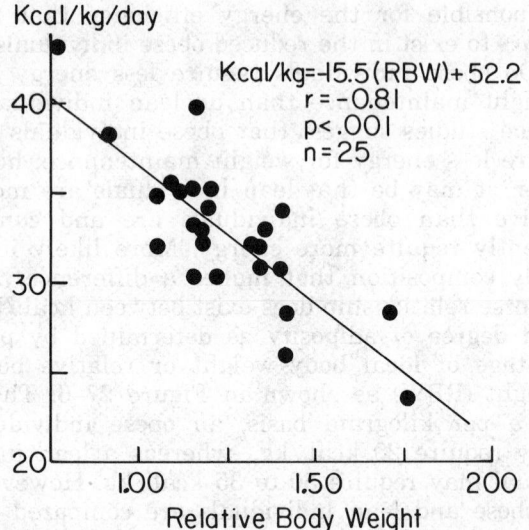

Figure 27–6. An inverse relationship exists between the energy requirement (kcal./kg.) and the degree of adiposity as determined by percentage ideal body weight or relative body weight in the obese.

and increases upon refeeding. Studies have demonstrated that severe caloric deprivation is associated with a decrease in metabolically active serum T_3 mirrored by an increase in metabolically inactive reverse $3,3',5'$-triiodothyronine (rT_3). The opposite occurs when lean or obese individuals are overfed.

The carbohydrate content of the diet may also play an important role in these dietary-induced changes in thyroid hormone metabolism. The increase in T_3 and decreased rT_3 produced by overfeeding is mimicked by increasing the amount of carbohydrate in the diet. Thus, it is clear that both the caloric content and composition of the diet affect thyroid metabolism.

The physiologic significance of nutritionally induced alterations in thyroid hormone metabolism is presently unknown. It is possible that thyroid hormone is associated with thermogenesis. Thus, changes in T_3 and rT_3 levels may play a role in energy balance and be one of many mechanisms involved in body weight regulation.

Treatment of Obesity

It is well established that obesity represents an imbalance between energy intake and energy expenditure. Thus, to counter the obese state, negative energy balance must be induced by increasing energy expenditure relative to energy intake.

The treatments for obesity fall into several categories: diet, psychotherapy, behavioral modification, pharmacology, exercise and surgery.

DIET

There are several dietary approaches to obesity treatment that are summarized in Table 27–4. Diets range from starvation to a high-protein–low-carbohydrate diet, to a high-carbohydrate–low-fat diet, to a low-calorie balanced diet. The lay literature abounds with reports of "scientific discoveries" that promise to help the obese shed pounds in a number of days as shown in Figure 27–7. These diets are followed by numerous overweight individuals, and the obese individual spends large amounts of money and potentially endangers health in the attempt to cure the affliction of obesity.

Starvation or Fasting

Fasting is a severe, aggressive treatment for obesity resulting in rapid weight loss. Losses of 4 to 8 lb. in the first 24 hours in the initial stages of a fast are largely due to loss of water and sodium. As the diet continues, nitrogen losses (from muscle catabolism) tend to increase while the loss of water and sodium decreases. By 2 to 3 weeks, the rate of nitrogen loss decreases as the body begins to use fatty acids for energy, and the person maintains a low steady nitrogen loss.

During fasting, the major metabolic fuel is from the adipose tissue. An adaptive process occurs in which tissues other than the brain derive their energy primarily from fatty acids, and even the brain can to some degree. This adaptive process is exerted principally by insulin, secondarily by insulin and glucagon interaction, and by "permissive" effects from a wide variety of other hormones. An absence of exogenous nutrients leads to lower insulin levels. This results in increased lipolysis in adipose tissue (reflected by increased circulating free fatty acids and glycerol) and release of amino acids from muscle protein. The liver takes up fatty acids and amino acids for ketogenesis and gluconeogenesis as shown in Figure 27–8. Glucose is utilized by the central nervous system and obligate glycolytic tissues; the rest of the body utilizes fatty acids and ketones to a lesser extent. Starvation is accompanied by increased serum uric acid levels resulting primarily from an increase of urinary ketones, which interfere with the renal clearance of uric acid.

Starvation treatment is used primarily for the morbidly obese individual. Individuals with a history of gout or cardiac, renal, cerebral or hepatic disorders are not suitable candidates for this strenuous treatment. This form of treatment is not recommended as a routine weight loss treatment; if prescribed, it should be given in a hospital under strict medical supervision.

Table 27–4. EVALUATION OF SOME COMMON DIETS

TYPE OF DIET	COMMENT
Dr. Atkins Revolutionary Diet	A variant of the low-carbohydrate, high-protein diet. An unlimited amount of protein and fat is allowed, while carbohydrate intake is severely limited. This high-protein diet may result in up to an 8 lb. weight loss within the first week; this is largely water. When carbohydrates are added to the diet, this lost weight is regained. This diet is high in total fat, saturated fats and cholesterol. It is harmful to people with undiagnosed kidney disease and may precipitate gout due to increased uric acid levels.
Dr. Atkins Super Energy Weight Reduction Diet	This diet is a variation of the Dr. Atkins Revolutionary Diet. Megavitamin and mineral supplements are added with the claim that they can prevent or cure abnormal sugar metabolism, hypoglycemia, allergies and other problems. There is no evidence these supplements aid in weight loss.
Banana Milk Diet (also known as The Johns Hopkins Diet)	This diet contains 6 bananas plus 3 glasses of milk/day. The diet provides less than 1000 kcal./day. It is nutritionally unbalanced; vitamin and mineral supplements are recommended. It is not endorsed by Johns Hopkins University.
Beverly Hills Diet	For the first 10 days of this diet, the dieter eats nothing but fruit in a specific order on specific days. Owing to the high fruit and fiber intake, this diet results in flatus and is also known as the "diarrhea diet." It is low in protein, vitamins and minerals, such as iron, zinc, calcium and magnesium. It is nutritionally unsound.
Calories Don't Count	This diet is extremely high in fat and protein. Emphasis is placed on consuming large amounts of meat and milk products, avoiding sugars and starches including most fruits, breads and cereals. The dieter must consume approximately 1/3 cup of vegetable oil high in polyunsaturated fat each day.
The Cambridge Diet	This is a formula diet sold by "Cambridge counselors." Total daily intake is 330 calories composed of 33 gm. protein, approximately 40 gm. carbohydrate and 3 gm. fat. It is too drastic of a diet to be used without medical supervision.
Kempner Rice Diet or Duke University Rice Diet	This diet consists of very large amounts of cooked rice, fruits and vegetables. It is very low in sodium and low in protein, vitamin A, riboflavin, Ca^{2+} and Fe^{2+}. No foods from the milk or meat groups of the Basic Four are permitted.
Last Chance Re-feeding Diet	This diet is very low in CHO. A special formula (Pro Linn, a high-protein powder) is required as well as food. The diet begins with a fast using Pro Linn. During the fast, vitamin and mineral supplements, K^+ and folic acid are prescribed with at least 2 quarts of non-caloric fluids/day. Gradually food is re-introduced. This is the re-feeding phase. The Pro Linn powder continues to be used twice/day. Intakes of vitamin A, riboflavin, thiamin, iron and calcium are inadequate. ***This diet is hazardous to use without medical supervision.***
Lecithin, B_6, Apple-Cider Vinegar and Kelp Diet	This low-calorie diet calls for 2 tbsp. lecithin/day to help emulsify body fat; B_6 to help metabolize body fat; 1 tbsp. apple-cider vinegar after each meal to add potassium to the diet and because vinegar and fat do not mix; kelp is used to provide iodine to speed up metabolism. This diet is an exaggeration of physiological reality; it does not speed up weight loss.
Macrobiotics	This is a system of diets that relies primarily on whole-grain cereal, fish and selected vegetables. This diet will result in a lack of nutrients such as protein, calcium and vitamins A, D and C, and may result in pronounced nutritional deficiencies such as scurvy.
The Magic Mayo Diet (or Grapefruit Diet)	This diet recommends half a grapefruit or grapefruit juice with every meal, allows unlimited amounts of meat, fish and eggs, and limits sugars and starches. The grapefruit is claimed to act as a catalyst to actively burn fat. This is untrue. The diet is high in saturated fats and cholesterol and may be excessively low in carbohydrates. It is not endorsed by the Mayo Clinic in Rochester, Minnesota.

Table continued on the following page

Table 27–4. EVALUATION OF SOME COMMON DIETS *(Continued)*

TYPE OF DIET	COMMENT
Pritikin Diet	This diet is extremely low in fat—only 10% of total kcal. It is also low in salt and refined CHO. The diet forbids butter, margarine, oils, grain-fed beef, sugar and products containing them. The types of food allowed meet the Basic Four but large emphasis is placed on fruits, vegetables, breads and cereals. Dairy products are forbidden unless made with skim milk. The diet is slightly low in iron.
Scarsdale Diet	This diet is a version of a crash diet that is to be used for 14 days only and is "guaranteed' to cause a weight loss of 20 lb. It is low in CHO (about 50 gm./day) and energy content, thus is ketogenic; constraints are made on fluid intake, which is limited to tea or coffee. The diet is low in iron, vitamin A, calcium and riboflavin. It is low in milk, breads and cereals. Danger of dehydration is high. *This diet is dangerous without medical supervision.*
Slim Chance in a Fat World	Balanced energy sources; this diet places heavy emphasis on behavior modification. If instructions are followed, nutrient needs other than energy will be met.
The Southampton Diet	This diet, developed by a physician, claims to be effective because the dieter is encouraged to eat "happy" foods and to avoid "sad" foods that may lead to depression. It is based on the information concerning the neurotransmitters and their precursors but there is no evidence yet that allows this information to be applied in this way. Although the basis for the diet has no validity, it is a well-balanced diet.
Stillman Diet or The Doctor's Quick Weight Loss Diet	This diet consists of low-fat cheeses, lean meat, fish, poultry, eggs and 8 glasses of water per day. Neither milk nor visible fats are permitted. The diet fails to meet the Basic Four for either fruits and vegetables or breads and cereals since none are allowed. Vitamins A, C, thiamin and iron are low in the diet. A multivitamin pill is suggested.
Weight-Watchers Diet Plan	This diet was developed by a noted nutritionist and physician. It is nutritionally sound and has 3 basic programs—reducing, leveling and maintenance. Techniques of behavior modification are used with weekly meeting groups; exercise is also incorporated into the program.

Protein-Sparing Modified Fast

Some fasting regimens include supplementation with 40 gm. to 100 gm. protein per day—1.3 to 1.5 gm./kg. ideal body weight. The rationale for this treatment is to replace muscle and visceral protein (i.e., lean body mass) that is being metabolized for energy. This dietary treatment is referred to as a "protein-sparing modified fast" (PSMF).[11,52,69] Supplementation with vitamins and minerals, especially potassium, is also included in the regimen. Some well-supervised regimens also include exercise in order to promote retention of protein in muscle tissue. After the first week, when weight loss is rapid because of fluid loss, the fasting person loses 1/3 to 1/2 lb. (0.1 to 0.2 kg./day) even with an intake of 100 gm. protein/day.

Reportedly, the advantages of the PSMF are that appetite is suppressed[5] and that lean body mass, positive mood and well-being, and neuromuscular performance in sedentary work are maintained.[5] However, recent evidence shows that the PSMF does not decrease appetite or elevate mood.[70] Suppression of appetite does not appear to be a sufficient reason alone for using diets of this type.

The safety of the PSMF has also been questioned.[85] A number of individuals on this diet died of ventricular arrhythmia. However, the cause of death could not be attributed to lack of potassium supplementation or absence of medical supervision and appears to be independent of the protein product used. Most of the subjects were consuming "liquid protein" (solutions of collagen hydrolysate to which varying amounts of tryptophan were added); however, two of the subjects had supplemented the liquid protein with protein products of higher biological value. The common features of the cases were marked obesity, extremely low energy intake (i.e., 300 kcal. per day) and sustained rapid weight loss. The consistent autopsy finding was

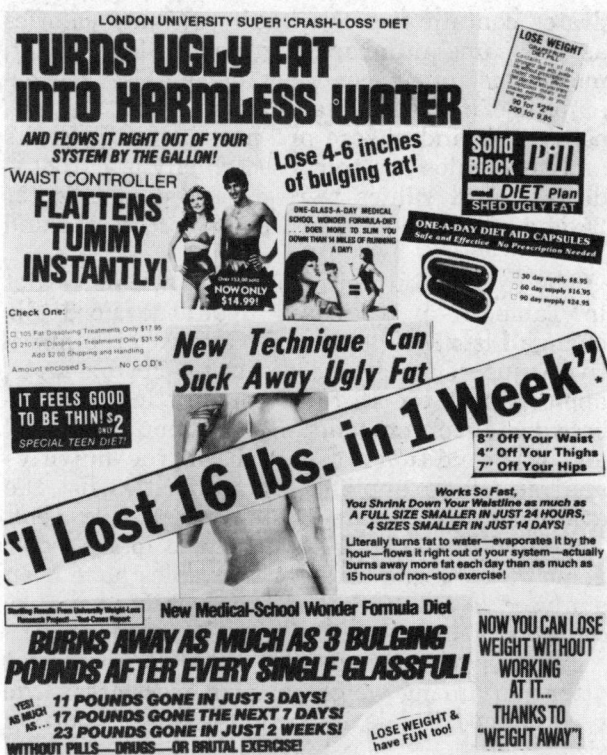

Figure 27–7. Examples of claims of weight loss products and programs featured in popular magazines. (From Story, M.: Adolescent Lifestyle and Eating Behavior, in Mahan, L. K., and Rees, J. M.: Nutrition in Adolescence. St. Louis, C. V. Mosby Company, 1984.)

myocardial atrophy, a condition fairly specific for protein-energy malnutrition. It is obvious that it is not known how much of an energy-protein deficit the obese body can tolerate for a period of time without side-effects. Could the deaths have been prevented by a modification of the diet, or were the deaths an inevitable outcome of prolonged periods of near starvation? Until these questions are fully answered, supplemented fasts should be implemented with great caution and prescribed only for the very obese.

High-Protein Diets

A diet that commonly reappears under different names is the high-protein, no- or low-carbohydrate, moderate- or high-fat diet. This type of diet usually contains 1000 kcal. or less with less than 50 gm. of carbohydrate and 120 gm. or more of protein. This nutrient composition coupled with energy restriction causes ketosis to develop. Individuals on these diets tend to lose weight rapidly during the first ten days to two weeks due to excessive water and sodium loss, and not all due to excessive fat loss.

Because such diets are very low in carbohydrate and calories, the body makes metabolic adjustments. In order to maintain blood glucose, the body metabolizes liver and muscle glycogen and muscle protein. Fat is also mobilized for energy, particularly after the first ten days. The liver is unable to oxidize fat completely, thus there is an accumulation of ketone bodies in the blood and urine as they are excreted. In addition, there is an increase in urinary nitrogen secondary to breakdown of muscle protein used for energy. A high water intake is required to enable the kidneys to excrete the increased levels of ketones and nitrogenous waste products properly. There is increased diuresis and water loss, which may be related to carbohydrate and insulin changes that affect renal sodium handling as well as excess ketone bodies; this diuresis is reflected in the initial rapid weight loss. As the body adapts in two to three weeks, water can be retained even to the point of causing a weight gain, while net losses of fat and protein continue.

The disadvantage of a diet that causes ketosis in the dieter is the risk of developing high uric acid levels and hypokalemia. The interaction of these two conditions with ketosis can lead to sudden death, as previously mentioned.

Balanced Energy Reduction

A balanced energy-restricted diet is the most reasonable method of weight reduction. Ideally, the diet should be nutritionally adequate except

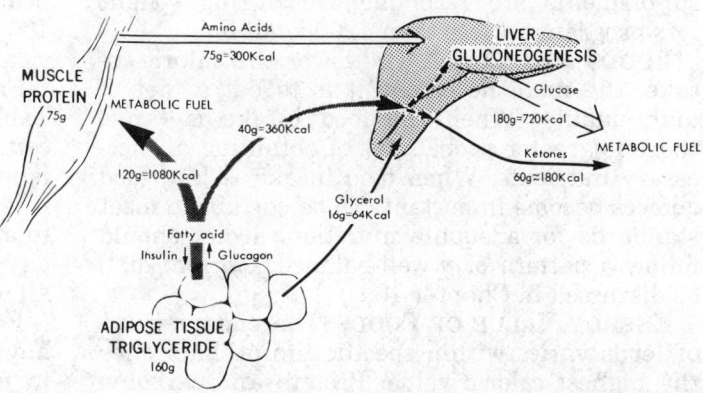

Figure 27–8. Summary of the fate of metabolic fuels during starvation. The liver takes up fatty acids and amino acids for ketogenesis and gluconeogenesis. (From Bray, G. (ed.): Recent Advances in Obesity Research: II. Proceedings of the 2nd International Congress on Obesity. Westport, Conn., Food and Nutrition Press, 1979.)

for energy. The number of calories must be decreased to the point where the body must mobilize fat stores to meet daily energy needs. The maximally restricted diet should have 100 gm. carbohydrate and 0.8 to 1.2 gm. protein/kg. ideal body weight. Fat should be restricted as much as possible, since, during weight loss, free fatty acids will be mobilized from adipose tissue. Weight loss on this type of regimen generally occurs at a rate of 0.5 to 2 lb. per week, but this is largely dependent on the energy intake. In such a dietary regimen, there is no increase in ketone bodies in the blood, thus minimizing serious side-effects as discussed previously.

The caloric value of body fat is approximately 3500 kcal./lb. Thus, if a person reduces daily caloric intake by 500 kcal./day, the weekly deficit will be 3500 kcal., or 1 lb. of weight loss. However, this 3500 kcal. figure is based on pure fat catabolism, which takes a while to develop.

Keys and others[45] found that while the energy deficit of 3500 kcal. is cited as being necessary to induce a 1 lb. weight loss, the average value in non-obese subjects was 1910 kcal./lb. during the first 11 weeks of semistarvation and 2460 kcal./lb. during the last 12 weeks of semistarvation, much below the cited figure of 3500 kcal. During the first 10 days of a fast, approximately 8 to 12 per cent of the expenditure is from protein with the balance (88 to 92 per cent) from fat. Later in starvation, up to 96 per cent of energy expenditure is from stored triglyceride. Thus, as energy restriction continues, the body adapts and more efficiently uses fat which contains more calories per gram than body glycogen or protein, which are used in the beginning of the semistarvation regimen or energy restriction regimen.

Table 27–5 presents a 1200 kcal. balanced diet, based on the exchange system discussed in Chapter 25. The energy content of the diet can be increased by adding midafternoon and evening snacks, or by increasing the number of vegetable, bread and fruit servings.

MINERALS AND VITAMINS. The foods selected for the diet should supply an adequate amount of minerals and vitamins. Vitamin and mineral supplements are recommended during weight loss programs of less than 1200 kcal.

FOODS TO INCLUDE. The lower the calorie intake, the more necessary it is to eat a diet of high quality. When the food intake is large, there is greater probability of obtaining all necessary nutrients. When food intake is low, food choices become important. To be certain to meet standards for adequate nutrition, a diet should follow a pattern of a well-balanced normal diet, as discussed in Chapter 10.

ENERGY VALUE OF FOODS. The energy value of foods varies within specific limits. Fats offer the highest caloric value. Protein and carbohydrates contain less than half as many calories as the same number of grams of fat. Butter, margarine, oil, bacon and mayonnaise are examples of foods that are primarily fat. Meats, eggs, milk and cheese are protein foods. Fruits and vegetables are composed chiefly of carbohydrates. Food values were discussed in Chapter 25 and may be found in Appendix Tables 1 and 2.

The calculation figures for the low calorie diet in Table 27–5 are based upon the Food Exchange Lists in Chapter 25. However, the nutritive value of specific foods varies. For example, apples vary from 12 to 35 per cent in their carbohydrate content, depending upon the kind and the conditions of growth. In the nutritive analysis of an apple, most authorities list the average carbohydrate content as 15 per cent. The cited example is applicable to many foods. Some of the foods listed in the tables have been analyzed in the uncooked form, while in reality cooked foods are eaten.

Size of portions and frequency require careful attention during weight loss. In most cases, the type of food is less important than the portion size.

ALCOHOL. Alcohol is relatively high in calorie content. One gram of alcohol yields about 7 calories or 200 kcal./oz.—almost as much as fat. In addition, sugar or some form of carbohydrate (such as Coke or ginger ale) is frequently added to alcoholic beverages, and they are often taken along with a snack (see Appendix Table 2).

A pint of beer (4 per cent alcohol) yields about 200 kcal.; a 4 oz. glass of wine (10 per cent alcohol) has about 75 kcal. and 1 oz. of distilled liquor, such as whiskey, brandy, gin or rum, yields from 75 to 80 kcal. See Table 1–1 for a method of calculating the caloric content of liquor.

One martini has about the same number of calories as 2½ slices of bread (a bread slice averages 60 to 75 kcal.). One whiskey highball has the same number of calories as 2 tbsp. of sugar and an old fashioned contains the same number of calories as 6 tbsp. of cream. Add potato chips at the rate of 100 kcal. for 8 to 10 of them; or peanuts, around 50 kcal. for 10; or almonds at 100 kcal. to the dozen, and one has a very calorically expensive cocktail hour.

SNACK FOODS AND BEVERAGES. In Appendix Table 2 is a list of other foods and beverages commonly consumed between meals. This table is included for the purpose of showing how easy it is to add calories, especially "empty" calories, to a day's intake. A few snacks taken during the day can equal or exceed the entire day's calorie allowance.

FOODS ALLOWED AS DESIRED. Foods that have little or no caloric value and can be taken in unrestricted amounts by diabetic and obese

Table 27–5. 1200 KCAL. DIET FOR AN ADULT (HIGH–PROTEIN, LOW–FAT, MODERATE–CARBOHYDRATE)

Diet Prescription: kcal., 1200; protein, 85 gm.; fat, 30 gm.; carbohydrate, 150 gm. Calculation based on Food Exchange Lists, Chapter 25. All diets are calculated with a leeway of 3 to 5 gm. above or below the diet order.

FOOD	FOOD EXCHANGES (no.)	LIST[b]	CARBO-HYDRATE (gm.)	PROTEIN (gm.)	FAT (gm.)
Milk, skim	2	1	24	16	—
Vegetables	2	2	10	4	
Fruits	4	3	40		
Bread	5	4	75	10	
Meat,[a] lean	8	5		56	24
Fat	1	6			5
			Totals 149	86	29

SAMPLE MEAL PLAN

Breakfast	List
Fruit, 1 exchange	3
Bread, 2 exchanges	4
Meat, lean, 2 exchanges	5
Milk, skim, 1 exchange	1

Lunch or Supper	
Vegetables, 1 exchange	2
Bread, 2 exchanges	4
Meat, lean, 3 exchanges	5
Fruit, 1 exchange	3
Milk, skim, 1 exchange	1

Dinner or Supper	
Meat, lean, 3 exchanges	5
Vegetable, 1 exchange	2
Bread, 1 exchange	4
Fat, 1 exchange	6
Fruit, 2 exchanges	3

SAMPLE MENU

Breakfast	Lunch	Dinner
½ grapefruit (small)	5 small oysters with catsup and horseradish	Bouillon
½ cup plain cottage cheese	Sandwich:	1 parsley potato
2 slices whole-wheat toast	2 slices rye bread	(2 in. diameter)
1 glass (8 oz.) skim milk	2 oz. cold sliced tongue	3 oz. roast veal, lean
Coffee or tea as desired	2 stalks celery	½ cup peas and carrots
	1 carrot	1 tsp. mayonnaise
	1 peach (medium)	1 cup applesauce
	1 glass (8 oz.) skim	(unsweetened)
	buttermilk	Tea or coffee as desired

[a]Lean meat with visible fat removed is used, reducing the fat content from 5 to 3 gm. per Meat Exchange. Limit eggs to 1 per day and omit peanut butter.

[b]From exchange lists, Table 25–8.

patients, unless the diet order specifies to the contrary, are listed in Table 25–8.

FORMULA DIETS. Formula diets for reducing weight come into vogue periodically. They are supplied by pharmaceutical, dairy and food companies and are in liquid, powder or solid (wafers, etc.) form. The recommended daily quantity supplies approximately 900 calories and consists of 20 per cent protein, 30 per cent fat and 50 per cent carbohydrate. With vitamins and minerals to meet the Recommended Dietary Allowances (RDA), these formulas are safe.

However, in the early 1980's there was introduction of very low calorie, 300 kcal./day liquid diets (i.e., Cambridge and others). These are so low in calories that they cannot be recommended as safe for any length of time.

The use of the formula diets is simple, since they require no meal planning and no decisions. However, liquid formulas soon become monotonous and are often discarded in favor of another fad. The person will most likely return to previous dietary habits and regain the pounds lost.

Formula diets may be of value in the early treatment of obesity or for those individuals who watch the scales and use formulas occasionally to lose a few pounds, but they should be restricted to a limited period. On a long-term basis, they may be useful as a substitute for one meal per day. They also have a limited use for patients with a serious medical disorder that requires immediate weight reduction, patients requiring surgery whose obesity poses a hazard, or patients who have become discouraged after many futile attempts at dieting. The formula diets are not a panacea for overweight, and the best approach to excessive weight still is a combination of reduced calories and increased exercise, carefully balanced to meet the individual's nutritional needs in terms of his sociological, cultural, economic, physiological and psychological requirements.

Fiber

The inclusion of dietary fiber in a weight reduction program may help prevent excessive energy consumption by performing the following functions: (1) reducing the caloric density of the diet; (2) slowing the rate at which energy is ingested, thus allowing the gastrointestinal satiety mechanism to work; (3) decreasing slightly the efficiency of absorption of dietary energy; and (4) promoting satiety by adding extra volume to the postprandial gastrointestinal contents.[93] However, further research is required to substantiate these speculations.

PSYCHOLOGY OF WEIGHT REDUCTION

It is of utmost importance to utilize the principles of learning in assisting the patient with the dietary program to lose weight. The plan is individualized to his needs and in terms of how he perceives his task and is developed from the dietary history.

The person may be *aware* of his need to change but not interested in losing weight. One who is *interested* in losing weight is usually ready to learn how the task can be achieved. He *evaluates* possible solutions and becomes involved in planning his regimen. He then gives the plan a *trial*. Satisfaction may or may not occur and adjustments are necessary before complete satisfaction with the program and its adoption take place. These are the stages that an individual undergoes to change former eating habits and dietary patterns. Some people do not progress beyond the awareness stage. They may "go on diets" but never become involved in a change of eating habits and dietary pattern.

Eating habits are acquired. The person who is overweight, regardless of age, may have poor food habits. If the past food habits have caused overweight, then the patient must change eating habits and not just restrict calories for a limited period of time. He should be informed that the weight maintenance process may mean lifelong attention to diet and restriction of intake. The overweight patient should be reminded that it took time to accumulate the excessive weight and that the effective changes occur gradually.

The process of re-education on the part of the individual is difficult. He has to make the necessary changes and adopt a pattern that he can reasonably follow. The greatest hurdle for the patient is to lose the first few of the accumulated pounds. The task seems quite hopeless if the excessive weight amounts to 70 to 80 or more pounds. Even for those individuals, the loss of 3 to 5 pounds will arouse enthusiasm and encourage them to continue to reach the goal.

The correction of obesity poses dual problems: (1) the balance between energy intake and energy expenditure and (2) the dependence upon food for satisfaction. Attempts at weight reduction are futile if a large share of food—and satisfaction—is denied and there is no compensatory replacement. Attention to other activities (away from eating) is necessary.

BEHAVIORAL MODIFICATION

Behavioral modification is commonly used in weight loss programs. The techniques address one or more of the three separate behaviors related to feeding: (1) those related to the initiation of eating, (2) those related to the selection of food and (3) those related to the cessation of eating. Behavioral treatment departs from alternative treatments (i.e., special diets, drugs, surgery) in that the primary goal is to alter the obese person's eating and activity habits, not just the weight. The emphasis is placed on changing behavior in order to reduce energy intake and increase energy expenditure. Behavior modification treatment is based upon the following assumptions about the nature of obesity:[55]

(1) Obesity is a learning disorder, created by and amenable to principles of conditioning; (2) obesity is a simple disorder resulting from excess calorie intake; (3) the obese individual is an overeater; (4) obese persons are more sensitive to food stimuli than are nonobese individuals; (5) there are important differences in the "eating style" of obese and nonobese persons; (6) training an obese person to behave like a nonobese one will result in weight loss.

These assumptions are being invalidated continuously. It is becoming increasingly apparent that genetic, metabolic and physiological factors have a profound influence on body weight regulation and possibly food intake. However, psychological factors are undoubtedly involved in weight regulation. Thus, behavior modification may benefit some individuals by assisting them in weight loss, as well as help a reduced obese person to tolerate a new low weight.

Several behavior modification techniques have been used in weight control therapy:

1. *Adverse control* involves a real or imagined stimulus, such as nausea, that is associated as a consequence to a favorite food or eating behavior. Whenever this food or eating behavior occurs, the aversive stimulus also occurs.

2. *Contingency management* involves a positive or negative consequence being attached to a desirable or undesirable eating behavior, depending on the need of the patient. The patient may be asked to leave a deposit that is "earned back" when weight is lost. Self-administered contingencies as opposed to therapist-administered or group-administered contingencies appear to be more effective for long-term weight control.[41]

3. *Stimulus control* involves learning ways to restructure the environment in order to reduce the saliency of cues that stimulate eating.

4. *Self-monitoring* involves keeping a record of eating behavior or weight change and of the antecedents and consequences of eating behavior.

The most effective programs include at least two of these four components.

The most important item for beginning modification of eating behavior is a record of that behavior—the *food record* or *food diary*. The food diary, kept by the client to record present eating behavior, may include (1) time of eating, (2) place of eating, (3) physical position during eating, (4) presence of others, (5) activity associated with eating, (6) mood or emotional state at time of eating, (7) degree of hunger just before eating and (8) type and amount of food eaten.

The record kept by the client is then shared with the counselor or therapy group, and the client is made aware of some of the factors that influence his eating behavior. Depending upon which individual behaviors are recognized as problems (that is, those that produce a high-caloric, rapid or frequent intake), behavioral changes may be decided upon by the client and the counselor.

Initial reports of behavior modification as an approach to weight control looked positive;[42,87] however, there are doubts about long-term results. While maintenance of treatment-produced weight loss appears to be good during the first year following treatment, evidence indicates that maintenance beyond 1 year is unsatisfactory.[89] Thus, the effectiveness of behavior modification is questionable in the long-term treatment of obesity, but its implementation as an adjunct to diet therapy is advised in receptive individuals or in individuals who have a specific problem related to feeding behavior.

PSYCHOTHERAPY

Psychotherapy has been used in both individual and group situations for the treatment of obesity.[68] The effectiveness of this therapy is not well validated, primarily because there is a lack of appropriate control studies. An important outcome arising from psychotherapy is the encouragement of a change in attitude toward obesity if weight reduction is not going to be possible. Overweight people may be helped to feel better about themselves in spite of their obesity, and this in itself is an important psychotherapeutic achievement. This, in turn, may lead to a change in eating behavior or activity level that may result in weight reduction.

PHARMACOLOGY

Hormonal Therapy

Hormonal therapy has been employed in obesity treatments over the years but it is fraught with incomplete understanding about its physiological effects, risks and long-term effectiveness.

Thyroid hormone has been the most commonly prescribed hormone for weight reduction based on the assumption that an obese person has a low basal metabolic rate (BMR), which causes decreased energy expenditure (i.e., increased metabolic efficiency) that leads to overweight. Thyroid hormone increases the BMR and this is the rationale for using it in obesity treatment. However, most obese individuals have normal thyroid hormone function and it is highly questionable if obese individuals should be prescribed thyroid hormone for weight loss. Large doses of thyroid hormone are necessary to overcome the suppression of endogenous thyroid release that occurs when exogenous thyroid is administered.

It is not clear if a hypermetabolic state can be achieved without undesirable side-effects. Thyroid hormone increases protein catabolism, which counteracts the goal of a successful weight loss program—loss of body fat with maintenance of lean body mass. Thus, thyroid hormone treatment is not recommended in obese individuals who are euthyroid; however, in obese individuals who are hypothyroid, treatment is indicated and may help such individuals in weight loss.

Human chorionic gonadotropin (HCG), a hormone found in the urine of pregnant women, was first used by Simeons in conjunction with a 500 kcal. diet to promote weight loss.[81] One study supports that HCG has more than a placebo effect in obesity treatment.[2] Subsequent studies have failed to demonstrate a significant effect.[37,86,98] Thus, the reduced caloric level associated with HCG injections promotes the weight loss, not the hormone. The use of repeated HCG injections is probably a psychological motivator forcing patients to see the physician and adhere to the diet.

Human growth hormone has recently been used in obesity because its action depletes body fat and does not produce excess protein depletion. It may be effective; however, the supplies of this hormone are small, and it is used only for limited research purposes, and does not assist in the problem of maintenance of weight loss.

Drugs

Various drugs are used in the treatment of obesity and can be divided into two categories: (1) anorectic drugs and (2) agents that interfere with intestinal digestion and absorption.

ANORECTIC DRUGS. Anorectic drugs are agents that act on the central nervous system to suppress appetite. These are the amphetamines and their derivatives as shown in Table 27–6. The amphetamines possess many properties of adrenergic hormones (i.e., epinephrine and norepinephrine). All amphetamines decrease appetite and increase sympathetic/motor activity. Adverse side-effects of amphetamine use include: insomnia, dysphoria, excitement, agitation, dizziness, tremor, headache, dry mouth, confusion, hypertension, palpitations and tachycardia. Thus, individuals taking anorectic drugs may experience severe agitation and nervousness, making continued use of the drug contraindicated. Recent research suggests that the hypothalamus may contain specific receptor sites that mediate the anorexic activity of amphetamines.[62] This finding may lead pharmaceutical firms to search for new drugs that suppress appetite without undesirable sympathetic side-effects.

Table 27–6.   POPULAR ANORECTIC DRUGS

GENERIC NAME	BRANDS
Amphetamine (racemic)	Benzedrine
Dextroamphetamine	Dexedrine
Amphetamine resin complex (racemic amphetamine plus dextroamphetamine)	Biphetamine
Benzphetamine complex	Didrex
Chlorphentermine	Pre-Sate
Clortermine	Voranil
Diethylpropion	Tenuate, Tepanil
Fenfluramine	Pondimin
Mazindol	Sanorex
Phendimetrazine	Plegine
Phenmetrazine	Preludin
Phentermine hydrochloride	Adipex
Phentermine resin	Ionamin

The effectiveness of anorectic drugs appears to decrease with time, as do the side-effects. Anorectic drugs are by no means the solution to weight loss, but they may help people in the beginning of weight loss programs by suppressing appetite.

BULKING AGENTS AND NON-PRESCRIPTION DIET AIDS. Bulk fillers, such as methylcellulose and other calorically inert bulk materials, have been used in experimental and clinical attempts to inhibit food intake. The rationale for the use of such agents is that they swell in the stomach and give a feeling of satiety. The use of such agents (e.g., Ayds candy works on this principle) has not proved to be effective in reducing feelings of hunger in patients on weight loss programs. See Table 27–7 for a summary of nonprescription diet aids.

EXERCISE AND PHYSICAL ACTIVITY

The word obesity is derived from *ab* (over) and *edere* (to eat). The emphasis of weight loss programs reflects the bias inherent in the etymology of the word describing the obese state—obesity develops primarily from overeating. However, it is becoming increasingly apparent that physical inactivity may be a major contributor to obesity.[12, 19] This has been continuously documented, but most vividly in a study which used time-lapse photography of obese and non-obese adolescents at camp. The obese adolescents were much less active than were the non-obese adolescents, as can be seen in Figure 27–9. Obese adults are usually less active than normal weight adults, as has been shown in a number of studies.

Physical activity is recommended as an adjunct to diet therapy owing to its effects on body weight, body composition, appetite and metabolic rate. Exercise has an effect on body weight as well as on the ratio of lean body mass to fat tissue. Exercise decreases body fat, but this does not necessarily mean a decrease in body weight. Initially, physical exercise increases muscle mass, and since lean body mass is more dense than the fat it replaces, body weight may not change. Eventually, with continued exercise, the capacity of muscle mass to increase is limited and is overcome by the fat decrease, resulting in a net decrease in body weight. It appears that a minimum of 2 months is needed to obtain any reduction of adipose tissue with training programs, providing they are strenuous enough.[6] Exercise should be aerobic and last 20 minutes and be performed three times per week.

Exercising at about 50 to 55 per cent of maximum intensity instead of at 60 to 75 per cent results in greater fat catabolism and more weight control benefits.[80] If the heart rate or in-

Table 27–7.   NON–PRESCRIPTION DIET AIDS*

PRODUCT	EXAMPLE	ACTION	COMMENT
Candies to curb appetite	Ayds Fructose tablets	Suppress appetite by raising blood glucose levels	Harmless; candies usually contain carbohydrate, fat, vitamins and minerals Expensive, since fruit juice before meal could have similar effect
Over-the-counter appetite suppressants	Appendrine Control Dexatrim Prolamine Dietac Dex-a-Diet II Anorexin	Most contain phenylpropanolamine (PPA) that reduces appetite temporarily Many also contain caffeine	PPA is mild stimulant, as is caffeine PPA can be dangerous to those with heart disease, high blood pressure, diabetes or hyperthyroidism CSPI, public interest group, has proposed banning PPA in diet aids
Local anesthetics	Reducets Spantrol Diet-trim	Benzocaine, local anesthetic, is the active ingredient Anesthetic presumably deadens taste buds	No controlled studies demonstrate efficacy
Bulking agents	Pretts Taper	Contain methylcelluose; due to affinity for water, increase in volume and supposedly trick stomach into feeling full	Methylcellulose does not swell until in intestine, rather than in stomach, so limited effectiveness
Diuretics	Diurex	Cause body to lose water and thus body weight reduces Weight loss short-lived	No loss of body fat Can be dangerous in that it can cause dehydration and loss of potassium Should be used only under direction of a physician
Exotic and secret cures	Spirulina extract	Questionable action	Not shown to be effective in controlled studies
Amylase inhibitors	Calorex	*In vitro* inhibit action of pancreatic enzyme amylase and thus thought to prevent digestion and absorption of starch *In vivo* cause diarrhea and GI distress	Not shown to be effective Banned from marketplace by FDA in 1982

* From Mahan, L.K., and Rees, J.M.: Nutrition in Adolescence. St. Louis, C.V. Mosby Co., 1984, p. 93.

tensity of the exercise is above 60 per cent of maximum intensity, the body shifts to using more carbohydrate and less fat. Fat catabolism should be promoted for weight loss.

Exercise produces fat loss in obese and non-obese individuals, although this loss is rarely greater than 5 per cent. Although the immediate effects of exercise appear negligible, physical activity may prove to be beneficial over the long term.

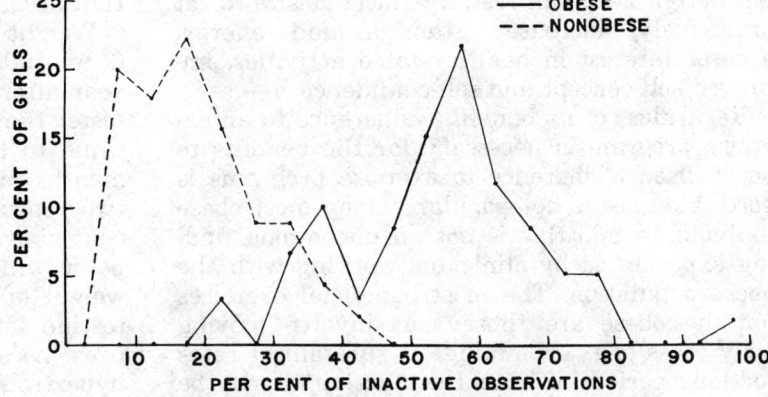

Figure 27–9. Activity of obese and lean girls playing tennis. Pictures taken with time-lapse photography were analyzed for the percentages of inactive frames. Obese girls had nearly 60 per cent inactive frames on average, while the average for the lean girls was only 15 to 20 percent. (From Bullen, B. A., et al.: Physical activity of obese and non-obese adolescent girls appraised by motion picture sampling. Am. J. Clin. Nutr., *14*:211, 1964.)

Fat cell size after physical training is smaller than that after dietary reduction. Furthermore, fat cells *in vitro* seem to become more sensitive to lipolytic (fat breakdown) stimuli after physical training.[3] In addition to decreasing fat, physical activity also produces decreased plasma insulin and triglycerides, increased tissue sensitivity to insulin and improved glucose tolerance.[8, 10]

In certain circumstances, studies in animals and humans suggest that physical activity may decrease appetite.[95, 96] Studies demonstrated that exercise did not increase spontaneous intake in obese females, suggesting that obese persons may profit in two ways from incorporating physical exercise into a weight reduction program: increased energy output along with decreased energy intake. See Table 1–4 for a summary of energy expended by physical activity.

Resting metabolic rate accounts for a large percentage of total daily energy expenditure. Exercise may facilitate weight loss by increasing metabolic rate, which may counteract the decrease in metabolic rate that occurs with energy restriction,[1, 14] as illustrated in Figure 27–6. Investigators claim that physical training can raise metabolic rate;[75] however, this claim requires further research and substantiation.

Exercise may have a number of other benefits in a weight reduction program. Physiologically, it results in improved cardiovascular functioning and changes in plasma lipid profiles. High density lipoprotein (HDL) cholesterol is negatively correlated with obesity and heart disease. Thus, high HDL appears to have a protective function against heart disease, as discussed in Chapter 28. Several studies have shown that HDL-cholesterol levels increase after exercise training, whereas levels of very low density (VLDL) and low density lipoproteins (LDL) may decrease.[4] Other physiological benefits already mentioned include increased energy expenditure and positive changes in body composition.[9] Psychologically, the effects can be profound. Some effects are reduction in tension and stress levels, better sleep and rest, a reduced desire to eat excessively, increased stamina and energy, greater interest in health-related activities, improved self-concept and self-confidence.

Regardless of its benefits, adherence to an exercise program is necessary for the benefits to be realized. Adherence to exercise programs is poor. Exercise is not popular among most obese individuals, and this is not an uncommon finding experienced by clinicians working with the obese population. The most beneficial exercises for the obese are those that involve moving body mass (e.g., swimming) at substantial rates for long periods of time. Such activities may be difficult for the obese individual. Thus, it is recommended that the obese person be continuously counseled about the benefits of exercise and encouraged to increase activity at a reasonable rate.

SURGERY

Three types of surgery have been used in obesity treatment: surgical removal of adipose tissue, the jejunoileal bypass and the gastric bypass or stapling. Surgical removal of adipose tissue has been ineffective, since the adipose stores return. The jejunoileal bypass has been found to have tremendous complications and is no longer a recommended treatment. The gastric bypass or stapling is presently the accepted surgery for weight reduction. However, either of these surgeries should be used in the treatment of only the very obese for whom the procedure is a last resort.

Jejunoileal Bypass Surgery

The jejunoileal bypass will be discussed because there are many people who have had this surgery and are doing fine or struggling with its consequences, many of which are nutritional.

As the term jejunoileal bypass implies, the surgery involves bypassing most of the absorptive capacity of the intestine by connecting the jejunum directly to the terminal ileum, as shown in Figure 27–10. The result is a tremendous reduction in the absorptive length of the small intestine, from about 22 feet (approximately 7 meters) to about 1 1/2 feet (about 1/2 meter). Consequently, the patient is put into a chronic state of malabsorption due to reduced absorptive area and reduced transit time (which may be as little as 45 minutes in some patients). Food nutrients, including energy, are "lost" in the feces. The patient is in energy deficit and loses weight even though he eats the same amount of food he was eating before. However, the person usually decreases his intake somewhat because of the discomfort and diarrhea that accompany overeating.

Weight losses are substantial, ranging from 60 to 100 lb. or more (27 to 45+ kg.) within a year after surgery. The heavier the patient, the faster the rate of weight loss. Most patients continue to lose at the rate of 8 lb. (3.6 kg.) per month, and usually their weight stabilizes about two years after surgery at a point 20 to 25 per cent above their ideal body weight. Where this point will be is determined by the presurgical weight of the patient and the length of the intestine left intact after surgery. Weight stabilizes because the remaining intestinal tract hypertrophies and is able to absorb enough nu-

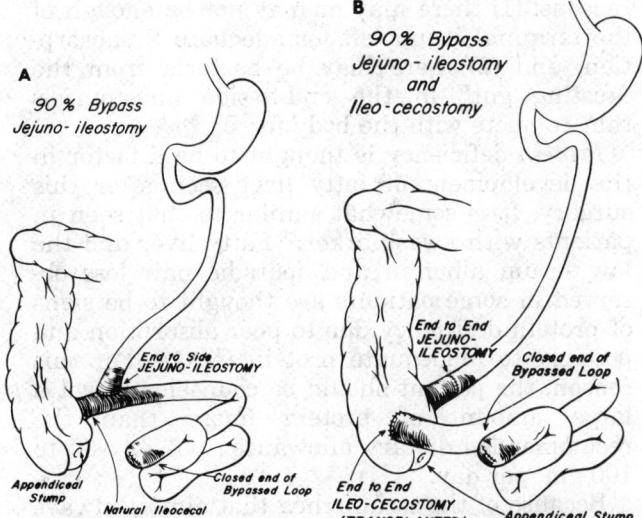

Figure 27–10. *A*, Intestinal bypass: end-to-side jejunoileostomy (Payne procedure). *B*, Intestinal bypass: end-to-end jejunoileostomy (Scott procedure). (From Soper, R. T., et al.: Gastric bypass for morbid obesity in children and adolescents. J. Pediatr. Surg., *10*:51, 1975. Reproduced by permission.)

trients to maintain this weight. For this reason and the fact that eating habits are rarely changed, the person who has his intestine reconnected will almost always regain the lost weight and perhaps gain more.

There are a number of complications of this surgery, as listed in Table 27–8. Liver failure is the most severe long-term complication, and the patient should be made aware of this and the other major complications that can occur and that are not clearly understood.

NUTRITIONAL CARE. Nutritional care is as important for these patients as it is for any other person with a malabsorption syndrome. Attention must be given to vitamin and mineral supplements and nutritional counseling to minimize discomfort from diarrhea, cramping, steatorrhea and gas, to prevent complications and to maintain body protein stores.

Food intolerances are very individual although some general advice may be helpful.[24] The patient must be supported and encouraged to try adding new foods as the intestine adapts. Jejunoileal bypass patients can receive a great deal of support from each other, and the organization of a group may be very helpful for them.

Potassium supplements (usually in the form of KCl) are necessary because of the very common problem of hypokalemia that results from excessive losses of K^+ because of the profuse diarrhea. As the intestine adapts to its new condition, the number of stools will slowly decrease from 10 to 20 per day right after surgery to 3 to 4 per day by the end of the year after surgery. After the patient is able to eat fruits and vegetables and other potassium-rich foods, the potassium supplements may be decreased and substituted with fruits and vegetables.

Calcium, magnesium and vitamin D may also need supplementation because of poor absorp-

tion. Vitamin D may be poorly absorbed as a result of fat malabsorption, and calcium can form calcium soaps with the fatty acids in the gut lumen, which prevents its absorption. The few reported cases of tetany following jejunoileal bypass may have been due to hypocalcemia or hypomagnesemia.

All *vitamins* should be given as supplements, usually in therapeutic doses, in anticipation of poor absorption. A liquid vitamin preparation may be more valuable, considering the reduced transit time in the gut. An encapsulated vitamin preparation may not be digested and absorbed fast enough. Although the terminal ileum remains after most of these surgeries and allows for the absorption of vitamin B_{12}, some authorities still suggest supplementation for two

Table 27–8.   COMMPLICATIONS OF INTESTINAL BYPASS SURGERY*

SURGICAL
    Operative death
    Wound infection or dehiscence
    Anastomotic leas
METABOLIC
    Hypocalcemia and tetany
    Hypokalemia and weakness
    Oxalate renal stones
    Risk of osteoporosis
    Dehydration
GASTROINTESTINAL
    Nausea and vomiting
    Diarrhea that may persist
    Abdominal distention
    Cirrhosis
    Malnutrition with risks of hypovitaminosis
MISCELLANEOUS
    Loss of hair
    Arthralgia and arthritis
    Anemia

*From Bray, G. A.: The overweight patient. Adv. Intern. Med., *21*:267, 1976.

reasons: (1) there may or may not be enough of the terminal ileum left for adequate B_{12} absorption, and (2) there may be bacteria from the "resting gut" in the end-to-side anastomosis that compete with the body for B_{12}.[64]

Protein deficiency is thought to be a factor in the development of fatty liver seen after this surgery. It is somewhat similar to that seen in patients with kwashiorkor.[58] Fatty liver and the low serum albumin and sporadic hair loss observed in some patients are thought to be signs of protein deficiency due to poor absorption and possibly to inadequate protein intake. For this reason, the patient should be counseled to eat a large amount of protein (more than the recommended dietary allowance), possibly 80 to 100 gm. per day.

Because of the steatorrhea that almost always occurs after a high-fat meal, a *low-fat* diet (less than 50 gm. of fat) is suggested for the patient. However, these patients were not amenable to diet changes before, so the counseling must be in the form of suggestion and encouragement.

Alcohol should be avoided for the first year after surgery and preferably avoided permanently. Alcohol may place a metabolic load on an already overtaxed liver, and these patients will become highly intoxicated after drinking just a small amount of alcohol. For most patients, giving up alcohol is no problem.

Medications are given to help reduce the diarrhea, and creams are recommended to alleviate the anal discomfort associated with diarrhea and frequent bowel movements.

These patients should be checked even after they have reached a stable weight and assessed periodically for nutritional status through biochemical measurements, dietary history, and clinical examination, as discussed in Chapter 9.

All investigators have reported that their patients are happy with the surgery and would never go back to their former condition. Solow reports an improvement in patients' self-confidence, self-esteem and body image after substantial weight loss. He found that these patients felt a relief of the constant guilt and helplessness that had accompanied every mouthful they had eaten before. The weight loss appeared to restore a more normal responsiveness to the internal cues of satiety and a sharpening of satiety mechanisms.[84]

Gastric Partitioning Surgery

Gastric partitioning surgery closes part of the stomach and thus reduces its reservoir capacity. There are several technical variations to achieve this effect. One is the *gastroplasty*, whereby the stomach is partitioned such that there is only a small opening (10–12 mm.) into the distal stomach. Using this procedure, the stomach can be stapled closed. The other is the *gastric bypass*, where the small opening is connected to the small intestine in a Roux-en-Y procedure as shown in Figure 27–11. The remaining portion is connected directly to the jejunum via a small opening about 2 cm. in diameter. The main cause of weight loss appears to be the reduced food intake due to the smaller stomach and to the nausea and vomiting that result if the person continues to eat. As with the jejunoileal bypass, patients usu-

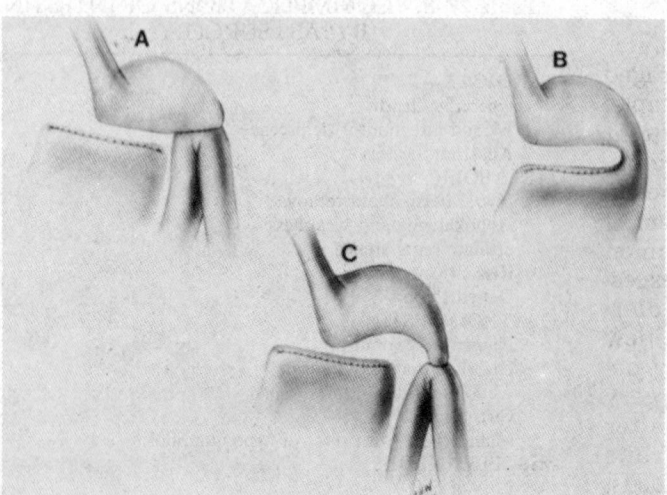
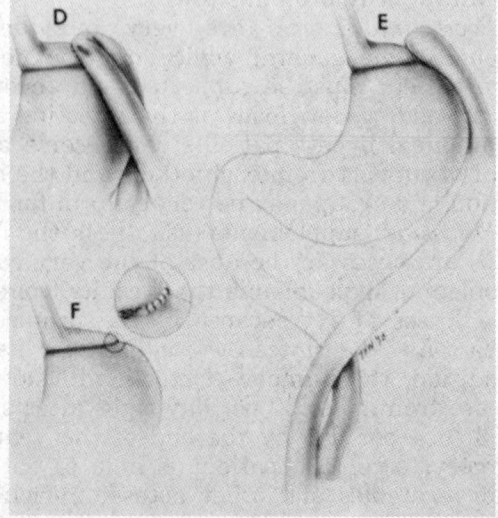

Figure 27–11. *Left,* The gastric bypass operation as performed in 1966–1970, *A*; 1971, *B*; and 1972–1974, *C. Right,* The operations in use since 1974 in which the specifications have been defined: loop gastroenterostomy, *D*; Roux-en-Y gastroenterostomy, *E*; and gastroplasty, *F.* (From Mason, E. E., Printen, K. J., Blommers, T. J., Lewis, J. W., and Scott, D. H.: Gastric bypass in morbid obesity. Am. J. Clin. Nutr., *33*:396, 1980.)

ally stabilize at a weight somewhat above their ideal weight. The gastric bypass is probably as effective as the jejunoileal bypass in producing and maintaining weight reduction, and the operation is not accompanied by the problems of the jejunoileal bypass surgery.

Gastric partitioning procedures are successful in achieving weight reduction in the vast majority of obese people. At present it appears that the gastric bypass is somewhat more effective in achieving weight loss, but the gastroplasty may be minimally safer in terms of operative morbidity and mortality.

NUTRITIONAL CARE. Most studies indicate that 90 per cent of weight loss following gastric partitioning occurs within the first 12 months postoperatively, and weight loss usually stops after 24 months. The ultimate success in terms of degree of weight loss and maintenance depends on changes in the patient's eating behavior and activity patterns established during the first 2 years following surgery. The anatomical barrier preventing excessive eating is transient, since the gastric pouch stretches and the opening enlarges over time. Nutritional counseling should be intensive and directed toward achieving desired weight within these 2 years when the anatomical barrier to overeating exists. Attention should be given to eating behavior and activity changes that will enable the patient to maintain the new low weight. There should also be attention to adequate protein intake and vitamin and mineral supplementation.

The most frequent complication of gastric bypass or gastroplasty is nausea and vomiting. Attention to a food record kept after surgery will give the counselor information on how much the patient is consuming, what is being consumed and tolerated, and what is being vomited. Patients should be counseled to eat slowly, chew food well and avoid swallowing chunks of meat or other food that cannot be completely liquefied. They should be instructed to eat small amounts frequently. However, patients can deter weight loss if they drink too much calorically dense liquid.

Jaw Wiring (Maxillomandibular Fixation)

Wiring the jaws closed is another method of reducing food intake through physical control rather than through a change in eating or activity habits. The result is that the person can no longer eat solid food but can only take liquids through a straw. Dental attention before wiring and oral hygiene and nutritional care while the jaws are wired are important. *Nutritional care* should include obtaining a dietary history to find out what types of liquids the person is taking. Counseling should include recommenda-

tions for liquids so that adequate protein, minerals and vitamins are ingested during the period of weight loss. Rather than only juices, Kool-aid and soda pop, the dieter should be taking nutritious soups, milk, formula diets and vitamin and mineral supplements. The patient should also be instructed how to cut the wires, and the proper position for vomiting should it happen.

This technique has been effective in producing weight loss during the time the jaws are wired. However, body weight generally returns to pretreatment levels following removal of the wires.

It has been proposed that it might be most effective as a preoperative weight reduction method in patients who will then undergo gastric partitioning.[32]

Prevention of Weight Gain

Despite a multitude of treatment programs designed to treat obesity, there is a depressing therapeutic failure rate. It has been shown that 95 per cent of patients who have lost weight on a variety of programs regain it within nine years,[27] as detailed in Figure 27–12. Most studies find similar recidivism rates in the ability to maintain weight loss; however, Schachter claims that these grim statistics may be explained in terms of self-selection—only people with the most difficult cases seek help. People who cure themselves do not go to therapists. He found that individuals who cure themselves are more able to lose and to keep off weight than are obese patients included in studies of therapeutic effectiveness.[73] However, the bulk of evidence supports the fact that most people regain lost weight. Of those who do maintain a reduced body weight, it may be at the expense of physical or psychological stress. It can be concluded that obesity is extremely resistant to treatment and long-term cure. This is, in part, influenced by social factors that promote physical inactivity and excess food intake, but, as already mentioned, there are some physiological mechanisms in the obese person that may work to maintain the obese state.

Successful treatment of obesity has, to date, not been developed. A major emphasis in the treatment of obesity has been placed on weight loss, which, in the long term, is unsuccessful. Thus, a preventive treatment program designed to prevent the development of obesity should be advocated.

In those individuals who are currently obese, perhaps more benefit might be derived by placing an increased emphasis on the prevention of

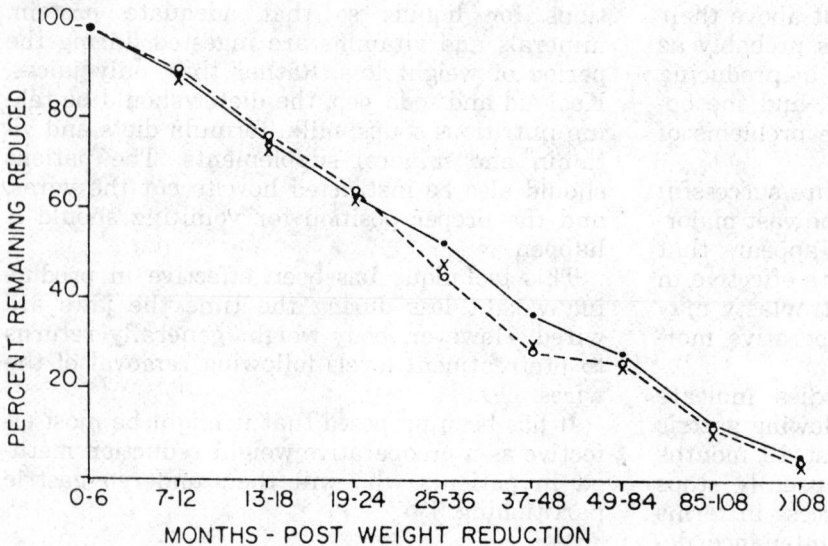

Figure 27–12. Per cent of patients remaining at reduced body weights at various time intervals following accomplished weight loss. Solid line represents 60 subjects with onset of obesity before age 21; broken line, 42 subjects becoming obese after age 21. X represents the mean. (From Johnson, D., and Drenick, E. J.: Therapeutic fasting in morbid obesity. Arch. Intern. Med., *137*: 1381, 1977.)

further weight gain rather than stressing weight loss. If no adverse symptoms associated with obesity are present, a primary goal of therapy might be maintenance of current weight. If weight loss is desired or medically indicated, weight loss goals must be set relative to the individual's usual weight rather than attempting to "normalize" body weight completely.

Prevention of Obesity

Health professionals must begin to develop techniques by which to identify individuals with a genetic propensity toward obesity and identify them prior to the onset of obesity. This may require an increased emphasis on family histories and patterns of weight gain in family members. Individuals so identified might benefit from being made aware of their propensity toward obesity and restricted in weight gain through adult life as opposed to attempting to decrease weight after obesity has developed.

The real hope for "curing" obesity seems to lie in prevention of the problem, efforts that usually begin in childhood. Some strategies for preventing obesity in children and adults are:

1. Early indentification of obesity by careful monitoring of height, weight and skinfold thickness in children and adults.

2. Early identification of eating and activity habits that will result in energy imbalance and weight gain.

3. Early education to change obesity-promoting activities and eating habits.

4. Careful control of the diet of the preschool child so that it does not include excessive amounts of concentrated sweets, fat and calories.

5. Restriction of food advertising that promotes excessive energy consumption.

6. Encouragement of regular aerobic exercise programs through low-cost classes for skill development and appropriate areas to do the activities.

7. Instruction of children and their parents about food and the proper role of food and nutrients in health and well-being.

Underweight

Almost eclipsed by all the attention focused on obesity in the United States is the effort of some persons to gain weight. The term *underweight* is applicable to persons who are 15 to 20 per cent or more below the normal accepted weight standard or desired weight. Because *underweight is often a symptom of a disease*, it should receive medical investigation. In underweight individuals the resistance to disease is lowered, and the growth during childhood and adolescence may be retarded. The person who is seriously underweight often tires easily, is sensitive to cold and complains of feeling weak.

ETIOLOGY

Underweight may be caused by (1) an insufficient intake in the quantity and quality of food to meet the needs of the person's activity, (2) excessive activity as in the case of compulsive athletes in training, (3) poor absorption and utilization of the food consumed, (4) a wasting disease such as tuberculosis or hyperthyroidism that increases the metabolic rate and (5) psychological or emotional stress or psychological abnormality (eating disorders) as discussed in

Chapter 32. Undernutrition itself may lead to multiple endocrine disturbances. Undernourished individuals may show signs of underfunction of the pituitary, thyroid, gonads and adrenals. Young women with anorexia nervosa, for instance, stop menstruating when they have lost a significant amount of weight.

ASSESSMENT

It is important to assess the extent of underweight before starting a treatment program. By using anthropometric data such as arm muscle area and arm fat area, as discussed in Chapter 9, it is possible to determine whether health-endangering underweight really exists. Then it is necessary to determine the basic cause of the patient's underweight. If a wasting disease is the cause then the disease must be treated, and the diet becomes part of the treatment. Faulty absorption of food is a medical problem and must be treated. If the problem is psychological, psychological therapy is needed for the patient. In cases of anorexia nervosa, the basic fears and anxieties need to be discovered and removed; at the same time, maximal food intake is encouraged.

It is frequently more difficult for an underweight individual to gain weight than it is for an obese patient to lose weight. The "setpoint" theory applies to thin people as well as to overweight individuals. However, this applies only to individuals for whom thinness is a natural state and not the result of excessive dieting or disease. The selection and service of food is important. Well-planned meals at scheduled hours instead of hastily planned, bolted meals are advised. Mealtimes should be periods of leisure and relaxation, since nervous tension is often part of the cause of underweight in some individuals.

HIGH-CALORIE DIETS FOR WEIGHT GAIN

Before a diet is planned with the patient, a careful dietary history should be taken. This history of the food intake most likely will reveal the good and poor dietary habits and inadequacies.

The Diet Plan

ENERGY. In addition to the calories needed to meet the total energy requirement of the body, an allowance of 500 to 1000 additional calories for muscle growth and storage of fat in the adipose tissues should be planned. An acceptable method of determining the patient's daily energy requirement is simply to calculate his needs on the basis of his present weight. If a person normally needs 2800 kcal. (11,700 kJ.) to maintain his present weight, his dietary needs would be 3300 to 3800 kcal. (13,800 to 15,900 kJ.) to gain weight. The intake should be gradually increased to avoid gastric discomfort and periods of discouragement. When a person is offered or expected to ingest more food than he can take at one time, he is apt to be overwhelmed by the amount and be unable to eat very much. The amount of food that could be ingested at one meal should be determined and the rest of the calories supplied in a concentrated supplemental form.

It has been found through experience with patients of both sexes and different ages that men seem to prefer to receive the additional calories through extra portions of the usual foods served at meals, children and adolescents prefer between-meal nourishment, and women seem to favor more concentrated foods, such as the addition of cream to milk when it is served as a beverage. The secret of a successful diet program is to *individualize* the treatment for each patient and to include foods which the patient really enjoys.

PROTEIN. In the average high-energy diet for the underweight, the daily protein allowance is maintained at the optimum level. A high protein intake of 100 gm. or more may be necessary for replacement and repair of the body tissues. In cases of severe malnutrition caused by the patient's inability to take sufficient food, crystalline amino acids are sometimes given orally or parenterally. It has been found that, after a certain period of malnutrition, the gastrointestinal tract is incapable of digesting a sufficient amount of protein foods, especially if edema of the gastrointestinal tract is present, and vomiting or diarrhea may result. Sparing the patient's digestion by giving amino acids (protein hydrolysates) will frequently alleviate the difficulty.

CARBOHYDRATE AND FAT. The amount of fuel foods, carbohydrates and fats, is increased in the high-calorie diet. The concentrated calorie foods such as butter, fortified margarine, cream, cereals, bread, potatoes and high-calorie desserts are especially advised. A moderate fat allowance is made to increase the palatability of the diet and increase the caloric value without dulling the appetite. Carbohydrates are digested easily and when taken in excess of body needs are readily used or stored as body fat.

MINERALS AND VITAMINS. The mineral and vitamin allowances should be maintained at an optimum level. Supplements of vitamins, especially the B vitamins, are given as a possible appetite stimulant and to meet the requirement when energy intake is increased.

For the high-calorie diet this food pattern provides about 3000 kcal., 130 gm. protein and generous amounts of vitamins and minerals. The normal protective diet, outlined in Tables 10–8 and 10–9, is the basis or pattern for the high-calorie diet. Increasing the amounts of the basic foods increases the intake of daily calories, minerals and vitamins. Additional foods such as desserts, candy and special dishes may be enjoyed by the patient if the protective foods are not sacrificed. Eating between meals is encouraged but should not interfere with the patient's appetite for regular meals.

To increase the patient's daily calorie intake, the 500 kcal. step-up is suggested, as outlined in Table 27–9.

SUGGESTIONS FOR INCREASING CALORIES IN THE DIET

Use light cream instead of milk whenever possible. Include cereal at breakfast with a banana or other fruit. This is a good source of additional carbohydrate calories.

Butter breakfast toast when it is hot because more butter or margarine can be used. Cinnamon toast, pancakes, waffles and French toast are good alternates for breakfast toast.

Serve jelly and jam along with bread and butter. Add jelly, jam and preserves to cheesecake, puddings and other desserts.

Add cream or undiluted evaporated milk to milk beverages. Malted milk and eggnogs can replace milk.

Add skim milk powder to milk, milk beverages, soups and puddings and on hot cereal.

Add ice cream or whipped cream to desserts and milk beverages.

Use cream soups instead of clear bouillon broth–based or tomato-based soups.

Eat dried fruits between meals because they are high in calories besides being good sources of minerals and vitamins.

Serve mayonnaise, oil and salad dressings whenever possible with sandwiches, salads and vegetables.

Serve gravy on meat and potatoes.

Add sauces to desserts such as puddings, molded gelatins, custards, rennet puddings, cakes and ice creams.

Have potatoes, spaghetti, rice, macaroni or noodles at least twice every day.

Eat nuts between meals. They are high in calories besides being good protein and vitamin additions.

Plan a definite eating schedule and then adhere to it.

It may be more difficult for an underweight person to gain 1 lb. a week than for an obese person to lose 1 lb. a week. It is not an easy

Table 27–9. SUGGESTIONS FOR INCREASING ENERGY INTAKE IN STEPS OF 500 KCAL.

ADDITIONAL FOODS	WEIGHT (gm.)	KCAL.	PROTEIN
Plus 500 kcal. (served between meals)			
1. 1 cup dry cereal	28	110	2
1 banana	100	80	
1 cup whole milk	244	159	8
1 slice toast	23	60	2
1 tbsp. peanut butter	15	86	4
		495	16
2. 8 saltine crackers	23	99	3
1 oz. cheese	28	113	7
1 cup ice cream	133	290	6
		502	16
3. 6 graham cracker squares	42	165	3
2 tbsp. peanut butter	30	172	8
1 cup orange juice	249	122	
2 tbsp. raisins	18	52	
		511	11
Plus 1000 kcal. (served between meals)			
1. 8 oz. fruit flavored yogurt	227	240	9
1 slice bread	23	60	2
2 oz. cheese	56	226	14
1 apple	150	87	
1/4 of 14" cheese pizza	130	306	16
1 small banana	140	81	1
		1000	42
2. Instant Breakfast with whole milk	276	280	15
1 cup cottage cheese	225	239	31
1/2 cup pineapple	128	95	
1 cup apple juice	248	117	
6 graham cracker squares	42	165	3
1 pear	180	100	1
		996	50
Plus 1500 kcal. (served between meals)			
1. 2 slices bread	46	120	4
2 tbsp. peanut butter	30	172	8
1 tbsp. jam	20	110	
4 graham cracker squares	28	110	2
8 oz. fruit flavored yogurt	227	240	9
3/4 cup roasted peanuts	108	628	28
1 cup apricot nectar	251	143	1
		1523	52
2. 1 baked custard	248	285	13
Instant Breakfast with whole milk	276	280	15
1 cup dry cereal	28	110	2
1 banana	100	80	
1 cup whole milk	244	159	8
1 cup orange juice	249	122	
4 tbsp. raisins	36	104	
1 bagel	55	165	6
2 tbsp. cream cheese	28	99	
2 tbsp. jam	40	110	2
		1514	46

task for the underweight person to add 500 kcal. to his daily intake of food. He should be involved in planning what and how much additional food he will take at one time and how often he will eat. He usually can suggest what can be added to make the plan appealing.

Behavior modification techniques can be applied to the process of weight gain just as they are used in weight reduction. The bases for thinness is the person's eating behaviors, which must be changed to result in a consistently higher caloric intake.

Problems and Suggested Topics for Discussion

1. Define (a) overweight and (b) obesity.
2. Explain how neural and hormonal factors may be interrelated in their control of food intake.
3. What techniques might be used to determine a person's level of body fatness? What are the advantages and disadvantages of each?
4. What are the problems with the height-weight tables that are so commonly used to dictate appropriate weight?
5. Discuss some of the factors that help the obese person maintain his overweight and make losing weight so difficult.
6. What is the role of exercise in weight loss and weight maintenance? Why should it be included in a weight reduction program?
7. What are the principles of a low-calorie diet?
8. Describe various reducing regimens and give the advantages and disadvantages of each.
9. Should all overweight individuals reduce? Explain.
10. Assist a person who is overweight with the necessary changes in her present dietary pattern to lose 1 lb. per week. Permit her to indicate the changes that she will make.
11. Interview a patient who is obese. How many calories is he consuming to maintain his present weight? How many excess calories is he consuming? How can he improve his diet? Try to follow the patient's progress in the outpatient clinic.
12. Keep a diary of your own eating for two days, making note of the items discussed in this chapter. If you had to lose or gain weight, which behavior would you attempt to change first?
13. How would you help a person who is underweight gain weight? How will he or she implement the changes?
14. Take a food-consumption history of an underweight patient who is in the hospital or in the outpatient clinic. Calculate the calories. How many calories does she need to reach her ideal or desired weight? How long will it take her to reach the desired weight?
15. List the foods that should be stressed or added to the normal diet to make it a high-calorie diet.

Cited References

1. Apfelbaum, J.T., et al.: Effect of caloric restriction and excessive caloric intake on energy expenditure. Am. J. Clin. Nutr., 24:1405, 1971.
2. Asher, W.L., and Harper, H.W.: Effect of human chorionic gonadotropin on weight loss, hunger, and feeling of well-being. Am. J. Clin. Nutr., 26:211, 1973.
3. Askew, E.W., et al.: Adipose tissue cellularity and lipolysis. Response to exercise and cortisol treatment. J. Clin. Invest., 56:521, 1975.
4. Ballantyne, D., et al.: Prescribing exercise for the healthy: assessment of compliance and effects on plasma lipids and lipoproteins. Health Bull., 36:169, 1978.
5. Bistrian, B.R.: Clinical use of a protein sparing modified fast. JAMA, 240:2299, 1978.
6. Björntorp, P.: Exercise in the treatment of obesity. Clin. Endocrinol. Metabol., 5:431, 1976.
7. Björntorp, P.: Development of Adipose Tissue. In Cioffi, L.A., James, W.P.T., and Van Itallie, T.B. (eds.): The Body Weight Regulatory System: Normal and Disturbed Mechanisms. New York, Raven Press, 1981.
8. Björntorp, P., et al.: The effect of physical training on insulin production in obesity. Metabolism, 19:631, 1970.
9. Björntorp, P., et al.: Physical training in human obesity. Effects of long term physical training on body composition. Metabolism, 22:1467, 1973.
10. Björntorp, P., et al.: Effects on plasma insulin in glucose intolerant subjects with marked hyperinsulinemia. Scand. J. Clin. Lab. Invest., 32:41, 1973.
11. Blackburn, G.L.: The liquid protein controversy—a closer look at the facts. Obesity Bariatric Med., 7:25, 1978.
12. Bloom, W.L., and Eidex, M.F.: Inactivity as a major factor in adult obesity. Metabolism, 16:679, 1967.
13. Borjeson, M.: The aetiology of obesity in children. Acta Pediatr. Scand., 65:279, 1976.
14. Bray, G.A.: Effect of caloric restriction on energy expenditure in obese patients. Lancet, 2:397, 1969.
15. Bray, G.A.: Metabolic effects of corpulence. In Howard, A. (ed.): Recent Advances in Obesity Research. Westport, Conn., Technomic Publishing Co., Inc., 1976.
16. Bray, G.A.: Definition, measurement, and classification of the syndromes of obesity. Int. J. Obesity, 2:99, 1978.
17. Bray, G.A., et al.: Evaluation of the obese patient. 1. An algorithm. JAMA, 235:1487, 1976.
18. Brook, G.G.D., et al.: Relation between age of onset of obesity and size and number of adipose cells. Br. Med. J., 2:25, 1972.
19. Bullen, B.A., et al.: Physical activity of obese and nonobese adolescent girls appraised by motion picture sampling. Am. J. Clin. Nutr., 14:211, 1974.
20. Davis, J.D., et al.: Inhibition of food intake by a humoral factor. J. Comp. Physiol. Psychol., 67:407, 1969.
21. Della-Fera, M.A., and Baile, C.A.: Cholecystokinin octapeptide: continuous picomole injections into the cerebral ventricles of sheep suppress feeding. Science, 206:471, 1979.
22. Della-Fera, M.A., et al.: Cholecystokinin antibody injected in cerebral ventricles stimulates feeding in sheep. Science, 212:687, 1981.
23. DeLuise, M., et al.: Reduced activity of the red-cell sodium-potassium pump in human obesity. N. Engl. J. Med., 303:1017, 1980.
24. DeWind, L.: Jejunoileal bypass surgery for obesity. In Bray, G.A., and Bethune, J.E. (eds.): Treatment and Management of Obesity. New York, Harper and Row, 1974, pp. 142–143.
25. Dore, C., et al.: Prediction of energy requirements of obese patients after massive weight loss. Br. J. Nutr., 36:41, 1982.
26. Drenick, E.J., and Dennin, H.F.: Energy expenditure in fasting obese men. J. Lab. Clin. Med., 81:421, 1973.
27. Drenick, E.J., and Johnson, D.: Weight reduction by fasting and semi-starvation in morbid obesity. Int. J. Obesity, 2:123, 1978.
28. Dugdale, A.E., and Griffiths, M.: Estimating body fat mass from anthropometric data. Am. J. Clin. Nutr., 32:2400, 1979.
29. Durnin, J.V.G.A., and Womersley, J.: Body fat assessed for total body density and its estimation from

the skin-fold thickness: measurements on 481 men and women aged from 16 to 72 years. Br. J. Nutr., *32*: 77, 1974.

30. Flack, R., and Grayer, E.A.: Consciousness-raising group for obese women. Social Work, *20*:484, 1975.

31. Food and Nutrition Board, National Research Council: Fetal and infant susceptibility to obesity. Nutr. Rev., *36*:122, 1978.

32. Fordyce, G.L., et al.: Jaw wiring and gastric bypass in the treatment of severe obesity. Obesity Bariatric Med., *8*:14, 1979.

33. Frisancho, A.R.: New norms of upper limb fat and muscle areas for assessment of nutritional status. Am. J. Clin. Nutr., *34*:2540, 1981.

34. Garn, S.M., and Clark, D.C.: Trends in fatness and the origins of obesity. Pediatrics, *57*:443, 1976.

35. Gibbs, J., et al.: Cholecystokinin decreases food intake in rats. J. Comp. Physiol. Psychol., *84*:488, 1973.

36. Gordon, T., and Kannel, W.B.: Obesity and cardiovascular disease: The Framingham study. Clin. Endocrinol. Metabol., *5*:367, 1976.

37. Greenway, F.L., and Bray, G.A.: HCG and placebo equivalent in obesity. West. J. Med., *127*:461, 1977.

38. Hager, A., et al.: Adipose tissue cellularity in obese school girls before and after dietary treatment. Am. J. Clin. Nutr., *31*:68, 1978.

39. Herman, C.P., and Mack, D.: Restrained and unrestrained eating. J. Pers., *43*:647, 1975.

40. Hirsch, J., and Knittle, J.L.: Cellularity of obese and non-obese adipose tissue. Fed. Proc., *29*:1516, 1970.

41. Jeffrey, D.J.: A comparison of the effects of internal control and self-control on the modification and maintenance of weight. J. Abnorm. Psychol., *83*:404, 1974.

42. Jordon, H.A., and Levitz, L.S.: Behavior modification in a self-help group. J. Am. Diet. Assoc., *62*:27, 1973.

43. Jung, R.T., et al.: Reduced thermogenesis in obesity. Nature, *279*:322, 1979.

44. Karam, J.H.: Obesity: fat cells—not fat people. West. J. Med., *130*:128, 1979.

45. Keys, A., et al.: The biology of human starvation. Minneapolis, University of Minnesota Press, 1950.

46. Keys, A., et al.: Indices of relative weight and obesity. J. Chronic Dis., *25*:329, 1972.

47. Khosla, T., and Lowe, C.R.: Indices of obesity derived from body weight and height. Br. J. Prev. Soc. Med., *21*:122, 1967.

48. Kissileff, H.R., et al.: C-terminal octapeptide of cholecystokinin decreases food intake in man. Am. J. Clin. Nutr., *34*:154, 1981.

49. Knittle, J.L., and Ginsberg-Fellner, F.: Can obesity be prevented? In Collipp, P.L. (ed.): Childhood Obesity. Acton, Mass., Publishing Services Group, 1975.

50. Knittle, J.L., et al.: Adipose tissue development in man. Am. J. Clin. Nutr., *30*:762, 1977.

51. Kupfermann, I.: Feeding behavior is regulated by a variety of signals. In Kandel, E.R., and Schwartz, J.H. (eds.): Principles of Neural Science. New York, Elsevier North Holland, Inc. 1982, pp. 453–457.

52. Lindner, P.G., and Blackburn, G.L.: Multidisciplinary approach to obesity utilizing fasting modified by protein-sparing therapy. Obesity Bariatric Med., *5*:198, 1976.

53. Lloyd, J.D., et al.: Childhood obesity—a long-term study of height and weight. Br. Med. J., *15*:145, 1961.

54. Lopez, A., et al.: Effect of exercise and physical fitness on serum lipid and lipoprotein. Atherosclerosis, *30*:1, 1974.

55. Mahoney, M.J.: Behavior modification in the treatment of obesity. Psychiatr. Clin. North Am., *1*:651, 1978.

56. Mann, G.V.: The influences of obesity on health. N. Engl. J. Med., *291*:178 and 226, 1974.

57. Metropolitan Life Insurance Co.: New weight standards for men and women. Stat. Bull., *40*:1, 1959.

58. Moxley, R.T., III., et al.: Protein nutrition and liver disease after jejunoileal bypass for morbid obesity. N. Engl. J. Med., *290*:291, 1974.

59. Newman, J.H., et al.: Twins, a study of heredity and environment. Chicago, University of Chicago Press, 1937.

60. Nisbett, R.E.: Hunger, obesity, and the ventromedial hypothalamus. Psychol. Rev., *79*:433, 1972.

61. Parizkova, J.: Total body fat and skinfold thickness in children. Metabolism, *10*:794, 1961.

62. Paul, S.M., et al.: (+) − Amphetamine binding to rat hypothalamus: relation to anorexic potency of phenylethylamines. Science, *218*:487, 1982.

63. Persson, B., et al.: Effects of prolonged fast on lipoprotein lipase activity eluted from human adipose tissue. Acta Med. Scand., *188*:225, 1970.

64. Pi-Sunyer, F.X.: Jejunoileal bypass surgery for obesity. Am. J. Clin. Nutr., *29*:409, 1976.

65. Porte, D., and Woods, S.C.: Regulation of food intake and body weight by insulin. Diabetologia, *20*:274, 1981.

66. Protein diets. FDA Drug Bull., *8*:2, 1978.

67. Pykalisto, O.J., et al.: Determinants of human adipose tissue lipoprotein lipase: effects of diabetes and obesity on basal and diet induced activity. J. Clin. Invest., *56*: 1108, 1975.

68. Rand, C., and Stunkard, A.J.: Obesity and psychoanalysis. Am. J. Psychiatry, *135*:547, 1974.

69. Robson, J.R.K.: Obesity, an overview. Professional Nutritionist, *10*:3, 1978.

70. Rosen, J.D., et al.: Comparison of carbohydrate-containing and carbohydrate-restricted hypocaloric diets in the treatment of obesity: effects on appetite and mood. Am. J. Clin. Nutr., *36*:463, 1982.

71. Salans, L.B., et al.: Studies of human adipose tissue: adipose cell size and number in non-obese and obese patients. J. Clin. Invest., *52*:929, 1973.

72. Salans, L.B., et al.: Glucose metabolism and the response to insulin by human adipose tissue in spontaneous and experimental obesity. J. Clin. Invest., *53*: 848, 1974.

73. Schachter, S.: Recidivism and self-cure of smoking and obesity. Am. Psychol., *37*:436, 1982.

74. Schachter, S., et al.: Effects of fear, food deprivation and obesity on eating. J. Pers. Soc. Psychol., *10*:91, 1968.

75. Scheuer, J., and Tipton, C.M.: Cardiovascular adaptations to physical training. Ann. Rev. Physiol., *39*:221, 1977.

76. Schwartz, R.B., and Brunzell, J.D.: Increased adipose tissue lipoprotein lipase activity in moderately obese men after weight reduction. Lancet, *1*:1230, 1978.

77. Schwartz, R.B., and Brunzell, J.D.: Increase of adipose tissue lipoprotein lipase activity with weight loss. J. Clin. Invest., *67*:1425, 1981.

78. Seltzer, C.C., and Mayer, J.: Body build and obesity—who are the obese? JAMA, *189*:677, 1964.

79. Seltzer, C.C., and Mayer, J.: A simple criterion of obesity. Postgrad. Med., *38*:101A, 1965.

80. Sharkey, B.J.: Physiology of fitness: prescribing exercise for fitness, weight control and health. Champaign, Ill., Human Kinetics Publishers, 1979.

81. Simeons, A.T.W.: The action of chorionic gonadotropin in the obese. Lancet, *2*:946, 1954.

82. Sims, E.A.H., et al.: Endocrine and metabolic effects of experimental obesity in man. Recent Prog. Horm. Res., *29*:457, 1973.

83. Smith, G.P., and Gibb, J.: Brain-gut peptides and the control of food intake. In Martin, J.B., Reichlin, S., and Bick, K.L. (eds.): Neurosecretion and Brain Peptides. New York, Raven Press, 1981, p. 389.

84. Solow, C., et al.: Psychological effects of intestinal bypass surgery for severe obesity. N. Engl. J. Med., *290*: 300, 1974.

85. Sours, H.E., et al.: Sudden death associated with very low calorie weight reduction regimens. Am. J. Clin. Nutr., *34*:453, 1981.

86. Stein, M.R., et al.: Ineffectiveness of human chorionic gonadotropin in weight reduction: a double blind study. Am. J. Clin. Nutr., *29*:940, 1976.

87. Stuart, R.B., and Davis, B.: Slim chance in a fat world: behavioral control of obesity. Champaign, Ill., Research Press, 1972, pp. 23–31.

88. Stunkard, A., and Koch, C.: The interpretation of gastric motility. I. Apparent bias in the reports of hunger by obese persons. Arch. Gen. Psychiatry, *11*:74, 1964.

89. Stunkard, A.J., and Penick, S.: Behavior modification in the treatment of obesity: the problem of maintaining weight loss. Arch. Gen. Psychiatry, *36*:801, 1979.

90. Sturdevant, R., and Goetz, H.: Cholecystokinin both stimulates and inhibits food intake. Nature, *261*:713, 1976.

91. Ten State Nutrition Survey, 1968–70, U.S. Department of Health Education and Welfare (H.S.M.) 72–8131, Washington, D.C., 1972.

92. Van, R.L.R., and Roncari, D.A.K.: Complete differentiation of adipocyte precursors. Cell. Tissue Res., *195*:317, 1978.

93. Van Itallie, T.B.: Dietary Fiber and Obesity. Am. J. Clin. Nutr., *31*(Suppl):S43, 1978.

94. Van Itallie, T.B.: Liquid protein mayhem. Editorial. JAMA, *240*:144, 1978.

95. Woo, R., et al.: Effect of exercise on spontaneous calorie intake in obesity. Am. J. Clin. Nutr., *36*:470, 1982.

96. Woo, R., et al.: Voluntary food intake during prolonged exercise in obese women. Am. J. Clin. Nutr., *36*:478, 1982.

97. Woods, S.C., et al.: Chronic intra-cerebroventricular infusion of insulin reduces food intake and body weight of baboons. Nature, *282*:503, 1979.

98. Young, R.L., et al.: Chorionic gonadotropin in weight control. A double blind cross-over study. JAMA, *236*:2495, 1976.

Additional References

Bennett, W., and Gurin, J.: The Dieter's Dilemma. New York, Basic Books, Inc., 1982.

Bray, G.A.: The Obese Patient. Volume 9. In Smith, L.H. (ed.): Major Problems in Internal Medicine. Philadelphia, W.B. Saunders Co., 1976.

Bray, G.A. (ed.): Kroc Foundation Symposium on comparative methods of weight control. John Libbey and Company, Ltd., 1979.

Cioffi, L.A., James, W.P.T., and Van Itallie, T.B. (eds.): The Body Weight Regulatory System: Normal and Disturbed Mechanism. New York, Raven Press, 1981.

Food intake, satiety and peptide hormones of brain-gut axis. Nutr. Rev., *41*:20, 1983.

Greenwood, M.R.C. (ed.): Contemporary Issues in Clinical Nutrition. Volume 4: Obesity. New York, Churchill, Livingstone, 1983.

Hirschman, G.H., and Burton, B.T.: Symposium on surgical treatment of morbid obesity. Am. J. Clin. Nutr., *33*:Suppl., 1980.

Mason, E.E.: Surgical Treatment of Obesity. Volume 26. Major Problems in Clinical Surgery. Philadelphia, W.B. Saunders Company, 1981.

Schemmel, R. (ed.): Nutrition, Physiology, and Obesity. Boca Raton, Florida, CRC Press, Inc., 1980.

Stunkard, A.J. (ed.): Obesity. Philadelphia, W.B. Saunders Company, 1980.

Thompson, C.Y.: Controls of Eating. New York, SP Medical and Scientific Books, 1980.

DISEASES OF THE CIRCULATORY SYSTEM AND ANEMIAS

Nutritional Care in Cardiovascular Disease

The United States is reported to have one of the highest death rates from cardiovascular disease in the world, and cardiovascular disease accounts for half of all deaths in the U.S. Coronary disease takes first place; with stroke in second place; combined they account for three fourths of all deaths from cardiovascular disease. However, since the 1950's there has been a steady and substantial decline in mortality from coronary heart disease (CHD), which is thought to be due in large part to changes in lifestyle. Proper functioning of the cardiovascular system depends upon good nutrition, and diet plays an important role in the management and prevention of heart disease.

Heart Disease

The severity of heart disease depends upon the extent to which the cardiovascular system is involved and its functions are affected. Symptoms of heart disease can have a sudden onset, as with a *myocardial infarction,* or an insidious onset with gradual loss of cardiac function as in *chronic heart disease.*

CHRONIC HEART DISEASE

While not causing immediate death, chronic heart disease can adversely affect other organs in the body (such as the liver, kidneys and brain) because of the decreased blood flow as cardiac function declines. In compensated heart disease the organ is able to maintain almost normal circulation, through its own efforts, by an enlargement of the heart and by an increased pulse rate. In decompensated heart disease the heart is unable to compensate for its disturbance; it is unable to maintain normal circulation to supply nutrients and oxygen to the tissues or to carry away the waste products. There is shortness of breath and chest pain with any activity. With continued decompensation there is circulatory congestion from abnormal salt and water retention and *congestive heart failure* develops as shown in Figure 28-1. The reduced cardiac output results in decreased blood flow through the kidney and causes increased tubular resorption of sodium and finally an increased retention of water.

Treatment

Treatment involves medication to improve the function of the heart muscle and medication to reduce blood pressure. If edema is present, diuretics are used to increase water and sodium excretion and a low-sodium diet is prescribed.

Nutritional Care

The purpose of the diet in cardiac disease is to give adequate nourishment with the least possible work effort and muscular strain on the heart and to prevent or eliminate edema.

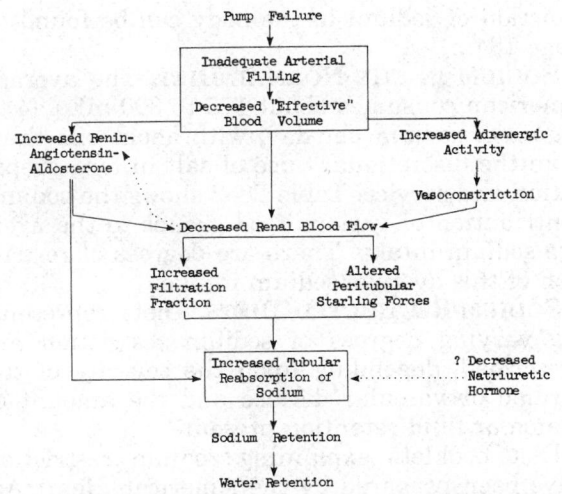

Figure 28–1. Pathogenesis of sodium and water retention in congestive heart failure. (From del Greco, F.: The kidney in congestive heart failure. Mod. Concepts Cardiovasc. Dis., 44:47, 1975.)

ACUTE CARDIAC DISEASE. In acute cardiac disease, which occurs in certain acute infections resulting in endocarditis or carditis, in cardiac failure, after myocardial infarction and after cardiac surgery, the diet is reduced to the minimum nutritional requirements. Dyspnea and chewing are incompatible in patients with severe congestive heart failure, since they often have to breathe through their mouths. Initially, these individuals should be given soft or liquid food that does not require chewing and should eat or be fed slowly in order to avoid aspiration of food. The frequency of feeding is also important; more frequent and smaller feedings are obviously indicated.

Stimulants. Since dietary stimulants such as caffeine and theobromine should be avoided in the acute phase of cardiac disease, the patient should not be allowed to have coffee, tea or cola drinks (which contain caffeine) or chocolate or cocoa (which contain caffeine and theobromine). Very weak tea or herb tea may be allowed but should be served warm rather than hot. Unfortunately, the caffeine content of these beverages varies widely depending on the strength, blend of coffee or tea and method of brewing as stated in Table 23–4. Individual coronary care units may have additional "coronary precautions" regarding stimulants.

Food Frequency and Consistency. Frequently the patient can tolerate five or six small meals a day much better than the usual three meals. Large meals can cause increased distention of the stomach and elevation of the diaphragm, thus displacing the heart upward and restricting breathing. Foods commonly considered bulky, gas-forming (see page 440), eas-

ily fermented and indigestible can have the same result and cause distress or an acute attack. Other foods may need to be restricted depending upon the individual. It is important to learn from the patient or his family which foods give him gas or gastrointestinal distress in order to avoid unnecessary restriction in the diet.[5]

The cardiac patient should not eat when upset, under stress or in a hurry, because at those times there may not be a sufficient supply of blood in the digestive organs to carry on good digestion. Each patient is different, and the dietary management should be planned according to the individual's needs.

CHRONIC CARDIAC DISEASE

Compensated Heart Disease. The patient's weight should be normal or 10 per cent underweight to help improve the functional state of the vascular system. *Slight underweight* lessens the burden on the heart and thereby improves its efficiency. However, this should be monitored because severe underweight and malnutrition can develop easily. The well-compensated heart may not require any diet modification other than to avoid obesity. However, mild restriction of sodium is sometimes prescribed to maintain fluid balance.

Decompensated Heart Disease. For patients with decompensated heart disease a rigid diet treatment is usually planned to relieve the present strain and prevent further damage to the organ. These patients, if obese, will experience symptomatic relief following *weight reduction.*

The protein allowance is kept a little high at 60 to 80 gm. Complex carbohydrates should furnish the bulk of the remaining calories, with fat adjusted to type and energy allowance.

When there is poor circulation to tissues in advanced cardiac disease, the tissues are deprived of nutrients, and the patient can become malnourished and may lose weight. This state of malnutrition can be masked by the concomitant weight gain that results from fluid retention and edema as the heart fails. The patient's face can continue to look puffy and the extremities edematous. For this patient it is important to record periodic anthropometric data and the daily weight both before and during therapy, so that as diuresis begins there will be an accurate determination of the person's dry body weight as a starting point for the nutritional care.

In severe heart failure the patient is also less likely to eat and may become malnourished from a decreased intake of nutrients, particularly protein. This problem is made worse by the fact that with greatly reduced renal blood flow, proteinuria may exist and can cause a significant loss of body protein.

Vitamins and minerals (except perhaps sodium) are given in normal amounts but may need some supplementation.

SODIUM AND FLUIDS. Edema is the result of impaired cardiac function that causes sodium (and therefore fluids) to accumulate in the tissues. Sodium and sometimes fluids are restricted and adjusted to the patient's individual needs. Theories regarding control of fluid balance emphasize the restriction of sodium, and fluid intake is usually not restricted except in the case of dilutional hyponatremia. When the sodium intake is limited the formation of edema fluid can be prevented, since the mechanisms that usually regulate the sodium concentration in extracellular fluid do not permit the retention of water without sodium. The effect of electrolytes upon the fluid balance is related primarily to the sodium ion rather than to the chloride ion, and dietary recommendations should refer to sodium rather than to salt.

Sodium restriction alone may be effective in reducing fluid volume by sodium depletion, but the use of diuretics may also be necessary. Since sodium restriction enhances the sodium-depleting effects of diuretics, the use of sodium restriction in conjunction with diuretics will give the best results.

Sodium Restriction

NOMENCLATURE. The diets commonly called "salt-restricted" are really *sodium restricted diets*. Each molecule of salt is approximately 40 per cent (39.3 per cent) sodium. To convert a specified weight of salt or sodium chloride to its sodium equivalent, multiply the weight of salt by 0.40 (0.393). In other words, 10 gm. of sodium chloride contains approximately 4 (3.93) gm. of sodium. Sodium is also measured in milliequivalents (mEq.). See Appendix Table 40 for an explanation of the conversion of mg. of sodium to mEq. of sodium. 1 gm. of sodium is equal to 43.5 mEq. of sodium, and Table 28–1 lists other conversions of sodium in mg. to sodium in mEq. One tsp. of salt contains approximately 2400 mg. or 104 mEq. of sodium. Discussion of the

Table 28–1. SODIUM AND SALT IN GRAM AND MILLIEQUIVALENT MEASUREMENTS

MEq. Na$^+$ (Approximate)	Mg. Na$^+$	Gm. NaCl (Approximate)
11	250	0.6
22	500	1.3
43	1000	2.5
65	1500	3.8
87	2000	5.0
130	3000	7.6
174	4000	10.2

function of sodium in the body can be found on page 184.

SODIUM IN THE NORMAL DIET. The average American consumes about 175 to 300 mEq. (4 to 7 gm.) of sodium per day, with about one third from the discretionary use of salt in food preparation and service. Table 28–2 shows the sodium contribution of various food groups to the average sodium intake. There are degrees of restriction of this average sodium intake.

SODIUM-RESTRICTED DIETS. Diets representing varying degrees of sodium restriction are prescribed, depending upon the severity of the cardiac or vascular disease and the amount of edema or fluid retention present.

Diet booklets explaining sodium restriction have been prepared by the American Heart Association's Nutrition Committee and are available from local heart association offices to use when counseling patients who need to restrict sodium in their diets. Sodium-controlled diets can be planned using an exchange list system similar to that used for patients with diabetes. Table 28–3 gives the average sodium values of the food exchanges. Table 28–4 gives the foods included in each exchange list. These lists are especially useful in designing a diet for someone who also needs to control energy intake.

Mild Sodium Restriction: 87 to 130 mEq. (2000 to 3000 mg.) Sodium Daily. For the patient with only moderate heart failure when some control of sodium intake is indicated, sodium restriction of this degree will probably not influence blood pressure. However, it will be useful in maintaining proper fluid and electrolyte balance. A *limited* amount of salt is allowed in cooking; however, no salt is added to the food after cooking. Salty foods such as those listed in Table 28–5 should be omitted.

Moderate Sodium Restriction: 43 to 87 mEq. (1000 to 2000 mg.) Sodium Daily. For the patient with edema or a tendency to develop edema when following only mild sodium restriction or for the patient taking diuretics to control blood pressure, no salt is added during the preparation of food or at the table, with the exception of allowing either 1/4 tsp. of salt daily or measured amounts of foods such as regular bakery bread (1 slice contains 150 mg. sodium) and salted butter (2 tsp. contains 100 mg. sodium) to make the diet more palatable. No salty foods (Table 28–5) are allowed. A diet providing these restrictions will usually increase urine output as body sodium is depleted.

Strict Sodium Restriction: 22 mEq. (500 mg.) Sodium or Less Daily. If edema and pulmonary congestion persist despite medication and moderate sodium restriction, sodium should be reduced to 22 mEq. (500 mg.) or less daily. For strict sodium restriction no salt is added

Text continued on page 555

Table 28–2. SODIUM CONTENT OF THE "TOTAL DIET" AND THE PER CENT CONTRIBUTION TO THE TOTAL CONTENT FOR INFANTS, TODDLERS, AND ADULTS, BY COMMODITY GROUP

COMMODITY GROUP	MG./DAY*	%	COMMODITY GROUP	MG./DAY*	%
Infants[†]			*Toddlers*[†] *(Continued)*		
Drinking water	10 ± 17	1.4	Oils and fats	75 ± 20	4.2
Whole milk, fresh	266 ± 92	37.7	Sugars and adjuncts[‡]	16 ± 6	0.9
Other dairy products and substitutes	82 ± 51	11.6	Beverages	5 ± 3	0.3
Meat, fish, and poultry	96 ± 73	13.6			
Grain and cereal products	94 ± 92	13.3	Total/day	1805 ± 226	
Potatoes	1 ± 1	0.1	Total/1,000 kcal.	1388	
Vegetables	110 ± 105	15.6	% maximum ESADDI[§]	185	
Fruits and fruit juices	14 ± 18	2.0			
Oils and fats	26 ± 55	3.7	*Adults*[†]		
Sugars and adjuncts[‡]	6 ± 4	0.8	Dairy products	647 ± 72	9.7
Beverages	1 ± 1	0.1	Meat, fish, and poultry	968 ± 139	14.5
			Grain and cereal products	1959 ± 537	29.3
Total/day	706 ± 304		Potatoes	77 ± 26	1.2
Total/1000 kcal.	802		Leafy vegetables	17 ± 6	0.3
% maximum ESADDI[§]	128		Legume vegetables	228 ± 21	3.4
			Root vegetables	15 ± 7	0.2
Toddlers[†]			Miscellaneous vegetables	291 ± 54	4.3
Drinking water	12 ± 16	0.7	Fruits	77 ± 40	1.2
Whole milk, fresh	215 ± 26	11.9	Oils, fats, and shortening	406 ± 64	6.1
Other dairy products and substitutes	150 ± 42	8.3	Sugars and adjuncts[‡]	1983 ± 429	29.6
Meat, fish, and poultry	459 ± 93	25.4	Beverages (including drinking water)	25 ± 16	0.4
Grain and cereal products	634 ± 197	35.1			
Potatoes	5 ± 5	0.3	Total/day (3900 kcal.)	6692 ± 767	
Vegetables	220 ± 63	12.2	Total/1000 kcal.	1,716	
Fruits and fruit juices	13 ± 14	0.7	% maximum ESADDI[§]	203	

* Mean ± standard deviation.

† The diets for infants, toddlers and adults contain 880, 1300, and 3900 kcal. respectively. The sodium and potassium intakes would be less in individuals consuming diets of fewer kcalories. The infant is 6 months old, the toddler is 2 years old and the adult is a 15- to 20-year-old male, chosen because he is likely to be the largest consumer of food and thus of sodium and potassium.

‡ Includes the discretionary salt added during preparation of foods and at the table. The amount varied slightly according to the geographic region but averaged about 4.5 gm. (1800 mg. sodium) per day.

§ Estimated safe and adequate daily dietary intake (ESADDI) established by the National Research Council, National Academy of Sciences. Since the study was to represent 6-month-old infants, the average of the two ESADDIs was used as the standard for this age group.

Data from the FDA Total Diet Studies. (From Shank, F.R., et al: Perspective of Food and Drug Administration on dietary sodium. J. Am. Diet. Assoc., *80*:29, 1982.)

Table 28–3. SODIUM AND NUTRIENT VALUES FOR FOOD EXCHANGE GROUPS

LIST	FOOD GROUP	AMOUNT	Na+ (mg.)	Na+ (mEq.)	PRO (gm.)	CHO (gm.)	FAT (gm.)	KCAL.
1	Milk	see list						
1A	whole milk	1 cup	120	5	8	12	10	170
	skim milk	1 cup	120	5	8	12	–	80
1B	Milk, low sodium	1 cup	7	–	8	12	10	170
	Buttermilk, salted	1 cup	280	13	8	12	3	110
2	Vegetables							
	cooked, raw, fresh, frozen	½ cup	9	–	2	5	–	25
	canned	½ cup	230	10	v a r i a b l e			
3	Fruits	see list	2	–	–	10	–	40
4	Bread or cereal	see list						
	low sodium or made without salt		5	–	2	15	–	70
	salted yeast bread	1 slice	150	7	2	15	–	70
5	Meat, poultry, fresh fish	1 oz. or						
	cooked without salt	see list	25	1	7	–	5	75
	Cheese, cottage (dry)	¼ cup	5	–	7	–	5	75
	cheddar	1 oz.	207	9	7	–	5	75
	Egg	1	70	3	7	–	5	75
6	Fat							
	unsalted	see list	–	–	–	–	5	45
	salted		50	2	–	–	5	45

Table 28–4. SODIUM CONTENT OF FOOD EXCHANGES
(PROCESSED OR PREPARED WITHOUT ADDED SALT)

MILK (LIST 1)

GROUP A *Regular Milk*		GROUP B *Low-sodium Milk*	

Each unit in both groups contains about 170 kcal., 8 gm. protein, 10 gm. fat and 12 gm. carbohydrate. Group A units contain 120 mg. sodium, whereas group B units contain 7 mg. sodium.

1 cup	Evaporated whole milk (reconstituted)	4 tbsp.	Low-sodium dry milk (powder)
[a]2 fat units and 1 cup	Non-fat buttermilk (unsalted–ask dairy)	1 cup	Low-sodium dry milk (reconstituted)
[a]2 fat units and 3 tbsp.[b]	Non-fat dry milk (powder)	[a]2 fat units and 3 tbsp.[b]	Low-sodium non-fat dry milk (powder)
[a]2 fat units and 1 cup	Non-fat dry milk (reconstituted)	[a]2 fat units and 1 cup	Low-sodium non-fat dry milk (reconstituted)
[a]2 fat units and 1 cup	Skim milk	1 cup	Low-sodium whole fresh milk
1 cup	Whole milk		
1 cup	Whole milk buttermilk (unsalted–ask dairy)		

Note: Two units from the meat list may be substituted for not more than one milk unit a day.
[a] If non-fat milk is used, 2 fat units can be added to the diet.
[b] Use the amount specified on package for making one cup of milk–usually 3 or 4 tbsp.
DO NOT USE: Any kind of milk not on list.
    Any commercial foods made of milk: ice cream, sherbet, milk shakes, chocolate milk, malted milk, milk mixes, condensed milk.

VEGETABLES (LIST 2)

Use fresh, frozen or dietetic canned vegetables only. Each unit contains about 9 mg. sodium, 25 kcal., 2 gm. protein, 5 gm. carbohydrate and negligible fat.

VEGETABLE UNITS *Each unit is a ½-cup serving.*	DO NOT USE:

Asparagus
Broccoli
Brussels sprouts
Cabbage
Cauliflower
Chicory
Cucumber
Eggplant
Endive
Escarole
Green beans
Lettuce
Mushrooms
Okra
Onions
Peas (fresh or low-sodium dietetic canned only)
Peppers, green or red
Pumpkin
Radishes
Rutabaga (yellow turnip)
Squash, summer (yellow, zucchini, etc.)
Squash, winter (acorn, Hubbard, etc.)
Tomato juice (low-sodium dietetic only)
Tomatoes
Turnip greens
Wax beans
	Canned vegetables or vegetable juices unless they are low-sodium dietetic.
	Frozen vegetables if processed with salt. (Watch out especially for frozen peas and lima beans.) *Read the label.*
	Do not use these vegetables in any form:
	    Artichokes
	    Beet greens
	    Beets
	    Carrots[c]
	    Celery[c]
	    Chard, Swiss
	    Dandelion greens
	    Hominy
	    Kale
	    Mustard greens
	    Sauerkraut
	    Spinach
	    Turnips, white
	
	Do not use salt or MSG in cooking or at the table.

From Your 500 Milligram Sodium Diet. New York, American Heart Association, 1970, pp. 38–53, and Appendix Table 12. Refer to Exchange Lists, Chapter 25.

[c] Even though carrots and celery are high in sodium to be used as vegetables, you may use them sparingly to season (for example, one stalk of celery or carrot to a pot of stew) or as garnish.

Table 28–4. SODIUM CONTENT OF FOOD EXCHANGES
(PROCESSED OR PREPARED WITHOUT ADDED SALT) (*Continued*)

FRUIT (LIST 3)

Use fresh, frozen, canned, or dried fruit. Each unit contains about 2 mg. sodium, 40 kcal., negligible protein and fat and 10 gm. carbohydrate.

FRUIT UNITS				DO NOT USE:
1 small	Apple	⅛ medium	Honeydew melon	Crystallized or glazed fruit.
⅓ cup	Apple juice or apple cider	½ small	Mango	Maraschino cherries.
½ cup	Applesauce	1 small	Orange	**Do not use salt or MSG in cooking or at the table.**
4 halves	Apricots (dried)	½ cup	Orange juice	
2 medium	Apricots (fresh)	⅓ medium	Papaya	
¼ cup	Apricot nectar	1 medium	Peach	
½ small	Banana	1 small	Pear	
1 cup	Blackberries	½ cup diced or 2 small slices	Pineapple	
⅔ cup	Blueberries			
¼ small	Cantaloupe			
10 large	Cherries	⅓ cup	Pineapple juice	Note: Read labels on packages of dried and frozen fruit. Sometimes sodium sulfite has been added to dried fruit and salt to frozen fruit.
1 tbsp.	Cranberries (sweetened)	2 medium	Plums	
		2 medium	Prunes	
⅓ cup	Cranberry juice (sweetened)	¼ cup	Prune juice	
		2 tbsp.	Raisins	
2	Dates	1 cup	Raspberries	
1 medium	Fig	2 tbsp.	Rhubarb (sweetened)	
½ cup	Fruit cup or mixed fruits			
½ small	Grapefruit	1 cup	Strawberries	
½ cup	Grapefruit juice	1 large	Tangerine	
12	Grapes	½ cup	Tangerine juice	
¼ cup	Grape juice	1 cup	Watermelon	

Note: Fresh lemons and limes (and their juice) may be used as desired. They do not count as a unit. Unsweetened cranberries and cranberry juice and unsweetened rhubarb may also be used as desired.

BREAD (LIST 4)

Low-sodium Breads, Cereals and Cereal Products

Each unit contains about 5 mg. sodium, 70 kcal., 2 gm. protein, negligible fat and 15 gm. carbohydrate.

BREAD UNITS	DO NOT USE:
Breads and rolls (yeast) made without salt.	Yeast breads or rolls made with salt, MSG or from commercial mixes.

1 slice	Bread
4 pieces (3½″ × 1½″ × ⅛″)	Melba toast (unsalted)
1 medium	Roll

Breads (quick) made with sodium-free baking powder or potassium bicarbonate and without salt or made from low-sodium dietetic mix.	Quick breads made with baking powder, baking soda, salt, MSG or made from commercial mixes.

1 medium	Biscuit
1 cube (1½″)	Cornbread
2 three-inch	Griddle cakes
1 medium	Muffin

Cereals (cooked), unsalted Each unit is a ½-cup serving	Quick-cooking and enriched cereals that contain a sodium compound. Read the label.

Farina
Grits
Oatmeal
Rolled wheat
Wheat meal

Table continued on following page

Table 28–4. SODIUM CONTENT OF FOOD EXCHANGES
(PROCESSED OR PREPARED WITHOUT ADDED SALT) (*Continued*)

BREAD (LIST 4) (*Continued*)
Low-sodium Breads, Cereals and Cereal Products
Each unit contains about 5 mg. sodium, 70 kcal., 2 gm. protein, negligible fat and 15 gm. carbohydrate.

BREAD UNITS		DO NOT USE:
	Cereals (dry)	Dry cereals except for those listed as allowed.
¾ cup	Puffed rice	
¾ cup	Puffed wheat	
⅔ biscuit	Shredded wheat	

(You may use other dry cereals—¾-cup serving—*if the label states* that there are no more than 6 mg. of sodium to each 100 gm. of cereal.)

1½ tbsp. uncooked	Barley	Self-rising cornmeal.
2 tbsp.	Cornmeal	Graham crackers or any other crackers except low-sodium dietetic.
2½ tbsp.	Cornstarch	
5 two-inch-square	Crackers (low-sodium dietetic)	Self-rising flour.
2½ tbsp.	Flour	
½ cup cooked	Macaroni	
1 five-inch-square	Matzo (plain, unsalted)	Salted crackers.
½ cup cooked	Noodles	Salted popcorn. Potato chips.
1½ cups	Popcorn	Pretzels.
½ cup cooked	Rice, brown or white	
½ cup cooked	Spaghetti	
2 tbsp. uncooked	Tapioca	Waffles containing salt, baking powder, baking soda.
1 three-inch-square section	Waffle, yeast or low-sodium baking powder, and/or your egg for the day	
½ cup cooked	Beans, lima or navy (fresh or dried)	**Do not use salt or MSG in cooking or at the table.**
¼ cup	Beans, baked (no pork)	
⅓ cup or 1 small ear	Corn	
½ cup cooked	Lentils (dried)	
⅔ cup	Parsnips	
½ cup cooked	Peas, split green or yellow, cowpeas, etc. (dried)	
1 small	Potato, white	
½ cup	Potatoes, mashed	
¼ cup or ½ small	Sweet potato	

Note: One unit from the bread list may be substituted for one unit from Group C.

Table 28–4. SODIUM CONTENT OF FOOD EXCHANGES
(PROCESSED OR PREPARED WITHOUT ADDED SALT) *(Continued)*

MEAT[d] (LIST 5)
Meat, Poultry, Fish, Eggs and Low-sodium Cheese and Peanut Butter
Units allowed per day will average about 25 mg. sodium, 75 kcal., 7 gm. protein, 5 gm. fat and negligible carbohydrate.

MEAT UNITS	DO NOT USE:
Meat or poultry (fresh, frozen or canned low-sodium dietetic)	Brains or kidneys
1 oz., cooked, of any of the following is a unit	Canned, salted, or smoked meat: bacon, bologna, chipped or corned beef, frankfurters, ham, meats koshered by salting, luncheon meats, salt pork, sausage, smoked tongue, etc.

MEAT UNITS			DO NOT USE:
beef	quail		
chicken	rabbit		
duck	tongue (fresh,		
lamb	cooked without salt)		
liver (beef, calf,	turkey		
chicken, pork)	veal		
pork			

(Beef or calf liver allowed not more than once in two weeks.)

Frozen fish fillets

Fish or fish fillets (fresh only)

Canned, salted, or smoked fish: anchovies, caviar, salted and dried cod, herring, canned salmon,[e] sardines, canned tuna,[e] etc. Shellfish: clams, crabs, lobsters, oysters, scallops, shrimp, etc.

1 oz., cooked, of any of the following is a unit

Cheese[e]

bass	eels	salmon
bluefish	flounder	sole
catfish	halibut	trout
cod	rockfish	tuna

Salted cottage cheese

Regular peanut butter

1 oz.	Canned low-sodium dietetic fish (tuna or salmon)	
¼ cup	Cottage cheese (unsalted)	
1	Egg (limit is 1 a day)	
1 oz.	Low-sodium dietetic cheese	
2 tbsp.	Low-sodium dietetic peanut butter	

Do not use salt or MSG in cooking or at the table.

[d]See List 5, Table 25–5 to select meats that are also low in fat.
[e]Unless it is low-sodium dietetic.

GUIDE TO BUYING MEAT, POULTRY AND FISH

An average serving of meat, poultry or fish is 3 oz. This is equal to three units.
Because these foods shrink during cooking, you will have to buy more than 3 oz. for a 3 oz. serving.
To have a 3 oz. serving of fish or lean meat without bone—for example, liver or ground beef—you will need to start with 4 oz. raw.
For meat with bone or fat, you will need to buy 5 to 6 oz. of raw meat to give you 3 oz. of lean cooked meat.
Here are some examples to guide you when you shop. One of these will usually give you three meat units:

> 1 pork chop
> 2 rib lamb chops
> leg and thigh of 3-lb. chicken
> half breast of chicken
> 2 meat patties, 2″ diameter, ½″ thick
> 2 thin slices roast meat, each 3″ × 3″ × ¼″

Table continued on the following page

Table 28–4. SODIUM CONTENT OF FOOD EXCHANGES
(PROCESSED OR PREPARED WITHOUT ADDED SALT) (*Continued*)

FAT (LIST 6)

Each unit contains negligible sodium, about 45 kcal. and 5 gm. fat.

FAT UNITS		DO NOT USE:
⅛ of four-inch	Avocado	Salted butter
1 tsp.	Butter, unsalted	Bacon and bacon fat
(1 small pat)		Olives
1 tbsp.[f]	Cream, heavy	Salt pork
	(sweet or sour)	Commercial French or other dressing[g]
2 tbsp.[f]	Cream, light	Salted margarine
	(sweet or sour)	Commercial mayonnaise[g]
1 tsp.	Fat or oil for cooking, unsalted	Salted nuts
1 tbsp.	French dressing, unsalted	
1 tsp.	Margarine, unsalted	
1 tsp.	Mayonnaise, unsalted	
6 small	Nuts, unsalted	

[f]Limit is 2 tbsp. a day because cream contains more sodium than the other fats.
[g]Unless it is low-sodium dietetic.

MISCELLANEOUS FOODS (LIST 7)

Each food listed contains small amounts of sodium.

	DO NOT USE:
Sugar, white or brown	Saccharin
Syrup, honey, jelly, jam, marmalade	Molasses
	Instant cocoa mixes
Alcoholic beverages	Beverage mixes, including fruit-flavored powder
Cocoa, made with milk from diet	Fountain beverages: Malted milk and their milk preparates
Coffee, regular and instant	Commercial candies
Coffee substitute	Commercially sweetened gelatin desserts
Tea	Regular baking powder
Postum	Regular baking soda
	Barbecue sauce
Candy, homemade without salt	Regular bouillon cubes
Cornstarch	Catsup and sauces
Gelatin	Celery, onion and garlic salts
	Meat sauces, extracts and tenderizers
Cream of tartar	MSG salt
Sodium-free baking powder	Soy or Worcestershire sauce
Potassium bicarbonate	Salt substitutes, unless recommended by physician
Yeast	Mustard, prepared
	Olives, pickles, relishes
Bouillon cube (Low-Na)	Celery leaves, dried or fresh
Spices	Cooking wine
Chives	Horseradish
Flavorings	
Vinegar	
Wine	

Table 28–5. DIETARY SUBSTANCES GENERALLY TO BE AVOIDED IN SODIUM RESTRICTION

1. Salt
2. Vegetable salts and flakes, such as onion, garlic or celery salt; celery and parsley flakes
3. Smoked, processed or cured meats and fish, such as ham, bacon, corned beef, cold cuts, frankfurters, sausage, tongue, salt pork, chipped beef, pickled herring and anchovies
4. Meat extracts, bouillon cubes and meat sauces
5. Salted foods, such as potato chips, nuts and popcorn
6. Prepared condiments, relishes, Worcestershire sauce, catsup, pickles, mustard and olives
7. Prepackaged frozen foods, packaged mixes for sauces, gravies, casseroles, and noodle, rice or potato dishes unless prepared without salt
8. Canned soup unless made without salt
9. Prepared flour mixes or packaged baking mixes unless prepared without salt
10. Frozen fish fillets and shellfish, except oysters
11. Frozen peas and lima beans; sauerkraut in any form
12. All canned meat and vegetable products unless prepared without salt (dietetic pack)
13. Butter, cheese and peanut butter unless prepared without salt

during the preparation of food or at the table, and foods listed in the "Do Not Use" column of Table 28–4 are avoided completely.

Table 28–6 shows the nutritive value of a dietary pattern for an adult that provides approximately 22 mEq. (500 mg.) of sodium daily. The foods included provide nutrients at levels that, except for total iron content for young women, and perhaps zinc for both men and women, equal or exceed those of the Recommended Dietary Allowances for the normal healthy adult. Adjustments and substitutions can be made from this basic pattern to design diets of higher or lower sodium content.

The energy content of this basic diet can also be increased or decreased to meet the individual requirements by using more or less of the foods low in sodium, such as unsalted cereal foods, bread, potatoes and fat. Sugar and jelly may be used as desired within the energy requirements.

Severe Sodium Restriction: 11 mEq. (250 mg.) Sodium Daily. Further reduction in sodium content of the basic diet pattern outlined in Table 28–6 can be accomplished by substituting appropriate amounts of low-sodium whole or non-fat milk (7 mg. sodium per cup) for the regular whole or skim milk (120 mg. sodium per cup). This is necessary to meet the protein and calcium requirements for this diet since meat, fish, poultry and eggs, which contain naturally occurring sodium, will also have to be restricted.

Sodium-deficient milk has been processed to remove most of the naturally occurring sodium. It is usually prepared in powder form, which can be reconstituted; however, a fluid milk preparation is also available. Within the last 10 years the palatability of this milk has been vastly improved. The fluid low-sodium milk is usually available from local dairies. Dietary adequacy is maintained so long as the sodium-deficient milk contains the other nutrients usually present in regular milk. For those who object to the taste of the milk, flavorings such as chocolate, honey, lemon, vanilla, maple and coffee can be added. The milk can also be used in preparing such dishes as soups, custards and puddings. Low-sodium cheeses are also available, and unlike the milk, these can be found in regular grocery stores. The difference between the sodium in an ounce of regular cheese and an ounce of a low-sodium cheese can be 210 mg. versus 6 mg.

LOW SODIUM SYNDROME. Severe sodium restriction is intended primarily for the hospitalized patient whose sodium tolerance is unusually low. Caution should be employed to avoid hyponatremia, hypochloremia and eventually sodium depletion azotemia as the glomerular filtration rate falls. Harmful results may follow severe and prolonged restriction of sodium intake, with continued water intake, and it is important that the patient be watched carefully for evidence of sodium depletion. Grave danger may exist in severely restricting sodium intake in cases of renal insufficiency in which the kidneys cannot excrete dilute urine. Some symptoms of potential salt depletion that must be evaluated are: (1) complaints of weakness, lassitude, anorexia and vomiting, (2) mental confusion, and (3) abdominal cramps and aching skeletal muscles. However, the possibility that the *low sodium syndrome* may occur does not contraindicate the use of a sodium-restricted diet when therapeutically indicated.

SODIUM IN FOODS. In their natural state, the majority of foods contain varying amounts of sodium, but the main source of sodium in the diet is salt added in food preparation, food preservation and processing, and at the table. Other sodium compounds are found in leavening agents (baking powder, baking soda), and some additives and preservatives as listed in Table 28–7.

The sodium content of water supplies must be known before it is possible to design effective sodium-restricted diets. The amount of sodium in drinking water may vary widely in different localities but unless it is greater than 1 mEq./liter it will probably not be a significant source of sodium in the diet. Water sodium content is apt to be relatively high where "softening" treatment is employed. Typical water softeners exchange Na⁺ ions for calcium and other ions that cause water hardness. Beverages and processed foods also reflect the sodium content of the drinking water where they are man-

Table 28-6. NUTRITIVE VALUE OF BASIC DIET PATTERN FOR A SODIUM-RESTRICTED DIET (500 MG. SODIUM)*

FOOD	MEASURE^a	WEIGHT (gm.)	KCAL.^b	PROTEIN (gm.)	FAT (gm.)	CARBOHYDRATE (mg.)	MINERALS			VITAMINS				
							Na^c (mg.)	Ca (gm.)	Fe (mg.)	A (I.U.)	THIAMIN (mg.)	RIBOFLAVIN (mg.)	NIACIN (mg.)	ASCORBIC ACID (mg.)
Milk	2 cups (1 pt.)	488	335	17	19	24	244	0.58	0.4	780	0.18	0.84	0.6	6
Meat, fish or poultry	5 oz. (raw) (cooked)	120	365	28	27		104	0.01	3.5	2280^d	0.30	0.40	6.9	1
Egg	1 medium	54	75	6	6		70	0.03	1.3	550	0.05	0.14	tr.	0
Whole-grain or enriched cereal^e	1 serving	20	75	2	tr.	16	tr.	0.01	0.6	0	0.11	0.03	0.7	0
Whole-grain or enriched bread (without added sodium)	3 slices	90	250	8	1	47	27	0.07	1.6	0	0.22	0.14	2.0	0
Potato	1 medium	150	125	3	tr.	29	4	0.02	1.0	30	0.14	0.05	1.5	21
Leafy green or yellow vegetable^f	1 serving	100	30	2	tr.	6	9	0.05	0.9	880	0.08	0.07	0.7	26
Other vegetable^g	1 serving	100	35	1	tr.	8	4	0.02	0.6	770	0.06	0.06	0.7	17
Citrus fruit	1 serving	100	45	1	tr.	12	1	0.03	0.4	120	0.07	0.03	0.2	47
Other fruit^h	2 servings	200	125	1	1	32	5	0.02	1.0	120	0.08	0.08	0.8	18
Butter, unsalted	2 tbsp.	30	215		24		3			990				
Totals			1675	69	78	174	471	0.84	11.3	6520	1.29	1.84	14.1	136
Recommended Dietary Allowances:† Woman (51+ years)			1800	44			1100-3300	0.8	10	4000^j	1.0	1.2	13^i equiv.	60
Man (51+ years)			2400	56			1100-3300	0.8	10	5000^j	1.2	1.4	16^i equiv.	60

*From Sodium-Restricted Diets. A Report of the Food and Nutrition Board. National Research Council. Publication 325, 1954.

† From Recommended Dietary Allowances. Washington, D.C. National Research Council. 1980.

^a Average values for each food group have been computed according to the percentage distribution of food supplies as described in "Planning Food for Institutions." Agriculture Handbook No. 16, Washington, D.C.: U.S. Dept. of Agriculture, 1951. Food values used are those published in "Composition of Foods—Raw, Processed, Prepared" by Bernice K. Watt and Annabel L. Merrill, Agriculture Handbook No. 8, Washington, D.C.: U.S. Dept. of Agriculture, 1950.

^b Calories have been rounded off to the nearest 5. The total calories should be adjusted to the patient's needs by using more or less of cereal foods, bread, potatoes or unsalted fat. Sugar and jelly may be used when there is no calorie restriction.

^c Values for sodium are those naturally occurring in food before any additions have been made through processing and cookery.

^d This vitamin A value is reduced to 0 if average of 1 oz. liver per week is omitted.

^e Includes farina, rolled oats, rolled wheat cereal, wheat meal, puffed wheat, puffed rice, shredded wheat. Quick-cooking cereals and other dry cereals omitted because of high sodium content.

^f Includes asparagus, green lima beans (not frozen), snap beans, broccoli, brussels sprouts, lettuce and escarole, okra, peas (not frozen), peppers, pumpkin, winter squash, turnip greens and products packed without added sodium. Excludes carrots, kale, beet greens, chard, spinach.

^g Includes cauliflower, corn, cucumber, eggplant, onion, parsnip, radishes, rutabagas, summer squash, tomatoes and products packed without added sodium. Excludes beets, celery, white turnips.

^h Includes all fruits other than citrus—fresh, canned or frozen according to consumption data.

^i Niacin equivalents include sources of the preformed vitamin and the precursor tryptophan. 60 mg. tryptophan equals 1 mg. niacin.

^j 4000 and 5000 I.U. vitamin A are more appropriately expressed as 800 RE and 1000 RE (retinol equivalents), respectively.

Table 28–7. SOME SODIUM-CONTAINING PRESERVATIVES

NAME	FOODS LIKELY TO CONTAIN
Disodium phosphate	Cereals, cheeses, ice cream, bottled drinks
Monosodium glutamate	Accent (a flavor enhancer), meats, condiments, pickles, soups, candy, baked goods
Sodium alginate	Ice cream, chocolate milk
Sodium benzoate	Breads
Sodium hydroxide	Pretzels, sour cream, cocoa products, canned peas
Sodium propionate	Breads
Sodium sulfite	Dried fruits
Sodium pectinate	Syrups and toppings, ice cream, sherbet, salad dressings, jams and jellies
Sodium caseinate	Ice cream, and other frozen products
Sodium bicarbonate	Baking powder, tomato soup, self-rising flour, sherbets, confections

ufactured. It may also be necessary to use distilled water or a natural water low in sodium.

The animal protein foods, namely, milk, cheese, eggs, meat, poultry and fish, are relatively high in sodium. Just like human muscle cells, cells of animal tissue are surrounded by sodium chloride—physiological saline. Thus, while nutritionally essential, these foods must be used in measured amounts unless they are processed so that most of the naturally occurring sodium is removed.

Meat and poultry may be a special problem for Jewish patients who follow orthodox dietary laws. In order to be kosher, freshly slaughtered meat and poultry is salted for one hour to remove the blood. Although it is thoroughly washed before it is cooked, some sodium is retained in the meat so that the sodium content may be 4 times higher—90 to 115 mg. per ounce.[32] Alternatives are to use ammonium chloride instead of sodium chloride for drawing out the blood or to boil the meat and discard the broth before eating it.

Fruit is low in natural sodium and its use should be encouraged, since frequently the sodium restricted patient also needs to lose weight, and fruits are generally low in calories. In addition most are high in potassium (Appendix Table 10), which is important for those patients taking potassium-wasting diuretics.

Certain vegetables—beets, beet greens, celery, kale, dandelion greens, carrots, chard, white turnips and spinach—are relatively high in natural sodium (50 to 80 mg. per serving). Baked goods such as breads, desserts, cakes, cookies and cereals contribute almost 30 per cent of the sodium in the average diet, as can be seen in Table 28–2. They vary appreciably in amounts of sodium. In these foods salt must be omitted, an appropriate non–sodium-containing leaven-

ing agent chosen and allowances made for milk and eggs used. Cream of tartar, sodium-free baking powder, potassium bicarbonate and yeast are leavening agents that may be used. Appendix Tables 1 and 10 give the sodium content of certain foods.

Availability of Special Low-Sodium Foods. Many of the more important food items are available as specially prepared low-sodium products. These include:

Low-sodium milk (whole and skimmed)
Unsalted canned meat
Unsalted canned vegetables
Unsalted cheese (cottage, cheddar)
Unsalted butter and margarine
Unsalted bakery products (bread, crackers, cake, cookies)
Low-sodium baking powder
Low-sodium soups

The term "salt free" does not imply necessarily that the product is low in sodium. The food may have natural sodium or sodium-containing additives such as those listed in Table 28–7. In the early 1980's the Food and Drug Administration (FDA) began revising food labeling regulations so that labeling of sodium content would be required on more foods and the terms "low sodium," "moderately low sodium" and "reduced sodium," would have legal definitions.

Commercial Salt Substitutes. Most salt substitutes are mineral bases consisting of salts other than sodium compounded to simulate sodium chloride in taste. Potassium chloride, calcium chloride and ammonium chloride are used, but it is conceivable that the administration of a substitute containing large amounts of potassium to patients with renal insufficiency or of ammonium to patients with severe liver disease could be harmful. However for patients requiring potassium supplementation because of diuretic therapy, the use of potassium chloride salt substitutes is an easy way to add potassium to the diet.

Some products advertised as being "low sodium" salt substitutes contain in fact another salt *and* sodium chloride. They contain *half* as much sodium as regular table salt, and this must be understood by the patient. *These are not salt substitutes.*

Other products classified as vegetized salts are available. They range somewhere between condiments and salt substitutes. Most products have powdered dehydrated vegetables as a base and varied additional ingredients. However, they may contain considerable quantities of sodium and should therefore not be used. Salt substitutes should be used only when recommended by a physician for a particular patient. Generally, it is advisable for the patient to learn to avoid the salt substitutes and to employ other methods, such as the use of herbs and spices, in making the sodium restricted diet more palatable.

IODINE. In areas of the country where iodine intake is largely dependent on the use of iodized salt, the sodium-restricted diet should be carefully evaluated for adequate iodine content when prolonged sodium restriction is required. The RDA for adults for iodine is 150 μg. per day, and one tsp. (5 gm.) of iodized salt contains approximately 380 μg. of iodine. Supplemental iodine in tablet form may have to be provided if the iodine content of the diet and local drinking water is inadequate. This is unlikely, however, considering the many other sources of iodine in our diet that are discussed on pages 170 and 511.

NON-FOOD SOURCES OF SODIUM. In addition to the sodium in food and water, incidental amounts may be ingested in the form of medicines and dentifrices. Barbiturates, sulfonamides, antibiotics and other drugs, cough medicines, stomach alkalizers, laxatives, tooth pastes and powders and mouthwashes may contain large amounts of sodium. For example, over-the-counter chewable antacid tablets can add between 1200 and 7000 mg. of sodium daily when used as therapy for ulcer or gastrointestinal distress.[6] Aspirin supplies about 50 mg. of sodium per dose. Labels on these items should be read carefully. Most medicines contain less than 5 mg. of sodium per dose; those that have 80 to 120 mg. per dose are the ones that contribute substantially to sodium intake. The San Francisco Heart Association has published a complete booklet of the sodium content of medicines.[53] The use of sodium saccharin or sodium cyclamate (in Canada) as the sole sweetener in the diet could contribute a small amount of sodium, 50 to 100 mg. per day, to the diet.

SUGGESTIONS FOR MAKING THE SODIUM-RESTRICTED DIET PALATABLE. Every possible means should be used to make the sodium-restricted diet palatable. The patient should be encouraged to enjoy the natural flavors of foods. The preparation of food for the sodium-restricted diet need not be complicated, but ingenuity should be exercised in developing flavorings that will compensate for the lack of salt. This is particularly important for the patient following a diet of 43 mEq. (1000 mg.) of sodium or less. In addition, these patients are frequently very sick and frightened. A number of recipe manuals and cooking suggestions are available and are listed at the end of this chapter. In general, as in the case of the diabetic diet, the recipes must be related to the daily food allowances from the diet, especially when energy intake is limited. For example, the milk and egg used in a custard will need to be deducted from the total day's food allowance of these foods.

Many spices, herbs and other seasonings can be used to improve the flavor of low sodium foods. According to Elvehjem and Burns, "Most of the values [of sodium in spices] are below 0.05%, and all are below 0.1% with the exception of allspice, celery seed, dehydrated celery flakes, whole mace and dehydrated parsley flakes. These figures indicate that, with the exception of celery flakes and parsley flakes, the amount of sodium contributed through the usual amount of spices used is insignificant and that most spices can be used safely in low-sodium diets.[18] However, any of the herb or spice "salts" such as garlic salt must be avoided.

INSTRUCTION OF THE PATIENT. If a sodium-restricted or modified fat diet is prescribed, it is not enough to give the patient a list of foods to avoid. The instructions should help the person secure an adequate diet. He must be given assistance in planning menus, in methods of preparing foods at home and in selecting food when eating away from home, since sodium is very prevalent in prepared and packaged foods.

The nurse, dietitian and physician can do much to encourage the patient concerning the necessary modifications in his diet, but real success depends upon the patient's understanding of the importance of the diet and of the need to adhere to it indefinitely. Changes probably will be made slowly over time as the patient adapts the diet to his lifestyle. Over time, he will also decrease his taste for salt, which makes further restriction of sodium possible if it is necessary.

The patient should be encouraged to experiment with seasoning and flavoring foods. Suggestions and recipe sources, such as those listed at the end of this chapter, will be stimulating and helpful. Cooking classes or demonstrations for a group of patients who need to control their sodium intake can be effective and enjoyable.

Vascular Disease

Vascular disorders can be classified as hypertensive vascular disease, various forms of arteriosclerosis, diseases of the aorta and vascular disorders of the extremities.

HYPERTENSION

Hypertension or high blood pressure occurs during the course of such maladies as thyrotoxicosis and hyperparathyroidism, in certain forms of cardiac disease, in atherosclerosis and kidney disease and during the course of pregnancy. In the majority of cases the cause is not known, and then it is called "essential" or primary hypertension.

Prevalence

It is estimated that 25 per cent of Americans, or 60 million, have hypertension; 95 per cent of these have essential hypertension, and 75 per cent have only mild hypertension. The prevalence is highest in the black population. This prevalence statistic depends upon the criteria used to define hypertension. A diastolic blood pressure greater than 90 mm. Hg at first screening has traditionally been used based on epidemiological studies correlating diastolic blood pressure with risk of developing coronary disease, strokes and other cardiovascular complications. However, data from the Framingham study show that risk of high blood pressure (HBP) is unevenly distributed and related to other factors. For this reason Kaplan suggests that an operational definition of HBP should be that level of blood pressure at which the benefits of action or treatment outweigh the costs of treatment.[31] Table 28–8 presents current thinking about hypertension and how it should be changed to be more in line with actual knowledge about the disease.

Etiology

Essential hypertension is a disease of altered regulation or control of arterial pressure and has a multifactorial origin. There is an imbalance of the many mechanisms that usually control arterial pressure. These interacting mechanisms are: the nervous system, specifically adrenergic function and catecholamines; the renin-angiotensin system; the excretory function of the kidney, including the handling of sodium and water; and other functions mediated through other hormonal, electrolytic and fluid balance mechanisms. Rise in blood pressure is caused by increased smooth muscle tone of the arterioles, which increases the vascular resistance to the forward flow of blood. This causes an increased afterload on the left ventricle of the heart, which is the pump responsible for perfusing blood through the system. The increased load on the left ventricle eventually will lead to its enlargement in order to compensate, and eventually if the increased vascular resistance is left untreated, the heart will fail.

RENIN-ANGIOTENSIN SYSTEM. In the evaluation of the hypertensive patient, *plasma renin activity (PRA)* frequently is measured to determine whether renin is a factor in the pathogenesis of the hypertension.[48] *Renin* is an enzyme secreted by the juxtaglomerular apparatus of the kidney in response to many cardiovascular factors, such as a fall in blood pressure, sodium depletion or a fall in plasma volume, and it indirectly increases blood pressure. It acts to increase the blood concentration of angiotensin, which is converted to angiotensin II when it circulates through the lungs. Angiotensin II causes an increase in aldosterone secretion, which increases peripheral vascular resistance, and hypertension develops. The PRA level is a useful measure for determining the necessary therapy.

In order to stimulate renin release and prepare the patient for the PRA test, the patient is told to follow a diet very low in sodium for three days prior to the test. The diet contains 10 to 20 mEq. (250 to 400 mg.) of sodium and is shown in Table 28–6. To adapt the diet to a 10 mEq. sodium restriction, omit the milk or substitute low-sodium milk. It is very important that the patient follow this diet closely, and the nurse must help the patient understand the necessity for compliance.

Patients with low renin levels respond best to salt depletion by either sodium restriction or diuretic therapy. Those with high renin levels do not respond to sodium restriction. Thus, with renin measurements the health practitioner is able to determine when sodium restriction is appropriate therapy.[39]

SODIUM. Dahl[13] has reported that sodium plays a primary role in causing essential hypertension

Table 28–8. CURRENT THINKING AND REINTERPRETATION OF THE EVIDENCE ON HYPERTENSION

	CURRENT THINKING	REINTERPRETATION
Prevalence of hypertension	Sixty million Americans have hypertension, of whom 75% have mild hypertension (diastolic blood pressure, 90 to 104 mm. Hg).	At least one third of patients with an initial diastolic blood pressure greater than 95 mm. Hg will be below 90 mm. Hg on repeated measurements, so that the prevalence of hypertension is probably much lower than current estimates.
Risks of hypertension	The risks for cardiovascular disease are significantly increased for all patients with any degree of elevated blood pressure.	Most patients with mild hypertension are not at high risk for cardiovascular disease. Patients at relatively high risk can be easily identified.
Benefits of therapy	The benefits of active drug therapy for mild hypertension have been proved.	The benefits of active drug therapy for those with diastolic blood pressure below 100 mm. Hg have not been proved. Patients with a diastolic blood pressure below 100 mm. Hg who are at relatively low risk should be provided with non-drug therapies.

From Kaplan, N. M.: Hypertension: prevalence, risks, and effect of therapy. Ann. Intern. Med., *98*(Suppl. 5, Part 2):705, 1983.

in rats. He also suggests that there is a genetic tendency toward hypertension that interacts with environmental factors such as kidney function, emotions and salt intake, particularly early in life, as diagrammed in Figure 28–2.

Tobian[61] has summarized the body of information linking hypertension to dietary sodium intake in humans. A working hypothesis is that at present it appears that only a fraction of humans are genetically susceptible to developing hypertension as adults. This varies between 9 and 20 per cent of the population depending upon which segment of the American population is under study. The remainder of the population, 80 to 91 per cent, could be considered as genetically resistant to developing essential hypertension. Genetically resistant individuals can consume as much as 200 mEq. of sodium chloride daily without developing an elevated blood pressure. However, if a person is among those genetically susceptible to hypertension, a lifelong modest restriction of sodium intake to levels less than 60 mEq per day in adults will probably prevent the onset of the hypertension indefinitely and may also prevent all subsequent hypertensive complications.

At present there is no technique that identifies those persons who are susceptible to developing hypertension in middle life, but individuals who are at great risk for developing subsequent essential hypertension are: (1) individuals with a family history of hypertension, (2) individuals with a blood pressure in the 80th percentile of the population or higher, (3) individuals whose resting heart rate is considerably more rapid than would be expected from their state of physical fitness, and (4) individuals who are more than 15 per cent above optimal body weight.[60]

It is also not known what fraction of the U.S. population is "salt sensitive" and how to recognize these individuals before they become hypertensive. About 17 per cent of adult Americans become hypertensive on the typical American intake of 150 to 250 mEq. of sodium per day.[60] Table 28–2 indicates salt and sodium intake by the American population.

It is still not understood how dietary sodium exerts its pressure-elevating effect. Is it a direct effect of the ion itself or an indirect effect on the activity of other ions?

In 1974 the Committee on Nutrition of the American Academy of Pediatrics recommended "actions that reduce or avoid increasing the present level of salt intake by children in the population at large," even though there is only enough evidence to *suggest* a relationship between salt consumption and hypertension.[11] In 1979 the National High Blood Pressure Education Program (HBPEP) of the National Heart, Lung, and Blood Institute stated that there is considerable evidence to indicate that dietary changes may help some hypertensive people control their blood pressure and that the two most promising aspects are weight reduction and restriction of sodium intake.[47]

OBESITY. Obesity is even more strongly correlated with the presence of hypertension than is sodium intake. Weight reduction will lower the blood pressure of both hypertensive and normotensive individuals, and weight gain tends to raise their blood pressure. It seems that the hypertensive effect of weight reduction is independent of a reduced sodium intake. Patients do not need to achieve ideal body weight to benefit from lowering of elevated blood pressure.[49]

In the Framingham study, a major 18-year epidemiological study of cardiovascular disease in Framingham, Massachusetts, it was shown that an increase in weight of 10 per cent resulted in a 6.5 mm. Hg rise in systolic blood pressure.[29]

The physiological mechanism relating weight and hypertension is unknown. It appears though, that it is related more to body fat mass rather than weight alone.[57] Suggested mechanisms of obesity in hypertension are increased cardiac output, increased blood volume or body sodium due to hyperinsulinemia or abnormal aldosterone/renin relationships, and neuroendo-

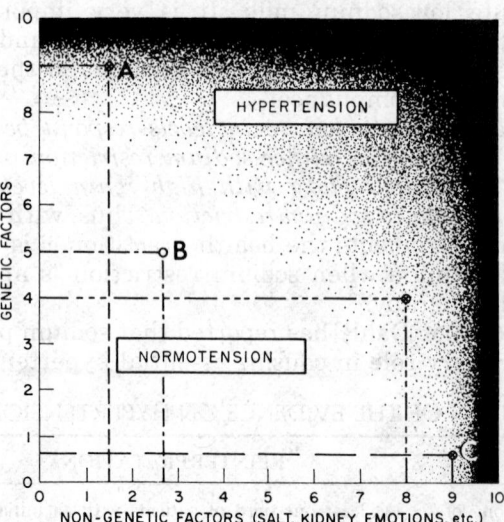

Figure 28–2. Possible relationship between genetic and non-genetic factors in hypertension. *A* represents the person with a strong genetic tendency who will develop hypertension when consuming large amounts of salt or who has abnormal kidney function or another medical problem. *B* represents the person with less of a genetic predisposition toward hypertension who requires a greater influence from environmental factors (more salt, for instance) before developing hypertension. *C* represents the person in whom the genetic tendency to develop hypertension is extremely low. He develops hypertension is extremely low. He develops hypertension only after several nongenetic factors are present. (Adapted from Dahl, L. K.: Salt and hpertension. Am. J. Clin. Nutr., *25 :231, 1972.*)

Table 28-9.   AVERAGE SODIUM AND POTASSIUM CONTENT OF TOTAL DIET, 1980

	SODIUM (MG./DAY)	POTASSIUM (MG./DAY)	RATIO Na:K
Infant*			
total/day	706	1684	
total/1000 kcal.	802	1913	.42
Toddler*			
total/day	1805	1938	
total/1000 kcal.	1388	1491	.93
Adult*			
total/day	6692	4682	1.43
total/1000 kcal.	1716	1200	

* Infant, toddler, and adult diets contain 880, 1300, and 3900 kcal. respectively. The infant is 6 months old, the toddler is 2 years old, and the adult is a 15-to 20-year-old-male, chosen because he is likely to be the largest consumer of food and thus of sodium and potassium.

Data from Shank, F. R., et al: Perspective of Food and Drug Administration on dietary sodium. J. Am. Diet. Asoc., *80*:29, 1982.

crine abnormalities due to increased nonadrenergic activity or opiate suppression, and these have been reviewed elsewhere.[17]

CALCIUM. As discussed, most of the attention to identify dietary components in the pathogenesis of hypertension has focused on sodium. Recently, however, calcium has come under scrutiny for a possible role in the development of hypertension. McCarron[42] studied the extracellular ionized calcium concentrations in 23 untreated hypertensive patients and an equal number of normotensive controls matched for age, sex and race. He found essentially identical serum total calcium concentrations, but the hypertensive patients had significantly lower concentrations of serum ionized calcium and phosphorus. These findings suggest that an abnormality in protein binding of extracellular calcium exists in hypertensive people. McCarron postulates that the depressed levels of serum ionized calcium trigger release of parathyroid hormone, which in turn increases renal phosphate excretion; hence the serum ionized phosphorus is lowered also.

The intriguing question from these findings is whether calcium supplementation will prevent hypertension or lower blood pressure in those already hypertensive. Studies using genetically hypertensive rats showed that calcium supplementation had a significant attentuating effect on elevated blood pressure.[3] When spontaneously hypertensive rats were fed three different levels of dietary calcium, animals who consumed the high-calcium diet were found to have significantly lower blood pressure and to develop hypertension more slowly compared with the other two diet groups.[41]

Epidemiological studies by McCarron suggest that the daily calcium intake of hypertensive individuals studied was significantly less than that of the normotensive individuals by 18 to 22 per cent.[40,43] He also found that the premenopausal middle-aged woman is relatively protected despite an average calcium intake of less than 650 mg. per day.[41]

Kesteloot and Geboers have reported similar findings—a significant positive correlation between serum calcium and systolic and diastolic blood pressure in 9321 men studied in Belgium, but no significant correlation in women.[34] These authors hypothesize the following for the role of calcium in pathogenesis of hypertension. Calcium is an essential component in normal functioning of vascular smooth muscle cells and along with magnesium contributes to blood pressure control through neurohumoral, renal and adrenal mechanisms. Recent studies have shown an abnormality in cell membrane binding or transport of calcium in hypertension.[19, 42] In subjects with genetic predisposition a high sodium consumption leads to volume overload, which leads to appearance of natriuretic hormone (NH). NH influences membrane permeability in a way that leads to an increase in intracellular sodium and, by inhibiting sodium-calcium exchange, causes accumulation of calcium in the vascular smooth muscle cells. This increase in intracellular calcium would lead to an increase in contractility and vascular tone, resulting in augmented peripheral vascular resistance and thus raised blood pressure.[34] However, just because serum calcium and blood pressure are correlated does not mean that this is of any significance or that a cause-and-effect relationship exists. McCarron's theory needs much testing and study before calcium supplementation should be recommended to people with hypertension.

POTASSIUM. Also controversial is the hypothesis relating potassium intake to hypertension. Epidemiological evidence and animal and human studies show that an acute increase of potassium will lower blood pressure. Increased potassium intake can partially negate the blood pressure–elevating effects of sodium. Langford suggests that the sodium:potassium ratio should be considered in the diet.[37]

Many studies have shown no correlation between sodium excretion and blood pressure. The strongest correlation is between hypertension and low-salt-intake populations. But the same populations with low sodium intake also have high potassium intake. Potassium intakes of 120 to 175 mEq. per day result in a modest 3 to 10 per cent lowering of blood pressure.[59] A potassium intake of this magnitude is not dangerous to those with normal renal function, but it could be a risk to those with compromised renal function. It is inappropriate to recommend high-potassium therapy widely at this time.[59]

However, a low-potassium diet also lowers blood pressure, as was shown 30 years ago in normotensive people. Thus it appears that a high potassium intake has no effect on the blood pressure of normotensive individuals and that a high potassium intake lowers blood pressure only in hypertensive people. The decline is modest, though. Scientists are still not completely sure of the mechanism of this effect, but it may involve alteration in salt and volume status, alteration in renin, neurogenic mechanisms and the resistance of vessels.[59]

Treatment

DRUGS. Antihypertensive drugs have been used extensively in the treatment of hypertension. Various agents are employed—alone and in combination—including those that act centrally, those that produce ganglionic blockade, those that exert peripheral sympatholytic and adrenolytic effects and those that act on the renin-angiotensin system. Unfortunately, side effects are common with the use of every agent currently available, but newer agents are appearing and it is hoped that these side effects can be eliminated.

In some patients, the diuretics lower blood pressure by promoting volume depletion and sodium loss. However, thiazide diuretics increase urinary potassium excretion, thus leading to potassium wasting and possibly hypokalemia, especially in the presence of a high salt intake. *Even in those patients taking diuretics, the sodium intake should be restricted to about 60 mEq. (1400 mg.) for the most effective lowering of blood pressure.*[60] The antihypertensive effect is related to sodium intake since sodium in excess of 350 mEq. per day can completely prevent diuretic-related lowering of blood pressure.[61] Except in the case of a potassium-sparing diuretic, such as spironolactone or triamterene, additional potassium usually is required. Appendix Table 10 gives the potassium values of various foods that contribute potassium to the diet. Fortunately, many of the foods that are high in potassium (fruits and vegetables, for instance) are also low in sodium. A KCl supplement can also be used. The sodium:potassium ratio is important, and Langford suggests that the most effective diet for patients using thiazide diuretics contains 50 mEq. each of sodium and potassium, although 100 mEq. of each is more realistic. He further has found that patients taking diuretics crave salt because of the increased excretion of sodium in the urine and will eat even more salt unless it is intentionally restricted.[38]

Other possible effects of the excessive use of diuretics are hyponatremia, hypochloremia, hyperuricemia and hyperglycemia. The use of drugs to treat mild hypertension is now being questioned. Are the risks and costs of lifelong medication really exceeded by the benefits of lowered blood pressure? Mortality data from the Multiple Risk Factor Intervention Trial (MRFIT) showed that among those patients who entered the trial with diastolic pressures between 90 and 94 mm. Hg there were more deaths among those who were more intensively treated.[46] It is now recommended that there should be more widespread use of non-drug therapies in mildly hypertensive patients. These therapies—moderate sodium restriction, weight reduction, isotonic exercise and relaxation—are of proven benefit in controlling hypertension. Even if less potent than drugs, they impose fewer risks.

NUTRITIONAL CARE

Sodium Restriction. In 1944 the *Kempner rice diet*[33] was introduced for treatment of both hypertensive vascular disease and kidney disease. The diet consists of 10 oz. of dry rice (approximately 1050 kcal.), which is cooked without salt. The remaining 900 to 1000 kcal. are supplied by liberal quantities of sugar and fresh or preserved fruits. Thus, the diet is high in carbohydrate, furnishes about 2000 kcal., 15 to 30 gm. of protein, 4 to 6 gm. of fat and 100 to 150 mg. of sodium daily. Salt and sodium preservatives are strictly forbidden. Fluids are limited to 700 to 1000 ml. of fruit juices. Iron and vitamin supplements are given. After reduction of blood pressure and alleviation of the symptoms, the diet is somewhat liberalized. However, it is difficult for a patient to live on this regimen for any length of time, and dietary restriction and manipulation may lead to nutritional deficiencies.

Kempner utilized this method in 213 patients with high blood pressure who exhibited various stages of the disease. After an average period of 62 days on the strict or modified diet, improvement was noted in 64 per cent of the patients.

Although it was long assumed from subsequent studies that it was the severe sodium restriction that caused lowering of blood pressure, it is now thought that the high potassium intake of this diet and the low sodium:potassium ratio may also be a factor.[22]

There is adequate evidence to show that about 20 to 50 per cent of hypertensive patients will respond with a lowered blood pressure to a severely restricted sodium diet. A reduction of sodium intake to less than 20 mEq. (460 mg.)

per day, such as that in the Kempner diet, will normalize blood pressure in about one third of patients with established hypertension.[39] However, the effectiveness of moderate sodium restriction has not been studied as well. There is only fragmentary evidence that a moderate restriction in dietary sodium (75 to 160 mEq. per day) might have a small antihypertensive effect in some patients. There is some evidence, however, that moderate sodium restriction can be effective particularly in reducing the need for hypertensive medication.[45]

The patient should be evaluated for renin to help determine if his hypertension might be responsive to sodium restriction, as mentioned on page 559. Assessment of present sodium intake by 24-hour urinary sodium or dietary intake record will give the clinician an idea of present sodium intake. The reduction in sodium intake should be gradual with the final goal of 60 to 75 mEq. (1400 to 1700 mg.) per day. Sodium restriction may begin at one of the levels described on page 548 with steps downward to lower levels as necessary. A common management plan is the use of diuretics with an 85 to 130 mEq. (1950 to 3000 mg.) daily sodium intake and weight reduction if necessary. However, it appears that for sodium restriction to be effective it should be 60 to 75 mEq. (1400 to 1700 mg.) per day in those patients who are sodium-sensitive.

Weight Reduction. As mentioned on page 560, obesity is a factor in the development of hypertension and there is general agreement that achieving normal weight is important in relieving symptoms of hypertension. It has been shown that weight reduction (body fatness reduction) alone can lower blood pressure.[49] Chapter 27 discusses nutritional care in weight reduction.

ATHEROSCLEROSIS

Atherosclerosis is a form of arteriosclerosis; that is, a thickening of the walls of the arteries. *Atherosclerosis* involves the intimal layer of the arteries, whereas *arteriosclerosis* involves primarily the medial layer. Normally, the blood vessels are smooth-lined tubes. In atherosclerosis small yellow flakes on the inner lining of arteries and arterioles represent deposits of fatty materials containing cholesterol, phospholipids and calcium. There is cellular and fibrous proliferation and the arteries become roughened and narrowed, the elasticity is lost and the flow of blood through the vessels is curtailed. The cholesterol deposited on the arterial wall is derived from plasma lipoproteins. Atherosclerosis results when the influx of cholesterol into the ar-

terial wall exceeds the outflow. The arteriosclerotic process does not develop at a uniform rate in all arteries.

Atherosclerosis interferes with the circulation, chiefly to the heart, kidneys and brain. These organs need blood to function efficiently, and when impairment occurs, the effect is noted throughout the system. Atherosclerosis of the coronary arteries—*coronary heart disease* (CHD) or *atherosclerotic heart disease* (ASHD)—underlies most heart attacks. *Stroke,* or *apoplexy,* is often caused by atherosclerosis, but it appears that the atherosclerosis causing stroke differs from that which causes heart attacks. The problem of preventing or retarding these attacks or diseases is largely one of preventing or retarding atherosclerosis.

Etiology

The mechanisms involved in the pathogensis of atherosclerosis have been the subject of much study for many years and there is still no complete answer. There are probably many environmental factors involved combined with a genetic predisposition.

Risk Factors

In trying to unravel the puzzling etiology of CHD, scientists have identified several risk factors. Summarizing the knowledge concerning risk factors, the Inter-Society Commission for Heart Disease Resources identified three *major* risk factors: hypercholesterolemia, hypertension and cigarette smoking.[50] Some other risk factors are diabetes mellitus, hypertriglyceridemia, obesity, sedentary living, psychosocial tensions and certain dietary factors.

1. *Hypercholesterolemia* in relation to CHD has been studied extensively, and this has led to development of the *lipid hypothesis.* This is based upon the assumption that since elevated serum cholesterol concentration is associated so closely with the progression of human atherosclerosis, it must be an intervening variable. This relationship has not been proved; however, much evidence suggests that an elevated serum cholesterol concentration is essential for the other risk factors to have an appreciable effect on either arterial lesions or clinical disease.[44] The correlate of this hypothesis is that reducing the level of plasma cholesterol in an individual or in a population group will lead to a reduction in the risk of coronary heart disease. This has not been proved. The fact that dietary factors affect the level of serum cholesterol, has been established however, and there is good evidence that gives validity to several dietary recommen-

dations for lowering blood cholesterol in some individuals.

The Framingham Study provided considerable evidence that the level of blood cholesterol is a powerful factor in development of major manifestations of CHD, myocardial infarction and angina pectoris. Elevated levels of blood cholesterol are not normal, and they do lead to a much higher rate of CHD.[14]

International studies have demonstrated that in populations in which the range of cholesterol levels is considerably below that observed in Western countries, there is a much lower incidence of CHD. The Framingham study and other similar studies have shown that the risk of CHD is also related to the individual cholesterol level compared with others in the same population. Not yet clearly established are the reasons for differences in cholesterol levels within a given population. Within the Framingham population the level of cholesterol in the blood proved to be a good predictor of the development of atherosclerotic disease.[14] However, total serum cholesterol loses some of its predictability in the older population. Determining high-density lipoprotein (HDL) and low-density lipoprotein (LDL) fractions may increase predictability only in the older population. The value of the measure as a predictor in younger people is unknown.

2. *Hypertension* seems to aggravate the atherosclerotic process, especially in the presence of elevated levels of blood lipid. As with the blood lipid level, the correlation between hypertension and risk of CHD is continuous—the higher the blood pressure, the greater the risk of CHD.

3. *Cigarette smoking* is positively correlated with CHD mortality. Carbon monoxide inhaled in cigarette smoke leads to a relative state of hypoxia, which results in an increase in serum lipid levels. Cholesterol-fed rabbits in which hypoxia was induced through inhalation of carbon monoxide showed an increase in lipid accumulation in the arterial walls.[2] Smoking is also accompanied by lowering of HDL levels, and this also may be a reason why it is a risk factor.[23, 62]

4. Evidence connecting *obesity* with increased risk of developing coronary heart disease is both consistent and substantial. This effect seems to come from the atherogenic traits promoted by obesity. It is not known whether obesity exerts an independent direct effect on CHD development or an indirect effect.

There is also some evidence to suggest that obesity acquired between the ages of 20 and 40 years may have a much greater effect on subsequent development of cardiovascular disease than obesity that occurs after age 40.[51]

The Framingham Study showed that for every 10 per cent increase in relative weight there was a 12 mg./dl. rise in serum cholesterol and a 6.5 mm. rise in systolic blood pressure—two known risk factors for CHD.[29] In several free-living populations it has been observed that as body weight decreases, HDL levels tend to increase.[9]

The Influence of Serum Cholesterol Reduction on Mortality from CHD

Four studies in the 1950's and 1960's attempted to establish the relationship between diet, blood lipids and CHD.[15, 52, 58, 61] All involved free-living populations in which strategies were used to change diet in ways known to influence serum cholesterol. In addition some involved methods to reduce smoking and overweight and to increase activity. The findings were encouraging regarding the effect of serum cholesterol reduction on CHD mortality, but not definitive because of small sample sizes and in some cases lack of control groups.

In 1974 the *Multiple Risk Factor Intervention Trial (MRFIT)* was initiated to study whether a large-scale multifactor intervention program with 12,866 high-risk men could affect mortality from CHD. The men were assigned to either a special intervention (SI) program consisting of drug treatment of hypertension, counseling to stop cigarette smoking and dietary advice for lowering blood cholesterol, or to their usual sources of health care (UC). Over the seven years of follow-up, the difference in mortality from CHD was not statistically significant between the two groups even though the risk factors declined to a greater extent in the SI men than in the UC men. Thus, it appeared that risk factor reduction had no effect on reducing CHD mortality.[46] However, the investigators suspect that measures to reduce cigarette smoking and to lower blood cholesterol levels may have reduced CHD mortality within subgroups of the SI population, but that there was an unfavorable response to antihypertensive drug therapy in some of the hypertensives in the same SI group, that changed the statistics.[46] Unfortunately, this unanticipated finding from the use of high doses of the diuretic hydrochlorothiazide to treat hypertension confounded the findings of the trial.

Another long-term study was the *Coronary Primary Prevention Trial (CPPT)* started in 1973. In this study, intervention to lower blood cholesterol was through dietary changes and medication. The results of the 10-year study showed that reducing serum total cholesterol and LDL-cholesterol caused a reduction in CHD incidence in men at high risk for CHD because of hypercholesterolemia.[39a]

Serum Lipids—Cholesterol and Triglyceride

INFLUENCE OF NON-DIETARY FACTORS. Increasing evidence suggests that blood cholesterol levels are directly related to exercise. This evidence thus favors a continued, active life of muscular work. Sex and hormones have also been mentioned as factors, and atherosclerosis is more common in young males than young females. During the childbearing years women have relatively little cardiovascular disease, and the blood fat levels are relatively low. After menopause there is a greater frequency of such disorders and higher blood cholesterol levels. This suggests that the female sex hormones are a protective factor. However, pregnancy and oral contraceptives containing estrogen can also cause hyperlipidemia. Alcohol ingestion can elevate serum triglycerides, as can thiazide diuretics.[26] In certain diseases such as hypothyroidism, nephrosis, diabetes, obstructive liver disease and pancreatitis there is more lipid in the blood than normally, and athersclerosis frequently is associated with these conditions.

INFLUENCE OF DIETARY FACTORS

Fat. The type and amount of fat in the diet influence the serum cholesterol level. Although epidemiological evidence shows that a low fat intake is associated with lower serum cholesterol levels and lower incidence of CHD, it appears that the *type* of fat is also important.

By *substituting highly unsaturated fats* (those with multiple double bonds, such as safflower, corn and cottonseed oils as described on page 40), for saturated fats (animal or hydrogenated vegetable fats) in human diets or, in some instances, by adding sufficient amounts of unsaturated fats to a normal fat intake, the total amounts of plasma lipids and serum cholesterol are consistently lowered in a high percentage of cases. It appears that the two types of polyunsaturated fatty acids, ω-6 (i.e., linoleic and arachidonic acids) and ω-3 (i.e., linolenic acid), have different functions in the body, as discussed in Chapter 3. In general, polyunsaturated fatty acids (PUFA) depress LDL concentrations. Omega-3 fatty acids appear to also reduce levels of plasma triglyceride, in particular VLDL. The mechanism by which PUFA in the diet lowers plasma lipid, especially cholesterol, is unclear.

The *removal of saturated fat* from the diet is twice as effective as adding an equal amount of polyunsaturated fat in lowering blood cholesterol. Grande and associates have shown that even when the total fat content of the diet remains the same, subtracting a certain amount of saturated fat has the same effect as adding twice that amount in polyunsaturated fat.[25] Monounsaturated fats were found to be neutral and do not cause a rise or fall of serum cholesterol. Apparently, it is the proportion of saturated to polyunsaturated fatty acids in the total diet consumed that determines the lipid level and, consequently, the vascular deposition of lipids. The Framingham study showed that the polyunsaturated fat to saturated fat ratio (P:S) for the American diet was between 0.3 and 0.4:1.[30] Connor recommends that it be increased to 1:1.[12]

Cholesterol. It appears that dietary cholesterol does not have as much influence on serum cholesterol level as does the intake of saturated or polyunsaturated fat, and some argue that it has very little effect.[9,44] Responses to dietary cholesterol are more variable and probably depend on genetic control as well as the type of dietary fat. In the Framingham study dietary cholesterol was found to have no significant effect on blood cholesterol concentration.[14] Perhaps it is a matter of the level of cholesterol intake. McGill states that a cholesterol intake above 600 mg. per day does not correlate with serum cholesterol.[44] Connor and Connor state that dietary cholesterol must be lowered to 100 mg. per day to have a lowering effect on serum cholesterol.[12]

A reduction of 100 mg. in dietary cholesterol results in a lowering of only 5 mg. in serum cholesterol when dietary fat is not also altered. However, dietary cholesterol becomes a significant factor when compared with the polyunsaturated fat in the diet, which has a greater lowering effect on serum cholesterol when dietary cholesterol is also reduced. For example, Hegsted and coworkers found that when the only fat in the diet was the highly saturated coconut oil, a 300 mg. cholesterol intake (reduced from the usual American intake of 800 mg.) had little effect, and serum cholesterol increased by 40 mg./dl. When the dietary fat was monounsaturated olive oil, a 300 mg. cholesterol intake did not affect the serum cholesterol level, and when the dietary fat was polyunsaturated safflower oil with the 300 mg. cholesterol intake, the serum cholesterol level was reduced 35 mg./dl.[27]

Carbohydrate. It is now generally accepted that whereas a high carbohydrate intake may lead to a temporary increase in serum triglycerides in some people, the long-term effect is no change in serum triglycerides. Some people are more sensitive to a carbohydrate load than others, but carbohydrate-induced hypertriglyceridemia seems to be closely related to an impaired glucose tolerance and diabetes mellitus and also to obesity.[54]

Dietary Fiber. Pectin, a form of dietary fiber found in fruits, has been found to lower serum cholesterol levels. Guar gum in synthetic diets, as well as the fiber in oats and soy beans, has also been shown to lower serum cholesterol. There is no substantial evidence for the lowering of blood cholesterol by cellulose (the fiber in wheat bran).[28]

Vegetables. Recent evidence suggests that vegetables, both leafy and root vegetables, and grains (wheat, corn and oats) taken in normal amounts in the diet will lower blood cholesterol. Consumption of vegetable leaves and stalks is associated with lower serum values of very low density lipoproteins (VLDL) and total cholesterol, and whole grains are associated with lower values of low density lipoproteins (LDL) and total cholesterol.[20] It is not clear whether it is only the fiber or other factors in the vegetables that are effective in lowering serum cholesterol.

Garlic is another vegetable that seems to affect serum cholesterol. The essential oil of garlic lowers serum total cholesterol and triglycerides and raises high density lipoproteins (HDL) significantly in both healthy and hyperlipidemic individuals. Garlic oil given in gelatin capsules in two doses to give 0.25 mg. of oil per kg. of body weight lowered total serum cholesterol by 17 to 18 per cent.[7] To illustrate, a 60-kg. person would need 15 mg. of garlic oil, which corresponds to approximately 30 gm. of raw garlic or about half of a head of garlic cloves. Garlic oil may also have a role in inhibiting blood coagulation.[8] Unfortunately, the amount of daily garlic necessary to cause a hypolipidemic effect is so large that it is not clinically practical. Most odorless garlic pills are probably not as potent as the actual oil.

Trace Elements. An interesting observation that may possibly link a trace element with coronary heart disease is the reported lower death rate from CHD in areas with a hard water supply.[55] When the water has been softened, the mortality from CHD has increased. A likely difference between hard and soft water that may be important is the increased calcium content of hard water, but this has not been proved.[16]

Klevay has suggested that the zinc:copper ratio in the body becomes abnormal as a result of food choices, hypertension, water hardness and lack of exercise. This zinc-copper imbalance results in an increased serum cholesterol level and thus, increased mortality due to CHD.[35]

Vitamin E. The function of vitamin E in ischemic heart disease is not clear, but at this time there is no evidence to implicate a deficiency of vitamin E.

Numerous attempts to alter blood total cholesterol with supplemental vitamin E have yielded equivocal results. One study showed significant increases in high density lipoproteins after vitamin E supplementation in women, but in men increases in HDL levels were minimal and were confined to those with initially low concentrations of HDL.[4] Further work is required to evaluate the long-range effects of vitamin supplementation on HDL levels and coronary heart disease. The use of vitamin E supplements is unfounded.

Vitamin C. Vitamin C may have a function in lipolysis and protection against atherosclerosis, but this is still unclear.

The Prudent Diet for the Prevention of Atherosclerosis

Because many Americans have elevated or moderately elevated blood lipid levels and because there is now greater knowledge about the dietary factors that influence blood lipid levels, the Inter-Society Commission on Heart Disease Resources and the American Heart Association have suggested some general guidelines to the public for dietary modification.[1] A diet following these guidelines will lower blood lipid levels and possibly help prevent coronary heart disease. These recommendations have been termed the "Prudent Diet."[1] Table 28–10 summarizes this diet and compares it with the present typical American diet. In the late 1970's the Senate Select Committee on Nutrition and Human Needs, in its report *Dietary Goals for the United States*, endorsed similar guidelines.[56] The statements of this and other groups are summarized in Table 17–11.

To translate these recommendations into eating habits means: (1) eating smaller portions of meat (6 oz. per day) that is lower in fat, (2) avoiding all whole-milk dairy products such as ice cream, hard cheeses, cream, butter and whole milk, (3) increasing the intake of fruits and vegetables, which contain virtually no fat, no salt (except in canned vegetables) and no cholesterol and are low in calories and high in fiber, (4) eating breads, cereals and grain products that do not contain large amounts of sugar, salt and fat, (5) restricting eggs and high cholesterol foods to three times per week, (6) using a polyunsaturated oil as listed in Figure 28–3 for cooking and baking and (7) cooking to avoid saturated fats and to include polyunsaturated fats. See Table 28–11 for exchange lists for the translation of these principles into a diet. The exchange lists are those presented in Table 25–8 with some modifications. Table 28–12 gives the nutritional analysis of the food exchange groups.

Table 28–10.   COMPARISON OF TYPICAL AMERICAN DIET, THE AHA PRUDENT DIET AND THE ALTERNATIVE DIET

NUTRIENT	APPROXIMATE COMPOSITION		
	Typical American Diet	*AHA Prudent Diet*	*Alternative Diet (Phase III)*
Cholesterol	600–700 mg.	≤ 300 mg.	100 mg.
Total Calories	Often overconsumption	Reduction to achieve and/or maintain ideal weight	
Total Fat (% of kcal.)	40–42%	30–35%	20%
Saturated	15%	10%	5%
Monounsaturated	16–17%	10–15%	8%
Polyunsaturated	5– 6%	10%	7%
P:S Ratio	0.3–0.4:1	1–1.5:1	1.3:1
Carbohydrate (% of kcal.)	40–45%	50–55%	65%
Starch	20–25%	Increased	40%
Simple sugars	15–20%	Decreased	25%
Protein (% of kcal.)	12–15%	12–15%	15%
Sodium	150–200 mEq.	Decreased	75–100 mEq.
Potassium	30–70 mEq.	Increased indirectly	120–150 mEq.
Dietary Fiber	10–12 gm.	Increased indirectly	48–60 gm.

Sources: U.S. Department of Agriculture, Agricultural Research Service, 1974; Connor, W. E., and Connor, S. L.: The dietary treatment of hyperlipidemia, rationale, technique and efficacy. Med. Clin. N. Am., *66*:485, 1982; Am. Heart Assoc. Nutrition Comm.: Rationale of diet-heart statement of the Amer. Heart Assoc. Arteriosclerosis, *4*:177, 1982; and Dahl, L. K.: Salt and hypertension. Am. J. Clin. Nutr., *25*:231, 1972.

The food industry has responded to the recommendations for dietary changes by making available leaner meats; processed meats, dairy products, frozen desserts and baked goods reduced in saturated fat, cholesterol and calories; and margarine, shortening, mayonnaise, salad dressing and oil of low saturated fat and cholesterol content. There are cholesterol-free egg substitutes, cheeses and breakfast meats, polyunsaturated margarines, and the fat content is listed on food labels. Appendix Table 5 lists the fatty acid and cholesterol content of some foods.

Even highly motivated individuals will find some of these changes difficult; the process of change will not be sudden and complete. Connor states that it takes two to ten years to make radical changes in one's eating habits and proposes "phases" of diet adjustment that should be individualized.[12] A reasonable change for some people may be the use of a soft or tub margarine instead of regular stick margarine or butter. As discussed in Chapter 18, it is important to know what is reasonable for patients when counseling and helping them to begin the process of dietary modification.

Hyperlipidemia

Hyperlipidemia, or an elevated blood lipid level, is either primary or secondary to other diseases such as diabetes, uremia, alcoholism or hypothyroidism. Primary hyperlipidemia is classified into one of the various types of *hyperlipoproteinemia*, based upon the amounts of various lipoproteins in the blood. All blood lipids (cholesterol, phospholipid and triglyceride) are bound to specific *apoproteins* that circulate in the plasma. There are several distinct apoproteins, and they have receptors in tissues that enable them to transport lipid and function properly. These proteins transport the lipids into and out of plasma in complexes called *lipoproteins*. An abnormally high level of one or more of these lipoproteins in the blood is called hyperlipoproteinemia.

These lipoproteins may be identified by zonal gel electrophoresis or by ultracentrifugation, which is now commonly preferred. Each lipoprotein contains cholesterol, phospholipid, triglyceride and protein in different and characteristic proportions. The blood lipoproteins are (1) *chylomicrons*, (2) *very low density lipoproteins* or VLDL, (3) *low density lipoproteins* or LDL and (4) *high density lipoproteins* or HDL. Normally most of the plasma cholesterol is found in the low density lipoproteins and most of the plasma triglyceride is in the very low density lipoproteins, as shown in Figure 28–4. An extensive review of lipoproteins and the lipid transport system can be found elsewhere.[26]

Dietary chylomicrons consist mostly of triglycerides absorbed from the diet. Chylomicrons

P:S Ratio

8.0—	Safflower Oil
7.0—	
6.0—	Sunflower oil
5.0—	
	Corn oil
4.0—	Soybean oil Mayonnaise
3.0—	Soft tub safflower oil margarines, sesame oil, sesame seeds Salad dressing, pecans, almonds
2.0—	Soft tub corn oil margarines, cube safflower oil margarines Cottonseed oil Cube corn oil margarines
1.0—	Peanut oil, peanuts, peanut butter, mixed nuts Soft tub vegetable oil margarines
0.9—	
0.8—	Cashews
0.7—	Avocado
0.6—	Cube vegetable oil margarines Olive oil, olives, all vegetable shortening
0.5—	
0.4—	
0.3—	Bacon, lard
0.2—	Macadamia nuts
0.1—	
	Butter, baking chocolate Coconut oil, palm kernel oil
0.0—	

Figure 28–3. Ratios of polyunsaturated to saturated fats. Information from *Nutritive Value of American Foods in Common Units.* Agriculture Handbook No. 456, U.S. Department of Agriculture, 1975. Courtesy of E. Burrows, Northwest Lipid Research Clinic, Seattle.

are synthesized in the intestine and transport mainly dietary triglycerides from the intestine into the plasma. They give a milky appearance to normal plasma after a fatty meal, but their presence in the fasting plasma is indicative of abnormal lipid levels.

The *VLDL* are composed largely of triglycerides (but also contain some cholesterol and apoproteins) and function to transport triglycerides of mainly endogenous origin, largely from the liver. Virtually all of the triglyceride that is not in chylomicrons is in VLDL. VLDL interact with lipoprotein lipase and release their triglyceride to be taken up as fatty acids by extrahepatic tissue, and the remnants are made into LDL.

The *LDL* represent the plasma residue of VLDL catabolism. They carry two thirds of the total blood cholesterol, which is derived mainly from the action of the hepatic enzyme lecithin-cholesterol acyltransferase (LCAT).

The fourth and smallest group in the lipoprotein family are the *HDL*. They contain the remainder of plasma cholesterol, and their cholesteryl esters are also formed from the action of LCAT. In fact, it appears that HDL contain LCAT, which esterifies cholesterol to cholesteryl esters that can then be carried to the liver, hydrolyzed and excreted in the bile. Thus, HDL are the carriers of cholesterol from body cells, including those of the arterial walls, to the liver. This function may be the reason for the apparent protectiveness of HDL levels against CHD. Many studies have shown an inverse relationship between HDL levels and the incidence of coronary heart disease.[10, 14]

Remnants are particles of chylomicrons or VLDL remaining in circulation after the triglycerides are removed by the extrahepatic tissues. They include apoproteins and some lipid and can be measured as *intermediate density lipoproteins (IDL)*.

When any of the blood lipid levels are abnormally elevated, particularly those of cholesterol or triglyceride, there will also be an elevation in the levels of the particular lipoproteins that transport them, and vice versa.

DIAGNOSIS. Total serum triglycerides and cholesterol can be measured by a blood test. For serum triglycerides the blood sample should be a fasting sample (10 to 15 hours) in order to avoid normal postprandial chylomicronemia, which could make serum triglycerides look falsely high. Authorities do not agree on the "cutoff" point used to define hyperlipidemia. The 5th, 50th and 95th percentiles for serum lipids are given in Table 28–13. However, there is evidence to show that when plasma cholesterol is above 220 mg./dl. in adults and 180 mg./dl. in children there is increased risk of developing premature CHD. The upper limit for plasma triglycerides is 150 mg./dl., although this limit is even hazier. An elevated triglyceride level alone warrants the "refrigerator test" to rule out hyperchylomicronemia (after chilling, chylomicrons rise and form a creamy fat layer on the top of the serum or plasma). If that is negative, then hypertriglyceridemia usually in-

Text continued on page 577

Table 28–11. FOOD EXCHANGES FOR DIETS TO CONTROL
HYPERLIPIDEMIA

MILK EXCHANGES

One Serving Contains:

80 calories, 12 gm. carbohydrate, 8 gm. protein, 5 mg. cholesterol, 0.2 gm. fat, 0.1 gm. saturated fat, trace monounsaturated fat, trace polyunsaturated fat

Serving Size	Foods to Choose	Avoid
1 cup	skim milk	whole milk
$^1\!/_3$ cup	powdered skim (undiluted)	
½ cup	evaporated skim (undiluted)	evaporated or condensed made with whole milk
1 cup	†skimmed buttermilk	†instant beverage drinks
8 oz.	plain yogurt (made with skim milk)—should contain no more than 2 gm. fat per cup	flavored yogurt, eggnogs, and malted beverage mixes, instant hot chocolate mixes

Note: If you use 2% low-fat milk, eliminate 1 Fat serving from the B list.

FAT EXCHANGES

FAT A

One Serving Contains:

45 calories, 5 gm. total fat, 0.5 gm. saturated fat, 3 gm. polyunsaturated fat, and negligible cholesterol

	OILS	
1 tsp.	corn, soybean, safflower, sunflower, cottonseed, or sesame oil	hydrogenated vegetable oil, coconut oil, palm oil

FAT B

One Serving Contains:

45 calories, 5 gm. total fat, 1 gm. saturated fat, 2 gm. polyunsaturated fat and negligible cholesterol

Serving Size	Foods to Choose	Avoid
	VEGETABLE FATS	
1 tsp.	margarine, with listed as the first ingredient either liquid corn, safflower, soybean, sunflower, cottonseed, or sesame oil	butter, lard, bacon,† chicken fat, cocoa butter, cream, half and half, margarine with unidentified vegetable oil on label
1 tsp.	mayonnaise, with listed first ingredient same as for margarine	mayonnaise with unidentified vegetable oil on label
	salad dressing: Thousand Island, tartar sauce, mayonnaise-type, French, and Italian with listed first ingredient same as for margarine	salad dressings containing cheese; salad dressings with unidentified vegetable oil on label
	†NUTS	
10	almonds, whole	cashews
6	pecans, halves	Macadamia nuts
6	walnuts, halves	
	peanuts, (occasionally):	
10	Virginia	
20	Spanish	
1 tbsp.	chopped peanuts	
20	pistachios	

†Item high in sodium.

Adapted from Stone, N. J., et al.: Fat Chance. Chicago, Year Book Medical Publishers, Inc., 1980, pp. 46–63.

Table continued on the following page

Table 28–11. FOOD EXCHANGES FOR DIETS TO CONTROL
HYPERLIPIDEMIA (*Continued*)

MISCELLANEOUS

⅛ slice	avocado, 4″ diameter	†cheese and cheese mixes, cream cheese, sour cream
5 small	†olives	

Limit salad dressings and mayonnaise to 2 exchanges per day.

Olive oil and peanut oil are not recommended, due to their low polyunsaturated fat content.

FRUIT EXCHANGES

Fruits may be fresh, dried, cooked, canned, or frozen with no sugar or syrup added. Read the labels carefully. Use fruit or juice labeled: unsweetened, no sugar added, artificially sweetened, or packed in its own juice.

One Serving Contains:

40 calories, 10 gm. carbohydrate, negligible protein, and no fat or cholesterol

Fruit	Serving size
apple	½ apple (3″ diameter)
	½ cup sauce (unsweetened)
	⅓ cup juice (cider)
apricot	2 medium, fresh
	4 halves, dried or canned
	¾ cup nectar (unsweetened)
	⅓ cup nectar (sweetened)
banana	½ banana (3″ long)
berries	½ cup blackberries
	½ cup blueberries
	½ cup boysenberries
	1 cup cranberries
	¾ cup cranberry juice (unsweetened)
	¼ cup cranberry juice (sweetened)
	½ cup gooseberries
	½ cup loganberries
	½ cup raspberries
	1 cup strawberries
cherries	10 large, fresh or canned
currants	1 tbsp. dried
dates	2 fresh
figs	1 large, fresh
	2 medium, canned
	1 small, dried
fruit cocktail	½ cup, fresh or canned
grapefruit	one half
	½ cup juice
	½ cup, sections (unsweetened)
	½ cup blended juice
grapes	12 large or 24 small, fresh
	¼ cup juice
lemon	1 large, fresh
	½ cup juice
lime	1 medium, fresh
	½ cup juice
mango	½ small, fresh
melon	¼ small cantaloupe (6″ diameter)
	⅛ medium honeydew (8″ diameter)
	1 slice watermelon (3″ × 1″)
	1 cup diced melon
nectarine	1 small, fresh
orange	1 small, whole
	½ cup, sections
	½ cup juice
papaya	¾ cup, diced
	⅓ medium
peach	1 medium, fresh
	2 medium halves, canned
	¾ cup nectar (unsweetened)
	½ cup, slices
	¼ cup nectar (sweetened)

†Item high in sodium.

Table 28–11.   FOOD EXCHANGES FOR DIETS TO CONTROL
HYPERLIPIDEMIA (*Continued*)

FRUIT EXCHANGES (*Continued*)

pears	1 small, fresh
	2 medium halves, canned
	¾ cup nectar (unsweetened)
	¼ cup nectar (sweetened)
persimmon	1 medium, fresh
pineapple	½ cup diced, raw
	1½ rings, canned
	⅓ cup juice
plums	2 medium, fresh
	4 halves, canned
prunes	2 medium, dried
	¼ cup juice
raisins	2 tbsp., dried
tangerine	1 medium, fresh

BREAD EXCHANGES

One Serving Contains:

70 calories, 15 gm. carbohydrate, 2 gm. protein, and negligible fat

Serving Size

	BREAD
1 slice	white, wheat, pumpernickel, rye, raisin, French, and Italian
2 (8½ " long)	bread sticks
1	*cornbread (2″ × 2″ × 1″)
½	pita
	ROLLS
½	bagel
1	bialy
½	bun, hamburger or frankfurter
½	English muffin (2 oz.)
½	hard Kaiser roll (25 gm.)
1	*muffin, biscuit (2″ diameter)
1	plain soft roll
	CRACKERS
10	animal
3	arrowroot
2	graham (2½ " square)
½	matzo (4″ × 6″)
5	melba toast
20	oyster (½ cup)
20	†pretzels, small sticks
3	pretzels, medium
5	*round (1½ " diameter)
2	rusk
3	rye crackers (2″ × 3½ ")
6	†saltines (2″ square)
4	†soda (2½ " square)
	CEREAL
½ cup	cooked, hot
¾ cup	unsweetened, dry (flake, puffed, biscuit type)
3 tbsp.	wheat germ
	PASTAS
½ cup	barley, cooked
½ cup	macaroni, cooked
½ cup	noodles, cooked (avoid egg noodles)
½ cup	rice, brown, cooked
½ cup	rice, white, cooked
½ cup	spaghetti, cooked
	PREPARED FOODS
1 cube	angel food cake (1½ " cube)
15	†**corn chips
2	corn tortillas (5″ diameter)
	flour tortillas (5″ diameter)
½ cup	gelatin, flavored
¼ cup	*ice milk

*Omit one B Fat Exchange.
**Omit two B Fat Exchanges.
†Item high in sodium.

Table continued on the following page

Table 28–11. FOOD EXCHANGES FOR DIETS TO CONTROL HYPERLIPIDEMIA (*Continued*)

BREAD EXCHANGES (*Continued*)

1	*pancake (5″ × ½″)
1½ cup	popcorn, popped (small kernels)
3 cups	popcorn, popped (large kernels)
15	†**potato chips
¼ cup	sherbet
1	taco shell
1	*waffle (5″ × ¼″)

SOUPS

1 cup	†vegetable or broth type
1 cup	†*cream soup (commercial, diluted with water)
1 cup	†cream soup (made with skim milk)

STAPLES

2½ tbsp.	pearled barley, dry
2½ tbsp.	bread crumbs, dry
2½ tbsp.	cornstarch, dry
2½ tbsp.	flour, dry
2½ tbsp.	tapioca, dry
2½ tbsp.	cornmeal

STARCHY VEGETABLES

POTATOES

8 pieces	*french fried (2″ × 3½″)
1 small	white baked or boiled, (2″ diameter)
½ cup	white, mashed
¼ cup	sweet potato or yam

BEANS

¼ cup	baked (no pork)
⅓ cup	dried (cooked)
½ cup	lima (baby)

CORN

⅓ cup	cooked
1 small	on cob (4″ long)

PEAS

½ cup	cooked (green pea)
½ cup	dried (cooked)

WINTER SQUASH

¼ large	acorn, Hubbard, or butternut, fresh
¼ cup	mashed

PARSNIPS

½ cup	cooked

PUMPKIN

¾ cup	cooked

MIXED VEGETABLES

½ cup	cooked

VEGETABLE EXCHANGES

One Serving Contains:

35 calories, 5 gm. carbohydrate, 1 gm. protein, and negligible fat and cholesterol

Serving Size: ½ cup cooked or 1 cup uncooked

artichokes	greens:	rhubarb
asparagus	beet	romaine
bamboo shoots	chard	rutabagas
bean sprouts	collards	†sauerkraut
beans, string	dandelion	summer squash
beans, wax	kale	yellow-crooked neck
beets	mustard	yellow-straight neck
broccoli	spinach	flat-scalloped
brussel sprouts	turnip	zucchini
cabbage	kohlrabi	tomatoes
carrots	mushrooms	†tomato juice
cauliflower	okra	tomato puree
celery	onions or leeks	†vegetable juice
chives	peppers, green	watercress
cucumbers	†pickles, unsweetened	water chestnuts
eggplant	pimento	

*Omit one B Fat Exchange.
**Omit two B Fat Exchanges.
†Item high in sodium.

Table 28–11.   FOOD EXCHANGES FOR DIETS TO CONTROL
HYPERLIPIDEMIA (*Continued*)

VEGETABLE EXCHANGES (*Continued*)

Free Vegetables:

These vegetables contain negligible amounts of carbohydrate, protein, or fat and may be used as desired.

chicory	lettuce
Chinese cabbage	parsley
endive	radishes
escarole	

Note: Starchy vegetables, such as potatoes, are found in the Bread Exchange list.

MEAT EXCHANGES

Serving sizes reflect cooked weight.

One Serving Contains:

40 calories, 7 gm. protein, 25 mg. cholesterol, 1 gm. fat, 0.5 gm. saturated fat and 0.5 gm. polyunsaturated fat

GROUP A

Serving Size	Foods to Choose	Avoid
1 oz.	poultry without skin: Cornish hen, white and dark meat of chicken and turkey	duck, goose, stewing hen
1 oz.	fish with fins: fresh or frozen; e.g., bass, brook trout, cod, flounder, haddock, halibut, perch, pike, red snapper, sole, whitefish	
5 individual or 1 oz.	shellfish: fresh or frozen; e.g., clams, lobster, oysters, scallops, shrimp	
¼ cup	†canned fish: e.g., crab, lake herring, mackerel, salmon, sardines, tuna (canned in water or in allowed oil, drained)	†caviar
2 medium	egg whites	egg yolks (max. 2 per week)
¼ cup	low-cholesterol (substitute) egg products	
1 oz. or ¼ cup	fat-free cheeses: (contain less than 5% butterfat) e.g., farmer's, gjetost, pot, and sapsago	
¼ cup	cottage cheese: dry and 1% low-fat	
1 oz. or ¼ cup	†94% fat-free: low-cholesterol cheeses and cheese products	

PLANT PROTEIN

½ cup (cooked)	**dried beans: all varieties; e.g., calico, common lima, kidney, pinto, red Mexican, or mung beans	†beans cooked with pork
½ cup (cooked)	**dried peas: e.g., chick peas (garbanzo), cowpeas, lentils, split peas	
1/3 cup (cooked)	soybeans, (also omit ¼ Bread Exchange)	
½ cup	*soybean curd	

Note: If plant protein only used, attention must be given to adequate high-quality protein from dairy products or protein complementation as discussed on pages 58 and 227.

---

*Omit 1 B Fat Exchange.
**Omit 2 Fruit Exchanges.
†Item high in sodium.

Table continued on the following page

Table 28–11. FOOD EXCHANGES FOR DIETS TO CONTROL HYPERLIPIDEMIA (*Continued*)

GROUP B

One Serving Contains:

55 calories, 7 gm. protein, 30 mg. cholesterol, 3 gm. fat, 1.0 gm. saturated fat, and no polyunsaturated fat

Serving Size	Foods to Choose	Avoid
¼ cup	COTTAGE CHEESE regular (4% creamed)	†other whole milk cheeses
1 oz.	TURKEY †processed turkey roll	
1 oz.	BEEF †chipped and wafered slices round: round steak (Swiss or minute steak)	organ meat, kidney, liver, sweetbread, †meats canned or frozen in gravy
	sirloin: sirloin tip steak and roast	regular hamburger—80% lean
	chuck: shoulder arm pot roast and arm steak	
	other: tongue	†cold cuts; e.g., bologna, head cheeses, hot dogs, luncheon loaf, and salami
1 oz.	VEAL veal leg: standing rump roast, rolled rump roast, (shank or heel end), round center-cut veal cutlet	
1 oz.	LAMB leg of lamb: roast (top rump) sirloin: boneless roast and sirloin chop	
1 oz.	PORK †pork leg: whole rump or ham roast (butt and shank ends), fresh ham, ham center-cut butt slice †canned: ham †smoked: center slices of ham, shoulder roll, loin chop	†sausage, †bacon

GROUP C

One Serving Contains:

80 calories, 7 gm. protein, 30 mg. cholesterol, 6 gm. fat, 2.5 gm. saturated fat, and no polyunsaturated fat

Serving Size	Foods to Choose	Avoid
1 oz.	BEEF chuck: boneless chuck pot roast, blade steak, and pot roast	
	flank: flank steak, boneless flank, stew meats	
	plate: plate skirt steak, short plate ribs	rolled plate
	loin: filet mignon, roast, tenderloin cubes	
	rib: rib eye steak (Delmonico cut)	
	rump: standing rump and rolled rump roast	
	†canned: corned beef round	corned beef brisket
	round: ground, 85% lean	shank
1 oz.	VEAL veal loin: chop and roast; sirloin steak and roast rib: crown rib roast, chop	

†Item high in sodium.

Table 28–11.   FOOD EXCHANGES FOR DIETS TO CONTROL HYPERLIPIDEMIA (*Continued*)

GROUP C (*Continued*)

1 oz.	shank: foreshank and hind shank shoulder: rolled roast, blade steak blade: roast, arm steak, arm roast	
1 oz.	**LAMB** loin: chop, rolled roast rib: crown rib roast or chop shank: foreshank, mock duck shoulder: rolled and bone-less roast, boneless shoul-der arm chop (Saratoga cut)	
1 oz.	**PORK** loin: tenderloin center-cut and rolled boneless roast, †Canadian style ba-con, sirloin roast rib: tenderloin, center-cut chop	†jowl, ham hock, back ribs, spare ribs, pig feet, liver-wurst
	shoulder: fresh or rolled picnic shoulder arm roast (boiled ham), center slice Boston butt (roast or rolled), center slice shoul-der blade arm steak and roast	†smoked picnic, shoulder butt, blade steak
1 slice (4½″ × ⅛″)	†**CHEESE** part skim milk base: Edam, Mozzarella, Gouda, Havarti, Neufchâtel, Ri-cotta	
	EGG yolk or whole egg	max. 2/week
1 oz.	**OTHER** pheasant, guinea hen, venison	†commercially fried chicken made with unidentified oil

GROUP D

One Serving Contains:

110 calories, 7 gm. protein, 30 mg. cholesterol, 9 gm. fat, 4 gm. saturated fat and 1 gm. poly-unsaturated fat

Limit choices to once a month.

Serving Size	Foods to Choose Sparingly
1 slice (4½″ × ⅛″)	†**CHEESES** whole-milk base: American blue, Swiss, brick, Camembert, Lim-burger, Roquefort, Parmesan, and cream cheese
3 tbsp.	processed cheese foods and spreads
1 oz.	**BEEF** loin: club steak, strip steak (New York or Kansas City strip steak), T-bone steak, Porterhouse steak sirloin: top or bottom butt steak and roast, pinbone steak rib: standing rib roast, steak
1 oz.	**LAMB** shoulder: cushion roast, blade chop
1 oz.	**PORK** rib: butterfly chop, loin chop and roast shoulder: blade loin roast and steak, cushion picnic shoulder
1 oz.	**POULTRY** capon
1 oz.	**FISH** ocean fresh: salmon, rainbow trout, †herring, lake trout
1 oz.	†**NUTS** *††cashew nuts
1 oz.	*††peanuts (2 tbsp.)

†Item high in sodium.
‡Omit 1 B Fat Exchange.
*Do not contain cholesterol.

Table continued on the following page

Table 28–11. FOOD EXCHANGES FOR DIETS TO CONTROL
HYPERLIPIDEMIA (*Continued*)

GROUP D (*Continued*)

1 oz.	*††pistachio nuts (60)
1 oz.	*††walnuts (16–20 small)

Note: Since nuts do not provide as good an assortment of amino acids as animal proteins, they should be supplemented with another plant or animal protein to insure an adequate high quality protein intake.

EGG EXCHANGES

One Serving (1 whole egg) contains:

80 calories, 7 gm. protein, 270 mg. cholesterol, 6 gm. fat, 1 gm. saturated fat, 5 gm. polyunsaturated fat. Limit whole eggs or egg yolks to two per week. 2 oz. of one of the following may be substituted for 1 egg: shrimp, sardines, liver or other organ meats.

FREE FOODS

The following items may be used as desired:

Artificial sweeteners
†Baking powder
†Baking soda
†Bouillon cubes
†Broth, bouillon or consomme—clear, without fat
Carbonated beverages, unsweetened or artificially sweetened
Carbonated or soda water
Celery seed or †celery salt
Chives
Coffee—brewed, instant, decaffeinated
Dill
Garlic, garlic powder, †garlic salt, garlic juice
Gelatin, unflavored or artificially sweetened
Herbs—sage, curry, oregano, thyme, etc.
Horseradish
Mint leaves
Mustard
Onion salt,†onion powder, onion flakes, onion juice
Parsley
Pepper, paprika
Pimento
Poppy seed
Poultry seasoning
Rhubarb, unsweetened or artificially sweetened
†Salt, seasoned salt, tenderizers
Spices—cloves, cinnamon, ginger, etc.
Tea
Vinegar

The following foods may be used in small amounts, but not more than 1 or 2 tsp. (5 or 10 gm.) per meal.

†Catsup
†Chili sauce
Cocoa
Jellies, artificially sweetened
Lemon or lime juice
Postum
Syrup, artificially sweetened
†Worcestershire sauce, A–1 sauce, soy sauce, Tabasco sauce

---

†Item high in sodium.
*Omit 1 B fat exhchange.
‡Do not contain cholesterol.

Table 28–12. NUTRITIONAL ANALYSIS OF FOOD EXCHANGES OF DIETS TO CONTROL HYPERLIPIDEMIA

FOOD EXCHANGE	KCAL.	PROTEIN (gm.)	CHO (gm.)	FAT (gm.)	SAT. FAT (gm.)	POLYUNSAT. FAT (gm.)	CHOLESTEROL (mg.)
Milk	80	8	12	0.2	0.1	tr.	5
Fat A	45	—	—	5	0.5	3	—
B	45	—	—	5	1	2	—
Fruit	40	—	10	—	—	—	—
Bread/starch	70	2	15	—	—	—	—
Vegetable	35	1	5	—	—	—	—
Meat A	40	7	—	1	0.5	0.5	25
B	55	7	—	3	1.0	—	30
C	80	7	—	6	2.5	—	30
D	110	7	—	9	4.0	1	30
Egg	80	7	—	6	1.0	0.5	270

dicates elevated VLDL. An elevated serum cholesterol alone is probably due to elevated LDL but may be due to elevated HDL and this should be assessed. If combined with hypertriglyceridemia, elevated cholesterol could reflect elevated VLDL, which contain cholesterol also.

Chylomicronemia is not atherogenic but can cause functional abnormalities such as pancreatitis. The atherogenicity of elevated VLDL is uncertain and may be related to the site of atherogenesis. Elevated LDL is correlated with premature atherosclerotic disease. However, this correlation is no stronger than that between total serum cholesterol and premature atherosclerosis. Increased levels of HDL appear to be related to resistance to atherosclerosis.[26]

CLASSIFICATION OF HYPERLIPOPROTEINEMIAS. Six types of hyperlipoproteinemias have been described. However, *five distinctions based on functional defects are evolving as more clinically useful.* These are outlined in Table 28–14. There is a genetic component in the development of hyperlipoproteinemia.

Types IIa, IIb and IV are associated with premature atherosclerosis and as a group are often called *familial combined hyperlipidemia.*[36] Because they are fairly common they deserve special attention, particularly now that type II is detectable in neonates by cord blood analysis. Thus, preventive dietary measures can be started early.[24]

The identification and classification of these primary hyperlipidemias may be useful with regard to optimal dietary and medical treatment.

NUTRITIONAL CARE FOR THE HYPERLIPOPROTEINEMIAS. A plan for dietary management of the hyperlipoproteinemias has been carefully formulated and is available upon request from the National Institutes of Health.[21] Appropriate suggestions for using, buying and cooking foods are included. See Table 28–15 for a summary of these diets, which will be discussed later.

However, more recent evidence suggests that in some cases a maximum change as a result of diet can be achieved with the use of a single diet rather than the multiple diets as originally suggested.[12] Table 28–16 lists the effects of dietary cholesterol reduction, dietary fat reduction and caloric restriction on the various lipoprotein fractions. Depending on which lipoprotein fractions need to be changed, those components of the diet would be changed. Thus, a single diet low in total fat, low in saturated fat and, if weight reduction is necessary, low in energy may be recommended. Additional considerations must be made for hyperchylomicronemia and for hyperlipidemia combined with diabetes.

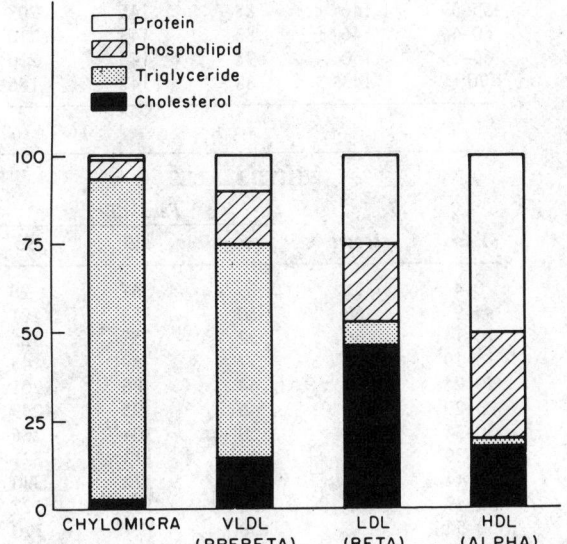

Figure 28–4 Approximate percentage of composition of the four lipoprotein families. VLDL= very low density lipoproteins, LDL= low density lipoproteins, HDL= high density lipoproteins. (Adapted From Levy, R. I., et al.: Dietary and drug treatment of primary hyperlipoproteinemia. Ann. Intern. Med., 77:267, 1972.)

Table 28–13. NORMAL PLASMA VALUES OF U.S. POPULATION (MG./DL.)

TOTAL CHOLESTEROL

Age (Years)	WHITE MALES Mean	Percentiles 5	50	95	Age (Years)	WHITE FEMALES (NON–SEX HORMONE USERS) Mean	Percentiles 5	50	95
0–4	155	114	151	203	0–4	156	112	156	200
5–9	160	121	159	203	5–9	164	126	163	205
10–14	158	119	155	202	10–14	160	124	158	201
15–19	150	113	146	197	15–19	157	120	154	200
20–24	167	124	165	218	20–24	164	122	160	216
25–29	182	133	178	244	25–29	171	128	168	222
30–34	192	138	190	254	30–34	175	130	172	231
35–39	201	146	197	270	35–39	184	140	182	242
40–44	207	151	203	268	40–44	194	147	191	252
45–49	212	158	210	276	45–49	203	152	199	265
50–54	213	158	210	277	50–54	218	162	215	285
55–59	214	156	212	276	55–59	231	173	228	300
60–64	213	159	210	276	60–64	231	172	228	297
65–69	213	158	210	274	65–69	233	171	229	303
70+	207	151	205	270	70+	228	169	226	289

LDL CHOLESTEROL

Age (Years)	WHITE MALES Mean	Percentiles 5	50	95	Age (Years)	WHITE FEMALES (NON–SEX HORMONE USERS) Mean	Percentiles 5	50	95
0–4	—	—	—	—	0–4	—	—	—	—
5–9	93	63	90	129	5–9	100	68	98	140
10–14	97	64	94	132	10–14	97	68	94	136
15–19	94	62	93	130	15–19	95	60	93	135
20–24	103	66	101	147	20–24	98	—	98	—
25–29	117	70	116	165	25–29	106	70	103	151
30–34	126	78	124	185	30–34	109	67	108	150
35–39	133	81	131	189	35–39	119	76	116	172
40–44	136	87	135	186	40–44	125	77	120	174
45–49	144	98	141	202	45–49	130	80	127	187
50–54	142	89	143	197	50–54	146	90	141	215
55–59	146	88	145	203	55–59	152	95	148	213
60–64	146	83	143	210	60–64	156	100	151	234
65–69	150	98	146	210	65–69	162	97	156	223
70+	143	88	142	186	70+	149	96	146	207

TOTAL TRIGLYCERIDES

Age (Years)	WHITE MALES Mean	Percentiles 5	50	95	Age (Years)	WHITE FEMALES (NON–SEX HORMONE USERS) Mean	Percentiles 5	50	95
0–4	56	29	51	99	0–4	64	34	59	112
5–9	56	30	51	101	5–9	60	32	55	105
10–14	66	32	59	125	10–14	75	37	70	131
15–19	78	37	69	148	15–19	72	39	66	124
20–24	100	44	86	201	20–24	72	36	64	131
25–29	116	46	95	249	25–29	75	37	65	145
30–34	128	50	104	266	30–34	79	39	69	151
35–39	145	54	113	321	35–39	86	40	73	176
40–44	151	55	122	320	40–44	98	45	82	191
45–49	152	58	124	327	45–49	105	46	87	214
50–54	152	58	124	320	50–54	115	52	97	233
55–59	141	58	119	286	55–59	125	55	106	262
60–64	142	58	119	291	60–64	127	56	105	239
65–69	137	57	113	267	65–69	131	60	112	243
70+	130	58	111	258	70+	132	60	111	237

From Havel, R. J.: Approach to the patient with hyperlipidemia. Med. Clin. N. Am., 66:319, 1982. Data from U.S. Department of Health and Human Services, Public Health Service, National Institutes of Health, Lipid Metabolism Branch, NHLBI: The Lipid Research Clinics. Population Studies Data Book, Vol. 1. Bethesda, Md., NIH Pub. No. 80–1527, 1980.

Table 28-14. TYPES OF PRIMARY HYPERLIPOPROTEINEMIA

TYPE	LIPID ABNORMALITIES	LIPOPROTEIN ABNORMALITIES[a]	USUAL AGE OF EXPRESSION	FAMILIAL FORMS	SOME CLINICAL FEATURES
I: Familial Hyperchylomicronemia	Cholesterol: normal or elevated; Triglyceride: elevated (>1000 mg./100 ml.)	Severe chylomicronemia	Infancy and childhood	Rare and usually familial (recessive)	Bouts of abdominal pain, pancreatitis, eruptive xanthomas, hepatosplenomegaly
IIa: Familial Hypercholesterolemia	Cholesterol: elevated (300–600 mg./100 ml.); Triglyceride: normal	LDL increased	At birth, if genetic	Most obvious genetic form is expressed in heterozygote, more severe in homozygote; many mild examples are not obviously familial	Premature vascular disease; in familial forms, tendon and tuberous xanthomas
IIb or III: Familial Combined Hyperlipidemia	Cholesterol: elevated (300–600 mg./100 ml.); Triglyceride: elevated (150–1000 mg./100 ml.)	IIb—LDL increased, plus excess VLDL; III—Increased ILDL	Adulthood (over age 20)	Frequently familial and if so appears recessive; sporadic	Glucose intolerance, tuberoeruptive or planar xanthomas, premature vascular disease (especially peripheral vascular disease); worsened by alcohol excess
IV: Familial Endogenous Hypertriglyceridemia	Cholesterol: normal or elevated; Triglyceride: elevated (400–1000 mg./100 ml.)	VLDL increased	Usually third decade or later; can occur in children	When genetic, is dominant; sporadic	Glucose intolerance in about 50%, excess caloric intake common; occasionally eruptive xanthomas, hyperuricemia; worsened by alcohol excess; accelerated by coronary vessel disease
V: Mixed Hyperlipemia	Cholesterol: elevated; Triglyceride: elevated (>1000 mg./100 ml.)	VLDL increased, chylomicrons present	Adulthood, very rare in children	When familial, more than half of close relatives have either type IV or type V	Bouts of abdominal pain and pancreatitis, eruptive xanthomas, hepatosplenomegaly, excess caloric intake common, hyperuricemia; most patients have glucose intolerance; worsened by alcohol excess

Adapted from Levy, R. I., et al.: Dietary and drug treatment of primary hyperlipoproteinemia. Ann. Intern. Med., 77:267, 1972; and Havel, R. J.: Approach to the patient with hyperlipidemia. Med. Clin. N. Am., 66:319, 1982.

[a]LDL = low density lipoproteins; VLDL = very low density lipoproteins; ILDL = intermediate low density lipoproteins.

Table 28–15. SUMMARY OF DIETS AND DRUGS FOR HYPERLIPIDEMIAS

	FAMILIAL HYPERCHYLOMICRONEMIA	FAMILIAL HYPERCHOLESTEROLEMIA OR COMBINED HYPERLIPIDEMIA	MIXED HYPERLIPIDEMIA
Diet Prescription	Low fat (25–35 gm. per day; 10–15 gm. for child per day)	Low cholesterol; low total fat; polyunsaturated to saturated fat ratio increased; weight reduction	Low cholesterol; low fat; polyunsaturated to saturated fat ratio increased; weight reduction.
Energy	Not restricted unless weight reduction necessary	Achieve and maintain "ideal" weight; reduction diet if necessary	Achieve and maintain "ideal" weight; reduction diet if necessary
Protein	Total protein intake not limited	Total protein intake not limited other than to achieve and maintain "ideal" weight	Total protein intake not limited other than to achieve and maintain "ideal" weight.
Fat	Restricted to 25–35 gm. per day; kind of fat not important.	Total fat limited to 30% or less; saturated fat intake limited to 10% of calories; polyunsaturated fat intake increased to 6 to 7% of calories; P/S ratio 1.0	Restricted to 20% or less of calories in addition to other recommendations
Cholesterol	Not restricted	As low as possible, preferably 100 to 200 mg./day	As low as possible, preferably 100 to 200 mg./day
Carbohydrate	Not limited	Not limited, but increased—if no reduction in lipids, then controlled; concentrated sweets restricted	Not limited, but increased—if no reduction in lipids, then controlled; concentrated sweets restricted
Alcohol	Not recommended	May be used with discretion	Not recommended

Adapted from Fredrickson, D. S., et al.: Dietary Management of Hyperlipoproteinemia. DHEW Publ. No. (NIH) 75–110. Bethesda, Md., National Heart and Lung Institute, 1974; and Connor, W. E., and Connor, S. L.: The dietary treatment of hyperlipidemia. Rationale, technique and efficacy. Med. Clin. N. Am., 66:485, 1982.

Generally, the purpose of the diets is to reduce the hyperlipidemia and keep the patient asymptomatic. A 15 per cent or greater reduction in serum cholesterol or triglyceride levels means that the diet is successful and should be continued. All persons on these diets should try to achieve or maintain ideal body weight.

Table 28–16. SUMMARY OF THE PHASES OF THE ALTERNATIVE DIET FOR LOWERING BLOOD LIPIDS

Phase I:	Avoid foods very high in cholesterol and saturated fat; delete egg yolk, butterfat, lard, and organ meat.
	Substitute soft margarine for butter; vegetable oils and shortening for lard; skim milk for whole milk; egg whites for whole eggs.
Phase II:	A gradual transition from using up to 16 ounces of meat a day to no more than 6–8 ounces a day.
	Use less fat and cheese.
	Acquire new recipes using whole grains, beans, and vegetables.
Phase III:	Eat mainly cereals, legumes, fruits, and vegetables.
	Use meat as a condiment.
	Use low-cholesterol cheeses.
	Save these foods for use only on special occasions: extra meats, regular cheese, chocolate, candy, and coconut.

From Connor, W. E., and Conner, S. L.: The dietary treatment of hyperlipidemia. Rationale, technique and efficacy. Med. Clin. N. Am., 66:485, 1982.

Weight loss in itself will cause a lowering of lipids in overweight patients. In designing these diets the exchange lists given in Table 28–11 can be used.

Diet for Familial Hyperchylomicronemia. In this lipid disorder there is an inability to clear chylomicrons from the blood due to a deficiency of adipose tissue lipoprotein lipase. As a result, the *serum triglyceride* concentration is *extremely high* (more than 1000 mg. per 100 ml.). A very low fat diet, 25 to 35 gm. of fat per day, is effective therapy and results in a clearing of the triglyceride from the serum and prevention of bouts of abdominal pain. Children should receive a 0.5 gm. of fat per kg. of body weight with special attention to essential fatty acids. Cholesterol in the diet does not need to be excessively low. Medium-chain triglycerides (MCT) can be used as supplementary fat, since they are absorbed directly into the portal vein and are transported to the liver without requiring chylomicron formation. This source of fat may help to make the diet more palatable. The exchange groups in Table 28–11 can be used. The goal of treatment is plasma triglyceride levels no greater than 1000 mg./dl. and optimally less than 400 mg./dl.

In the acute phase of severe chylomicronemia a minimal-fat diet is most effective in relieving vomiting and abdominal pain. A low-fat, high-

EXAMPLE OF A DIET FOR THE CHILD WITH FAMILIAL HYPERCHYLOMICRONEMIA

(4–6 Years of Age, 15–18 kg.) 1400–1600 kcal.[21]

DAILY FOOD PLAN

1 qt. skim milk (fortified with vitamins A and D)
2 oz. cooked poultry, fish or lean trimmed meat[a] (Meat Group A or B, Table 28–11)
4 servings of vegetable and fruit
4 or more servings of bread or cereal
1 or more servings of potato, rice, etc.
Allowed desserts[b] and sweets

[a] Add one additional ounce of meat for the child 6 to 12 years old.
[b] Desserts made with skim milk; also Jello, fruit, fruit ices. MCT oil may be used.

EXAMPLE OF A DIET FOR THE ADULT WITH FAMILIAL HYPERCHYLOMICRONEMIA

1700–2000 Kcal.[21]

DAILY FOOD PLAN

1 qt. skim milk (fortified with vitamins A and D)
4 oz. cooked poultry, fish or lean trimmed meat (Meat Group A or B, Table 28–11)
5 servings of vegetable and fruit including 1 serving citrus fruit, and 1 serving dark green or deep yellow vegetable
6 or more servings whole-wheat or whole-grain bread or cereal
1 or more servings potato, rice, noodles, grits
Desserts[a]
Sugars, sweets
Beverages (non-dairy)
1–2 fat servings

[a] Made with skim milk; Jello, fruit, fruit ices. Medium chain triglycerides (MCT) may be used if prescribed by a physician, in which instance adjustment in calories is necessary.

carbohydrate formula (0 to 5 per cent fat, 20 per cent protein, and 75 to 80 per cent carbohydrate) may be useful (see Table 35–7). A rice and fruit diet may also be useful because it is very low in fat and easy to prepare.

Diet for Familial Hypercholesterolemia or Combined Hyperlipidemia. Familial hypercholesterolemia is characterized by an increase in LDL due to either overproduction or inadequate removal. It is thought to be transmitted as an autosomal dominant trait and is easily diagnosed in the first or second year of life. VLDL levels may also be elevated, leading to an elevated serum triglyceride level; this condition is usually called familial combined hyperlipidemia. *For all of these situations (the old designations of types IIa, IIb, III and IV) the nutritional care is the same.* Nutritional care involves lowering the intake of cholesterol to as low as possible with 100 to 200 mg. per day preferred (100 to 150 mg. per day for children) and modifying the fat intake to produce a high polyunsaturated to saturated fatty acid ratio (P:S of about 1.0). (See Figure 28–5 for calculation of P:S ratio.) The to-

$$\frac{\text{gm. of linoleic acid}}{\text{gm. of saturated fat}} = \text{P:S ratio}$$

Example:

$$\text{P:S ratio for vegetable fat} = \frac{0.4 \text{ gm. linoleic acid}}{1 \text{ gm. saturated fat}} = 0.4$$

$$\text{P:S ratio for corn oil} = \frac{2.7 \text{ gm. linoleic acid}}{0.5 \text{ gm. saturated fat}} = 5.4$$

Figure 28–5. Calculation of polyunsaturated: saturated fat ratio (P:S).

tal fat content of the diet is limited to 20 to 30 per cent of total kcalories.[12] The saturated fat is limited to 5 to 10 per cent, the polyunsaturated to 6 to 7 per cent, and the monounsaturated fat to 9 to 13 per cent. Complex carbohydrate is increased, as is dietary fiber.

To follow this diet the patient must eat lean meat, including fish and poultry (without skin), limited to not more than 9 oz. per day, and beef, lamb, ham and pork, limited to a 3 oz. portion three times a week. Whole-milk dairy products and eggs are omitted. Many cookbooks are available from local heart associations and bookstores for low-fat cooking. The exchange lists in Table 28–11 should be used in designing the diet. Connor and Connor suggest approaching the necessary dietary changes in phases and propose the scheme in Table 28–16.[12] The following is an example of a diet for a person with elevated LDL.

EXAMPLE OF A DIET FOR THE ADULT WITH FAMILIAL HYPERCHOLESTEROLEMIA

1700–2000 Kcal.[21]

1 pt. or more skim milk (fortified with vitamins A and D)
6 oz. cooked poultry, fish or lean trimmed meat[a] (preferably from Meat Group A or B, Table 28–11)
5 servings of vegetable and fruit[b] including 1 serving dark green or deep yellow vegetable[c]
7 or more servings of bread or cereal[d]
1 or more servings of potato, rice, etc.
2–3 fat servings, fat A or B group
Desserts and sweets made with skim milk, egg whites, oil and sugar substitute[e]

[a] Limit beef, lamb and pork to 3 oz. portions 3 times per week. Fish and poultry without skin are naturally lower in fat and should be used in place of meat as often as possible.
[b] One serving of citrus fruit is recommended daily to provide adequate ascorbic acid.
[c] One dark green or deep yellow vegetable is recommended daily to provide adequate vitamin A.
[d] Enriched cereal or bread should be included in the diet to provide adequate vitamin B complex and iron. Use Exchange lists, Table 28–11, for calculation.
[e] To maintain calories at this level, it will be necessary to omit additional desserts and sweets.

Those with combined hyperlipidemia (elevated LDL and VLDL) will also be helped by this diet and weight reduction. For those who do not experience satisfactory reduction of serum triglycerides and VLDL after achievement and maintenance of ideal body weight, omission of alcohol and curtailment of simple sugars may be necessary.

Hyperlipidemia is frequently associated with diabetes mellitus and may be the reason for the premature atherosclerosis seen in this population. Nutritional care focuses first on diabetic control. If hyperlipidemia persists after the plasma glucose is under control, then attention should turn to weight reduction and achievement of ideal body weight. At ideal body weight the individual nearly always has lower (or normal) triglyceride concentrations than when he or she was heavier. The other aspects of nutritional care for hyperlipidemia already outlined should be also followed. If there is still no response, carbohydrate and alcohol restrictions are recommended. See Chapter 25 for nutritional care in diabetes.

Diet for Mixed Hyperlipemia. Mixed hyperlipemia (previously designated type V) is usually secondary to acute metabolic disorders such as diabetic acidosis, pancreatitis, alcoholism and nephrosis. Both exogenous triglyceride (chylomicrons) and VLDL accumulate in the fasting plasma. Plasma triglyceride levels are markedly elevated, and there is frequently abnormal glucose tolerance. Nutritional care stresses caloric restriction and maintenance of desired body weight. The amount of fat is restricted to 25 to 30 per cent of the calories, with unsaturated fats predominating. The same principles discussed for familial hypercholesterolemia and combined hyperlipidemia are followed. Lack of adherence to the diet and eating a high-fat meal will result in chylomicronemia and abdominal pain. To relieve pain it may be necessary to reduce the fat in the diet to 5 to 10 per cent of total kcalories.

SUMMARY OF DIETS FOR HYPERLIPIDEMIA. It is important to keep all nutrient requirements in mind, not just those nutrients that must be restricted when designing diets to manage hyperlipidemia. If certain nutrients are lacking, appropriate supplements are indicated. For example, the diet can be low in the fat-soluble vitamins, essential fatty acids and iron. Dark green and deep yellow vegetables three to four times per week are recommended, as well as liver occasionally. In fact, water-soluble forms of the fat-soluble vitamins may have to be given to remedy the lack of absorption in the absence of fat in hyperchylomicronemia.

In summary, the practical nutritional care for patients with hyperlipidemias includes a weight-controlling diet that is low in total fat, saturated fat and cholesterol and more liberal in polyunsaturated fat. Naturally, the carbohydrate, particularly complex carbohydrate, must

be high. Dietary fiber intake (water soluble fiber) should be as high as possible. If serum triglyceride levels do not come down after several months on this diet, restriction of simple sugars and alcohol may be necessary. Medication may also be required.

Problems and Suggested Topics for Discussion

1. Interview cardiac patients to learn the foods that cause distention. What is your conclusion?
2. Name some substitutes for salt that can be used safely in flavoring a low-sodium diet.
3. When is salt restricted for a cardiac patient? Study the diet prescribed for cardiac patients in your institution.
4. What is the average sodium intake of the U.S. population? Which food groups contribute to this intake? What percentage of the normal intake comes from added salt?
5. Obtain a diet history from a patient with congestive heart failure. Determine how much a 500 mg. sodium diet would deviate from his usual pattern.
6. Check the food intake of a patient in the hospital who is recovering from an acute heart attack. Is it adequate? What dietary changes would you recommend for long-term nutritional care?
7. Obtain a dietary history from a patient who is suffering from hypertension. What is her usual sodium intake? How high is her potassium intake? Is she overweight, and if so, by how much? What nutritional care would you plan for her?
8. Interview a patient with hypercholesterolemia. Does he have any other problems? Plan his nutritional care. Will the dietary changes be extensive? Plan a sequence of changes for the next few years.
9. Plan the nutritional care for a child with familial hyperchylomicronemia. Assess his present nutritional status and growth. What will the new diet changes mean for the family?

Cited References

1. American Heart Association Nutrition Committee: Rationale of diet-heart statement of the American Heart Association. Arteriosclerosis, *4*:177, 1982.
2. Astrup, P., and Kjeldsen, J.: Carbon monoxide, smoking, atherosclerosis. Med. Clin. North. Am., *58*:323, 1974.
3. Ayachi, S. Increased dietary calcium lowers blood pressure in the spontaneously hypertensive rat. Metabolism, *28*:1234, 1979.
4. Barboriak, J.J., et al.: Vitamin E supplements and plasma high-density lipoprotein cholesterol. Am. J. Clin. Pathol., *77*:371, 1982.
5. Barnes Hospital: Handbook of Nutrition Care. 5th ed., St. Louis, Barnes Hospital, 1975, p. 166.
6. Bennett, D.R., and Smith, S.J.: Sodium content of prescription and nonprescription drugs. In White, P.L., and Crocco, S.C. (eds.): Sodium and Potassium in Foods and Drugs. Chicago, American Medical Association, 1980.
7. Bordia, A.: Effect of garlic on blood lipids in patients with coronary heart disease. Am. J. Clin. Nutr., *34*: 2100, 1981.
8. Bordia, A.: Effect of garlic on human platelet aggregation in vitro. Atherosclerosis, *30*:355, 1978.
9. Brisson, G.J.: Lipids in Human Nutrition. Englewood, N.J., Jack K. Burgess, Inc., 1981.
10. Castelli, W.P., et al.: HDL cholesterol and other lipids

in coronary heart disease. The cooperative lipoprotein phenotyping study. Circulation, *55*:767, 1977.

11. Committee on Nutrition, American Academy of Pediatrics: Salt intake and eating patterns of infants and children in relation to blood pressure. Pediatrics, *53*:115, 1974.

12. Connor, W.E., and Connor, S.L.: The dietary treatment of hyperlipidemia. Rationale, technique, and efficacy. Med. Clin. N. Am., *66*:485, 1982.

13. Dahl, L.K.: Salt and hypertension. Am. J. Clin. Nutr., *25*:231, 1972.

14. Dawber, T.R.: The Framingham Study. The Epidemiology of Atherosclerotic Disease. Cambridge, Mass., Harvard Univ. Press, 1980.

15. Dayton, S., et al.: Controlled clinical trial of a diet high in unsaturated fat in preventing complications of atherosclerosis, Circulation *39/40*(Suppl. 2):1, 1969.

16. Diet and coronary heart disease. Report of the Advisory Panel of the British Committee on Medical Aspects of Food Policy (Nutrition) on Diet in Relation to Cardiovascular and Cerebrovascular Disease. Nutr. Today, *10*(1):16, 1975.

17. Duston, H.M.: Mechanisms of hypertension associated with obesity. Ann. Intern. Med., *98*(Suppl. 5, Part 2): 860, 1983.

18. Elvehjem, C.A., and Burns, C.H.: Sodium content of commercial spices. JAMA, *148*:1033, 1952.

19. Folkow, B.: Physiological aspects of primary hypertension. Physiol. Rev., *62*:347, 1982.

20. Fraser, G.E.: The effect of various vegetable supplements on serum cholesterol. Am. J. Clin. Nutr., *34*: 1272, 1981.

21. Fredrickson, D.S., et al.: Dietary Management of Hyperliproproteinemia: A Handbook for Physicians and Dietitians. DHEW Publ. No. (NIH) 75–110. Bethesda, Md., National Heart and Lung Institute, 1974.

22. Fregly, M.J.: Estimates of sodium and potassium intake. Ann. Intern. Med., *98*(Suppl. 5, Part 2):792, 1983.

23. Garrison, R.J., et al.: Cigarette smoking and HDL cholesterol. The Framingham offspring study. Atherosclerosis, *30*:17, 1978.

24. Glueck, C.J., et al.: Neonatal familial type II hyperlipoproteinemia: cord blood cholesterol in 1800 births. Metabolism, *20*:597, 1971.

25. Grande, F., Anderson, J.T., and Keys, A.: Diets of different fatty acid composition producing identical serum cholesterol levels in man. Am. J. Clin. Nutr., *25*:53, 1972.

26. Havel, R.J.: Approach to the patient with hyperlipidemia. Med. Clin. N. Am., *66*:319, 1982.

27. Hegsted, D.M., et al.: Quantitative effects of dietary fat on serum cholesterol in man. Am. J. Clin. Nutr., *17*:281, 1965.

28. Jenkins, D.J., et al.: Effect of pectin, guar gum and wheat fiber on serum cholesterol. Lancet, *1*:1116, 1975.

29. Kannel, W.B., and Gordon, T.: Physiological and medical concomitants of obesity: the Framingham Study, In Bray, G.A. (ed): Obesity in America. NIH Publ. No. 79–359. Washington, D.C., National Institutes of Health, Public Health Service, 1979. pp. 125–163.

30. Kannel, W.B., and Gordon, T. (eds.): The Framingham Study: Diet and the Regulation of Serum Cholesterol. Section 24. Washington, D.C., Public Health Service, 1970.

31. Kaplan, N.M.: Hypertension: prevalence, risks and effect of therapy. Ann. Intern. Med., *98*(Suppl. 5, Part 2):705, 1983.

32. Kaufman, M.: Adapting therapeutic diets to Jewish food customs. Am. J. Clin. Nutr., *5*:676, 1957.

33. Kempner, W.: Compensation of renal metabolic dysfunction: treatment of kidney disease and hypertensive vascular disease with rice diet. N. Carolina Med. J., *6*:61 and 117, 1945.

34. Kesteloot, H., and Geboers, J.: Calcium and blood pressure. Lancet, *2*:813, 1982.

35. Klevay, L.M.: Coronary heart disease: The zinc/copper hypothesis. Am. J. Clin. Nutr., *28*:764, 1975.

36. Kuo, P.T.: Hyperlipidemia and coronary artery disease. Med. Clin. North Am., *53*:351, 1974.

37. Langford, H.G.: Dietary potassium and hypertension: epidemiologic data. Ann. Intern. Med., *98*(Suppl. 5, Part 2):770, 1983.

38. Langford, H.G., Watson, R.L., and Thomas, J.G.: Salt intake and treatment of hypertension. Am. Heart J., *93*:531, 1977.

39. Laragh, J.H., and Pecker, M.S.: Dietary sodium and essential hypertension: some myths, hopes, and truths. Ann. Intern. Med., *98*(Suppl. 5, Part 2):735, 1983.

39a. Lipid Research Clinics Program: The Lipid Research Clinics Coronary Primary Prevention Trial results. Parts 1 and 2. JAMA, *251*:351 and 365, 1984.

40. McCarron, D.A.: Calcium and magnesium nutrition in human hypertension. Ann. Intern. Med., *98*(Suppl. 5, Part 2):800, 1983.

41. McCarron, D.A.: Development and maintenance of elevated blood pressure in the spontaneously hypertensive rat based upon dietary calcium. Clin. Res., *30*: 338a, 1982.

42. McCarron, D.A.: Low serum concentrations of ionized calcium in patients with hypertension. N. Engl. J. Med., *307*:226, 1982.

43. McCarron, D.A., Morris, C.C., and Cole, C.: Dietary calcium in human hypertension. Science, *217*:267, 1982.

44. McGill, H.C.: The relationship of dietary cholesterol to serum cholesterol concentration and to atherosclerosis in man. Symposium report of task force on the evidence relating six dietary factors to the nation's health, Am. J. Clin. Nutr., *32*(Suppl.):2664, 1979.

45. Morgan, T., et al.: Hypertension treated by salt restriction. Lancet. *1*:278, 1978.

46. MRFIT Research Group: Multiple risk factor intervention trial: risk factor changes and mortality results. JAMA, *248*:1465, 1982.

47. National High Blood Pressure Education Program Coordinating Committee: Statement on the Role of Dietary Management in Hypertension Control. Bethesda, Md., National Heart, Lung, and Blood Institute, 1979.

48. Peart, S.W.: Renin-angiotensin system. N. Engl. J. Med., *292*:302, 1975.

49. Reisen, E., et al.: Effect of weight loss without salt restriction on the reduction of blood pressure in overweight hypertensive patients. N. Engl. J. Med., *298*:1, 1978.

50. Report of the Inter-Society Commission for Heart Disease Resources. Circulation, *42*, December 1970, revised April 1972.

51. Rabkin, S.W., Mathewson, F.A.L., and Hsu, P.-H.: Relation of body weight to development of ischemic heart disease in a cohort of young North American men after a 26-year observation period. The Manitoba study. Am. J. Cardiol., *39*:452, 1977.

52. Rinzler, S.H.: Primary prevention of coronary heart disease by diet. Bull. N.Y. Acad. Med., *44*:936, 1968.

53. San Francisco Heart Association: Sodium in Medicinals. San Francisco, SFHA, 1973.

54. Scheig, R.: Diseases of lipid metabolism. In Bondy, P.K., and Rosenberg, L.E. (eds.): Duncan's Diseases of Metabolism. 7th ed., Philadelphia, W.B. Saunders Company, 1974, p. 382.

55. Schroeder, H.A.: Municipal drinking water and cardiovascular death rates. JAMA, *195*:81, 1966.

56. Select Committee on Nutrition and Human Needs of

the U.S. Senate: Dietary Goals for the United States. Washington, D.C., U. S. Government Printing Office, 1977.

57. Siervogel, R.M., et al.: Blood pressure, body composition, and fat tissue cellularity in adults. Hypertension, 4:382, 1982.

58. Stamler, J., et al.: Prevention and control of hypertension by nutritional-hygienic means. JAMA, 243:1819, 1980.

59. Tannen, R.L.: Effects of potassium on blood pressure control. Ann. Intern. Med., 98(Suppl. 5, Part 2):773, 1983

60. Tobian, L.: The relationship of salt to hypertension. Am. J. Clin. Nutr., 32(Suppl.):2739, 1979.

61. Turpeinen, O., et al.: Dietary prevention of coronary heart disease: the Finnish mental hospital study. Int. J. Epidemiol., 8:99, 1979.

62. Williams, P., Robinson, D., and Bailey, A.: High density lipoprotein and coronary risk factors in normal men. Lancet, 1:72, 1979.

Additional References

American Spice Trade Association: The art of seasoning low sodium diets. Hospital Management, 89:80, 1960.

Bierman, E.L.: Carbohydrates, sucrose, and human disease. Symposium: Report of task force on the evidence relating six dietary factors to the nation's health. Am. J. Clin. Nutri., 32(Suppl.):2712, 1979.

Comstock, G.W.: Water hardness and cardiovascular disease. Am. J. Epidemiol., 110:375, 1979.

Connor, W.E., et al.: The plasma lipids, lipoproteins, and diet of the Tarahumara Indians of Mexico. Am. J. Clin. Nutr., 31:1131, 1978.

Crocco, S.C.: The role of sodium in food processing. J. Am. Diet. Assoc., 80:36, 1982.

Dawberg, T.R., et al.: Eggs, serum cholesterol and coronary heart disease. Am. J. Clin. Nutr., 36:617, 1982.

Del Greco, F.: The kidney in congestive heart failure. Mod. Concepts Cardiovasc. Dis., 44:47, 1975.

Eder, H.A., and Gidez, L.I.: The clinical significance of the plasma high density lipoproteins. Med. Clin. N. Am., 66:431, 1982.

Ederer, F., et al.: Cancer among men on cholesterol-lowering diets: experience from five clinical trials. Lancet, 2:203, 1971.

Engstrom, A.M., and Tobelman, R.C.: Nutritional consequences of diet modification to reduce sodium intake. Ann. Intern. Med., 98:870, 1983.

Food and Drug Administration: Preliminary Data: FY 77. Selected Minerals in Food Survey Total Diet Studies. Washington, D.C., Department of Health, Education and Welfare, 1977.

Glueck, C.J.: Dietary fat and atherosclerosis. Am. J. Clin. Nutr., 32:2703, 1979.

Goodnight, S.H., et al.: Polyunsaturated fatty acids, hyperlipidemia and thrombosis. Arteriosclerosis, 2:87, 1982.

Gordon, T., et al.: High density lipoprotein as a protective factor against coronary disease. The Framingham Study. Am. J. Med., 62:707, 1977.

Harper, A.E.: Coronary heart disease—an epidemic related to diet. Am. J. Clin. Nutr., 37:669, 1983.

Havel, R.J. (ed.): Symposium on lipid disorders. Med. Clin. N. Am., 66(2), 1982.

Hegsted, D.M., et al.: Quantitative effects of dietary fat on serum cholesterol in man. Am. J. Clin. Nutr., 17:281, 1965.

Hulley, S.B., Cohen, R., and Widdowson, G.: Plasma high density lipoprotein cholesterol level. JAMA, 238:2269. 1977.

Johnson, B.G., and Nilsson-Ehle, P.: Alcohol consumption

and high density lipoprotein. N. Engl. J. Med., 298:633. 1978.

Kaplan, N.M.: Mild hypertension: when and how to treat. Arch. Intern. Med., 143:255, 1983.

Kark, R.M., and Oyama, J.H.: Nutrition, hypertension, and kidney disease. In Goodhart, R.S., and Shils, M.E. (eds.): Modern Nutrition in Health and Disease. 6th ed., Philadelphia. Lea & Febiger, 1980.

Keys, A., Anderson, J.T., and Grande, F.: Prediction of serum-cholesterol responses of man to changes in fats in the diet. Lancet, 2:959, 1957.

Laubusch, E., and McCammon, C.S.: Water as a sodium source and its relation to sodium restriction therapy patient response. Am. J. Publ. Health, 45:1337, 1955.

Levy, R.I., and Moskowitz, J.: Cardiovascular research: decades of progress, a decade of promise. Science, 217:121, 1982.

Marsh, A.C., and Koons, P.C.: The sodium and potassium content of selected vegetables, J. Am. Diet. Assoc., 83:24, 1983.

Meneely, G.R., and Battarbee, H.D.: Sodium and potassium. Nutr. Rev., 34:225, 1976.

Ponsati, L.P., et al.: Comprehensive evaluation of fatty acids in foods. J. Am. Diet. Assoc., I. Dairy products, 66:482, 1975; II. Beef products, 67:35, 1975; III. Eggs and egg products, 67:351, 1975; V. Unhydrogenated fats and oils, 68:224, 1976; VIII. Finfish, 69:243, 1976; IX. Fowl, 69:517, 1976; X. Lamb and veal, 70:53, 1977.

Schonfeld, G., et al.: Alterations in levels and interrelations of plasma apolipoproteins induced by diet. Metabolism, 25:261, 1976.

Stamler, J.: Diet and coronary heart disease. Biometrics, 38 (Suppl.):95, 1982.

Thelle, D.S., Arnesen, E., and Forde, O.H.: The Tromso Heart Study . Does coffee raise serum cholesterol? N. Engl. J. Med., 308:1454, 1983.

Van Itallie, T.: Obesity: adverse effects on health and longevity. Am. J. Clin. Nutr., 32:2723, 1979.

Vermeulen, R.T., Sedor, J.A., and Kimm, S.Y.S.: Effect of water rinsing on sodium content of selected foods. J. Amer. Diet. Assoc., 82:394, 1983.

Wynder, E.L., and Reddy, B.S.: Dietary fat and colon cancer. J. Natl. Cancer Inst., 54:7, 1975.

Recipes and Meal Planning for Sodium-Restricted Diets

American Heart Association, local office or 44 East 23rd St., New York, N.Y. 10010. Booklets: Your Sodium-Restricted Diet 500 mg.; 1000 mg.; Mild Restriction.

Claiborne, C.: Craig Claiborne's Gourmet Diet. New York, Times Books, 1980.

James, J., and Goulder, L.: The Dell Color-Coded Low Salt Living Guide. New York, Dell Publishing Co., 1980.

Payne, A.S., and Callahan, D.: The Fat-Sodium Control Cookbook, Boston, Little, Brown and Co., 1975.

Recipes and Meal Planning for Fat-Controlled Diets

American Heart Association booklets: Planning Fat-Controlled Meals for Unrestricted Calories; Planning Fat-Controlled Meals for 1200 and 1800 Kcalories.

Brown, W.J., Liebowitz, D., and Olness, M.: Cook to Your Heart's Content on a Low-Fat, Low-Salt Diet. New York, Van Nostrand Reinhold, 1976.

Connor, W.E., et al.: The Alternative Diet Book. Iowa City, Iowa, Univ. of Iowa Publications, 1976. Order Dept., 17 W. College Street, Iowa City, 52240

Consumers' Guide to Fat, Cholesterol-Controlled Food Products. American Heart Association, Greater Los Angeles Affiliate, 2405 W. Eighth St., Los Angeles, Ca., 90057, 1981.

Cutler, C.: Haute Cuisine For Your Heart's Delight. New York, Clarkson N. Potter, Inc., 1973.

Eshleman, R., and Martin, M.: American Heart Association Cookbook. 3rd ed. New York, David McKay Co., Inc. 1979.

James, J., and Goulder, L.: The Dell Color-Coded Low-Fat Living Guide. New York, Dell Publishing, Inc., 1980.

Jones, J.: Diet For A Happy Heart. San Francisco, 101 Productions, 1975.

Keys, M., and Keys, A.: The Benevolent Bean. New York, Farrar, Straus, and Giroux, 1972.

MacRae, N.M.: How to have your cake and eat it too!, 2nd ed. Anchorage, Alaska, Alaska Northwest Publishing Co., 1982

Stead, E.S., and Warren, G.K.: Low Fat Cookery. 2nd ed., revised. New York, McGraw-Hill, 1968.

Williams, J.B.: No Salt No Sugar, No Fat Cookbook. Concord, Calif., Nitty Gritty Productions, 1981.

CHAPTER 29

Nutritional Care in Anemias

Physiology and Function of the Blood

Blood transports nutrients, oxygen, hormones, electrolytes, cellular excreta and other substances to and from all parts of the body. It is life itself, and any anemia affects the body as a whole.

In the normal, healthy individual the blood amounts to approximately 5 to 6 per cent of the body weight. The concentration of red blood cells (erythrocytes) is approximately 4,500,000 per cu. mm. in women and 5,000,000 per cu. mm. in men. The white blood cells (leukocytes) are fewer in number than the erythrocytes; the ratio is approximately 1 to 500.

The Anemias

Anemia is a condition in which there is a deficiency in the size or number of erythrocytes or in the amount of hemoglobin they contain. Nutritional factors of greatest importance in anemias are deficiencies of iron, vitamin B_{12} and folic acid.

CLASSIFICATION. Formerly, the anemias were classified into primary and secondary types; however, it is known now that anemia is never primary. It is always secondary to some pathological state in the patient. As shown in Table 29–1, anemia may be classified according to cell size and hemoglobin content.

ANEMIAS RESULTING FROM ACUTE HEMORRHAGE

Following an acute hemorrhage in a formerly healthy individual, a normochromic-normocytic anemia can appear (Table 29–1). The body replaces plasma within a few days. However, the speed with which the hemoglobin is restored depends largely upon the type of diet ingested. An adequate normal diet rich in foods containing iron, ascorbic acid and protein is essential. Liquids are mandatory to replace the fluid lost through hemorrhage and consequently lost from the tissues. In cases of very serious hemorrhage, restoration of blood volume by transfusion may be necessary.

NUTRITIONAL ANEMIAS

The anemias that result from an inadequate intake of iron, protein, certain vitamins (B_{12}, folic acid, pyridoxine, ascorbic acid), copper and other heavy metals are frequently termed nutritional anemias. The deficiency may be caused by inadequate ingestion, defective absorption, imperfect utilization, injury to the bone marrow or increased requirement, as in pregnancy or adolescence. Stores of these nutrients may be reduced, and in periods of increased need there may be biochemical or clinical effects. A further reduction in nutrient stores may result in anemia, the final stage of deficiency. The most common types of nutritional anemias in this country are due to iron deficiency or folic acid deficiency. However, not infrequently a com-

Table 29–1. MORPHOLOGICAL CLASSIFICATION OF ANEMIA

MORPHOLOGICAL TYPE OF ANEMIA[a]	UNDERLYING ABNORMALITY	CLINICAL SYNDROMES	TREATMENT
I. Macrocytic (MCV>94, MCHC>31)			
Megaloblastic	Vitamin B_{12} deficiency	Pernicious anemia, etc.	Vitamin B_{12}
	Folic acid deficiency	Nutritional megaloblastic anemias, sprue and other malabsorption syndromes.	Folic acid
	Inherited disorders of DNA synthesis	Orotic aciduria, etc.	According to nature of disorder
	Drug-induced disorders of DNA synthesis	Chemotherapeutic agents	Stop offending drug
		Anticonvulsants, oral contraceptives	Folic acid
Non-megaloblastic	Accelerated erythropoiesis	Hemolytic anemia	Treatment of underlying disease
	Increased membrane surface area		
	Obscure		
II. Hypochromic-microcytic (MCV<80, MCHC<31)			
	Iron deficiency	Chronic loss of blood, inadequate diet, impaired absorption, increased demands, etc.	Ferrous sulfate and correction of underlying cause
	Disorders of globin synthesis	Thalassemia, along or with a hemoglobinopathy	Non-specific
	Disorders of porphyrin and heme synthesis	Pyridoxine-responsive anemia, etc.	Pyridoxine
	Other disorders of iron metabolism		
III. Normochromic-normocytic (MCV 82–92, MCHC>30)			
	Recent blood loss	Various	Transfusion, iron Correct underlying condition
	Overexpansion of plasma volume	Pregnancy Overhydration	Restore homeostasis
	Hemolytic diseases		According to nature of disorder
	Hypoplastic bone marrow	Aplastic anemia Pure red cell aplasia	Transfusions Androgens
	Infiltrated bone marrow	Leukemia, multiple myeloma, myelofibrosis, etc.	Chemotherapy, etc.
	Endocrine abnormality	Hypothyroidism, adrenal insufficiency, etc.	Treatment of underlying disease
	Chronic disorders		Treatment of underlying disease
	Renal disease	Renal disease	Treatment of underlying disease
	Liver disease	Cirrhosis	Treatment of underlying disease

From Wintrobe, M. M., et al.: Clinical Hematology. 7th ed. Philadelphia, Lea & Febiger, 1974, p. 547.

[a]MCV (mean corpuscular volume) = volume of one red cell expressed in femtoliters (fl.).

MCHC (mean corpuscular hemoglobin concentration) = concentration of hemoglobin expressed in gm. per deciliter (dl.).

bined type of anemia is present. There appears to be an interdependence between iron deficiency and folic acid deficiency. Iron deficiency precipitates folic acid deficiency, possibly by increasing the folic acid requirement. The increased hemolysis of red blood cells that occurs in iron deficiency would increase the amount of folate needed to regenerate them.

Iron deficiency anemia, as will be explained, is the last stage of an iron-deficient state. Using the level of circulating hemoglobin as the criterion for diagnosing the iron-deficient state identifies only the severely iron-deficient person in the late stages of the disease. This leads to the difficulty in defining the prevalence of iron deficiency. Iron deficiency is now recognized as the most common deficiency state in man and affects 10 to 20 per cent of the world population.[6] For further discussion of iron deficiency, see page 163. This chapter will deal mainly with iron deficiency anemia, which is still the most common way that iron deficiency is detected.

Iron Deficiency Anemia

ETIOLOGY. This form of anemia is characterized by a reduced concentration of hemoglobin in the blood and a depletion of total body iron content. The three causes of iron deficiency anemia are (1) chronic blood loss, such as from a chronically bleeding peptic ulcer, bleeding hemorrhoids or from parasites or malignancy, (2) faulty iron intake or absorption and (3) increased iron requirement for growth of blood volume, which occurs in infancy, puberty, pregnancy and lactation. Another cause of iron deficiency anemia is defective release of iron into the plasma from the iron stores as occurs in chronic inflammation and other chronic disorders. However, this is not true iron deficiency anemia.

During infancy, a close relationship exists between diet and iron deficiency. At puberty, as well as in infancy, there is an acceleration of growth and an increased requirement for iron. The anemia that can develop when this increased requirement is not met is often present in growing children or adolescents.

In the adult male, iron deficiency anemia is, with few exceptions, ascribed to blood loss, usually resulting from disease or treatment for disease. While loss of menstrual blood is a natural process in females, if losses are large, iron deficiency anemia can result. Many women are unaware of the extent of their menstrual losses and a method has been developed to quantify them.[13]

During pregnancy, there is an increased need for iron to supply the growing fetus. During lactation, there is a loss of iron in milk secretion, which probably is similar in quantity to the loss in the menstrual flow. Unless iron is provided to replace the amount lost or to build new hemoglobin, iron deficiency anemia will develop. Sometimes gastrointestinal disturbances such as diarrhea, achlorhydria or intestinal disease, which interfere with the absorption, will prevent iron from entering the blood stream in the required amount, even though the dietary intake of iron is adequate. When such a condition

exists, the individual may maintain a low hemoglobin level for years.

CLINICAL FINDINGS. Iron deficiency has been categorized by the stages of deficiency: (1) iron stores depletion, (2) deficient erythropoiesis and (3) iron deficiency anemia.

In the early stage, ferritin and hemosiderin (storage forms of iron) are depleted, and iron absorption increases. The *total iron binding capacity (TIBC)* of transferrin (or transferrin iron binding capacity) rises as iron stores in the bone marrow and liver decrease. When iron stores are depleted, the level of plasma iron falls. There may also be depletion of iron-containing enzymes in the tissues. Finally, in stage three the hemoglobin falls, and the erythrocytes become smaller *(microcytic)* and contain less hemoglobin *(hypochromic)*. Figure 29–1 outlines the progression of iron deficiency. The mean corpuscular volume (MCV), mean corpuscular hemoglobin (MCH) and mean corpuscular hemoglobin concentration (MCHC) are all below normal (Table 29–1).

When there is not enough iron entering the plasma, plasma iron concentration falls from its normal levels. When it is less than 60 μg./dl., it is probable that the needs of the bone marrow for making hemoglobin and red blood cells (RBC) are not being met. The percentage of saturation of transferrin, the plasma iron binding protein, decreases to low levels. Once it falls below 15 per cent, the delivery of iron to the marrow is compromised. When the supply of iron to the developing RBC in the marrow is suboptimal, not all porphyrin can be used to make heme, so the level of protoporphyrin in circulating RBC rises above normal.

DIAGNOSIS. The hemoglobin concentration alone is definitely unsuitable for diagnosing iron deficiency because it is affected late in the disease. It alone is incomplete in diagnosing anemia because it does not indicate what type of anemia exists. Lastly, hemoglobin concentration is an unreliable indicator because of the wide scatter of values in normal subjects. Even iron-replete women may have low hemoglobin.

Thus, the proper diagnosis of iron deficiency anemia, or any anemia for that matter, must include other data as mentioned in Table 29–1, including cell morphology assessment. *Serum or plasma ferritin is the most sensitive parameter of iron status.* It falls only with true iron deficiency, whereas transferrin saturation (TS), free erythrocyte protoporphyrin (FEP) and hemoglobin levels are affected by chronic infection and other factors that may cause an anemia that looks like iron deficiency anemia when in fact iron is adequate. One μg./liter serum ferritin (SF) is equivalent to between 8 and 21 mg. iron stores with a weighted mean of 9.9 mg. Thus, in

Sequential Changes in the Development of Iron Deficiency	Normal	Iron Depletion	Iron Deficient Erythropoiesis	Iron Deficiency Anemia
Iron Stores →				
Erythron Iron →				
RE Marrow Fe (0-6)	2-3+	0-1+	0	0
Transferrin IBC (µg/dl)	330±30	360	390	410
Plasma Ferritin (µg/l)	100±60	20	12	<12
Iron Absorption	normal	↑	↑	↑
Plasma Iron (µg/dl)	115±50	115	<60	<40
Transferrin Saturation (%)	35±15	30	<15	<10
Sideroblasts (%)	40-60	40-60	<10	<10
RBC Protoporphyrin (µg/dl RBC)	30	30	100	200
Hgb (gm./dl)	>12	>12	>12	<12
Erythrocytes	normal	normal	normal	microcytic and hypochromic

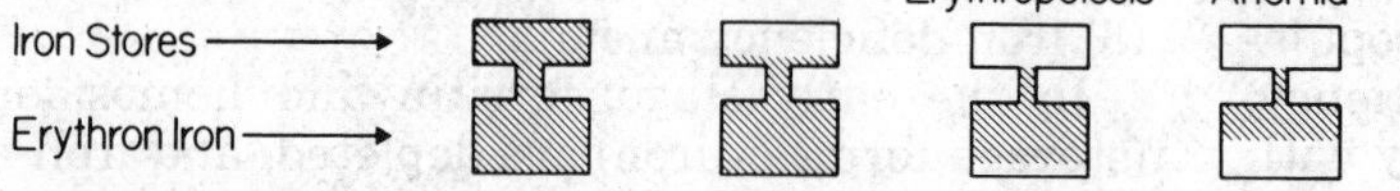

Figure 29–1. The sequence of changes induced by a gradual reduction in the iron content of the body. (Adapted from Bothwell, T. H., et al.: Iron Metabolism in Man. Oxford, Blackwell Scientific Publications, 1979.)

individuals with a normal TS, normal FEP and normal hemoglobin concentration, iron stores can be calculated by multiplying SF by 10.[6] However, once iron stores are exhausted, the SF falls below 12 µg./liter and then no longer reflects the true body iron stores because now there is also a deficit in circulating iron.

When plasma ferritin is less than 12 µg./dl. and if the hemoglobin is above 12 gm./dl. and either transferrin saturation or red cell protoporphyrin is abnormal, then no storage iron is present. When both are abnormal and the plasma ferritin is 12 µg./dl. and the hemoglobin is 12 gm./dl., then there is a hemoglobin iron deficit of 150 mg. When the hemoglobin concentration is less than 12 gm./dl., the iron deficit can be calculated because 1 gm./dl. hemoglobin in a 70 kg. woman is equivalent to 150 mg. iron. A hemoglobin value of 12 when normal is 14 gm./dl. indicates a hemoglobin iron deficit of 300 mg.

The transferrin saturation, free erythrocyte protoporphyrin and serum ferritin must be incorporated into the clinical evaluation of iron deficiency anemia. Cook and Finch conclude that the cause of anemia can reasonably be attributed to iron deficiency only when at least two of these iron parameters fall within the deficient range.[6] It may be best to perform all four tests—SF, TS, FEP and hemogloin—when assessing the iron status of a population.[6]

The World Health Organization has identified the following hemoglobin concentrations as being those below which anemia is likely: adult males 13 gm./dl., adult females 12 gm./dl., and adult pregnant females 11 gm./dl.[23]

SYMPTOMS. A symptom that is possibly a sign of early iron deficiency is a reduction in immunocompetence and therefore an increased propensity to infection. However, the association of immunological changes with iron deficiency is still controversial. The dispute centers on the fact that iron is required for microbial growth. Serum with a high iron content enhances microbial growth; therefore, it seems likely that iron deficiency would protect the host. On the other hand, several investigators have observed that cell-mediated immunity and the phagocytic activity of neutrophils are impaired in iron-deficient subjects.[4, 17] However, others have found no change in phagocytic activity in such cases.[16] Chandra suggests that the outcome of the exposure of an iron-deficient person to an infective challenge probably depends upon the host defense mechanisms as well as upon the effect of the person's iron status on the growth of the infecting organism.[3]

Patients with iron deficiency usually adapt to their slowly progressing disease, and frequently seek health care only when another symptom or problem arises. Most patients develop symptoms from anemia when their hemoglobin level approaches 8 to 11 gm./dl. Fatigue, although popularly thought to be an early symptom of iron deficiency anemia, has not been correlated with decreased hemoglobin levels.[9] Several behavioral symptoms of iron deficiency, such as fatigue, weakness, anorexia and pica (which seem to respond to iron therapy much before the anemia is cured), may be due to tissue depletion of iron-containing enzymes and not to the decreased level of blood hemoglobin,[24] as discussed on page 163.

As iron deficiency anemia becomes more severe, defects develop in the structure and function of the epithelial tissues, especially of the tongue, nails, mouth and stomach. Fingernails become thin and flat, and eventually *koilonychia* (spoon-shaped nails) develops as shown in Figure 29–2. Mouth changes include atrophy of the lingual papillae, burning and redness and, in severe cases, a completely smooth, waxy and glistening appearance to the tongue. Angular stomatitis may also develop, as well as a form of dysphagia (difficulty in swallowing). Gastritis occurs frequently and may result in achlorhydria. Progressive, untreated anemia results in cardiovascular and respiratory changes that can eventually end in cardiac failure.

TREATMENT. Treatment should focus primarily on the underlying disease leading to the anemia. This may be very difficult to determine. Repletion of iron stores, not just alleviation of the anemia, should be the goal.

MEDICATION. The chief treatment for iron deficiency anemia consists of oral administration of inorganic iron, preferably ferrous iron, in adequate dosage over a proper time interval. Absorption of ferrous iron at a dose of 30 mg. iron is three times greater than if the same amount is given of a ferric form of iron; with larger doses, the difference is even more marked. The most widely used preparation is *ferrous sulfate,* and the dose is calculated in terms of the amount of elemental iron provided. Other ferrous salts absorbed to about the same degree as the sulfate are ferrous lactate, fumarate, glycine sulfate, glutamate and gluconate. Ferrous succinate may be absorbed 30 per cent better than the sulfate, and all others are less well absorbed.[12]

Iron is best absorbed when the stomach is empty; however, it also causes the greatest gastric irritation at this time. The degree to which absorption is inhibited by food depends upon the composition of the meal, as discussed on page 591; however, it is still preferable to administer iron between meals. Gastrointestinal side-effects of nausea, epigastric discomfort and distention, heartburn, diarrhea or constipation can also be minimized by increasing the dose slowly over a few days until the required amount is reached and by giving the iron in at least three doses per day. The side-effects are dose-related, so one option is to reduce the daily dosage and plan that the therapeutic program will take longer. However, patients tolerate iron supplements much better than is generally believed. In one study, lactose tablets labeled "Iron Pills" produced symptoms in the same percentage of subjects as did genuine iron pills labeled "Iron Pills," whereas identical lactose tablets labeled "Control Pills" did not.[15]

Adults should take 100 to 225 mg. of iron as a ferrous salt daily, and children should receive 1.5 to 2.0 mg. iron per kg. of body weight, depending upon the severity of the anemia and their tolerance of the iron. Table 29–2 gives recommended oral preparations. Sustained-release iron preparations reduce gastrointestinal side-effects by preventing rapid dissolution of iron, but at the same time they may allow the iron to bypass the jejunum, which is the most active site of iron absorption. However, some recently developed preparations are showing absorption equivalent to ferrous sulfate without the gastrointestinal side-effects. Ascorbic acid greatly increases iron absorption through its capacity to maintain iron in the reduced state, as discussed in Chapter 7.

The response to iron treatment usually occurs in one to three weeks, with an increased number of reticulocytes being the first sign. Blood hemoglobin level increases, and then epithelial

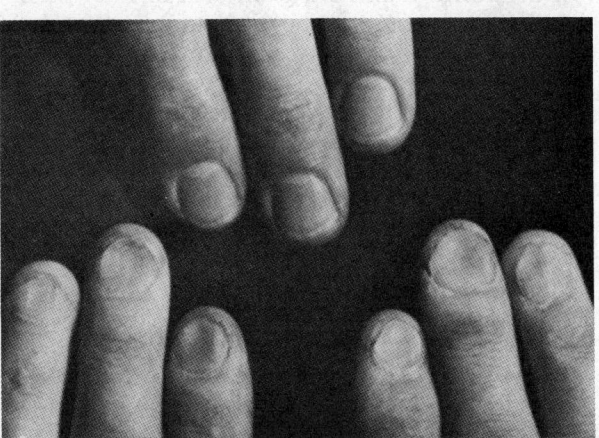

Figure 29–2. Fingernails of an iron-deficient adult (below) compared with those of a normal subject. (From: Rosenbaum, E., and Leonard, J. W.: Nutritional iron deficiency anemia in an adult male. Ann. Intern. Med., *60:683,* 1964, p. 684.)

Table 29–2. RECOMMENDED ORAL IRON PREPARATIONS

| Preparation | gm./tablet | IRON CONTENT | | ACCEPTABLE ADULT DOSE |
		%	mg. Fe/tablet	tablets/day
Ferrous sulfate • 7H$_2$O	0.32	20	60	4
Ferrous sulfate, exsiccated	0.2	29	60	4
Ferrous gluconate	0.32	12	40	4 or 5
Ferrous fumarate	0.2	33	66	4
	0.32	33	105	2 or 3
Ferroglycine sulfate	0.25	16	40	5

From Beutler, E.: Iron. In Goodhart, R. S., and Shils, M. E.: Modern Nutrition in Health and Disease. 6th ed. Philadelphia, Lea & Febiger, 1980, p. 346.

changes are corrected. Iron therapy should be continued for 6 to 12 months, even after hemoglobin levels have been restored, to allow for repletion of body iron reserves. The absorption of 40 to 50 mg. iron per day will permit a red cell production rate of about three times normal and, if there is not blood loss, a hemoglobin concentration rise of 0.2 gm./dl./day, although it may be less in cases of mild anemia.[1]

The rate of iron absorption depends on the severity of the anemia so that in the beginning of treatment more will be absorbed than toward the end when iron stores are being replenished.

If iron supplementation fails to correct the iron deficiency anemia, there are three possible reasons that should be investigated. By far the most common is that the patient is not taking the medication, most likely because of unpleasant side-effects. The patient should be questioned carefully. The second possibility is that bleeding is continuing at a rate faster than the erythroid marrow can replace blood cells. Last is the possibility that the iron is not being absorbed, which, if the bioavailability of the iron is not in question, could be due to malabsorption possibly due to idiopathic steatorrhea or celiac sprue.

Parenteral administration of iron may be necessary for patients who are unable to take it orally because of gastrointestinal symptoms or an inability to absorb iron or who lose iron (blood) too rapidly to be replaced by oral intake. Although replenishment of stores by this route is faster, it is more expensive and less safe.

NUTRITIONAL CARE. In addition to medication, attention should be given to the amount of absorbable iron in food. Liver, kidney, beef, tripe, egg yolk, dried fruits (apricots, peaches, prunes, raisins), dried peas and beans, nuts, green leafy vegetables (beet greens), molasses, whole-grain breads and cereals and fortified cereals rank highest among foods in their iron content. (See Appendix Table 11 for a more complete list; also see Table 10–7.) However, their contribution of absorbable iron needs to be considered in the context of the entire meal or snack.

Since the content of iron in typical Western diets is 6 mg./1000 kcal. with surprising consistency, it is apparent that the bioavailability of the iron in the diet is of greater importance than the total dietary iron in correcting or preventing iron deficiency. The nutritional counseling of individuals should focus on this.

Iron absorption and the factors influencing it are discussed generally in Chapter 7. Here in this section, specific information is provided on the method for quantifying the influence of meal composition on the absorption of the iron from that meal. This knowledge will enable the nutrition counselor to recommend to the patient very specific and effective ways to modify the diet in order to increase the amount of absorbable iron in the diet.

BIOAVAILABILITY OF DIETARY IRON. It is estimated that 1.8 mg. of iron must be absorbed daily to meet the needs of 80 to 90 per cent of adult women and adolescent males and females.

As already mentioned, the rate of absorption of iron depends on the iron status of the individual, and this is reflected in the level of iron stores. The lower the iron stores, the greater the rate of iron absorption. Secondly, the absorption rate is influenced by the form of iron in the diet, whether it is *heme* iron (present in *meat, fish, and poultry* [MFP]) or *non-heme* iron (present in grains, vegetables, and also MFP). Heme iron is much better absorbed than is non-heme iron. Thirdly, non-heme iron absorption is influenced by several dietary enhancing factors. The two that are most well-defined on a quantitative basis are ascorbic acid and MFP. *One milligram of ascorbic acid is approximately equivalent in enhancing power to 1 gm. of cooked MFP or 1.3 gm. of raw MFP.* The sum of these enhancing factors (ΣEF) has been correlated with iron absorption and a logarithmic function defined as shown in Table 29–3.[19]

Not only is ascorbic acid a powerful reducing agent, but it also binds iron in equimolar concentrations to form a readily absorbed complex. By an unknown mechanism MFP potentiates the absorption of non-heme iron in other foodstuffs. It may be that (MFP) digestion leads to the release of amino acids and polypeptides in the upper small bowel, which then form soluble, absorbable complexes with non-heme iron.[7]

An individual with no iron stores may be expected to absorb about 35 per cent of the heme iron and 8 per cent of non-heme iron (if enhancers are present) in the diet, while an individual with replete iron stores (1000 mg.) would probably absorb only 15 per cent of heme iron and 3 per cent of non-heme iron (with no enhancers present). So even though the percentage of absorption of non-heme iron is below that of heme iron, its absorption is greatly influenced by enhancing factors or inhibitors. The rate of absorption of non-heme iron is between 3 and 8 per cent, depending upon the number of enhancing factors. More important, the vast majority of the iron in the diet is non-heme iron; thus, the enhancement of its absorption is very important. Table 29–3 gives a method for calculating the bioavailable dietary iron in a meal,

snack or total day's intake. Table 29–4 shows how the total absorbable iron can vary by as much as 300 per cent in four different meals, all of which contain the same amount of iron. The enhancing substances must be consumed with the non-heme iron to have an effect. If ascorbic acid is given four hours prior to a meal, no enhancing effect has been seen.[8]

In addition to these enhancing factors are other factors mentioned in Chapter 7. In contrast are inhibiting factors, which include carbonates, oxalates, phosphates and phytates (unleavened bread, unrefined cereals and soybeans). However, the degree to which such complexes inhibit iron absorption is variable, depending upon other unknown factors. These may be factors in vegetable fiber that inhibit non-heme iron absorption. Tea (which contains tannic acid) when taken with meals, reduces iron absorption, and the effect is shown to be due to the formation of insoluble iron tannates. Tea at meals can decrease the absorption of iron from the meal by 50 per cent.[29] Phosvitin in egg yolk also inhibits non-heme iron absorption. Ethylenediamine tetraacetic acid (EDTA), which is used as a food preservative, causes a 50 per cent reduction in the absorption of non-heme

Table 29–3. CALCULATING BIOAVAILABLE DIETARY IRON

1. For each individual meal or snack, determine:
   a. Total iron
   b. Heme iron (40% of meat, fish and poultry iron)[1]
   c. Non-heme iron (60% of meat, fish and poultry iron, *and* all other food iron)
   d. mg. ascorbic acid of foods as ingested[2]
   e. gm. cooked meat/fish/poultry (MFP)
      Note: gm. raw MFP ÷ 1.3 = gm. cooked MFP
2. Mg. heme iron × 23%[3] = mg. heme iron bioavailable.
3. Sum mg. ascorbic acid (ld, above) + gm. cooked MFP (le) = enhancing factors (Σ EF) for non-heme iron bioavailability.
   Consult table (*right*) for % non-heme iron bioavailability.
   Mg. non-heme iron × % for Σ EF = mg. non-heme iron bioavailable.
4. Sum (2) and (3) to determine total bioavailable iron for the individual meal or snack.
5. Sum individual meal and snack bioavailable iron for day's bioavailable iron.[4]

% BIOAVAILABLE NON-HEME DIETARY IRON FOR INDIVIDUAL WITH 500 MG. BODY IRON STORES*

Σ EF	%	Σ EF	%	Σ EF	%	Σ EF	%	Σ EF	%
0	3.00	16	4.33	31	5.41	46	6.38	61	7.26
1	3.09	17	4.40	32	5.48	47	6.44	62	7.31
2	3.18	18	4.48	33	5.55	48	6.50	63	7.37
3	3.26	19	4.55	34	5.61	49	6.56	64	7.42
4	3.35	20	4.63	35	5.68	50	6.62	65	7.47
5	3.44	21	4.70	36	5.75	51	6.68	66	7.53
6	3.52	22	4.78	37	5.81	52	6.74	67	7.58
7	3.60	23	4.85	38	5.88	53	6.80	68	7.64
8	3.69	24	4.92	39	5.94	54	6.86	69	7.69
9	3.77	25	5.00	40	6.01	55	6.92	70	7.74
10	3.85	26	5.06	41	6.07	56	6.97	71	7.79
11	3.93	27	5.14	42	6.13	57	7.03	72	7.85
12	4.01	28	5.21	43	6.20	58	7.09	73	7.90
13	4.09	29	5.28	44	6.26	59	7.14	74	7.95
14	4.17	30	5.34	45	6.32	60	7.20	75	8.00
15	4.25								

*for Σ EF < 75: % = 3 + 8.93 log n $\frac{EF + 100}{100}$
for Σ EF ≥ 75: % = 8

Developed by Elaine R. Monsen, Ph.D., R.D., Professor, Dept of Nutritional Sciences, University of Washington, Seattle, Washington.

[1] Although the proportion of heme iron contained in various tissues probably varies, it is probably not significant enough to warrant separate factors for each type of animal tissue. A heme iron content of 40 per cent is assumed as is 60 per cent for non-heme iron.

[2] Because much or all of the ascorbic acid contained in a meal may be inactivated by heating and oxidation during storage and preparation, estimates of ascorbic acid ideally should be based on the actual amount contained in the meal as eaten. However, this usually is not possible to determine so that the food composition table amount can be used.

[3] Percentage absorption of heme iron will depend upon the iron status of the individual in an inverse logarithmic function. In subjects with 0, 250, 500 and 1000 mg. of iron stores, absorption of heme iron is estimated to be 35, 28, 23 and 15 per cent, respectively. In this table factors for non-heme iron absorption are based on 500 mg. iron stores because iron stores of about 500 mg. are desirable if women are to meet requirements of pregnancy without supplemental iron. The bioavailable iron would be twice as high in a person with 0 stores.

[4] The calculated amount of absorbable iron for the day can be related to the RDA by multiplying the value by a factor of 10 because the RDA are based on the assumption that 10 per cent of the total iron intake is absorbed. Thus 1.8 mg. absorbable iron would meet the RDA for adult women and adolescent males and females regardless of the total dietary iron from which this figure was derived.

Table 29–4. COMPARISON OF ABSORBABLE IRON FROM DIFFERENT SINGLE MEALS

FOOD	WT. (GM.)	TOTAL IRON (MG.)	HEME FACTOR	HEME IRON	NON-HEME IRON (MG.)	ASCORBIC ACID (AS SERVED)
I. Meat, poultry, fish-containing, high ascorbic acid (26 gm protein; 650 kcal.)						
Beef-vegetable stew						
Beef, lean, cooked, 3 oz.	85	2.7	0.4	1.1	1.6	0
Potatoes, ½ cup	78	0.4			0.4	13
Carrots, 2 tablespoons	20	0.1			0.1	1
Onions, 2 tablespoons	15	0.1			0.1	2
Green pepper, raw, 2 slices	20	0.2			0.2	26
Breadstick, 2 medium	35	0.3			0.3	Trace
Margarine, 2 teaspoons	10	0			0	0
Peaches, canned, ½ cup	128	0.4			0.4	4
Gingerbread	63	1.0			1.0	Trace
Totals		5.2		1.1	4.1	46
Ascorbic acid 46 mg.						
Meat, fish, poultry cooked, 85 gm.						
Σ Enhancing factors = 131		% absorbable iron		23%	8%	
		Absorbable iron (mg.)		0.25	0.33	
		Total absorbable iron (mg.)		0.58		
II. Meat, poultry, fish-containing, low ascorbic acid (27 gm protein; 700 kcal.)						
Macaroni, tuna fish, and cheese casserole						
½ cup macaroni and cheese	120	0.9			0.9	Trace
Tuna, drained, 1 oz.	29	0.6	0.4	0.2	0.4	0
Green peas, ½ cup	80	1.5			1.5	10
Cucumber, 3 large slices	14	0.2			0.2	1
Molasses cookies, 2	65	1.4			1.4	0
Blueberry muffin, 1	40	0.6			0.6	Trace
Totals		5.2		0.2	5.0	11
Ascorbic acid 11 mg.						
Meat, fish, poultry raw, 29 gm (cooked = 22)						
Σ Enhancing factors = 33		% absorbable iron		23%	5.55%	
		Absorbable iron (mg.)		0.05	0.28	
		Total absorbable iron (mg.)		0.33		
III. Nonmeat, -poultry, or -fish containing, low ascorbic acid (22 gm protein; 730 kcal.)						
Beans, navy, cooked ½ cup	95	2.6			2.6	0
Rice, brown, cooked ½ cup	98	0.5			0.5	0
Cornbread, 1 piece	78	0.9			0.9	1
Margarine, 1 tablespoon	14	0			0	0
Apple slices, ½ cup	55	0.1			0.1	1
Walnuts, black, raw, 1 tablespoon	8	0.5			0.5	0
Almonds, raw, 1 tablespoon	8	0.4			0.4	Trace
Yogurt, skim milk, 1 cup	226	0.1			0.1	2
Totals		5.1			5.1	4
Ascorbic acid 4 mg.						
Meat, fish, poultry, 0						
Σ Enhancing factors = 4		% absorbable iron			3.35%	
		Absorbable iron (mg.)			0.17	
		Total absorbable iron (mg.)		0.17		
IV. Nonmeat, -poultry, or -fish containing, high ascorbic acid (23 gm. protein; 650 kcal.)						
Red kidney beans, ½ cup	93	2.2			2.2	
Tomato sauce, 2 tablespoons	30	0.2			0.2	4
Broccoli, ⅔ cup	120	0.9			0.9	70
French bread, 1 slice	35	0.8			0.8	Trace
Margarine, 1 tablespoon	14	0			0	0
Cottage cheese, ¼ cup	55	0.2			0.2	0
Pineapple, canned, 2 large slices	210	0.6			0.6	14
Banana, sliced, ¼ cup	37	0.3			0.3	4
Totals		5.2			5.2	92
Ascorbic acid 92 mg.						
Meat, fish, poultry, 0						
Σ Enhancing factors = 92		% absorbable iron			8%	
		Absorbable iron (mg.)			0.42	
		Total absorbable iron (mg.)		0.42		

Adapted from Monsen, E.R., et al.: Estimation of available dietary iron. Am. J. Clin. Nutr., *31*:134, 1978.

iron. Soy products also inhibit non-heme iron absorption, as do calcium phosphate salts. For example, orange juice increases the absorption of iron from bread and eggs, but if an egg is eaten with bread, the poor absorption of the iron in bread is further reduced.

In general, the following recommendations can be made: (1) include a source of vitamin C at every meal, (2) include MFP at every meal if possible, (3) avoid the drinking of tea or coffee with meals (both contain tannic acid), (4) avoid high quantities of EDTA by checking food labels for its presence in foods and (5) improve food choices to increase amount of total dietary iron.

Anorexia, if present, must be considered when selecting food or planning the diet. Gastrointestinal side-effects from concurrent iron medication should also be considered.

Iron Toxicity and Iron Overload

An overdose of iron medication, seen occasionally in children who eat iron tablets thinking they are candy, can be fatal in doses of 3 to 10 gm.[11] Death can occur in 12 to 48 hours from the irritative action of iron—mucosal ulceration and bleeding, hypoxia, metabolic acidosis, alveolar and hepatic damage and renal failure. Treatment consists of oral or intravenous administration of deferoxamine, which chelates with iron and allows its excretion by the kidneys. Calcium disodium EDTA can also be used.

An excessive amount of iron in the body can also occur from parenteral iron administration, transfusional overload or greater than normal gastrointestinal absorption. Idiopathic hemochromatosis, excessive intake (such as from prolonged iron therapy in non–iron-deficient individuals), chronic alcoholism, chronic liver disease and certain types of refractory anemia can lead to excessive gastrointestinal absorption.

Excess iron is stored as hemosiderin in reticuloendothelial cells in the liver or in parenchymal cells of certain tissues. *Hemosiderosis* is increased iron storage without tissue damage, whereas *hemochromatosis* refers to increased storage with associated tissue damage. It is still not clear whether excess iron accumulation results in the tissue damage of hemochromatosis or whether an additional process is going on.

Anemia of Protein-Energy Malnutrition (PEM)

Protein is essential for the proper production of hemoglobin and red blood cells (RBC). It appears that in PEM, because of the reduction in the cell mass and thus oxygen requirements, the person requires fewer RBC to oxygenate the tissue. Since blood volume remains the same, this reduced number of RBC can look like an iron deficiency anemia with a low hemoglobin. In acute PEM, where the loss of active tissue mass may be greater than the reduction of RBC number, the person may be polycythemic, with the result that the body responds to this with suppression of RBC production. RBC production is reduced as a consequence of polycythemia, not of protein and amino acid deficiency. Iron released from normal RBC destruction is not reused in RBC production and is stored so that often there will be adequate iron stores.

The anemia of PEM may be complicated by deficiencies of iron and other nutrients and by associated infections, parasitic infestation and malabsorption. Patients usually suffer from multiple deficiencies, such as iron, folic acid and, less frequently, vitamin B_{12}, when their diet is lacking in protein. In such cases, administration of folic acid, iron, vitamin B_{12} or a combination, along with a normal, well-balanced diet, will usually bring good response. Iron deficiency anemia can reappear with rehabilitation when there is a rapid expansion of RBC mass.

Copper Deficiency Anemia

While copper and other heavy metals are essential for the proper formation of hemoglobin, the amounts needed are so minute that they are usually amply supplied by the normal adequate diet.

Copper plays a role in iron metabolism. The copper-containing protein *ceruloplasmin* is essential for normal mobilization of iron from its storage sites to the plasma. In the copper-deficient state iron cannot be released, and this leads to low serum iron and hemoglobin levels even in the presence of normal iron stores. Serum copper and ceruloplasmin concentrations are low. Other consequences of copper deficiency suggest that copper proteins are also needed for utilization of iron by the developing erythrocyte and for optimal functioning of the erythrocyte membrane.

Copper deficiency is likely only in infants who are fed cow's milk or a copper-deficient infant formula instead of human milk, in an adult or child with a malabsorption syndrome or in an adult or child receiving long-term total parenteral nutrition where copper is not present in the solution.

Pyridoxine-Responsive Anemia

A sideroblastic anemia that responds to vitamin B_6 therapy has been reported. This is a severe microcytic, hypochromic anemia in the presence of high serum iron and tissue iron levels. Transferrin saturation is increased. Frequently, this condition is not due to a pyridoxine deficiency but is an inherited sex-linked anemia. The synthesis of heme appears to be impaired because of an inherited defect in the formation of ALA (D-aminolevulinic acid), a substance involved in heme synthesis. Pyridoxal-5-phosphate is necessary in this reaction. The iron that cannot be used for heme synthesis is stored in the mitochondria of immature red blood cells, which are then called *sideroblasts*. These iron-laden mitochondria do not function normally, and the development and production of red blood cells becomes ineffective. The symptoms are those of anemia and iron overload. The neurological and cutaneous manifestations of vitamin B_6 deficiency are not observed. The anemia responds to the administration of pyridoxine.

TREATMENT. Treatment consists of a therapeutic trial dose of pyridoxine of 50 to 200 mg. per day, which is 25 to 100 times the RDA. If the anemia responds, pyridoxine therapy is continued for life. However, the anemia is only partially corrected; normal red blood cell morphology is never achieved. Patients respond to this treatment in varying degrees, and some may achieve normal hemoglobin levels.

Pyridoxine is widely distributed in foods as shown in Table 10–6. Meat, liver, vegetables and whole-grain cereals and breads are good sources.

Vitamin E–Responsive Hemolytic Anemia

Hemolytic anemia in the newborn which responds to vitamin E is discussed on pages 114 and 764.

Vitamin Deficiency Megaloblastic Anemias

There is an interrelationship between the metabolism of folic acid to folinic acid, and vitamin B_{12} and folic acid; a deficiency of either one will interfere with the normal development of erythrocytes and lead to anemia. Vitamin B_{12} and folic acid are essential for the synthesis of nucleoproteins required in the development of erythrocytes. Ascorbic acid is believed to function as a protector of reduced folates from oxidative destruction in the body. Ascorbic acid also influences the rate of iron absorption and the release of iron from transferrin to the tissues.

FOLIC ACID DEFICIENCY ANEMIA

Etiology. This anemia is present in tropical sprue (Chapter 23), in some pregnant women (Chapter 11) and in infants born to mothers who have the deficiency. Poor eating habits of long duration, faulty absorption and utilization of folic acid and increased requirements due to

growth are believed to be the most frequent causes of the disorder. Additional causes are shown in Table 29–5. Normal body stores of folate are depleted rapidly (within two to four months) on a folate-deficient diet, and anemia is soon evident.

Clinical Findings. Because of their interrelated roles in protein synthesis, a deficiency of either vitamin B_{12} or folic acid will result in the same clinical sign—a megaloblastic bone marrow and anemia. In the deficient state red blood cell protein cannot be synthesized properly, and a large (*macrocytic*) immature (*megaloblastic*) blood cell is the result. This state is characterized by a decreased number of erythrocytes, leukocytes and platelets.

Folate deficiency anemia is manifested by very low serum folate and red blood cell folate levels, less than 3 ng./ml. and less than 140 ng./ml., respectively. Serum levels of vitamin B_{12} are lowered moderately. To differentiate B_{12} deficiency anemia from folate deficiency anemia, both serum folate and B_{12} levels should be measured. There are several other tests that can be used, among which is the *FIGLU (formiminoglutamic acid) urinary excretion test.* Excretion of FIGLU is increased in folic acid deficiency and to a lesser extent in B_{12} deficiency. (See Chapter 9.) Other symptoms of folate deficiency and B_{12} deficiency, as listed in Table 29–6, can be used to differentiate between them.

Treatment. Before initiating treatment it is important that the megaloblastic anemia be properly diagnosed. administration of folate in the presence of a B_{12} deficiency could correct the megaloblastic anemia, but it will not correct the B_{12} deficiency, which will continue and cause progressive nerve disease.

To replenish folate stores, 1 mg. of folate given orally every day for two to three weeks is recommended. To maintain repleted stores, the person should have an intake of at least 50 to 100 μg. of pure folic acid every day, either in his food or in a supplement. One half to 1 cup of orange juice supplies between 50 and 100 μg. of folic acid. See Appendix Table 7 for the folate content of some other foods.

When folate deficiency is complicated by conditions that either suppress hematopoiesis, increase folate requirement or reduce folate absorption, therapy should begin with 500 μg. to 1000 μg. daily.

Symptomatic improvement, such as increased alertness, cooperativeness and appetite, may be apparent before the hematological values are back to normal. After the anemia is corrected, the patient should be instructed about ways to include folate in the diet. Liver, asparagus, dried beans, brewer's yeast, spinach, wheat bran, dark green vegetables and whole-wheat bread are all good sources of folate. Since folate

Table 29–5. PATHOGENETIC CLASSIFICATION OF THE CAUSES OF MEGALOBLASTIC ANEMIA

I. Vitamin B_{12} deficiency
  A. Dietary deficiency (rare)
  B. Lack of Castle's intrinsic factor
    1. Pernicious anemia
      a. Congenital form
      b. Adult form
    2. Gastrectomy
      a. Total
      b. Partial
    3. Ingestion of caustic materials
  C. Functionally abnormal intrinsic factor
  D. Biologic competition
    1. Small-bowel bacterial overgrowth
      a. Small-bowel diverticulosis
      b. Anastomoses and fistulae
      c. Blind loops and pouches
      d. Strictures
      e. Scleroderma
      f. Achlorhydria
    2. Fish tapeworm disease
  E. Familial selective vitamin B_{12} malabsorption (Imerslund's syndrome)
  F. Drug-induced vitamin B_{12} malabsorption
  G. Chronic disease of the pancreas
  H. Zollinger-Ellison syndrome
  I. Diseases especially affecting the ileum
    1. Ileal resection and bypass
    2. Regional enteritis
II. Folate deficiency
  A. Dietary deficiency
  B. Increased requirements
    1. Cirrhosis
    2. Pregnancy
    3. Infancy
    4. Diseases associated with rapid cellular proliferation
  C. Congenital folate malabsorption
  D. Drug-induced folate malabsorption
    1. Anticonvulsants
    2. Oral contraceptives
  E. Extensive intestinal resection, jejunal resection
III. Combined folate and vitamin B_{12} deficiency
  A. Tropical sprue
  B. Gluten-sensitive enteropathy
IV. Inherited disorders of DNA synthesis
  A. Orotic aciduria
  B. Lesch-Nyhan syndrome
  C. Thiamin-responsive megaloblastic anemia
  D. Deficiency of enzymes required for folate metabolism
    1. N^5-methyl tetrahydrofolate transferase
    2. Formiminotransferase
    3. Dihydrofolate reductase
  E. Congenital megaloblastic anemia responsive to large doses of folate and vitamin B_{12}
V. Drug-induced disorders of DNA synthesis
  A. Folate antagonists (e.g., methotrexate)
  B. Purine antagonists (e.g., 6-mercaptopurine)
  C. Pyrimidine antagonists (e.g., cytosine arabinoside)
VI. Erythroleukemia

From Wintrobe, M. M., et al.: Clinical Hematology. 8th ed. Philadelphia, Lea & Febiger, 1981.

is destroyed by heat, fruits and vegetables should be eaten fresh, if possible, or with very little cooking.

SCURVY. The macrocytic anemia of scurvy may be the result of the ascorbic acid deficiency, which interferes with the conversion of folic acid to folinic acid. In such cases, ascorbic acid and folic acid therapy plus an adequate diet high in protein and ascorbic acid are indicated. Not all anemia in scurvy is true macrocytic anemia requiring folic acid therapy. Some scorbutic anemia will respond to ascorbic acid therapy alone, while some may be the result of iron deficiency. The normal adequate diet with increased amounts of protein of high biological value will carry the necessary vitamins, unless there is also evidence of vitamin deficiency.

PERNICIOUS AND OTHER MACROCYTIC ANEMIAS

Etiology. Macrocytic megaloblastic anemia due to vitamin B_{12} deficiency is only rarely caused by inadequate B_{12} intake. One example is the strict vegetarian who has no intake of vitamin B_{12} because B_{12} is found only in foods of animal origin or in plants contaminated by microorganisms which synthesize vitamin B_{12}. Other causes are shown in Table 29–5.

A more common cause of B_{12} deficiency is pernicious anemia. *Pernicious anemia* is attributed to a deficiency of vitamin B_{12} due to the lack of the *intrinsic factor* (IF), a glycoprotein in the gastric juice, which is necessary for absorption of this vitamin from food. Since B_{12} is involved in DNA synthesis, its lack results in defective synthesis and defective maturation of red blood cells. Although the disease was formerly considered fatal, it can now be treated successfully and controlled.

The most popular method for testing B_{12} absorption is the *Schilling urinary excretion test.* After an oral dose of radioactive B_{12} is given, excretion of B_{12} will be low in patients with pernicious anemia, because the B_{12} was not absorbed. When the same test is repeated with IF also given orally, the urinary excretion becomes almost normal, because the B_{12} is absorbed. A deficiency of vitamin B_{12} due to factors other than pernicious anemia, such as defective bile metabolism due to a malabsorption syndrome, will be reflected in decreased urinary excretion of B_{12} in the Schilling test that will remain unchanged upon administration of IF.

Clinical Findings. Pernicious anemia affects not only the blood but the gastrointestinal tract and the peripheral and central nervous systems as well. The symptoms are paresthesia, especially numbness and tingling in the hands and feet, diminution of senses of vibration and position,

Table 29–6. CLINICAL PICTURE OF THE MEGALOBLASTIC ANEMIAS*

SYMPTOMS

Weakness, tiredness
Dyspnea
Sore tongue
Paresthesia (B_{12} deficiency only)
Diarrhea (especially folate deficiency)
Constipation (especially B_{12} deficiency)
Irritability and forgetfulness (especially folate deficiency)
Anorexia
Syncope
Headache
Palpitation

SIGNS

Megaloblastic bone marrow (orthochromatic megaloblasts, giant metamyelocytes)
Anemia, leukopenia, thrombocytopenia, with macroovalocytes (normal MVC = 87 ± 5 cu. μ) and "hypersegmented polys" (normal Arneth count 2 lobes = 20 to 40 per cent, 3 lobes = 40 to 50 per cent, 4 lobes = 15 to 25 per cent, 5 lobes = 0 to 5 per cent, 6 lobes = 0 to 0.1 per cent, more than 6 lobes = 0) (normal "lobe average" = 3.17 ± 0.25). (Rule of fives: When 100 neutrophils counted, the presence of 5 or more with 5 or more lobes means hypersegmentation.)
Morphological red herrings: congenital hypersegmentation (approximately 1 per cent of population), hypersegmentation with renal disease; twinning deformities; macrocytes of pyruvate kinase deficiency, aplastic anemia, reticulocytosis, hypothyroidism, neoplasia.
Fever
Icterus plus pallor (lemon-yellow skin)
Glossitis
    Acute
    Chronic atrophic
Neurologic damage (only proven in B_{12} deficiency, which damages myelin)
    Vibration sense diminished
    Position sense diminished, ataxia, "combined systems disease"
    Impaired mentation, paranoid ideation (seen in both deficiencies)
Malabsorption
Achylia gastrica (primary with B_{12} deficiency, secondary with folate deficiency) (reduced intrinsic factor)
Splenomegaly (in approximately one third of cases, if looked for radiologically)
Weight loss (especially folate deficiency)
Pigmentation; vitiligo
Postural hypotension (especially B_{12} deficiency)
Low serum vitamin B_{12} or folate level
Elevated serum lactic dehydrogenase (LDH)
Elevated urine formiminoglutamate
Methylmalonic aciduria (B_{12} deficiency only)
High serum iron, increased saturation of iron-binding capacity of serum, increased bone marrow iron stores, normal free erythrocyte protoporphyrin
Low red cell folate is present in either deficiency
Circulating antibody to intrinsic factor in two-thirds of pernicious anemia patients
Circulating antibody to gastric parietal cells in most patients with gastric damage, regardless of cause
Abnormal "dU suppression test"
Abnormal liver function tests
Subnormal intestinal absorption
Low red cell B_{12} or folate level; low lymphocyte B_{12} or folate

* From Herbert, V., Colman, N., and Jacob, E.: Folic acid and vitamin B_{12}. In Goodhart, R. S., and Shils, M. E.: Modern Nutrition in Health and Disease. 6th ed. Philadelphia, Lea & Febiger, 1980, p. 252.

poor muscular coordination, poor memory and hallucinations. This B_{12} neuropathy is due to inadequate myelinization of the nerves. If it continues long enough it may be irreversible, even with treatment.

Vitamin B_{12} deficiency has been reported to impair the microbicidal activity of leukocytes, the cells involved in phagocytosis. The function of leukocytes in folic acid–deficient individuals is not impaired. Therefore, B_{12} appears to play a specific role separate from that of folic acid in the production of the intermediates necessary for normal cell metabolism and function.[14]

Methylfolate Trap. Deficiency of vitamin B_{12} can result in a deficiency of folic acid by causing the entrapment of folate as 5-methyltetrahydrofolate as shown in Figure 29–3. The lack of B_{12} means that methyltetrahydrofolate is unable to release its methyl group and become tetrahydrofolate (THFA), the optimal substrate for folate polyglutamate synthesis in the cell. The cells are thus deprived of tetrahydrofolate, and other folate coenzymes cannot be synthesized. Hence, a folic acid deficiency results.

Treatment. In 1926 Minot and Murphy[18] reported the effectiveness of liver therapy in per-

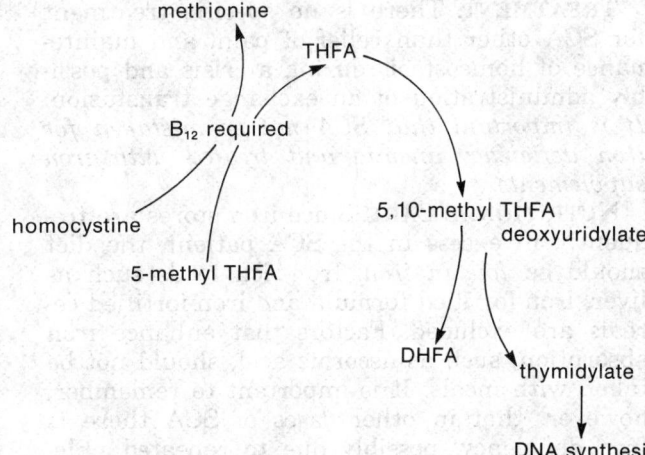

Figure 29–3. Methylfolate trap. Deficiency of vitamin B_{12} can result in a deficiency of folic acid because folate is trapped in the form of 5-methyltetrahydrofolate (5-methyl THFA), which cannot be converted to tetrahydrofolate (THFA) by the vitamin B_{12}–dependent pathway.

nicious anemia. Soon after, active concentrates of liver suitable for clinical use were developed, and by 1936 relatively purified extracts of liver were available for intramuscular injection, in addition to those preparations that had been developed earlier for oral administration. Since preparations of liver extract contain hematopoietic materials other than B_{12} (i.e., folic acid, folinic acid), they constitute shotgun therapy and should not be used and are no longer available for injection. Far more appropriate is administration of B_{12} itself either orally or parenterally. Today, treatment usually consists of intramuscular or subcutaneous injections of 1 μg. vitamin B_{12} daily for one week. After response, the frequency of injection is reduced until remission can be maintained with monthly injections. Oral doses of B_{12} without intrinsic factor may also be effective in very large doses, because about 1 per cent of B_{12} is absorbed by diffusion without the presence of IF.

When vitamin B_{12} deficiency is complicated by debilitating illness such as infection, hepatic disease, uremia, coma, severe disorientation or marked neurological damage, initial dosages should be higher—30 μg. given parenterally for 5 to 10 days.

Response is evidenced by improved appetite, alertness and cooperativeness followed by improved hematological results, as seen by marked reticulocytosis. Neurological improvement may take six months or more. The shorter the duration of the B_{12} deficiency, the greater the neurological response. Neurological manifestations of B_{12} deficiency that have been present less than three months before treatment are usually reversible.

Nutritional Care. A well-balanced diet, with increased amounts of protein, iron and vitamins, is advised for pernicious anemia in addition to vitamin B_{12} administration. The high-protein diet (1.5 gm. of protein per kg. of body weight) is desirable both for liver function and blood regeneration. Since the green leafy vegetables contain both iron and folic acid, the diet should contain increased amounts of these necessary components. Liver should be included frequently because it carries a good supply of iron, vitamin B_{12}, folic acid and other important nutrients. Meats (especially beef and pork), eggs, milk and milk products are particularly rich in vitamin B_{12}. (See Table 10–6.) Diarrhea may also be present and will have to be treated as discussed in Chapter 23. Also refer to Appendix Table 7 and the material on folic acid and vitamin B_{12} in Chapter 6.

SICKLE CELL ANEMIA

Sickle cell anemia (SCA) is an inherited hemolytic anemia in which the hemoglobin is defective and the erythrocytes are sickle-shaped. It occurs most frequently in populations that can trace their origins to areas of endemic malaria (such as the black population), and it manifests itself clinically in persons homozygous for the gene. It is usually diagnosed toward the end of the first year of life and has degrees of severity that depend upon the amount of abnormal hemoglobin and the number of erythrocytes with the characteristic odd shape.

CLINICAL FINDINGS. In addition to the usual symptoms of anemia, sickle cell anemia is characterized by "crises." These are painful occlusions of the small blood vessels due to the abnormal shape of the erythrocytes. The occlusions frequently occur in the abdomen, causing acute, severe abdominal pain. The hemolytic anemia and vaso-occlusive disease result in impairment of liver function, hepatitis, jaundice, gallstones and deteriorating renal function. Growth slows to below normal. Because of the constant hemolysis of erythrocytes and release of iron, iron stores in the liver are increased.

TREATMENT. There is no specific treatment for SCA other than relief of pain, and maintenance of homeostasis during a crisis and possibly administration of an exchange transfusion. *It is important that SCA not be mistaken for iron deficiency anemia and treated with iron supplements.*

NUTRITIONAL CARE. Since iron stores are frequently in excess in the SCA patient, the diet should be *low in iron*. Iron-rich foods such as liver, iron-fortified formula and iron-fortified cereals are excluded. Factors that enhance iron absorption, such as ascorbic acid, should not be taken with meals. It is important to remember, however, that in other cases of SCA there is iron deficiency, possibly due to repeated phlebotomies, hematuria due to renal papillary necrosis or other unknown mechanisms.[22]

The diet should be *high in folate* (400 to 600 μg.) because the increased production of erythrocytes needed to replace the cells being continuously destroyed also increases the body's folic acid requirements. Administration of folate supplements (250 μg. per day) is also recommended.[30]

The symptoms of sickle cell disease, such as delayed onset of puberty and hypogonadism in males, low body weight, rough skin and poor appetite, are similar to those seen in people with zinc deficiency. Prasad and colleagues examined 36 men and women with SCA and found significantly decreased levels of *zinc* in erythrocytes, plasma and hair as compared with normal subjects. They also found an increased urinary excretion of zinc. They postulate that the decreased zinc nutriture could be due to the hemolysis of erythrocytes, which contain zinc, and to the resulting hyperzincuria. When a dose of 660 mg. of zinc sulfate (more than 20 times the RDA for zinc) was given daily to these patients, the young men grew and developed sexually, all but one patient gained weight and the healing of ulcers was improved.[25] It has also been shown that zinc can increase the oxygen affinity of both normal and sickle-shaped erythrocytes.[2] Thus, a *deficiency of zinc* in SCA patients may intensify the anemia of sickle cell disease.

Zinc supplementation appears to be beneficial in the management of sickle cell disease, but the long-term effects of such high doses are unknown. For example, since zinc competes with copper for binding sites on proteins, the use of high doses of zinc may precipitate a copper deficiency, and this possibility should be kept in mind.[26]

Some researchers have observed decreased plasma and RBC levels of *vitamin E* (alpha-tocopherol) in sickle cell anemia.[5, 20] When six patients were given 450 I.U. of alpha-tocopherol daily for 6 to 35 weeks there was a decrease of 30 to 84 per cent in the number of irreversibly sickled cells (ISC), and plasma tocopherol levels rose to normal levels in five of the six patients.[21] Natta postulates that since there is some evidence that formation of ISC is related to changes in the erythrocyte membrane rather than hemoglobin structure, vitamin E may have a protective effect against sickling by stabilizing the erythrocyte membrane against oxidative stress.[21] Whether this effect on the number of ISC can be related to the rate of hemolysis and course of the disease cannot be determined but warrants further research.

BETA–THALASSEMIA MAJOR

Beta–thalassemia major is an inherited disorder characterized by a hypochromic-microcytic anemia due to a disorder in hemoglobin synthesis. As in sickle cell anemia there also seems to be a disorder in erythrocyte membrane.[27] Supplementation with high oral doses of alpha-tocopherol caused decreased peroxidative damage and improved red cell survival after an average of 16 months of vitamin E therapy. Unfortunately, this was not associated with decreased requirement for transfusions.[28] Giardini reported better results when vitamin E was given parenterally rather than orally.[10] Obviously, the relationship of vitamin E to beta-thalassemia major needs considerably more study.

Problems and Suggested Topics for Discussion

1. Discuss the functions of hemoglobin.
2. Study the effect of iron deficiency on the metabolic processes of the body. What are the causes of iron deficiency?
3. Describe the absorption, transport and storage of iron.
4. Describe the stages of iron deficiency and the tests used to diagnose each stage.
5. Interview a patient with iron deficiency anemia. How much absorbable iron does she presently have in her diet? How could she increase the amount?
6. Obtain a dietary history from a person with pernicious anemia or from a postgastrectomy patient. What would you recommend for nutritional care?
7. What role does vitamin B$_{12}$ play in the treatment of pernicious anemia? How does the treatment of pernicious anemia differ from that of folic acid deficiency anemia?

Cited References

1. Bothwell, T.H., et al.: Iron Metabolism in Man. Oxford, Blackwell, 1979.
2. Brewer, G., and Oelshlegal, F.J., Jr.: Antisickling effects of zinc. Biochem. Biophys. Res. Commun., *58*:854, 1974.
3. Chandra, R.K.: Iron and immunocompetence. Nutr. Rev., *34*:129, 1976.
4. Chandra, R.K., and Saraya, A.K.: Impaired immunocompetence associated with iron deficiency. J. Pediatr., *86*:899, 1975.

5. Chiu, D., and Lubin, B.: Abnormal vitamin E and glutathione peroxidase levels in sickle cell anemia: evidence for increased susceptibility to lipid peroxidation. J. Lab. Clin. Med., 94:542, 1979.

6. Cook, J.D., and Finch, C.A.: Assessing iron status of a population. Am. J. Clin. Nutr., 32:2115, 1979.

7. Cook, J.D., and Monsen, E.R.: Food iron absorption in human subjects. III. Comparison of the effect of animal proteins on non-heme iron absorption. Am. J. Clin. Nutr., 29:859, 1976.

8. Cook, J.D., and Monsen, E.R.: Vitamin C, the common cold, and iron absorption in man. Am. J. Clin. Nutr., 30:235, 1977.

9. Elwood, P.C.: Evaluation of the clinical importance of anemia. Am. J. Clin. Nutr., 26:958, 1973.

10. Giardini, O., Cantani, A., and Donfrancesco, A.: Vitamin therapy in homozygous β-thalassemia. N. Engl. J. Med., 305:644, 1981.

11. Greenblatt, D.J., Allen, M.D., and Koch-Weser, J.: Accidental iron poisoning in children. Clin. Pediatr., 15:835, 1976.

12. Hallberg, L., Norrby, A., and Sölvell, L.: Oral iron with succinic acid in the treatment of iron deficiency anaemia. Scand. J. Haematol., 8:104, 1971.

13. Hallberg, L., et al.: Menstrual blood loss—a population study. Variation at different ages and attempts to define normality. Acta. Obstet. Gynecol. Scand., 45:320, 1966.

14. Kaplan, S.K., and Basford, R.E.: Effect of vitamin B_{12} and folic acid deficiencies on neutrophil function. Blood, 47:801, 1976.

15. Kerr, D.N.S., and Davidson, S.: Gastrointestinal intolerance to oral iron preparations. Lancet, 2:489, 1958.

16. Kulapongs, P., et al.: Cell mediated immunity and phagocytosis and killing function in children with severe iron-deficiency anemia. Lancet, 2:689, 1974.

17. Macdougall, L.G., et al.: The immune response in iron-deficient children: impaired cellular defense mechanisms with altered humoral components. J. Pediatr., 86:833, 1975.

18. Minot, G.R., and Murphy, W.P.: Treatment of pernicious anemia by special diet. JAMA, 87:470, 1926.

19. Monsen, E.R., et al.: Estimation of available dietary iron. Am. J. Clin. Nutr., 31:134, 1978.

20. Natta, C., and Machlin, L.: Plasma levels of tocopherol in sickle cell anemia subjects. Am. J. Clin. Nutr., 32:1359, 1979.

21. Natta, C.L., Machlin, L.J., and Brin, M.: A decrease in irreversibly sickled erythrocytes in sickle cell anemia patients given vitamin E. Am. J. Clin. Nutr., 33:968, 1980.

22. Natta, C., et al.: Sickle cell anemia and iron deficiency. JAMA, 247:1442, 1982.

23. Nutritional Anaemias. Report of a World Health Organization Scientific Group, World Health Technical Report Series, No. 405, 1968.

24. Pollitt, E., and Leibel, R.L.: Iron deficiency and behavior. J. Pediatr., 88:372, 1976.

25. Prasad, A.S., et al.: Zinc deficiency in sickle cell disease. Clin. Chem., 21:582, 1975.

26. Prasad, A.S., et al.: Trace elements in sickle cell disease. JAMA, 235:2396, 1976.

27. Rachmilewitz, E.A., Lubin, B.H., and Shobet, S.B.: Lipid membrane peroxidation in β-thalassemia major. Blood, 47:495, 1976.

28. Rachmilewitz, E.A., Shifter, A., and Kahane, I.: Vitamin E deficiency in β-thalassemia major: changes in hematological and biochemical parameters after a therapeutic trial with α-tocopherol. Am. J. Clin. Nutr., 32:1850, 1979.

29. Rossander, L., Hallberg, L., and Björn-Rasmussen, E.: Absorption of iron from breakfast meals. Am. J. Clin. Nutr., 32:2484, 1979.

30. Trubowitz, S.: The management of sickle cell anemia. Med. Clin. North Am., 60:933, 1976.

Additional References

Control of Nutritional Anemia with Special Reference to Iron Deficiency. WHO Technical Report Series No. 580, Geneva, WHO, 1975.

Dallkman, P.R.: Iron deficiency: diagnosis and treatment. West. J. Med., 134:496, 1981.

Herbert, V.: Folic acid and vitamin B_{12}. In Goodhart, R.S., and Shils, M.E. (eds.): Modern Nutrition in Health and Disease. 6th ed. Philadelphia, Lea & Febiger, 1980.

International Nutritional Anemia Consultative Group (INACG): Iron deficiency in women. Washington, D.C., The Nutrition Foundation, 1981.

International Nutritional Anemia Consultative Group (INACG): The effects of cereals and legumes on iron availability. Washington, D.C., The Nutrition Foundation, 1982.

Lukens, J.N.: Iron deficiency and infection. Am. J. Dis. Child., 129:160, 1975.

Monsen, E.R., and Balintfy, J.L.: Calculating dietary iron bioavailability: refinement and computerization. J. Am. Diet. Assoc., 80:307, 1982.

Moore, C.V.: Iron and hypochromic anemia. Prog. Food Nutr., 1:245, 1975.

Morck, T.A., Lynch, S.R., and Cook, J.D.: Reduction of the soy-induced inhibition of non-heme iron. Am. J. Clin. Nutr., 36:219, 1982.

Nutritional Anemias. WHO Technical Report Series No. 503, Geneva, WHO, 1972.

Review: Zinc deficiency in sickle cell disease. Nutr. Rev., 33:266, 1975.

Serjeant, G.R., Galloway, R.E., and Gueri, M.C.: Oral zinc sulfate in sickle cell ulcers. Lancet, 2:891, 1970.

Wintrobe, M.M., et al.: Clinical Hematology. 8th ed. Philadelphia, Lea & Febiger, 1981.

UNIT 10

RENAL DISEASE

CHAPTER 30

Nutritional Care in Diseases of the Kidney

Revised by
KATY G. WILKENS, R.D.

Physiology and Function of Normal Kidneys

The kidneys maintain the chemical homeostasis of all body fluids. Their chief functions are to regulate and conserve nutrients and water and to excrete waste products. Blood entering the kidneys reaches the arterioles and enters the nephrons. Approximately 1.2 liters of whole blood pass through the kidneys each minute, about one fourth of the total cardiac output.

Each nephron is composed of a *glomerulus* surrounded by a membrane (Bowman's capsule) and the *tubule* (which includes the proximal convoluted tubule, Henle's loop and the distal tubule) as shown in Figure 30–1. Blood is supplied through the capillaries. Approximately one fifth of the water from plasma is filtered through the nephron, forming a glomerular filtrate of fluid, electrolytes and low-molecular-weight proteins and carbohydrates. At various points along the tubules, certain elements are selectively reabsorbed or secreted. A number of factors influence the selection of elements to be reabsorbed. The final fluid leaving the nephron is water that contains a high concentration of waste metabolites. The reabsorbed essential elements are returned to the blood.

Ultimately, the waste products proceed into large channels and finally arrive in the funnel-shaped central edge of the area known as the renal pelvis. Now the waste products are ready to be sent to the bladder for accumulation and then elimination as urine.

Water makes up the greatest percentage of the waste products. The quantity is related to the amount taken into the body and the amount excreted through the skin and lungs in the process of temperature regulation, but normally it averages 1 to 2 liters daily. Urine usually consists of approximately 95 per cent water and 5 per cent solutes.

Water reabsorption from the distal tubules and collecting ducts is controlled by the small peptide hormone *vasopressin,* or *antidiuretic hormone (ADH),* which is made by the cells of the hypothalamus and stored in the pituitary. When there is a fall in the body water content or the total blood volume, the hypothalamus stimulates the secretion of ADH, which increases the reabsorption of water. The hormone is not released when the body water or blood volume is high and thus allows diuresis to take place.

A minimum urinary volume of approximately 600 ml. (obligatory fluid) is required for the excretion of the average load of solids. A greater volume is required for the excretion of an increased load.

About 60 per cent of the solute load is nitrogenous wastes, and inorganic salts make up the other 40 per cent. Of the *nitrogenous wastes,* urea predominates; uric acid, creatinine and ammonia are present in small amounts. The amount of urea present depends upon the diet. A high protein intake increases the urea output. A lower consumption of protein decreases the urea content. If these normal waste products

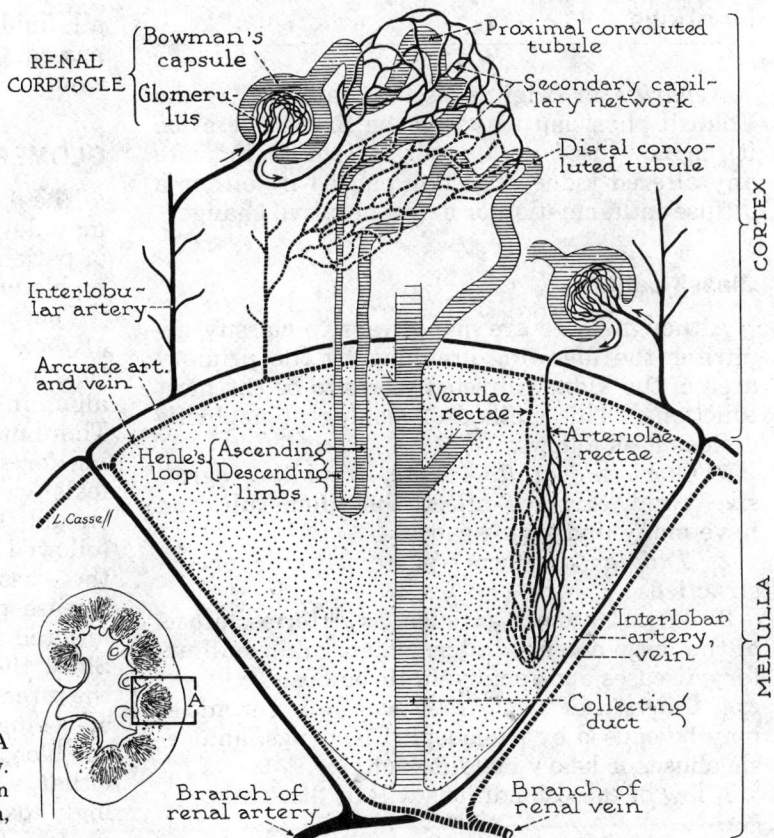

Figure 30–1. Diagram of a nephron. Inset A shows the location of the nephron in the kidney. (From King, B. G., and showers, M. J.: Human Anatomy and Physiology. 6th ed. Philadelphia, W. B. Saunders Company, 1969.)

are not eliminated appropriately, they collect in abnormal quantities in the blood.

Of the *inorganic salts,* sodium chloride predominates; phosphate and sulfate salts of calcium, sodium, potassium and magnesium are present in small amounts. In the balance of minerals, some sodium is reabsorbed from the distal tubules and is exchanged for potassium or hydrogen ion (H+).

Through this process of waste elimination, the kidney maintains a chemical homeostasis in the body, balances the amounts of body fluids, and maintains the normal pH of body fluids, thus keeping an acid-base balance. In addition, the kidney performs some non-excretory functions:

1. Through the *renin-angiotensin* mechanism the kidney exerts one of the controls on blood pressure. Cells of the glomerulus (known as the juxtaglomerular apparatus) react to decreased blood volume and secrete renin, a proteolytic enzyme. Renin acts in the plasma to form angiotensin I, which is converted to angiotensin II, a powerful vasoconstrictor and a potent stimulus of aldosterone secretion by the adrenal gland, as discussed on page 559. Thus aldosterone is secreted, sodium is reabsorbed, and blood pressure is returned to normal.

2. The kidney produces *erythropoietin,* which is a critical determinant of erythroid activity in the bone marrow. A deficiency of erythropoietin is a factor in the severe anemia present in chronic renal disease.

3. The kidney maintains *calcium-phosphorus-bone homeostasis* and equilibrium by making the active form of vitamin D_3, 1,25-$(OH)_2$ D_3, which is needed for regulation and maintenance of the system. For this reason, osteodystrophy is a common, complex and usually inevitable outcome of renal disease. This will be discussed later in the chapter.

Diseases of the Kidney

Diseases of the kidney, whether acute or chronic, have many causes. The origin of the disease and the structures in the kidney affected will determine the effects and subsequently the treatment. Depending on the type, kidney diseases may produce (1) nephrotic syndrome, with significant protein loss, (2) decreased overall renal function, in which the remaining nephrons cannot handle the metabolic load, or (3) a combination of the two. Objectives of nutritional care will depend on the abnormality to be treated.

Nephritis

Nephritis, or Bright's disease (named after the English physician who was the first to describe it), is now used as a general term to indicate any altered kidney function caused by either a diffuse inflammation or a degenerative change.

Classification

Although there are many ways to classify nephritis, the following grouping by the primary area of the kidney affected seems to be the most functional. This method of looking at nephritis divides it as follows:

1. *Glomerulopathies*—acute, "rapidly progressive" and chronic—affect the glomeruli and have many underlying causes.

2. *Tubular disorders*—acute, chronic or obstructive.

3. *Vascular diseases,* such as arteriosclerosis of the large arteries, intermediate and small artery diseases and renal vein thrombosis.

4. *Interstitial nephritis*—acute or chronic—may be caused by pyelonephritis, drugs, analgesic abuse, or heavy metal toxicity.

A few of these conditions will be discussed.

GLOMERULONEPHRITIS (ACUTE)

Etiology and Characteristics

Acute glomerulonephritis is characterized by inflammation of the capillary loops in the glomeruli of the kidney, with varying degrees of hematuria, edema, hypertension and nitrogen retention *(azotemia)*. A decreased amount of urine is excreted *(oliguria)* and it is dilute since the kidney loses its concentrating ability. Red blood cells appear in the urine. Anorexia and lethargy are present; nausea and vomiting are usual. Edema of the soft tissues may be either minimal or massive.

The disorder occurs most frequently in children and young adults and is often a sequel to a *streptococcal* infection.

Objectives and Principles of Nutritional Care

The treatment of acute glomerulonephritis attempts to maintain good nutritional status while allowing time for the disease to resolve spontaneously. There is no reason to restrict protein or potassium intake unless significant uremia or hyperkalemia develops. Sodium is restricted to 22 to 33 mEq. daily if there is extracellular volume excess (edema), and this is continued until there is no evidence of congestion or edema. When diuresis occurs, it is important to replace all fluid lost. The sodium-retaining phase has passed; thus, sodium restriction is no longer necessary.

GLOMERULONEPHRITIS (CHRONIC)

The "rapidly progressive" form of nephritis may develop into a chronic form. The majority of patients with chronic glomerulonephritis give no history of having had the acute condition.

The patient may be symptomless, but he usually exeriences headaches and frequent urination during the night. Variable amounts of albumin and casts are present in the urine. There may be a "slowly progressive" period lasting for several years, during which the patient feels well. In this period optimum nutrition should be maintained. This period may be followed by a nephrotic stage, depending upon the disease causing the kidney problem. As the disease progresses, hypertension, proteinuria, a lowered serum protein level and edema develop. Since the kidneys are unable to excrete all of the urea and the other metabolic wastes that are being formed, these products are retained in the blood. Eventually, uremic symptoms such as lethargy and anorexia result from the increasingly toxic levels of waste products.

Objectives and Principles of Nutritional Care

The primary objectives of nutritional care are (1) to minimize the production of urea and metabolic waste products, (2) to restore good nutritional status, replace protein lost in urine and return serum protein to normal levels by providing adequate protein and energy, (3) to prevent edema and control hypertension and (4) to maintain potassium balance. Depending upon the stage of the disease, nutritional care is the same as that for nephrotic syndrome or chronic renal failure.

Nephrotic Syndrome (Nephrosis)

Nephrotic syndrome is a term used to designate a variety of pathological conditions characterized by edema, proteinuria, hypoalbuminemia and, usually, hypercholesterolemia. Hypertension may also occur, depending on the diseased state of the kidney. There is an *increased capillary permeability* in the glomeruli and probably throughout the body. Its effect on the kidney is such that there is *massive proteinuria* (3 gm. per 24 hours or greater), which leads to the other symptoms of nephrotic syndrome. Clinically, the kidneys are usually able to function adequately in the excretion of urea and other metabolic waste products, but the severe loss of protein from the plasma continues. Sometimes the protein deficit is so great that tissue wastage and malnutrition result, and plasma albumin concentrations of less than 1 gm. per 100 ml. are common. The reduced serum albumin level causes a transudation of fluid from the circulating blood into the surrounding tissue, resulting in edema and decreased blood volume. The decreased volume, in turn, causes an increased reabsorption of sodium.

Objectives and Principles of Nutritional Care

The primary objective of the diet treatment in nephrotic syndrome is to replace the albumin and other protein that is lost from the plasma into the urine. Patients with a severe protein deficiency already established who have a continued protein loss may require months of carefully supervised nutritional care.

The diet should provide sufficient protein and calories to maintain a positive nitrogen balance, with an increase in the plasma albumin concentration and the disappearance of edema. Thus the diet should be designed to provide 1.5 gm. protein per kg. body weight per day and to replace the protein lost in the urine in a 24-hour period. There are rare times when the amount of protein in the urine is greater than the maximum daily plasma albumin regeneration, and in such cases it becomes virtually impossible to make up the protein deficit.

Eighty per cent of the protein should be from sources of high biological value to allow for optimal use of the protein. Fuel sources should be provided to prevent utilization of protein for energy. Therefore, energy intake should be from 35 to 50 kcal. per kg. body weight per day for adults. Energy intake for children should be 100 to 150 kcal. per kg.

Because of the tubular reabsorption mentioned previously, it is essential to restrict sodium in the diet. The level of intake can be established by measuring the patient's 24-hour output and merely replacing the daily loss. The amount may vary from 40 to 90 mEq. per day. Table 30-1 gives a high-protein, sodium-restricted diet for nephrotic syndrome. Sodium restriction is discussed further in Chapter 28. In addition, the patient may be given diuretics, including aldosterone antagonists, fluid expanders, such as albumin, and steroids.

There is little evidence to suggest that dietary control of cholesterol and fat alters the patient's hyperlipidemia, since it seems to be related to the protein loss. The extent of the hypercholesterolemia and hyperlipidemia in the individual

---

Table 30-1. HIGH-PROTEIN, LOW-SODIUM DIET FOR NEPHROTIC SYNDROME[a]

(Approximately 120 gm. protein, 74 mEq. [1700 mg.] sodium, 2800 kcal.)

SAMPLE MENU

Breakfast

Stewed prunes
Cooked Wheatena
Poached eggs, 2
Toasted whole-wheat bread, 1 slice
Sweet butter
Milk, 8 oz.
Coffee

Lunch

Cream of pea soup
Cold sliced roast lamb, 4 oz.
Cooked spinach
Sliced tomato salad
Whole-wheat bread, 1 slice
Sweet butter
Vanilla ice cream
Milk, 8 oz.

Dinner

Swiss steak, 4 oz.
Mashed potatoes
Baked squash
Whole-wheat bread, 1 slice
Sweet butter
Fresh fruit cup
Milk, 8 oz.

Bedtime

Eggnog

[a]This diet is prepared and served without added salt.

---

patient will determine whether fat and cholesterol modification is necessary.

PARENTERAL PROTEIN. In some circumstances, particularly in the presence of pronounced anorexia, nausea or vomiting, oral administration of protein in sufficient amounts to correct the protein deficit may not be possible. In these cases protein hydrolysates or amino acids may be given parenterally.

Uremia in Renal Failure

Uremia is a toxic condition caused by the retention of urinary constituents in the blood: urea, creatinine, uric acid, potassium, organic acids and other end-products of protein metabolism. The name indicates that urea is the waste product retained in the greatest amount. The term *azotemia* refers only to excess urea and other nitrogenous products in the blood. Uremia is a result of the severe loss of renal function that is seen in acute and chronic renal failure, and it is characterized by weakness, anorexia, nausea, vomiting, pruritus, twitching, neuropathy, mental disturbances and, in advanced cases, stupor and coma. The symptoms are not dependent on a specific level of blood urea nitrogen (BUN) but rather on how rapidly the BUN level rises and on the individual's tolerance of the chemical changes. Some patients may have severe uremic symptoms at BUN levels of 50 mg./dl., while others show few symptoms at levels greater than 100 mg./dl.

A more accurate and specific indicator of renal function is the *serum creatinine,* since BUN may be inappropriately low due to nausea and vomiting, poor intake or liver disease despite severe renal failure.

History and General Principles of Protein Nutrition in Renal Failure and Uremia

The primary problem in managing the uremia of kidney failure is to reduce the amount of nitrogenous waste that must be excreted by the kidney and yet maintain a positive nitrogen balance. Nitrogenous wastes are reduced by restricting the intake of protein enough so that there is no "extra" protein to be metabolized and no excess nitrogen to be removed. Ideally, all the protein or nitrogen will be used by the body for enzyme and hormone synthesis, muscle and tissue repair and general body maintenance. The second and more difficult phase is to provide enough protein to maintain nitrogen balance. This problem was first investigated by three Italian researchers, Giordano, Giovannetti and Maggiore, who showed that it was possible to produce positive nitrogen balance and yet reduce blood urea nitrogen levels in uremic patients. These doctors fed their patients a high-calorie diet containing 24 gm. of protein, of which at least 70 per cent was complete protein of high biological value (HBV) containing all of the essential amino acids. Protein of low biological value (LBV), which contains mostly non-esssential amino acids, was kept to a minimum. Unfortunately the diet was very unpalatable and patient compliance was poor.

Present research is seeking better methods of providing the essential amino acids in a low-protein diet. One such attempt involves supplementing the diet with the carbon skeletons of the essential amino acids (the *alpha-hydroxy* and *alpha-keto acids*). It is known that only the skeleton structure of essential amino acids is needed and that the uremic person can use the excess nitrogen in urea to form not only the non-essential amino acids but the essential ones as well. The deterrents to using this method at present are the cost, availability and palatability of the alpha-hydroxy and alpha-keto acids.

It is now accepted that *histidine* is an essential amino acid for the uremic adult; therefore, any essential amino acid supplements would need to include histidine for optimal nitrogen balance. *Arginine* has also been found to produce a more positive nitrogen balance in uremic patients, but it is not yet available in essential amino acid supplements. Methods of providing essential amino acids separate from the diet have been sought, so that dietary protein does not have to be restricted to those containing mostly essential amino acids (eggs, meat, poultry, fish and milk). If the essential amino acids are provided in liquid (Amin-Aid, McGaw Labs) or tablet form (Aminess, Cutter Labs),[14] then the diet may contain more incomplete proteins (vegetables, cereals, bread) making it more acceptable to the patient. Again, the problem is one of cost and palatability, but the future should bring improvement. Use of these products in addition to a low-protein diet might enable uremic patients to be managed with less frequent dialysis.

Adequate energy is essential in the dietary treatment of uremia to prevent oxidation of protein for energy and allow use of protein for tissue maintenance. Providing calories at the level of 35 to 55 kcal. per kg. IBW is difficult because of protein, sodium and potassium restrictions. In addition, the anorexia and nausea that occur with uremia deter the patient from consuming sufficient calories. Insuring adequate energy intake requires special attention by nurses, dietitians and nutritionists and physicians caring for patients with renal diseases.

Acute Renal Failure

Acute renal failure (ARF) is characterized by a sudden reduction in glomerular filtration rate (GFR) and an alteration in the ability of the kidney to excrete waste products and preserve the internal milieu. It is usually associated with oliguria (defined as excretion of less than 400 ml. of urine in 24 hours). Its duration varies from a few days to several weeks, and it may develop in previously healthy kidneys from a number of causes. These causes are usually divided into three categories: (1) inadequate renal perfusion (pre-renal), (2) diseases within the renal parenchyma (intrinsic) and (3) obstruction (post-renal), as shown in Table 30–2.

Acute renal failure has two distinct phases. The first is the *oliguric phase,* during which extensive catabolism and tissue destruction take place. Hemodialysis is used to reduce the acido-

Table 30–2. SOME CAUSES OF ACUTE RENAL FAILURE

Pre-renal

Severe dehydration
Circulatory collapse

Intrinsic

Acute tubular necrosis
  Trauma, surgery
  Septicemia
Nephrotoxicity
  Antibiotics, contrast agents and other drugs
Vascular disorders
  Bilateral renal infarction, etc.
Acute glomerulonephritis of any cause
  Post-streptococcal infection
  Systemic lupus erythematosus

Post-renal

Obstruction
  Benign prostatic hypertrophy
  Carcinoma of bladder or prostate
  Ureterovesical stricture

sis, correct the uremia and lower the rapidly increasing hyperkalemia.

This oliguric phase is followed by a recovery period, referred to as the *diuretic phase,* during which the urinary volume may double each day. For several days renal function remains poor, and uremia continues to be a problem, with rising BUN levels. Dialysis may still be necessary for treatment. The major concern during this period is the excessive loss of fluid, sodium and potassium. It is of utmost importance to assess extracellular volume (ECV) and potassium balance in order to provide for appropriate replacements.

Nutritional Care

Nutritional care in acute renal failure is particularly important, because the patient is suffering not only from uremia, metabolic acidosis, and fluid and electrolyte imbalance, but usually also from physiological stress (e.g., infection, tissue destruction or poisoning), which increases protein needs. The problem of balancing protein and energy needs with treatment of acidosis and excessive nitrogenous waste is a complicated and delicate one.

FLUID AND SODIUM BALANCE. The diet should be planned to help regulate the water balance and the adjustment of the various mineral salts, especially sodium and potassium. In both the oliguric and diuretic phases, fluid intake is extremely important and is regulated according to the volume of urine excreted. Intake therefore should replace the output in urine, vomitus or diarrhea, with an additional amount to account for the usual daily insensible losses

due to skin and respiratory evaporation. Table 30–3 outlines this calculation.

While the steps in calculating the fluid intake are relatively simple, fluid balance continues to be a difficult daily management problem due to the variation in the patient's status. His insensible fluid loss, for instance, may be very high because of infection and high fever. On the other hand, the patient may easily become overloaded with fluid as a result of a catabolic decrease in lean body weight and the consequently greater endogenous production of water or, more likely, because of excessive fluid intake due to medical treatment. The patient's weight and serum sodium should be measured frequently.

During the diuretic phase it is often very difficult to keep up with the patient's water and sodium excretion. The amounts lost in 24 hours must be carefully monitored, and replacements should be given to avoid hypovolemic shock. Often intravenous administration of normal saline is required.

Sodium is restricted depending on the level of urinary excretion. In the oliguric phase when the output is very low, the intake is kept as low as possible, about 20 to 40 mEq. per day depending upon the dialysis treatment.

POTASSIUM BALANCE. In ARF potassium is not excreted, and its level in serum may also rise because of tissue destruction and the movement of K^+ out of the cells. For this reason, potassium intake must be restricted as much as possible, to 30 to 50 mEq. per day. Exchange resins such as Kayexalate in sorbitol can be used to treat the high K^+ concentration but it is unpleasant. It is important to remember that this drug exchanges sodium for potassium. For every gram of Kayexalate used, 1 mEq. of K^+ is removed and 1 mEq. of Na^+ is added. This increased sodium intake could aggravate edema that is already present. Sorbitol is used because it is an unabsorbed sugar that induces diarrhea and so aids the removal of the resin and K^+

Table 30–3. SAMPLE CALCULATION OF FLUID REQUIREMENTS FOR A TYPICAL PATIENT IN ACUTE RENAL FAILURE

Measured urine output of previous 24 hr.	−200 ml.
Insensible water loss in 24 hr.	−1000 ml.
(Varies with room temperature, room humidity and body temperature)	
Water loss in vomitus	−100 ml.
Total water loss in 24 hr.	−1300 ml.
Water produced by metabolism in 24 hr.	+500 ml.
(Provided catabolism and weight loss are not occurring)	
Water requirements for 24 hr.	800 ml.
Water in usual diet in 24 hr.	500 ml.
Additional fluid intake needed in 24 hr.	300 ml.

from the body. Insulin may also be used since insulin forces the movement of potassium out of the serum and into the cell. Peritoneal dialysis or hemodialysis is used when the need to reduce the serum potassium level is urgent.

PROTEIN. At the onset of acute renal failure, when few patients can tolerate oral feedings because of vomiting and diarrhea, I.V. preparations have been used to reduce protein catabolism. Giving carbohydrate alone (for example, 100 gm. over a 24-hour period) will only reduce protein breakdown by 50 per cent. The preferred treatment is parenteral administration of essential amino acids such as Nephramine (McGaw Labs) in glucose. This will reduce protein catabolism and urea production to a minimum until the patient can tolerate oral feeding. Since aggressive treatment using dialysis can rapidly reduce uremic symptoms, this parenteral nutritional support may only be necessary for a short period of time, if at all.

At this point, regulation of the protein content of the diet is important, but authorities differ regarding the amount of protein to include. Some recommend 0.2 to 0.3 gm. protein per kg. per day,[2] but others feel that this is too low. A good method is to limit protein to the minimum of 0.5 gm. per kg. IBW per day in the beginning to reduce uremia by decreasing nitrogen metabolism and retention. Gradually the amount is increased as the kidneys show signs of improvement and the GFR returns to normal. The protein intake eventually reaches the RDA of 0.8 gm. per kg. IBW per day or even higher if there has been much tissue wasting.

Reducing protein intake to 0.6 gm. per kg. per day means that a 70-kg. man will eat only 42 gm. of protein per day. Eighty per cent, or 34 gm., should be HBV protein, which means that the diet should include 5 oz. of meat, fish or poultry or 1 egg, 3 oz. of meat, fish or poultry and 1 cup of milk. Consequently, this allows only 8 gm. of protein to be obtained from other protein-containing foods in a diet—breads, cereals, vegetables and fruits. Exchange lists such as those given in Table 30–8 may be used to aid in the planning of the diet.

ENERGY. Energy needs are high (approximately 50 kcal. per kg. IBW per day) in order to provide positive nitrogen balance under stress situations. Alternative fuel sources that will prevent the use of protein for energy production must come from a high intake of carbohydrate and fat. In addition to the usual dietary sources of refined sweets and fats, special high-calorie, low-protein and low-electrolyte formulas have been developed to add to the diet. Borst was the first to develop such a product when he concocted the butterball (butter and sugar).[5] Some of the modern products are Controlyte

Table 30–4. NUTRITIONAL CARE DURING ACUTE RENAL FAILURE

NUTRIENT	AMOUNT
Protein	0.5 gm./kg. IBW, increasing as GFR returns to normal. 80% should be HBV protein.
Energy	40–55 kcal./kg. body weight.
Potassium	20–50 mEq./day in oliguric phase (depending on urinary output, dialysis and serum K^+ level); replace losses in diuretic phase.
Sodium	20–40 mEq./day in oliguric phase (depending on urinary output, edema, dialysis and serum Na^+ level); replace losses in diuretic phase.
Fluid	Replace output from the previous day plus 750 ml.

(Doyle), Polycose (Ross), Cal-Power (General Mills) and Hycal (Beecham) (see Table 35–8). The liquid products contain 70 to 85 kcal. per oz., and the powders contain approximately 140 kcal. per oz. Special recipes that are low in protein and electrolytes and extremely high in calories have been developed and several cookbooks are listed at the end of this chapter. Table 30–4 summarizes nutritional care during acute renal failure.

Chronic Renal Failure

Renal disease can progress relentlessly until chronic renal failure develops and finally uremia appears. As illustrated in Figure 30–2, a person may lose almost 85 per cent of renal function before experiencing symptoms of uremia and renal failure. Frequently, by the time the person sees a physician or the diagnosis has been made, disease has been raging in the kidneys for years. With chronic renal failure comes a myriad of problems related to the kidney's inability to excrete waste products, reabsorb nutrients, maintain fluid and electrolyte balance, produce hormones and perform other metabolic functions. As the failure grows more severe and as more nephrons die, the kidney can no longer compensate for their loss, and symptoms become apparent.

Medical Treatment

Treatment of chronic renal failure requires one of two therapies, either transplantation or dialysis.

TRANSPLANTATION. Transplantation involves the surgical implantation of a kidney from a living related donor or a cadaver. The recipient's rejection of the foreign tissue is a major compli-

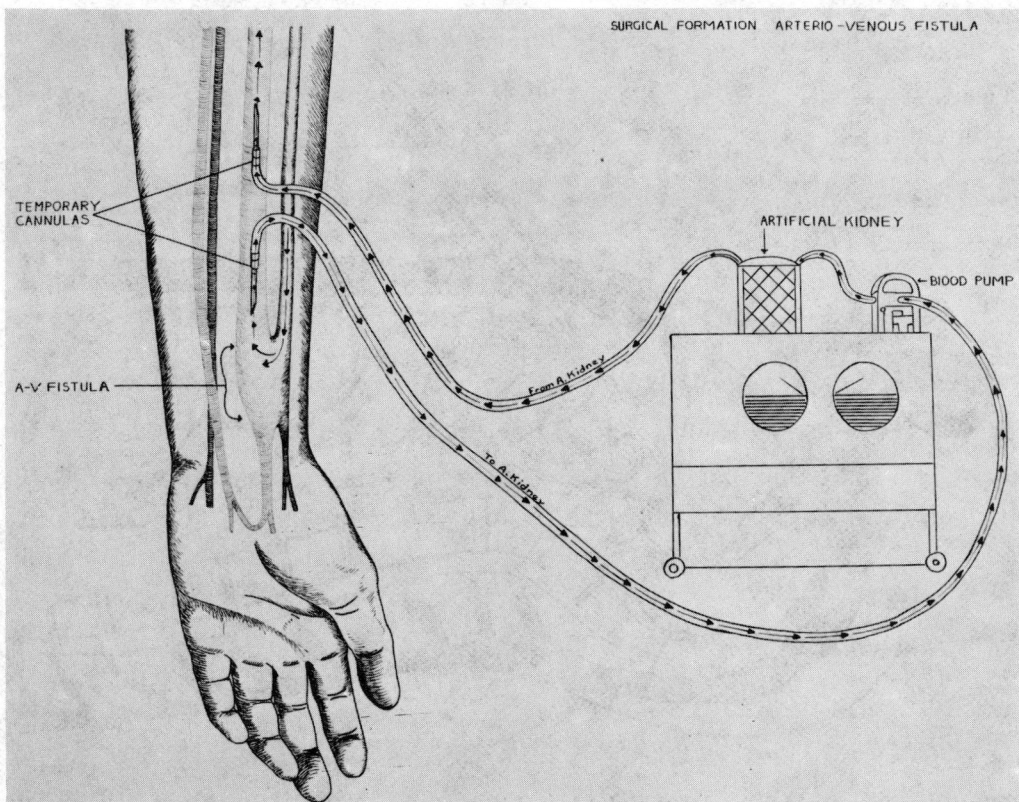

Figure 30–2. Arteriovenous fistula with temporary cannulas in place and blood circulating to and from the artificial kidney. Arrows show the direction of blood flow. (Photograph courtesy of Northwest Kidney Center, Seattle, Washington.)

cation of transplantation. Immunosuppressive therapy, such as corticosteroids, is used to decrease the immune response. To limit problems of rejection, tissue typing to determine histocompatibility antigens is done before transplantation. Currently there are far more patients awaiting transplantation than there are donated kidneys.

DIALYSIS. Dialysis can be done by two methods, hemodialysis or peritoneal dialysis. The most common method is hemodialysis, in which blood passes by the semipermeable membrane of the artificial kidney and waste products are removed by diffusion.

Hemodialysis. Hemodialysis requires a permanent access to the blood stream through a fistula created by surgery to connect an artery and a vein. Often fistulas are made near the wrist, causing the forearm veins to become greatly enlarged. Large needles are inserted into the fistula prior to each dialysis and then removed after dialysis.

The dialysis fluid is similar to that of normal plasma. Waste products and electrolytes move by osmosis from the blood into the dialysate and are removed. Hemodialysis usually requires 4 to 6 hours three times per week. Dietary protein needs are about 1 gm./kg. to make up for some losses through dialysate.

Peritoneal Dialysis. The second type of dialysis, peritoneal dialysis, takes place using the semipermeable membrane of the patient's peritoneum. A tube, or catheter, is surgically implanted in the abdomen and into the peritoneal cavity, as shown in Figure 30–3. Dialysate containing a high dextrose concentration is instilled into the peritoneum, where diffusion carries waste products from the blood through the peritoneal membrane and into the dialysate. This fluid is then withdrawn and discarded and new solution added.

Peritoneal dialysis is a less efficient method of removing waste products from the blood, so treatments usually last longer than hemodialysis, about 10 to 12 hours per day, three times per week. Peritoneal dialysis patients have higher protein needs than do hemodialysis patients, about 1.2 to 1.5 gm. of protein per kg. because of greater protein losses from peritoneal dialysis.

Continuous ambulatory peritoneal dialysis (CAPD) is similar to peritoneal dialysis, except that the dialysate is left in the peritoneum and exchanged manually so that no machine is required. Exchanges of dialysis fluid are done four to five times daily, making it a 24-hour treatment. Protein losses are similar to those from regular peritoneal dialysis.

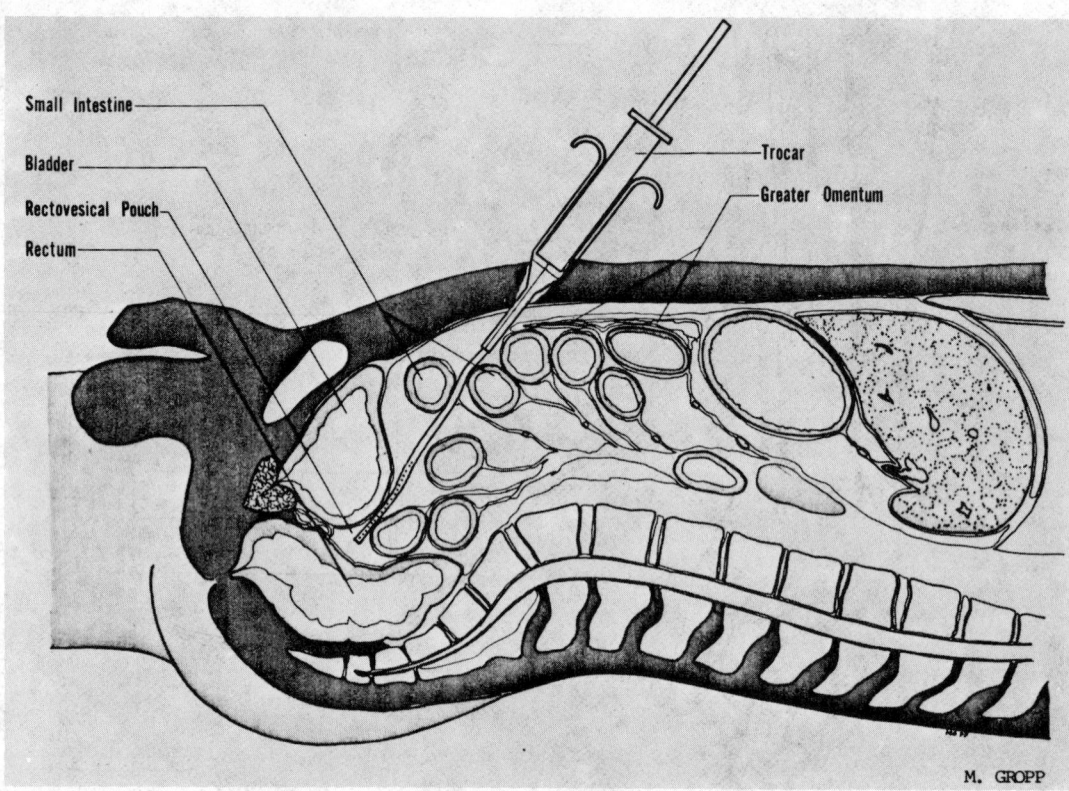

Small Intestine

Bladder

Rectovesical Pouch

Rectum

Trocar

Greater Omentum

M. GROPP

Figure 30–3. Catheter position for peritoneal dialysis. (Adapted from Shapter, R. K., and Yonkman, F. K.: The Kidneys, ureters and urinary bladder. CIBA, 1973.)

CAPD patients are on more liberal fluid, sodium and potassium restrictions since the therapy is continuous and more of these products are removed. The loss of sodium can be as much as 6 gm. per day, so these patients may need high sodium intakes as shown in Table 30–5. Complications associated with CAPD include peritonitis, hypotension requiring additional fluid and sodium replacement, and tissue weight gain. The weight gain is experienced by most CAPD patients because they absorb and metabolize about 600 to 800 calories from the glucose dialysate per day. These extra calories can quickly lead to tissue gain if the patient maintains his normal energy intake. This may be desirable for some period of time in patients who are underweight, but eventually dietary caloric intake may have to be modified to account for calories absorbed from dialysate.

Psychological Support

Patients with renal failure must deal not only with conflicting feelings about prolonging their lives with a machine but also with the fact that their lives are no longer the same. They become "marginal" people who are partially ill and partially well. They must take certain medications, can no longer eat what they please and must devote several hours per week to being dialyzed as shown in Figure 30–4. Even then, they do not feel "perfect" or completely well and have to live with progressive bone disease, problems with the fistula or peritonitis, and anorexia or nausea. By being especially sympathetic to their feelings of thirst, their anorexia when faced with eating, the taste changes due to uremia, and the tedium of the diet, the nurse, dietitian, physician and social worker can help dialysis patients cope with their new way of life.

Those who work with renal dialysis patients must be aware of both the often-present depression and the frequent denial of illness and overindependence of these patients, who are trying to live with chronic illness and the threat of death.

Nutritional Care

Nutritional care aims to make up for the work no longer being done by the non-functioning nephrons. The goals of nutritional care in chronic renal failure are:

1. To prevent deficiency and maintain good nutritional status (and growth, in the case of children) through adequate protein, calorie, vitamin and mineral intake.

2. To minimize uremia by controlling the pro-

Table 30–5. NUTRIENT REQUIREMENTS FOR ADULTS WITH RENAL DISEASE BASED ON TYPE OF THERAPY

THERAPY	ENERGY	PROTEIN	FLUID	SODIUM	POTASSIUM	PHOSPHORUS
Impaired renal function (pre-dialysis)	40–50 kcal./kg. IBW*	0.6 gm./kg. IBW	ad lib.	Variable, 2–3 gm./day	Variable, usually ad lib. or increased to cover losses with diuretics	1–1.2 gm./day
Hemodialysis	35 kcal./kg. IBW	1 gm./kg. IBW (1.2–1.5 gm./kg. for repletion)	750 ml./day + urine output	2–3 gm./day	2–3 gm./day	1–1.2 gm./day
Intermittent peritoneal dialysis (IPD)	30 kcal./kg. IBW (40–50 kcal./kg. for repletion)	1.2 gm./kg. IBW (1.5 gm./kg. for repletion)	750 ml./day + urine output	2–3 gm./day	2–3 gm./day	1–1.2 gm./day
Continuous ambulatory peritoneal dialysis (CAPD)	25 kcal./kg. IBW (40–50 kcal./kg. for repletion)	1.2 gm./kg. IBW (1.5 gm./kg. for repletion)	ad lib. (minimum of 2000 ml./day + urine output)	6–8 gm./day	3–4 gm./day	1.5–2 gm./day
Diabetic on hemodialysis, IPD, or CAPD	35 kcal./kg. IBW (40–50 kcal./kg. for repletion)	1.5 gm./kg. IBW	Same as for hemodialysis, IPD, or CAPD. Monitor thirst, blood sugar, and weight changes		Same as for hemodialysis, IPD, or CAPD. (Increased blood sugar may cause increased potassium.)	1–1.2 gm./day (Often liberalized due to other restrictions.)
Transplant	30 kcal./kg. IBW Low carbohydrate (35–45% of calories, low saturated fat)	1.5–2.0 gm./kg. IBW	ad lib.	Variable, 2–3 gm./day	Variable, usually ad lib.	ad lib.

* IBW = Ideal body weight.
Developed by Katy Wilkens, R.D., Northwest Kidney Center, Seattle, Washington.

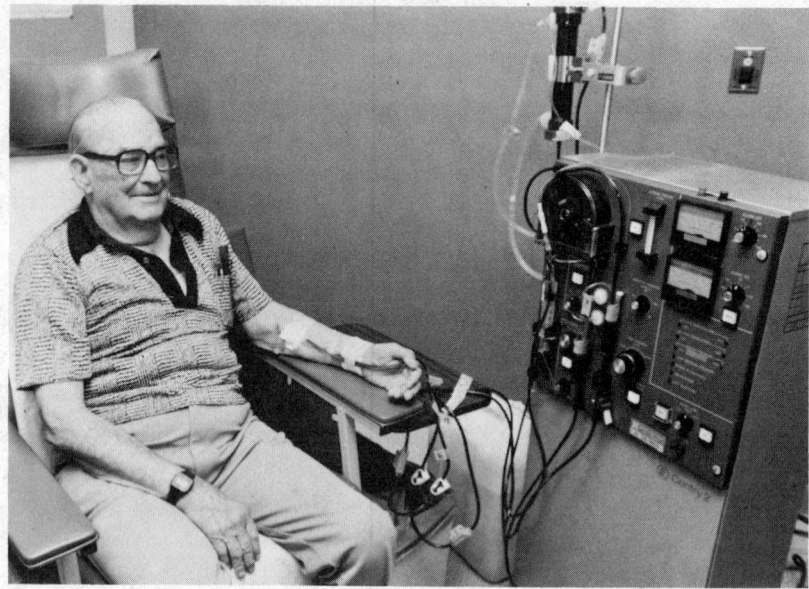

Figure 30–4. A man with chronic renal failure receiving hemodialysis.

tein intake while still maintaining a positive nitrogen balance.

3. To control edema and electrolyte imbalance by controlling sodium, potassium and fluid intake.

4. To prevent or retard the development of renal osteodystrophy by controlling calcium, phosphorus, magnesium and vitamin D intake.

5. To enable the patient to eat a palatable, attractive diet that fits into his lifestyle as much as possible.

Even with the development of dialysis methods and transplantation techniques, nutritional care remains an important therapy for patients with chronic renal failure. Such care is essential to enhance dialysis, maintain optimal nutritional status and prevent complications.

People with chronic renal failure have a unique role in the treatment of their disease. Unlike those with acute renal failure, these people assume much of the responsibility for their care. Since treatment is on an outpatient basis or dialysis is done at home, these patients assume all responsibility for their diet.

Most chronic renal failure patients know their diets very well, having been instructed by a dietitian or nutritionist prior to each hospital discharge. In addition, all dialysis units have dietitians or nutritionists whose main responsibility is educating the patient and family. As in any chronic disease, the patient who does best is the patient who fully understands his disease and therapy. Table 30–6 is a guide for teaching patients about their blood values and control of their disease. Education of the patient is the primary role of the dietitian; monitoring the patient's long-term nutritional status becomes the secondary but still very important role. Long-

term compliance with a difficult diet regimen is a major problem chronic renal failure patients face.

FLUID AND SODIUM. The kidney's ability to handle sodium and water in the patient with chronic renal failure changes and must be assessed frequently through measurement of urinary sodium excretion, urine output, blood pressure, presence of edema, serum sodium level and dietary intake. The diet and fluid intake are then modified accordingly. In the early stages of renal failure, nephrons may not be able·to concentrate urine, and large quantities of fluid and sodium may be lost daily and will have to be replaced. As the failure worsens, the kidney may only be able to produce 400 to 500 ml. of dilute urine per day (oliguria). At this point, fluid restriction is necessary.

Although most patients with chronic renal failure retain sodium, some may be *losing* sodium. Examples of diseases with a salt-losing tendency are polycystic disease of the kidney, chronic obstructive uropathy, chronic pyelonephritis and analgesic nephropathy. Other renal diseases, such as chronic glomerulonephritis, can have a *salt-losing phase*. To prevent hypotension, hypovolemia, cramps and further deterioration of renal function, extra sodium may be required. Measurement of the urinary sodium excretion of patients receiving a known amount of sodium should be made several times to assess the sodium excretion of patients who are still excreting urine.

The diet should be matched to the sodium and fluid excretion. Usually this is 87 to 130 mEq. (2 to 3 gm.) or higher of sodium per day, which may be found in a normal diet without added salt. In some cases sodium intake will need to

Table 30–6. DIALYSIS PATIENT'S GUIDE TO BLOOD VALUES

This guide is to help you understand your lab reports. The normal values are for people with good kidney function. Acceptable values for dialysis patients are given in the next column. Your blood values should fall within the range for dialysis patients. Many things affect your blood values. Diet is one of these. Understanding the chemistry of your blood will help you control your diet. Be sure to ask the dietitian or nurse if you have questions.

SUBSTANCE	NORMAL VALUES	VALUES FOR DIALYSIS PATIENTS	FUNCTION	DIET CHANGES
Sodium	136–145 mEq./l.	Same	Found in salt and many preserved foods. A diet high in sodium will make you thirsty. When you drink too much fluid, it may dilute the sodium and it will look low. If you eat too much sodium and do not drink water, it may be high. Always check your weight gains against your sodium value.	High: Eat less salt and salty foods. Make sure you are gaining about 1.5 kg. between dialyses and are not dehydrated. Low: Probably drinking too much fluid. Limit weight gains to 1.5 kg. between dialyses. Eat less salt and fewer salty foods.
Potassium	3.5–5.5 mEq./l.	Same	Found in most high-protein foods, fruits and vegetables. It affects muscle action, especially the heart. High levels can cause your heart to stop. Low levels can also cause symptoms such as weakness.	High: Avoid foods with over 250 mg. potassium per serving and limit daily intake to 2000 mg. Consult dietitian. Low: Add one 250 mg. potassium food per day and recheck blood level.
Chloride	97–108 mEq./l.	Same	Usually associated with amount of sodium in the blood.	No dietary changes.
Total CO₂	23–30 mEq./l.	Lower than normal	Total carbon dioxide is a measure of how acidic your blood is. Your kidneys normally keep this normal. When they fail, your blood becomes more acidic and your CO₂ is lower.	No dietary changes.
Creatinine	0.7–1.5 mg./dl.	10–15 mg./dl.	A normal waste product of muscle breakdown. This value is controlled by dialysis. You have a higher amount because the artificial kidney is not working all the time like the normal kidney does.	No dietary changes. Normally dialysis controls creatinine.
Glucose	60–125 mg./dl.	Same (higher for diabetic)	This sugar in the blood is made from the food that you eat, especially the starches and sugars. The body uses glucose for energy. For diabetics: a high blood sugar can make you thirsty; be sure to follow diet.	You need a *minimum* of 4 servings of breads/starches or cereals and 2–3 servings of fruit to provide energy. For diabetics: Avoid concentrated sweets unless your blood sugar is low.
Calcium	8.5–10.5 mg./dl.	8.5–11.0 mg./dl.	Found in dairy products, meats and green vegetables. It is used by the body to make bone and help muscle movement. It is closely related to phosphorus; vitamin D is needed for its absorption. Calcium and phosphorus are 2 minerals needed for strong bones. They have a "see-saw" relationship, so when phosphorus is up, calcium is down. The ratio should be kept within normal for strong bones.	High: Eat fewer milk products. Check with doctor if you are taking calcium supplement like Tums or vitamin D (DHT or Rocaltrol). Low: Increase calcium in diet (if phosphorus is normal) by adding more milk products. You may need a calcium supplement like Tums or vitamin D. Check with your doctor before taking.
Phosphorus	2.3–4.3 mg./dl.	Same	Found in milk products, dried beans and peas, nuts and meat. It is also used to build bones.	High: Limit milk and milk products to 1 serving per day. Take phosphate binders as prescribed. Low: Add 1 serving milk product or other high-phosphorus food per day.

Table continued on the following page

611

Table 30-6. DIALYSIS PATIENT'S GUIDE TO BLOOD VALUES (*Continued*)

SUBSTANCE	NORMAL VALUES	VALUES FOR DIALYSIS PATIENTS	FUNCTION	DIET CHANGES
Urea nitrogen (blood urea nitrogen or BUN)	4–22 mg./dl.	Less than 100 mg./dl.	Waste product of protein breakdown. Unlike creatinine, this is affected by the amount of protein in your diet. Dialysis removes urea nitrogen.	High: Limit intake of meat, fish, chicken and dairy products to about 3 servings per day and contact dietitian. Low: May be low if you are not eating and are losing weight. May also increase with loss of muscle. Contact dietitian.
Uric acid	4.0–8.5 mg./dl.	Same	A waste product of purine. A high level may be related to symptoms of gout. Purines are found in a variety of foods.	No dietary changes. Since purines are found in most foods, you would have to stop eating! If you have gout your doctor can prescribe a medicine to lower it.
Alk Phos (alkaline phosphatase)	30–115 I.U./l.	Same	Found in normal bone. Released from bone when calcium is being removed.	Keep calcium and phosphorus within normal range.
LDH (lactic dehydrogenase)	80–220 I.U./l.	Same	Enzymes released when tissue is damaged. Increased in infection, heart problems, liver damage and damage of any tissue.	No dietary changes.
SGOT (serum glutamic oxaloacetic transaminase)	0–41 I.U./l.	Same		
Cholesterol	150–330 mg./dl.	Often lower	Found in high-fat foods from animal sources: e.g., meat, milk, eggs. Your body can also make its own if there is not enough in your diet. Within normal levels, cholesterol is not harmful.	Usually no dietary changes are necessary.
Total protein	6.0–8.2 gm./dl.	Same	Proteins make up all body cells. Albumin is a type of protein. Both are needed by the body. Protein is lost with dialysis. Peritoneal dialysis protein loss is much more than hemodialysis, so you need even more protein. If albumin is low, fluid will "leak" from blood vessels into tissue, causing edema. When fluid is in the tissue, it is more difficult to remove with dialysis.	Low: Increase intake of protein-rich foods: meat, fish, chicken, eggs. Ask your dietitian for high-protein recipes.
Albumin	3.5–5.0 gm./dl.	Same		
HCT (hematocrit)	35–45%	Usually lower	This is the percentage of red blood cells in the blood. Red blood cells carry oxygen to the cells. Everyone's value is different; learn what is normal for you.	If hematocrit is dropping, check with your doctor.
Serum Ferritin	15–200 µg./l. (men) 12–150 µg./l. (women)	Same Same	Ferritin is the form of iron stored in the liver. If iron stores are low, you cannot make new red blood cells.	Iron in food is not well enough absorbed. Ask your doctor about an iron supplement. Do not take iron with your phosphate binders.
Hep B surface antigen (hepatitis)	Negative		A protein in your body if you have serum hepatitis, a liver disease.	No dietary changes.

Developed by Linda Peterson, R.N., and Katy Wilkens, R.D., Northwest Kidney Center, Seattle, Washington.

be increased above normal. Sodium can be increased by adding salt or salty foods such as bouillon (one cube contains 20 mEq. of sodium).

Patients with hypertension and edema may need a restricted sodium and fluid intake. Again, intake should be matched to the urinary sodium excretion. Since fluid in solid foods is approximately 500 to 800 ml., these foods will replace the 500-ml. insensible water loss (insensible water loss of 1000 ml. offset by water of metabolism of 500 ml.) as shown in Table 30–3. Additional fluid is given to replace urinary loss.

In the *anuric* patient (without urine) who is maintained with dialysis sodium intake and fluid intake are regulated to allow for a weight gain from increased fluid in vasculature of 3 lb. (1.5 kg.) between dialyses. This means a sodium intake of 87 to 90 mEq. (2 gm.) per day and a fluid intake of 750 ml. per day plus the amount equal to the urine output. An 87- to 90-mEq. sodium diet allows for light salting of foods during cooking but no additional salt at the table and no salted, smoked or cured meat or fish, salted snack foods, bouillon and canned soups or foods canned in brine. Chapter 28 gives the details of the 87- to 90-mEq. (2-gm.) sodium diet plan.

In educating patients about fluid balance, the dietitian must deal with their constant complaints of thirst. Suggestions to suck on a few ice chips, cold sliced fruit or sour candies, to use a spray mouth wash, or to chew "sports gum" containing citric acid may help to take away the dryness.

Patients must be taught to measure their fluid intake and urine output, to examine their eyelids and ankles for edema, to weigh themselves regularly each morning and to record their weight. Occasionally (in about 10 per cent of patients), hypertension is not alleviated even after meticulous attention is paid to fluid and water balance. Usually in these cases hypertension is being perpetuated by the presence of a high level of renin secreted by the kidney and requires medication for control.

Fluid and sodium requirements can increase in the presence of perspiration, vomiting or fever. Hypotension and the possibility of clotting at the shunt site must be avoided by scrupulous attention to fluid and sodium intake.

POTASSIUM. Potassium usually requires restriction, depending upon the individual's body size, the 24-hour urinary potassium excretion, the serum K^+ level and the frequency of dialysis. The patient receiving less frequent dialysis cannot tolerate a high potassium intake. Potassium intake is usually 40 to 65 mEq. (1.5 to 2.5 gm.) per day. For the patient with no urine excretion who is maintained with dialysis, the diet usually includes 51 mEq. (2 gm.) of potassium. This is a moderate restriction from the usual intake of 75 to 100 mEq. (3 to 4 gm.) of potassium for most Americans. Appendix Table 10 gives the potassium content of foods. The exchange lists in Table 30–8 show the potassium content for groups of food.

Rarely, a chronic renal failure patient may require additional potassium. Those who are taking diuretics may be losing potassium in the urine. The amount lost in a 24-hour period should be measured and replaced. The potassium may be added to the diet, added to the dialysate or given as potassium supplements.

PROTEIN. In chronic renal failure, as the GFR decreases and fewer nitrogenous waste products are excreted, it becomes necessary to control the level of protein intake while continuing to maintain a positive nitrogen balance. A mild protein restriction is usually initiated when the kidney function has decreased to about 25 per cent of normal, and protein is decreased further as renal function continues to decline, as measured by creatinine clearance. Therefore, the renal failure patient may restrict his protein intake in stages as failure progresses. Authorities do not agree on the exact amount of protein recommended at each stage of deterioration, but the plan shown in Table 30–7 is representative.

At least 75 per cent of the protein intake should be of high biological value (HBV) or complete proteins to assure that the essential amino acid requirements are met. The body then uses its extra nitrogen to synthesize the non-essential amino acids and thus reduces the amount of urea that must be removed.

Dialysis is a drain on protein in the body, and the daily protein intake should be increased to compensate for this. Losses of 10 to 30 gm. of protein can occur during a 24-hour peritoneal dialysis, with an average of 1 gm. per hour. Hemodialysis results in a similar loss of approximately 1 gm. of protein for every hour of dialysis. Patients receiving peritoneal dialysis three times per week or continuous ambulatory dialysis should have an intake of at least *1.2 to 1.5 gm. protein per kg. body weight* per day, while those receiving hemodialysis three times per week should ingest *1 gm. protein per kg.*

Table 30–7. RECOMMENDED PROTEIN INTAKE ACCORDING TO DEGREE OF RENAL FAILURE

GLOMERULAR FILTRATION RATE (ml./min.)	PROTEIN INTAKE (gm./day)
20–25	60–90
15–20	50–70
10–15	40–55
5–10	35–40
less than 5	Dialysis or transplantation

body weight per day. Protein requirements for patients on different types of dialysis are summarized in Table 30–5. However, the patient's serum BUN and serum creatinine levels, uremic symptoms and weight should be monitored and the diet adjusted accordingly.

An example of a dietary protein calculation is as follows:

Example: A 60-kg. anuric female receiving hemodialysis three times per week should be eating 60 gm. of protein per day. If 75 per cent of this protein is to be of high biological value, then 46 gm. of protein should be in the form of eggs, meat, fish, poultry, milk or cheese. A likely combination of these foods to *contribute 46 grams of HBV protein* would be the following:

FOOD	GM. PROTEIN
1 egg	7
2 oz. chicken	14
3 oz. beef	21
½ cup milk	4
Total	46

The remaining 14 gm. is obtained from the LBV protein sources: breads and cereals, vegetables, fruit, potatoes, pasta and desserts. An example of a combination of foods that would provide this *14 gm. LBV protein allowance* is the following:

FOOD	GM. PROTEIN
3 slices bread	6
¾ cup cereal	3
½ cup mashed potatoes	2
½ cup carrots	1
½ cup peas	1
1 small glass orange juice	0.5
1 large apple	0.5
Total	14

While the intake of HBV and LBV proteins is important, most patients find it difficult, if not impossible, to consume adequate calories and still have a palatable diet. In addition, the uremia itself causes some taste aberrations, noticeably to red meats, making the HBV/LBV ratio difficult to achieve.

Table 30–8 contains the exchange lists quantified for protein, sodium, potassium and calories that are used in designing a diet for patients who must have controlled intakes. Table 30–9 shows how these exchanges might be combined to construct diets to meet various requirements. Table 30–10 presents a sample menu.

Although the exchange lists may make the calculation of the diet easier, they may not make following the diet easier. Some patients may prefer to learn the actual protein, potassium and sodium content of foods and adjust their intake accordingly. Sodium and potassium values of foods are given in Appendix Table 10, and protein values are given in Appendix Table 1.

ENERGY. Energy intake must be adequate in order to spare protein for tissue protein synthesis and prevent its metabolism for energy. Energy provided by foods other than protein is very important for patients with chronic renal failure, just as it is in cases of acute renal failure. Depending on the patient's present nutritional status and degree of stress, between *35 and 50 kcal. per kg. body weight* should be provided.

Patients with chronic renal failure who require tube feeding may be given a product such as Amin-Aid (McGaw), which contains only the essential amino acids plus histidine in the amount required and which when mixed with water provides amino acids, carbohydrate and a few electrolytes. Another possible source of protein may be electrodialyzed whey (milk protein [lactalbumin] treated to remove the electrolytes), which when combined with glucose and water provides HBV protein with adequate calories and few electrolytes. The palatability of these products is low, and as soon as possible the patient should be encouraged to eat a moderate protein, high-calorie diet with controlled sodium and potassium intake. A third possible means of nutritional support is parenteral administration of the essential amino acids as discussed in Table 30–11.

CALCIUM, PHOSPHORUS AND VITAMIN D. A major complication of chronic renal failure is metabolic bone disease or renal osteodystrophy. The disease is essentially of three types: *osteomalacia*, or bone demineralization; *osteitis fibrosa cystica*, caused by hyperparathyroidism; and *metastatic calcification* of joints and soft tissues.

As the GFR decreases, phosphorus is retained in the plasma, resulting in a decrease in serum calcium. Normally, a low calcium level with a high phosphorus level would trigger: (1) the release of parathyroid hormone (PTH) from the parathyroid glands and (2) the release of 1,25-dihydroxycholecalciferol (1,25-[OH]$_2$ D$_3$), the chief active metabolite of vitamin D from the kidney. The PTH would act with 1,25-(OH)$_2$D$_3$ (a calcium mobilizer) to reabsorb calcium from the bone, raising the serum level to normal. Simultaneously, the 1,25-(OH)$_2$D$_3$ would be enhancing the absorption of Ca^{++} in the gut to replace the calcium ions lost from the bone and to keep serum Ca^{++} within normal range. The activities of 1,25-(OH)$_2$D$_3$ are discussed more fully in Chapter 6.

Cholecalciferol is first converted in the liver to 25-hydroxycholecalciferol, and 1-hydroxylation occurs in the kidney to make it an active vitamin (1,25-[OH]$_2$D$_3$). Renal failure prevents

Table 30–8. EXCHANGE LISTS FOR DIETS CONTROLLED FOR PROTEIN, SODIUM AND POTASSIUM

FOOD	APPROXI-MATE AMOUNT	PRO-TEIN (gm.)	CAL-ORIES	SODIUM (mEq.) Unsalted	SODIUM (mEq.) Salted	POTAS-SIUM (mEq.)
Egg	1	7	75	3.0	5.0	2.0
Meat	1 oz.	7	75	1.0	3.0[a]	2.5
Fat	Varies	–	35	–	2.0	–
Milk Product	Varies	4	Varies	2.5	2.5	4.0
Bread	1 slice	2	70	0.5	6.0	1.5
Potato	½ cup	2	70	0.5	10.0[b]	7.0
Cereal	½ cup	2	70	0.5	10.0[b]	1.5
Vegetable						
Group 1	Varies	1	20	0.3	10.0[b]	3.0
Group 2	Varies	1	20	0.8	11.0[b]	5.0
(Average value)				(0.5)		(4.0)
Fruit						
Group 1	Varies	0.5	60	–	–	2.5
Group 2	Varies	0.5	60	–	–	5.0
(Average value)						(3.0)
CHO Supplement	Varies	–	120	–	–	1.0
Beverage (coffee, tea)	1 cup	–	–	–	–	2.0
Salt	1 tsp.	–	–	–	86	–

[a] Moderately salted during preparation, approximately ½ tsp. salt per lb. of meat.
[b] Moderately salted during preparation or processing, approximately ⅛ tsp. salt per ½ cup.

Meat Group (Unsalted)

Protein	7.0 gm.
Sodium	1.0 mEq.
Potassium	2.5 mEq.
Calories	75

FOOD	AMOUNT	WEIGHT (gm.)
Meat (unsalted)		
Beef, lamb, liver, pork, veal	1 oz.	30
Fowl (unsalted)		
Chicken, duck, turkey	1 oz.	30
Fish (unsalted, fresh or frozen)		
Fish	1 oz.	30
Clams	2 oz.	50
Oysters	2½ oz.	50
Shrimp	1 oz.	30
Egg (unsalted, 3 mEq. sodium)	1 medium	50
Cheese (unsalted)		
Cheese	1 oz.	30
Cottage cheese	¼ cup	50
Peanut butter (unsalted)	2 tbsp.	30

Omitted: Salted meat, fish, fowl, cheese, peanut butter; other organ meats; other shellfish.

Fat Group (Unsalted)

Protein	–
Sodium	–
Potassium	–
Calories	35

Table continued on the following page

Table 30–8.   EXCHANGE LISTS FOR DIETS CONTROLLED FOR PROTEIN, SODIUM AND POTASSIUM (*Continued*)

FOOD	AMOUNT	WEIGHT (gm.)
Margarine	1 tsp.	5
Mayonnaise	1 tsp.	5
Cooking fats or oils	1 tsp.	5

Omitted: Salted butter or margarine; commercial salad dressings.

Milk Group

Protein	4.0 gm.
Sodium	2.5 mEq.
Potassium	4.0 mEq.
Calories	Varies
Phosphorus	110 mg.

FOOD	AMOUNT	WEIGHT (gm.)
Milk	½ cup	120
Evaporated or condensed milk	¼ cup	60
Yogurt	½ cup	120
Powdered whole milk	2 tbsp.	14
Half and half (coffee cream)	½ cup	120
Light whipping cream	⅔ cup	160
Heavy whipping cream	¾ cup	180
Sour cream	½ cup	120
Ice cream	½ cup	100
Ice milk	⅓ cup	80
Sherbet	1 cup	240
Custard	¼ cup	60

Omitted: Commercial buttermilk, powdered skim milk, instant dairy mixes, non-dairy cream substitutes

Bread Group (Unsalted)

Protein	2.0 gm.
Sodium	0.5 mEq.
Potassium	1.5 mEq.
Calories	70

FOOD	AMOUNT	WEIGHT (gm.)
Bread (unsalted)	1 slice	25
Cereal (unsalted; calcium = 5 mg.)		
Cooked	½ cup	100
Dry, flake	⅔ cup	20
Dry, puffed wheat or rice	1½ cups	20
Dry, biscuit	1	25
Crackers (unsalted)		
Crackers	6	20
Melba toast	4	15
Flour Products (unsalted)		
Flour	2 tbsp.	20
Cornmeal	2 tbsp.	25
Macaroni, noodles, spaghetti		
Dry	½ oz.	15
Cooked	¼ cup	50
Rice		
Dry	1 oz.	30
Cooked	½ cup	100
Vegetable (unsalted)		
Brussels sprouts	¼ cup	50
Corn[c]	⅓ cup	80

Table 30–8. EXCHANGE LISTS FOR DIETS CONTROLLED FOR PROTEIN, SODIUM AND POTASSIUM (*Continued*)

FOOD	AMOUNT	WEIGHT (gm.)
Corn grits	½ cup	100
Lima beans	¼ cup	50
Parsnips[e]	½ cup	100
Peas	¼ cup	50
Potato[e]	½ cup	100
Sweet potato, fresh or canned[e]	½ cup	100
Miscellaneous		
Milk or sweet chocolate	1 oz.	30
Pie crust (unsalted)	⅛ pie (9″)	135
Popcorn	1 cup	14

Omitted: Breads, rolls or crackers made with salt, baking powder or baking soda; self-rising flour; instant, quick-cooking or ready-to-eat cereals processed with salt or sodium compound; commercially prepared mixes; dried beans or peas, commercially frozen peas.

[e]Potassium = 3–9 mEq.

Vegetable Groups (unsalted)

Group 1	Protein	1.0 gm.
	Sodium	0.3 mEq.
	Potassium	3.0 mEq.[d]
	Calories	20

VEGETABLE	AMOUNT	WEIGHT (gm.)
Asparagus, fresh, frozen, canned	¼ cup	50
Bean sprouts	½ cup	50
Beans (green or wax), canned	½ cup	100
Broccoli, fresh or frozen	¼ cup	50
Carrots, canned	½ cup	100
Cauliflower, fresh or frozen[e]	¼ cup	50
Collards, cooked	¼ cup	50
Dandelion greens, cooked	¼ cup	50
Endive[e]	½ cup	50
Escarole[e]	4 leaves	50
Lettuce[e]	¼ small head	100
Mustard greens, cooked	¼ cup	50
Okra	¼ cup	50
Onions[e]	½ cup	50
Pepper, green, cooked	¼ cup	50
Radishes	10	100
Rutabaga, fresh or frozen	⅓ cup	80
Spinach, cooked	¼ cup	50
Squash	⅓ cup	80

[d]Potassium restrictions: cooked vegetables, drained.
[e]May be eaten raw in amounts specified.

Vegetable groups (unsalted)

Group 2	Protein	1.0 gm.
	Sodium	0.8 mEq.
	Potassium	5.0 mEq.[d]
	Calories	20

VEGETABLE	AMOUNT	WEIGHT (gm.)
Beans (green or wax), fresh or frozen	½ cup	100
Beets, fresh, frozen, or canned	½ cup	100
Cabbage, fresh[e]	½ cup	100

Table continued on the following page

Table 30–8.   EXCHANGE LISTS FOR DIETS CONTROLLED FOR PROTEIN, SODIUM AND POTASSIUM (*Continued*)

VEGETABLE	AMOUNT	WEIGHT (gm.)
Carrots, fresh or frozen	¼ cup	50
Cucumber[e]	½ cup	100
Eggplant[e]	½ cup	100
Mushrooms, fresh[e]	2 large or 5 small	50
Pepper, green, fresh[e]	⅓ cup	80
Pumpkin	⅓ cup	80
Tomato, fresh or canned[e]	½ cup or 1 small	100
Tomato juice, canned	½ cup	120
Turnip greens, cooked	⅓ cup	80
Watercress[e]	10 sprigs	50

Omitted: Vegetables processed or prepared with salt, sodium, or sodium compound; any vegetable not listed.

[d]Potassium restrictions: cooked vegetables, drained.
[e]May be eaten raw in amounts specified.

Fruit Groups

Group 1	Protein	0.5 gm.
	Sodium	–
	Potassium	2.5 mEq.
	Calories	60

FRUIT	AMOUNT	WEIGHT (gm.)
Apple	1 (2″ diameter)	80
Apple juice	½ cup	120
Applesauce	½ cup	100
Blackberries	¼ cup	50
Blueberries	½ cup	100
Cantaloupe	¼ small	50
Cherries, canned or frozen	⅓ cup	80
Coconut, fresh or dried	½ oz.	15
Cranberries, fresh	½ cup	100
Cranberry juice	2 cups	480
Dates	2	15
Grapefruit, fresh	½ small	100
Grapefruit sections, canned	½ cup	100
Grapes, canned	⅓ cup	80
Grapes, fresh	⅓ cup or 10	50
Grape juice	¼ cup	60
Grape juice drink	1 cup	240
Honeydew melon	¼ small	50
Lemon juice	½ cup or 1 lemon	100
Loganberries	⅓ cup	80
Mango, fresh	1 medium	70
Orange-apricot drink	½ cup	120
Peach, frozen	½ cup	100
Peach nectar	⅔ cup	160
Pear, fresh	1 small	80
Pear, canned	¾ cup	150
Pear nectar	¾ cup	180
Pineapple, canned	½ cup	100
Pineapple, fresh or frozen	⅓ cup	80
Pineapple-grapefruit drink	⅔ cup	160
Pineapple-orange drink	⅔ cup	160
Plums, canned	3	80
Raisins	2 tbsp.	15
Raspberries, frozen	⅓ cup	80
Strawberries, frozen	½ cup	100
Tangerine	2 small	80
Watermelon	½ cup	100

Table 30–8. EXCHANGE LISTS FOR DIETS CONTROLLED FOR PROTEIN, SODIUM AND POTASSIUM (*Continued*)

Group 2	Protein	0.5 gm.
	Sodium	–
	Potassium	5.0 mEq.
	Calories	55

FRUIT	AMOUNT	WEIGHT (gm.)
Apricots	1 medium	80
Apricot nectar	½ cup	120
Banana, fresh	½ small	60
Blackberries, fresh	⅓ cup	80
Figs, canned	½ cup	100
Figs, fresh	1 large	50
Fruit cocktail, canned	½ cup	100
Grapefruit juice	½ cup	120
Melon balls, frozen	⅓ cup	80
Nectarines, fresh	1 small	80
Orange, fresh	1 small	80
Orange juice, fresh, frozen or canned	½ cup	120
Papaya, fresh	⅓ cup	80
Peaches, fresh or canned	2 halves	100
Persimmon, fresh	½ small	60
Pineapple juice	½ cup	120
Plums, fresh	2 small	80
Prune juice	½ cup	120
Prunes	2 small	15
Raspberries	⅓ cup	80
Rhubarb	⅓ cup	80
Strawberries, fresh	½ cup	100

Omitted: Any fruit not listed.

Carbohydrate Supplement Group
(CHO Supplement)

Protein	–
Sodium	–
Potassium	1 mEq.
Calories	120

FOOD	AMOUNT	WEIGHT (gm.)
Sugar and syrups		
Sugar	2½ tbsp.	30
Honey	2 tbsp.	40
Jelly or jam	2 tbsp.	40
Syrup (table blends)	2 tbsp.	40
Candy		
Fondant or sugar mints	3	30
Gumdrops	3 large	30
Hard candy, unfilled	6 pieces	30
Jelly beans	20	60
Lollipops, unfilled	1 medium	30
Fruit desserts		
Cranberry (sauce or relish)	2 tbsp.	80
Fruit ice	⅔ cup	140
Popsicle	1 twin bar	130
Flavored beverages		
(carbonated, fruit flavored; Kool Aid; lemonade)	1 cup (8 oz.)	240
Flour products		
Cornstarch or tapioca	¼ cup	30

Table continued on the following page

Table 30–8.   EXCHANGE LISTS FOR DIETS CONTROLLED FOR PROTEIN, SODIUM AND POTASSIUM (*Continued*)

Beverage (Values Should Be Calculated Individually)

BEVERAGE	AMOUNT	WEIGHT (*gm.*)	POTASSIUM (*mEq.*)
Coffee, tea	1 cup	240	2

Miscellaneous

ALLOWED	OMITTED
Pepper; spices and herbs except "Omitted"; fresh celery (no more than 2 tbsp.); fresh garlic, onion powder or juice; horseradish root, powdered mustard; vinegar; unsalted white sauce made with milk allowance; flavoring extracts.	Salt[g], seasoned salts, mixed spices; baking powder, baking soda; parsley, dried celery products; bottled meat sauces, catsup, prepared mustard or horseradish, meat extracts, meat tenderizers, monosodium glutamate; pickles; gravy; commercial soups; commercially prepared dessert mixes; cocoa; nuts; olives; salt substitutes unless approved by physician.

[g]Allowed when specifically calculated.
Adapted from Mayo Clinic Diet Manual. 5th ed. Philadelphia, W. B. Saunders Co., 1981.

this process from being completed. In fact, it has been shown in patients with renal failure that there is reduced absorption of calcium from the intestine, supposedly because of inadequate amounts of 1,25-$(OH)_2D_3$.[6] Therefore, the active role that vitamin D_3 plays in maintaining serum Ca^{++} levels is reduced, and PTH is constantly being secreted. Furthermore, PTH usually works with vitamin D_3 to mobilize the bone Ca^{++}. In the absence of the vitamin, more PTH is required, and the end result is hyperparathyroidism and osteomalacia, or bone demineralization. The excessive action of PTH results in osteitis fibrosa cystica, with its characteristic dull, aching bone pain. Figure 30–5 outlines a theory to explain the development of hypocalcemia, hyperphosphatemia and resulting bone disease in chronic renal failure.

Even though the serum calcium level is elevated in response to PTH, the serum phosphate concentration will remain high as the GFR falls lower. If the product of the serum calcium level (mg. per 100 ml.) multiplied by the serum phosphate level (mg. per 100 ml.) is greater than 70, *metastatic calcification* is imminent. Clinical management aims to keep the product below 70 by preventing transient elevations in serum phosphate concentration.

In essence, calcium and phosphorus intake must be controlled to as great a degree as possible in order to avoid aggravation of the delicate situation posed by hyperparathyroidism, phosphate retention and hypocalcemia in renal failure. In practical terms, *calcium intake* is kept *high* and *phosphorus intake* is kept *low*. This is

a problem as far as food is concerned, since most of the high-calcium foods—milk and milk products—are also high in phosphorus. Consequently, methods other than dietary ones must be relied upon.

Calcium is increased by giving calcium supplements in the form of calcium carbonate (for example, Tums), lactate or gluconate along with the 300 to 500 mg. of calcium provided in the diet. For dialysis patients, calcium is added to the dialysate bath so that a smaller amount of serum calcium is drawn off during dialysis. The earlier calcium supplementation is started, the better it is for the patient in order to prevent hyperparathyroidism.

Phosphate intake is lowered by restricting it in the diet to 1200 mg. or less and by using phosphate-binding resins such as Basaljel or Amphojel. These aluminum hydroxide products (also used as antacids) bind with phosphate and prevent its absorption from the gut. Frequently, patients have to take large amounts (20 tablets per day) of the resins in order to keep their serum phosphate levels in control. Taken by themselves the resins may be distasteful, so recipes for cookies and other products that incorporate the aluminum hydroxide products have been developed.

A potential risk of excessive consumption of these phosphate binders is severe constipation leading to intestinal impaction. Occasionally this may lead to perforation of the intestine, with resultant peritonitis and death.

Constipation is often the reason why patients will not take the prescribed aluminum hydrox-

Table 30–9. FOOD EXCHANGE COMBINATIONS FOR CONTROLLED PROTEIN, SODIUM AND POTASSIUM DIETS

DIET	MEAT	FAT	MILK OR MILK PRODUCTS[a]	BREAD	VEGE-TABLE	FRUIT	CARBO-HY-DRATE SUPPLE-MENT	BEVER-AGE	SALT (Shaker)[b]
40 Gm. Protein: 50 mEq. potassium, 1500 ml. fluid									
20 mEq. Na	4	11	1	2	2[c]	4	6	3	–
40 mEq. Na	4	11	1	2	2[c]	4	6	3	¼ tsp.
90 mEq. Na	4[c]	11[c]	1	2[c]	2[c]	4	6	3	¼ tsp.
50 Gm. Protein: 65 mEq. potassium, 1800 ml. fluid									
20 mEq. Na	5(4[c])	8	1	2	3	6	5	3	–
40 mEq. Na	5(4[c])	8	1	2	3	6	5	3	¼ tsp.
90 mEq. Na	5[c]	8[c]	1	2[c]	3(1[c])	6	5	3	¼ tsp.
70 Gm. Protein: 85 mEq. potassium, 2200 ml. fluid									
20 mEq. Na	5	6	4	6	4	6	6	3	–
40 mEq. Na	5(4[c])	6[c]	4	6	4	6	6	3	–
90 mEq. Na	5[c]	6[c]	4	6[c]	4	6	6	3	–
100 Gm. Protein: 95 mEq. potassium, 2200 ml. fluid									
30 mEq. Na	9	6	4	6	4	5	4	3	–
40 mEq. Na	9	6[c]	4	6	4	5	4	3	–
90 mEq. Na	9	6[c]	4	6[c]	4	5	4	3	⅛ tsp.
120 Gm. Protein: 95 mEq. potassium, 2300 ml. fluid									
90 mEq. Na	11[c]	6[c]	6	7	3	4	2	3	¼ tsp.

Adapted from Mayo Clinic Diet Manual. 5th ed. Philadelphia, W. B. Saunders Co., 1981.

[a]A half cup of half-and-half is included in all diets (4 gm. protein, 14 gm. fat, 6 gm. carbohydrate, 165 kcal.). When other milk products are included, the nutritive composition of the diet should be re-evaluated.

[b]In place of salt allowance, the equivalent in salted foods may be given.

[c]Foods salted in preparation or processing.

ide gels. Suggestions for using bran or other high-fiber foods and regular light exercise may help patients to be more compliant.

As with calcium supplementation, the initiation of these phosphate reduction therapies as soon as possible is advantageous in order to delay hyperparathyroidism and bone disease. Unfortunately, most patients do not have any symptoms during the early phase of hyperparathyroidism and are not attentive about following a modified diet, taking the calcium supplements or taking the phosphate binders. However, they should be encouraged to do so.

Because of potential *hypermagnesemia*, which can exacerbate the already existent bone disease, magnesium-containing antacids such as Maalox, Gelusil or Mylanta should not be used.

Vitamin D is given only when the hypocalcemia of renal failure is severe or causing osteomalacia. However, because so little vitamin D_3 is changed into its active form $(1,25-[OH]_2D_3)$ in the renal failure patient, large amounts (10,000 to 30,000 I.U. daily) must be given. The dangers inherent in the use of these large doses of vitamin D_3 are hypercalcemia and hypomagnesemia from overdosage and metastatic calcification

Table 30–10. SAMPLE MENU FOR PROTEIN-, SODIUM-, AND POTASSIUM-CONTROLLED DIET

(60 gm. protein, 2000 mg. (87 mEq.) sodium, 2000 MG. (51 mEq.) potassium, 1500 ml. fluid, 2500 + kcal.)

MEAL	PROTEIN (gm.)	KCAL.	Na (mg.)	K (mg.)	FLUID (ml.)	P (mg.)
Breakfast						
½ cup orange juice	0.5	60	–	250	110	15
½ cup oatmeal	2.0	70	197	25	85	20
½ cup light coffee cream	3.5	250	52	150	95	95
1 poached egg	7.0	88	130	70	35	110
2 slices regular toast	4.0	140	260	50	20	40
6 tsp. unsalted butter or margarine	–	270	–	–	–	–
1 tbsp. jelly	–	48	–	–	–	–
6 oz. coffee	–	–	–	–	180	–
3 tsp. sugar	–	48	–	–	–	–
10:00 A.M. Snack						
4 oz. high-calorie supplement[a]	–	273	–	–	60	–
Lunch						
2 oz. unsalted beef patty	14.0	146	50	270	40	100
1 hamburger bun	2.0	70	130	25	10	20
1 tbsp. mayonnaise	–	106	84	28	–	–
Sliced tomato and lettuce	2.0	35	5	200	100	50
1 tbsp. French dressing	–	88	210	10	–	–
1 sugar cookie	1.0	35	65	12	5	10
5 oz. lemonade	–	50	–	–	150	–
3:00 P.M. Snack						
4 oz. high-calorie supplement	–	273	–	–	60	–
Dinner						
2 oz. unsalted broiled chicken	14.0	146	50	270	40	100
⅓ cup mashed potatoes	2.0	35+	300	200	100	50
2 slices bread	4.0	140	260	50	20	40
4 tsp. unsalted butter or margarine	–	180	–	–	–	–
1 tbsp. jelly	–	48	–	–	–	–
½ cup fruit cocktail	0.5	60	–	175	110	15
6 oz. lemonade	–	60	–	–	180	–
Bedtime Snack						
¾ cup orange sherbet	2.0	70+	7	25	100	20
1 slice poundcake	2.0	70	130	25	10	20
Totals	60.5	2859	1930	1835	1510	705

From Manual of Clinical Dietetics, 2nd ed. 1981. Researched and Approved by Chicago Dietetic Association and South Suburban Dietetic Association of Chicago. W. B. Saunders Co., Philadelphia

[a]Cal-Power is used as a high-calorie supplement. If the patient desires water instead of a high-calorie supplement, the calorie level of the diet will be decreased.

from combined hypercalcemia and hyperphosphatemia. Vitamin D and its metabolites should be used carefully, with attention to the development of hypercalcemia. Such hypercalcemia could be difficult to treat because of the accumulation of vitamin D in the body, and the long half-life of vitamin D_3, which would perpetuate the condition and the vitamin D toxicity even after discontinuing its administration.

Far more effective is the administration of $1,25\text{-}(OH)_2D_3$ directly. This hormone is available as *calcitriol* (Rocaltrol, Roche Labs). Analogues such as $1\text{-}\alpha\text{-}OHD_3$ and $1\text{-}\alpha,25\text{-}(OH)_2D_3$ (DHT, Roxane Labs), which have similar configurations, have been produced and are also available.

Hemodialysis or peritoneal dialysis does not alleviate osteodystrophy. However, it can reduce the progression of the disease because the infused calcium results in decreased PTH secretion. Patients must still be responsible for following a low-phosphorus diet and for taking the aluminum hydroxide binders.

FLUORIDE. High levels of fluoride in the serum of the uremic patient seem to aggravate the existing bone disease, possibly by enhancing bone demineralization. Increased serum fluoride levels in dialyzed uremic patients have been reported and may possibly be attributed to the fluoride content of the dialysate bath. It is recommended that water from fluoridated supplies be deionized before using it in dialysis.[18]

ALUMINUM. There is evidence that aluminum can be absorbed from the gut, and in fact it is found in increased concentrations in the tissues of uremic patients taking aluminum hydroxide

Table 30–11. REGIMEN FOR PARENTERAL NUTRITION BY PERIPHERAL VEIN FOR DIALYSIS PATIENTS

INFUSION	QUANTITY	CALORIES	VOLUME
10% Glucose	50 gm. glucose	170 kcal.	500 ml.
8.5 or 10% Amino acids	40–50 gm. protein	160 kcal.	500 ml.
10% Lipid emulsion	50 gm. fat	550 kcal.	500 ml.
Total		880 kcal.	1500 ml.*

Monitor serum glucose, sodium, potassium, bicarbonate and phosphate.

REGIMEN FOR PARENTERAL NUTRITION BY SUBCLAVIAN VEIN FOR DIALYSIS PATIENTS

INFUSION	QUANTITY	CALORIES	VOLUME
70% Glucose	700 gm. glucose	2380 kcal.	1000 ml.
8.5 or 10% Amino acids	40–50 gm. protein	160–200 kcal.	500 ml.
20% Lipid emulsion	100 gm. fat	1100 kcal.	500 ml.
Total		3640–3680 kcal.	2000 ml.*

Monitor serum glucose, sodium potassium, bicarbonate and phosphate.

*Additional volume may include insulin and vitamins.
Developed by Katy Wilkens, R.D., Northwest Kidney Center, Seattle, Washington.

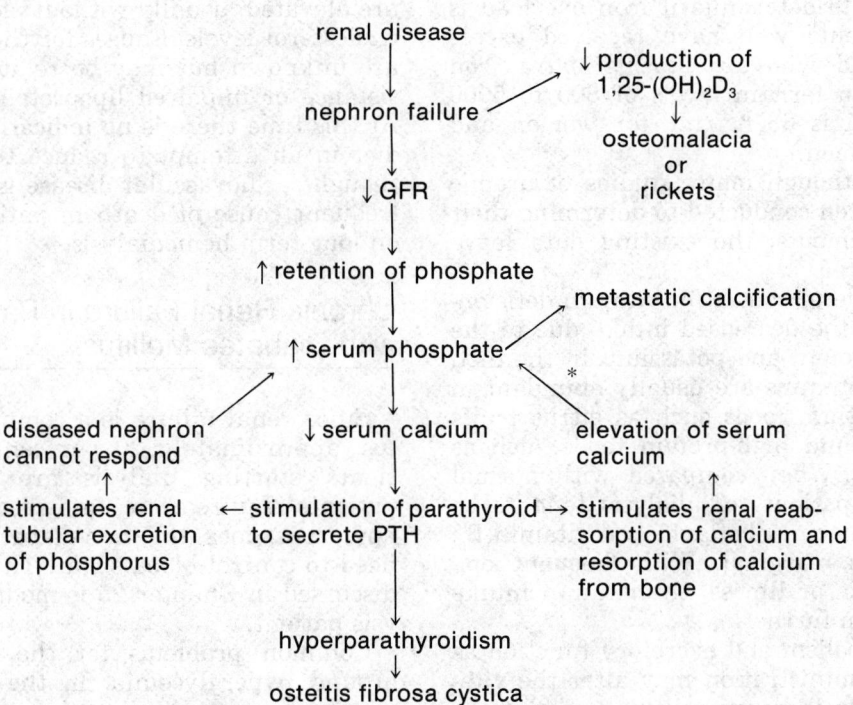

*As the disease worsens, the elevation in serum calcium level no longer causes a drop in serum phosphate level.

Figure 30–5. Development of renal osteodystrophy in chronic renal failure. (Adapted from Bricker, N. S.: The pathogenesis of the uremic state. An exposition of the "trade off" hypothesis. N. Engl. J. Med., *286*:1093, 1972.)

phosphate-binding resins.[4, 9] It has been postulated that the increased levels of aluminum found in the brain tissue of these patients *may* be a cause of the encephalopathy occasionally seen in renal patients.[1] It is also suggested that a hypochromic anemia is due to high serum aluminum levels.[16] However, until more proof is available, aluminum-containing phosphate resins continue to be used for lack of a better therapy. However, all water used in hemodialysis should be treated so that it is low in aluminum.[16]

IRON. The anemia of chronic renal failure usually stabilizes and is relatively asymptomatic, manifesting itself only in complaints of fatigue. It is treated with oral or parenteral iron supplementation and androgens or anabolic steroids that stimulate erythropoiesis. In addition, sources of iron in the diet such as liver, meat (particularly beef), eggs and some dark green vegetables may be used, as discussed further on page 590.

Blood transfusion is not recommended for most patients with chronic renal failure because of (1) its depression of erythropoiesis in the bone marrow, (2) the possibility of overexpansion of the blood volume, (3) the risk of hepatitis and (4) hemochromatosis and hemosiderosis due to increased iron stores and administration of parenteral iron.

Serum ferritin is an accurate measure of iron stores in order to determine if iron overload is occurring. Patients who have received excess transfusions and who are storing extra iron may have serum ferritin levels of 800 to 5000 ng./ml. (Normal is 68 ng./ml. for women and 150 ng./ml. for men.)

VITAMINS. Although many studies of uremic patients have been conducted to determine their vitamin requirements, the existing data leave much to be desired.

One of the several causes for vitamin deficiency in uremia is the decreased intake due to the restriction of protein and potassium in the diet. Water-soluble vitamins are usually abundant in both high-potassium foods such as citrus fruits and vegetables and high-protein foods such as meat and milk. When compared with normal diets, diets for patients on dialysis tend to be low in folacin, niacin, riboflavin and vitamin B_6; ascorbic acid is marginal. With frequent episodes of anorexia or illness, the vitamin intake is decreased even further.

Altered metabolism and excretory function as well as drug administration may alter the vitamin levels. Little is known about gastrointestinal absorption in uremia, but it may be significantly decreased. It is possible that uremic toxins interfere with the activity of some vitamins. For example, the phosphorylation of pyridoxine (vitamin B_6) and its analogues may be inhibited.

Water-soluble vitamins are also lost during dialysis. In general, most of the B-complex vitamins, i.e., folic acid, thiamin, riboflavin, nicotinic acid, pantothenic acid and biotin, as well as ascorbic acid, are dialyzable. Since vitamin B_{12} is protein-bound, losses during dialysis are minimal.

At present, no vitamin supplement is available that fits the needs of the uremic patient or of the patient receiving dialysis. A supplement of vitamin B complex and vitamin C is often used. Additional supplements of folic acid and pyridoxine may be given.

CARBOHYDRATE. Glucose intolerance with both hyperglycemia and hypoglycemia is frequently observed in patients with chronic renal failure. It seems to reflect a delayed and erratic action of insulin due to a resistance by the tissues to the action of insulin or to an insulin antagonism by the products of uremia. In any case, this glucose intolerance rarely requires administration of insulin and never requires control of the carbohydrate in the diet. If there are problems with hypoglycemia, dextrose can be added to the dialysate and usually alleviates the problem.

LIPID. There are lipid changes in renal failure patients. Concentrations of serum triglycerides are elevated, usually without elevation of serum cholesterol levels. Causes for the hyperlipidemia are unknown but may be related to insulin resistance or impaired lipoprotein lipase activity. At this time there is no indication to modify the diet in an attempt to reduce the lipemia, even though cardiovascular disease is by far the most frequent cause of death in patients maintained on long-term hemodialysis.

Chronic Renal Failure in Patients with Diabetes Mellitus

Since renal failure is a complication of diabetes, approximately 20 per cent of all new patients starting dialysis are diabetic. These patients require even more specialized diet therapy than does the non-diabetic owing to the need to control blood sugar. The diabetic diet as discussed in Chapter 25 is modified for the dialysis patient.

Common problems for the diabetic revolve around hyperglycemia. In the presence of hyperglycemia, most diabetics experience thirst, with fluid overload becoming a serious problem. Increased osmolarity due to high levels of glucose may cause water and potassium to be pulled out of cells with resultant hyperkalemia.

In addition, the diabetic dialysis patient often has other complications, such as retinopathy (leading to blindness), neuropathy and amputation (due to infection or poor circulation). All these complications can place the diabetic at high nutritional risk.

Often diabetics on dialysis develop gastropathy, with delayed gastric emptying, nausea, vomiting and diarrhea. The delayed gastric emptying and vomiting may result in hypoglycemia, since the food the patient eats does not enter the intestine for absorption within a normal time span. In addition, prolonged vomiting or diarrhea can lead to loss of fluid and electrolytes, leading to hypokalemia and dehydration.

With regard to therapy for the diabetic with gastropathy, little can be done except to treat symptoms that appear. Avoidance of nutritional deficiencies and hyperglycemia or hypoglycemia is the goal of nutritional therapy. Small, frequent feedings are recommended to avoid problems with gastric stasis. Foods usually offered are high in carbohydrate and low in fat to permit increased gastric emptying. Blood sugar and insulin requirements need to be monitored closely in order to avoid hyperglycemia. Close nutritional supervision of these patients is required in order to control symptoms and allow adequate intake.

A new drug, metoclopramide, seems to provide some hope of helping diabetics with gastric and intestinal stasis. The drug decreases gastric emptying time and intestinal transit time.

Chronic Renal Failure in Children

The child who develops chronic renal failure requires all the diet restrictions of the adult but is often unable to understand or unwilling to comply with complicated regimens. Renal failure in children ranges from the newborn infant through the adolescent. Parents and health care staff who deal with these patients must deal with all the additional problems of following a complicated diet.

Each child's diet should be individualized to meet his food preferences, family eating patterns and biochemical needs. Often this is not an easy task. In addition, care must be taken not to place too much emphasis on the diet to avoid its becoming a manipulative tool and attention-getting device by the child.

The same need to restrict sodium, fluid and potassium exists in the child as in the adult patient. Problems with hyperkalemia are much more common in children, and the family needs to be well informed about sources of potassium in the diet.

Growth in children with chronic renal failure is retarded owing to chronic acidosis, hypernatremic dehydration, hypertension, undernutrition and osteodystrophy. However, growth can be renewed or maintained if the child consumes enough calories (100 kcal. per kg. per day) and enough protein. The recommendation for dietary protein is at least 1 to 2 gm. per kg. per day, although this may not be possible in cases of severe uremia. It has been suggested that children's diets be routinely supplemented with the essential amino acids because their needs for them for growth are greater on a per kilogram basis than are those of adults.[3, 11] Table 30–12 presents the nutritional requirements of children with renal failure.

Special encouragement, creativity and attention are required to help the child with chronic renal failure consume the necessary calories. CAPD appears to be a viable therapy for young children, but little is known about the long-term effects.

Transplantation

For the patient who has received a transplanted kidney, nutritional care consists of controlling carbohydrate intake to counteract the effect of taking corticosteroids and controlling sodium intake to counteract the fluid retention tendencies of steroid therapy. There may also be some weight gain due to the steroid therapy.

During periods of rejection and compromised function, uremia may develop, requiring dietary management. In transplant patients hyperparathyroidism may continue to be a problem, and severe bone disease may develop.

Nephrolithiasis or Renal Calculi

Nephrolithiasis is a condition characterized by the presence of renal calculi. Renal calculi may form in either the kidney or the bladder. They look like pebbles, although their appearance varies depending upon their constituents. Some have a smooth surface and others are jagged. They vary in size from fine gravel to a small stone. Kidney stones appear to be a disease of affluent or industrially developed societies, but bladder stones are common in children in less developed countries.

Etiology

How renal calculi develop continues to be a mystery, although many theories have been suggested. Certain diseases seem to favor the

Table 30–12. NUTRIENT REQUIREMENTS BASED ON TYPE OF THERAPY FOR CHILDREN WITH RENAL DISEASE

THERAPY	ENERGY	PROTEIN	FLUID	SODIUM	POTASSIUM	PHOSPHORUS
Impaired renal function (pre-dialysis)	Infant (under 1 yr.): 120–150 kcal./kg. Child: First 10 kg. = 100 kcal./kg. Second 10 kg. = 50 kcal./kg. Every kg. thereafter: 20 kcal./kg.	Creatinine Clearance / Protein Requirement: 10–50 / 1.5 gm./kg.; <10 / 1 gm./kg.; <5 / 0.3–0.5 gm./kg.	35 ml./100 kcal. + urine output	23–69 mg./kg./day (1–3 mEq./kg./day)	29–87 mg./kg./day (1–3 mEq./kg./day)	0.5–1 gm./day
Hemodialysis	Same as above	Weight of Child / Protein Requirement: 10–20 kg. / 2 gm./kg.; 20–30 kg. / 1.5 gm./kg.; 30–40 kg. / 1.0–1.5 gm./kg.; 40+ kg. / 1.0 gm./kg.	Same as above, plus losses from dialysis. Child's fluid gains should be about 5% of body weight.	57 mg./kg./day (2.5 mEq./kg./day)	Same as above	0.5–1 gm./day
Intermittent peritoneal dialysis (IPD)	Same as above	Weight of Child / Protein Requirement: 10–20 kg. / 2 gm./kg.; 20–40 kg. / 1.5 gm./kg.; 40+ kg. / 1.0–1.5 gm./kg.	Same as above	Same as above	Same as above	0.5–1 gm./day
Continuous ambulatory peritoneal dialysis (CAPD)	100–120 kcal./kg.	Weight of Child / Protein Requirement: 10–20 kg. / 2–3 gm./kg.; 20–40 kg. / 1.5–2 gm./kg.; 40+ kg. / 1.0–1.5 gm./kg.	100–160 ml./kg./day + urine output	Same as above	Same as above	0.5–1 gm./day
Transplant	Normal energy requirement for age. Tendency toward obesity due to steroids. Low carbohydrate (35–45% of calories), low saturated fat.	2 gm./kg.	ad lib.	Variable	Variable, usually ad lib.	ad lib.

Developed by Katy Wilkens, R.D., Northwest Kidney Center, Seattle, and Anne Hetrick, R.D., Shands Teaching Hospital, University of Florida, Gainesville.

precipitation of gravel. Systemic infections, metabolic disturbances, hormone imbalances, inadequate fluid intake and lesions that obstruct the flow and produce stasis of urine are considered causative factors. Immobilization favors the formation of calcium stones because of large increases in the excretion of calcium.

Types of Stones

Vermooten[21] divides renal calculi into three basic types: (1) *organic calculi,* such as uric acid, cystine and xanthine stones, which result from some metabolic disturbance, (2) *alkaline earth stones,* such as calcium or magnesium ammonium phosphates or carbonates, which are generally secondary to urinary tract infection and (3) *calcium oxalate stones,* which usually are not associated with infection.

The types of stones that may develop depend largely upon the concentration of the constituent in the urine and the acidity or alkalinity of the urine. Normally, urine is slightly acid. The pH of urine depends upon the character of the diet. If the diet consists largely of acid-forming foods, a very acid urine is produced. Diets consisting mainly of base-forming foods yield an alkaline urine. Stones composed chiefly of uric acid and cystine appear most frequently in an abnormally acid urine. Stones appearing in an alkaline urine are composed of phosphates, carbonates and oxalates.

Nutritional Care

Although medication has largely replaced the use of therapeutic diets for the treatment of renal calculi, specific diets are still recognized and advocated by a number of authorities as a preventive measure against the recurrence of stones, especially following surgical removal. Urinary calculi recur in a significant number of patients; therefore, prophylactic programs are desirable.

The type of diet prescribed is determined by the acidity or alkalinity of the urine and by the variety of stone. Fluids are encouraged (3000 to 4000 ml. or more daily) to prevent concentration of the urine, which is believed to favor precipitation of the stone-forming minerals.

Regardless of the diet prescribed, it must be an adequate one. Renal calculi are a chronic condition, and the diet treatment must be carried on indefinitely.

CALCIUM-CONTAINING CALCULI. Of all renal calculi, 90 to 95 per cent contain calcium salts as the predominant crystalline component. A urine that is high in calcium (*hypercalciuria,* or a urine calcium level greater than 4 mg. per kg. body weight in 24 hours with a dietary intake of 1000 mg. calcium) predisposes to the formation of calcium oxalate, calcium phosphate and calcium carbonate stones. Causes of hypercalciuria are given in Table 30–13.

Idiopathic hypercalciuria is found in approximately 40 per cent of patients with calcium stones, possibly due to faulty renal tubular reabsorption of calcium (calcium "leak"). Other causes are increased absorption of calcium from the intestinal tract and primary parathyroidism. Thiazide diuretics have been used to treat idiopathic hypercalciuria. They reduce the renal excretion of calcium and thus the possibility of a calcium renal stone.[13] Cellulose phosphate or aluminum hydroxide gel can be used to reduce gastrointestinal absorption of calcium.[17] Milk, cheese and other milk products are limited (1 to 2 cups of milk daily), and the diet usually contains 400 mg. or less of calcium. There is some danger of calcium deficiency if this diet regimen is continued indefinitely. Fortified vitamin D milk is excluded, as well as other D-fortified dairy products.

The protein content of the diet should be moderate because urinary calcium excretion rises as dietary protein increases, as discussed on page 150. The high protein intake leads to increased acid production and increased urinary calcium.[15] Acid ash foods favoring production of an acid urine might help to keep the calcium salts in solution.

Calcium Oxalate Stones. When oxalates predominate, the condition is known as hyperoxaluria. *Hyperoxaluria* commonly results from ileal disease or intestinal resection or bypass due to increased absorption of oxalates.[8, 20] Large doses of vitamin C (about 4 gm. per day) taken regularly result in increased oxaluria and potential oxalate stones. Seventy-five per cent of the renal stones in patients in the U.S. are calcium oxalate.

There is no generally accepted dietary regimen for patients with recurrent calcium oxalate stones. The diet therapy is to avoid large quantities of foods listed in Appendix Table 9 as be-

Table 30–13.   POTENTIAL CAUSES OF
HYPERCALCIURIA

Excessive calcium intake
   "Milk-alkali syndrome"
Excessive vitamin D or vitamin A intake
Phosphate deprivation
High carbohydrate intake
High sodium intake
High protein intake
General body immobilization
Idiopathic hypercalciuria

Table 30–14. LOW OXALATE MEAL PLAN

(40–50 mg.)

FOODS	LITTLE OR NO OXALATE < 2 mg. oxalate/serving Eat as desired.	MODERATE OXALATE CONTENT 2–10 mg. oxalate/serving Limit: two (1/2 cup) servings/day from each of the 8 food groups.	HIGH OXALATE FOODS > 10 mg. oxalate/serving Avoid completely.
Beverages/Juices	Apple juice Beer, bottled Coca-Cola (12 oz. limit/day) Distilled alcohol Grapefruit juice Lemonade or limeade, no peel Wine, red, rose Pepsi-Cola (12 oz. limit/day) Pineapple juice Tap water (preferred for extra calcium)	Coffee, any kind (8 oz. serving) Cranberry juice Grape juice Orange juice Tomato juice Nescafe powder (1 tsp.)	Draft beer Stout, Guiness Draft Lager, Tuborg Pilsner Juices containing berries not allowed Ovaltine and other beverage mixes Tea, cocoa
Milk (2 or more cups)	Buttermilk Low-fat milk Low-fat yogurt with allowed fruit Skim milk		
Meat Group	Eggs Cheese, cheddar Lean lamb, beef or pork Poultry Seafood	Sardines	Baked beans canned in tomato sauce Peanut butter Soybean curd (tofu)
Vegetables	Avocado Brussels sprouts Cauliflower Cabbage Mushrooms Onions Peas, green Potatoes (Irish) Radishes	Asparagus Broccoli Carrots Corn, sweet white, sweet yellow Cucumber, peeled Green peas, canned Lettuce, iceberg Lima beans Parsnips Tomato, 1 small Turnips	Beans: green, wax, dried Beets: tops, root, greens Celery Chard, Swiss Chive Collards Dandelion greens Eggplant Escarole Kale Leeks Mustard greens Okra Parsley Peppers, green Pokeweed Potatoes, sweet Rutabagas Spinach Summer squash Watercress
Fruits	Avocado Banana Cherries, bing Grapefruit Grapes, Thompson seedless Mangoes Melons Cantaloupe Casaba Honeydew Watermelon Nectarines Peaches Plums, green or golden gage	Apple Apricots Black currants Cherries, red sour Orange, edible portion Peaches, Alberta Pears Pineapple Plums, Damson Prunes, Italian	Blackberries Blueberries Concord grapes Red currants Dewberries Fruit cocktail Gooseberries Lemon peel Lime peel Orange peel Raspberries Rhubarb Strawberries Tangerine
Bread/Starches	Cornflakes Macaroni Noodles Oatmeal Rice Spaghetti White bread	Cornbread Sponge cake Spaghetti, canned in tomato sauce	Fruit cake Grits, white corn Soybean crackers Wheat germ

Table continued on the following page

Table 30–14. LOW OXALATE MEAL PLAN (*Continued*)

(40–50 mg.)

FOODS	LITTLE OR NO OXALATE <2 mg. oxalate/serving Eat as desired.	MODERATE OXALATE CONTENT 2–10 mg. oxalate/serving Limit: two (1/2 cup) servings/day from each of the 8 food groups.	HIGH OXALATE FOODS >10 mg. oxalate/serving Avoid completely.
Fats and Oils	Bacon Mayonnaise Salad dressing Vegetable oils		Nuts: Peanuts Pecans
Miscellaneous	Jelly or preserves (made with allowed fruits) Lemon, lime juice Salt, pepper (1 tsp./day) Soups with ingredients allowed Sugar		Chocolate, cocoa Pepper (in excess of 1 tsp./day) Vegetable soup Tomato soup

Adapted from Ney, D.M., et al: The Low Oxalate Diet Book for the Prevention of Oxalate Kidney Stones. San Diego, University of California, 1981.

gAllowed when specifically calculated.

Adapted from Mayo Clinic Diet Manual. 5th ed. Philadelphia, W. B. Saunders Co., 1981.

ing high in calcium and high in oxalates, but attention to oxalate in the diet is more important, since oxalate excretion has more effect on calcium oxalate solubility than similar increases in urinary calcium.[7] In addition, it may be useful to reduce animal protein intake, which has been shown to increase urinary excretion of calcium, oxalate and uric acid.[19] Lastly, a diet low in fat is recommended because the hyperabsorption of oxalate from the gut seems to be related to fat malabsorption.

The oxalate content of foods is given in Appendix Table 13. The total dietary oxalate content in order to prevent oxalate stone formation should be 40 to 50 mg. per day; a low oxalate meal plan is given in Table 30–14. A good resource for patient education is given at the end of this chapter.

Oxalate stones are extremely resistant to treatment, and clinical experience has demonstrated that oxalate calculi may recur even after strict elimination of dietary oxalate intake. This may be due to endogenous production, independent of an exogenous food supply. Fluids are forced in order to reduce the concentration of calcium and oxalate ions in the urine.

According to studies by Gershoff,[12] vitamin B_6 (pyridoxine) deficiency causes increased production of oxalates. The administration of this vitamin to individuals on diets that presumably were adequate in vitamin B_6 sharply decreased oxalate production. Experimentally, calcium oxalate stones have been produced in animals fed a low pyridoxine and magnesium diet and prevented by increasing the dietary levels of these two nutrients. It is believed that magnesium aids in keeping the oxalate in solution and prevents precipitation of oxalates and stone forma-

tion. Vitamin B_6 increases citric acid secretion, and this may keep oxalates in solution.

Calcium Phosphate Stones. Dietary treatment for calcium phosphate stones is the normal adequate diet moderate in calcium and phosphorus. Foods generally considered high in phosphate that should be limited are: milk and milk products, eggs, organ meats (brain, heart, liver, sweetbreads, kidney), sardines, fish roe, whole-grain bread and cereal, bran, oatmeal, brown and wild rice, wheat germ, nuts, soybeans and meat in general. Table 7–2, gives the phosphorus content of foods.

Zinsser,[22] however, warns that in using low-phosphorus diets there is a possibility that citrate stones can form as a result of a rise in citrate excretion in the presence of inadequate phosphorus intake. Thus, the reduction in phosphorus intake as a treatment for the condition is fraught with hazard.

URIC ACID STONES. When kidney stones containing uric acid—an end-product of purine metabolism—have been found to occur in an acid medium, the *high alkaline ash diet* is sometimes prescribed. While acidifying or alkalinizing medications are more effective and have largely replaced the high-alkaline and high-acid diets, the diet should support the medication used.

An attempt is made to keep the pH of the urine above 7, or alkaline, as discussed on page 630. If urinary alkalinization alone does not prove adequate, purine intake restriction may be tried, along with anabolic drugs. The low purine diet is given on page 678. Proteins may be restricted to 0.8 gm. per kg. ideal body weight.

Allopurinol, a drug that prevents the synthesis of uric acid, has been used with success.

CYSTINE STONES. If the sulfur-containing amino acid cystine is not broken down in the body and appears in the urine (cystinuria), it may form stones. Cystine stones, formed because of an inborn error of metabolism, are very rare.

A low-protein diet is sometimes used but has not been shown to be very effective. All protein contains cystine (and methionine, from which cystine may be formed) in varying amounts, and it is especially high in milk and milk products. Alkalinizing agents or the high alkaline ash diet, or both, are recommended to keep the urine at pH of 7.2 or above. D-penicillamine has been used because it dissolves cystine stones but it can also be toxic in some patients.

Acid and Alkaline Ash Diets

ACID-BASE BALANCE IN FOODS. The potential acidity or alkalinity of foods refers to the reaction the food will ultimately yield after being burned in the body. The acids of most fruits and vegetables are utilized in the body and yield an alkaline or basic ash, owing to their high potassium, calcium and magnesium contents. Thus, a diet rich in vegetables and fruits will form bicarbonate and hence decrease urine acidity. Hence, fruits and vegetables, except prunes, plums, cranberries and corn, are restricted in an acid ash diet. On the other hand, a diet containing large amounts of proteins, which in their course of metabolism yield acids such as sulfuric and phosphoric, will increase the urine acidity. Foods that are not acid in taste, such as cereals, meat, fish, egg and bread, become strongly acid when their end-products reach the blood and urine owing to their high phosphorus, iron and sulfur contents. However, the normal, healthy individual always maintains a slightly alkaline reaction in the blood and other tissues regardless of the diet. Appendix Table 14 lists alkali-producing, acid-producing and neutral foods.

Salt (sodium) is sometimes restricted in the acid ash diet because sodium is alkaline, and some authorities believe it has a buffering action. Baking powder and soda products may also be prohibited. Salt substitutes contain an alkaline radical and cannot be used. Foods high in acid ash include eggs, meat, fish, poultry, bread, cereal and cereal products. Milk is fairly high in acid ash.

Cranberry juice has been recommended as a urine acidifying agent because it contains a precursor of hippuric acid. However, investigation of the literature behind this claim shows that in fact cranberry juice and products do not consistently and reliably lower urinary pH. If there is a lowering it is after consumption of a large amount of cranberry juice (at least 1.2 liters), and most cranberry juice is one third cranberry juice mixed with water and sugar.[10]

Acid-base reactions of foods are also discussed in Chapter 8.

Problems and Suggested Topics for Discussion

1. What are the functions of the kidneys? Describe the "functioning units." What does the urine from a normal, healthy individual contain?
2. What are the objectives and principles of dietary treatment in glomerulonephritis? When is fluid restriction indicated? When is sodium restriction indicated? When is potassium restriction indicated?
3. Why are most salt substitutes not allowed in the diets of patients with renal disease?
4. What are some of the nutritional problems in patients with uremia?
5. Outline a diet for the following amounts of protein, in each case keeping the calories to at least 2500 daily: (a) 40 gm., (b) 60 gm., (c) 100 gm. and (d) 150 gm.
6. Obtain a diet history from a patient with nephrotic syndrome. Analyze the food history, noting the amount of fat, protein, sodium and calories. What are the objectives and principles of diet therapy? How would you suggest that the patient change his diet?
7. Plan a diet with a person who is receiving hemodialysis. The diet ordered is 60 gm. protein, 2000 mg. sodium and 2000 mg. potassium. Fluids are restricted to 1000 ml. What would you do about the patient's calcium and phosphorus intakes?
8. Plan a menu pattern with a patient who has kidney stones. Observe the urine analysis made by the laboratory and note the pH of the urine. Compare with the adverage normal pH of the urine. What are the principles of the dietary treatment?
9. Outline a typical diet for a man with calcium oxalate kidney stones. What is the purpose of the diet?
10. List foods restricted and foods allowed in a high-acid ash diet; do the same for a high-alkaline ash diet. When might each diet be used?

Cookbooks and Manuals for Patients with Renal Disease

Cost, J.S.: Dietary Management of Renal Disease. Charles B. Slack, Inc. 6900 Grove Road, Thorofare, N.J., 08086, 1975.

Georgia Council on Renal Nutrition: Kidney Kooking: A Family Recipe Book. National Kidney Foundation of Georgia, 3330 Peachtree, Atlanta, Ga., 30326.

Jones, W.O.: Diet Guide for Patients on Chronic Dialysis. DHEW Publ. No. (NIH) 76–685. Artificial Kidney–Chronic Uremia Program, National Institute of Arthritis, Metabolism and Digestive Diseases, National Institutes of Health, Bethesda, Md., 1976.

Kidney Foundation of Illinois: Fun with Food for Dialysis Patients. Illinois Council on Renal Nutrition, 127 N. Dearborn, Chicago, Ill., 60602, 1977.

Koh, M., and Johnson, B.: Halt! No Salt. Dietary Research, 5201 16th Avenue, NE, Seattle, Wash., 98105.

Lenox Hill Hospital: Gourmet Renal Nutrition Cookbook. Dialysis Unit, Lenox Hill Hospital, 100 E. 77th Street, New York, N.Y., 10021.

Ney, D.M., et al.: The Low Oxalate Diet Book. General Clinic Research Center, (H203), The University of California, San Diego Medical Center, 225 Dickenson Street, San Diego, Cal., 92103.

Robinson, S.: The Hillcrest Happy Kidney Cookbook. Hillcrest Medical Center, Utica on the Park, Tulsa, Okla., 74104.

Spitzer, M.E., et al.: A Renal Failure Diet Manual Utilizing the Food Exchange System. Springfield, Ill., Charles C Thomas, 1976.

Wilkens, K., Schiro, K., and Wold, S.: Nutrition, the art of good Eating. A Workbook for People on Dialysis. Northwest Kidney Center, 700 Broadway, Seattle, WA. 98122, 1983.

Cited References

1. Alfrey, A.C., Le Gendre, G.R., and Kaehny, W.D.: The dialysis encephalopathy syndrome: possible aluminum intoxication. N. Engl. J. Med., 294:184, 1976.

2. Anderson, C.F., et al.: Nutritional therapy for adults with renal disease. JAMA, 223:68, 1973.

3. Aronson, S.A., et al.: Essential amino acids in the treatment of advanced uremia: 22 months experience in a 5 year old girl. Pediatrics, 56:538, 1976.

4. Berlyne, G.M., et al.: Hyperaluminaemia from aluminum resins in renal failure. Lancet, 2:494, 1970.

5. Borst, J.G.G.: Protein katabolism in uraemia: effects of protein-free diets, infections, and blood transfusions. Lancet, 1:824, 1948.

6. Brickman, A.S., et al.: Impaired calcium absorption in uremic man: evidence for defective absorption in the proximal small intestine. J. Lab. Clin. Med., 84:791, 1974.

7. Broadus, A., and Thier, S.O.: Metabolic basis of renal-stone disease. N. Engl. J. Med., 300:839, 1979.

8. Chadwick, V.S., Modha, K., and Dowling, R.H.: Mechanism for hyperoxaluria in patients with ileal dysfunction. N. Engl. J. Med., 289:172, 1973.

9. Clarkson, E.M., et al.: The effect of aluminum hydroxide on calcium, phosphorus and aluminum balances, the serum parathyroid hormone concentration and the aluminum content of bone in patients with chronic renal failure. Clin. Sci., 43:519, 1972.

10. Cranberries and urinary infections. Nutr. M.D., 8 (8):3, 1982.

11. Diaz, M., Kleinknecht, C., and Broyer, M.: Growth in experimental renal failure. Kidney Int., 8:349, 1975.

12. Gershoff, S.N., and Prien, E.L.: The effect of daily MgO and vitamin B_6 administration to patients with recurring calcium oxalate kidney stones. Am. J. Clin. Nutr., 20:393, 1967.

13. Kaplan, R.A., and Pak, C.Y.C.: Diagnosis and management of renal calculi. Tex. Med., 70:88, 1974.

14. Lee, H.A., et al.: Amino acid tablet substituted diets in the management of chronic renal failure. Nutr. Metab., 17:154, 1974.

15. Lemann, J., Adams, N.D., and Gray, R.W.: Urinary calcium excretion in human beings. N. Engl. J. Med., 301:535, 1979.

16. O'Hare, J.A., and Murnaghan, D.J.: Reversal of aluminum-induced hemodialysis anemia by a low-aluminum dialysate. N. Engl. J. Med., 306:654, 1982.

17. Pak, C.Y.C., Delea, C.S., and Bartter, F.C.: Successful treatment of recurrent nephrolithiases (calcium stones) with cellulose phosphate. N. Engl. J. Med., 290:175, 1974.

18. Rao, T.K.S., and Friedman, E.A.: Fluoride and bone disease in uremia. Kidney Int., 7:125, 1975.

19. Robertson, W.G., et al.: Should recurrent calcium oxalate stone formers become vegetarians? Br. J. Urol., 51:427, 1979.

20. Stauffer, J.Q., Humphreys, M.H., and Weir, G.J.: Acquired hyperoxaluria with regional enteritis after ileal resection. Ann. Intern. Med., 79:383, 1973.

21. Vermooten, V.: Some aspects of the medical management of renal calculi. JAMA, 157:783, 1955.

22. Zinsser, H.H.: Urinary calculi. JAMA, 174:2062, 1960.

Additional References

Abram, H.S.: Psychiatric reflections on adaptation to repetitive dialysis. Kidney Int., 6:67, 1974.

Aiken-Thor, E., Goodard, B., and O'Nion, J.: Hypogeusia and zinc depletion in chronic dialysis patients. Am. J. Clin. Nutr., 31:1948, 1978.

Bergstrom, J., et al.: Improvement of nitrogen balance in uremic patients by addition of histidine to essential amino acid solutions given intravenously. Life Sci., 9:787, 1970.

Blackburn, S.: Dietary compliance of chronic dialysis patients. J. Am. Diet. Assoc., 70:31, 1977.

Close, J.H.: The use of amino acid precursors in nitrogen accumulation diseases. N. Engl. J. Med., 290:663, 1974.

Cobrun, J.W.: Renal osteodystrophy. Kidney Int., 17:677, 1980.

Coe, F.L., and Kavalach, A.G.: Hypercalciuria and hyperuricosuria in patients with calcium nephrolithiasis. N. Engl. J. Med., 291:1344, 1974.

Cummings, M., Becker, H., and Kirscht, J.: Psychosocial factors affecting adherence to medical regimens in a group of hemodialysis patients. Med. Care, 6:567, 1982.

Curtis, J.R., and Williams, G.B.: Clinical Management of Chronic Renal Failure. Oxford, England, Blackwell Scientific Publications, 1975.

Davis, M., Comty, C., and Shapiro, F.: Dietary management of patients with diabetes treated by hemodialysis. J. Am. Diet. Assoc., 75:265, 1979.

Feinstein, E., Bleimenkvantz, M., and Healy, M.: Clinical and metabolic responses to parenteral nutrition in acute renal failure. Medicine, 60:124, 1981.

Freund, H., Atamian, S., and Fischer, J.: Comparative study of parenteral nutrition in renal failure using essential and nonessential amino acid solutions. Surg. Gynecol. Obstet., 151:652, 1980.

Giovannetti, S., and Maggiore, Q.: A low-nitrogen diet with proteins of high biological value for severe uraemia. Lancet, 1:1000, 1964.

Harlan, W.R., Jr., et al.: Proteinuria and nephrotic syndrome associated with chronic rejection of kidney transplants. N. Engl. J. Med., 277:769, 1967.

Hetrick, A., and Gilman, C.: Nutrition in renal disease when the patient is a child. Am. J. Nurs., 79:2152, 1979.

Hetrick, A., and Shah, R.: Dietary management of infants on CAPD. Am. Assoc. Neph. Nurs. Techs., 8:46, 1982.

Kark, R.M., and Oyama, J.H.: Nutrition and cardiovascular-renal diseases. In Goodhart, R.S., and Shils, M.E. (eds.): Modern Nutrition in Health and Disease. 6th ed. Philadelphia, Lea & Febiger, 1980.

Kensit, M.: Appetite disturbances in dialysis patients. J. Am. Neph. Nurs. Techs., 6:194, 1979.

Keto analogs of essential amino acids in treatment of human diseases. Nutr. Rev., 34:41, 1973.

Kopple, J., and Massry, S.: Symposium on nutrition in renal disease. Proceedings of second international congress on nutrition in renal disease. (Entire volume is on various aspects of renal disease and nutrition.) Am. J. Clin. Nutr., Vol. 33, 1980.

Kopple, J.D., and Swendseid, M.E.: Histidine deficiency anemia in renal failure. Clin. Res., 21:266, 1973.

Kopple, J.D., and Swendseid, M.E.: Nitrogen balance and plasma amino acid levels in uremic patients fed an essential amino acid diet. Am. J. Clin. Nutr., 27:806, 1974.

Levine, S.: Nutritional care of patients with renal failure and diabetes. J. Am. Diet. Assoc., 81:261, 1982.

Lindner, A., et al.: Accelerated atherosclerosis in prolonged maintenance hemodialysis and renal transplant patients. Am. J. Dis. Child., *130*:957, 1976.

Niwa, R., et al.: Plasma level and transfer capacity of thiamin in patients undergoing long-term hemodialysis. Am. J. Clin. Nutr., *28*:1105, 1975.

Pennisi, A. J., et al.: Hyperlipidemia in pediatric hemodialysis and renal transplant patients. Am. J. Dis. Child., *130*:957, 1976.

Possible aluminum intoxication. Nutr. Rev., *34*:166, 1976.

Roberts, C.: Nutritional management of the diabetic patient on hemodialysis. Dial. Trans., *7*:946, 1978.

Schoolwerth, A.C., and Engle, J.E.: Calcium and phosphorus in diet therapy of uremia. J. Am. Diet. Assoc., *66*:460, 1975.

Silverberg, D.S., et al.: Effects of 1,25-dihydroxycholecalciferol in renal osteodystrophy. Can. Med. Assoc. J., *112*: 190, 1975.

Wolfson, M.: Pharmacologic management of adult patients on chronic hemodialysis. Dial. Trans., *8*:52, 1979.

ALLERGY

Nutritional Care in Food Allergy and Food Intolerance

ELIZABETH J. ADAMS, B.S. ● L. KATHLEEN MAHAN, M.S., R.D.

Adverse reactions to foods are caused by many different mechanisms and elicit a wide variety of symptoms. Food allergy is thought to play a role in some but not all of these adverse responses. Responses not caused by food allergy are classified as food intolerances.

Definition of Food Allergy

The spectrum of disorders that should be included in the definition of food allergy is currently an area of controversy. *Food allergy* has been broadly defined as any abnormal response to foods that normally are tolerated by most people. Most narrowly, food allergy has been defined as including only those reactions that produce an anaphylactic response. With the broadest definitions, overdiagnosis of food allergy resulting in failure to identify and treat alternative underlying disorders may occur. With very narrow definitions, underdiagnosis and inadequate treatment of food allergy is likely. *In this text, food allergy will refer to an immunologically mediated reaction to food.* When this definition is applied, clinically significant food allergy is actually documented much less frequently than it is reported.

Because the criteria for diagnosis of food allergy have not been clearly defined or universally accepted, the true incidence of food allergy is unknown. Reported incidence ranges from 0.3 to 50 per cent of the population.[4, 18] Others have estimated that food allergy may affect 20 per cent of the population at some time in their lives but persists in only 1 to 2 per cent.[15] Generally food allergy is thought to be most common in infancy, less common in childhood and even less common in adults.[20]

Symptoms of Food Allergy

Symptoms that have been attributed to food allergy are extensive. However, symptoms actually documented to be caused by allergy to food are limited to the gastrointestinal tract, respiratory tract or skin, as listed in Table 31–1. The response produced by allergic reactions may be mild or severe, the most severe being anaphylactic reactions, which can result in shock, respiratory failure and death.

Behavioral, psychological and neurological manifestations of food allergy suggested by unorthodox practitioners are controversial and have not been objectively documented. The *allergic tension fatigue syndrome (ATFS)* has been described to include hyperactivity, fatigue, lethargy, muscle and joint aches and behavioral learning disorders. This has been claimed by some clinicians to be associated with food allergy.[23] However, the role of food allergy in this syndrome is unproven; it is possible that these symptoms may develop as a result of discomfort associated with an allergic response in general.

Similarly, enuresis, rheumatoid arthritis and migraine headaches have been reported in association with food consumption. There is little evidence at this time supporting a casual association with food allergy. Other mechanisms may be involved if these types of reactions to food ingestion actually exist.

Table 31–1. MANIFESTATIONS OF FOOD ALLERGY

CONFIRMED MANIFESTATIONS OF FOOD ALLERGY

Reaginic

abdominal pain	asthma	rhinitis
allergic dermatitis	diarrhea	urticaria
anaphylaxis	pruritus	vomiting
angioedema	rash	

Non-reaginic

allergic dermatitis	enteropathies	urticaria
asthma	malabsorption	vomiting
contact dermatitis	occult or gross bleeding	
diarrhea	pneumonitis	

UNCOMFIRMED POSSIBLE MANIFESTATIONS OF FOOD ALLERGY

arthralgia	enuresis	neuralgias
arthritis	epilepsy	personality changes
canker sores	idiopathic fever	serous otitis media
cheilitis	intermittent hydroarthrosis	vertigo (Meniere's syndrome)
colic	menstrual irregularity	visual (amblyopia)
deafness	migraine headache	

Compiled from May C. D., and Bock, S. A.: A modern clinical approach to food hypersensitivity. Allergy, *33*:166, 1978; and Tuft, L.: Allergy Management in Clinical Practice, St. Louis, C.V. Mosby Company, 1973, p. 143.

Food Allergy Versus Food Intolerance

The majority of adverse food responses are not mediated by the immune system but instead are caused by food intolerance. Although an extensive discussion of food intolerance is beyond the scope of this chapter, recognition of the broad spectrum it may cover is essential for the differential diagnosis and appropriate management of food-related disorders. Food intolerances may be caused by chemical idiosyncrasies, contamination, gastrointestinal disorders, enzyme deficiencies or psychological factors. Manifestations of food intolerances include abdominal pain, diarrhea, asthma, urticaria and headaches and often mimic those of food allergy, as Table 31–2 indicates.

Responses to pharmacological agents in foods and lactase deficiency are food intolerances frequently confused with food allergy. Natural pharmacological agents in foods such as histamine, tyramine and phenylethylamine and those added to foods such as monosodium glutamate, sodium metabisulfite, sodium nitrate and tartrazine are thought to affect a small portion of the population. For example, individuals who take monoamine oxidase inhibiting drugs, which block the metabolism of tyramine, may be especially susceptible to the vasoactive effects of this substance (See page 420). Asthma episodes have been induced in asthmatic patients by monosodium glutamate or metabisulfite when consumed in the amounts often provided by a restaurant meal.[1,28] Chinese restaurant meals may provide 0.5 to 2.5 gm. of monosodium glutamate.[1] When potassium or so-

dium metabisulfite is added to salads and vegetables to preserve their fresh appearance, a single meal may result in consumption of up to 100 mg. of metabisulfite, 30 to 50 times the average daily consumption estimated from other food sources.[28] Tartrazine in yellow food dye number 5 and sodium nitrite, a preservative in smoked pork products, have been associated with asthma and urticaria, respectively, in a small portion of the population.

The association of food additives, dyes and sugars with hyperactivity is a popularly accepted notion. However, this relationship has not been supported by controlled studies. Food additives may elicit behavioral changes that may be due to toxicity rather than food allergy in a small subgroup of the population.[6] See Chapter 32 for further discussion of this topic.

Lactose intolerance may be easily confused with cow's milk protein allergy. Symptoms of diarrhea and abdominal pain are common to both and resolve with elimination of milk from the diet. However, lactose intolerance is caused by a deficiency of lactase in the small intestine. Sources of lactose-free cow's milk protein should be tolerated by the patient with lactose intolerance. Common in Blacks, Asians and Middle Eastern populations, lactose intolerance develops with increasing age. It may also develop following damage to the gastrointestinal mucosa caused by disease or allergy; this form is often transient, lasting two to three weeks. Occasionally, congenital lactose intolerance is reported. A history suggesting lactose intolerance can be confirmed by a lactose tolerance test or a hydrogen breath test. Mild cases can be diagnosed with a challenge test with milk treated with

Table 31-2. SPECTRUM OF FOOD INTOLERANCES

CAUSE	ASSOCIATED FOODS	SYMPTOMS DESCRIBED
Reaction to Pharmacological Agents in Foods		
Phenylethylamine	Chocolate, aged cheese, red wine	Migraine headaches
Tyramine	Cheddar cheese, French cheeses, brewers yeast, chianti, canned fish	Migraine headaches, cutaneous erythema, urticaria
Histamine	Fermented cheeses, fermented foods (e.g., sauerkraut), pork sausages, canned tuna, anchovy filets, sardines	Erythema, headaches, decreased blood pressure
Histamine releasing agents	Shellfish, chocolate, strawberries, tomatoes, peanuts, pork, ethanol, pineapple	Urticaria, eczema, pruritus
Methylxanthines	Coffee, tea, cola, chocolate	Neurological or hypertensive symptoms
Other foods taken in excess	Legumes, berries, apples, Jerusalem artichokes	Diarrhea, abdominal pain, flatulence
Reactions to Food Additives		
Monosodium glutamate	Oriental foods (esp. those prepared in restaurant)	Asthma, dizziness
Metabisulfites	Restaurant salads and potatoes, avocado dips, beer, wine, cordials, dried fruits and vegetables, vinegar, shrimp	Asthma
Tartrazine	FD&C yellow no. 5 in orange drinks, cake mixes, cheese curl snacks, macaroni and cheese dinner, gelatin, instant pudding, lemon candies	Asthma, urticaria, rhinitis, edema
Sodium nitrate	Cooked pork products, cheese	Urticaria, gastrointestinal disorders, headaches
Others (controversial)	Food additives, coloring, salicylates or sugar	Varied, includes hyperactivity, behavioral and psychological symptoms
Reactions to Toxins in Foods		
Endogenous	Specific mushrooms (*Amanita, Gyromira esculenta*)	Abdominal pain, vomiting, diarrhea, death
	Shellfish, mussels, clams, scallops, oysters	Numbness of fingers, paralysis, death
	Tropical fish including puffer fish, snapper, grouper, moray eel, sturgeon	Neurologic symptoms, death
Bacterial, e.g., botulism (one of many)	Improperly canned foods	Dysphagia, muscular weakness, difficulty breathing, death
Fungal, e.g., aflatoxin	Stored cassava beans, peas, cereals, ground nuts	Inhibited protein synthesis, death
Trace metals, e.g., mercury	Fish from contaminated water	Mental confusion, muscular disorders, numbness of extremities, death
Gastrointestinal Disorders		
Enzyme deficiency		
Lactase	Foods containing lactose (milk)	Bloating, flatulence, diarrhea, abdominal pain
Maltase	Foods containing maltose	
Sucrase	Foods containing sucrose	
G-G-PD*	Fava or broad beans	Hemolytic anemia
Disease		
Parasitic infection, cystic fibrosis, gallbladder disease, peptic ulcer, enteropathy, malignancy	Symptoms may be precipitated by any foods	Abdominal distention, abdominal pain, flatulence, diarrhea, vomiting
Physical disorders		
Obstruction hiatal hernia, dysphagia, feeding technique	Symptoms may be precipitated by any foods or by specific type or texture	Abdominal distention, diarrhea, constipation, abdominal pain, vomiting, aspiration
Inborn Errors of Metabolism†		
Phenylketonuria	Foods containing phenylalanine	Elevated serum phenylalanine levels, mental retardation
Maple syrup urine disease	Foods containing branched chain amino acids	Urine smells like maple syrup, increased BCAA ‡
Galactosemia	Foods containing lactose or galactose	Vomiting, lethargy, failure to thrive
Von Gierke's disease (lack of G-6-PD)§	Foods containing lactose or sucrose	Acidosis, hypoglycemia
Psychological Reactions	Symptoms may be precipated by any food	Wide variety, any system may be involved

* G-6-P = glucose-6-phosphatase.
† See Chapter 39.
‡ BCAA = branched chin amino acids.
§ G-6-PD = glucose-6-phosphate dehydrogenase.

Lactobacillus acidophilus. Treatment requires avoidance of lactose in milk. Lactose intolerance is further discussed in chapter 23.

Mechanisms of Food Allergy

An overview of the immune system is provided to help in understanding the disorders of the system that lead to allergic reaction to foods. The reader is referred to a text on immunology for a more complete discussion.[5]

The immune system functions to clear the body of foreign substances. A substance that elicits an immune response is an *antigen*. There are two principal parts of the immune system, humoral and cellular, as Figure 31–1 indicates. The *humoral system* involves immunoglobulins. *Immunoglobulins* or *antibodies* are produced by the host's B lymphocytes in response to the presence of an antigen. The interaction of immunoglobulins and antigens causes the production of direct cellular damage or chemical mediators, which are responsible for the effects of the humoral branch of the immune system. Five immunoglobulins (Ig) have been identified and seem to have different roles in the immune response: IgA, IgD, IgE, IgG and IgM. *IgA,* found in mucous secretions of the gastrointestinal and respiratory tracts, provides localized protection; it seems to block antigen penetration and so may be protective against food allergy. *IgM* is the antibody produced in early immune reactions. *Maternal IgG* crosses the placenta and plays a role in the immune protection of newborns. *IgM and IgG* may be involved in complement-mediated reactions. *IgE* is the antibody classically associated with allergic responses, although other antibodies are thought to play important roles as well. The role of *IgD* is as yet uncertain.

Cellular immunity or delayed hypersensitivity is accomplished by the action of T lymphocytes. When sensitized and activated by antigens, these cells enlarge, divide and release *lymphokines,* which participate in the attack on foreign proteins and are responsible for the effects of cellular immunity. T cells may also interact with the B cells, other T cells or macrophages to enhance or suppress antibody formation. *Macrophages* are white blood cells involved in the destruction of invading bacteria or foreign material.

Under normal conditions the antigen either interacts with an antibody and is cleared from the blood or is destroyed by lymphocyte action and no adverse response occurs. The presence of antigen-antibody complex or sensitized T cells in the blood does not necessarily indicate that an allergy exists, since these may represent normal response of the immune system to the antigen presented.

REAGINIC REACTIONS TO FOOD

Allergic reactions to food may be divided into two groups that reflect current understanding of the mechanisms involved. *Reaginic* responses are those that have been associated with specific IgE or IgG antibody. IgE antibodies are thought to interact with the antigen and then bind to the surface of mast or basophil cells, causing degranulation and the release of chemical mediators such as histamine. These mediators are responsible for the effects of immediate hypersensitivity reactions. Manifestations most often involve the skin, the gastrointestinal tract or the respiratory system and may include the following: anaphylaxis, abdominal pain, diarrhea, vomiting, angioedema, urticaria, rhinitis and asthma, as listed in Table 31–1. This response, usually evident within minutes to hours after food is ingested, is often referred to as an *immediate reaction.*

NON-REAGINIC REACTIONS TO FOOD

The mechanisms and manifestations of *non-reaginic* or *non–IgE-mediated* reactions have been less clearly defined than those of reaginic mechanisms. *Antigen–antibody complex–mediated reactions* and the cell-mediated immune response are two mechanisms that have been implicated in non-reaginic food allergy. In the

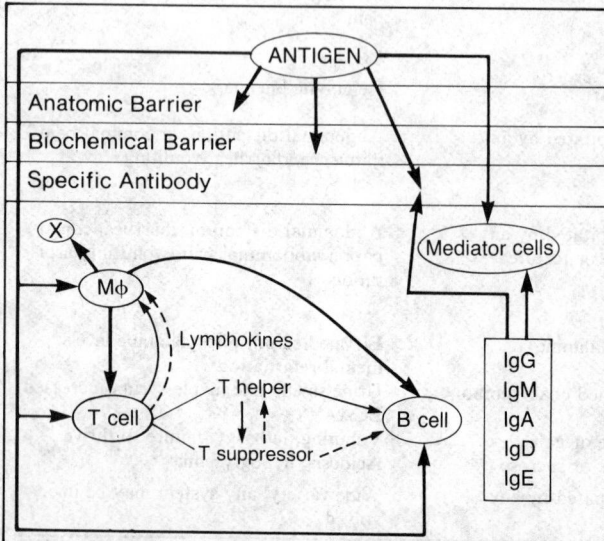

Figure 31–1. The immune system's response to an antigen. Mφ indicates macrophage. (Redrawn from Bierman, C. W., and Furukawa, C. T.: Food allergy. Ped. Rev., *3*(7):212, 1982.)

first, formation of a circulating antigen-antibody complex is thought to activate the complement system, a series of interacting enzymes, and result in cellular damage. *Cell-mediated immune responses*, or delayed hypersensitivity, involves the interaction of antigen and T cells. T cells multiply and produce lymphokines, which act through macrophages or other T cells or by direct cytotoxicity to produce the effects of delayed hypersensitivity. Manifestations of the non-reaginic reactions are most often gastrointestinal and include vomiting, diarrhea, occult blood loss and protein-losing enteropathy. Urticaria, allergic dermatitis, pneumonia and hemosiderosis have also been demonstrated.[8] Symptoms are often evident from 4 to 24 hours after the ingestion of food but may appear after 2 to 72 hours. Owing to the timing of the symptoms, this has been referred to as a *delayed response*. A delay in reaction may occur during digestion if the antigen is a breakdown product of a larger structure. In other cases it may be only the onset of a clinically observable symptom that is delayed; the reaction itself may be initiated immediately.[8, 20] The time lag between ingestion of food and the onset of symptoms often makes it difficult to identify the food causing a non-reaginic reaction.

Non-reaginic reactions are thought to be involved in the food-sensitive gastroenteropathies such as gluten-sensitive enteropathy (celiac disease) or cow's milk–sensitive enteropathy (CMSE), which cause mucosal damage and histological changes in the gastrointestinal tract.[8] Except for the gluten-sensitive form, non-reaginic reactions seem to be transient and occur most often in children less than three years old.[16]

Factors Influencing the Development of Allergic Reactions

Several steps must be completed to produce an allergic reaction with clinically significant symptoms. The extent of this process may explain some of the variability demonstrated in individuals' responses to antigens. An immune cell must be sensitized to the antigen before a reaction can occur (Fig. 31–3). In food allergy this is thought to happen primarily when the antigen enters the body by crossing the gastrointestinal mucosa and interacts with the lymphoid cell. Antigens may also cross the oral, nasal or respiratory mucosa or the skin. Because sensitization is a prerequisite, a food cannot cause an allergic reaction the first time it is introduced. With subsequent presentation the antigen must again cross the mucosa and then interact with the sensitized antibody or lympho-

cyte and produce chemical mediators, direct cellular damage or lymphocyte proliferation. Ultimately the development of clinically significant symptoms depends upon adequate response by the target organ. Antigens may invoke a response locally in the gastrointestinal tract or may be carried by the blood to a distant site in the body, and so manifestations of food allergy may affect any part of the body. Specific manifestations and the course of the reaction observed will vary with the amount of antigen absorbed, the types of reactions that occur and the sensitivity of the end organ.

Many additional factors are thought to influence the development and manifestations of food allergy. These include overstimulation of the normal immune system by excessive antigen contact, disorders of the immune system, antigen characteristics and the physiological or environmental conditions at the time of antigen presentation.

ANTIGEN PENETRATION

Infancy, immunodeficiency, malnutrition and gastrointestinal disorders may all lead to excessive antigen uptake and increase the risk of sensitization and an immune reaction. Secretory IgA retained in the mucous coat of the intestine may play a protective role by blocking antigen penetration. IgA deficiency associated with infancy or other immunodeficient states may be predisposing to antigen entry and food allergy. Permeability of the gut is thought to be greatest in infancy and to decrease after six months.[6] Permeability may be further increased by prematurity, since gut closure appears to increase with gestational age.[24] Gut permeability may also be increased by ischemia, infection, malnutrition or disease such as gastroenteritis in which the gastrointestinal cells have been damaged and the mucus destroyed. Gastrointestinal IgE-mediated reactions may cause increased capillary permeability and permit increased antigen penetration.

HEREDITY

Atopy, the tendency to develop IgE reactions, appears to be familial. In atopics the development of allergies may be increased due to a disorder of the immune system rather than increased antigen penetration.[11,12] Disorders of the immune system that promote increased IgE production are thought to include decreased T suppressor cell activity, increased T helper cell activity, or decreased macrophage action and antigen clearance.[6]

INDIVIDUAL VARIATION

Despite the familial nature of atopy, the specific food allergies and symptoms that develop often differ within a family, suggesting that additional factors cause individual variation. Patterns of antibody response to antigens and the tendency to form antigen-antibody complexes are individualized[15] and may affect the response demonstrated. Variation in the production of mediators, in end-organ response and in an individual's response to discomfort will also influence the symptoms demonstrated. Mechanical disorders of the gastrointestinal tract or disorders that favor aspiration may also increase the chance of development of food allergy.[15]

THE ANTIGEN

The characteristics of antigens presented seem to influence their tendency to elicit allergic responses although properties determining allergenicity have not been clearly identified. Food antigens are thought to be glycoproteins with a molecular weight of 18,000 to 36,000 daltons.[7] Foods contain many proteins, of which only a few may be associated with food allergy. For example, cow's milk contains over 20 proteins; alpha-lactalbumin, beta-lactoglobulin, casein, bovine serum albumin, and alpha-globulin appear to be the most sensitizing. Additional proteins characterized as antigens include egg white ovomucoid, allergen M of fish and kunitz soybean trypsin inhibitor in soy beans.[6] Foods frequently implicated in allergic reactions include cow's milk, soy, chicken eggs, peanuts, wheat, corn, peas, nuts, fish, shellfish, tomatoes, oranges, strawberries and chocolate. Nuts, cow's milk, chicken eggs and soy may be responsible for the majority of allergic reactions demonstrated.[8] Regional variation in foods commonly reported as allergens may be influenced by the presentation of different antigens or by environmental factors. Allergenicity seems to vary with the form of antigen presented and may be increased or decreased by cooking or by partial digestion. For example, demonstrated sensitivity to heated milk is sometimes less than sensitivity to unheated milk.

Cross-reactivity between antigens, especially within biological food families, may occur in some but not all individuals. An individual allergic to peanuts may also be sensitive to soy, and one allergic to cow's milk may be sensitive to goat's milk. Cross-reactivity between biological families is also thought to occur, although it has not been proven. The biological classifications of common foods are listed in Table 31–3.

Table 31–3. THE BIOLOGICAL CLASSIFICATION OF COMMON FOODS

PLANT FAMILIES

Apple (Pomaceae): apple, crab apple, loquat, medlar, pear, quince
Citrus (Rutaceae): bengal quince, citron, grapefruit, lemon, orange, tangerine
Cola nut (caffeine): coffee, chocolate, cola, cola drinks, tea
Goose foot (Chenopodiaceae): beet, spinach, Swiss chard
Gourd (Cucurbitaceae): cantaloupe, citron, cucumber, melon, pumpkin, squash, vegetable marrow
Grass (Graminaceae): barley, corn, oats, rice, rye, wheat
Heath (Ericaceae): blueberry, cranberry, huckleberry, loganberry
Laurel (Lauraceae): avocado, bay leaf, cinnamon
Lily (Liliaceae): asparagus, garlic, leek, onion, sarsaparilla
Mint (Labiatea): balm, basil, bergamot, marjoram, peppermint, oregano, sage, savory, spearmint, thyme
Morning glory (Convolvulaceae): sweet potato
Mustard (Cruciferae): broccoli, cabbage, cauliflower, mustard, Brussels sprout, horseradish, radish, turnip
Nightshade (Solanaceae): cape gooseberry, cayenne pepper, aubergine (eggplant), potato, tomato
Palm (Palmae): cabbage, coconut, date, palm oil
Parsley (Apiaceae): anise, caraway, carrot, celery, coriander, cumin, fennel, parsley
Pea: bean (including soybean), lentil, pea, peanut, alfalfa, clover, liquorice, tamarind
Pepper (Piperaceae): black pepper, white pepper
Plum (Amygdalaceae): almond, apricot, blackberry, cherry, peach, plum, sloe (gin)
Rose (Rosaceae): blackberry, black raspberry, raspberry, red raspberry, strawberry
Seaweeds: agar, longan
Sunflower (Compositaceae): artichoke, camomile, cardoon, celtuce, chicory, endive, lettuce, sunflower, tansy, tarragon
Walnut (Juglandaceae): black walnut, English walnut, hickory nut, pecan

ANIMAL CLASSES

Amphibia: frog
Birds: chicken, egg, duck, goose, pheasant, etc.
Crustaceans: crab, crayfish, lobster, prawn, shrimp
Fish (fish with fins): cod, flounder, halibut, salmon, sole, trout, tuna, etc.
Mammals: cow (milk), goat, lamb, pig, pork, rabbit, sheep, squirrel, etc.
Mollusks: abalone, clam, cockle, oyster, scallop, mussel

ADDITIVE EFFECT OF ALLERGENS AND IRRITANTS

The amount of antigen presented can also influence the response elicited. The effects of food and other allergens may be additive. Some foods may be tolerated in small amounts or when eaten infrequently but in large amounts may produce clinically significant symptoms. Food or non-food allergens that produce mild symptoms individually often cause a severe response collectively. Common non-food allergens include house dust mites, feathers, animal dander, pollens, molds and grain dust. Seasonal variation of food allergy is often reported; foods otherwise tolerated may produce symptoms at times when pollen allergies are exacerbated. Food allergies not manifested since early childhood may again become evident if new allergies develop in later life. Similarly, the effects of antigens that cross-react, such as peas and beans, may be additive. The effects of non-specific irritants such as tobacco smoke, stress, exercise and cold also appear to be additive and to enhance the clinical response to allergens.

Diagnosis of Food Allergy

Foods that cause severe allergic reactions with immediate onset of symptoms are usually readily identified. As the time between the ingestion of food and the onset of symptoms increases, or when symptoms are mild or subjective in nature, identification of the causative food becomes more of a challenge. The relationship between specific foods and symptoms may be obscured when the symptoms of illness or food intolerance are superimposed on those of food allergy or when the pattern of response is altered by environmental factors such as additional allergens or stress. Psychological components or firmly held beliefs may strongly influence the clinical response demonstrated, and it may be difficult to separate physiological from psychosomatic responses. Objective diagnosis of food allergy is needed to correctly identify foods causing an adverse response and to assure that foods are not removed from the diet unnecessarily. Diagnosis of food allergy requires identification of suspected foods, proof that the food causes an adverse response and verification of immunological involvement. Non-allergic causes of adverse responses must be ruled out.

HISTORY

A history is the first tool used in diagnosis. The collected information helps to characterize the nature of the response and to identify prob-

lem foods. Information gathered should include a description of symptoms from their onset to the time the history is taken. The frequency and duration of the reaction and patterns of response related to time or location should be noted. Foods consumed up to 72 hours before the reaction should be recorded and environmental and psychosocial conditions described. If a particular food is suspected, the amount of that food thought to cause the reaction should be determined.

Factors often associated with the development of food allergy should also be investigated. A food allergy may be initiated with the introduction of new foods. Delayed growth is often associated with untreated allergy. Therefore, early feeding history, patterns of growth and development and their relationship to the onset of symptoms should be explored. Current medical status and medical history should be reviewed. Conditions often associated with the development or manifestation of food allergy should be investigated. These include gastroenteritis, chronic ear infections, vomiting, diarrhea, atopic dermatitis (Fig. 31–2), rhinitis or asthma. Dark circles under the eye, called allergic shiners (Fig. 31–3) or the "allergic crease", a line on the nose caused by frequent nose rubbing, may also be apparent. Family history of allergy should be reviewed, since this may help to identify susceptible individuals.

FOOD RECORD

A record of all foods eaten and symptoms observed should be kept for at least two weeks. A chart such as that shown in Figure 31–4 may be

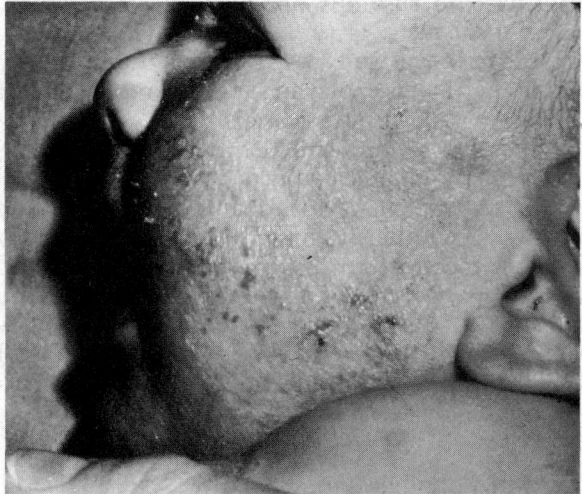

Figure 31–2. Eight-month-old infant with atopic dermatitis. (From Bierman, C. W., and Pearlman, D. S. (eds.): Allergic Diseases of Infancy, Childhood and Adolescence. Philadelphia, W. B. Saunders Company, 1980.)

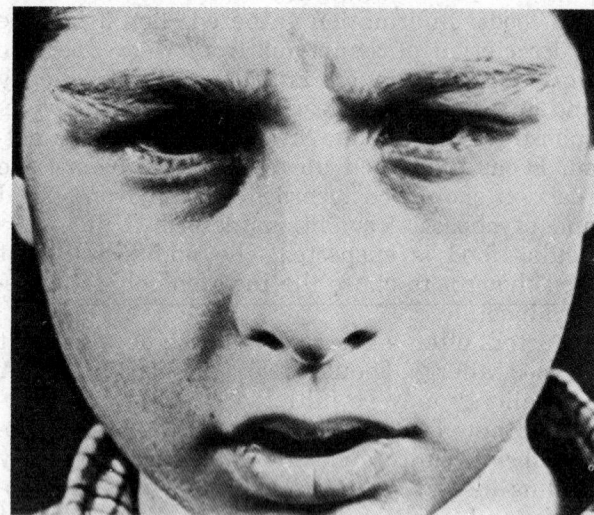

Figure 31–3. Allergic shiner. (From Leiberman, P. L., and Crawford, L. V.: Management of the Allergic Patient. New York, Appleton-Century-Crofts, 1982.)

used. Medications should also be recorded, since their effects may mask or mimic symptoms. This food symptom diary helps to document specific symptoms and may suggest relationships between diet and symptoms that are not evident upon recall. The diary will serve as a baseline for the evaluation of future intervention.

BIOCHEMICAL TESTS AND IMMUNOTESTING

When the history and food symptom diary do not clearly implicate specific foods, several laboratory tests may help to reveal problem foods and to establish an immunological basis for the adverse response reported. General screening tests used to rule out non-allergic disorders include blood tests; tests of stool for pH, reducing substances, ova and parasites or occult blood; xylose and lactose tolerance tests; and the sweat chloride test for cystic fibrosis.

The value of immunotesting to detect sensitization in the diagnosis of food allergy is controversial. Although no tests can be used alone to diagnose food allergy, some tests help to identify problem foods when properly administered and interpreted. Misuse of test results is potentially dangerous. Protein-energy malnutrition has been described in a child following the removal of 200 foods from the diet on the basis of demonstrated skin test reactivity alone.[26]

Tests of Reaginic Sensitization

The *scratch test* measures specific skin-fixed IgE. A small scratch is made on the skin and a drop of antigen applied. Development of a red wheal and flare indicates sensitization. *Puncture* or *prick tests* are similar to the scratch test, except that antigen is applied to the skin surface and the skin is then pricked, which allows antigen to enter the body. Currently skin testing appears to be the most reliable and cost-effective test of sensitization in food allergy. However, confirmation of positive skin tests by subsequent demonstration of adverse reaction to food has been described in less than half of the cases studied.[20] The usefulness of skin test results is limited by positive skin tests that may be associated with no evident clinical response (false positive) and by negative skin tests that may be associated with clinical symptoms (false negative). These discrepancies may occur for several reasons: (1) the skin tests can detect levels of sensitization that are less than that needed to cause clinically significant symptoms, (2) the single antigen isolated from the food being tested may not be the antigen causing the reaction and (3) the skin test detects only IgE and histamine mediated responses; others are undetected.

The *intradermal skin test* is similar to the scratch test except that antigen extract is injected intracutaneously. Because this test is approximately 100 times more sensitive than the skin test, it may detect antigen sensitivity too low to produce an adverse response of clinical significance. The intradermal test is the most sensitive available indicator of reaginic sensitization. It has the same limitations as the scratch test.

The *radioallergosorbent test (RAST)* is an *in vitro* assay to detect circulating antigen-specific IgE in blood. Circulating IgE may be subject to wide fluctuation and so be a less stable indicator of sensitization than skin testing.[20] RAST testing is no more reliable than skin testing, is more expensive and appears to be most useful in experimental rather than clinical situations.[20] However, one advantage of RAST over the skin test is that only a single blood sample is taken, and for some it may be less painful.

Total serum IgE levels are often elevated in atopic disease and may help to identify allergic individuals. However, determination of serum IgE is of limited diagnostic value since levels may be normal in some allergic individuals or may be elevated in non-allergic individuals with parasitic infections.

Tests of Non-Reaginic Sensitization

Gastrointestinal biopsy reveals histological changes of the small intestine and is used in combination with a food challenge to confirm a diagnosis of food-sensitive enteropathy. Other indicators of non-reaginic sensitization are currently used in research but are not of use clini-

Name _____

	DAY 1 DATE __	DAY 2 DATE __	DAY 3 DATE __	DAY 4 DATE __	DAY 5 DATE __	DAY 6 DATE __	DAY 7 DATE __
B R E A K F A S T							
SYMPTOMS							
SNACK SUPPLEMENTS							
L U N C H							
SYMPTOMS							
SNACK SUPPLEMENTS							
D I N N E R							
SYMPTOMS							
SNACK							
SYMPTOMS							
MEDICATION							

Figure 31–4. Food and symptom diary.

cally. These include quantitative serum levels of IgA, IgM and IgG measured after ingestion of specific foods, lymphocyte proliferative response tests, changes in complement level and the presence of circulating antigen-antibody complexes.[8]

Tests of Unproven Value in Diagnosis

Additional tests may be used but have no proven value in the diagnosis of food allergy. The *cytotoxic test* is an *in vitro* test in which white blood cells are incubated with a specific antigen and observed for changes in morphology. Evaluation is subjective and susceptible to error, and results frequently include many false positives. The cytotoxic test is not recommended.[3] *Intracutaneous or sublingual provocative testing* requires administration of the antigen under the skin or the tongue in sufficient quantity to provoke mild symptoms. There is no known immunological basis for this method of diagnosis.[3] The accelerated *pulse test* is performed by recording the pulse rate at specific time intervals after a suspected food is eaten. This test is based on claims that the heart rate increases after the ingestion of allergenic foods. There is little evidence that this is effective for diagnosis.

FOOD ELIMINATION AND CHALLENGE

History and skin test results are sometimes not compatible with the food response actually demonstrated. Diagnosis of clinically significant food allergy ultimately depends upon the demonstration of an adverse response when a food is eaten. This relationship is most reliably established by systematic *elimination* of suspected foods followed by their reintroduction or *challenge*. Symptoms will clear when foods that cause an adverse response are removed from the diet and will return when they are reintroduced. A food and symptom diary like that shown in Figure 31–4 should be kept throughout the evaluation period to document symp-

toms. Because the risks associated with anaphylactic reactions are great, foods thought to cause such a response are generally omitted from the diet without further challenge.

Trial Elimination Phase

Foods identified as possible allergens by history, food diary or positive skin tests are removed from the diet for 14 days. This allows time for symptoms to clear and may enhance the response observed upon reintroduction. Avoidance of all foods containing the selected food or its derivatives is required. For example, when cow's milk is eliminated, all dairy products must be avoided, including foods that contain ingredients such as non-fat dry milk solids, whey and sodium caseinate. Table 31–4 lists foods to be avoided in trial elimination tests for various allergies. Label reading and careful product selection are essential.

If symptoms do not clear with the elimination of foods initially implicated and food allergy is still suspected, progressively more restrictive elimination diets are implemented, as outlined in Table 31–5. Diet 1 omits the most common allergens including cow's milk, chicken eggs, and wheat. Diet 2 is a minimal elimination diet that excludes additional common allergens. On this diet all animal products except lamb and all cereals except rice are excluded, as are nuts, legumes, strawberries and citrus fruits. If symptoms persist additional foods can be omitted one by one. Some patients find it more effective and acceptable to create their own elimination diet consisting of only one or two foods from each food group that are known to be tolerated.

A nutritionally adequate hypoallergenic elemental diet such as Vivonex can be used as an alternative to the trial elimination diet (see also Table 35–7). It can be used to reduce testing time normally required for the elimination phase or when symptoms have persisted with the minimal elimination diet. A four- to five-day fast in which the patient receives only bottled

Table 31–4.   FOOD SELECTION IN FOOD ALLERGY

RESTRICTED FOODS	MAY BE LISTED ON LABEL	FOODS TO AVOID	SUBSTITUTES
Milk	Casein	Cheese	Mocha mix
	Caseinate	Cottage cheese	Coffee Rich
	Whey	Ice cream, yogurt	Soy formulas (Isomil, Prosobee)
	Lactalbumin	Creamed soups & sauces	Tofu
	Sodium caseinate	Butter & many margarines	Milk-free baked goods (often french bread)
	Lactose	Baked goods made with milk	
	Non-fat milk solids	Some "non-dairy" products	Nut milk*
	Cream	Candy (creams & milk chocolate)	Coconut milk
	Calcium caseinate	Custards & puddings	Supplement for calcium & vitamin D

Table continued on the following page

Table 31–4. FOOD SELECTION IN FOOD ALLERGY (*Continued*)

RESTRICTED FOODS	MAY BE LISTED ON LABEL	FOODS TO AVOID	SUBSTITUTES
Egg	Albumin Egg whites Egg yolks	Many baked goods Egg noodles Custards, pudding Mayonnaise, some salad dressings Hollandaise sauce Meringues Many egg substitutes (Eggbeaters) Some batter fried foods	Egg-free baked goods[†] Spaghetti Rice Some egg substitutes[†] (read label)
Wheat	(Enriched) flour Wheat germ Wheat bran Wheat starch Gluten Food starch Vegetable starch Vegetable gum	Baked goods made with wheat flour Crackers Macaroni Spaghetti Noodles Gravies, thickened sauces Fried food coating Baking mixes Soy sauce Hot dogs with wheat filler Batter fried foods Some sausages	Wheat-free breads,[†] crackers (rice cakes, special breads) Certain cold cereals (corn, barley, rice) Oatmeal or cream of rice Corn pasta[†] Bean threads (oriental) Rice Corn tortillas Popcorn Wheat-free cereal crumbs for "breading" Thickeners: cornstarch, rice flour, tapioca Flours: rye, rice, potato
Soy	Soy flour Soybean oil Vegetable oil Soy protein Soy protein isolate Textured vegetable protein (TVP) Vegetable starch Vegetable gum	Soy sauce Teriyaki sauce Worcestershire sauce Tuna packed in vegetable oil Tofu Baked goods or cereals that include soy Soy nuts Soy infant formulas (Isomil, Prosobee) Many margarines	Nut milk Coconut milk
Corn	Cornmeal Corn starch Corn oil Corn syrup (solids) Corn sweetener Corn alcohol Vegetable oil Vegetable starch Vegetable gum Food starch	Some baked goods Corn tortillas (chips, tacos) Popcorn Some cold cereals Corn syrup Pancake syrup Many candies Most baking powders	Wheat flour tortillas Thickeners: wheat, potato or rice flour Beet or cane sugar Maple syrup or honey Baking soda and cream of tartar (for leavening agent)
Chocolate	Cocoa Cocoa butter	Candy Baked goods Colas	Carob products
Beef	Shortening Lard Gelatin	Soups Bouillon Beef gravies and sauces Hot dogs Cold cuts	Pure vegetable shortening Turkey hot dogs
Pork	Shortening Lard	Bacon Sausage Hot dogs Baked beans and soups with pork	All-beef hot dogs and cold cuts Vegetarian baked beans Pure vegetable shortening

* See Table 31–7 for soy or cashew milk recipes.
† Products available from Ener-g Foods, 6901 Fox Avenue South, P.O. Box 24723, Seattle, Wash.

Table 31–5. TWO STAGES OF ELIMINATION DIETS

ELIMINATION DIET 1
(Milk-, Egg- and Wheat-Free)

	Allowed	Avoid
Animal protein sources	Lamb, chicken, turkey, beef, pork	Cow's milk, chicken eggs
Vegetable protein sources	Soy milk, soy beans, peas, other beans, lentils, peanuts	
Grains or alternate	White potato, sweet potato, yams, rice, tapioca, arrowroot, buckwheat, corn, barley, rye, millet, oats	Wheat
Vegetables	All vegetables	
Fruits	All fruits and juices	
Sweeteners	Cane or beet sugar, maple syrup, corn syrup	
Oils	Soy oil, corn oil, safflower oil, coconut oil, vegetable oil, olive oil, peanut oil, milk-free margarines	Butter and margarines that include milk
Other	Salt, all spices	

ELIMINATION DIET 2
(Minimal Elimination Diet)

	Allowed	Avoid
Animal protein sources	Lamb	All other animal protein: meat, fish, poultry, eggs and milk
Vegetable protein sources		Soy milk, soy beans, peas, other beans, lentils, peanuts, bean sprouts, all nuts
Grains or alternate	White potato, sweet potato, yams, rice, tapioca, buckwheat, arrowroot	Wheat, oats, corn, barley, millet, rye
Vegetables	All vegetables* except corn, peas	Corn, peas (tomatoes)
Fruits	All fruits and juices* except citrus fruits, strawberries, tomatoes	Citrus fruits, strawberries, tomatoes
Sweeteners	Cane or beet sugar, maple syrup	Corn syrup, corn syrup solids
Oils	Safflower oil, coconut oil, olive oil, sesame oil	Butter, margarine, vegetable oils, soy oil, corn oil, peanut oil, non-specific shortening or fats of animal origin
Other	Salt, pepper, all spices,* vanilla or lemon extract, baking soda and cream of tartar	Chocolate, coffee, tea, colas and other soft drinks, alcoholic beverages Corn starch, baking powder with corn-starch

* Suggest limiting number to five to minimize dietary variables.

water has also been used in diagnosis of food allergy. However, because of the dangers associated with fasting, this is contraindicated for children and must be carefully supervised in adults.

Elimination diets must be planned carefully for nutritional adequacy. Extensive elimination programs may be nutritionally inadequate and should be continued only as long as necessary. Alternative causes should be thoroughly investigated before restrictive diets are implemented, especially for children. If the diet is continued for several weeks, appropriate vitamin or mineral supplementation will be necessary.

A symptom-free baseline must be established in the elimination phase to make the evaluation of future food challenges possible. Ideally, the elimination process should be carried out in the absence of symptoms thought to be caused by other allergens or illness.

Challenge Phase

When symptoms have cleared, suspected foods can be reintroduced one at a time while the response is carefully observed and recorded. The return of symptoms confirms a positive history of an adverse response. A *double blind food challenge (DBFC)*, in which the patient and observer are unaware of the food being given, is the optimal form of challenge because it provides unbiased confirmation of adverse food response.[8, 20] A *single blind food challenge (SBFC)*, in which only the patient is unaware of the food being offered, is prone to observer bias but may still be informative. Foods for blind challenges can be concealed in opaque capsules or masked in another food for children not able to swallow capsules. In addition to the challenge food, a placebo must be offered in order to identify any response to the testing procedure itself. *Open*

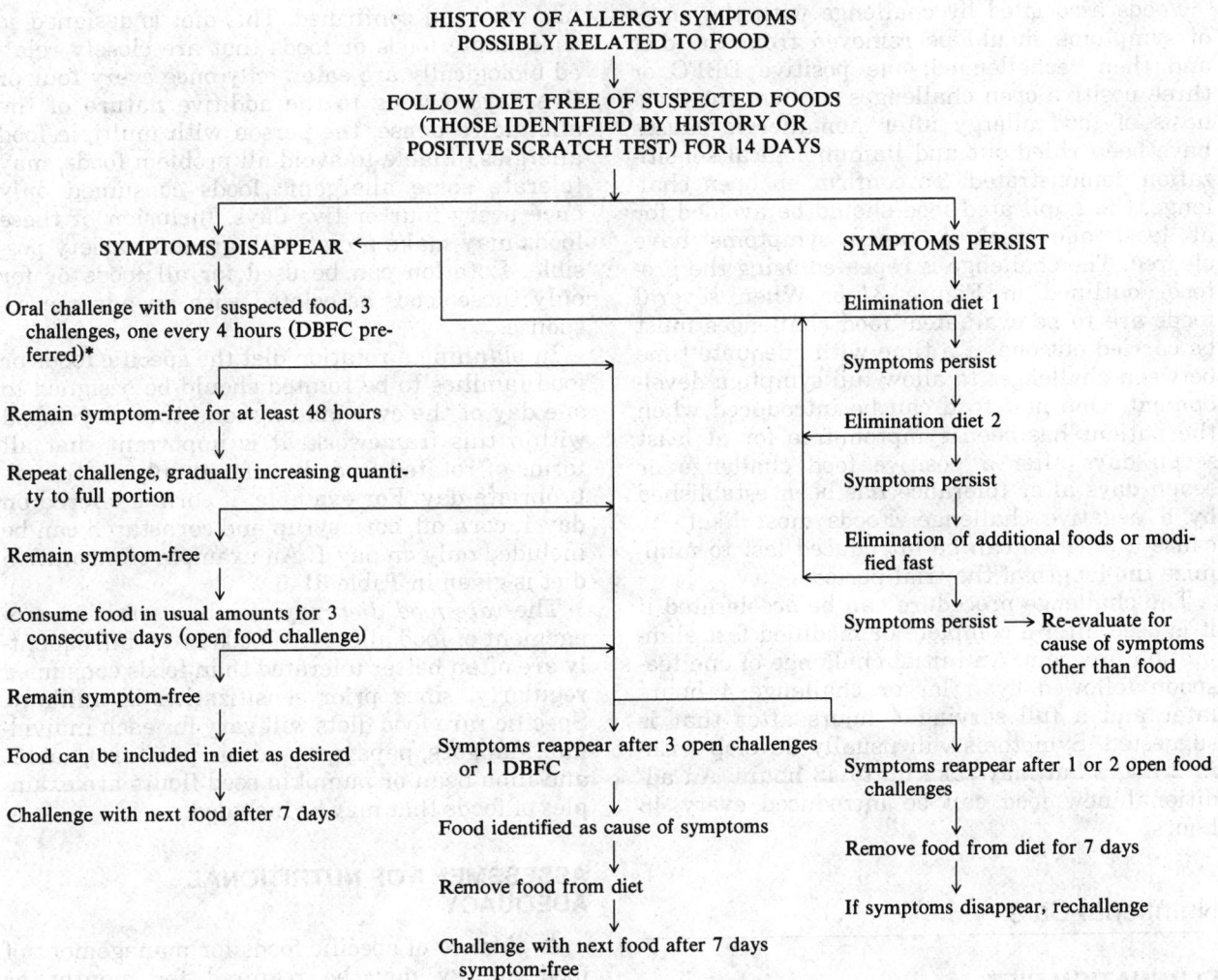

HISTORY OF ALLERGY SYMPTOMS POSSIBLY RELATED TO FOOD

FOLLOW DIET FREE OF SUSPECTED FOODS (THOSE IDENTIFIED BY HISTORY OR POSITIVE SCRATCH TEST) FOR 14 DAYS

SYMPTOMS DISAPPEAR

Oral challenge with one suspected food, 3 challenges, one every 4 hours (DBFC preferred)*

Remain symptom-free for at least 48 hours

Repeat challenge, gradually increasing quantity to full portion

Remain symptom-free

Consume food in usual amounts for 3 consecutive days (open food challenge)

Remain symptom-free

Food can be included in diet as desired

Challenge with next food after 7 days

Symptoms reappear after 3 open challenges or 1 DBFC

Food identified as cause of symptoms

Remove food from diet

Challenge with next food after 7 days symptom-free

SYMPTOMS PERSIST

Elimination diet 1

Symptoms persist

Elimination diet 2

Symptoms persist

Elimination of additional foods or modified fast

Symptoms persist ⟶ Re-evaluate for cause of symptoms other than food

Symptoms reappear after 1 or 2 open food challenges

Remove food from diet for 7 days

If symptoms disappear, rechallenge

Figure 31–5. The protocol for food challenge. *Challenge is not recommended for those foods associated with anaphylactic response, wheezing or asthma.

challenges in which the patient and observer are informed of the food being challenged can be used when resources preclude a blind food challenge. In open challenges the tester must be careful not to bias the patient toward positive findings.

The procedure for food challenge presented in Figure 31–5 is one that has been used effectively in a clinical setting. Details of the procedures suggested by different authors vary.[6, 15, 20]

Only those foods known to be well tolerated are included in the diet throughout the challenge period. The first food challenge is made after a six-hour fast. One suspected food is offered in the amount suggested by history to cause an adverse response. If that quantity is unknown, a small amount is used; 10 mg. to 2 gm. of dried food can be offered in capsule form[20]

and up to 1 tsp. offered in masked or open form. If no reaction is observed, two successively larger challenges are made at four-hour intervals. If the patient remains symptom-free for 48 hours the food is then provided daily, and portions are gradually increased to a full standard serving or the equivalent amount of dried food. After 8 gm. of dried food have been offered in double blind fashion without evidence of adverse reaction, open food challenges are instituted.[20] Standard-sized portions of the suspected food are then offered on three consecutive days and symptoms monitored carefully. If no symptoms are observed the food can be ruled out as the cause of the adverse response and incorporated into the diet as tolerated. Symptoms not evident at this point rarely develop after long-term exposure to the food.

Foods associated by challenge with the onset of symptoms should be removed from the diet and then rechallenged; one positive DBFC or three positive open challenges confirm the diagnosis of food allergy after non-allergic causes have been ruled out and immunological sensitization demonstrated. To confirm an open challenge, the implicated food should be avoided for at least one week or until symptoms have cleared. The challenge is repeated using the protocol outlined in Figure 31–5. When several foods are to be evaluated, food challenges must be carried out one at a time with adequate time between challenges to allow full symptom development. One new food can be introduced when the patient has been symptom-free for at least seven days after a positive food challenge or seven days after tolerance has been established by a negative challenge. Foods most likely to cause a reaction can be introduced last to minimize the length of the trial period.

The challenge procedure can be accelerated if it is used after a complete or modified fast elimination program. An initial challenge of one teaspoon followed by a larger challenge 4 hours later and a full serving 4 hours after that is suggested. Symptoms will usually develop within 2 hours but may take up to 48 hours. An additional new food can be introduced every 48 hours.

Nutritional Care

ELIMINATION DIET

Basic management for food allergy calls for elimination of the offending food from the diet. This may be accomplished easily if only a few foods must be avoided. The planning and implementation of an adequate diet to accommodate multiple food allergies is more difficult. All foods containing the identified food allergens or their derivatives are omitted from the diet. As in the trial elimination diet, it is important to select foods carefully. The elimination diet may be modified on an individual basis to include specifically tolerated forms of otherwise untolerated foods. A wide range of tolerances is likely to exist, since many factors influence the immune response. Some individuals develop symptoms after any contact with the food allergen, while others tolerate small amounts of the food in the cooked form or when eaten infrequently.

ALTERNATIVE DIETS

The *rotation diet* may be clinically useful for management of dose-related food reactions. However, the scientific basis for its effectiveness has not been confirmed. This diet is designed so that single foods or foods that are closely related biologically are eaten only once every four or five days. Owing to the additive nature of the allergic response, the person with multiple food allergies, unable to avoid all problem foods, may tolerate some allergenic foods consumed only once every four or five days. Inclusion of these foods may make a diet with greater variety possible. Rotation can be used for all foods or for only those foods associated with an adverse response.

In planning a rotation diet the specific foods or food families to be rotated should be assigned to one day of the cycle and a menu then developed within this framework. It is important that all forms of rotated foods be offered only on the appropriate day. For example, if corn is offered on day 1, corn oil, corn syrup and cornstarch can be included only on day 1. An example of a rotation diet is given in Table 31–6.

The *rare food diet* may also be useful in management of food allergy.[14] Foods eaten infrequently are often better tolerated than foods consumed regularly, since prior sensitization is unlikely. Specific rare food diets will vary for each individual. Mangoes, papayas, venison, poi (taro), rabbit and lima bean or pumpkin seed flours are examples of foods that may be included.

ASSESSMENT OF NUTRITIONAL ADEQUACY

Avoidance of specific foods for management of food allergy may be required for months or years. Therefore, after a diet change has been made, follow-up care is essential to assure that the diet is nutritionally adequate, effective for the control of symptoms and well accepted by the individual.

When a food is removed from the diet, alternative sources for the nutrients previously provided by that food must be planned. For example, the calcium, vitamin D, protein and energy previously supplied by milk must be replaced when a milk-free diet is implemented. Evaluation of food records and monitoring of nutritional status and growth patterns are all important in assessing the adequacy of the diet.

When the appropriate diet is followed carefully, an individual should remain symptom-free. If symptoms persist or reappear although identified food allergens have been carefully avoided, additional sources of allergens or alternative non-allergic causes for the symptoms should be investigated. If symptoms that initially improved with the removal of a specific food later reappear, the possibility of allergy or intolerance to its replacement food should be considered.

Table 31–6. FOUR-DAY ROTATION DIET

	DAY 1	DAY 2	DAY 3	DAY 4
B R E A K F A S T	Wheatina Fresh peaches Peanut butter Wheat toast	Oatmeal Banana Oat muffin* Orange juice Corn oil margarine	Chicken eggs Fresh strawberries Rye Krisp Grapes Soy oil margarine	Cow's milk Cream of rice Pineapple Butter
S N A C K	Peach nectar	Pear nectar or banana	Grapes	Plain yogurt with pineapple or plums

L U N C H	Sandwich
	  Wheat bread†
	  Peanut butter
	  or
	  Chicken, lettuce
	Fresh peach or apple
		Corn tortilla
		Chopped tomato
		Hamburger patty
		Orange or pear
			Rye Krisp
			Tuna salad made with soy
			  oil mayonnaise
			Strawberries
			Sliced carrots
				Sandwich
				  Rice bread
				  Turkey or cheese
				Pineapple

S N A C K	Apple juice Wheat crackers with peanut butter	Orange Corn chips made with corn oil	Grape juice Rye Krisp	Pineapple juice Cheese

D I N N E R	Sweet potato
	Broccoli
	Chicken
	Lettuce salad
	Vinegar and safflower oil
	  dressing
	Safflower margarine
		Corn pasta
		Tomato sauce with ham-
		  burger
		Tomato/cucumber salad
		Lemon juice/corn oil
		  dressing
			Chopped carrots
			Pork chops
			Spinach salad with
			  chopped egg
			Soy oil mayonnaise
			Rice
				Pineapple with cottage
				  cheese salad
				Roasted turkey
				Potatoes
				Peas
				Rice-cranberry muffin‡

S N A C K	Applesauce	Popcorn	Strawberries	Plums

*Made without eggs and milk; egg and milk substitutes and corn oil used.
† Made without milk and with safflower oil.
‡ Made with egg substitute.

METHODS FOR LONG-TERM ELIMINATION OF SPECIFIC FOODS

A treatment diet is effective only when implemented. It may be difficult to eliminate specific foods from the diet, especially favorite foods or those that appear frequently in the food supply such as wheat, chicken egg, or cow's milk. Specific suggestions about how to implement the required diet, as well as consideration of the psychological and social impact of following a special diet, may help an individual to follow the diet successfully.

First, it is essential to identify the dietary sources of the foods to be eliminated. Many of these are not easily recognized, so tips for label reading and information about the specific foods to be avoided and acceptable alternatives as listed in Table 31–4 may be helpful for the patient. Ingredients used in baking and cooking and those found in prepared foods may be the most difficult to identify and eliminate. For example, non-specific vegetable shortenings, starches and gums as well as cornstarch, corn oil, corn sweeteners and baking powder that contains cornstarch may not be tolerated by the person who is allergic to corn and should be excluded from a corn-free diet. Suggestions for cooking without specific foods such as wheat, milk, eggs and chocolate are shown in Tables 23–11 and 31–7.

Dietary changes also have psychological and social impacts. Persons following a special diet may need support to cope with feelings of being different. They may experience social pressures to eat the foods they are allergic to in order to be accepted or to avoid offending a host or hostess. They may need to respond to those who insist that "a little bit won't hurt." When an individual is not responsible for his own food supply or receives food from a variety of

Table 31–7.   COOKING FOR THE ALLERGIC PERSON: ALTERNATIVE INGREDIENTS

Milk: Use herbal tea or fruit juice in recipes calling for milk. They add a spicy fragrance to cookies, cakes, puddings and breads.

Use soy or cashew milk for milk replacement. Combine 1 cup soy powder or ground cashews with 3 cups water in a large saucepan. Whisk until well dissolved. Bring to a boil over high heat, stirring constantly. Lower heat and simmer for three minutes. Serve hot or cold. Makes 3 cups.

Corn: If a recipe calls for cornstarch, substitute equal amounts of arrowroot or potato starch or double the amount of whole wheat, soy or barley flour.

Most baking powders include cornstarch. Make corn-free baking powder by combining ¼ tsp. baking soda with ½ tsp. cream of tartar. This is equivalent to 1 tsp. baking powder.

Egg: In baking, you can achieve the emulsifying effect of one egg by combining 2 tbsp. whole wheat flour, ½ tsp. oil, ½ tsp. baking powder and 2 tbsp. milk, water or fruit juice. Egg substitutes are also available.

Chocolate: Use carob powder measure for measure when substituting for cocoa. As a substitute for one square of chocolate, use 3 tbsp. carob powder plus 2 tbsp. milk, water, or butter or margarine.

Wheat: Wheat flour replacements and tips for cooking with wheat are listed in Table 23–11.

sources, planning and coordination are necessary to assure that the diet can be consistently followed. For example, if a child spends the day at school or under the care of a babysitter it is essential that all caretakers and food providers understand and accommodate special dietary needs.

Medications

Medications may aid in the management of food allergies that cannot be controlled by diet alone. Oral administration of *sodium cromoglycate* before ingestion of food allergens decreases clinical and histological symptoms of food allergy for some patients; this medication is thought to act locally on the gastrointestinal mucosa to block mast cell degranulation and may inhibit an increase of intestinal permeability.[29] *Aspirin* taken before eating or drinking has also been used effectively to minimize gastrointestinal symptoms of food allergy. However, aspirin is known to induce asthma episodes in some asthmatics and so may not be appropriate for many allergic patients. *Antihistamines* and *theophylline* can be useful for symptomatic treatment of food allergy. Corticosteroids may be necessary in severe cases. Associated side effects include weight gain, delayed growth in stature and increased nutrient requirements as well as gastrointestinal and psychological disturbances (see Chapter 21).

Additional treatments for food allergy have been reported. However, their efficacy is not documented and their use is not widely accepted. Alkali salts such as *sodium carbonate* have been described to neutralize the effects of food allergy.[22, 23] The mechanism is unknown but may involve psychological components. Beneficial effects of large doses of *ascorbic acid* to alleviate common symptoms of allergy have been de-

scribed but not substantiated in controlled trials.[13] Anecdotal reports suggesting that *lysine* tablets relieve the symptoms of food allergy for some individuals are also undocumented.

Desensitization with food extracts administered orally or subcutaneously has been described. There is no evidence to support the effectiveness of desensitization, and it is contraindicated in reaginic food allergy. Reports of successful oral desensitization in the past may have been due to psychological factors or a natural decrease in sensitivity unrelated to treatment.

Prognosis

Many food allergies tend to resolve with age. Allergies to peanuts, fish, shrimp and nuts appear to be the least likely to resolve with age.[9] Children less than three years old when food allergy is confirmed are more likely to be able to ingest that food without symptoms when they become older than children over three years old when the allergy is confirmed.[9] Food sensitive enteropathies are often transient and tend to resolve by two to three years of age. In IgE-mediated reactions, if a food is avoided, serum IgE may decrease and in some cases sensitivity is decreased. Positive skin tests may persist even when a food is tolerated and so may not be useful for identification of changes in tolerance. Individuals who attach firmly to their food beliefs may not be willing to investigate or recognize a change in sensitivity.[9]

Since food sensitivity may decrease with age, it is important to rechallenge with avoided foods after 6 to 12 months to assure that foods are not restricted unnecessarily. Generally, foods that have caused anaphylactic reactions are not rechallenged. However, if the restriction of a specific food is difficult for an individual to accept or implement, a food challenge can be done. The challenge with foods previously associated with an anaphylactic response should be carried out in the presence of a trained medical staff, in facilities equipped to treat the symptoms of anaphylaxis. A small amount of food should just contact the tongue for the initial challenge; if no symptoms develop, a small amount of food can be ingested on the second challenge and then the amount gradually increased as tolerated.

Food Allergy in Infancy

Allergy to cow's milk protein is the most common food allergy in infancy, followed by allergy to soy protein. Although only cow's milk protein allergy (CMPA) will be reviewed here, many of the manifestations and principles of management for CMPA can be applied to soy protein allergy as well.

Cow's milk protein allergy (CMPA) is thought to affect from 0.3 to 12 per cent of the pediatric population.[16] The average age of onset is approximately three months.[16] CMPA commonly occurs in infants with a family history of atopy or CMPA. Disorders of the immune system, increased gastrointestinal permeability, transient IgA deficiency or gastrointestinal damage secondary to gastroenteritis may all facilitate sensitization to cow's milk protein.

Reaginic and non-reaginic mechanisms are thought to be involved in CMPA. However, because evidence of an immunological reaction is not always available in clinical practice, the term cow's milk protein intolerance is preferred to cow's milk protein allergy by some clinicians.[16]

Manifestations of CMPA can vary greatly. Gastrointestinal symptoms such as vomiting, abdominal pain and diarrhea are common. Similar symptoms are caused by lactase deficiency. Untreated, either condition may lead to persistent diarrhea and malabsorption causing malnutrition and growth failure. Differential diagnosis is essential for appropriate treatment. Cutaneous, respiratory or systemic responses may occur as well. These include eczema, urticaria, wheezing, asthma and anaphylaxis. Diseases such as cow's milk–sensitive enteropathy and Heiner's syndrome may have an immunological basis and be a part of CMPA as well.

Cow's milk–sensitive enteropathy (CMSE) is a disease of the small intestine that may be caused by a non-reaginic immunologic reaction to cow's milk protein. CMSE can occur in acute or chronic form, and acute CMSE is thought to be more common than the chronic form. CMSE is characterized by a flattening of the jejunal villi, similar to that seen in celiac disease. Manifestations include the onset of diarrhea and vomiting 12 to 48 hours after ingestion of cow's milk.

Symptoms of chronic CMSE include iron-unresponsive hypochromic anemia, edema, hypoalbuminemia, peripheral eosinophilia, intermittent vomiting and diarrhea, and failure to thrive associated with occult blood and protein loss from the small intestine. A secondary enzyme deficiency such as lactase deficiency may occur and may persist after the symptoms of CMSE have cleared.

In the past, diagnosis of CMSE has been made through clinical evaluation and improvement with the removal of cow's milk and recurrence with multiple challenges. Definitive diagnosis of CMSE can now be made with a single milk challenge and serial gastrointestinal biopsies. The biopsy will be abnormal upon initial presentation and challenge and normal after the elimination of cow's milk. Laboratory tests such as serum levels of antibodies have not been found to correlate well with symptoms.[20]

Similar transient food-sensitive enteropathies have been described in association with soy and wheat,[16] and less often in association with chicken, fish and rice.[2] CMSE may be characteristic of other food-sensitive enteropathies.[16]

Heiner's syndrome is a rare syndrome of unknown etiology characterized by recurrent pulmonary disease, gastrointestinal symptoms, iron deficiency anemia, failure to thrive, eosinophilia, and serum precipitins to cow's milk protein.[4] This disorder has resolved with avoidance of cow's milk in some infants. Reaginic and non-reaginic immunological mechanisms may be involved.[20]

The management of CMPA, as well as CMSE and Heiner's syndrome, calls for the elimination of cow's milk from the diet. For the infant a cow's milk replacement should be of high nutritional quality and designed to meet estimated nutritional needs. Substitutes for cow's milk are listed in Table 31–8. Homemade formulas, banked human milk and pasteurized goat's milk are additional alternatives. The replacement should be selected on the basis of demonstrated tolerance and individual preference. Clearly, infants with allergy to soy should avoid soy-based formulas. The source of carbohydrate should be taken into account for infants with disaccharidase deficiencies. Protein hydrolysate formulas (e.g., Pregestimil) and elemental diet formulas (Table 31–8) may also be alternatives. Cow's milk and soy formulas appear to be equally allergenic;[21] soy intolerance is reported in up to 40 per cent of the infants demonstrating CMPA.[16] Cross-reactivity between goat's milk and cow's milk has been demonstrated and some infants

Table 31–8. SOME ALTERNATIVES TO COW'S MILK FORMULAS FOR INFANTS*

FORMULA	KCAL./OZ.	PROTEIN SOURCE	CARBOHYDRATE SOURCE	FAT SOURCE	INDICATION
Infant Formulas					
Human milk	22	Lactalbumin, casein	Lactose	Human milk	Cow's milk protein allergy (CMPA), soy allergy
Isomil	20	Soy protein	Sucrose, corn syrup solids	Coconut oil, soy oil	CMPA, lactose intolerance, galactosemia
Prosobee	20	Soy protein	Corn syrup solids	Soy oil	CMPA, lactose intolerance, galactosemia, post-gastroenteritis
Soyalac	202	Soy protein	Soybean, sucrose, corn syrup	Soy oil	CMPA, lactose intolerance
Nutramigen	20	Casein hydrolysate	Modified tapioca, sucrose	Corn oil	CMPA, lactose intolerance, soy allergy, multiple food allergies, galactosemia
Pregestimil	22	Casein hydrolysate	Modified tapioca, corn syrup solids	MCT oil, corn oil	CMPA, soy allergy, multiple food allergies, disaccharidase deficiencies
CHO-Free	20	Soy protein		Soy oil, corn oil	Disaccharidase deficiencies, carbohydrate malabsorption
Meat Base Formula	20	Beefhearts	Modified tapioca, sucrose	Sesame oil	CMPA, soy allergy, galactosemia
Elemental Formulas					
Flexical	30	Casein hydrolysate, amino acids	Tapioca starch, corn syrup solids	Soy oil, MCT oil	Multiple food allergies, disorders of digestion and absorption
Precision	30	Egg albumin, sodium caseinate	Glucose oligosaccharides, sucrose	Vegetable oil	Multiple food allergies, disorders of digestion and absorption
Vital	30	Partially hydrolyzed whey, soy and meat protein, free amino acids	Glucose oligosaccharides, glucose polysaccharides	MCT oil, safflower oil	Multiple food allergies, disorders of digestion and absorption
Vivonex	30	Amino acids	Glucose, glucose oligosaccharides	Safflower oil	Multiple food allergies, disorders of digestion and absorption

* Also see Table 12–1 and Table 35–7 for complete analysis.

may react to both. Use of goat's milk requires supplementation with vitamins A, D, C and B$_{12}$ and folic acid. Its high solute load makes it inappropriate for young infants. Feedings of casein hydrolysate or elemental formula are recommended following the acute phase of CMSE to minimize the risk of sensitization to alternative feedings. However, the osmolarity of elemental formulas as listed in Table 35–7 is high and tolerance may have to be built up gradually.

The clinical symptoms of CMPA in infancy, including CMSE, often resolve by three years of age.

COLIC

Food allergy, especially CMPA, has been suggested as one of many possible causes of infantile colic. However, its role remains controversial. Maternal diet seems to influence the development of colic in breast-fed infants; the rate of colic may increase with increased vari-

ety in the mother's diet.[10] However, symptoms of colic have not been unequivocally linked to maternal milk intake.[10, 16] Diet also appears to influence symptoms of colic in some formula-fed infants. Symptoms of colic have been associated with cow's milk or soy feedings.[19] Infants who clearly demonstrate atopy or exhibit a return of symptoms with milk challenge may benefit from a trial milk-free diet. However, the treatment of colic by elimination of cow's milk may have primarily a placebo effect and be unwarranted for most other infants.[16]

INTOLERANCE TO BREAST MILK

Although uncommon, sensitivity to breast milk has been reported and may be suspected when a breast-fed infant does not tolerate feedings. Adverse responses may be caused by allergic reactions or by intolerances to substances consumed by the mother that pass into the breast milk. Prenatal sensitization to foods ingested during pregnancy may occur.[25] Breast milk allergy is most likely to develop in infants with a family history of atopy.

Cow's milk and chicken eggs appear to be the most common allergens in breast milk. Adverse responses, not necessarily documented to be allergic reactions, have been associated with the following foods: apples, bananas, coffee, tea, strawberries, cabbage, onions, garlic, turnips, radishes, rhubarb, spinach and spices.

Causes for adverse response should be investigated before discontinuation of breast-feeding is considered. If breast feedings are supplemented by food or formula, adverse response to these should first be ruled out. A hypoallergenic protein hydrolysate formula is suggested if a supplement is required to meet nutritional needs during this time. If symptoms persist or if no supplement is used, suspected foods, including cow's milk and eggs or those foods frequently eaten by the mother prior to the onset of symptoms, should be eliminated from the mother's diet for one week.[25] If the infant's symptoms clear, return with maternal food challenge, and clear again with the second elimination, the suspected food is thought to be the cause of symptoms. If symptoms persist, alternative antigen sources or non-allergic causes should be investigated as in the standard elimination/challenge format. Supplementation may be necessary to meet the mother's nutritional needs if dietary eliminations are extensive.

Identified food allergens should be avoided by the mother while breast-feeding continues and eliminated from the infant's diet for six months.[25] If the infant remains asymptomatic for six months, foods can be reintroduced. If symptoms are not resolved by the elimination of suspected foods and other causes of adverse response have been ruled out, an alternative to breast milk such as a hypoallergenic protein hydrolysate formula may be tolerated.

Prevention of Food Allergy

Initial feeding practices may influence the development of allergic disease, especially for infants with a family history of atopy. Whether the development of allergic diseases can be avoided or simply delayed is unknown.

Exclusive breast-feeding appears to be protective against the development of atopic disease and is recommended for the potentially atopic child.[27] The IgA provided in breast milk may protect against antigen entry. Alternative feedings of cow's milk may promote the development of allergy through alterations of intestinal flora[27] or by causing altered humoral and cell mediated responses to antigens.[17] Although the optimal duration of breast-feeding as the sole nutrient source may vary for each infant, four to six months is suggested.[4, 6, 27] When breast-feeding is impossible, expressed human milk or a hypoallergenic hydrolyzed cow's milk formula may be the optimal alternatives.

Avoidance of supplemental foods is recommended for the first four to six months of life.[6] Introduction of solid foods thought to be least allergenic is suggested, starting with rice, barley or oats followed by fruits, vegetables and finally meats. The addition of cow's milk, chicken eggs, wheat, fish and meats should be delayed until 9 to 12 months of age.[4, 6, 27] Foods should be added to the diet individually, with a new food added no more frequently than every two weeks. The sensitizing potential of foods is not thought to be proportional to the quantity of food presented. In fact, small amounts of milk supplements given to a breast-fed infant appear to be more sensitizing than large amounts.[12, 27] Small doses of antigen may stimulate T helper cells, whereas large doses may stimulate T suppressor cells and inhibit IgE production. Susceptibility to antigen-specific sensitization may be increased following episodes of gastroenteritis, so potentially sensitizing feedings should be avoided at these times; breast milk or a hydrolyzed cow's milk formula is recommended.

Summary

Food allergy has been defined as an adverse response to foods mediated by immunological reactions. Food allergy must be differentiated from food intolerance, an adverse response not mediated by the immune system, so that treatment can address the underlying disorder. Food intolerances may be caused by enzyme deficiencies, chemical idiosyncrasies and physiological or psychological disorders.

Symptoms of food allergy cover a wide range and can be systemic, gastrointestinal, cutaneous or respiratory. The development and manifestations of food allergy are shaped by a multitude of factors which include individual variations, genetic predisposition and physical status as well as antigen characteristics, environmental conditions and the nature of the immunological reaction that occurs.

The diagnosis of food allergy requires demonstration of a relationship between food eaten and symptoms displayed, and identification of immunologic involvement after other causes for the adverse response have been ruled out. Food allergy must be evaluated in a systematic way to assure that foods are not removed from the diet arbitrarily. It is important to assure that modifications implemented for the treatment of food allergy do not compromise nutritional adequacy of the diet. Since sensitivity to foods may change with age, food allergy should be re-evaluated periodically to assure that dietary restrictions are not continued unnecessarily.

Although much is known about food allergy, toxins and pharmacological agents in food, controversy exists about foods related to certain chronic illnesses and vague somatic complaints. A wide variety of approaches to diagnosis and management exist. It is important for clinicians to distinguish between acceptable practices compatible with current scientific knowledge and those apparently not based on scientific understanding and not acceptable to traditional allergists. As the understanding of food allergy improves, definitive methods for diagnosis and management may become more evident and the controversy that surrounds food allergy may diminish.

Problems and Suggested Topics for Discussion

1. An eight-year-old is allergic to wheat and eggs.
   a. What foods should be avoided?
   b. What are likely to be "hidden" sources of wheat or eggs that may be hard to identify?
   c. What alternatives for wheat and egg products would you suggest for breakfast, a packed lunch, dinner and snacks?
2. Outline the procedure for diagnosis of food allergy.
3. An eight-month-old infant has experienced intermittent diarrhea and vomiting since solid foods were introduced at six months. What information should be collected in the initial interview to help with evaluation of possible food allergy?
4. Which laboratory tests are useful for investigation of food allergy and which are not? What are the limitations for each test?
5. Allergies to 35 foods diagnosed by RAST are reported in a six-year-old. These foods have been excluded from the diet for the past two years. The current diet includes only chicken, rice, vegetables and fruit.
   a. What are likely nutritional concerns?
   b. How would you explain the need for further investigation of food allergy to this patient and his or her family?
   c. Devise a plan for the initial investigation of reported allergies.
6. Cow's milk protein intolerance has been confirmed for a one-year-old and a five-year-old child. For each patient:
   a. What are the calcium and vitamin D needs?
   b. How can these needs be met?
   c. What is the prognosis?
7. What are common food allergens? What foods are often associated with food intolerances?
8. An atopic woman is concerned about possible food allergies in her infant. What feeding recommendations would you make for the infant at birth, 6 months and 1 year?

Cited References

1. Allen, D.H., et al.: Monosodium glutamate induced asthma. J. Allergy Clin. Immunol., 71:98, 1983.
2. Allergy to other dietary proteins in infants with intolerance to cow's milk protein. Nutr. Rev., 40:334, 1982.
3. American Academy of Allergy: Position statements—controversial techniques. J. Allergy Clin. Immunol., 67:333, 1981.
4. Bahna, S.L., and Heiner, D.C.: Allergies to Milk. New York, Grune & Stratton Inc., 1980.
5. Beall, G.N.: Allergy and Clinical Immunology. New York, John Wiley & Sons, Inc., 1983.
6. Bierman, C.W., and Furukawa, C.T.: Food allergy. Pediatr. Rev., 3:213, 1982.
7. Bierman, C.W., and Pearlman, D.S.: Allergic Diseases of Infancy, Childhood and Adolescence. Philadelphia, W.B. Saunders Company, 1980.
8. Bock, S.A.: Food sensitivity: A critical review and practical approach. Am. J. Dis. Child., 134:973, 1980.
9. Bock, S.A.: The natural history of food sensitivity. J. Allergy Clin. Immunol., 69:173, 1982.
10. Evans, R.W., et al.: Maternal diet and infantile colic in breast-fed infants. Lancet 1:1340, 1981.
11. Ferguson, A., and Strobel, S.: Immunology and physiology of digestion. In Lessof, M.H. (ed.): Clinical Reactions to Foods. New York, John Wiley & Sons, Inc., 1983.
12. Firer, M.A., Hosking, C.S., and Hill, D.J.: Effect of antigen load on the development of milk antibodies in infants allergic to milk. Br. Med. J. 283:693, 1981.
13. Fortner, B.R., et al.: The effect of ascorbic acid on cutaneous and nasal response to histamine and allergen. J. Allergy Clin. Immunol., 69:484, 1982.
14. Gerrard, J.W.: Food allergy: New Perspectives. Springfield, Ill., Charles C Thomas Publishing Co., 1980.
15. Heiner, D.C., and Singer, A.D.: Food allergy. In Beall, G.N.: Allergy and Clinical Immunology. New York, John Wiley & Sons, Inc., 1983.
16. Hutchins, P., and Walker-Smith, J.A.: The gastrointestinal system. Clin. Immunol. Allergy, 21:43, 1982.
17. Juto, P., et al.: Influence of type of feeding on lymphocyte function and development of infantile allergy. Clin. Allergy 12:409, 1982.
18. Leiberman, P.L., and Crawford, L.V.: Management of the Allergic Patient. A Text for the Primary Care Physician. New York, Appleton-Century-Crofts, 1982, p. 254.
19. Lothe, L., Lindberg, T., and Jacobsson, I.: Cow's milk formula as a cause of infantile colic: a double blind study. Pediatrics, 70:7, 1982.
20. May, C.D., and Bock, S.A.: A modern clinical approach to food hypersensitivity. Allergy, 33:166, 1978.
21. May, C.D., Fomon, S.J., and Remigio, L.: Immunologic consequences of feeding infants with cow's milk and soy products. Acta Paediatr. Scand., 71:43, 1982.
22. Radcliff, M.J.: Clinical methods for diagnosis. Clin. Immunol. Allergy, 21:205, 1982.
23. Rapp, D.J.: Allergies and Your Family. New York, Sterling Publishing Company, Inc., 1980, pp. 214, 352.
24. Robertson, D.M., et al.: Milk antigen absorption in the preterm and term neonate. Arch. Dis. Child., 57:369, 1982.
25. Shacks, S.J., and Heiner, D.C.: Allergy to breast milk. Clin. Immunol. Allergy, 2:121, 1982.
26. Silverman, S.H., and Lecks, H.L.: Protein-calorie deficiency and vitamin indiscretion in an atopic child who developed hypervitaminosis A. Clin. Pediatr., 21:172, 1982.
27. Soothill, J.F.: Prevention of food allergy. Clin. Immunol. Allergy, 2:243, 1982.
28. Stevenson, D.D., and Simon, R.A.: Sensitivity to ingested metabisulfites in asthmatic subjects. J. Allergy Clin. Immunol., 68:26, 1981.
29. Zanussi, C.: Food allergy treatment. Clin. Immunol. Allergy, 2:221, 1982.

Additional References

Dockhorn, R.J., and Smith, T.C.: Use of a chemically defined hypoallergenic diet (Vivonex) in the management of patients with suspected food allergy/intolerance. Ann. Allergy, 47:264, 1981.

Lessof, M.H. (ed.): Clinical Reactions to Foods. New York, John Wiley & Sons Inc., 1983.

McCarty, E.P., and Frick, O.L.: Food sensitivity: keys to diagnosis. J. Pediatr., 102:645, 1983.

National Dairy Council: Food sensitivity. Dairy Council Digest, 54(4):7, 1983.

Rowe, A.H., and Rowe, A., Jr.: Food Allergy: Its Manifestations and Control and the Elimination Diets. Springfield, Ill. Charles C Thomas, Publisher, 1972.

Sampson, H.A., and Albergo, R.: Comparison of results of skin rash and double blind food challenge (DBFC) food test in children with atopic dermatitis, J. Allergy Clin. Immunol., 71:473, 1983.

Sapeika, N.: Food Pharmacology. Springfield, Ill., Charles C Thomas, Publisher, 1969.

Patient Education Materials

1. Asthma and Allergy Foundation of America: The Asthma and Allergy Advance. 9604 Wisconsin Avenue, Suite 100, Bethesda, Md. 20814.
2. Hills, H.C.: Good Food, Milk Free, Grain Free. New Canaan, Conn., Keats Publishing, Inc, 1980.
3. Meals Without Milk. Nutritional Division, Mead Johnson and Co., Evansville, Ind., 47721, 1981.
4. Williams, M.L.: Cooking Without: Recipes for the Allergic Child and His Family. Bluebell, Pa., Tri-Cor Inc, 1981.
5. Young, P.: Asthma and Allergies: An Optimistic Future. U.S. Department of Health and Human Services, NIH Publ. No. 80–388, Washington, D.C., U.S. Government Printing Office, 1980.

DISEASE OF THE NERVOUS SYSTEM AND BEHAVIORAL DISORDERS

Nutritional Care in Disease of the Nervous System and Behavioral Disorders

The state of the nervous system is largely dependent upon the state of nutrition of the individual. Minor disturbances, such as forgetfulness, irritability, uneasiness and disorderly thinking, as well as gross mental changes, may develop from poor nutrition. Following prolonged nutritional inadequacy, lesions appear in both the central and peripheral nervous systems. For the most part these changes are reversible when the nutritional deficiency is corrected. However, there is very little evidence that increasing the intake of nutrients to hundreds of times the RDA will enhance mental functioning. Several mental disorders that can be relieved by proper nutritional care in conjunction with other forms of therapy will be discussed in this chapter.

Neuritis and Polyneuritis

Etiology

Polyneuritis is a term applied to any condition in which there is a symmetrical involvement of the peripheral nerves, and it is usually believed to be the result of some nutritional, toxic or metabolic disturbance. It is inflammatory in nature. Frequently, the cause is unknown, and most of the treatment must be of the symptoms only. Polyneuropathy may result from a deficient intake or absorption of any one of the B vitamins: thiamin, niacin, pyridoxine, vitamin B_{12} or pantothenic acid, as indicated in Table

32–1. There is some evidence that folate deficiency may also cause neuropathy rather than only causing hematological changes as previously thought.[32, 43]

Nutritional Care

Treatment is dependent on the basic disorder. Biochemical assessment of the status of suspected nutrients as described in Chapter 9 will determine which nutrient deficiency is causing the neuritis. In most cases the cause will be multiple deficiencies that have existed for a long time. If the diet is inadequate in one nutrient, it is usually deficient in many. In addition, if malabsorption is causing the neuritis, it will usually affect many nutrients.

The diet must be adequate and contain liberal amounts of vitamins. Supplementary vitamins, particularly of the B complex, are supplied as indicated. Parenteral vitamin B_{12} is of value in some cases, for example, for the neurological involvement in pernicious anemia. In a thiamin deficiency the administration of thiamin hydrochloride (100 mg. a day) should be beneficial. The mental symptoms of pellagra respond specifically to administration of niacin.

Establishment of a diet with high intake of the protective foods is the important aim in therapy of any of the neurological manifestations of nutritional deficiencies. Many of the patients are elderly, with early personality deterioration; some are impoverished and others have chronic disease or drug use that leads to the nutrient deficiency state. Understanding,

654

Table 32–1. NEUROLOGICAL AND BEHAVIORAL EFFECTS OF SOME VITAMIN DEFICIENCIES

| VITAMIN | EFFECTS OF DEFICIENCY | | | SITUATIONS WHERE INTAKE MAY BE INADEQUATE |
	Somatic	*Neurological*	*Behavioral*	
Thiamine (B₁)	Poor appetite Loss of tone of gastrointestinal tract Constipation Cachexia Edema Cardiac failure Beriberi	Wernicke's encephalopathy Peripheral neuropathy Polyneuritis	Mental depression Apathy Anxiety Irritability Korsakoff's psychosis	Alcohol abuse Poor diet, particularly one low in whole grain and fortified carbohydrates and high in refined carbohydrate and sugar
Riboflavin (B₂)	Cheilosis (cracks at corners of lips) Scaly shedding around nose and ears Nasolabial seborrhea Sore tongue and mouth Burning and itching of eyes Light sensitivity Ocular lesions Angular stomatitis	EEG abnormalities	No specific behavioral effects reported	Poor diet, particularly if other B vitamins are inadequate

Niacin, nicotinic acid, niacinamide (B₃)	Anorexia
	Glossitis
	Diarrhea
	Dermatitis
	Pellagra
		Neurological degeneration
		Tremor
		Loss of position sense
		Spasticity
		Exaggerated tendon reflexes
		Progressive paralysis of lips, tongue, mouth, pharynx and larynx
		Abnormally increased skin sensitivity
		Abnormal sensations such as burning or prickling
			Associated with pellagra:
			  apathy
			  depression
			  anxiety
			  hyperirritability
			  mania
			  memory deficits
			  delirium
			  organic dementia
			  emotional lability
				Poor diet, particularly if very low in protein

Pyridoxine, pyridoxal, pyridoxamine (B₆)	Weakness Abdominal pain Cutaneous lesions Lymphocytopenia	Lack of muscle coordination Convulsions EEG changes	Depression Nervous irritability Hyperacousia	Use of oral contraceptives or other estrogen-containing medication Poor diet Use of isoniazid or cycloserine, used to treat tuberculosis Pregnancy

Pantothenic acid	Deficiency seen only with severe multiple B-complex deficits:
	  gastrointestinal disturbance
	  burning feet
	  muscle cramps
		Neuritis
		Lack of motor coordination
		Staggering gait
		Numbness
		Paresthesia
			Restlessness
			Irritability
			Depression
			Fatigue
				Very poor diet, especially one low in all B vitamins

Biotin	Deficiency only seen with excessive raw egg white consumption:
	  dermatitis
	  anorexia
	  anemia
	  EKG changes
	  muscle pain
		Abnormally increased skin sensitivity	Depression
			Extreme lassitude
			Somnolence
				Consumption of many raw egg whites (about 24) daily for a long time

Cyanocobalamin (B₁₂)	Macrocytic anemia	Combined systems diseases:
		  diminished vibratory and position sense
		  abnormal EEG
		  motor weakness
			No specific behavioral effects reported
			Symptoms may occur as with other deficiency states:
			  irritability
			  depression
			  confusion
			  memory loss
			  hallucinations
			  delusions
			  paranoia
				Strict vegetarian diet
				Pernicious anemia
				Chronic consumption of large doses of vitamin C

Table continued on the following page

Table 32–1.   NEUROLOGICAL AND BEHAVIORAL EFFECTS OF SOME VITAMIN DEFICIENCIES (*Continued*)

| VITAMIN | EFFECTS OF DEFICIENCY | | | SITUATIONS WHERE INTAKE MAY BE INADEQUATE |
	Somatic	*Neurological*	*Behavioral*	
Folic acid, folacin, pteroylglutamic acid	Megaloblastic anemia of tropical sprue	No CNS symptoms reported after 2nd year of life In infants: mental retardation lack of muscle coordination continuing writhing movements	Forgetfulness Insomnia Apathy Irritability Depression Psychosis Delirium Dementia	Severe, chronic gastrointestinal disorders Use of anticonvulsants (diphenylhydantoin) Use of oral contraceptives Use of cancer treatment drugs Poor diet, especially one lacking fresh fruits and vegetables
Vitamin C (ascorbic acid)	Weakened cartilage and capillary walls Cutaneous hemorrhage Sore, bleeding gums Anemia Poor wound healing Poor bone and tooth development Scurvy	No CNS symptoms reported	Lassitude Personality changes such as those occurring in physically ill persons, such as hypochondriasis, depression and hysteria	Poor diet, especially one lacking fresh fruits and vegetables Hyperthyroidism Pregnancy Neoplastic disease Wound healing Tuberculosis Stress

From Mahan, L. K., and Rees, J. M.: Nutrition in Adolescence. St. Louis, C. V. Mosby Company, 1984. Adapted from Lipton, M. A., Mailman, R. B., and Nemeroff, C. B..: Vitamins, megavitamin therapy and the nervous system. In Wurtman, R. J., and Wurtman, J. J. (eds.): Nutrition and the Brain. Vol. 3. New York, Raven Press, 1979.

patience and skill are required to cope with the patient's psychological, financial and other problems in order to change eating habits and promote a more adequate nutrient intake.

Migraine Headache

Migraine headache is a severe headache often accompanied by nausea and vomiting. It is intermittent and lasts for a few hours to a few days. It usually is unilateral and throbbing. It is often disabling and may cause the sufferer to remain in a darkened room or in bed.

Tyramine, an amine in foods, is often blamed for a migraine attack, but the relationship of tyramine to migraine is controversial. Kohlenberg reviewed the studies of migraine and tyramine and concluded that the tyramine hypothesis appears to have some validity.[28] Hanington, who did the original work linking tyramine intake to migraine headache, stated that it applied to only about 5 to 10 per cent of the migraine patients.[18] See Table 21–7 for a list of tyramine-containing foods.

Another pharmacological agent in food that has been linked to migraine headache is the vasoactive amine *phenylethylamine,* which is found in chocolate.[39, 49] However, this area is still controversial, since other studies have shown no relationship between diet and migraine headaches.[35] Lastly, *monosodium glutamate* in large amounts may set off headaches in susceptible persons.[47]

Epilepsy

Epilepsy is one of the oldest known and most dreaded diseases. The name comes from the Greek word for "seizure," and in ancient times the seizing was believed to be the work of spirits. It is defined as a chronic functional disease of nervous origin, characterized by seizures or attacks in which there is sometimes loss of consciousness with a succession of tonic or clonic convulsions. The attacks vary in frequency, occurring several times daily in some instances. With other patients, a year or two may elapse between episodes. If severe convulsions appear, the disorder is labeled *grand mal,* which is French for "great sickness" or "major attack." When seizures are mild, the condition is called *petit mal,* meaning "little sickness" or "minor attack." Other types of seizures are jacksonian, psychomotor, simple febrile or myoclonic. The attack may last from a few seconds to 20 minutes. Epilepsy may be the result of a variety of lesions of the central nervous system, which are still not understood. It is estimated that approximately 1 per cent of the total population of the United States have epilepsy. Most diagnosed as children will "outgrow" their seizures and be seizure-free after removal of their medication. Electroencephalography has helped physicians to a better understanding of the disease.

Nutritional Care

Anticonvulsant medication has largely superseded diet therapy in the treatment of epilepsy. An adequate, well-balanced diet in addition to use of anticonvulsants is the treatment of choice. However, for a few individuals who do not tolerate drugs well or who do not respond to anticonvulsant medication, the ketogenic diet may be helpful in controlling *petit mal* seizures. It is more effective in young children, possibly because the brain of a younger individual has a greater capacity to oxidize ketone bodies than does the brain of an adult.

KETOGENIC DIET. This is a diet designed to produce a state of ketosis in the patient. It is now thought that the anticonvulsant effect of the diet is due to the high plasma levels of ketone bodies.[25] The diet is extremely low in carbohydrate and high in fat, so that the ketogenic-antiketogenic ratio, the ratio of calories from fat to calories from protein and carbohydrate, is 3:1. In older children the ratio may need to be 4:1 to keep them in ketosis.

The ketogenic diet can be calculated using either regular dietary fat or medium-chain triglycerides (MCT), which are discussed in Chapter 3. Using dietary fat to construct a diet with a ketogenic-antiketogenic ratio of 3:1 or 4:1 means that the fat content of the diet must be 80 to 90 per cent of the calories. (The usual diet contains 40 per cent of the calories as fat.) Protein and carbohydrate each contribute about 7 per cent of the calories. These extremely high-fat diets are unpalatable and difficult for a child to follow.

The more effective method is to use medium-chain triglycerides. Unlike dietary fat, MCT oil is more rapidly absorbed and is transported directly to the liver. This accounts for its more rapid induction of ketosis in the child. As a result, a smaller amount of fat is needed, and dietary fat need not be so high. MCT oil should make up 50 to 70 per cent of the total kcalories and other fats 11 per cent. Carbohydrate and protein provide the remainder of the kcalories. The diet using MCT is more flexible and palatable because more protein and carbohydrate are allowed, and yet the diet is still as effective.[25] Another advantage is that serum cholesterol levels are not elevated, as happens frequently with the traditional ketogenic diet.

The method for calculating the ketogenic diet is given in Table 32–2. Calories are determined first; most children require 75 to 90 kcal./kg./day, depending on their activity. After the energy requirement has been determined, the amount of MCT oil needed is calculated, then the dietary fat, protein and carbohydrate allowances are computed. Protein should be 1.2 to 1.7 gm./kg., depending upon the age of the child, as listed in Table 10–1. It can be lower in the adult. A source of linoleic acid in the diet must be provided in order to avoid essential fatty acid deficiency.

To simplify the choosing of food to contribute the necessary nutrients, the diabetic exchange

---

Table 32–2.   CALCULATION OF KETOGENIC DIET USING MCT FOR AN EPILEPTIC FOUR-YEAR-OLD CHILD

Child: age = 4 yr., weight = 20 kg.

1. Establish caloric requirement:
     20 kg. × 80 kcal./kg./day = 1600 kcal./day
2. Determine amount of MCT oil to be given—50 to 70% of total calories, depending on the amount needed
     to induce ketosis in the individual child:
     60% of 1600 = 960 kcal. from MCT
     1 gm. MCT = 8.3 kcal.
     960 ÷ 8.3 = approximately 116 gm. MCT (115.6)
     116 × 8.3 = 963 kcal.
     15 ml. (1 tbsp.) MCT = 14 gm.
     116 ÷ 14 = 8.3 tbsp. (8 tbsp. + 1 tsp.) MCT
3. Determine calories to be provided by foods exclusive of MCT:
     1600 − 960 = 640 kcal.
4. Establish protein intake according to recommended allowance and patient's desires:
     RDA = 1.5 gm./kg./day
     20 kg. × 1.5 gm./kg./day = 30 gm. protein
   For this child, protein intake is set at 41 gm./day.
     41 gm. protein × 4 kcal./gm. = 164 kcal. from protein
5. Estimate maximum calories to be given in form of carbohydrate:
     19% of 1600 = no more than 304 kcal.
     304 kcal. ÷ 4 = no more than 76 gm. carbohydrate
     74 gm. carbohydrate × 4 kcal./gm. = 296 kcal.
6. Estimate maximum calories to be given in form of protein and carbohydrate combined:
     29% of kcal. × 1600 kcal. = no more than 464 kcal. from protein and carbohydrate
     164 + 296 kcal. = 460 kcal. from protein + carbohydrate
7. Estimate minimum calories to be given as fat exclusive of MCT oil:
     10% × 1600 kcal. = 160 kcal. from other fats
     20 gm. of fat × 9 kcal./gm. = 180 kcal. from fat exclusive of MCT
8. After determining above dietary requirements, the dietary pattern can be calculated using the Exchange
     Lists, as shown in Table 25–8. See Table 32–3.

Adapted from Signore, J. M.: Ketogenic diet containing medium-chain triglycerides. J. Am. Diet. Assoc., *62*:285, 1973.

lists given in Table 25–8 are used. Table 32–3 gives an example of the food exchanges included in a ketogenic diet using MCT oil for a four-year-old child. The oil can be used in skim milk, fruit juice, casseroles, salad dressings and sandwich spreads.

The child may feel hungry during the first few days while growing used to the diet, but weight should be the criterion used to judge whether the diet is adequate. He or she may also experience nausea and vomiting if ketosis becomes excessive. This condition can be relieved by giving fruit juice. Symptomatic hypoglycemia is rare, but all children should be tested for a tendency to ketotic hypoglycemia before starting the diet.

If rapid ketosis is desired, the treatment starts with a period of fasting. During the two to three days of fasting, the patient is permitted a very restricted daily diet of water, broth, tea and 6 to 8 oz. of orange juice. After the fasting period the prescribed ketogenic diet is given.

If no further attacks are noticed after the diet has been followed for a period of three months, then the carbohydrate intake may be increased gradually in steps of 5 gm., until 50 to 60 gm. of carbohydrate are tolerated daily. Of course, the fats in the diet are reduced proportionately to maintain the desired level of energy intake. A state of ketosis must always be maintained, as shown by diacetic acid and acetone in the urine. Urinalysis will indicate the effectiveness of the diet. Ketogenic diets, and even anticonvulsive medication, lose some of their anticonvulsant effect over time.

MINERALS AND VITAMINS. Great care must be exercised to prevent any nutritional deficiencies, especially in calcium, iron and the water-soluble vitamins (B vitamins and vitamin C) and vitamin D. A daily dose of a supplement containing vitamin D, calcium, the vitamin B complex and vitamin C should be given.

Drugs

When the ketogenic diet has been used exclusively in cases of epilepsy, it has been reported to be only partially successful. Several years ago more progress was noted if the sedative phenobarbital was prescribed. Some patients showed more improvement with a combination of the ketogenic diet plus medication.

There are now several drugs that are effective and safe for controlling epileptic seizures. They are somewhat selective in the way they work, and different ones are used to control different kinds of seizures. Phenytoin, for example, is more effective in controlling convulsions, whereas trimethadione is used to prevent blackouts in petit mal epilepsy. Each new drug has been used to control seizures in some individuals who were helped only a little or not at all by previous medications. The currently available medications can enable 80 to 85 per cent of epileptics to lead an essentially normal life. Evaluation of the effectiveness of the drugs continues.

NUTRITIONAL IMPLICATIONS. The anticonvulsants, when taken for periods of time ranging from several months to several years, affect the nutritional status of the child or adult. An osteomalacia, *anticonvulsant rickets,* is frequently seen in children taking phenobarbital, primidone, or phenytoin. It is thought that these drugs, through hepatic enzyme induction, decrease the activation of 25-hydroxy vitamin D_3 so that it cannot be further converted to 1,25-dihydroxy vitamin D_3 in the kidney. Since 1,25-$(OH)_2D_3$ acts on the gut to facilitate calcium absorption, calcium absorption is reduced. The inadequate calcium absorption leads to osteomalacia. It is thought that phenytoin also affects calcium absorption directly, and the drug does lower serum folate levels. Low serum folate and vitamin B_{12} levels and megaloblastic anemia may be present.[33] Chapter 21 has further discussion of this drug-nutrient interaction.

The person taking anticonvulsants should probably receive at least 1000 I.U. of vitamin D per day or whatever amount is required to maintain normal serum levels of 25-OHD$_3$. Regular exposure to sunlight will also help. If folic acid is given to correct low serum folate levels, there may be a deterioration of seizure control. Although the reason is not clear, anticonvulsive agents in the presence of folate supplements are less effective in some people. The relationship between folate metabolism, anticonvulsive drugs and epileptic seizures needs further study.[6, 48]

Multiple Sclerosis

Multiple sclerosis (MS) is a central nervous system disease of unknown etiology affecting the myelinated nerve fibers and the muscles they innervate. It develops as an acute disease without warning and runs an intermittent course characterized by exacerbations at intervals of weeks, months or years. There is destruction of the fatty myelin sheaths that surround the nerves in different parts of the brain and spinal cord. This insulating material is replaced by scar tissue, and there are many such areas (multiple) of nerve degeneration (sclerosis). The condition may appear at any age but usually does so between the ages of 20 and 40. It is more common in temperate climates, especially in the northern European countries such as the British Isles, Iceland, the Low

Table 32–3.   KETOGENIC DIET USING MCT OIL FOR A FOUR-YEAR-OLD CHILD[a]

FOOD	EXCHANGES	PROTEIN (gm.)	FAT (gm.)	CHO (gm.)
Skim milk	2	16	–	24
Lean meat	2½	17	8	–
Fruit	1	–	–	10
Vegetable	2	4	–	10
Bread	2	4	–	30
Fat	2½	–	12.5	–
MCT oil[b] 116 gm. = 8 T. + 1 tsp.				
Total MCT = 116 gm.		41	20.5	74

[a]Calories from foods exclusive of MCT = 960. Total calories including MCT = 1600.
[b]1 gm. MCT oil = 8.3 kcal.

Countries, northern and central France, Germany, Poland and Czechoslovakia. The northern U.S., southern Canada, southern Australia and New Zealand are also regions of high prevalence. Groups at high risk of developing MS are Caucasians, females, those of high socioeconomic status, urban residents and those with high measles antibody titer.

Etiology

Many theories have been advanced about the cause of multiple sclerosis. The most promising one seems to be that it is a slow viral disease or, more likely, a virus-induced immune disease.[54] However, it also seems that many other factors are involved, such as vascular condition, heredity, metabolic alterations and disturbed immune mechanisms.

A metabolic alteration involving fatty acid metabolism in this disease has attracted attention for over 20 years. In a well-controlled study, investigators found that the clinical course of the disease was improved if the diet was supplemented with linoleic acid rather than oleic acid (a saturated fatty acid).[37] However, because remissions are characteristic of this disease, it is difficult to document therapeutic effectiveness.

Nutritional Care

The patient should have a well-balanced and adequate diet to meet all the requirements of normal nutrition for age, activity and desired weight. When activity is limited owing to nerve degeneration, the patient should carefully control his weight. Because of the crippling nature of the disease, every opportunity for rehabilitation should be taken to make life more livable and worthwhile. Present capabilities and potentialities of each patient should be developed to the maximum. The patient should be given feeding aids and taught to use them, rather than be made to feel helpless by being fed.

FAT. There is no proven nutritional care that will improve the course of multiple sclerosis; however, Swank reported convincing evidence from a 20-year study that a low-fat diet maintained over a long period of time tends to retard the disease process and to reduce the incidence of new attacks.[52] He recommends a fat intake of 10 gm. of saturated (animal) fat and 40 to 50 gm. of a polyunsaturated oil (8 to 10 tsp.) daily. At least 1 tsp. should be cod liver oil. A 10 gm. saturated fat diet is given in Table 32–4. Protein is kept at normal levels (60 to 70 gm.), and carbohydrate is supplied to meet energy needs. At this time there is not enough evidence to say definitely that a low-saturated-fat diet will improve the course of multiple sclerosis. However, it probably would not hurt a patient to follow such a diet after receiving some dietary counseling to assure that the diet is adequate. A diet very low in animal fat restricts meat, usually to less than 2 oz. per day, and therefore less than adequate intakes of protein, iron, B vitamins and trace minerals such as zinc may result from it.

Excessive physical and emotional stress should be avoided. Currently no medication is proven to be consistently beneficial, although steroid treatment during periods of exacerbation or relapse may be helpful.

Hyperkinetic Behavior Syndrome

Hyperkinetic behavior in children is an ill-defined disorder. When is an active child hyperactive? Although there is disagreement on the precise definition of hyperkinetic behavior, most authorities agree that the following are major features of such behavior: excessive gross motor activity, impulsiveness, low tolerance to frustration, short attention span and easy distraction. Any or all of these can be present in the hyperkinetic or hyperactive child.

A child may be hyperkinetic for a variety of

Table 32–4.   TEN GRAM ANIMAL FAT DIET

(Polyunsaturated vegetable oils are allowed; animal fats are restricted.)

FOOD CLASS	FOODS INCLUDED	FOODS OMITTED
Beverages	Coffee, coffee substitutes, tea, skim milk, buttermilk made from skim milk. At least 4–5 glasses of milk per day.	Whole milk, 2% milk, low-fat milk, chocolate milk, cream, half and half.
Breads	Enriched white, rye, whole-wheat breads; Italian or French breads; hard rolls, saltines, graham crackers, melba toast.	Commercial pancakes, waffles, hot breads, snack crackers.
Cereals	Hot and ready-to-eat.	None
Condiments	All	None
Desserts	Angel food cakes, white cake, fruit whips, gelatin and rennet desserts, puddings made with skim milk; sherbets, fruit ices and other desserts made with allowed foods.	Ice cream, pastries and other desserts made with butter, cream, half and half, whole milk, 2% milk or egg yolks.
Fats	Corn oil, safflower oil, soybean oil, cottonseed oil only; soft or liquid margarines; non-dairy creamers.	Butter, stick margarine, lard, shortenings, hydrogenated vegetable oils; coconut oil and all others not allowed.
Fruits and fruit juices	Canned, cooked, fresh or frozen.	Avocado.
Meats and substitutes	2 oz. daily of lean meats, fish, poultry without skin, and eggs only; one egg is equal to 1 oz. of meat. Use as desired: egg whites, cottage cheese made from skim milk, dry cottage cheese, fat-free cheeses or those made with skim milk or allowed oils; vegetable protein substitutes; egg substitutes; dried beans, lentils and peas.	Fatty meats, fish and poultry, such as duck, goose, luncheon meats; canned fish packed in oils; bacon, sausages, frankfurters and organ meats; all cheeses except those allowed.
Potatoes and substitutes	White and sweet potatoes; macaroni, rice, noodles and spaghetti.	Potato chips; pastas made with eggs, such as egg noodles.
Soups	Fat-free broths, consommés and bouillons; cream soups made with skim milk; other soups made with allowed foods.	All others.
Sweets	Hard candies, gum drops, marshmallows, jams, jellies, sugars and syrups.	Candies made with chocolate, coconut, cream, fats and nuts.
Vegetables and vegetable juices	Canned, cooked, fresh or frozen.	Any vegetables prepared with a butter, cream or cheese sauce.
Miscellaneous	Vinegar, fat-free gravies, salad dressings made with allowed oils, pickles, olives; nuts: hazel, hickory, pecans, walnuts; cocoa.	Coconut; rich gravies and sauces; nuts, except those allowed.

physiological or psychological reasons and should always be thoroughly examined and evaluated before any kind of treatment is started. Therapies encompass stimulant medication, behavior modification, psychotherapy, family therapy, special classroom situations and educational techniques, and several dietary manipulations. Dietary manipulations include allergy elimination diets, which are discussed in Chapter 31, omission of sugar, megavitamin therapy and the Feingold diet. All of these have been tried with various degrees of success, but claims for the Feingold diet have probably attracted the most attention.

The Feingold Diet

In 1973 Feingold proposed that some children are hyperactive because they are sensitive to salicylates and artificial flavors and colors in their food. His hypothesis seems to have originated from his observations that in some people salicylates cause allergic reactions such as urticaria and asthma. When he treated the allergy by removing the salicylates from the diet, he noted a behavior change in addition to the disappearance of the allergic symptoms. Since many patients who are allergic to salicylates also react to artificial colors, specifically FD & C yellow no. 5, he postulated that the food colors may also have a behavioral effect similar to that of the salicylates in those people sensitive to them. He applied this hypothesis to children with hyperkinetic behavior. Based upon his anecdotal clinical observations, he published a popular book in which he presented both the hypothesis and the salicylate-free, artificial color–free and artificial flavor–free diet, which he claimed had been successful in improving behavior in 30 to 50 per cent of the hyperactive children he had treated.[13] Since the first book, he has modified his diet so that now the preservatives butylated hydroxyanisole (BHA), butylated hydroxytoluene (BHT), monosodium glutamate (MSG) and sodium benzoate are also omitted.

No convincing experimental work is available to confirm Feingold's claims of success with his diet. Harley and colleagues have conducted a controlled study to test the Feingold hypothesis.[20] They found that the Feingold diet did not cause a consistent or significant reduction in hyperactive behavior in the children, as assessed from the observations of parents, teachers and trained classroom observers or the results of neuropsychological tests. Nine of the 46 children who showed the best, although not significant, response to the diet were then challenged with special candy bars and cookies containing all of the certified artificial food colors and others without artificial coloring, in an attempt to "turn on" and "turn off" their hyperactive behavior. Again, the results were negative.[19] In addition, many of the foods that Feingold eliminates from the diet because they contain salicylates are in fact salicylate-free.[2] Others have also shown negative results similar to Harley's.[16,34] Connors, who also tested the hypothesis but under less rigorous conditions, concluded that the diet may be effective in a small subgroup of hyperactive children, but he also reported that the diet produced poorer nutritional intake than the child's regular diet, particularly for vitamin C, since the diet omits many fruits.[8] Others have also shown small but significant improvement in behavior or learning in a small percentage of hyperactive children when on the Feingold diet.[53, 57] The percentage of children who do respond to the Feingold diet with a reduction in hyperactive behavior seems to be around 10 per cent, and it appears that most of these are the younger (preschool) children.

To help explain the conflicting results in controlled studies, investigators have suggested that the sensitivity is a matter of degree and that the amount of food additives is important.[40] It may be that there is a tolerance level below which a child will not react. In addition, the time elapsed after the additive is eaten may be important.

The Nutrition Foundation Advisory Committee Panel and the Interagency Collaborative Group of the Department of Health, Education and Welfare have made statements to the effect that the Feingold diet has no efficacy in the treatment of hyperactivity and that the role of artificial colors and flavors is unclear.[26,40] However, parents and families continue to claim fabulous results with the use of the diet, so the National Institute of Health formed a panel to study the situation. Their report states that the diet seems to have a beneficial effect in a small percentage of children and if the physician and family agree, the diet could be used as a first treatment trial in the management of hyperkinesis.[10]

It is important to consider the placebo effect when evaluating the effect of the Feingold diet or any other dietary change on behavior. Besides the effect from knowing that the dietary change might make a difference, there also is an effect on behavior from the changed interaction between the child and the family. If a child has been behaving badly in a bid for more attention, the new diet, which requires increased attention to food preparation for the child, can become the focus for increased positive family attention, and the child's behavior may improve. Parents, teachers or counselors claim that the diet "works" when actually it is the positive interaction around the diet that has "worked."[31]

Another outcome of the diet is a change in the approach to the child's behavior. Instead of assigning the responsibility to the child for choosing to be bad, the questioning of the child concentrates on what the child had to eat. The motivation for the behavior is transferred from the child to the suspect food that made the child behave inappropriately. This shift alone can have an effect on the child's behavior.[31]

Feingold's hypothesis has not been experimentally confirmed, and the claims for its success by Feingold and the press may be primarily attributable to a placebo effect rather than to the characteristics of the diet. However, if the diet is to be used, attention should be paid to its possible nutritional inadequacies, and there should be some nutritional counseling and vitamin supplementation, if necessary.

Sugar

Sugar is another dietary component that has been implicated as a cause of hyperactive behavior in children. It is known that consumption of carbohydrate can increase the brain level of serotonin, as discussed on page 666, but the behavioral result of this change is not known.

Some postulate that sugar consumption may affect behavior when it is metabolized abnormally as may be the case in some individuals, but there is no controlled study supporting this. One study showed that of 261 hyperkinetic children who had five-hour oral glucose tolerance tests (OGTT) performed on them, 74 per cent had glucose tolerance curves that were abnormal, and the predominant abnormality accounting for 50 per cent of the results was a low, flat curve. The low, flat curve is typical of that seen in hypoglycemia. Hypoglycemia is a potent stimulus for an increased production of epinephrine, which could certainly affect behavior. Recognizing the shortcomings of the OGTT, the authors suggest that glucose metabolism in hyperkinetic children is an area that requires further investigation.[30]

Findings by Rapoport, presented at a recent National Institute of Mental Health conference, are interesting. In boys whose parents were convinced that they were made hyperactive by sugar intake, a double-blind test of sugar showed that the boys slowed down rather than becoming more active after sugar consumption. The effect was seen in three hours for the normal boys and in one hour for the psychiatrically disturbed boys.[29] The area of sugar intake, glucose metabolism and behavior certainly requires much more investigation before any recommendations can be made.

Food Allergy

Food allergy as a cause of hyperactive behavior or other behavioral disturbances is receiving widespread attention in the popular press. Unfortunately there is a paucity of well-controlled studies in this area. If there is a role for food allergy in hyperactive behavior, it is probably due to a delayed-onset reaction, and this is very difficult to define with our present knowledge of food allergy. See Chapter 31 for further discussion of food allergy and hyperkinetic behavior.

Eating Disorders

Jane M. Rees, M.S., R.D.

Knowledge about this spectrum of disorders has greatly increased in recent years. A list of currently used terms appears in Table 32–5.

This section will include discussion of anorexia nervosa and bulimia; the behavioral aspects of obesity are discussed in Chapter 27.

ANOREXIA NERVOSA

Anorexia nervosa (AN) is a disorder usually seen among adolescent females that seems to be becoming more common.[9] However, it has also been seen in males and in females at other ages. Typically, AN occurs among middle socioeconomic level families in affluent societies. Most of these families appear to be stable and happy, but a characteristic pattern of unresolved conflicts generally lies beneath the surface. The occurrence of the syndrome is reinforced in a culture where slimness is highly valued while at the same time food is used for recreation as well as for survival and health. The developmental problems of the affected young women make them extremely vulnerable to these mixed messages.[15]

Although this disorder has been recognized since the 19th century (Gull described it in 1874), there is still some uncertainty as to whether it is primarily a psychological disorder, primarily a physical disorder of hypothalamic or pituitary function, or a combination of both. The current thinking is that the hypothalamic-pituitary dysfunction may result from psychogenic stress or may be secondary to the malnutrition and starvation that result from the condition.

These patients develop bizarre food habits and refuse to eat. They may lose 25 per cent or more of body weight (many lose up to 35 per cent of their body weight). They usually exercise vigorously and may abuse laxatives or diuretics and voluntarily vomit to decrease the energy they retain in their system. Without intervention, the disorder may progress to starvation, at which time the symptoms listed in Table 32–6 will be evident. While *amenorrhea* (cessation of menstruation) is a natural occurrence in starvation, it is usually seen in these patients initially as a consequence of psychological stress.[45, 46]

Psychologically, anorectics have an abnormal fear of being fat.[9] They exhibit distortions of body image and other perceptions. This is probably a combination of altered physical state, distorted perception, and denial of perceptions in order not to gratify themselves. Anorectics experience an arrested development so that they do

Table 32–5. TERMINOLOGY OF EATING DISORDERS

Anorexia nervosa	Voluntary starvation in the absence of an identifiable physiological or psychological disorder and accompanied by characteristics of the syndrome as described in the text
Bulimarexia	Bingeing/gorging followed by vomiting and/or purging, accompanied also by starvation
Bulimia	Bingeing/gorging followed by vomiting and/or purging, without starvation
Binge/gorge	Eating abnormally large quantities of food as defined by the bulimic (actual quantities may be small or large)

Table 32–6. PHYSICAL SIGNS OF ANOREXIA NERVOSA

Fat store depletion
Muscle wasting
Amenorrhea
Cheilosis
Desquamation
Dry skin
Hirsutism
Thin, dry, brittle hair
Alopecia
Degradation of fingernails
Acrocyanosis
Postural hypotension
Dehydration
Edema
Bradycardia
Bradypnea
Hypothermia
Constipation
Sleep disturbance

From Rees, J. M.: Eating disorders. In Mahan, L. K., and Rees, J. M.: Nutrition in Adolescence. St. Louis, C. V. Mosby Company, 1984.

not develop a normal sense of "self" nor complex advanced patterns of thinking. Thus, their interactions with their total environment are interrupted.[4, 14]

Etiology

The earliest theories proposed that disturbed sexuality was the cause of AN. Later it was thought to be due to a hypothalamic abnormality. Presently, it is seen as arising from disturbed patterns of family interactions. In early life the patient has generally functioned as a cooperative participant in the "anorexigenic" family until an event or phase of life precipitated the physical manifestation of symptoms.[38] Figure 32–1 shows the usual progression of this disease.

The change in body functions other than food intake, such as thermoregulation, menstruation, basal metabolic rate and activity, have led to the speculation that the disorder may be due to an organic cause. On the other hand, the hypothalamic dysfunction and other endocrine abnormalities may be secondary to the starvation, malnutrition or psychiatric illness. Many have pointed to the parallel with starvation. Besides amenorrhea, slowed heart rate, dry skin, disturbance in hair growth and disinterest in sex are seen in starvation as they are in AN. The psychological stress is an additional complication.[27] The study of physiological factors continues, however, and may eventually show there are contributing physical factors that are not caused by malnutrition.[55, 56]

Treatment

Both anorectics and their families are very resistant to treatment. Great skill is usually needed to convince them of the need for professional help. Treatment incorporates psychotherapeutic, nutritional and medical components.

PSYCHOTHERAPY. Both family and individual psychotherapy should be initiated as soon as AN becomes apparent. When the situation is diagnosed early, therapy can turn the focus away from food to the underlying interactional and developmental problems before a severe physical state develops. If the disorder has reached an advanced stage, the patient may need to be hospitalized. In the crisis of starvation, the psychological problems of starvation, including mental dullness, apathy and constant preoccupation with food, will compound the psychological state. Psychotherapy may not be effective until the patient is renourished, but psychological factors are considered uppermost in the design of in-hospital treatment plans. Hospitalization may also provide needed separation of

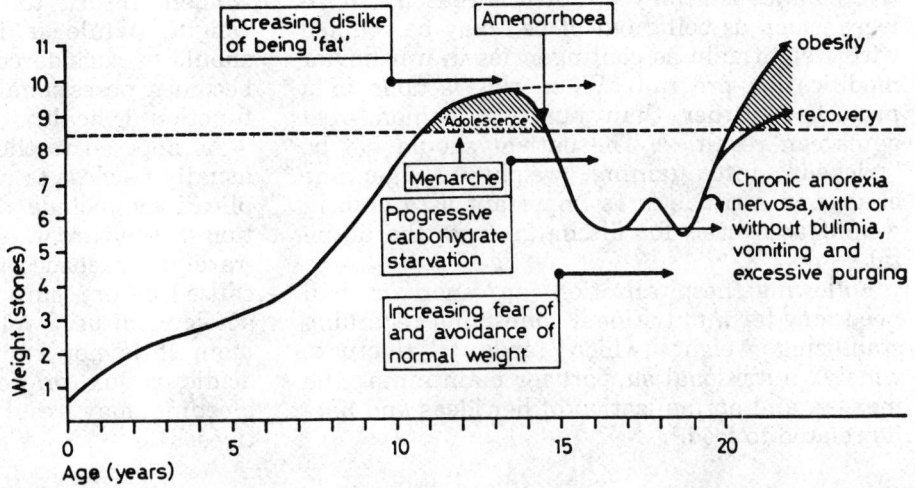

Figure 32–1. Some typical developments found in a series of 82 patients with primary anorexia nervosa or weight phobia. One stone equals 14 lb. (From Crisp, A. H.: Anorexia nervosa. In: Silverstone, T., and Barraclough, B. (eds.): Contemporary Psychiatry. Br. J. Psychiatry, Special Publication No. 9, 1975.)

the anorectic patient from her family. Following hospitalization, long-term psychotherapy must address the developmental and psychological problems.[4, 9, 38]

NUTRITIONAL CARE. The importance of health professionals being able to recognize AN cannot be overemphasized. During the initial stage, the goal will be to establish the patient and her family in psychotherapy. Nutritional care at this time will consist of providing information and helping the anorectic to change her ideas about food. This can be done only at a pace acceptable to the patient, which will depend in great part on the success of psychotherapy.[46]

If the physical state deteriorates, the need for hospitalization to manage the patient's rehabilitation will be indicated by fainting spells, insufficient strength to carry out normal activities, slowed speech and muscle wastage. (See Chapter 9 for assessment of extent of muscle depletion.) Specific nutritional problems in individuals will be related to their specific habits. Most of these appear to be subclinical and are only now being investigated.

The hospital atmosphere should be protective and non-punitive. The method by which the patient is encouraged to eat varies depending on the overall protocol, but it is generally possible to succeed in oral feeding. Highly nourishing liquids may be given if the patient will not eat solid food. Parenteral, enteral or nasogastric feeding routes are reserved for life-threatening states and are usually unnecessary. An imbalance of fluid and electrolytes, severe cardiac abnormalities in the absence of electrolyte imbalances, an absence of ketone bodies in the urine, and concurrent infection are signs that a life-threatening state has been reached.

The diet should be made up of foods acceptable to the patient, and ideally should be moderate in protein, carbohydrate and fat. The goal will be to increase the dietary intake gradually while energy output is decreased so that a positive balance is achieved. For this reason, "privileges" such as being out of bed may be coupled with weight gain as contingencies in a behavior modification program. When this is done in a protective rather than punitive fashion, real gains can result.[7, 51] The patient should not be "tricked" into gaining weight. A genuine change in attitude is as important as a gain in weight as a basis for discharge from the hospital.[3]

Following hospitalization an anorexic will need long-term nutritional counseling regarding stabilizing weight (which tends to fluctuate widely), nutritional support for maintaining the menses, and normalization of her ideas and habits related to food.[9]

Prognosis

Early and more knowledgeable treatment of AN in recent years has led to a decline in mortality from around 10 to 2 per cent. Present emphasis on the broad range of treatment issues should contribute to a similar improvement in the other outcomes of the disorder. A 1980 review showed that to that point evaluation of progress was very inconsistent. Weight and dietary habits (including food intake, weight and shape ideation and weight for height proportion), menstruation, adjustment of sexual, psychological and social characteristics, and occupational status have been recognized as outcome criteria. They must be assessed several years after a crisis to signify true outcome.[24]

BULIMIA

While gorging and vomiting have been seen as part of the syndrome of AN, these symptoms in combination have recently been recognized as making up a separate syndrome known as bulimia. It has been estimated that as many as 20 per cent of college women have this disorder. It seems to affect women who are slightly older and to some extent of lower socioeconomic groups than those most often affected by AN.[17]

Definition

Bulimics periodically stuff themselves with food and then force themselves to vomit or take laxatives to purge themselves. At present some workers in the field interchange the terms *bulimia* and *bulimarexia*, whereas others make the distinction, Table 32–5. Because the bulimic's total concept of food is distorted, it is often possible to discern that what some bulimics consider a binge would be a normal amount of food to the unrestricted eater. Vomiting or purging after a normal intake of food may later come to be known as a variant of the principal disorder. It should also be pointed out that many young women resort to vomiting to control their weight. While it is always inappropriate, it should be considered a serious problem only if it becomes obsessional or interferes with normal function or health.

As opposed to the anorectic, the bulimic will usually be close to normal weight. Physical complications include damage to the teeth, irritation of the throat, esophageal inflammation and (rarely) tracheoesophageal fistula; these are caused by exposure of the unprotected tissue to acidic vomitus. Swollen salivary glands are common. It is not known whether this is due to acidic reflux or constant stimulation. Rectal bleeding may result from an overuse of laxatives.

The bulimic is afraid of gaining too much weight, and her feeling of self-worth is tied to her feelings about her body. Like the anorectic, her psychosocial development to mature adulthood is delayed. One of the chief psychological characteristics is guilt over the cycle of bingeing and vomiting she carries out in secret, even while her life may seem ideal to those around her. She is usually unable to tolerate frustration and attempts to dull various feeling states by the gorging and vomiting behavior.[1] As opposed to the more calm anorectic, the bulimic tends to have poor impulse control, misuses substances, and shoplifts.[44]

Etiology

It is proposed that disturbed family interaction patterns are the cause of bulimia. Some patients have been previously anorectic or obese.

Treatment

PSYCHOTHERAPY. Bulimics will be treated most like recovering anorectics. Facilitation of normal development is a primary goal. Because they are often older and separated from their families, they are more commonly involved in individual counseling, though the family should be included if they are living together. Bulimics are often able to make gains within therapy groups.[44]

NUTRITIONAL CARE. A smaller number of bulimics than anorectics are seen in poor physical condition. Those who have severe fluid and electrolyte imbalances or cardiac irregularities will need to be hospitalized.[1] In nutritional counseling during long-term recovery the underlying philosophy of the bulimic about weight and food clearly need to be assessed and the dis-

torted beliefs replaced.[12] Often the bulimic attempts to restrict her intake below that which will reasonably maintain her. Thus, not only psychologically but physiologically she sets herself up for gorging. As she makes psychological gains she will be able to accept her body (including reasonable weight for height and body structure), give up vomiting or purging, and adapt a more physiologically normal dietary ideal.[45] An important breakthrough comes with being able to separate the goal of ceasing to vomit from that of losing weight. This cannot be imposed upon the patient but must come from within, facilitated by skillful counseling.[46]

Prognosis

The outcome data are beginning to indicate that bulimics in treatment make gains. Disclosure appears to be an important issue for these patients, occurring when disgust with the habit outweighs their fear of fatness.[12]

Neurotransmitters and Neurological Factors

Considerable research has shown that the concentrations of some of the neurotransmitters in the brain are influenced by diet. *Neurotransmitters* are the substances present in the neurons of mammals that, when released, will transmit signals across synapses to other neurons in the brain or to muscle cells or secretory cells outside the brain. Successful functioning of the nervous system depends on the release of sufficient quantities of neurotransmitters into the synapse, which is shown in Figure 32–2. Four primary amines, serotonin, dopamine, nor-

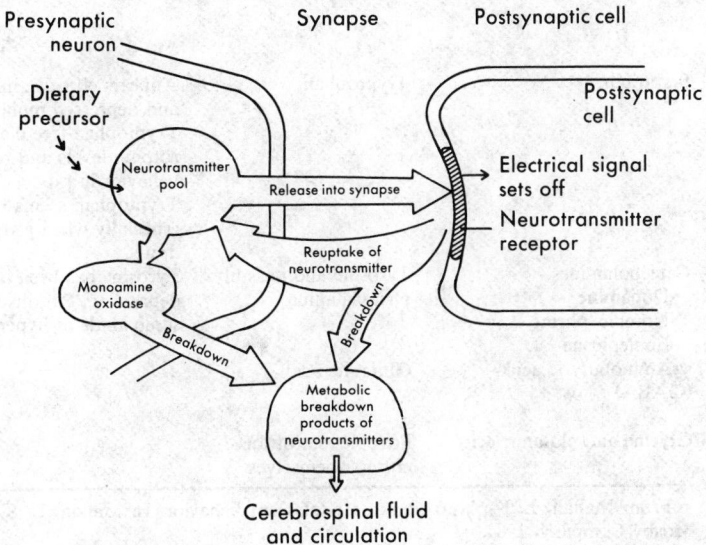

Figure 32–2. Neurotransmitter formation and metabolism at a synapse in the nervous system. (From Mahan, L. K., and Rees, J. M.: Nutrition in Adolescence. St. Louis, C. V. Mosby Company, 1984.)

epinephrine, and acetylcholine, are synthesized from amino acid precursors and appear to be under dietary control. (Other possible neurotransmitters are epinephrine, gamma-aminobutyric acid (GABA), glycine and glutamic acid.) *Dopamine* and *norepinephrine* are synthesized from tyrosine and phenylalanine (phenylalanine is metabolized to tyrosine), *serotonin* is synthesized from tryptophan, and *acetylcholine* is synthesized from choline.

Food consumption influences the levels of tyrosine, choline and tryptophan in the brain, and the brain's synthesis of the neurotransmitters depends on the level of these precursors. However, the relationships are not direct, since insulin is involved in the control of serum levels of amino acids.

The relationship of dietary choline content to brain choline levels and acetylcholine formation is straightforward: choline in a meal increases brain choline levels and thus increases brain acetylcholine levels. When lecithin has been used as the source of choline, it is in highly purified form, not the form of most commercially available lecithin that health food stores promote. Choline is discussed further on page 44. Table 32–7 summarizes what is presently known about the actions of acetylcholine.

The synthesis of the neurotransmitters serotonin, norepinephrine and dopamine is also affected by the diet, but the relationship is not a direct one as it seems to be with choline and acetylcholine.

Tryptophan, tyrosine and other large neutral amino acids, such as phenylalanine, are passed into the brain by a common transport system. These amino acids all compete with one another for entry into the brain. Since most food proteins contain small amounts of tryptophan and much larger proportions of the other amino acids, a high-protein meal, although increasing blood tryptophan levels, retards the uptake of tryptophan into the brain by disproportionately increasing the plasma concentrations of the other amino acids that compete with tryptophan. On the other hand, a high carbohydrate meal, which causes the release of insulin, results in elevated brain tryptophan and serotonin concentrations. The blood tryptophan's entry into the brain is facilitated because the release of insulin leads to a reduction in the blood levels of the other large neutral amino acids that compete with tryptophan for brain uptake. Thus, tryptophan can pass into the brain without competition.

The precursor of norepinephrine and dopa-

Table 32–7. NEUROTRANSMITTERS AND THEIR PRECURSORS AND THEIR POSSIBLE RELATIONSHIP TO DIET

NEUROTRANSMITTER	METABOLIC PRECURSOR	EXPERIMENTAL EVIDENCE AND RELATIONSHIPS	REMARKS
Acetylcholine	Choline or lecithin, which contains choline	Has been used to treat manic depressive illness, Friedreich's ataxia, Huntington's chorea, tardive oral dyskinesia, and Alzheimer's disease.	Choline in meal leads to elevated brain acetylcholine. Effects do not appear to be long lasting. Commercially available lecithin does not contain phosphatidylcholine in high enough amounts to affect brain choline levels. Lecithin is found in eggs, meat, fish, and legumes.
Serotonin	Tryptophan	Appears effective in improving sleep and depressed mood. Tryptophan-free diet reduces brain serotonin levels and reduces aggressive behavior in rats. Tryptophan seems to promote sleep, especially when given with carbohydrate.	Protein in almost all foods contains 0.5% to 1.5% tryptophan. High-carbohydrate meal leads to elevated brain tryptophan and brain serotonin.
Catecholamines Dopamine Norepinephrine Epinephrine	Tyrosine and possibly phenylalanine	Tyrosine has been used in treatment of depression, Parkinson's disease, and some kinds of hypertension.	High-protein meal results in increased brain tyrosine.
γ-Aminobutyric acid (GABA)	Glutamic acid		A part of monosodium glutamate that in large amounts causes "Chinese restaurant syndrome" in some people.
Glycine and glutamic acid	Possible neurotransmitters themselves		

From Mahan, L. K.: Nutrition and adolescent behavior. In Mahan, L. K., and Rees, J. M.: Nutrition in Adolescence. St. Louis, C. V. Mosby Company, 1984.

mine is tyrosine. Like tryptophan, tyrosine is a large neutral amino acid that must compete with other similar amino acids for transport into the brain. However, unlike tryptophan, brain tyrosine and norepinephrine are increased after a high-protein meal.

Lastly, it is important to remember that the precursors of the neurotransmitters interact with each other. For example, treatments designed to increase serotonin synthesis, such as tryptophan administration or a high-carbohydrate meal, may also decrease tyrosine uptake into the brain and thus brain synthesis of norepinephrine.[31]

Large amounts of precursors may also be toxic. For example, as a reaction to the preliminary research reported in the press that lecithin can affect atherosclerosis, memory and cognition, many are taking large amounts of choline or lecithin. Besides possible disturbance in concentrations of neurotransmitters there are known effects of acute gastrointestinal distress, sweating, salivation and anorexia.

An increase in the level of a brain neurotransmitter will be physiologically significant only if it is also correlated with a change in the amount of neurotransmitter secreted into synaptic clefts. Whether or not this occurs is still not known.

However, concentrations of brain neurotransmitters are already being manipulated with clinical effect, as outlined in Table 32–7. Tryptophan, tyrosine and choline themselves, as isolated substances rather than as part of the diet, are being used as "precursor therapy." Tryptophan at bedtime appears to be an effective sleep-promoting agent.[21] Perhaps drinking the traditional glass of hot milk (carbohydrate) increases the tryptophan level in the brain and is really a rather scientific practice.

Orthomolecular Psychiatry

The term *megavitamin therapy* was coined in the early 1950's to describe a treatment for schizophrenia that employed large doses (3 to 30 gm. daily or 200 to 2000 times the RDA) of nicotinic acid or nicotinamide. Niacin was chosen because it is a non-toxic methyl acceptor, not because of its value as a nutrient. Although anecdotal clinical reports of success have been given by its proponents,[23,41] in clinically controlled trials other investigators have been unable to reproduce their results.[58]

The term *orthomolecular psychiatry,* coined by Linus Pauling in 1968, means "the achievement and preservation of good mental health by the provision of the optimum molecular environment for the mind, especially the optimum concentrations of substances normally present in the human body, such as the vitamins."[42] He claims that certain people require larger quantities of some vitamins than others do for optimal mental function. Orthomolecular psychiatry takes a broader approach than megavitamin therapy and relies on several therapeutic components: nicotinic acid, vitamin C, vitamin B_6, other water-soluble vitamins such as vitamin B_{12}, trace minerals, an antihypoglycemia diet, electroconvulsive therapy (ECT) and administration of hormones such as thyroid. Large doses of vitamins (10 to 500 times the RDA) are used. Many authorities argue that these are not physiological doses and that, when used in these amounts, vitamins should be considered drugs.

Orthomolecular psychiatrists and physicians proclaim that their treatments are effective in a variety of mental and physical illnesses including autism, reading disabilities, hyperactivity, mental retardation and drug addiction. However, none of these statements have been confirmed in well-controlled studies.

In 1973 an American Psychiatric Association (APA) Task Force report rejected orthomolecular psychiatry on the grounds that it is unsubstantiated by scientific evidence and uses questionable clinical methods and that its results are non-reproducible in controlled studies.[36]

Do large doses of vitamins taken orally increase the brain levels of vitamins? There is considerable evidence that this is not the case and that the blood-brain barrier and other mechanisms maintain close control of brain levels of vitamins.[50] Do vitamins have a role in the nervous system outside of their role as cofactors or coenzymes that catalyze metabolic steps? Can large doses of vitamins have pharmacological effects?[11] The answers to these questions are not known, but it is known that our present concept of nutrient toxicity is very narrow and includes only short-term megadose effects. Even less is known about chronic nutrient toxicity where the effects develop slowly over time. The potential for toxicity is further reason to question the use of orthomolecular psychiatry.

Mental Illness

Patients in psychiatric hospitals or on psychiatric or mental units of hospitals are often in a poor nutritional state and require sympathy and understanding on the part of the entire hospital team—nurse, dietitian and physician—to encourage the ingestion of a balanced diet. Food served in an attractive and pleasant environment will often stimulate the patient to eat. Many psychiatric disorders follow prolonged periods of tension, worry and anxiety, during which intelligent and adequate food intake was neglected. The patient may be overweight as a result of compulsive eating during anxiety periods or thin and emaciated from lack of interest in eating. Both types of patients require discerning guidance to meet their emotional needs and metabolic requirements.

As previously pointed out, mental symptoms such as forgetfulness, confusion, depression and anxiety may result from dietary inadequacies. For example, deficiencies of folate and vitamin B_{12} are associated with sleeplessness, forgetfulness and irritability, and these symptoms disappear within 24 hours of starting therapy.[22]

Nutritional status of the psychiatric patient should be assessed whenever possible. One study showed that 53 per cent of the people admitted to a British district general hospital psychiatric unit were deficient by biochemical analysis for at least one B vitamin and 12 per cent for more than one.[5] See Table 32–1 for the possible neurological consequences of vitamin deficiencies.

Many of the drugs used to treat psychiatric disorders interact with nutrients to cause nutritional deficiencies or metabolic problems. For example, *monoamine oxidase inhibitors* used to treat depression can interact with tyramine in food and cause a hypertensive reaction, as discussed in Chapter 21.

Food has many meanings for people. These vary with individuals in health and illness. From early childhood food can form the basis of many motives and behaviors. Emotions can be expressed in how one responds to food. Feelings of defiance, helpless submission or self-contempt, demands for love and affection and many other underlying emotions may be expressed or acted out through overeating or rejection of food. Fears and anxieties can be associated with eating certain foods that will "hurt" or "poison." These feelings may be relieved by permitting the patient to discuss the problem, to participate in the preparation of food or to select his food along with others in whom he has confidence.

Feeding patients means a good deal more than simply offering a well-balanced diet rich in protein and vitamins and balanced in minerals, fats, and carbohydrates. It offers a way to reach them on the level of satisfying a simple human need and thereby also offering them in an unthreatening way the opportunity of rebuilding relationships with others.

Problems and Suggested Topics for Discussion

1. Obtain a food intake history from a patient suffering with neuritis. Calculate the vitamin content of the diet. Compare the calculation with the Recommended Dietary Allowances. What changes are needed to correct low intakes of nutrients? Are the energy and protein intakes appropriate?

2. What is the objective of the ketogenic diet for epilepsy? Plan a food prescription for an epileptic patient who is going on a ketogenic diet. The patient is a 14-year-old schoolgirl who weighs 135 pounds, and her height is 5 feet 2 inches. Using the food prescription as a basis, make out a meal plan.

3. Talk with a patient who has anorexia nervosa. Describe what she looks like and how she acts. What is her weight? How much is she underweight for her height? What is her family like? How much does she exercise?

4. Interview a person who has bulimia or bulimarexia. Describe her dietary habits and purging activity.

5. Plan a menu for one day for a 35-year-old woman with multiple sclerosis who has difficulty in chewing and in feeding herself.

6. Talk with the family of a hyperactive child. What have they tried to control their child's behavior? Have they tried any dietary changes? Would you recommend any dietary changes?

7. List typical dietary problems encountered in the mentally ill patient.

Cited References

1. Anderson, A.E.: Anorexia nervosa and bulimia: a spectrum of eating disorders. J. Adol. Health Care, *4*:15, 1983.

2. Ashoor, S., and Chu, F.S.: Analysis of Salicylic Acid and Methyl Salicylate in Fruits and Almonds (unpublished manuscript). Madison, Wisconsin, Food Research Institute, University of Wisconsin, 1977.

3. Bruch, H.: Perils of behavior modification in treatment of anorexia nervosa. JAMA, *230*:1419, 1974.

4. Bruch, H.: Eating Disorders. New York, Basic Books, Inc., 1973.

5. Carney, M.W.P., et al.: Thiamine, riboflavin and pyridoxine deficiency in psychiatric in-patients. Br. J. Psychiat., *141*:271, 1982.

6. Cerebrospinal folate levels in epileptics and their response to folate therapy. Nutr. Rev., *32*:70, 1974.

7. Collins, M., Hodas, G.R., and Liebman, R.: Interdisciplinary model for the inpatient treatment of adolescents with anorexia nervosa. J. Adol. Health Care, *4*: 3, 1983.

8. Connors, C.K.: Food Additives and Hyperactivity. New York, Plenum Press, 1980.

9. Crisp, A.H.: Anorexia Nervosa: Let Me Be. New York, Grune & Stratton, 1980.

10. Defined diets and childhood hyperactivity. JAMA, *248*: 290, 1982.

11. Dreyfus, P.M.: The nutritional management of neurological disease. In Miller, S.A. (ed.): Nutrition and Behavior. Philadelphia, Franklin Institute Press, 1981.

12. Fairburn, C.: A cognitive behavioral approach to the treatment of bulimia. Psychol. Med., *11*:707, 1981.

13. Feingold, B.F.: Why Your Child is Hyperactive. New York, Random House, 1974.

14. Garfinkel, P.E.: Some recent observations on the pathogenesis of anorexia nervosa. Can. J. Psychiat., *26*: 218, 1981.

15. Garner, D.M., et al.: Cultural expectations of thinness in women. Psychol. Reports, *47*:483, 1980.

16. Goyette, C.H., et al.: Effects of artificial colors on hyperkinetic children: a double-blind challenge study. Psychopharmacol. Bull., *14*:39, 1978.

17. Halmi, K.A., Falk, J.R., and Schwartz, E.: Binge-eating and vomiting: a survey of a college population. Psychol. Med., *11*:697, 1981.

18. Hanington, E.: Preliminary report on tyramine headache. Br. Med. J., *2*:550, 1967.
19. Harley, J.P., and Matthews, C.G.: Food additives and hypersensitivity in children. Knights, R., and Bakker, D.J. (eds.): In Treatment of Hyperactive and Learning-Disordered Children, Baltimore, University Park Press, 1980.
20. Harley, J.P., et al.: Hyperkinesis and food additives: testing the Feingold hypothesis. Pediatrics, *61*:818, 1978.
21. Hartmann, E.: L-tryptophan: a rational hypnotic with clinical potential. Am. J. Psychiat., *134*:366, 1977.
22. Herbert, V., and Tisman, G.: Effects of deficiencies of folic acid and vitamin B_{12} on central nervous system function and development. In Gaull, G.E. (ed.): Biology of Brain Dysfunction. Vol. 1. New York, Plenum Press, 1973, pp. 380 and 387.
23. Hoffer, A.: Niacin Therapy in Schizophrenia. Springfield, Ill., Charles C Thomas, 1962.
24. Hsu, L.K.G.: Outcome of anorexia nervosa. Arch. Gen. Psychiat., *37*:1041, 1980.
25. Huttenlocher, P.R.: Ketonemia and seizures: metabolic and anticonvulsant effects of two ketogenic diets in childhood epilepsy. Pediatr. Res., *10*:536, 1976.
26. Interagency Collaborative Group on Hyperkinesis: First Report of the Preliminary Findings and Recommendations of the Interagency Collaborative Group on Hyperkinesis. U.S. Department of Health, Education and Welfare, 1976.
27. Keys, A., et al.: The Biology of Human Starvation. Vol I and II. Minneapolis, University of Minnesota Press, 1950.
28. Kohlenberg, R.J.: Tyramine sensitivity in dietary migraine: a critical review. Headache, *22*:30, 1982.
29. Kolata, G.: Food affects human behavior. Science, *218*:1209, 1982.
30. Langseth, L., and Dowd, J.: Glucose tolerance and hyperkinesis. Food Cosmet. Toxicol., *16*:129, 1978.
31. Mahan, L.K.: Nutrition and behavior. In Mahan, L.K. and Rees, J.M.: Nutrition in Adolescence. St. Louis, C.V. Mosby Company, 1984.
32. Manzoor, M., and Runcie, J.: Folate responsive neuropathy: report of 10 cases. Br. Med. J., *1*:1176, 1976.
33. March, D.C.: Handbook: Interactions of Selected Drugs with Nutritional Status in Man. Chicago, American Dietetic Association, 1976, pp. 49–53.
34. Mattes, J.A., and Gittelman, R.: Effects of artificial food colorings in children with hyperactive symptoms. Arch. Gen. Psychiat., *38*:714, 1981.
35. Medina, J.L., and Diamond, S.: The role of diet in migraine headache (abstract). Headache, *17*:93, 1977.
36. Megavitamin and orthomolecular therapy in psychiatry: excerpts from a report of the American Psychiatric Task Force on Vitamin Therapy in Psychiatry. Nutr. Rev., *32* (Suppl. 1):44, 1974.
37. Millar, J.H.D., et al.: Double-blind trial of linoleate supplementation of the diet in multiple sclerosis. Br. Med. J., *1*:765, 1973.
38. Minuchin, S., Rosman, B.L., and Baker, L.: Psychosomatic Families: Anorexia Nervosa in Context. Cambridge, Mass., Harvard University Press, 1978.
39. Moffett, A.M., Swash, M., and Scott, D.F.: Effect of chocolate in migraine: A double-blind study. J. Neurol. Neurosurg. Psychiat. *37*:445, 1974.
40. National Advisory Committee on Hyperkinesis and Food Additives: Report to the Nutrition Foundation, New York, The Nutrition Foundation, 1975.
41. Osmond, H., and Hoffer, A.: Massive niacin treatment in schizophrenia: review of nine year study. Lancet, *1*:316, 1962.
42. Pauling, L.: Orthomolecular psychiatry. Science, *160*:265, 1968.
43. Pincus, J.H., Reynolds, E.H., and Glaser, G.H.: Sub-acute combined system degeneration with folate deficiency. JAMA, *221*:496, 1972.
44. Pyle, R., Mitchell, J.E., and Eckert, E.D.: Bulimia: a report of 34 cases. J. Clin. Psychiatry, *42* (2):60, 1981.
45. Rees, J.M.: Eating disorders. In Mahan, L.K., and Rees, J.M.: Nutrition in adolescence. St. Louis, C.V. Mosby Company, 1984.
46. Rees, J.M.: Nutritional counseling in adolescence. In Mahan, L.K., and Rees, J.M.: Nutrition in adolescence. St. Louis, C.V. Mosby Comapny, 1984.
47. Reif-Lehrer, L.: Possible significance of adverse reactions to glutamate in humans. Fed. Proc., *35*:2205, 1976.
48. Reynolds, E.H.: Folate and epilepsy. In Bradford, H.F., and Marsden, C.D. (eds.): Biochemistry and Neurology. New York, Academic Press, 1976, pp. 247–252.
49. Sandler, M., Youdim, M.B.H., and Hanington, E.: A phenylethylamine oxidising defect in migraine. Nature, *250*:335, 1974.
50. Spector, R.: Vitamin homeostasis in the central nervous system. N. Engl. J. Med., *296*:1393, 1977.
51. Stordy, B.J., et al.: Weight gain, thermic effect of glucose and resting metabolic rate during recovery from anorexia nervosa. Am. J. Clin. Nutr., *30*:138, 1977.
52. Swank, R.L.: Multiple sclerosis; twenty years on a low fat diet. Arch. Neurol., *23*:460, 1970.
53. Swanson, J.M., and Kinsbourne, M.: Food dyes impair performance of hyperactive children in a laboratory learning test. Science, *207*:1485, 1981.
54. Symposium on multiple sclerosis. Br. Med. Bull., *33*:2, 1977.
55. Vigersky, R.A. (ed.): Anorexia Nervosa. New York, Raven Press, 1977.
56. Vigersky, R.A., et al.: Anorexia nervosa: behavioral and hypothalamic aspects. Clin. Endocrin. Metab., *5*:517, 1976.
57. Weiss, B., et al.: Behavioral responses to artificial food colors. Science, *207*:1481, 1980.
58. Wittenborn, J.R., Weber, E.S.P., and Brown, M.: Niacin in the long-term treatment of schizophrenia. Arch. Gen. Psychiat., *28*:308, 1973.

Additional References

Epilepsy

Dodson, W.E., et al.: Management of seizure disorders: selected aspects. Part II. J. Pediatr., *89*:695, 1976.
Lasser, J.L., and Brush, M.K.: An improved ketogenic diet for treatment of epilepsy. J. Am. Diet. Assoc., *62*:281, 1973.
Schaefer, K., von Herrath, D., and Kraft, D.: Disordered calcium metabolism during anticonvulsant treatment. Ger. Med., *3*:140, 1973.
Signore, J.M.: Ketogenic diet containing medium-chain triglycerides. J. Am. Diet. Assoc., *62*:285, 1973.

Multiple Sclerosis

Alter, A., Yamoor, M., and Harshe, M.: Multiple sclerosis and nutrition. Arch. Neurol., *31*:267, 1974.
Maugh, T.H., III.: Multiple sclerosis: genetic link, viruses suspected (research news). Science, *195*:667, 1977.
McFarlin, D.E., and McFarland, H.F.: Multiple sclerosis. N. Engl. J. Med., *307*:1183, 1982.
Mertin, J., and Meade, C.J.: Relevance of fatty acids in multiple sclerosis. Br. Med. Bull., *33*:67, 1977.
Olson, W.H.: Diet and multiple sclerosis. Postgrad. Med., *59*:219, 1976.

Hyperkinetic Behavior Syndrome

Feingold, B.F.: Hyperkinesis and learning disabilities linked to artificial food flavors and colors. Am. J. Nurs., 75:797, 1975.

Ribon, A., and Joshi, S.: Is there any relationship between food additives and hyperkinesis? Ann. Allergy, 48:275, 1982.

Ross, D.M., and Ross, S.A.: Hyperactivity: Research, Theory and Action. New York, John Wiley & Sons, 1976.

Eating Disorders

Baker, L., and Lyen, K.R.: Anorexia nervosa. In Winik, M., (ed.): Adolescent Nutrition. New York, John Wiley & Sons, 1982.

Beumont, P.J.V., George, G.C.W., and Smart, D.E.: "Dieters" and "vomiters and purgers" in anorexia nervosa. Psychol. Med., 6:617, 1976.

Boskind-Lodahl, M., and White, W.C.: The definition and treatment of bulimarexia in college women—a pilot study. J. Am. College Health Assoc., 27:84, 1978.

Drossman, D.A., Ontjes, D.A., and Heizer, W.D.: Anorexia nervosa. Gastroenterology, 77:1115, 1979.

Dunn, P.K., and Ondercin, P.: Personality variables related to compulsive eating in college women. J. Clin. Psychology, 37:43, 1981.

Eckert, E.D., et al.: Behavior therapy in anorexia nervosa. Brit. J. Psychiat., 134:55, 1979.

Fransella, F., and Crisp, A.H.: Comparisons of weight concepts in groups of neurotic, normal and anorexic females. Brit. J. Psychiat., 134:79, 1979.

Garfinkel, P.E., and Garner, D.M.: Anorexia nervosa: a multidimensional perspective. New York, Brunner/Mazel, 1982.

Hasan, M.K., and Tibbetts, R.W.: Primary anorexia nervosa (weight phobia) in males. Postgrad. Med. J., 53:146, 1977.

Maxmen, J.S., Silverfarb, P.M., and Ferrell, R.B.: Anorexia nervosa: practical initial management in a general hospital. JAMA, 229:801, 1974.

Vigersky, R.A. (ed.): Anorexia nervosa symposium. J. Adol. Health Care, 4:1, 1983.

Walker, J., et al.: Caloric requirements for weight gain in anorexia nervosa. Am. J. Clin. Nutr., 32:1396, 1979.

White, W.C., Jr., and Boskind-White, M.: An experiential-behavioral approach to the treatment of bulimarexia. Psychotherapy: Theory, Research and Practice, 18:501, 1981.

Nutrition and Mental Function

Fernstrom, J.D.: Effects of the diet on brain neurotransmitters. Metabolism, 26:207, 1977.

Fernstrom, J.D., and Lytle, L.: Corn malnutrition, brain serotonin and behavior. Nutr. Rev., 34:257, 1976.

Fernstrom, J.D., and Wurtman, R.J.: Nutrition and the brain. Sci. Am., 230:84, 1974.

Growdon, J.H.: Neurotransmitter precursors in the diet: their use in the treatment of brain disease. In Wurtman, R.J., and Wurtman, J.J. (eds.): Nutrition and the Brain. Vol. 3. New York, Raven Press, 1979.

Growdon, J.H., Cohen, E.L., and Wurtman, R.J.: Treatment of brain disease with dietary precursors of neurotransmitters. Ann. Intern. Med., 86:337, 1977.

Miller, S.A. (ed.): Nutrition and Behavior. Philadelphia, Franklin Institute Press, 1981.

Rosenberg, G.S., and Davis, K.L.: The use of cholinergic precursors in neuropsychiatric diseases. Am. J. Clin. Nutr., 36:709, 1982.

Wurtman, R.J., and Fernstrom, J.D.: Control of brain neurotransmitter synthesis by precursor availability and nutritional state. Biochem. Pharmacol., 25:1691, 1976.

Orthomolecular Psychiatry

Committee on Nutrition, American Academy of Pediatrics: Megavitamin therapy for childhood psychoses and learning disabilities. Pediatrics, 58:910, 1976.

Hawkins, D., and Pauling, L. (eds.): Orthomolecular Psychiatry: Treatment of Schizophrenia. San Francisco, W.H. Freeman & Co., 1973.

Leff, D.N.: Megavitamins and mental disease. Med. World News, 16:71, 1975.

Pauling, L., et al.: On the orthomolecular environment of the mind: orthomolecular theory. Am. J. Psychiatry, 131:1251, 1974.

Winter, S.L., and Boyer, J.L.: Hepatic toxicity from large doses of vitamin B$_3$ (nicotinamide). N. Engl. J. Med., 289:1180, 1973.

Wittenborn, J.R.: Premorbid adjustment and response to nicotinic acid. In Serban, G. (ed.): Nutrition and Mental Functions. New York, Plenum Press, 1975, pp. 213–224.

DISEASE OF THE MUSCULOSKELETAL SYSTEM

Nutritional Care in Disease of the Musculoskeletal System

Diseases of the musculoskeletal system usually affect the nutritional status of the individual by altering dietary intake. Arthritis can make the processes of food preparation and eating very difficult and painful. Dental caries and periodontal disease can make the afflicted individual omit foods that require mastication and thus jeopardize the adequacy of his dietary intake. Immobilization, also discussed in this chapter, can affect food intake but also affects body metabolism and nutritional requirements. Nutritional intake can also affect the development of disease of the musculoskeletal system. Osteoporosis progression appears to be influenced by the dietary intake over the lifetime. Dental caries development is influenced by the timing of meals and snacks and their sugar content. Although there is little scientific literature to support it, many believe that arthritis is influenced by dietary intake.

Arthritis

Arthritis may be defined as inflammation of the joints. It has been estimated that at least 20 million people in the United States are afflicted with arthritis of one kind or another. About 5 million suffer from rheumatoid arthritis and another 12 million have some type of osteoarthritis.[3]

Arthritis may be acute or chronic. Any acute attack is of short duration but may recur and develop into a chronic condition. When acute arthritis involves multiple joints, rheumatic fever is a likely cause, particularly in a young person.

Arthritis may also be secondary to another disease, such as systemic lupus erythematosus, inflammatory bowel disease, celiac sprue, intestinal bypass surgery or malabsorption. Rheumatoid and degenerative arthritis are the most common forms of chronic arthritis, and of these two rheumatoid is the more severe.

RHEUMATOID ARTHRITIS

The etiology of rheumatoid or atrophic arthritis is unknown. It is a chronic, debilitating and frequently crippling disease that has tremendous personal, social and economic effects.

Any joint may be affected, but multiple involvement of the small joints of the extremities, most frequently the proximal interphalangeal joints, hands and feet, is the rule. Pain, stiffness and swelling are the common complaints. The swelling or puffiness shown in Figure 33–1 is caused by the accumulation of fluid in the lining membranes of the joints and inflammation of the surrounding tissues. Several cellular and chemical mediators, including prostaglandins, are probably involved in the inflammatory process.

The incidence of rheumatoid arthritis is reported to increase twofold in the later decades of life and may reach 15 per cent in females over 60 in some population studies. The average age of onset is 35 years, followed generally by numerous remissions and exacerbations. It occurs much more frequently in females than in males, the proportion averaging three to one. While patients with rheumatoid arthritis are frequently underweight, those with osteoarthri-

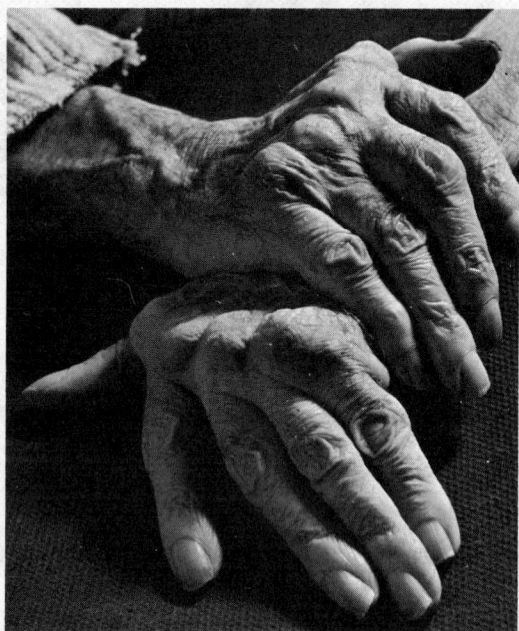

Figure 33–1. A patient with advanced rheumatoid arthritis. Note the twisted hands and the puffiness of the metacarpal joints, typical of the disease. (Courtesy of George E. Pickow, Three Lions, Inc.)

tis are often overweight. Because of the chronic disability and pain that accompany arthritis, these individuals are often given unwise or even harmful dietary advice. They become easy prey to the solicitous neighbor, food faddist or charlatan who offers quick and easy cures. The nurse, nutritionist and physician must be alert to this and use every opportunity available to stress good health habits, including a well-balanced diet.

Nutritional Care

Rheumatoid arthritis can affect the nutritional status of individuals in several ways. First, there can be malabsorption of nutrients due to gastrointestinal mucosal changes resulting from the inflammatory process of arthritis. Second, the inflammatory process can increase nutritional requirements. Third, the peptic ulcer and gastritis that are often present, due to either the disease or necessary medication, may decrease the person's desire to eat. Fourth, a complication of rheumatoid arthritis, *Sjögren's syndrome*, which is a deficiency in saliva and other secretions, makes swallowing difficult and severe dental decay occurs. Fifth, the condition is a chronic disease that frequently hinders the preparation and eating of adequate meals. Because of these factors, the nutritional status of patients with rheumatoid arthritis is frequently poor and their nutritional intake needs special

attention. With control of the disease, nutritional status usually improves. The teaching is focused on how the person's intake may be improved in order to have a well-balanced diet and to maintain weight at the desired level.

Low serum pyridoxal (vitamin B_6) levels have been reported in these patients.[27, 32] The low levels may be due to the drug therapy, or the gastric mucosal lesions commonly seen in rheumatoid arthritis patients may increase the need for pyridoxal-5-phosphate.[27] However, when serum pyridoxal levels were raised after B_6 supplementation, clinical symptoms of arthritis did not change.[32]

Low levels of ascorbic acid in white blood cells are also frequently seen in rheumatoid arthritis patients. Possibly this is due to their ingestion of large quantities of aspirin, although how this occurs is unclear.[26] A vitamin C deficiency state may exist in some individuals with cutaneous bruising that improves when they begin to take a vitamin C supplement.[17]

Hypochromic anemia is found frequently associated with arthritis, but it does not always respond well to the administration of iron. There is a defect in the metabolism of iron in people with rheumatoid arthritis. It involves the process by which iron is reused and appears to be an inherent characteristic of the disease itself. It has been reported that ingestion of ferrous sulfate in large amounts (600 mg./day) resulted in a clinical flare-up of arthritis.[6]

Copper has also been scrutinized in rheumatoid arthritis. Serum and joint fluid levels of copper are higher in people with rheumatoid arthritis than in normal people. Treatments such as cortisone and penicillamine, which lower serum copper levels, also improve rheumatoid arthritis. However, the conclusion is that the elevated copper levels are a result of the disease rather than a cause. The same situation exists for osteoarthritis.

In contrast to copper, serum zinc levels are lower than normal in individuals with rheumatoid arthritis. In one study, patients treated with zinc sulfate for three months were moderately better than those not receiving it, but this is still controversial.[34]

Numerous diets have been devised for the treatment of rheumatoid arthritis. At one time or another a low-carbohydrate diet, a high-protein diet, the B-complex vitamins, vitamin C, vitamin A and sulfur have been advocated with no real long-term success.

The use of massive therapeutic doses of vitamin D is not recommended because this form of treatment can result in severe and sometimes fatal calcification of the kidneys. Potent vitamin D preparations are capable of causing damage because of the effect of vitamin D on calcium and phosphorus metabolism. However, adequate amounts of calcium and vitamin D are recommended to prevent *osteopenia,* which often accompanies rheumatoid arthritis.

It is reported that up to 50 per cent of people with rheumatoid arthritis overcome the disease process spontaneously. This is encouraged through a well-directed daily pattern of living, including a well-balanced diet.

Hormones and Drugs

The symptoms of rheumatoid arthritis are usually controlled by large daily doses of aspirin, which is the mainstay of treatment. The side-effects of chronic aspirin ingestion are gastrointestinal problems, audiological problems and increased bleeding time (slowing of the clotting mechanism). The gastrointestinal problems can frequently be alleviated by taking the aspirin with food, milk or an antacid.

In 1949 rheumatoid arthritis was found to respond dramatically to two hormones, corticotropin (ACTH) and cortisone. Corticotropin is released by the pituitary gland and acts by stimulating the adrenal cortex to release cortisone, which relieves pain and stiffness in patients with rheumatoid arthritis. Since then, several synthetic variations of cortisone or of the adrenocorticosteroids, have been produced. They are very effective in reducing inflammation and can be given as local injections or taken orally. However, side-effects such as cushingoid symptoms, sodium retention, and potassium excretion, gastrointestinal complications, diabetes mellitus, osteoporosis and others are common. Oral corticosteroids are used only after aspirin and other nonsteroidal anti-inflammatory drugs such as indomethacin have not proved to be effective. Nutritional care, in the form of sodium restriction, potassium supplementation or a diabetic diet, may be needed for patients taking steroids. See page 509, for a discussion of the nutritional implications of steroid therapy.

Gold salt therapy can also cause a remission of rheumatoid arthritis. At least six months of therapy are necessary, and toxicity must be continually monitored by measurement of serum gold levels. There are significant dermatological, hematological and renal side-effects of this treatment.

OSTEOARTHRITIS (DEGENERATIVE ARTHRITIS)

Osteoarthritis, also known as hypertrophic or degenerative arthritis, is the most common form of arthritis and is almost universal among older people. It probably does not have a single cause but seems to develop from the stresses and strains experienced during the course of one's life. It may follow injuries and other diseases of the joints and be influenced by congenital and mechanical derangements of the joints. Numerous studies have established that the primary lesion is degeneration of the articular cartilage.

The joints most likely to be attacked are the distal interphalangeal joints, the thumb joint and especially the joints that bear the bulk of the weight: the knees, hips, ankles and spine. In the beginning there is stiffness, usually on arising from a chair or after standing. Later definite soreness may be experienced, which is worse when motion is first attempted but, after warming up, is less noticeable. One or more joints may be affected, and usually symptoms are confined to the afflicted parts. In this respect, the condition differs from rheumatoid arthritis, in which the general health may suffer.

Nutritional Care

Diet is important, especially if weight reduction is necessary. Excess weight means an added burden for the weight-bearing joints. However, it seems that weight reduction helps osteoarthritis in more than just the weight-bearing joints. It is not known why obesity should affect arthritis in other joints, but symptoms have been known to disappear completely after weight loss. Thus, the main dietary treatment is to achieve and maintain normal weight by the methods described in Chapter 27. Weight reduction is especially difficult for these patients because the disease limits their exercise potential and energy expenditure.

Drugs

Except for the oral corticosteroids, the same medications used for rheumatoid arthritis are used to treat osteoarthritis. Corticosteroids may be given as local injections.

Rest, Heat and Physical Therapy

For both osteoarthritis and rheumatoid arthritis the patient should be encouraged to lie down at least once during the day. This takes weight off the joints and allows them to rest. There should also be a regular exercise period, and massage and heat can also relieve pain.

Osteoporosis

Osteoporosis is a metabolic disorder which may be defined as *a reduction in the amount of bone without any changes in its chemical compo-*

sition. That is, the absolute amount has been diminished, but the bone remaining is normal in chemical composition. With bone loss, skeletal strength cannot be maintained and fractures occur with just minimal stress. Osteoporosis (deossification) is frequently confused with *osteomalacia* (demineralization). Table 33–1 outlines the differences between the two conditions.

Incidence and Etiology

Osteoporosis is encountered in persons after age 50 and especially in women after the menopause. Osteoporosis is more common in women by a ratio of about four to one. Practically all people begin to lose bone at about age 55. Although the reasons are unclear, it seems to be physiologically normal.

Osteoporosis can be detected by measuring the cortical thickness of the long bones, particularly the femur, by x-ray examination. The disease is either idiopathic (unknown etiology) or secondary to some known disorders. There are four types of *idiopathic osteoporosis*: (1) juvenile, (2) presenile, (3) postmenopausal and (4) senile, depending upon the age and sex of the patient. *Secondary osteoporosis* is usually endocrine, gastrointestinal, or renal induced. The majority of osteoporosis is the idiopathic type. Table 33–2 lists the causes of osteoporosis.

The most common type is osteoporosis of aging (senile) in females (postmenopausal). In these women and men the estrogen that is pres-

Table 33–2. SUSPECTED CAUSES OF OSTEOPOROSIS

PRIMARY DISEASE	SECONDARY DISEASE
Common causes	
Estrogen deficiency	Hyperparathyroidism
Inactivity	Hypercortisolism
High phosphate intake	Renal osteodystrophy
	Multiple myeloma
Uncommon causes	
Calcium deficiency	Hyperthyroidism
Vitamin D deficiency	Acromegaly
Immobilization	Heparin therapy
	Gastrectomy
	Anticonvulsant therapy
	Celiac disease
	Cirrhosis
	Scurvy
	Steatorrhea

Adapted from Jowsey, J.: Osteoporosis. It's nature and role of diet. Postgrad. Med., *60*:75, 1976.

ent is not effective, and the consequent lack of estrogen activity leads to the pathogenesis of the bone. Probably, osteoporosis is the result of a variety of factors, of which hormonal change is one. General consensus is that osteoporosis does not come on suddenly in old age, but develops over a lifetime. Clinical manifestations are seen only after bone loss is well advanced, as in Figure 33–2.

CALCIUM. Whether deficient calcium intake is a factor in the etiology of osteoporosis is not

Table 33–1. THE DIFFERENTIAL DIAGNOSIS OF OSTEOMALACIA AND OSTEOPOROSIS

	OSTEOMALACIA	OSTEOPOROSIS
Clinical features		
Skeletal pain	A major complaint and usually persistent	Episodic and usually associated with a fracture
Muscle weakness	Usually present and producing disability and, when severe, a characteristic gait	May be present
Fractures	Relatively uncommon; healing delayed	The usual presenting feature; heals normally
Skeletal deformity	Common, especially kyphosis	Only occurs where there is a fracture
Radiographic features		
Loss of density of bone	Widespread	Irregular and often most marked in the spine
Loss of bone detail	Characteristic	Not a feature
Looser's zones	Diagnostic	Absent
Biopsy		
Histological changes	Excess osteoid tissue with bone present in normal quantity	Bone reduced in quantity but fully mineralized
Biochemical changes		
Plasma Ca and P	Often low	Normal
Plasma alkaline phosphatase	Often high	Normal
Urinary calcium	Often low	Normal or high
Response to treatment		
Vitamin D	Dramatic	Small, unless active form of vitamin D

Adapted from Davidson, S., et al.: Human Nutrition and Dietetics, 7th ed. Edinburgh, Churchill Livingstone, 1979.

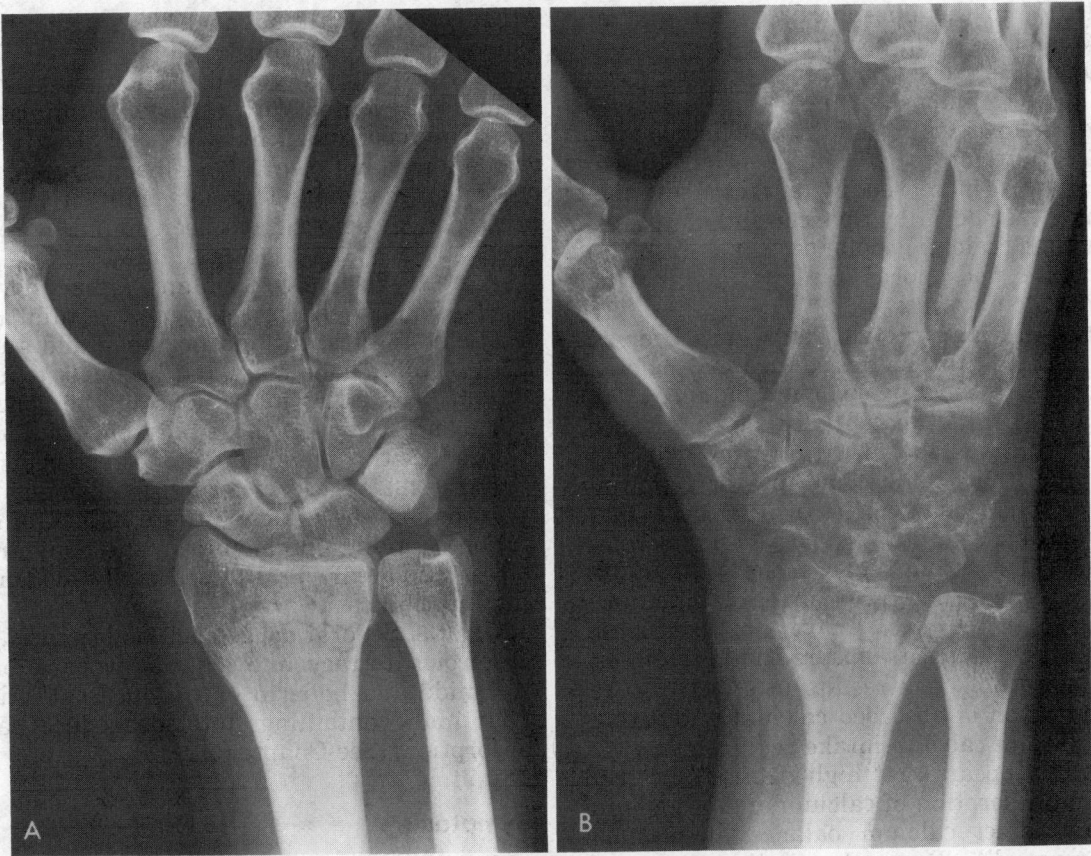

Figure 33–2. *A,* Roentgenogram of the carpal area shortly after fracture of the distal radius. The part was immobilized by a plaster cast. *B,* Roentgenogram of the same area several weeks after immobilization. Note the disuse atrophy of the carpal bones. (From Aegerter, E. E., and Kirkpatrick, J. A.: Orthopedic Diseases: Physiology, Pathology, Radiology, 4th ed. Philadelphia, W. B. Saunders Co., 1975, p. 32.)

clear. Persons with osteoporosis are in negative calcium balance, and the daily calcium loss may be as high as 90 mg./day.[21] Over a lifetime this could result in a significant loss of skeleton.

Individuals attain their adult complement of bone by their early twenties and the amount of bone attained at this point is probably nutritionally and genetically determined. Research suggests that bone formation (osteoblastic activity) remains the same with age, whereas the opposite bone activity, resorption, increases. The result is a gradual loss of bone. It has been presumed that this rate of bone loss after the fourth decade of life is a linear one and the same among all individuals. That would imply that individuals with the lowest bone mass at maturity are at the greatest risk for developing low mass and osteoporosis over time. However, prospective studies have shown that individuals lose bone at different rates and that the rate of loss slows in the eighth decade. It has also been shown that those with the greatest bone mass at the time when bone loss begins lose at a greater rate than those with less initial mass.[15]

Also, calcium absorption from the intestine decreases with age, as does the usual dietary intake of calcium. The role of factors such as level of protein intake, which alters calcium absorption, and excretion may also be important in determining calcium balance.

VITAMIN D. Nordin postulates that decreased calcium absorption with aging and in postmenopausal osteoporosis could be due to inadequate vitamin D or to a vitamin D "resistance." This vitamin D resistance could result from an increased sensitivity of bone to parathyroid hormone. This would elevate serum calcium and lead to less gastrointestinal absorption of calcium. Another cause may be impaired renal function, which accompanies aging. Decreased renal function results in less production of $1,25\text{-}(OH)_2D_3$ by the kidney and a decreased intestinal absorption of calcium. These suppositions have support in the fact that the elderly require large doses of vitamin D_2 but will respond to small doses of 1 α-OHD_3, the analogue of 1-OHD_3, the active vitamin D hormone.[22]

CALCIUM:PHOSPHORUS RATIO. The ratio of

the calcium to the phosphorus in the diet appears to be a factor in bone remodeling in growing youngsters. However, it does not at present appear to be an important factor in the development of osteoporosis in adults. Calcium balance does not deteriorate in adults when dietary phosphorus is increased by a factor of more than three, as shown by Spencer and coworkers, who studied calcium balance as a result of changing the phosphorus intake at low, normal and high calcium intakes.[36]

PROTEIN. A high protein intake has been reported to result in increased urinary calcium excretion, and a negative calcium balance could occur since calcium absorption is not increased. However, this was shown with a very high protein intake that came from purified protein fractions. When using meat to produce a high protein intake, one study reported no increase in calcium excretion because the phosphorus content of meat decreases urinary calcium.[35] Other studies, however, have not confirmed these findings. Thus it appears that protein intake in excess of need results in effectively reduced retention of absorbed calcium and a relative increase in calcium intake requirement.

FIBER. It appears that high fiber intakes can reduce the absorption of calcium and other minerals and affect calcium balance at least in short-term studies. Researchers estimate that an increase in dietary fiber of 26 gm. per day increases calcium requirements by 150 gm/day.[28]

PARATHYROID HORMONE (PTH). Berlyne and associates show that in osteoporosis in the aging, serum PTH levels are sometimes increased and can be related to the degree of osteoporosis. He explains the increased PTH by the fact that normal aging produces nephron death and decreased glomerular filtration rate. BUN rises and the decreased renal function causes an increase in parathyroid hormone and mineral resorption from the bone. The normal aging process then stimulates PTH secretion, and the low postmenopausal level of estrogen makes the bone sensitive to the action of PTH, which contributes to the osteoporotic process along with dietary factors.[5]

CALCITONIN. Calcitonin is a hormone that inhibits bone resorption or osteoclastic activity. Postmenopausal females have lower calcitonin levels than younger women and the levels continue to decrease with age.[9] Women have lower levels than men do.[12] Also, the calcitonin response to a calcium infusion is less in postmenopausal osteoporotic women than in normal women.[38] Since calcitonin acts to inhibit bone resorption, the decreased levels in postmenopausal osteoporosis result in increased bone resorption. This combined with the increased levels of PTH may be a very important factor in the bone loss

that occurs with advancing age and in postmenopausal osteoporosis.

ESTROGEN. Many studies show that bone loss can be prevented with estrogen administration, but the mechanism by which estrogen prevents bone loss is not clear. It has been suggested that estrogen may have its effect indirectly, since no estrogen receptors have been found in bone tissue.

OTHER HORMONES. Many other hormones such as androgens, progestogens, insulin, adrenocortical steroids, thyroid hormone and glucagon also regulate bone mass, but probably to a lesser extent. There are alterations in the concentrations and actions of these hormones that coexist to produce the phenomenon of osteoporosis.

EXERCISE. Lack of exercise of many aging persons may be a factor; there is lack of stimulation to maintain calcium in the bony areas of stress and wear. This is especially evident during immobilization.

DRUGS. Several drugs such as isoniazid, corticosteroids, tetracycline, thyroid preparations, furosemide and heparin can induce calcium loss. Aluminum-containing antacids reduce calcium absorption. (See Chapter 21.)

Symptoms

Osteoporosis is acquired slowly, and many years may elapse before the individual is aware of the change. Weakness is the initial manifestation, along with loss of appetite and pain in the back and hips associated with fractures. Fractures often occur easily; for example, individuals may break a hip from tripping over a rug or stepping down a low curb. The hip (femoral neck), vertebrae and distal radius are the common fracture sites. Involvement of leg bones is followed by pain, tenderness and muscle cramps. Bowing occurs when bone tissue becomes too soft to support the weight of the body. Deformity such as stooped posture is frequently marked, along with decrease in height due to shrinkage of the spine. Hypercalciuria may occur in the beginning stage, and renal stones frequently develop.

Medical Treatment

Androgens and estrogens have been shown to be protective against osteoporosis and have been used in therapy. Because of the risk of virilization, however, androgens are not used over the long term, and estrogen is the therapy of choice.

EXERCISE. Exercise should be included daily and the amount should be the most that the person can tolerate. It should involve movement of the large bones and muscles. Exercise results in more effective utilization of dietary calcium intake.

Nutritional Care

CALCIUM. The calcium intake should be increased to about 1500 mg. daily either from food or through calcium supplements. Calcium can be supplemented as calcium gluconate or lactate (10 per cent calcium) or calcium carbonate (50 per cent calcium). It has been shown that women with osteoporosis who did not yet have symptoms or x-ray evidence of osteoporosis were in negative calcium balance on 800 mg./day of calcium, but almost all could remain in balance on 1200 mg./day.[37]

VITAMIN D. The diet should be adequate in all respects to assure normal, or increased, calcium availability. Sufficient vitamin D must be present to permit utilization of the calcium taken into the body. Vitamin D intake may have to be 10,000–20,000 I.U. in order to achieve a response if there is any "vitamin D resistance." However, if this is the case, it is more effective to use an analogue of the active metabolite or the active metabolite itself (1,25-[OH]$_2$D$_3$).

FLUORIDE. Beneficial effects of fluoride in therapeutic doses (20–60 mg./day) have been reported but are still controversial. Some feel that the bone formation stimulated is of inferior quality. Others have produced good bone formation when the fluoride treatment (15–45 mg./day) is combined with calcium (1000 mg./day) and vitamin D (50,000 I.U. twice weekly).[16, 24] It is believed that the effect in bone is similar to that which helps prevent dental caries. However, long-term use of these high levels of fluoride can cause skeletal fluorosis, evidenced by bone spurs, and ligamentous calcification. The adverse rheumatic and also gastrointestinal reactions lead to fluoride discontinuation by some. The effects of fluoride in therapeutic doses are not completely understood, and the patient taking fluoride should be monitored closely.

Gout

Gout is one of the oldest diseases recorded in medical history. Even Hippocrates mentioned gout in his writings. It is a disorder of purine metabolism, in which an *excess of uric acid* appears in the blood, and the sodium urates are deposited as *tophi* in the small joints and the surrounding tissues; their most common site in chronic gout is the helix of the ear (Fig. 33–3). For some unknown reason, individuals with

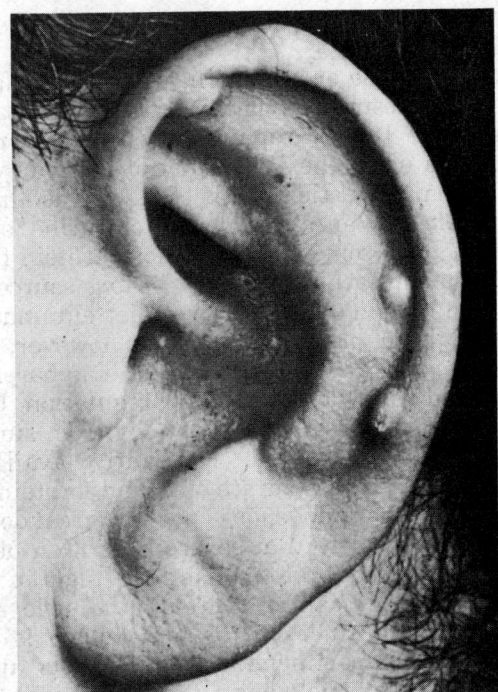

Figure 33–3. Tophi on the ear of a patient who had had gout for many years. (Courtesy of Dr. John H. Talbott. From Seminar Report, Merck, Sharp and Dohme, Div. of Merck and Co., Inc., Fall 1956.)

gout have trouble eliminating uric acid, an end-product of *purine* metabolism formed in the breakdown of *nucleoproteins*, chiefly those of animal origin. The normal person eliminates 700 mg. of uric acid daily via the kidneys. The body maintains a reserve pool of at least 1000 mg. in solution in body fluids. In gout, not only is there overproduction of uric acid, so that the amount in the pool increases from 3 to 15 times normal, but excretion is decreased.

Characteristics

The disease resembles arthritis. Sudden pain in the big toe, with the pain continuing up the leg, is characteristic of the disease.

Gout usually occurs after the age of 35 and is characterized by specific heritable metabolic defects. The ailment manifests itself in attacks, which in the beginning may last but a few days and then disappear for a period of months. With the advancement of the disease, the symptoms occur more frequently and are more prolonged. Trivial injury or unaccustomed exertion may encourage the episodes, and questions arise as to whether the attacks are related to excessive eating, drinking and exercise. Occasionally, the disturbance is a sequel to an operation. Obesity is usually associated with a gouty condition. Ketosis associated with fasting or a low-carbohydrate diet can also precipitate an attack.

Nutritional Care

PURINES. The emphasis that should be placed on purine restriction in the diet is debatable. Drugs have largely replaced the need for rigid restriction of purine in the diet of patients with gout. From a practical point of view, it is almost impossible to plan a diet devoid of purine, since all foods have some traces of nucleoprotein from which purines are derived. *Exogenous* sources of uric acid can be decreased by a diet eliminating foods high in preformed purine; however, the *endogenous* formation of uric acid is apparently influenced very little by dietary regulation. Uric acid is also synthesized in the body from simple metabolites, which are constantly available from dietary carbohydrate, fat and protein as well as from endogenous purine breakdown. Thus, it is unlikely that severe limitation of dietary purines or proteins that are high in purines will significantly decrease the uric acid pool. However, since purine metabolism is disturbed, it is recommended that patients avoid those foods extremely high in purines in order to avoid metabolic stress.[2a]

Excessive use of *fats* should be avoided, since fats are believed to reduce the normal excretion of urates. *Protein* intake should be adequate but not excessive. The calories should be maintained with *carbohydrates*, which have a tendency to increase uric acid excretion.

ACUTE STAGE. Rigid restriction of foods containing purines is generally recommended in the acute stage of gout so as not to add exogenous purines to the existing high uric acid load. Usually a diet that is relatively high in carbohydrate, moderate in protein and low in fat is indicated. Fluids such as water and fruit juice (up to 3 liters per day) should be forced to assist the excretion of uric acid and to minimize the possibility of calculi formation. Sodium bicarbonate or trisodium citrate can also be given to alkalinize the urine and increase the solubility of uric acid in the urine. Patients with a sodium restriction would require a potassium salt of carbonate or citrate instead.

INTERVAL STAGE. Dietary management during intervals between attacks is used, along with medication, to achieve negative uric acid balance and control the urate deposits and serum uric acid level. The current dietary treatment for patients who are maintained on medication for gout is a normal adequate diet adjusted so that the patient achieves his or her ideal weight. The diet should be moderate in protein (50 to 70 gm., or 0.08 gm. to 1.0 gm./kg./day), increased in carbohydrate and relatively low in fat, and should exclude foods of high purine content such as liver, kidney, sweetbreads, meat extracts, smoked meat, anchovies, sardines and leguminous vegetables. In the majority of patients, further dietary restriction does not seem to be justified. Protein intake is limited because it has been shown that endogenous uric acid biosynthesis may be accelerated in both normal and gouty patients by a high intake of protein. Most of the proteins in the therapeutic diet come from *cheese, eggs, milk and vegetables, which are low in nucleoproteins.* Fluids should be adjusted to produce a normal urinary output (2000 ml.).

ALCOHOL. It is now believed that mild or moderate use of alcohol by the patient with gout will not necessarily induce an acute attack. However, ethanol does increase uric acid production.[10] Ideally the patient would be wise not to consume alcohol, but moderate infrequent consumption could be allowed depending upon the patient's condition.

OBESITY. It is advisable that the obese patient reduce and then maintain a body weight that is 10 to 15 per cent below ideal weight. However, weight loss should not be drastic but should occur gradually over a period of several months. A sudden reduction of calories that results in the development of ketonemia is recognized as a precipitating factor of acute attacks. It may be that ketones compete with uric acid for excretion and therefore less uric acid is excreted and hyperuricemia develops.

LOW-PURINE DIET. Foods grouped according to purine content are listed in Table 33–3. The normal diet contains from 600 to 1000 mg. of purines daily. In cases of severe or advanced gout the purine content of the daily diet is restricted to approximately 100 to 150 mg. Fat is kept to 40 per cent of the energy intake. The diet may be prescribed according to these groupings, allowing for considerable individualization among patients. Nutritional care for gout is summarized in Table 33–4.

Use of Drugs

Gout is usually treated with a urate eliminant such as *probenecid* (Benemid) or sulfinpyrazone, which decreases the uric acid level in the blood by increasing the elimination of the acid through the kidneys. Another useful drug is allopurinol, which inhibits uric acid production. Both probenecid and sulfinpyrazone are frequently used with colchicine. Colchicine has proved helpful in relieving the joint pains of gouty arthritis but has no effect on uric acid metabolism. It is of more value during the acute stage but may be needed during symptom-free periods as a preventive. The nutritional effects of long-term colchicine ingestion are discussed in Chapter 21. In some instances, anti-inflammatory agents such as indomethacin or phenylbutazone may be used in the acute stage.

Table 33–3. FOODS GROUPED ACCORDING TO PURINE CONTENT

GROUP 1: HIGH PURINE CONTENT
(100 to 1000 mg. of purine nitrogen per 100 gm. of food)

Anchovies	Mackerel
Bouillon	Meat extracts
Brains	Mincemeat
Broth	Mussels
Consommé	Partridge
Goose	Roe
Gravy	Sardines
Heart	Scallops
Herring	Sweetbreads
Kidney	Yeast, baker's and
Liver	brewer's

Foods in this list should be omitted from the diet of patients who have gout (acute and remission stages).

GROUP 2: MODERATE PURINE CONTENT
(9 to 100 mg. of purine nitrogen per 100 gm. of food)

Meat and Fish *(except those in Group 1):*	*Vegetables*
Fish	Asparagus
Poultry	Beans, dried
Meat	Lentils
Shellfish	Mushrooms
	Peas, dried
	Spinach

One serving (2 to 3 oz.) of meat, fish or fowl or 1 serving (½ cup) vegetable from this group is allowed each day or five days a week (depending upon condition) during remissions.

GROUP 3: NEGLIGIBLE PURINE CONTENT

Bread, enriched white and crackers	Fruit
Butter or fortified margarine (in moderation)	Gelatin desserts
Cake and cookies	Herbs
Carbonated beverages	Ice cream
Cereal beverage	Milk
Cereals and cereal products (refined and enriched)	Macaroni products
	Noodles
	Nuts
Cheese	Oil
Chocolate	Olives
Coffee	Pickles
Condiments	Popcorn
Cornbread	Puddings
Cream (in moderation)	Relishes
Custard	Rennet desserts
Eggs	Rice
Fats (in moderation)	Salt
	Sugar and sweets
	Tea
	Vegetables (except those in Group 2)
	Vinegar
	White sauce

Foods included in this group may be used daily.

Table 33–4. SUMMARY OF NUTRITIONAL CARE FOR GOUT

1. Elimination of foods high in purines as shown in Table 33–3.
2. Moderate protein intake with large proportion of protein coming from milk, cheese, vegetables and bread.
3. Liberal carbohydrate intake (at least 100 gm./day) to prevent tissue catabolism and ketosis.
4. Low to moderate fat intake.
5. Maintenance of, or gradual reduction to, ideal body weight.
6. Restriction or elimination of alcohol.
7. Liberal fluid intake to keep urine dilute.

Prolonged Immobilization

Nutritional Implications

PROTEIN. Prolonged bed rest can result in the development of negative nitrogen balance. Immobilization of a healthy person leads to an appreciable increase in nitrogen loss. Nitrogen losses in healthy, immobilized subjects average 55 gm. over a six-week period or as much as 2 to 3 gm. of nitrogen per day when the diet would normally be adequate in protein and calories. To replace the 2 to 3 gm. of nitrogen lost, an additional 15 to 20 gm. of protein is needed (N lost × 6.25). On the other hand, debilitated, chronically ill patients will excrete less nitrogen because their bodies adapt to the stress, but they will still be in negative nitrogen balance and nutritionally depleted, as discussed in Chapter 35.

During immobilization the prevention of skin breakdown, decubitus ulcers, infection and negative nitrogen balance requires a nutritious diet adequate enough in energy and protein to put the patient into nitrogen balance or positive nitrogen balance. A minimum of 1.2 gm. protein per kg. per day is recommended for the average patient, and some patients may require more.

Helping the immobilized patient to avoid skin breakdown is a challenge to nursing care. Adequate dietary management, turning and positioning of the patient and provision of passive exercise for him will help to prevent the adverse metabolic effects of immobility. For more discussion of metabolic response to stress and the necessary nutritional care, see Chapter 35.

ENERGY. The energy requirement of the individual is of prime importance and is adjusted from time to time according to energy needs. The energy requirement in the acute phase following bone fractures or other types of accidents is usually high. There is a loss of weight due largely to anorexia and the failure of food intake and to the catabolic response on the part of the body to the noxious, toxic or mechanical agents that produced the condition. In the chronic phase and when weight has reached the ideal level, the energy intake is adjusted to meet requirements for activity. For instance, during physical therapy, which is often required for the rehabilitative process, hard work is involved, and energy should be sufficient to meet the metabolic demands.

On the other hand, the patient with hemiplegia, quadriplegia or another type of paralysis has a tendency to gain weight. Besides having a decreased energy expenditure, his intake may be increased because of a need for alternative means of gratification, which may be found in food. Both factors lead to obesity. Once the patient becomes obese, it is difficult to get him to be mobile again. Weight loss is necessary to facilitate physical rehabilitation and mobilization.

POTASSIUM. It has been observed that patients with chronic illness or under stress lose potassium, a mineral important to muscle contraction and strength. It should be liberal in the diet, or may need to be supplemented frequently in intravenous fluid.

CALCIUM. Calcium is lost from the bones (osteopenia) following a fracture and during periods of complete bed rest of a few weeks or more. Normally, bone integrity and homeostatic balance are maintained by the weight-bearing and muscle tension produced by normal motion and activity. With immobilization, hypercalcemia, hypercalciuria from bone resorption and osteopenia occur. On full bedrest the daily calcium loss is 200 to 300 mg./day. This also occurs in weightlessness and was observed in astronauts on the Skylab and Gemini space flights. There may be calcification of soft tissues such as the kidney. In addition kidney and bladder calculi can result. Hypercalcemia, although an unusual complication, seems to be more frequent in the immobilized child or adolescent. This is not surprising considering the bone growth activity of this age group. The clinical symptoms of hypercalcemia are more apparent in a patient who also has a low level of serum albumin, which normally binds calcium. When not bound, more calcium is available in its biologically active form.

The bone loss from immobilization is due to both reduced calcium absorption and increased urinary loss. The negative calcium balance may be even greater in individuals who are also ill or in a catabolic state. At the end of 3 to 6 months of immobilization, skeletal calcium content may be reduced by 30 per cent.[20] It appears that in most the loss can be repaired after mobilization providing nutritional sources of calcium, phosphorus and vitamin D are present in the diet.

The symptoms of immobilization hypercalcemia can occur immediately or insidiously and include anorexia, nausea and vomiting, abdominal cramps, constipation, headache, malaise, lethargy and sometimes polydipsia and polyuria. If these symptoms are not treated, renal insufficiency, hypertension, seizures and hearing loss can result. Hyman and colleagues hypothesize that immobilization hypercalcemia may be more common than is now realized and that vague complaints of anorexia, nausea and abdominal cramps from immobilized patients may be due to hypercalcemia.[14]

The treatment of choice for serum hypercalcemia is mobilization as soon as possible. A diet low in calcium does not seem to be effective in decreasing serum calcium concentration.[14] The calcium intake should remain at a normal level of 600 to 800 mg./day.

Phosphate supplements have been shown to decrease the level of serum calcium in immobilized patients in the first weeks following immobilization but not after that.[13] Phosphate therapy also does not decrease the bone resorption. It still is not clear whether this therapy is of any value for treating hypercalcemia.

Other therapy includes the use of diuretics and of up to 3 or 4 liters per day of saline fluids to dilute the calcium concentration. Hypomagnesemia and hypokalemia must be watched for when using this therapy.

Bowel and Bladder Training

Calciuria may precipitate the formation of urinary calculi, which is discussed in Chapter 30. Poor bladder function may cause urinary infection and may influence the formation of urinary calculi by alkalinizing the urine. An acid ash diet can be used to keep the urine acid. (The acid ash diet is described in Chapter 30.) A high fluid intake is necessary in the prevention and treatment of infection and urinary calculi. Diminished thirst sensation has been observed in these patients. Therefore close attention must be paid to be sure that the person has sufficient fluid intake.

During bladder training for the immobilized patient, fluid is given at regularly spaced intervals throughout the day, and recording of the time, type and amount given must be a routine procedure.

During bowel training, a high-fiber diet served at regular intervals is desirable, but too much fiber may cause fecal impaction. Foods causing watery stools should be avoided. A regular time should be set for defecation. For constipated individuals, prune juice given in large amounts may be helpful, as mentioned in Chapter 23.

Feeding the Disabled Patient

All the suggestions of ways to encourage the appetite and provide the essential nutrients apply here. The psychology of feeding is especially important, since most chronically ill and disabled individuals are limited in activity and hence have a greater amount of leisure time to focus attention on meals. Planning the diet with the patient around his customary eating pattern usually attracts his interest and motivation. A review of his food intake periodically discloses how well the person is following the principles of therapy recommended.

One of the aims in the rehabilitation of the person is to help him become as self-sufficient and productive as possible. The training process usually begins in the hospital or rehabilitation center, depending upon the nature of the illness or injury. Follow-up nursing care in the home may be supervised by the community health nurse. The importance of nutrition is stressed from the beginning. Persons who have difficulty in feeding themselves and in swallowing are often depressed because of this handicap. Food placed on the unaffected side of the mouth beyond the tip of the tongue in paralyzed patients can usually be tasted and swallowed. If the patient is unable to swallow or ingest enough food, tube feedings or liquid supplements may be necessary to supply adequate nutrition. Mechanical devices are available for those individuals who have difficulty in using ordinary eating utensils. The Additional References by Hargrave and by Lowman and Klinger provide helpful information about feeding techniques for the disabled patient. Kitchens have been renovated to heights that are convenient for people in wheelchairs. Guides for streamlining kitchen tasks are available.

Dental Caries

Tooth decay is the most prevalent chronic disease in the United States and occurs among all populations throughout the world. Some primitive peoples such as older Eskimos, some Pacific islanders, Greenlanders and South Africans, who live in remote areas of the world under native or natural conditions, are freer from dental caries than are more civilized peoples. When these persons come into contact with civilization, they frequently experience an increased incidence of tooth decay. This is believed to be due, in major degree, to a change in their diets, specifically to an increase in their consumption of simple sugar.[30]

Etiology

Dental caries are characterized by demineralization of the inorganic portion and dissolution of the organic substance of teeth. There are several types: pit and fissure caries, smooth surface caries, root caries and deep detinal caries. The role of diet in root caries and deep detinal caries

is not as well understood as it is in the other two, which are also called *coronal caries*. Dental caries are recognized as an infection caused by the bacterium *Streptococcus mutans*. The carious process begins with the production of acid by bacterial enzymatic action on carbohydrates in the dental plaque, and these organic acids cause decalcification of the enamel. Proteolytic degradation and demineralization of the dentin follow as shown in Figure 33-4. It has been shown that three factors must be present simultaneously for dental caries to develop: (1) food, particularly fermentable carbohydrate, in the oral environment; (2) a caries-prone tooth; and (3) bacteria on the surface of the tooth in the *plaque*, an adherent microbial matrix on the tooth surface.

No one knows why some individuals are more afflicted with dental caries than others. Hereditary influences have been demonstrated in experimental animals. Among humans some families have good teeth, whereas others do not. As yet ill-understood hormonal, immunological and nutritional factors in both the pre-eruptive and post-eruptive phases of tooth development affect later caries development.

CARBOHYDRATE. The current, dominant theory is that decay is caused by a chemical-bacterial action, acting from outside directly upon the enamel and dentin of the teeth. The cariogenic bacteria apparently prefer sucrose, but they can also act upon other sugars to produce extracellular polysaccharides, glucans, levans and acids. The acids dissolve the calcium in the tooth to form a cavity. Honey is just as cariogenic as sucrose.[33] Because of the knowledge of the destructive effects of the acids on the tooth, the latest techniques for measuring cariogenicity of foods measure the pH changes in the plaque.

An extensive experiment on the relationship between tooth decay and the form in which carbohydrate is taken was carried out in Vipeholm, Sweden.[11] Under institutional circumstances, patients were given a variety of carbohydrate supplements to the basic, highly nutritious diet. When sucrose in solution was added to the diet over prolonged periods of time, there was practically no increase in the incidence of dental

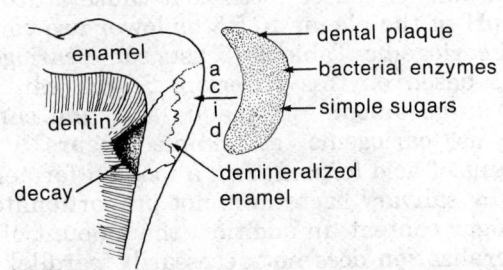

Figure 33–4. Formation of dental caries.

caries. However, when the sugar was fed in the form of sticky candies that adhered to the teeth, the incidence of dental caries increased far above that during the preliminary control period. As soon as these candy supplements were stopped, tooth decay quickly dropped to the control level. In other groups of patients, the sugar was fed in breads, or in less sticky candies. More severe effects were observed than with sugar in solution, but the effects were less severe than with the sticky candies. It is logical to conclude from these observations that the longer the carbohydrate is retained in the oral cavity and available to bacteria for fermentation, the greater the possibility of tooth decay. Thus, the physical characteristics of the carbohydrates determine to a large extent their influence on dental caries.

Frequency of eating is an important factor in caries causation, and between-meal eating is to be discouraged unless noncariogenic foods are consumed. Unfortunately this is not the usual pattern of children in the U.S. The 1977–1978 Nationwide Food Consumption Survey showed that one-fourth of the children surveyed ate five or more times during the day, so snacking is popular.[7] Of the most popular items for snacks —soft drinks, bakery products, milk, milk desserts, fruits and candy—five contain substantial amounts of sugar. It should be emphasized to parents and their children that a marked increase in caries development occurs when sweets are consumed between meals.

The rate at which carbohydrate and other bacterial substrate is cleared from the teeth is also important in determining the extent of caries formation. Adequate salivary secretion is an important factor and vigorous mastication promotes salivary production. For example, patients with damaged salivary function, such as those receiving radiotherapy for cancer, usually develop an increased number of dental caries.

When nothing is eaten, the pH of plaque stays relatively constant; when food or drink is ingested, the bacteria ferment the available carbohydrate to acids and the pH of the plaque drops. Dental scientists propose that once the pH of the plaque drops below about 5.5 (the critical pH) there is enough acid to begin to dissolve tooth enamel. Those foods that cause a drop in the pH of the plaque to 5.5 or lower are considered cariogenic. Table 33–5 lists some cariogenic foods based on this criterion. Starch can produce large amounts of plaque acid and can be just as cariogenic as simple sugars.[29] The amount of acid formed from a food on fermentation by salivary bacteria is not proportionate to its sugar content. In addition, the amount of demineralization does not necessarily parallel the amount of acid produced from the food. This ob-

Table 33–5. SOME FOODS THAT CAUSE THE pH OF HUMAN INTERPROXIMAL PLAQUE TO FALL BELOW 5.5

Apples, dried	Gelatin, flavored dessert
Apples, fresh	Grapes
Apple drink	Milk, whole
Apricots, dried	Milk, 2%
Bananas	Milk, chocolate
Beans, baked	Oatmeal, instant, cooked
Beans, green, canned	Oats, rolled
Bread, white	Oranges
Bread, whole wheat	Orange juice
Caramel	Pasta
Carrots, cooked	Peanut butter
Cereals, non-presweetened	Peas, canned
Cereals, presweetened	Potato amylose
Chocolate, milk	Potato, boiled
Cola, beverage	Potato chips
Cookies, vanilla sugar	Raisins
Cornflakes	Rice, instant, cooked
Cornstarch	Sponge cake, cream filled
Crackers, soda	Tomato, fresh
Cream cheese	Wheat flakes
Doughnuts, plain	

From Schachtele, C.F.: Changing perspectives on the role of diet in dental caries formation. Nutr. News, *45*:13, 1982.

servation may be due to the formation of different types of fermentation products or the presence in the food of substances that retard or accentuate the caries-producing action of their sugar content.

It is also known that following eating, the pH can remain low for prolonged periods of time depending upon the stimulation of saliva. The potential for decay continues for longer than 20 to 30 minutes, as previously thought. In summary, then, a food with low cariogenic potential should have a relatively high protein content with polypeptides rich in the basic amino acids, a moderate fat content to facilitate oral clearance, a minimal concentration of fermentable carbohydrate, a strong buffering capacity, a high mineral content including calcium and phosphorus, and a pH greater than 6. In addition, it should stimulate saliva flow. Certain cheeses (especially cheddar), meats and nuts have many of these characteristics and in fact have low cariogenic potential.[29] Factors influencing the cariogenicity of food are given in Table 33–6.

PROTEIN. Protein is important in dental health because of its role in the development of teeth, salivary glands, oral epithelium, lips, palate and maxillary and mandibular bone. Because tooth development involves the formation of a protein matrix that becomes mineralized, adequate protein must be available during the critical periods of tooth formation. These periods of increased protein need probably occur throughout gestation and during periods of childhood and adolescence, but their exact tim-

Table 33–6. FACTORS INFLUENCING THE CARIOGENICITY OF A FOOD AND EATING SITUATION

Plaque-forming ability
Adherence
Viscosity
Acid-producing ability
Ingestion time
Intraoral clearance time
Plaque pH response
Caries-modifying factors in food that reduce cariogenicity
  calcium and phosphorus
  organic substances such as phosphates and casein
  fats and oils
  flavoring agents
    cinnamon
    licorice

ing is not known. Protein and minerals must be adequate during these times to permit proper development, tooth mineralization and maximum resistive capabilities to later microbial challenge. Figure 33–5 illustrates the effect of malnutrition on tooth development.

Menaker and Navia have shown that the offspring of rats who received a protein-deficient diet during pregnancy had increased susceptibility to caries due to dental and salivary gland abnormalities that could be attributed to protein deficiency during gestation.[19] Part of the salivary gland abnormality was a decrease in the ability to synthesize and secrete salivary proteins, some of which may be antimicrobial agents such as secretory IgA and lysozyme, which are defense mechanisms against microbial invasion.

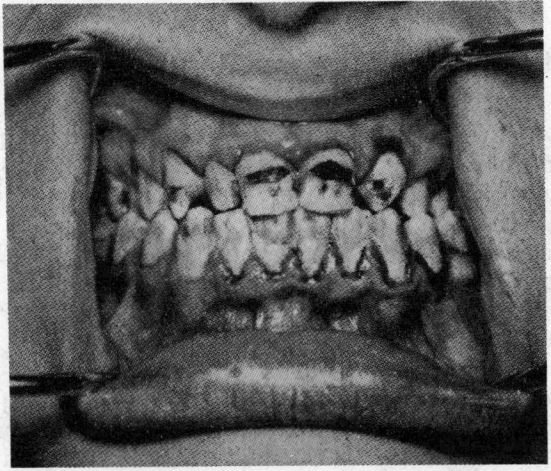

Figure 33–5. Excessive enamel hypoplasia of the anterior teeth of a 16-year-old girl caused by severe malnutrition at the age of 6 months. The marked gingivitis on lower anterior gingiva cleared up quickly as a result of vitamin C therapy. (From Cahn, L. R.: Pathology of the Oral Cavity. Baltimore, The Williams & Wilkins Co.)

FAT. Fats form a protective film on the surface of the tooth, have an antimicrobial action and thereby decrease the caries-producing potential of carbohydrates.

CALCIUM AND PHOSPHORUS. The importance of minerals in the diet, more specifically calcium and phosphorus, has been discussed in Chapter 7. Since these minerals make up a large percentage of the enamel and dentin of teeth, an ample amount must be supplied in the diet if the teeth are to be sound. Since major calcification of bones and teeth takes place during the last two months of gestation, it is important that the mother's calcium and phosphorus intake be adequate during this period. It appears that the calcium:phosphorus ratio is important, and phosphorus seems to have a protective effect.

FLUORIDE. The incidence of dental caries and its relation to the fluoride content of the drinking water has been studied. It appears from extensive studies that fluoride taken during the first 8 to 12 years of life (the period when the dentin and enamel of the permanent dentition are being formed) will reduce the incidence of dental caries by as much as 50 to 60 per cent.[1] This increased resistance is believed to be carried over into later life to an appreciable degree. Before the eruption of teeth, fluoride is incorporated into the enamel matrix. After eruption it can be applied to the tooth surface, where it is absorbed and so increases the fluoride content of the superficial layers of enamel. The mechanisms by which fluoride prevents caries development are not fully understood. It is probably a combination of its alteration of the morphology of teeth so that less plaque is retained, its interference with the adherence or metabolism of plaque bacteria, and its retardation of the demineralization and enhancement of remineralization of enamel. It converts the crystal hydroxyapatite normally present in teeth to fluoroapatite, which is much more resistant to acid demineralization.

During gestation the infant does not benefit from the fluoride intake of the mother because fluoride does not cross the placenta in sufficient amounts.[8] The optimal effect of fluoride ingestion is achieved when it is taken in from birth to 18 years of age.

Following favorable results from years of water fluoridation in well-controlled studies[4] in Evanston, Illinois, Newburgh, New York, and elsewhere, fluoride is now being added to the drinking water in a number of cities and communities as a prophylactic agent to reduce the incidence of dental caries. Virtually every authoritative public health and medical organization recommends fluoridation, including the American Medical Association, the American

Dental Association and the American Academy of Pediatrics. The level considered to be most protective is 0.7 to 1.2 parts fluoride per million parts of drinking water in the U.S. Since factors such as climate, usual water consumption, diet, nutritional status of the population and geochemical background affect fluoride intake and utilization, this may not be appropriate for other countries.[31] When fluoride exceeds 1.5 parts per million, as occurs naturally in some areas, mottling of the enamel is apt to occur, as shown in Figure 7–8. Fluoride is also discussed in Chapter 7.

It may be that the fluoride intake of some individuals is too high, leading to mild fluorosis due to increasing amounts of fluoride in the food chain.[18] Fluoride content of the diet in communities with fluoridated water is three times that in communities without fluoridated water. Fresh spinach, gelatin, and bone and fish meal concentrates are potent sources of fluoride. Mechanically deboned meat can contain a significant amount of fluoride. The generally regarded safe intake of fluoride is 0.05 to 0.07 mg. fluoride per kg. body weight, and the determined average intake of fluoride in typical diets of infants between two and six months of age living in a community with fluoridated water was 0.1 mg./kg. body weight. Fluorosis can occur at this level of intake. The level of intake of two-year-olds was lower, 0.049 mg./kg.[23] Increasing amounts of fluorosis have been reported in children in communities without fluoridated water. The fluorosis is mild and the level of mottling is not usually discernible by the lay person. However, because of the incorporation of fluoride into the food chain, perhaps there should be reconsideration of the levels of optimal fluoride use both in water and in dentifrices.[18]

VITAMINS. There is no definite evidence that vitamin A is concerned directly with dental caries, but it is a vital factor in the formation of dental enamel and dentin.

There is also no conclusive evidence that lack of any of the B-complex vitamins brings increased susceptibility to decay; however, pain in teeth may be due to a neuritis that is secondary to vitamin B deficiency.

Vitamin C is known to be important in building teeth and in maintaining health of gums and other structures, and changes in gum tissue are characteristic of scurvy. However, there has not been satisfactory evidence that susceptibility to decay is reduced by giving vitamin C to individuals on a diet that is partially deficient in vitamin C. Nor has it been found that scurvy makes a person more subject to tooth decay.

Vitamin D may help in caries prevention because it is involved in the calcification of teeth. It promotes greater deposition of calcium and phosphorus, the minerals in teeth.

Prophylactic Nutritional Care

There seems to be agreement that diet and the incidence of dental caries are closely related. The adequate normal diet (Chapter 10) should be followed, with restriction of foods containing readily adherent, fermentable carbohydrates such as sticky candy or other concentrated sweets. Jams, jellies, candies, sugar, heavily sugared beverages or soft drinks and all excessive sweets should be discouraged. Table 33–7 lists the sugar content of some popular foods. Acid-producing foods as listed in Table 33–5 should also be controlled. The chewing of nonadherent, rough, coarse foods such as raw carrots, lettuce, celery, apples and most fruits and vegetables causes saliva production and a cleansing of the teeth and is suggested to aid control of dental caries. The longer food is in contact with the teeth, the greater the reaction. Thus, it is claimed that the thicker and more gelatinous foods are more likely to cause dental caries than those of thinner consistency.

Since an acid mantle is formed on the teeth after every food ingestion, the decalcification from the acid's presence can be inhibited for the most part if proper oral hygiene is followed and if the "acid bath" exposures are not too frequent. The number of eating times throughout the day should be limited. Brushing the teeth or rinsing the mouth, or both, immediately after each meal or snack will remove the food particles and reduce the reactions. Dentists have discovered that most of the chemical reaction takes place within 15 minutes after the meal is started.

Also important is daily flossing, which removes plaque buildup and food from between the teeth and from between the gum and tooth.

Nursing Bottle Caries

This syndrome is commonly seen in children who are given a bottle of milk or sugared liquid to nurse when they go to bed. There is rampant decay of the upper front teeth that begins shortly after the teeth erupt, and if uncontrolled, decay may spread throughout the upper jaw. The lower front teeth usually are spared due to the protective position of the tongue and lip during sucking.

As the child falls asleep with the nipple of the bottle resting against the palate, the liquid spreads over the upper and the lower back teeth. As it covers the teeth it forms a medium that encourages the growth of bacteria. In addition, when the child is asleep the salivary secretion and swallowing decrease, thus adding to the cariogenic environment.

Parents should be told very early about the possibility of caries development caused by a

Table 33–7.   SUGAR CONTENT OF SOME POPULAR FOODS

FOOD	SERVING SIZE	TOTAL TSP. SUGAR IN SERVING	TOTAL SUGAR % WEIGHT	TOTAL SUGAR % CALORIES
Beverages				
Frozen concentrate grape juice	6 oz.	1	2	15
Coke	12 oz.	9.2	10	99
Welch's grape juice drink	6 oz.	3.9	9.3	55
Hi-C orange (Welch's)	6 oz.	4.8	11.4	81
Kool aid (sugar-sweetened flavors)	6 oz.	4.3	10	98
Sprite (Coca Cola)	12 oz.	9	9.8	100
Bright & Early Frozen Concentrate Imitation OJ	6 oz.	5.4	13	84
Cereals				
General Mills Cheerios	1¼ cup	0.2	3.6	3.5
GM Wheaties	1 cup	0.7	11	11
GM Total	1 cup	0.7	11	11
GM Kix	1½ cup	0.5	7.1	7
GM Lucky Charms	1 cup	2.7	39.3	39
GM Nature Valley Granola Cin & Raisin	⅓ cup	1.7	25	21
Post Alphabits	1 cup	2.7	39	39
Post Raisin Bran	½ cup	2.2	32	39
Ralston Purina Cookie Crisp (choc chip)	1 cup	3	46	42
Kellogg's Fruit Loops	1 cup	3.5	50	49
Kellogg's Sugar Pops	1 cup	3.2	46	46
Kellogg's Special K	1¼ cup	0.5	7.1	7
Kellogg's Corn Flakes	1 cup	0.5	7	7
Kellogg's Raisin Bran	½ cup	0.7	10.7	11
Kellogg's All Bran	⅓ cup	1	14.3	26
Kellogg's Apple Jacks'	1 cup	4	57	56
Kellogg's Sugar Frosted Flakes	⅔ cup	2.7	39	39
Kellogg's Country Morning	⅓ cup	1.5	21	18
Kellogg's Rice Krispies	1 cup	0.7	11	17
Kellogg's Sugar Smacks	¼ cup	4.0	57	56
GM Boo-Berry	1 cup	3.2	46	46
GM Cocoa Puffs	1 cup	2.7	39	39
GM Count Chocula	1 cup	3.2	46	46
GM Golden Grahams	1 cup	2.7	39	39
GM Crazy Cow	1 cup	3.0	43	42
Nabisco 100% bran	½ cup	1.5	21.4	33
Instant Quaker Oatmeal with cin & spice	1⅝ oz.	4	35.2	35
Quaker Captain Crunch	¼ cup	3	43	42
Quaker Life	⅔ cup	1.2	18	18
Quaker 100% Natural Cereal	¼ cup	1.5	21	17
Shredded Wheat	1 biscuit	—	—	—
Condiments				
Bleu cheese salad dressing	1 tbsp.	0.2	6.7	5.0
French salad dressing	1 tbsp.	0.7	18.8	18
Hellman's Spin Blend salad dressing	1 tbsp.	0.7	18.8	19
Italian dressing	1 tbsp.	0.2	6.7	4.5
Cranberry sauce	½ cup	11.7	35.1	90
Catsup	1 tbsp.	0.6	17	61
Protein				
Bacon (Oscar Mayer)	2 slices	0.0	1.7	1.1
Beef bologna (OM)	2 slices	0.3	3	4
Canadian style bacon (OM)	2 slices	0.0	0.4	1.0
Canned ham (OM)	3 oz.	0.1	0.4	1.1
Luncheon meat (OM)	2 slices	0.3	3	3
Peanut butter	2 tbsp.	0.3	4	3
Pork sausage	3 links	0.3	2	2
Hard salami	6 slices	0.1	1	1
Cotto salami	2 slices	0.1	1	2
Spam	3 oz.	0.8	4	5
Weiners (OM)	one	0.3	3	4
Vanilla ice cream, hard	½ cup	3.1	19	36
Vanilla ice milk	½ cup	3.4	15	47
Yogurt, lowfat flavored	8 oz.	4.1	7	33
Yogurt, fruit	8 oz.	7.5	13	50

Table continued on the following page

Table 33–7. SUGAR CONTENT OF SOME POPULAR FOODS (*Continued*)

FOOD	SERVING SIZE	TOTAL TSP. SUGAR IN SERVING	TOTAL SUGAR % WEIGHT	TOTAL SUGAR % CALORIES
Snacks				
Applesauce	½ cup	4.3	14	57
Columbo frozen yogurt (whole milk)	8½ oz.	5.3	22	60
Canned pears, heavy syrup	½ cup	3.1	10	50
Canned pineapple, heavy syrup	½ cup	3.1	10	52
Chocolate pudding	4 oz.	3.9	12	37
Cool Whip	1 tbsp.	0.2	23	28
Dannon frozen yogurt (vanilla)	½ cup	2.8	11	48
Gino's vanilla milkshake	12.1 oz.	7.5	9	37
Graham cracker	2 crackers	0.9	25	25
Hershey's milk chocolate	1.2 oz.	4.4	51	37
Hunt's vanilla Snackpack	5 oz.	4.4	13	36
Jello, cherry	½ cup	4.5	15	87
Kellogg's brown sugar cinnamon Poptarts	1 tart	3.8	31	28
Vegetables				
Beets, pickled (Delmonte)	½ cup	2.1	9.9	57
Sweet peas (canned)	½ cup	0.9	4.5	20
Tomato sauce	4 oz.	0.7	2.4	35

Adapted from: A nation sweet on sugar. Nutr. Action, *8*(5):9, 1979. Center for Science in the Public Interest, 1755 S. St., N.W. Washington, DC 20009.

bedtime bottle and should be counseled against this practice. A bottle of water or a pacifier can be given if the child insists. It is important not to start the nursing bottle habit; Rosenstein found that many children who have nursing bottle syndrome as infants develop the later habit of eating carbohydrate snack foods continually throughout the day.[25]

DIETARY FACTORS IN DENTAL DEVELOPMENT

There is an important relationship between nutrition and the development of the teeth. In both humans and animals deficiencies of energy, protein, iron, zinc, calcium, phosphorus, vitamin D, folic acid and ascorbic acid have all been associated with tooth and jaw abnormalities. The greatest hope in preventive dentistry lies in developing strong teeth that have a high resistance to deterioration and tooth decay—highly mineralized teeth with a low solubility of enamel. Close adherence to an adequate diet throughout the period of tooth development is of major importance in attaining this goal. This applies both to children and to women during pregnancy and lactation. The minerals from the mother's reserves are drawn upon to meet the demands of the growing, calcifying teeth and bones of the child.

It has been demonstrated that the early development of the teeth is influenced by the amount of calcium, phosphorus, fluoride and vitamins in the diet. Consequently, these substances should be supplied in adequate amounts in the diet during pregnancy and for the infant, the growing child and the adult. An ample supply of vitamin D should be provided daily throughout the period of growth and development. A highly desirable factor in the overall diet planning for the attainment of maximum caries resistance is the availability of a fluoridated water supply.

THE INFLUENCE OF DENTAL STATUS ON NUTRITIONAL INTAKE

The status of teeth is often reflected in the general health of an individual. Poorly formed, missing or painful teeth may result in the consumption of an inadequate diet and the bolting of food, followed by impaired digestion and poor health.

Denture patients are apt to avoid foods that are difficult to chew and will resort to soft foods. They tend to avoid meat, raw vegetables, fruit and salads. In counseling these patients the person's dietary pattern is obtained, an evaluation of the adequacy of the dietary practice is determined and a plan within his limitations is developed that will enable him to consume a more adequate diet.

Periodontal Disease

Etiology

Much of the confusion about the role of nutrition in the etiology of periodontal disease is due to the fact that a great deal of the research in this area has not been well conducted because of the many-faceted nature of the disease and its slow progression. It appears that the primary etiological factor in the development of periodontal disease is plaque, which progresses to dental calculus. This acts as a local irritant to the periodontium, which becomes inflamed. Also important are several host factors such as age; immunological, nutritional and endocrinological status; local oral irritants; faulty tooth restorations; poor tooth alignment and traumatic occlusion of the teeth. It has been suggested that a low calcium intake and high phosphorus intake may cause a secondary hyperparathyroidism that results in mobilization of calcium from the alveolar bone and periodontal disease. It is unlikely that this is a primary etiological factor, but it might contribute to the progression of the disease.[2]

Unlike dental caries disease, which is closely associated with Western civilization and dietary sucrose, periodontal disease is seen more frequently in malnourished, underprivileged populations. Although periodontal disease is not a nutritional deficiency disease, all would agree that malnutrition may predispose the host to periodontal disease or modify its severity and progression. The defense mechanisms of the gingival tissue, epithelial barrier and saliva can be affected by nutritional intake and status. Healthy epithelial tissue prevents the penetration of bacterial endotoxins into subgingival tissue. Deficiencies of vitamin C, folate and zinc in animals increase the permeability of the gingival barrier at the gingival sulcus, making the animals more susceptible to periodontal disease.

It is impossible to say that there is no role for nutrition in periodontal disease, yet is is equally wrong to say that the nutritional status of the host is always a factor. Nutrition seems to affect tissue resistance, the interaction between tissues and oral microbial agents and the chemical environment of the oral tissues. Each patient should be evaluated individually, and evaluation of host factors should include assessment of nutritional status as described in Chapter 9.

Nutritional care is particularly important in preparation for and after periodontal surgery, when adequate nutrients are needed to regenerate tissue and maintain an immune response to prevent infection. Vitamin C, vitamin A, zinc and protein appear to be important. Chapter 34 discusses the nutritional requirements for wound healing in more detail. If the procedure or the wound prevents normal dietary intake for longer than three days, a complete, nutritional liquid diet should be designed and recommended for the patient.

Problems and Suggested Topics for Discussion

1. Make a survey in your hospital of patients who are suffering with arthritis. Classify the types of arthritis. Obtain a diet history from a patient with rheumatoid arthritis. Analyze the diet history for carbohydrate, protein, fat, calories, minerals (calcium, phosphorus and iron) and vitamins. Calculate a meal plan based on the diet treatment outlined in this text for rheumatoid arthritis.
2. Plan a high-calorie diet with an underweight patient who has rheumatoid arthritis with extensive crippling of the hands. Use easy-to-handle and easy-to-eat foods.
3. Plan a reduction diet with an obese patient in your clinic who is suffering with osteoarthritis. Follow his or her progress.
4. Discuss the effects of prolonged immobilization on nutritional status and requirements.
5. Visit the dental clinic in your hospital and obtain a diet history from a patient with severe dental caries. Analyze the diet. Assist the patient to plan the correct nutritious diet and include suggestions for tooth decay prevention.
6. Find out the fluoride content of the water in your community and give a report. Is it low, adequate or excessive?
7. Interview a patient with chronic gout who is in an acute flare-up stage. What are his complaints? How much does he weigh? Obtain a diet history. What recommendations would you make?

Cited References

1. Adler, P.: Fluorides and dental health. In: Fluorides and Human Health., Vol. 9. Geneva, World Health Organization, 1970, p. 323.
2. Alfano, M.C.: Controversies, perspectives, and clinical implications of nutrition in periodontal diseases. Dent. Clin. North Am., 20:519, 1976.
2a. American Dietetic Association: Handbook of Clinical Dietetics. New Haven, Yale University Press, 1981.
3. Arthritis—The Basic Facts. New York, The Arthritis Foundation, 1976.
4. Ast, D.B., and Fitzgerald, B.: Effectiveness of water fluoridation. J. Am. Dent. Assoc., 65:581, 1962.
5. Berlyne, G.G., et al.: The etiology of osteoporosis. The role of parathyroid hormone. JAMA, 229:1904, 1974.
6. Blake, D., and Bacon, P.A.: Iron and rheumatoid disease (letter). Lancet, 1:623, 1982.
7. Consumer Nutrition Center: Eating patterns and food frequencies of children in the United States. Spring, 1977, Nationwide Food Consumption Survey, 1977–1978. Nutrition Science and Education Administration. Hyattsville, Md., U.S. Department of Agriculture, 1980.
8. De Paola, D.P., and Kuftinec, M.M.: Nutrition in growth and development of oral tissues. Dent. Clin. North Am., 20:441, 1976.
9. Deftos, L.J., et al.: Influence of age and sex on plasma calcitonin in human beings. N. Engl. J. Med. 302:1351, 1980.
10. Faller, J., and Fox, I.H.: Ethanol-induced hyperuricemia. N. Engl. J. Med., 307:1598, 1982.
11. Gustafsson, B.E., et al.: The Vipeholm dental caries study. The effect of different levels of carbohydrate intake on caries activity in 436 individuals observed for five years. Acta Odontol. Scand., 11:232, 1954.
12. Heath, H., and Sizemore, G.W.: Plasma calcitonin in normal man. Differences between men and women. J. Clin. Invest., 60:1135, 1977.
13. Hulley, S.B., et al.: The effect of supplemental oral phosphate on the bone mineral changes during prolonged bed rest. J. Clin. Invest., 50:2506, 1971.
14. Hyman, L.R., et al.: Immobilization hypercalcemia. Am. J. Dis. Child., 124:723, 1972.
15. Johnston, C.C., and Epstein, S.: The endocrinology of

osteoporosis. In Parsons, J.A. (ed.): Endocrinology of Calcium Metabolism. New York, Raven Press, 1982.

16. Jowsey, J., Riggs, B.L., and Kelly, P.J.: Long term experiences with fluoride and fluoride combination treatment of osteoporosis. In Kuhlencordt, F., and Kruse, H. (eds.): Calcium Metabolism, Bone and Metabolic Bone Disease. New York, Springer-Verlag, 1973.

17. Katz, W.A.: Rheumatic Diseases: Diagnosis and Management. Philadelphia, J.B. Lippincott Co., 1977, p. 429.

18. Leverett, D.H.: Fluorides and the changing prevalence of dental caries. Science, 217:26, 1982.

19. Menaker, L., and Navia, J.M.: Effect of undernutrition during the perinatal period on caries development in the rat. Parts, II, III and IV. J. Dent. Res., 52:680, 1973.

20. Minaire, P., et al.: Quantitative histological data on disuse osteoporosis: comparison with biological data. Calcif. Tissue Res., 17:57, 1974.

21. Nordin, B.E.C.: Metabolic Bone and Stone Disease. Baltimore, Williams & Wilkins Co., 1973.

22. Nordin, B.E.C., et al.: Calcium absorption in the elderly. In Nielsen, S.P., and Hjorting-Hansen, E. (eds.): Calcified Tissues, 1975. Copenhagen, Fadl Publishing Company, 1976.

23. Ophaug, R.H., Singer, L., and Harland, B.F.: Estimated fluoride intake of average two year old children in four dietary regions of the United States. J. Dent. Res., 59:777, 1980.

24. Riggs, B.L., et al.: Effect of the fluoride/calcium regimen on vertebral fracture occurrence in postmenopausal osteoporosis. N. Engl. J. Med., 306:446, 1982.

25. Rosenstein, S.H.: Systemic and environmental factors in rampant caries. N.Y. State Dent. J., 32:400, 1966.

26. Sahud, M.A., and Cohen, R.J.: Effect of aspirin ingestion on ascorbic acid levels in rheumatoid arthritis. Lancet, 1:937, 1971.

27. Sanderson, C.R., Davis, R.E., and Bayliss, C.E.: Serum pyridoxal in patients with rheumatoid arthritis. Ann. Rheum. Dis., 35:177, 1976.

28. Sandstead, H.H., et al.: Effects of dietary fiber and protein level on mineral element metabolism. In Inglett, G.E., and Falkenhaged, S.I. (eds.): Dietary Fibers, Chemistry and Nutrition. New York, Academic Press, 1979.

29. Schachtele, C.F.: Changing perspectives on the role of diet in dental caries formation. Nutr. News, 45(4):13, 1982.

30. Schaeffer, O.: When the Eskimo comes to town. Nutr. Today, 6(6):8, 1971.

31. Schamschula, R.G., and Barnes, D.E.: Fluoride and health: dental caries, osteoporosis, and cardiovascular disease. Annu. Rev. Nutr., 1:427, 1981.

32. Schumacher, H.R., Bernhart, F.W., and György, P.: Vitamin B$_6$ levels in rheumatoid arthritis: effect of treatment. Am. J. Clin. Nutr., 28:1200, 1975.

33. Shannon, I.L., Edmonds, E.J., and Madsen, K.O.: Honey: sugar content and cariogenicity. J. Dent. Child., 46: 29, 1979.

34. Simkin, P.A.: Oral zinc sulfate in rheumatoid arthritis. Lancet, 2:539, 1976.

35. Spencer, H., et al.: Effect of a high protein (meat) intake on calcium metabolism in man. Am. J. Clin. Nutr., 31:2167, 1978.

36. Spencer, H., et al.: Effect of phosphorus on the absorption of calcium and on calcium balance in man. J. Nutr., 108:7, 1978.

37. Spencer, H., et al.: Calcium loss, calcium absorption and calcium requirement in osteoporosis. In Barzel, U.S. (ed.): Osteoporosis II. New York, Grune & Stratton, 1979.

38. Taggart, H.M., et al.: Deficient calcitonin response to calcium stimulation in postmenopausal osteoporosis. Lancet, 1:475, 1982.

Additional References

ARTHRITIS

Aegerter, E.E., and Kirkpatrick, J.A.: Orthopedic Diseases. 4th ed. Philadelphia, W.B. Saunders Co., 1975.

Bienenstock, H., and Fernando, K.R.: Arthritis in the elderly. An overview. Med. Clin. North Am., 60:1173, 1976.

Grennan, D.M., et al.: Serum copper and zinc in rheumatoid arthritis and osteoarthritis. N. Z. Med. J., 91:47, 1980.

Katz, W.A.: Rheumatic Disease: Diagnosis and Management. 2nd ed. Philadelphia, J.B. Lippincott Co., 1984.

Kaye, R.L., and Pemberton, R.E.: Treatment of rheumatoid arthritis. Arch. Intern. Med., 136:1023, 1976.

Robinson, W.D.: Nutrition and rheumatic disease. In Kelley, W.N., et al.: (eds.): Textbook of Rheumatology. Philadelphia, W.B. Saunders Co., 1980.

Symposium on arthritis in older persons. J. Am. Geriatr. Soc., 25:49, 1977.

OSTEOPOROSIS

Heany, R.P., et al.: Calcium nutrition and bone health in the elderly. Am. J. Clin. Nutr., 36:986, 1982.

Ireland, P., and Fordtran, J.S.: Effect of dietary calcium and age on jejunal calcium absorption in humans studied by intestinal perfusion. J. Clin. Invest., 52:2672, 1973.

Marie, J.P., et al.: Histological osteomalacia due to dietary calcium deficiency in children. N. Engl. J. Med., 307:584, 1982.

Spencer, H.: Osteoporosis: goals of therapy. Hosp. Pract., 17 (3): 131, 1982.

GOUT

Boss, G.R., and Seegmiller, J.E.: Hyperuricemia and gout. N. Engl. J. Med., 300:1459, 1979.

Maclachan, M.J., and Rodnan, G.P.: Effects of food, fast and alcohol on serum uric acid and acute attacks of gout. Am. J. Med., 42:38, 1967.

IMMOBILIZATION

Hargrave, M.: Nutritional Care of the Physically Disabled. Publications-Audiovisuals Office, Sister Kenny Institute, 2727 Chicago Avenue, Minneapolis, Minn. 55407.

Lowman, E.W., and Klinger, J.L.: Aids to Independent Living: Self Help for the Handicapped. New York, McGraw-Hill Book Co., 1969, Chapters 1 and 2.

Stewart, A.F., et al.: Calcium homeostasis in immobilization: an example of resorptive hypercalciuria. N. Engl. J. Med., 306:1136, 1982.

Tilton C.N.: Diagnosing the dietary problems in stroke. Am. J. Nurs. 82:596, 1982.

Wolf, A.W., et al.: Immobilization hypercalcemia. A case report and review of the literature. Clin. Orthop., 118:124, 1976

DENTAL HEALTH

Brown, W.E., and König, K.G. (eds.): Cariostatic mechanisms of fluorides. Caries Res., 11(1), 1977.

Freeland, J.H., Cousins, R.J., and Schwartz, R.: Relationship of mineral status and intake to periodontal disease. Am. J. Clin. Nutr., 29:745, 1976.

Mellanby, M.: The chief dietetic and environmental factors responsible for the high incidence of dental caries: correlation between animal and human investigations. Br. Dent. J., 49:769, 1928.

Newbrun, E.: The safety of water fluoridation. J. Am. Dent. Assoc., 94:301, 1977.

Newbrun, E.: Sugar and dental caries: a review of human studies. Science, 217:418, 1982.

Nizel, A.E.: Nutrition in Preventive Dentistry: Science and Practice. 2nd ed. Philadelphia, W.B. Saunders Co., 1980.

Protein deficiency and tooth and salivary gland development. Nutr. Rev., 32:24, 1974.

Symposium on nutrition. Dent. Clin. North Am., 20(3), 1976.

Walsh, D.C.: Fluoridation: slow diffusion of a proved preventive measure. N. Engl. J. Med., 296:1118, 1977.

PHYSIOLOGICAL STRESS

Nutritional Care for Patients Having Surgery, Trauma or Burns

Revised by
JAYNE WILLIAMSON, R.D.

Research suggests that nutritional care before and after surgery plays an important role in the success of the operation as well as in the welfare and comfort of the patient. The duration of disability following surgery, trauma or burns may be significantly shortened, wound healing improved, the number of infections and complications lessened and mortality reduced by providing adequate nutritional support to the patient.[12, 22, 26, 48, 50, 56, 57, 68, 73]

Preoperative Nutritional Care

The actual preoperative nutritional care given a patient will depend largely upon the situation in which the operation is to be performed. If it is an emergency operation, there is little or no time for preliminary dietary treatment. In elective cases, particularly for patients having recent previous surgery, malabsorption, prolonged immobilization, chronic alcoholism, or bizarre eating habits, a nutritional assessment should be made. The patient should be brought to the best possible nutritional state before the operation. Illness and disease prior to surgical intervention may cause patients to restrict their food intake for days or weeks, predisposing them to nutritional depletion and weight loss. In some instances vomiting, diarrhea and bleeding may have contributed further to the patient's depletion, with marked losses of sodium, chloride, potassium and iron. In other cases

there may have been a long period of malabsorption due to disease, and the patient may be depleted in protein, vitamins and minerals.

Preoperative diagnostic procedures and blood tests frequently require that the patient fast or receive clear liquids only, a situation that acts against optimal nutritional intake. This is particularly detrimental to the already depleted or underweight patient. Supplements available to boost the energy and protein content of the preoperative clear liquid diets for these patients are listed in Table 35–7. However, more aggressive repletion may be required before an elective operation.[11]

On the other hand, it may be important for an overweight patient to lose weight prior to elective surgery. Special attention needs to be paid, though, to the rate and composition of weight loss, since losses of lean body mass exceeding 10 per cent over a short period of time may delay healing.

ENERGY AND PROTEIN. Although it is believed that malnourished patients have an increased surgical risk, no well-controlled, randomized clinical trials have documented this conclusively. Several multiparameter prognostic indexes have been developed to help identify those patients who might benefit from preoperative nutrition intervention.[52] Those patients determined to need preoperative repletion will need to receive energy and protein at levels 30 to 50 per cent above maintenance. Providing energy and protein much beyond these levels has not proved beneficial. Repletion occurs at a much slower rate than depletion. A depleted patient can be expected to gain a maximum of 50 to 100 mg. of lean tissue per day.[63]

Full repletion may take months and is not required to decrease operative risk. The critical determinant of reduced operative risk seems to be related more to the status of protein metabolism. Patients who show positive nitrogen balance and improving visceral protein status or immune status have been shown to have fewer operative complications. The length of time it takes for each patient to show improvement tends to vary. For this reason it has been suggested that the patient's nutritional status be evaluated every 7 days after starting nutritional support in order to determine if he or she is ready for surgery. Those who show no improvement after 14 days may be suffering from sepsis, which precludes anabolism.[11]

VITAMINS AND MINERALS. The method of nutritional support selected must provide adequate minerals and vitamins (fat-soluble and water-soluble). See Chapter 6 for further discussion of these requirements, which are basically those for normal good nourishment.

FOOD. It is important that the stomach be empty of food at the time of the operation. If food remains in the stomach there is danger of aspiration of vomitus during the induction of anesthesia or upon awakening. In elective cases no food is allowed by mouth for at least six hours prior to surgery. This is usually managed routinely by allowing a light meal the night before the operation and nothing after midnight. In emergency cases it is advisable to perform gastric lavage to remove the stomach contents before starting the anesthesia.

For intestinal surgery the colon should be free of residue to prevent postoperative infection, since colonic bacteria are reduced when less food residue is present. Low-fiber foods or liquid diet is given for two to three days preceding the operation, and the patient is given an enema a few hours before going to the operating room. A chemically defined or elemental liquid diet with minimal residue can be used preoperatively for patients at nutritional risk. Unpalatability and expense preclude its use with every patient. Recent studies have shown that the use of non-elemental products is just as effective for bowel preparation.[14]

FLUIDS. It is of utmost importance to the safety of the patient that no operation be attempted when the patient is dehydrated. In an emergency fluids can be given parenterally if there is insufficient time to administer them orally or if the patient is not tolerating oral fluids.

In general, intravenous infusions (preoperative, during the operation and postoperative) are administered to maintain fluid and electrolyte balance.

Postoperative Nutritional Care

Since it should be individualized and related to the type of surgery performed, the nutritional care for patients following surgery will vary. For example, a patient who has had a major stomach operation receives different care from that given to a patient who has undergone a limb amputation.

Whereas the importance of adequate postoperative nutrition is well recognized, oral feeding is often delayed for the first 24 to 48 hours following surgery to await the return of bowel tones. Recent evidence suggests, however, that the small intestine regains motility within hours and the stomach begins to empty at 24 hours after surgery, so bowel tones may not be a good measure of return of bowel function. Feeding may be well tolerated earlier postoperatively than is generally practiced.[28, 55]

Blood, fluids and electrolytes are lost from the body during surgery and further loss could occur through vomiting and drainage. To prevent dehydration and shock during the immediate postoperative period, fluid and electrolytic balances are maintained by intravenous, subcutaneous or rectal infusion. Although some surgeons may be very specific about the postoperative diet orders for their patients, there are some general principles applicable to all patients who have undergone surgery.

ENERGY AND PROTEIN. Ideally, actual energy requirements can be measured using direct or indirect calorimetry as discussed in Chapter 1. Although accurate non-invasive equipment is available for measuring gas exchange and calculating energy expenditure for critically ill patients, its use is often confined to the research setting. Mobile bedside measurement carts for determining energy expenditures are increasing in popularity but are not available in all institutions.

When it is not possible to make actual measurements, estimates of energy expenditure can be made using standard tables or formulas to calculate resting energy expenditure (REE) and adding a percentage increase for trauma. The most common methods for assessing resting energy expenditure were developed by Harris and Benedict or Boothby and are discussed in Chapter 1.

The extent to which energy expenditure increases above the REE varies with the nature and extent of injury. For the elective surgical patient the energy requirement postoperatively will increase by only 10 per cent providing that there are no complications. However, if the surgery was preceded by multiple fractures or trauma, the energy requirement can be increased from 10 to 25 per cent. See Table 35–5 for the increased energy requirements of stressful clinical situations, such as infection, surrounding surgery. Additional calories may also need to be added for hospital activity.

It must be kept in mind, though, that more is not always better. There seems to be a maximum amount of carbohydrate that the body is able to handle. Intakes beyond this level require lipogenesis with resultant increases in CO_2 production and respiratory demand, and fatty deposition in the liver. Excessive carbohydrate intakes should be suspect in patients with respiratory quotients greater than 1.0.[10, 29, 35, 41] The respiratory quotient is discussed on page 12.

Moderate or severe tissue damage caused either by injury or surgery also leads to an increased excretion of nitrogen and often to considerable loss of body protein. Sepsis, fever, infection and trauma accelerate nitrogen loss further. If there are exudates or discharges, such as occur in peritonitis or open wounds, additional nitrogen may be lost daily (6.25 gm. of protein is required to replace 1 gm. of nitrogen lost). There may be some loss of nitrogen through hemorrhage or through excretion from the kidneys.

If enough non-protein calories are not provided, body protein will be broken down to provide energy. The goal of nutritional support is to supply enough protein to promote anabolism, along with sufficient calories to assure that protein will not be used as a source of energy. The rate of nitrogen excretion varies for different trauma states,[61] which suggests that one level of protein intake cannot be appropriate for every patient. Several investigators support the use of calorie-to-nitrogen ratios anywhere from 100 to 200 kcal. per gm. of nitrogen for assessing protein needs. Others feel protein needs should be based on the patient's weight and recommend from 1.0 to a maximum of 2.0 gm. per kg. of usual body weight.[7, 23, 53, 63]

Depletion of body protein is very serious. It causes edema, inhibits wound healing, makes the body more vulnerable to infection, renders the liver more liable to toxic damage, impedes regeneration of hemoglobin, prevents resumption of normal gastrointestinal activity and delays the return of muscular strength. It is largely responsible for postoperative weakness and slow recovery.

VITAMINS. Ascorbic acid deficiency is associated with the delay or prevention of wound healing and with chronic, non-healing cutaneous ulcers. Vitamin C is required for the formation of collagen precursors and collagen. The amount of vitamin C to supplement is still a controversial subject. Megadoses of vitamin C have been associated with diarrhea, renal calculi and lowered serum B_{12} levels.[4, 31, 34] It is suggested that levels of 100 to 300 mg. will maintain adequate plasma levels postoperatively.[13]

Vitamin A deficiency may also interfere with wound healing because vitamin A is necessary for normal epithelialization. It may also help to prevent gastric stress ulceration.

Vitamin K deficiency is characterized by a decrease in prothrombin content of the blood, with a resultant defect in clotting. It is therefore of particular interest in surgery. An increased prothrombin time may be an indicator for vitamin K supplementation.

The B vitamins (thiamin, riboflavin and niacin) provide essential coenzyme factors to metabolize carbohydrate and protein and can be rapidly depleted after major trauma. It is believed that their requirements are increased in hypermetabolic states, but the extent to which they are increased is uncertain. It appears that thiamin deficiency during wound healing impairs collagen synthesis and decreases the breaking strength of the wound.[1, 71] However, the exact mechanism is not known. It may become important to assess thiamin status in postsurgical patients.

A healthy person having minor surgery usually does not require vitamin supplements. Patients fasting for long periods before or after surgery and those having major surgery, especially if poorly prepared for it or after a long debilitating illness, may need therapeutic doses of vitamins. However, there are no data that prove that patients who receive vitamins do better or at what levels vitamins should be given.

ZINC. There is evidence that the administration of zinc helps the process of wound healing in patients who have low serum zinc levels. Although its specific role in wound healing is unclear, zinc seems to be necessary for amino acid metabolism and synthesis of collagen precursors.[54, 59] The role of zinc and other minerals is discussed more fully in Chapter 7.

FLUIDS. Immediately following an operation the patient should be supplied with sufficient fluids to maintain normal water and electrolyte balance. At this time, the patient may experience more or less difficulty with the intake of large quantities of water by mouth, and fluids are usually administered intravenously. In some instances, fluids can be given by mouth as soon as the patient has recovered from the anesthesia.

FOOD. The introduction of food following surgery will depend upon the condition of the patient's gastrointestinal tract.

A general practice has been to start with

clear liquids for several meals postoperatively and then advance to full liquids for several meals before advancing to solid foods. However, there is no physiological reason that patients cannot be advanced to solid foods once the gastrointestinal tract is functioning and tolerance of a few liquids is established.

Many patients will be able to meet their energy and protein needs with the standard hospital diet. Those with small appetites or drastically increased nutritional needs may require supplemental oral liquids, tube feeding, or parenteral support.

Surgery of the Alimentary Tract

GASTRIC SURGERY

After gastric surgery, some varieties of which are diagrammed in Figure 34–1, all fluids and foods by mouth are withheld for three to five days and the patient is fed with a nasogastric tube. The use of total parenteral nutrition (TPN) is usually reserved for patients with poor preoperative nutritional status or postoperative complications that delay enteral feeding for an extended period of time.

The first type of fluids allowed by mouth are ice, which is held in the mouth, or infrequent sips of water. Some patients tolerate warm water better than iced or cold water. When vomiting ceases, larger amounts of fluids may be served. Bland foods can be started, but more important is offering the patient foods that are liked and well tolerated. By the fifth to seventh postoperative day, most patients can tolerate solid foods.

Nutritional impairment frequently occurs after gastrectomy, and many patients have difficulty regaining normal preoperative weight owing to one or both of the following: (1) inadequate food intake related in most instances to the dumping syndrome and (2) malabsorption of ingested food, specifically fat and protein. Patients who have had a total or nearly total gastrectomy often have difficulty in taking large amounts of food and may need to make a permanent habit of eating several small meals a day.

The Dumping Syndrome

The dumping syndrome is a complex physiological response to the presence of undigested food in the jejunum. Following gastric surgery, some patients who have had two thirds or more of the stomach removed (or some whose procedure has included a vagotomy[2, 38, 70]) and have advanced to the full diet regimen may experience the dumping syndrome. After food is swallowed, it is "dumped" into the jejunum about 10 to 15 minutes after ingestion instead of being gradually released in small amounts. Most patients who undergo this type of surgery develop a new pouch through nature's stretching of the remaining stomach tissue. However, many patients may continue to have chronic symptoms of the dumping syndrome.

SYMPTOMS. Some individuals complain of abdominal fullness, nausea and, at times, crampy abdominal pain followed by diarrhea within 15 minutes after eating. Others feel warm, dizzy, weak and faint; their pulse races and they break into a cold sweat. Lying down immediately after eating lessens these symptoms because food remains longer in the stomach pouch. Physiologically, the changes are explained by Figure 34–2.

Rapid entry of ingested nutrients into the jejunum and their subsequent hydrolysis lead to hypertonic intestinal contents. This hypertonic material is rapidly diluted by fluid drawn from the plasma and extra-cellular fluid and leads to a sharp drop in circulating blood volume. Drop in blood volume, decrease in cardiac output and perhaps dilatation of the jejunum lead to a sympathetic vasomotor response producing sweating, tachycardia, electrocardiographic changes and weakness. Serotonin, a vasoconstrictor, and vasoactive kinins, histamine and prostaglandins are thought to be released because of the hyperosmolarity of the jejunal chyme. These substances may be the cause of the cramping, hypermotility and diarrhea of the dumping syndrome.

Alimentary Hypoglycemia

Symptoms of hypoglycemia, such as weakness, perspiration, hunger, nausea, anxiety and tremors, can occur from one to two hours after the meal is ingested, in patients who have had gastrectomies or vagotomies. This hypoglycemia is due to the rapid digestion and absorption of the food (especially of carbohydrate) that has been dumped into the duodenum. The glucose rapidly enters the blood stream and causes a postprandial elevation in blood glucose and an overproduction of insulin, which results later in hypoglycemia.

Malabsorption

Following the Billroth II procedure in particular, there may be steatorrhea in addition to dumping and hypoglycemia. About 10 per cent of these patients have clinically significant steatorrhea. This is due to pancreatic insufficiency

COMMON GASTRIC SURGERIES

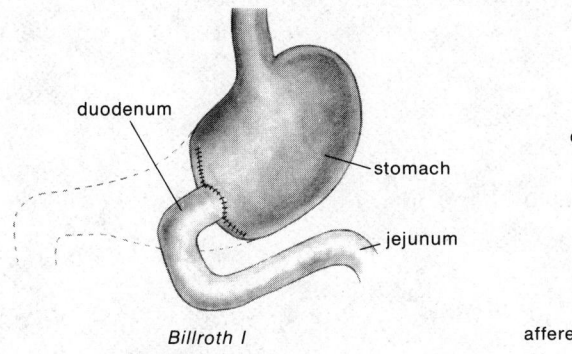

Billroth I

gastroduodenostomy
Less dumping than
with Billroth II.

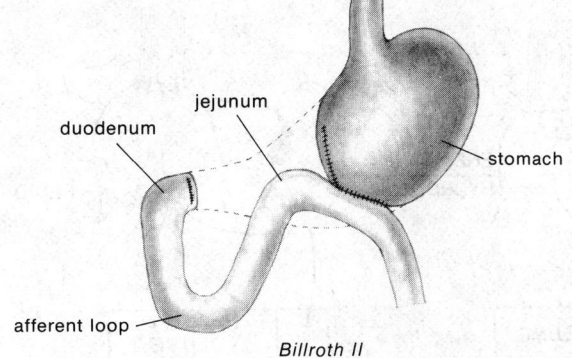

Billroth II
gastrojejunostomy

Sequelae such as steatorrhea, weight
loss, dumping, vomiting and bacterial
overgrowth occur more often with the
Billroth II procedure.

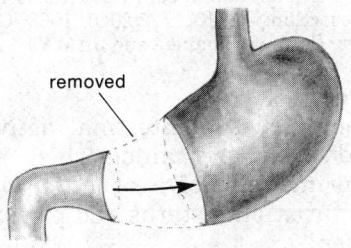

Partial Gastric Resection

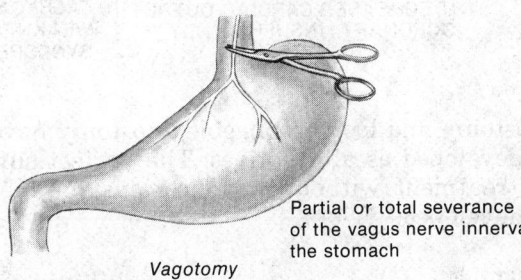

Vagotomy

Partial or total severance
of the vagus nerve innervating
the stomach

Depending on the extent of the
vagotomy, HCl secretion is reduced
and gastric emptying is slowed.
Dumping syndrome often follows
this surgery.

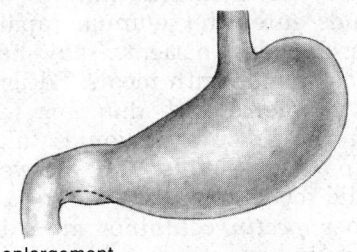

enlargement
of pyloric sphincter

Pyloroplasty

Duodenal reflux frequently
follows this surgery.

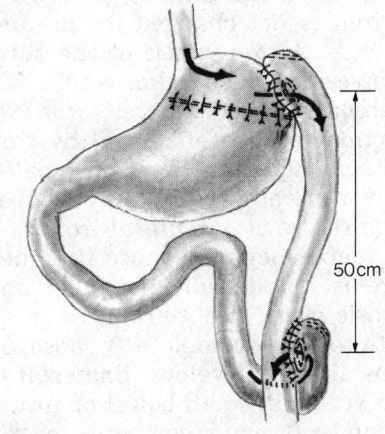

Roux-en-Y procedure

Figure 34–1. Gastric surgical procedures.

and defective digestion. Because food bypasses the duodenum, the secretion of secretin and pancreozymin by the duodenal mucosa is reduced. Since these two hormones stimulate the pancreas to secrete its enzymes and bicarbonate, there is little pancreatic exocrine secretion when they are not present. Furthermore, pancreatic atrophy and some fibrosis occur.[74]

Because of the complications with the Billroth II procedure, many other procedures including truncal, selective or parietal cell vagotomy, pyloroplasty, antrectomy, Roux-en-Y esophago-

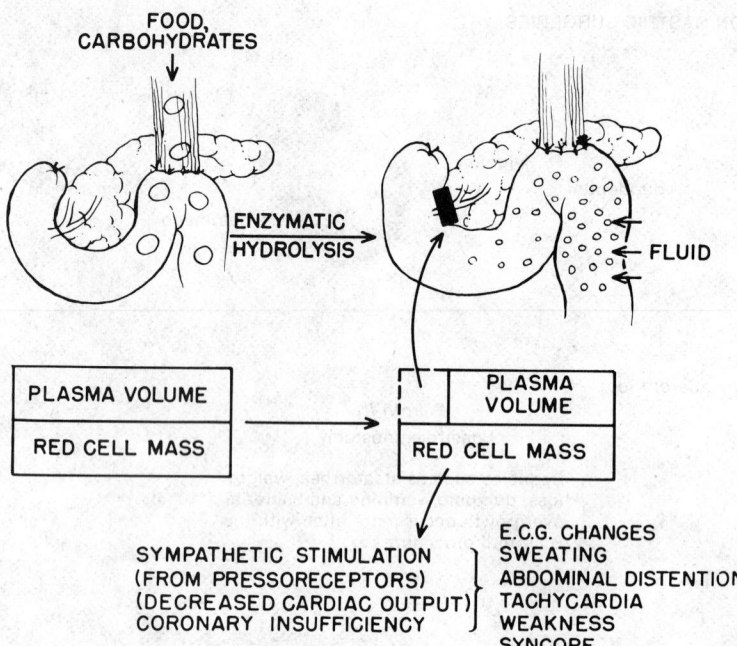

Figure 34-2. Changes occurring in dumping syndrome. (From: Vanamee, P.: Nutrition after gastric resection. JAMA, *172*:2045, 1960. Courtesy of Dr. Parker Vanamee and JAMA.)

jejunostomy and loop esophagojejunostomy have been developed as alternatives. The perfect surgical treatment without complications has yet to be developed.[8, 40]

Anemia

Anemia may develop after gastric surgery, possibly due to iron deficiency caused by bleeding from recurrent ulcers or by impaired iron absorption. Because of rapid stomach emptying, which prevents thorough mixing of food with gastric HCl, iron is not changed to the absorbable ferrous form. Also, because of the surgery, the iron bypasses the duodenum, where 50 per cent of iron absorption takes place.

Iron absorption may be enhanced by concurrent ascorbic acid ingestion. For some patients, however, poor iron absorption may be severe enough to require use of parenteral iron.[58]

Vitamin B_{12} deficiency may cause the anemia. Because there is a reduced amount of gastric mucosa, intrinsic factor is not produced in quantities adequate to allow complete B_{12} absorption, and pernicious anemia develops. Bacterial overgrowth in the proximal small bowel or in the afferent loop binds B_{12} and competes with the body for absorption. The result is a macrocytic anemia that should be treated with B_{12} injections.

Anemia can also result from folate deficiency as part of the general malabsorption syndrome.

Nutritional Care

Because of the problems that accompany eating, post-gastrectomy and post-vagotomy patients frequently do not eat enough, have diarrhea from the increased intestinal activity and become underweight, malnourished and frustrated. The prime objective of nutritional care is to restore nutritional status and pleasant living for the patient.

Protein and fats are better tolerated than carbohydrates because they are more slowly hydrolyzed into osmotically active substances. Simple carbohydrates—lactose, sucrose and dextrose—are rapidly hydrolyzed and should be limited, but complex carbohydrates such as starches can be included. Liquids enter the jejunum rapidly, and for that reason some patients may have problems tolerating liquids with meals. Patients who have severe problems with dumping may do better to limit the amount of liquids taken with meals or to take liquids only between meals, without solid food.

The dietary fiber *pectin* contained in fruits and vegetables may be useful in treating dumping syndrome. It seems to slow down carbohydrate absorption and reduce the glycemic response and thus insulin response. An *alpha-glucoside hydrolase inhibitor (acarbose)*, which reduces the digestion and absorption of starch, sucrose and maltose, may also reduce the blood glucose response and subsequent hypoglycemia.

Basically, the diet is moderate in fat (30 to 40 per cent of calories), low in simple carbohydrates and high in protein (20 per cent of calories), with the purpose of achieving or maintaining the optimal weight and nutritional status of the patient. The diabetic exchange lists given in Table 25–8 can be used to calculate the carbohydrate intake and to teach the patient about carbohydrate control.

Milk in small amounts is apt to be tolerated

Table 34–1. NUTRITIONAL CARE FOR PATIENTS SUFFERING FROM DUMPING SYNDROME AND ALIMENTARY HYPOGLYCEMIA

DUMPING SYNDROME

High-protein, moderate-fat, high-calorie diet adequate for weight maintenance near ideal body weight (IBW)
About 1.5–2 gm. protein per kg. ideal body weight (IBW) and 35–45 kcal. per kg. IBW
Use medium-chain triglycerides if steatorrhea is present
Lie down for about an hour after eating
Avoid taking liquids with meals or solids
Avoid those foods known to cause individual problems
Eat small meals of 4–5 oz. in size

ALIMENTARY HYPOGLYCEMIA

Avoid concentrated sweets such as candy, sugar, cola drinks, cookies, cakes and ice cream unless made with sugar substitutes
Have concentrated forms of sugar available in the event of hypoglycemia 1–2 hr. after meals
Eat small meals six times per day

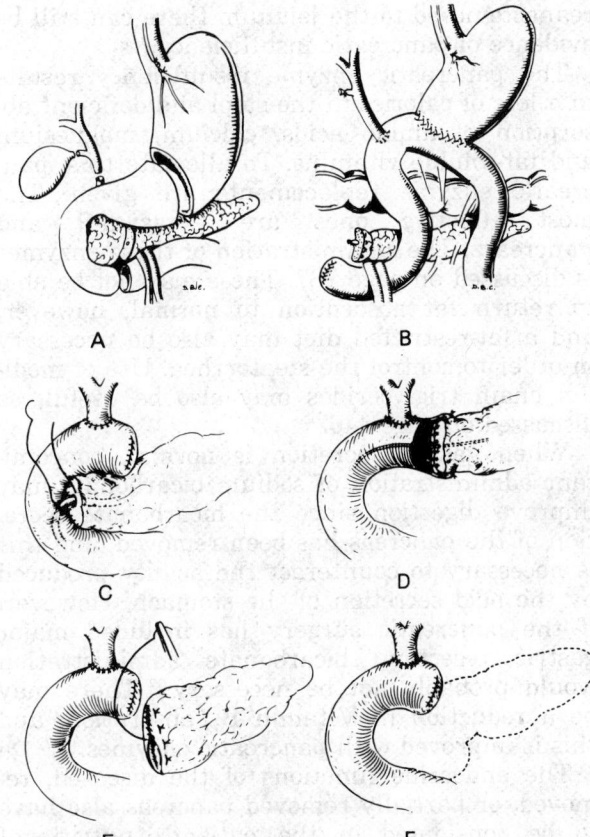

Figure 34–3. Pancreatoduodenectomy. *A,* Lines of section of stomach, pancreas, duodenum and common bile duct are shown; a vagotomy and cholecystectomy are indicated. *B,* Anastomoses after resection and reconstruction using an antecolic loop of jejunum. The head of the pancreas has been removed, and its stump and duct have been closed. *C* to *F,* Four methods of pancreatoduodenectomy used in the management of the pancreas. *C,* Anastomosis of the pancreatic duct to the mucosa of the jejunum. *D,* Inversion of the cut end of the pancreas into the jejunum. *E,* Ligation of the pancreatic duct with oversewing of the transected end of the pancreas. *F,* Total pancreatectomy. (*A* and *B* from Powis, S. J. A., and Young, H. B. A.: Modified pancreaticoduodenectomy. Surg. Gynecol. Obstet., *137:*259, 1973. *C* to *F* from Aston, S. J., and Longmire, W. P., Jr.: Management of the pancreas after pancreatoduodenectomy. Ann. Surg., *179:*322, 1974.)

better than in large amounts, although some patients may not tolerate it at all. Dried skim milk or various casein hydrolysates may be used and be well tolerated. Patients with minimal or no intake of milk or dairy products may need vitamin D and calcium supplementation.

If milk intolerance is due to lactose intolerance, various lactose-free commercial formulas that have high calorie and protein densities and low osmolalities are available. When steatorrhea is a problem, those formulas with more of the fat as medium chain triglycerides might be better tolerated. Supplemental formulas are described in Table 35–7. Table 34–1 gives the general nutritional care required for patients after gastric surgery. However, each diet must be adjusted to the patient, based on a careful dietary and social history.

GALLBLADDER AND COMBINED ABDOMINOPERINEAL RESECTIONS

Gallbladder

Following surgery such as removal of the gallbladder or combined abdominoperineal resections, oral feedings are usually resumed with the return of bowel sounds, and the patient gradually progresses to a regular diet as tolerated. If enteral feeding, either by tube or by mouth, is not possible by the seventh postoperative day, some form of intravenous nutritional support should be started. For patients at nutritional risk, nutritional support may have to be started sooner. Some patients who have had the gallbladder removed may be more comfortable on a low-fat diet if they are still having symptoms and discomfort. The usual full liquid diet, moderate in fat (70 to 100 gm. per day), may

have to be modified. However, most patients can be expected to tolerate fat in their diet after gallbladder surgery.

Pancreas

A common pancreatic surgical procedure is a *pancreatoduodenectomy,* often called a *Whipple procedure* after the surgeon who first described it in 1935. Figure 34–3 diagrams the Whipple procedure. A cholecystectomy and a vagotomy are often done at the same time. Partial or complete pancreatic insufficiency can result depending upon the surgical repair of the pancreatic stump. Even when the pancreatic duct is reanastomosed to the jejunum there can still be evidence of pancreatic insufficiency.[3]

The pancreatic enzyme insufficiency results in a loss of calories in the stool and deficient absorption of amino acids, calcium, magnesium and fat-soluble vitamins. To alleviate this, pancreatic enzyme replacements are given. The most effective ones are Cotazym-R and Pancrease. The administration of these enzymes is discussed on page 787. These may not be able to return fat absorption to normal, however, and a fat-restricted diet may also be necessary in order to control the steatorrhea. Use of medium chain triglycerides may also be useful, as discussed on page 446.

When gastric secretion is normal, concomitant administration of sodium bicarbonate may improve digestion since the bicarbonate secretion of the pancreas has been removed, and this is necessary to counteract the acidity produced by the acid secretion of the stomach. However, if the pancreatic surgery has included major gastric resection, bicarbonate administration would probably not be necessary.[62] There may be a reduction in Vitamin B_{12} absorption, and this is improved with pancreatic enzymes.[49, 72]

The endocrine functions of the diseased, removed, or partially removed pancreas also have to be considered in the patient's nutritional care. When there is evidence of insulin deficiency, a diabetic diet with frequent feedings and limited simple sugars should be started (see Chapter 25). Insulin administration may also be necessary. The inadequate endocrine function of the pancreas may be due to the fact that part was removed or to the fact that the remaining portion is diseased. In some patients with severe resulting malabsorption, diarrhea, anorexia or fistula, TPN may be necessary.

Liver

Liver resection is fairly frequent now that surgeons are able to preoperatively locate the liver problem area through tomography and arteriography. Since many patients with primary or secondary liver involvement are undernourished, it is necessary that these patients be nutritionally repleted before surgery, if possible.

After major hepatic resection it is necessary to manage biochemical and metabolic changes to permit recovery and rapid regeneration of liver tissue. Severe hypoglycemia has been noted in patients having hepatic resections of 70 per cent or more.[46] Therefore, it is necessary to monitor blood glucose and infuse 10 per cent glucose solution continuously for the first few days following surgery, or until adequate enteral intake of carbohydrate is achieved.[62]

Hypoalbuminemia will occur also since the liver is the site of albumin synthesis. Albumin should be supplied parenterally in order to prevent a progressive fall in osmotic pressure in the vascular compartment, which leads to accumulation of interstitial fluid, increased vascular load, and the danger of pulmonary edema. The need for supplementary albumin persists for one to three weeks postoperatively.[62]

Vitamin K should be administered pre- and postoperatively, since coagulation factors that are synthesized by the liver will fall in the postoperative phase. They will return to normal with liver regeneration.

Adequate nutritional support is important for optimal liver regeneration. Should liver insufficiency continue following surgery and the regeneration phase, nutritional care will need to continue. For a discussion of nutritional care for the patient with liver disease, see page 466.

SMALL BOWEL RESECTION

Patients undergo small or large bowel resection for treatment of cancer, diverticulitis, ileitis, local abscess, perforation, mesenteric vascular accidents or obstruction. When more than two thirds of the small bowel is removed, severe metabolic problems and malnutrition are very likely to occur. Weight loss, muscle wasting, diarrhea, rapid gastrointestinal transit time and malabsorption of calcium, zinc, magnesium, fats and iron are common. The syndrome is commonly referred to as "short bowel syndrome." The nutritional care for this condition is complex and must be aggressive and anticipatory. Figure 5–9 shows the sites of absorption of various nutrients and may be helpful in formulating proper nutritional care for these patients.

Effects of Decreased Intestinal Length

Protein nutrition is usually not a problem because protein absorption is efficient even in short lengths of otherwise normal intestine. Absorption may be decreased initially but improves with time. Glucose is also easily absorbed if adequate amounts of intestinal enzymes are present.

Fats are poorly absorbed, and malabsorption may exist for some time, in contrast with the adaptation exhibited by carbohydrate and protein absorption. Besides causing steatorrhea, the unabsorbed fatty acids may saponify calcium and magnesium in the intestine, form "soaps" and prevent the absorption of these two minerals. Fat-soluble vitamins are also thought to be poorly absorbed. However, recent research suggests that perhaps the absorptive capacity for fat is preserved and that these patients may benefit from high-fat diets.[64]

Certain other nutrients, such as vitamin B_{12}, which are absorbed mainly in the ileum, will have to be given parenterally if too much of the ileum has been removed.

Other Effects

Three conditions are secondary to small bowel resection and also contribute to the malabsorption. First, there is *hypersecretion of gastric acid* because there is no inhibitory effect on gastric acid secretion by small intestinal secretions. The gastric acid hypersecretion injures the remaining proximal mucosa and reduces absorption. It also inactivates pancreatic lipase and trypsin, so that fat and protein maldigestion and malabsorption result, and cause an acidic diarrheal stool. Second, *gastrointestinal motility and peristalsis are increased.* Third, in some patients there is *bacterial overgrowth* of unknown etiology.[16] These three complications should be considered in planning nutritional care.

Adaptation of the Remaining Small Bowel

Provided that adequate nutrition is maintained both parenterally and enterally for a period of several months, the remaining small bowel will increase its absorptive surface area through dilatation and cellular hypertrophy and hyperplasia.[60] It appears that the nutritional support cannot be entirely parenteral and that nutrients in the gastrointestinal tract stimulate the beginning of the hyperplasia. Gastrin may also be involved in this process.[66]

If 15 to 18 in. (38 to 46 cm.) or more of the small bowel is remaining, most likely the person will eventually be able to support himself nutritionally by oral intake alone. If he has less than this remaining, he will probably require permanent parenteral nutrition to supplement his oral intake. Chapter 35 discusses permanent parenteral nutrition for patients living at home.

Nutritional Care

In the *first stage* after surgery, nutritional support is totally by parenteral means and may be the only nutritional intake for several months. Oral or enteral feedings at this stage promote hypermotility, diarrhea and fluid and electrolyte loss. The diarrheal stool in this stage is acidic and frequent, and good perianal hygiene is necessary to prevent excoriation.

The *second stage* after surgery begins when the volume of the daily fecal output is about 1 liter per day. The first enteral feeding in this stage is a cautious trial of isotonic fluid about four weeks postoperatively, if 20 to 30 per cent (48 to 72 in.) of the small bowel remains. If less than this of the bowel remains, oral intake may have to be postponed another month or so. In this stage small bowel adaptation will take place as the bowel is presented with nutrients by the enteral route. Liquids are taken first and then, with a great deal of support from the dietitian and nurse, the patient begins the slow return to a normal diet. At this point, dilute feedings of an elemental diet or other complete liquid diet are appropriate if the patient can tolerate them. More liquids are added, then some solid foods and later a greater variety of foods. The patient should be told that there will be temporary setbacks and that he or she may not tolerate some foods one week that were tolerated the week before. The patient should not get discouraged, and the diet should just be simplified for a while. If a food is not tolerated at one time, it should be tried again several weeks later. As the oral intake increases, parenteral nutritional support is decreased, but only to the level where the patient can still maintain weight or gain weight if necessary. Antidiarrheal agents and potassium supplements may be necessary.

Within five months after the bowel resection, it is usually possible to provide the entire intake by mouth, and the patient enters *stage three*. More foods are introduced into the diet. It is helpful if the patient keeps a food diary that can be shared with the nurse and dietitian, who can help to correlate the patient's digestive problems with possible dietary causes. During this stage it is advisable to avoid alcohol and caffeine for at least a year following surgery, because they stimulate gastrointestinal activity. Six to eight small meals daily are usually better tolerated than three larger meals.

Many of these patients receive narcotics for several months postoperatively to decrease gastrointestinal motility. They can become addicted to these drugs, and this should be monitored; narcotic requirements should decrease progressively after surgery. Excessive use of narcotics manifests itself as abdominal distention, cramping, vomiting, poor dietary intake and progressive weight loss. The situation must be differentiated from dietary intolerance and treated accordingly.

ILEOSTOMY OR COLOSTOMY

An opening from the surface of the body to the intestinal tract is frequently created surgically in the treatment of patients with severe ulcerative colitis, Crohn's disease, colonic cancer or intestinal trauma. The purpose of the opening is to allow defecation from the intact portion of the intestine. An *ileostomy* is an opening into the ileum; a *colostomy* is an opening into the colon. An ileostomy is performed if the entire colon, rectum and anus must be removed, and a colostomy is performed if only the rectum and anus are removed. In some cases, a tempo-

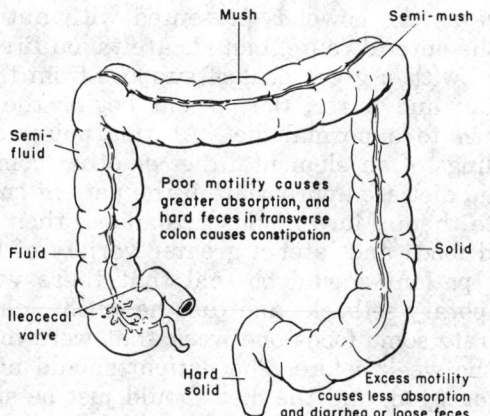

Figure 34–4. As the feces move from the ileocecal valve to the anus, water is absorbed and the feces become more solid. The characteristics of the output from a colostomy will depend on its location in the colon. (From: Guyton, A. C.: Textbook of Medical Physiology, 6th ed. Philadelphia, W. B. Saunders Co., 1981.)

rary opening may be made to allow surgery and healing of more distal parts of the intestinal tract. The opening, or *stoma*, eventually becomes about the size of a nickel. The output from the stoma will depend on its location in the colon, as explained in Figure 34–4. The consistency of the stool from an ileostomy will be liquid, while that from a colostomy can range from mushy to fairly well-formed.

One of the biggest concerns of the patient with an ileostomy or colostomy is odor. The usual ileostomy stool has a weakly acidic odor that is not unpleasant. A malodorous stool is usually caused by steatorrhea or by bacteria acting on particular foodstuffs to produce odorous gas. Patients learn to observe their stools to determine which foods to eliminate in order to minimize odor and gas production, and this differs with individuals. Items that seem to be particular odor-causers are corn, dried beans, onions, cabbage, highly spiced foods, fish, antibiotics and some vitamin-mineral supplements. Persistent odor may be due to poor stoma hygiene or to an ileostomy complication that allows bacterial overgrowth in the ileum. Deodorants are available and fortunately pouch appliances today are also odor-proof.

Gas production may cause the pouch to become tense and distended, and accidental dislodgment is likely. The nutritional recommendations in Chapter 23 for reducing flatulence may be helpful.

Ileostomy adaptation does occur, and fecal losses will lessen and stools will become firmer. This usually happens in seven to ten days. It does not happen to the same extent in patients who have an ileal resection in addition to the ileostomy. Their ileal output will be about two

to five times greater than that of the patient who has only an ileostomy.[33]

Patients who also have Crohn's disease and thus lose excessive quantities of salt and water need above average intakes of salt and water.[6] The high water intake is also necessary to prevent renal calculi. Because of water losses through the ileostomy, these patients have small urine volumes, which makes them prone to renal calculi.[47]

The patient with a normal, well-functioning ileostomy will not usually become nutritionally depleted. However, in instances of high ileal output and chronic ileostomy diarrhea, fluid and electrolyte losses can occur and will need replacement. Patients who also have an ileal resection will need vitamin B_{12} supplementation. A B_{12} depletion may result in patients with only an ileostomy if there is an imbalance in small bowel flora and vitamin B_{12} absorption. One study showed that ileostomy patients have vitamin C intakes below the recommended amount, because of their low vegetable and fruit intakes.[6] This should be monitored.

Since it is possible for a food bolus to get caught in the ileum at the point where it narrows as it enters the abdominal wall, it is important to caution the patient to avoid very fibrous vegetables and to chew all food well. Other than this, ileostomy and colostomy patients should be encouraged to follow their normal diet, omitting only those particular foods known to cause them problems.

Patients with a permanent colostomy or ileostomy require considerable sympathetic understanding from the nurse and the entire medical, surgical and dietary team. It is difficult for the person to accept his condition and the problems involved in maintaining bowel regularity. Plans to have these patients meet other people who have undergone similar surgery will help them to adjust to the new problems by comparing and discussing the difficulties involved. Eventually most patients are aided by the realization that in the future they will not have frequent gastrointestinal illness, multiple hospitalizations or chronic disabilities.

RECTAL SURGERY

Following rectal surgery such as hemorrhoidectomy, nutritional care should be directed toward maintaining an intake that will allow for wound repair, prevent frequent stools so that the wound can heal, and prevent infection of the wound by feces. A minimal-residue diet and the use of constipating drugs are indicated. Elemental diets, chemically defined diets and some complete liquid diets[14] are effective because they are low in residue. Using these diets, stool volume and frequency can be reduced to as little as 50 gm. every six days. Such diets can make the surgical construction of a temporary diverting colostomy unnecessary.[27] Chapter 35 discusses chemically defined diets. The minimal-fiber diet in Table 23–3 can be started by about the tenth day postoperatively, depending on the severity of the surgery. A normal diet is resumed after complete healing and the patient is instructed about eating a high-fiber diet in order to avoid constipation in the future. Table 23–2 gives a high-fiber diet.

FISTULA OF THE INTESTINAL TRACT

A *fistula* is an abnormal passage between two internal organs or from an internal organ to the surface of the body. Fistulas occur as a result of prenatal developmental error or are caused by trauma or inflammatory or malignant disease processes. Fistulas of the intestinal tract can be serious threats to the nutritional status of the patient because large amounts of fluid and electrolytes are lost, and malabsorption and infection can occur. Fluid and electrolyte balance must be restored, infection brought under control and aggressive nutritional support provided to allow for surgical closure of the fistula and wound.

Total parenteral nutrition or minimal-residue diets have been used successfully to allow spontaneous closure of fistulas without surgery. The success rate of either method depends on the location and cause of the fistula and the overall condition of the patient.[39]

TONSILLECTOMY

Following a tonsillectomy, very cold and very mild-flavored foods bring the most comfort to the patient and offer the most protection against bleeding of the surgical area. Because the convalescent period is comparatively short, the nutritional adequacy of the diet is not so important.

For the first 24-hour postoperative period, these foods are often preferred or best tolerated:

Cold milk
Milk beverages, such as malted milk and eggnogs
Chocolate and vanilla ice cream
Fruit ice
Pear, peach or prune juice

The following foods are usually added to the diet by the second day. Warm fluids and food may be started and cautiously replaced by hot foods as healing progresses and the patient can tolerate them.

Strained soups
Enriched refined cooked cereals

Soft-cooked or poached egg
Milk toast
Soft puddings, custard, and gelatin desserts
Mashed potatoes and strained vegetables
Finely ground chicken or meat in broth or gravy
Fruit purée (whips)

The patient will gradually return to the normal diet within a week to ten days.

SURGERY OF THE MOUTH OR ESOPHAGUS

After extensive surgery of the mouth or esophagus, it may be necessary to provide total nutritional support using parenteral feeding, nasogastric tube feeding or tube feeding directly into the stomach or jejunum, depending on the operative area. Since the patient may have to stay on such a schedule for a long period of time or even permanently, it is of utmost importance that the formula be adequate in all nutrients. For patients who are able to tolerate an oral liquid diet, variety can be obtained by liquefying normally solid foods, such as potatoes, chopped meat, vegetables and fruit purees, in a food blender or by forcing them through a sieve and adding liquids (see Table 35–9). This method may also be used for preparing tube feedings for the long-term patient at home. Commercial preparations of strained baby foods can be used when labor or the special devices needed for preparation are lacking. Although preparing tube feedings by these methods may save money, the time involved in preparation and the care needed to prevent contamination may warrant the use of a commercial, ready-to-use complete liquid diet.

Fractures and Other Mechanical Trauma

Following fractures of the long bones there is an increase in protein breakdown in well-nourished individuals, which is aggravated still further by prolonged immobilization. The loss of protein (loss of nitrogen) is accompanied by losses of phosphorus and sulfur.[19] Development of osteoporosis may coincide with loss in calcium due to immobilization. Severe functional imbalance and loss of fluids and electrolytes may take place.

In addition, there is a 20 to 25 per cent increase in energy requirements, which may go as high as 50 per cent if the patient also has an infection.[61] Figure 34–5 summarizes the metabolic changes that take place after an injury or burn.

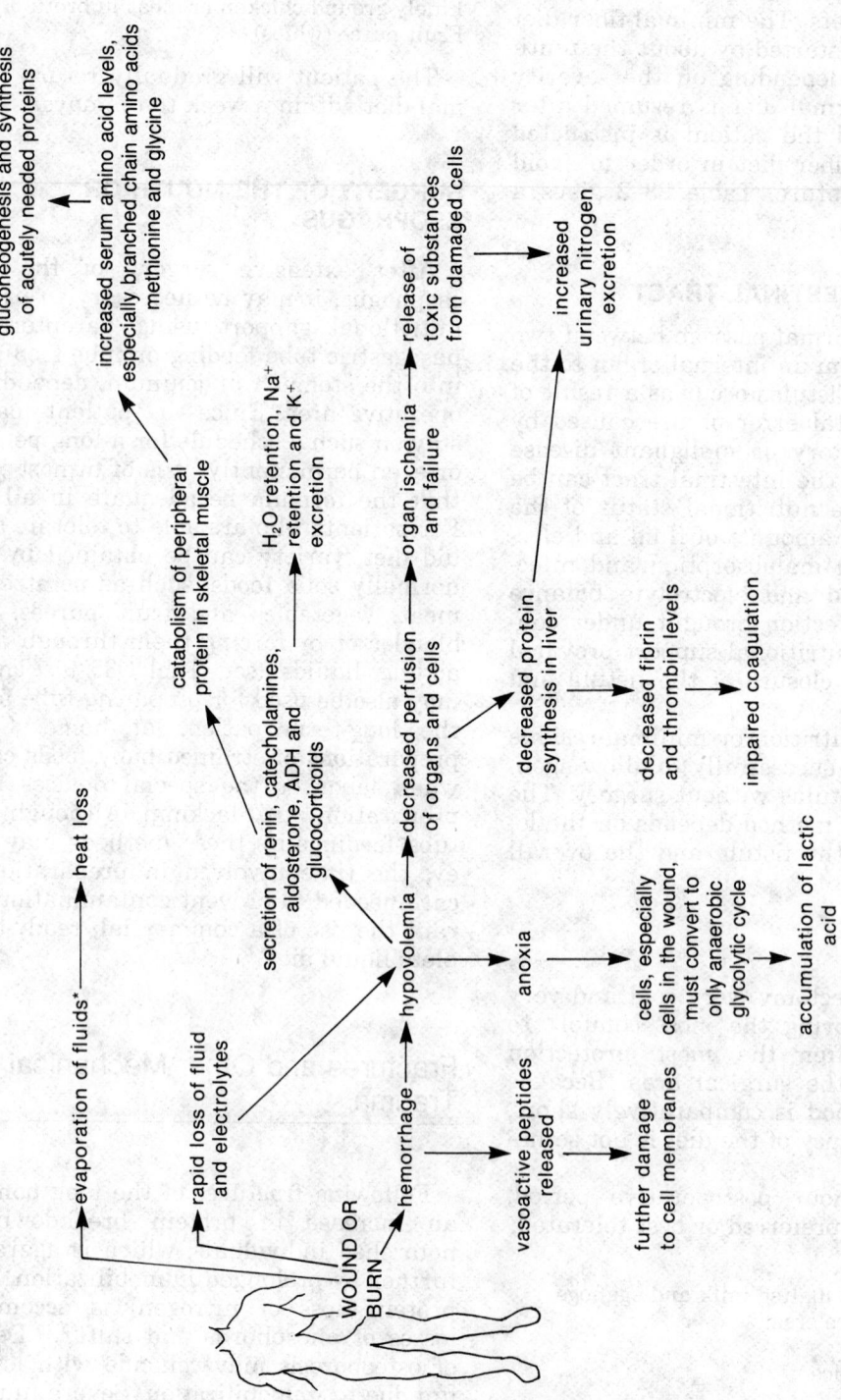

use of amino acids for
gluconeogenesis and synthesis
of acutely needed proteins

increased serum amino acid levels,
especially branched chain amino acids
methionine and glycine

catabolism of peripheral
protein in skeletal muscle

H_2O retention, Na^+
retention and K^+
excretion

secretion of renin, catecholamines,
aldosterone, ADH and
glucocorticoids

release of
toxic substances
from damaged cells

increased
urinary nitrogen
excretion

decreased perfusion
of organs and cells

decreased protein
synthesis in liver

organ ischemia
and failure

decreased fibrin
and thrombin levels

impaired coagulation

hypovolemia

anoxia

cells, especially
cells in the wound,
must convert to
only anaerobic
glycolytic cycle

accumulation
of lactic
acid

evaporation of fluids* ——→ heat loss

rapid loss of fluid
and electrolytes

hemorrhage

vasoactive peptides
released

further damage
to cell membranes

WOUND OR
BURN

*Mainly occurs in the patient with extensive burns

Figure 34-5. Physiological and metabolic changes immediately after an injury or burn. The extent of these changes depends on the severity of the trauma.

700

Nutritional Care

Replacement of losses and promotion of healing are the aims of diet therapy. During the first 24 to 48 hours after the injury it is necessary to maintain blood volume and electrolyte balance, and aggressive nutritional support is not important in this period. After this time, attention should be focused on nutritional support to help the patient resist infection, heal the wounds, regain muscular strength and prevent weight loss. Adequate protein and calories should be supplied to meet the patient's estimated needs (see Table 35–4 and Chapter 1). Special attention needs to be given to the intakes of calcium and vitamin D. Recent evidence suggests that calcium intakes in excess of the RDA of 800 mg. may be necessary to achieve optimal bone health and healing. Excessive intakes of protein increase calcium requirements as well.[21]

If the patient cannot eat an adequate amount at meals, high-protein, high-calorie beverages can be served between meals. A tube feeding is necessary for comatose patients or for patients unable to take food by the normal route. In cases of gastrointestinal injury, the tube will have to be placed at a point below the injury so that food can still be absorbed.

Parenteral nutrition is indicated if adequate nutrition by the gastrointestinal route is impossible. It may be given as either peripheral vein supplementation or central vein total nutrition, as discussed in Chapter 35. The number of calories that can be administered peripherally is limited owing to the fragility of peripheral veins. Therefore, peripheral parenteral nutrition is not indicated for long-term support of the severely stressed, catabolic patient. It may be a useful adjunct, however, to oral or tube feeding during a transitional phase.[75]

Extensive Burns

Extensive burns are one of the most severe traumas the body can sustain. Hypermetabolism due to neurohormonal changes can increase energy requirements up to 100 per cent above resting metabolic expenditure, depending upon the size of the burn. This hypermetabolism is accompanied by exaggerated protein catabolism and increased urinary nitrogen excretion as shown in Figure 34–5. Further protein is lost through wound exudate. With infection, energy and protein needs can be even greater. Since patients with major burns usually develop an ileus (a condition manifested by loss of intestinal peristalsis or lack of effective coordinated peristalsis) and experience anorexia, their nutritional support becomes a real challenge.

Fluid and Electrolyte Replacement

Because of tremendous fluid and electrolyte losses through the burn wound, the initial consideration in treatment is fluid and electrolyte replacement. The first 24 to 48 hours after the burn are devoted to fluid resuscitation. The volume of fluid needed is based on the patient's age, weight and extent of burn. Variations of the Lund and Browder chart[42] using the "rule of nines" can be used to determine the percentage of total body surface area (TBSA) burned. A variety of formulas have been developed to calculate the volume of resuscitation fluid needed. Most agree that half of the calculated volume for the first 24 hours be given over the first 8 hours, since this is the period of the greatest intravascular losses. The composition of the resuscitation fluid, however, remains controversial. Solutions containing water, electrolytes and albumin in varying proportions have all been advocated. The patient's general appearance, clear sensorium and adequate urinary output will help determine if the patient has received sufficient resuscitation. Once resuscitation is completed, ample fluids need to be given to cover both maintenance requirements and the evaporative losses that continue through open burn wounds. The early provision of adequate fluids and electrolytes is paramount for maintaining circulatory volume and preventing acute renal failure.

Wound Management

There are many approaches to treatment of burn wounds, including various topical antimicrobial agents and temporary or artificial skin grafts. The only permanent graft, however, is one's own skin. The current trend for wound management is early excision and grafting.[9, 17, 24, 43, 51] The main goal is to get wounds covered as early as possible to help reduce evaporative and nitrogen losses and prevent infection. The method of wound management chosen for a patient will depend upon the depth and extent of burn and could influence the type of nutritional support a patient receives. Patients receiving early excision and grafting may require total parenteral nutrition to help them meet their estimated nutritional needs consistently through a series of operations, whereas patients not requiring surgery may rely on enteral support.

Nutritional Care

Along with early wound coverage and infection control, nutritional support has been recognized as one of the most important aspects of the burn patient's care. Although patients may be severely catabolic initially, and not be readily converted to positive nitrogen balance, it is important to begin nutritional support soon after resuscitation is complete. Early initiation of nutritional support allows time to assess tolerance and change support if necessary without having extended periods of inadequate intake. Patients should be able to meet their estimated energy and protein needs consistently by the fifth to seventh day after the burn.

ENERGY. It is generally agreed that the burn patient's energy needs are increased and that increases vary according to the size of the burn. Various formulas have been developed for estimating energy needs ranging from using the Harris-Benedict equation given on page 15, with varying increases according to the percentage of burn, to using differing calorie levels per square meter of burned and unburned skin. One of the simplest and easiest to use formulas is the following:[18]

25 kcal./kg. usual body weight + 40 kcal. (% TBSA burned) = kcal. needed per day

The following example illustrates the application of the formula to the case of a 70-kg. man who has been burned over 25 per cent of his body:

Calorie requirements = 25 kcal. × 70 kg. + 40 kcal. × 25 = 1750 kcal. + 1000 kcal. = 2750 kcal. per day

One weakness of several of the formulas is that there is no upper limit to the number of calories that a patient may require. Recent literature suggests, however, that there is a maximum caloric load that the body can handle, somewhere near 100 per cent above resting metabolic expenditure.[76] This needs to be taken into account when using any of these formulas. Additional calories may need to be added beyond the burn formulas for fever, sepsis, multiple trauma or stress of surgery or to promote weight gain in the severely underweight. Weight maintenance is also the goal for overweight patients until they are completely healed. Current research suggests that estimated energy needs may be excessive if the obese patient's actual weight is used to calculate needs, but that using ideal weight may underestimate those needs; actual energy needs for the obese probably fall somewhere between these two values.[25]

The pediatric patient presents an additional challenge, in that since basic nutritional needs already differ so much for each age group because of growth requirements, it is not as easy to come up with one formula that will cover all age groups. Also there is less agreement as to the percentage of increased requirements for pediatric patients. Some authors feel there is no increase in requirements above the Recommended Daily Allowance, since children are less active when they are burned,[69] while others propose a 50 per cent increase above the RDA.[5, 36] An accurate formula for calculating the nutritional needs of the pediatric patient with a burn still needs to be developed.

PROTEIN. Protein recommendations for burn patients are also not well defined.[30, 65, 67] Curreri advocates using a calorie to nitrogen ratio (Cal:N) of 150 kcal. to 1 gm. of nitrogen.[15] More recent literature is suggesting that 100 kcal. per gm. of nitrogen may be necessary to meet the burn patient's needs.[32] Others have suggested giving 20 to 25 per cent of the total calories as protein or 2 to 4 gm. of protein per kg. of body weight. Yet, some researchers believe there is also a maximum protein intake the body can handle which is near 2 gm. per kg. of body weight. For children, protein recommendations are even less clear, because of varying growth requirements. It is generally agreed that protein needs are increased above the RDA. Calorie to nitrogen ratios between 130:1 and 200:1 have been recommended for children.[20] Pediatric patients' ability to tolerate protein will depend on their renal function and fluid balance. Current studies are evaluating whether specific amino acids or proteins in general are required in increased amounts, and there is some suggestion that branched-chain amino acids should be increased.[61, 63]

ASSESSING ADEQUACY OF ENERGY AND PROTEIN INTAKE. The best way to help assess whether energy and protein recommendations are appropriate and intakes adequate is by following wound healing and graft take along with basic nutritional assessment parameters. Wound healing or graft take may be delayed if weight losses exceed 10 per cent of usual weight. An exact percentage of weight loss may be difficult to assess, because of fluid shifts or excessive edema common to the burn patient, but trends can be identified. Nitrogen balance may give a rough estimate of protein needs, but cannot be considered accurate unless wound losses are accounted for. Nitrogen excretion should begin to decrease as wounds heal or are covered. Serum albumin usually remains depressed in the patient with major burns until wounds are healed. The turnover proteins with shorter half-lives show more promise for helping assess the protein status of burn patients.

VITAMINS. There is general agreement that vitamin needs are increased for burn patients, but exact requirements have not yet been established. Most patients on tube feeding or total parenteral nutrition will be receiving more than the RDA already. Supplements may be needed for patients on oral intakes.

MINERALS. Electrolyte imbalances involving sodium or potassium are usually corrected by adjusting the patient's fluid therapy. Hyponatremia may be seen in patients whose evaporative losses are drastically reduced with application of dressings or grafts without changing their maintenance fluids, or who are treated with silver nitrate soaks, which tend to draw sodium from the wound. For these patients, restricting the oral consumption of non–sodium-containing fluids or free water may help to correct the hyponatremia.

Depression of serum calcium levels may be seen in patients with burns involving greater than 30 per cent of TBSA. Calcium losses may be exaggerated if the patient is immobile or being treated with silver nitrate soaks. Early ambulation and exercise, which is promoted for most burn patients, should help decrease these losses. Administration of calcium supplements may be necessary to treat symptomatic hypocalcemia. A depressed serum zinc level has been reported in burn patients, but it is unclear whether this is representative of total body zinc levels. Zinc supplementation has been recommended to treat post-burn anorexia and impaired wound healing.[37, 59] Zinc supplementation may not be warranted for every patient, but those patients receiving total parenteral support for an extended period of time should have zinc included.[45]

Hypophosphatemia has also been identified in patients with extensive burns. This occurs most commonly in those patients receiving large volumes of resuscitation fluid along with parenteral infusion of glucose solutions and large amounts of antacids for stress ulcer therapy. Serum levels need to be monitored and appropriate phosphate supplementation provided, usually parenterally.

The anemia seen following a burn is usually not related to iron deficiency and is treated by giving packed red blood cells.

METHODS OF NUTRITIONAL SUPPORT. Most patients with minor burns should be able to meet their estimated energy and protein needs with a regular hospital diet as shown in Figure 34–6. High-calorie, high-protein snacks and supplemental beverages may be enough to augment the regular diet for some patients. Those with more extensive burns, severely exaggerated nutritional needs or poor appetites may require tube feeding or total parenteral nutrition to help meet their needs more consistently. Enteral feeding is usually preferred, but with early excision and grafting parenteral nutrition may be necessary initially to avoid the frequent interruptions in enteral nutritional support that

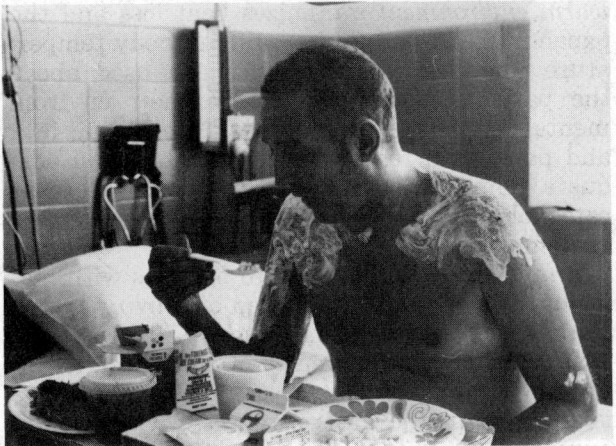

Figure 34–6. Most patients with minor burns should be able to meet their estimated energy and protein needs with the regular hospital diet. Note that the meal is served in disposable containers in order to maintain as sterile an environment as possible. (Courtesy of Regional Burn Center, Harborview Medical Center, Seattle, Washington.)

are required in giving anesthesia. TPN may also be the method of choice for patients with persistent ileus, who are not tolerating their tube feeding or who have a high risk of aspiration. Central lines for TPN can even be maintained through burn wounds with careful monitoring. In general, it is better to provide all of the nutritional support via one method or the other, to avoid doubling the risk of complications. Although most patients with burns greater than 40 per cent of TBSA cannot meet their estimated energy and protein needs with oral intakes alone, the appropriate method of support needs to be individually assessed for each patient. Table 34–2 summarizes nutritional care for burned patients.

Ancillary Measures

Physical therapy helps to prevent contractures along with helping to facilitate the incorporation of nitrogen into muscle. Provision of a

Table 34–2. NUTRITIONAL CARE FOR BURNED PATIENTS

1. Hospitalization in a warm environment
2. Covering of wounds to prevent fluid loss
3. Calorie allowance adequate to prevent weight loss of greater than 10 per cent of usual body weight
4. Protein allowance adequate for positive nitrogen balance
5. Vitamin and mineral supplementation
6. Physical therapy to promote muscle nitrogen retention
7. Antacids and frequent feedings to prevent development of Curling's ulcers
8. Use of supplements, tube feedings or parenteral nutrition necessary to meet the patient's requirements
9. Service of attractive, appetizing food in a pleasing, supportive environment

warm environment minimizes heat loss and the expenditure of energy to maintain body temperature. Individual heat shields are used above the patients' beds to maintain their environmental temperature near 30°C. Minimizing fear and pain, with reassurance from staff and adequate pain medication also helps to decrease catecholamine stimulation and hence energy requirements.

Antacids should be given to patients with major burns to prevent formation of *Curling's ulcer* in the gastric or duodenal mucosa. Although the reason for the development of this ulcer is unknown, it appears that through ischemia there is a break in the gastric mucosa, which when aggravated by excessive gastric acid secretion develops into an ulcer. The administration of antacids has been shown to be effective in preventing these ulcers.[44]

Problems and Suggested Topics for Discussion

1. List the principles of preoperative and postoperative nutritional care and give the reasons for this care.
2. Interview a patient who has had a partial or total gastrectomy. Does he or she have symptoms of the dumping syndrome? Alimentary hypoglycemia? Malabsorption? Describe the patient's symptoms. What changes would you recommend in the present diet?
3. Keep a record of the food ingested in one day by a patient who has had a colostomy. Is the intake meeting the patient's nutritional requirements? What changes will need to be made? Are there any nutrients that this patient may not be absorbing properly because of the surgery?
4. Follow a patient who has had the Whipple operation. Identify any nutritional problems. Design a nutritional care plan to manage these problems.
5. Prepare a nutritional care plan for a female patient with burns over 25 per cent of her body. Define the nutritional requirements and how they will be met. What teaching will be necessary?

Cited References

1. Alvarez, O.M., and Gilbreath, R.L.: Thiamine influence on collagen during the granulation of skin wounds. J. Surg. Res., *32*:24, 1982.
2. Artz, C.P., and Hardy, J.D.: Management of Surgical Complications. 3rd ed. Philadelphia, W.B. Saunders Company, 1975.
3. Aston, S.J., and Longmire, W.P., Jr.: Management of the pancreas after pancreatoduodenectomy. Ann. Surg., *179*:322, 1974.
4. Barness, L.A.: Safety considerations with high ascorbic acid dosage. Ann. N. Y. Acad. Sci., *258*:523, 1975.
5. Becker, J.M., and Artz, C.P.: The treatment of burns in children. Report No. 5, Surgical Research Unit, Brooke Army Hospital, Ft. Sam Houston, Texas, 1965.
6. Bingham, S., Cummings, J.H., and McNeil, N.I.: Diet and health of people with an ileostomy. 1. Dietary assessment. Br. J. Nutr., *47*:399, 1982.
7. Blackburn, G.L., and Bistrian, B.R.: Nutritional care in trauma and sepsis. Surg. Clin. N. Am., *56*:1195, 1976.
8. Blalock, J.B.: History and evolution of peptic ulcer surgery. Am. J. Surg., *141*:317, 1981.
9. Burke, J.F., Quinby, W.C., and Bondoc, C.C.: Early excision and prompt wound closure supplemented with immunosuppression. Surg. Clin. N. Am., *58*:1141, 1978.
10. Burke, J.F., et al.: Glucose requirements following burn injury. Ann. Surg., *190*:274, 1979.
11. Buzby, G.P.: Preoperative nutritional support: nutritional indications for delaying surgery. Clinical Consultations in Nutritional Support (Ross Laboratories). *2*(2):1, 1982.
12. Cahill, G.F.: Starvation in man. N. Engl. J. Med., *282*:668, 1970.
13. Caldwell, M.D., and Kennedy-Caldwell, C.: Normal nutritional requirements. Surg. Clin. N. Am., *61*:489, 1981.
14. Crossland, S.S., et al.: Preoperative nutritional support for bowel surgery patients. Contemp. Surg., *16*:37, 1980.
15. Curreri, P.W., and Luterman, A.: Nutritional support of the burned patient. Surg. Clin. N. Am., *58*:1151, 1978.
16. Curreri, P.W., and Richmond, D.: Nutritional management following massive small bowel resection. Dietetic Currents, *1*(4), 1974.
17. Curreri, P.W., et al.: Burn injury—analysis of survival and hospital time. Ann. Surg., *192*:472, 1980.
18. Curreri, P.W., et al.: Dietary requirements of patients with major burns. J. Am. Diet. Assoc., *65*:415, 1974.
19. Cuthbertson, D.P.: Observations on the disturbance of metabolism produced by injury to the limbs. Q. J. Med., *1*:233, 1932.
20. Derganc, M.: Parenteral nutrition in severely burned children. Scand. J. Plast. Recon. Surg., *13*:195, 1979.
21. Diet and bone disease. Dairy Council Digest, *53*(5):1, 1982.
22. Efron, G.: Abdominal wound disruption. Lancet, *1*:1287, 1965.
23. Elwyn, D.H., et al.: Changes in nitrogen balance of depleted patients with increasing infusions of glucose. Am. J. Clin. Nutr., *32*:1597, 1979.
24. Feller, I., Tholen, D., and Cornell, R.G.: Improvements in burn care 1965–1979. JAMA, *244*:2074, 1980.
25. Feurer, I., et al.: Resting energy expenditure in morbid obesity (Abstract No. 28) JPEN *5*:562, 1981. 6th Clinical Congress of ASPEN: Specialized Nutritional Support: The Standard of Care. San Francisco, Feb. 1982.
26. Fischer, J.E.: Nutritional assessment before surgery. Am. J. Clin. Nutr., *35*:1128, 1982.
27. Gordon, P.H.: The chemically defined diet and anorectal procedures. Can. J. Surg., *19*:511, 1976.
28. Graber, J.N., et al.: Relationship of duration of postoperative ileus to extent and site of operative dissection. Surgery, *92*:87, 1982.
29. Gump, F.E., Martin, P., and Kinney, J.M.: Oxygen consumption and caloric expenditure in surgical patients. Surg. Gynecol. Obstet., *137*:499, 1973.
30. Heibert, J.M., Anderson, G.R., and Rodeheaver, G.T.: Fueling the burn patient; when does enteric nitrogen to Calorie ratio influence nitrogen balance? Abstr. No. 34. Presented at American Burn Association 13th Annual Meeting, 1981.
31. Herbert, V., and Jacobs, E.: Destruction of vitamin B_{12} by ascorbic acid. JAMA, *230*:241, 1974.
32. Hill, G.: Studies of body composition and muscle enzymes in injury and sepsis. Presented at 6th Clinical Congress of ASPEN: Specialized Nutritional Support: The Standard of Care. San Francisco, Feb. 1982.
33. Hill, G.L.: Impairment of "ileostomy adaptation" in patients after ileal resection. Gut, *15*:982, 1974.

34. Hodges, R.E.: Vitamin C and cancer. Nutr. Rev., 40: 289, 1982.

35. Kinney, J.M., et al.: Tissue fuel and weight loss after injury. J. Clin. Pathol., 23(Suppl.) 4:65, 1970.

36. Klein, C.L., et al.: Increased rates of whole body protein synthesis and break down in children recovering from burns. Ann. Surg., 187:383, 1978.

37. Kohen, I.T., et al.: Hypogeusia, anorexia and altered zinc metabolism following thermal burn. JAMA, 223: 914, 1973.

38. Lawrence, W.: Nutritional consequences of surgical resection of the gastrointestinal tract for cancer. Cancer Res., 37:2379, 1977.

39. Levine, G.M.: Nutritional support in gastrointestinal disease. Surg. Clin. N. Am., 61:701, 1981.

40. Linner, J.H.: Comparative effectiveness of gastric bypass and gastroplasty. Arch. Surg., 117:695, 1982.

41. Long, C.L., et al.: Metabolic response to injury and illness: estimation of energy and protein needs from indirect calorimetry and nitrogen balance. JPEN, 3:452, 1979.

42. Lund, C.L., and Browder, N.C.: The estimation of areas of burns. Surg. Gynecol. Obstet., 79:352, 1944.

43. MacMillan, B.G.: Closing the burn wound. Surg. Clin. N. Am., 58:1205, 1978.

44. McAlhany, J.C., Czaja, A.J., and Pruitt, B.A.: Antacid control of complications from acute gastroduodenal disease after burns. J. Trauma, 16:645, 1976.

45. McCain, C.J.: Trace metal abnormalities in adults during hyperalimentation. JPEN, 5:424, 1981.

46. McDermott, W.V., Jr., and Ackroyd, F.W.: Nutrient demands imposed by surgery of the liver. Am. J. Clin. Nutr., 23:652, 1970.

47. McNeil, N.I., et al.: Diet and health of people with an ileostomy, 2. Ileostomy function and nutritional state. Br. J. Nutr., 47:407, 1982.

48. Meakins, J.L., et al.: Delayed hypersensitivity: indicator of acquired failure of host defenses in sepsis and trauma. Ann. Surg., 186:241, 1977.

49. Morishita, R., et al.: Effect of pancreatin on vitamin B_{12} malabsorption in patients with total pancreatectomy. Digestion, 11:240, 1974.

50. Mullen, J.L.: Consequences of malnutrition in the surgical patient. Surg. Clin. N. Am., 61:465, 1981.

51. Munster, A.: Early management of thermal burns. Surgery 87:32, 1980.

52. Nazari, S., et al.: Cluster analysis of nutritional and immunological indicators for identification of high risk surgical patients. JPEN, 5:307, 1981.

53. Peters, C., and Fischer, J.E.: Studies on calorie to nitrogen ratio for total parenteral nutrition. Surg. Gynecol. Obstet., 151:1, 1980.

54. Pories, W.J., et al.: Acceleration of healing with zinc sulfate. Ann. Surg., 165:432, 1967.

55. Rennie, J.A., et al.: Neural and humoral factors in postoperative ileus. Br. J. Surg., 67:694, 1980.

56. Rhoads, J.E., and Alexander, C.E.: Nutritional problems of surgical patients. Ann. N.Y. Acad. Sci., 63(2):268, 1955.

57. Rhoads, J.E., et al.: The mechanism of delayed wound healing in the presence of hypoproteinemia. JAMA, 118:21, 1942.

58. Ross, G.: Iron metabolism: perspectives. Nutr. Supp. Serv., 2(6):28, 1982.

59. Sandstead, H.H., et al.: Zinc and wound healing. Am. J. Clin. Nutr., 23:514, 1970.

60. Scheflan, M., et al.: Intestinal adaptation after extensive resection of the small intestine and prolonged administration of parenteral nutrition. Surg. Gynecol. Obstet., 143:757, 1976.

61. Scrimshaw, N.S.: Effect of infection on nutrient requirements. Am. J. Clin. Nutr., 30:1536, 1977.

62. Shils, M.E.: Effects on nutrition of surgery of the liver, pancreas, and genitourinary tract. Cancer Res., 37: 2387, 1977.

63. Shizgal, H.M.: Body composition and nutritional support. Surg. Clin. N. Am., 61:729, 1981.

64. Simko, V., et al.: High-fat diet in a short bowel syndrome: intestinal absorption and gastroenteropancreatic hormonal responses. Dig. Dis. Sci., 25:333, 1980.

65. Snelling, C.F.T., et al.: Amino acid metabolism in burn patients. Surg., 91:474, 1982.

66. Stimulus for hyperplasia of the small bowel. Nutr. Rev., 34:345, 1976.

67. Stinnett, J.D., et al.: Plasma and skeletal muscle amino acids following severe burn injury in patients and experimental animals. Ann. Surg., 195:75, 1982.

68. Studley, H.O.: Percentage of weight loss: a basic indicator of surgical risk. JAMA, 106:458, 1936.

69. Sutherland, A.B., and Batchelor, A.D.R.: Nitrogen balance in burned children. In Wilkinson, A.W. (ed.): International Congress on Research in Burns. Edinburgh, Livingston, Ltd., 1966, pp. 147–157.

70. Taylor, T.V.: Postvagotomy and cholecystectomy syndrome. Ann. Surg., 194:625, 1981.

71. Thiamin and wound repair. Nutr. Rev., 40:316, 1982.

72. Toskes, P.P., et al.: Vitamin B_{12} malabsorption in chronic pancreatic insufficiency. N. Engl. J. Med., 284: 627, 1971.

73. Tui, C.O., et al.: Studies on surgical convalescence. Ann. Surg., 120:99, 1944.

74. Tympner, F., et al.: The function of the exocrine pancreas after exogenous and endogenous stimulation in Billroth II patients. Acta Hepatogastroenterol., 23:444, 1976.

75. Watters, J.M., and Freeman, J.B.: Parenteral nutrition by peripheral vein. Surg. Clin. N. Am., 61:593, 1981.

76. Wolfe, B.M., and Chock, E.: Energy sources, stores and hormonal controls. Surg. Clin. N. Am., 61:509, 1981.

Additional References

SURGICAL CONDITIONS

American College of Surgeons, Committee on Pre and Postoperative Care: Manual of Surgical Nutrition. 3rd ed., Philadelphia, W. B. Saunders Company, 1983.

Gurry, J.F., and Ellis-Pegler, R.G.: An elemental diet as preoperative preparation of the colon. Br. J. Surg., 63:969, 1976.

Haley, J.V.: Zinc sulfate and wound healing. J. Surg. Res., 27:168, 1979.

Himal, H.S., et al.: The importance of adequate nutrition in closure of small intestinal fistulas. Br. J. Surg., 61:724, 1974.

Jenkins, D.J.A., et al.: Low dose acarbose without symptoms of malabsorption in dumping syndrome. Lancet, 1:109, 1982.

Lee, P.W.R., et al.: Zinc and wound healing. Surg. Gynecol. Obstet., 143:549, 1976.

Leeds, A.R., et al.: Pectin in the dumping syndrome: reduction of symptoms and plasma volume changes. Lancet, 1: 1075, 1981.

McClelland, R.N.: Surgical treatment of peptic ulcer and postgastrectomy complications. In Dietschy, J.M., and Sanford, J.P. (eds.): Disorders of the Gastrointestinal Tract, Disorders of the Liver, Nutritional Disorders. New York, Grune & Stratton, 1976, pp. 102–111.

Muller, J.M., et al.: Preoperative parenteral feeding in patients with gastrointestinal carcinoma. Lancet, 1:68, 1982.

Scott, H.W., et al.: The dumping syndrome. Gastroenterology, 37:194, 1959.

Tilston, W.J.: The effects of environmental conditions on the metabolic requirements after injury. In Lee, H.A. (ed.): Parenteral Nutrition in Acute Metabolic Illness. New York, Academic Press, 1974, pp. 167–177.

Webster, M.W., and Corey, L.C.: Fistulae of the intestinal tract. Curr. Probl. Surg., 13(6), 1976.

Wilmore, D.W.: The Metabolic Management of the Critically Ill. New York, Plenum Med. Book Co., 1980.

BURNS

Alexander, J.W., et al.: Beneficial effects of aggressive protein feeding in severely burned children. Ann. Surg., 192:505, 1980.

Artz, C.P.: Guide to assessment and management of burns. Hosp. Med., 14:105, 1977.

Baxter, C.R.: Fluid therapy. In Practical Approaches to Burn Management. Deerfield, Ill., Flint Lab. 1977, pg. 13–16.

Davies, J.W., et al.: The effect of environmental temperature on the metabolism and nutrition of burned patients. Proc. Nutr. Soc., 30:165, 1971.

Dudrick, S.J.: Nutritional therapy in burned patients. J. Trauma, 19:908, 1979.

Feller, I., et al.: The team approach to total rehabilitation of the severely burned patient. Heart Lung, 2:701, 1973.

Haynes, W.B.: Management of burns in children. J. Trauma, 5:267, 1955.

Long, C.: Energy expenditure of major burns. J. Trauma, 19:904, 1979.

MacMillan, B.G.: Burns in children. Clin. Plast. Surg., 1:633, 1974.

Moncrief, J.A.: Burns. N. Engl. J. Med., 288:444, 1973.

Mullen, J.L., et al.: Reduction of operative morbidity and mortality by combined preoperative and postoperative nutritional support. Ann. Surg., 192:604, 1980.

Mullen, J.L., et al.: Prediction of operative morbidity and mortality by preoperative nutritional assessment. Surg. Forum, 30:80, 1979.

Newsome, T.W., Mason, A.D., and Pruitt, B.A.: Weight loss following thermal injury. Ann. Surg., 178:215, 1973.

Parks, D.H., Carvajal, H.F., and Larson, D.L.: Management of burns. Surg. Clin. N. Am., 57:875, 1977.

Pruitt, B.A.: Fluid and electrolyte replacement in the burned patient. Surg. Clin. N. Am., 58:1291, 1978.

Schenk, W.G. and Moylan, J.A.: Nutritional aspects of burn care. In Practical Approaches to Burn Management. Deerfield, Ill., Flint Lab., 1977.

Shakespeare, P.G.: Studies on the serum levels of iron, copper and zinc and the urinary secretion of zinc after burn injury. Burns, 8:358, 1982.

Wilmore, D.W., et al.: Catecholamines: mediator of the hypermetabolic response to thermal injury. Ann. Surg., 180:653, 1974.

Wilmore, D.W.: Nutrition and metabolism following thermal injury. Clin. Plast. Surg., 1:603, 1974.

CHAPTER

35

The Metabolic Stress Response and Methods of Providing Nutritional Care for Stressed Patients

In the previous chapter the physiological stress associated with surgery, trauma and burns and the nutritional care necessary for these conditions were discussed. In this chapter we will explore the metabolic response to physiological stress and the effect of infection or starvation added to this stress. Parenteral and enteral feeding techniques to meet the nutritional requirements of these conditions and others will also be discussed. These techniques can be used to meet the nutritional needs of patients who are either unable or unwilling to take regular food or who cannot meet their nutritional requirments with the usual oral intake.

Starvation

Adaptive Response to Starvation

The normal response to starvation must be understood before discussing the response when physiological stress is also present. In the nor-mal adult the available stored energy amounts to about 200 gm. of glycogen, 6000 gm. of protein and 15,000 gm. of fat. Obviously, the fat component varies the most among individuals. When a person starves, the glycogen stores are used first as glycogenolysis takes place for the synthesis of blood glucose. These stores, which supply about 800 kcal., are usually exhausted within 15 to 20 hours. After that, protein from skeletal muscles is mobilized, converted to glucose in the liver and released into the blood stream to maintain the blood glucose level. Initially, the body may use as much as 75 gm. of protein per day in maintaining the blood glucose concentration. This protein must have the nitrogen (N) removed before it can be converted into glucose, and this nitrogen is excreted in the urine. Consequently, urinary nitrogen excretion is increased, which reflects a negative nitrogen balance of about -12 gm. N per day (1 gm. N = 6.25 gm. of protein). (Chapter 4 discusses nitrogen balance and its calculation.) Shown below is a method for estimating nitrogen balance:

ROUGH ESTIMATION OF NITROGEN (N) BALANCE

Nitrogen balance = nitrogen intake − nitrogen output

$$\text{Nitrogen intake} = \frac{\text{protein in gm. consumed by patient in 24 hr.}}{6.25 \text{ gm. protein}/1 \text{ gm. nitrogen}}$$

Nitrogen output = gm. urinary urea N in 24 hr. + 4.0 gm.

Nitrogen intake > nitrogen output = *positive* nitrogen balance = patient in state of anabolism with synthesis of body tissue protein exceeding breakdown of tissue protein

Nitrogen intake = nitrogen output = nitrogen *balance* = build-up of tissue protein is equal to breakdown of tissue protein

Nitrogen intake < nitrogen output = *negative* nitrogen balance = patient in state of catabolism with breakdown of tissue protein exceeding synthesis of tissue protein

In the fasting body, muscle protein is metabolized first, then the protein in digestive enzymes and last, liver protein. This use of body protein for energy is very costly, so the body adapts by using a more dispensable body energy store—fat. This process of adaptation takes 3 to 4 days, but soon the body is mobilizing fatty acids for energy and using only about 25 gm. of protein per day for energy. A look at the patient's daily negative nitrogen balance at this point shows that it has decreased to −4 gm. N.

Besides using fatty acids directly for energy and converting some to glucose, the liver also converts some fatty acids to ketone bodies. In the next stage of adaptation, all tissues of the body, including the brain, can metabolize ketones for energy. Seventy per cent of the brain's energy needs can be supplied by the oxidation of ketones rather than of glucose. In this stage, the urinary nitrogen loss will become even less, and the negative nitrogen balance will decrease further, to −2 to −4 gm. N per day. In the final phase of starvation, fat stores are used up, and the entire energy requirement must be met by visceral organ and plasma proteins. Depletion of these proteins is signaled by edema and finally results in death.

Healthy humans of normal weight will not tolerate the loss of more than 35 to 40 per cent of their body weight. Losses of this size (about 300 gm. of nitrogen in the male and 200 gm. of nitrogen in the female) represent a loss of 1200 to 1800 gm. of body protein, about one third of the total body protein. This is fatal. In a person who is depleted or underweight prior to starvation, a lesser body weight loss will be fatal.

The process of conversion to the economical utilization of stored fat for energy depends on a progressive decrease in circulating insulin, which falls from a basal level of 16 to 20 μU. per ml. to less than 12 μU. per ml. When this happens, fatty acid mobilization and ketone body production are promoted. Severe ketonemia will stimulate insulin secretion, however, and since insulin strongly inhibits ketogenesis,

a feedback control exists that prevents ketosis from reaching pathological levels. This is not the situation with diabetics, who have no insulin to control the ketogenesis when it becomes excessive. Table 35–1 summarizes the phases of starvation and the changes that take place in a person who is fasting completely but is otherwise healthy. Table 35–2 summarizes the effects of prolonged undernutrition on organic function.

Starvation Added to Physiological Stress

While the totally fasting healthy person adapts to an economical utilization of body fat with a conservation of body protein to the greatest possible extent, the person who has had trauma, burns, surgery, infection or shock does not adapt as well to starvation. In this situation, the body exhibits a *stress response* that is protective and necessary for the body yet is very catabolic. Eventually the body adapts to both the stress and the starvation so that the nitrogen loss decreases, but it never decreases as much as it will in a starving person who has no other stress.

Nutrition and the Immune Response
Dorice Czajka-Narins, Ph.D.

Laboratory, clinical and field observations have demonstrated that the severity and outcome of infection are frequently worsened by malnutrition. This is due to the fact that the nutritional status of the host influences its production of antibodies and lymphocytes, which play an important role in both natural and acquired immunity. A complete discussion of the immune response is beyond the scope of this text, but the reader is encouraged to consult other references on this subject.

For several decades clinicians and public health professionals working with malnourished children in developing countries have known

Table 35–1. STAGES OF STARVATION

STAGE I (Days 2–4)		STAGE II (Days 20–40)		STAGE III (Ketoadaptation)
Increase in urinary N loss from use of tissue protein for gluconeogenesis	A D A P T A T I O N	Decrease in urinary N loss as protein conservation takes place	A D A P T A T I O N	Decrease in urinary N loss as glucose-burning tissues adapt to ketone metabolism
Negative nitrogen balance: −12–15 gm. N/day		Negative nitrogen balance: −4 gm. N/day		Negative nitrogen balance: −2 to −4 gm. N/day
		Reduction in BMR		In absence of dietary intake, total urinary N is a measure of gluconeogenesis
		Body fat utilization at maximum		
		Serum fatty acids ↑		
		Serum ketones ↑		
		Serum insulin (basal) ↓		

that infections not only are more frequent in these children but are also more fulminant and lethal. Measles in children with protein-energy malnutrition (PEM) can be fatal. Furthermore, an infectious episode can precipitate the development of symptoms of severe malnutrition. During the past few years researchers have learned much about the interaction between immunology and nutrition, but there is still much

Table 35–2. IMPACT OF PROTEIN-ENERGY UNDERNUTRITION ON ORGAN FUNCTION

RESPIRATORY SYSTEM
—deterioration of performance in standard pulmonary function testing
—decreased sensitivity of oxygen receptors to hypoxic stimuli
—marked blunting of ventilatory response to hypercapnia
—in animals: decreased tissue elasticity of the lung and increased lung surface elastic forces

CARDIAC SYSTEM
—decrease in cardiac mass
—congestive heart failure with refeeding and resulting increased basal metabolic rate
—animals: decreased myocardial contractility with protein depletion

GASTROINTESTINAL SYSTEM
—a marked thinning of gastrointestinal tract with loss of both muscular and mucosal components
—shortened mucosal villi with loss of absorptive surface and brush-border enzyme activity
—decrease in gastric motility
—in severe PEM, there is a decrease in stomach HCl secretion and worsening of resultant malabsorption

LIVER
—in early stage of PEM can see drug metabolism and protein synthesis changes. Significant prolongation of drug clearance from blood. Decreased albumin synthesis
—in late stage liver failure may result

RENAL SYSTEM
—decreased ability to concentrate urine and diuresis occurs
—decreased ability to excrete titratable acid
—altered glomerular filtration rates and renal plasma flow in children

From Grant, J. P.: Impact of protein-calorie undernutrition on organ failure. Clin. Consult., 3(1):1, 1983.

to be learned, particularly of the more subtle effects of moderate rather than severe malnutrition. It is the latter that is seen in patients suffering from a variety of disorders such as malabsorption, in the elderly and very poor, who may not be eating well, and in those who follow fad diets.

Nutrition and Cell-Mediated Immunity

PEM and deficiencies of many specific nutrients impair various aspects of cell-mediated immunity. Since PEM is a multiple deficiency, not just of protein and/or energy, many micronutrients are also deficient. Therefore, specific nutrients may cause changes in cell-mediated immunity, which interact to produce the effects seen in patients with PEM. A consistent impairment of cutaneous delayed hypersensitivity reactions, which are reduced both in the number of positive responses and diameter of induration, is evident in PEM patients. Any of the steps of this reaction—sensitization, antigen recognition, proliferation and elaboration of lymphokines by T cells, vascular changes, and migration of cells to local site—may be altered in patients with PEM. These patients also have a reduced number of circulating lymphocytes, depending upon the degree of malnutrition. The decrease in the number of T cells in peripheral circulation reflects the reduction in total lymphocytes. Cell-mediated immunity is most commonly assessed by total lymphocyte count and cutaneous delayed hypersensitivity.

Some experimental evidence appeared to suggest that normal maturation and differentiation of T cell precursors was retarded by the lower levels of thymic hormones seen in children with PEM. However, more recent studies have indicated that children with moderate to severe PEM do not necessarily have reduced levels of circulating thymic hormone. The high levels seen in some children with PEM may be explained by the stimulating effect of concurrent infection or be related to their zinc status.

Zinc, vitamin A and pyridoxine have been shown to be important in maintaining adequate cell-mediated immunity. *In vitro*, cell-mediated immunity is decreased in patients with acrodermatitis enteropathica, a manifestation of zinc deficiency as mentioned in Chapter 7. Several aspects of cell-mediated immunity normalize when dietary zinc is increased, with a concurrent rise in serum zinc.

Lymphoid tissue also requires an adequate amount of iron. Delayed hypersensitivity skin responses are also impaired in patients who are iron deficient, and lymphocyte stimulation *in vitro* is reduced. The number of circulating lymphocytes is slightly reduced.

Isolated vitamin deficiencies are rare in clinical practice. Until information is available on the effects of marginal vitamin deficiency on cell-mediated immunity, most of the effects of specific vitamin deficiencies will be seen only as part of a total protein or energy deficiency.

Nutrition and Humoral Immunity

Serum immunoglobulin concentrations are usually normal or increased in children with PEM. Adult levels of circulating immunoglobulins are often seen in children about two years of age owing to this elevation. The degree of malnutrition is inversely correlated with immunoglobulin levels. With nutritional rehabilitation and antimicrobial therapy, circulating immunoglobulin concentrations may return to normal. Infants under two with severe marasmus, low serum albumin and infections, sometimes have hypoimmunoglobulinemia.

Serum IgE is extremely high in children with PEM, but allergy is uncommon. The elevation of serum IgE can be explained in part by the higher frequency of infestation with intestinal parasites. Another reason for the elevated IgE levels in malnourished patients is an abnormality of T cell regulation. T cells both initiate and suppress IgE synthesis.

Animal studies have shown that specific dietary deficiencies may also impair humoral immunity. Magnesium, zinc, pyridoxine, pantothenic acid and folate appear to be important.

Surface Immunity—Mucocutaneous Integrity

Tissue barriers to infection are damaged by a variety of deficiencies. Deficiencies of vitamins A and C and of niacin impair tissue integrity, wound healing, fibroblastic response to trauma, walling off of abscesses, collagen formation and thus the body's resistance to the invasion of infective organisms. Lysozymes, which help to destroy pathogenic microorganisms, are present in tears, sweat and saliva, and their levels in the body are reduced in malnutrition, particularly when vitamin A is deficient.

Infection reduces blood levels of vitamin A. Considerable research has been carried out on the relationship between vitamin A and the common cold, pulmonary tuberculosis and other infectious diseases. Apparently, vitamin A deficiency may play a role in reducing natural resistance, but the administration of the vitamin during the course of an infection has little, if any, beneficial effect unless a deficiency is present.

Vitamin C may have a role in the white blood cell response to infection, but this is only a speculation. It seems to depend on the timing and type of infection. See page 134 for a discussion of this theory.

No doubt future research will support current evidence that people who have inadequate diets also have a decreased resistance to infection and will elucidate the mechanisms whereby nutritional deficiencies influence the body's resistance to infectious diseases.

Effect of Infection on Nutritional Requirements

INCREASED METABOLIC RATE. Fever is usually present with infection. According to DuBois,[7] there is an elevation of approximately 7.2 per cent in the metabolic rate for each 1°F, or 13 per cent for each 1°C. Sometimes the increase is as much as 40 per cent when a patient has a temperature of 104°F (40°C). If the patient is restless, delirious or coughing, the total energy need is increased further because of increased activity.

An easy method to determine the metabolism of a patient with fever, suggested by DuBois, is:

1. Determine the normal basal metabolic rate (1400 to 1800 kcal. per day) and then add 7 per cent of the BMR for each degree Fahrenheit (13 per cent for each degree Celsius) of elevation of temperature above normal.

2. If there is sepsis, add another 10 per cent of the BMR.

3. If the patient is restless, add another 10 to 30 per cent of the BMR. This method will give a sufficiently accurate energy requirement for a patient with fever.

CATABOLISM. During the early part of the century it was established that severe bacterial infections, such as typhoid fever, pneumonia, malaria and tuberculosis, cause severe and prolonged loss of nitrogen, chiefly as a result of the toxic destruction of intracellular protein. Studies have shown that mild and asymptomatic viral invasion, such as that produced by yellow fever vaccine or mild chickenpox in children, will produce adverse nitrogen balance effects, even when the patient is receiving an apparently adequate protein intake.[23]

The catabolic response to infection, which is discussed in detail on page 711 begins after the onset of fever, as Figure 35–1 indicates. This catabolism is reflected in negative nitrogen, potassium, magnesium, phosphate, sulfate and zinc balances that persist into convalescence. If the infection is severe and prolonged there will be muscle wasting and weight loss as muscle protein is catabolized for energy. Eventually, however, a stable negative nitrogen balance is reached.

In addition to the wastage of nutrients caused by this catabolic response, there are additional gastrointestional losses from vomiting and diarrhea. Nutrient intake is diminished because of anorexia and the common practice of withholding food from an ill person and possibly because of malabsorption, as in the case of gastrointestinal infection. Demands on the host's defense system to synthesize phagocytes, leukocytes, immunoglobulins and nonspecific proteins further increase protein requirements.

Nutritional Care

ENERGY AND PROTEIN. During the acute phase of infection it is difficult to maintain positive nitrogen balance because of the patient's anorexia and the catabolic stress response, which promotes tissue protein breakdown. However, after the body adapts in three to four days it may be possible to achieve positive nitrogen balance, depending upon the severity of the infection.[2] Protein must be supplied at levels of at least 0.8 to 1.0 gm. per kg. ideal body weight per day. Orally, protein can be supplied in the form of meat, fish, poultry, eggs, milk, cheese or soups and broths made from proteins such as casein, soy isolate and hydrolyzed protein. Nutritional support should be started as early as possible.

After the catabolic phase subsides, an anabolic phase follows, during which energy and protein should be provided at higher than normal levels. Protein should be increased to 1.2 to 2.0 gm./kg. and energy to 35 to 45 kcal./kg. to restore nitrogen losses. The nutritional goal is to put the patient into positive nitrogen balance.

FLUIDS. Fluids are of major importance in the treatment of infections. Any fluids that appeal to the patient are satisfactory. As a rule, very sweet liquids are not appealing and frequently cause gastric disturbance as well as distention in the abdominal region. Carbonated beverages (such as ginger ale) and lemonade that is not too sweet seem to be favorites. Protein-containing fluids would be preferable because they help to spare body protein. If the patient is nauseated and vomiting and too ill to take fluids by mouth, fluid may be given parenterally. Often 3 to 4 liters of fluids are required daily to keep the patient well hydrated.

VITAMINS. Fevers increase vitamin requirements, especially of the B-complex vitamins, ascorbic acid and vitamin A. As the energy need increases, thiamin, riboflavin and niacin re-

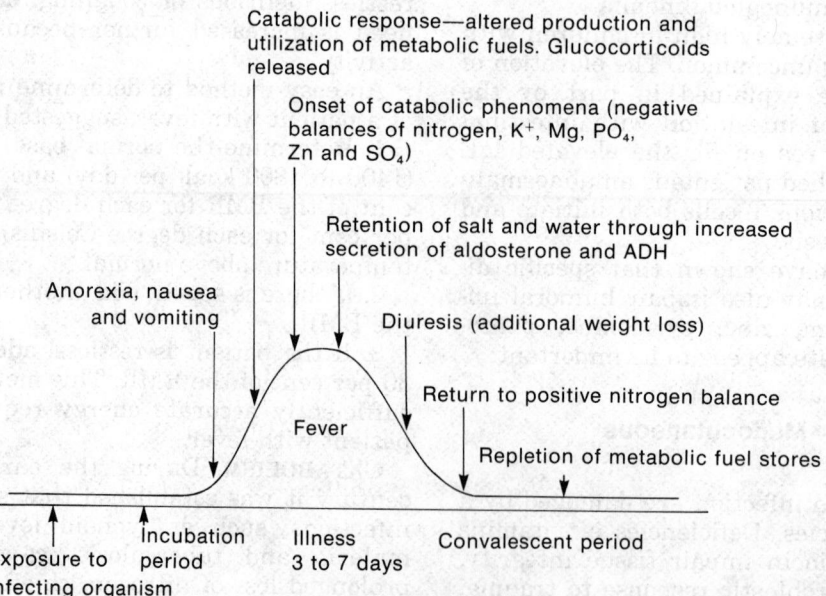

Figure 35–1. Timing of catabolic response to infection. (Adapted from Beisel, W. R.: The influence of infection or injury on nutritional requirements during adolescence. In McKigney, J. I., and Munro, H. N. (eds.): Nutrient Requirements in Adolescence. Cambridge, Mass., MIT Press, 1976, p. 259.)

quirements also increase. Antibiotics and drugs may interfere with the intestinal synthesis of the B-complex vitamins. Vitamin supplements are usually advised during the illness and convalescence.

MINERALS. Loss of sodium and potassium because of fever may be considerable during the acute phase of illness. The serum levels of these electrolytes should be monitored. Unless contraindicated, salty broth, soups and additional sodium and potassium in foods usually replenish the loss. A full liquid or regular diet usually supplies enough potassium. An inadequate intake of food may be supplemented by fruit juices and milk, which are good sources of potassium. If oral intake is inconsistent, parenteral supplementation of sodium or potassium may be necessary.

Sometimes patients with infections develop anemia, but this is due to a redistribution of iron in the body's defense against infection rather than to a deficient iron intake.

MEAL PLAN. Frequent small liquid feedings are usually best tolerated in the beginning. Occasionally, tube feedings as described on page 715 may be necessary if the patient has no appetite. The full liquid diet given in Table 19–10 can be served to the patient as soon as it is tolerated. Such a diet contains food that is easily and quickly digested. Protein supplements may be added in varying amounts to fruit juice, milk or soup. Many patients do better when they eat a regular diet with protein and calorie adjustments to meet the individual requirements. They experience less anorexia, nausea and vomiting. See Table 35–3 for increased protein content of the daily meal plan.

Since most patients with fevers have poor appetites, it is important that special attention be given to the selection of food. An attempt should be made to appeal to the appetite through the careful choice of color, temperature and texture of different foods. Often the person can suggest a food or foods that are appealing. The foods should be easily digested, good sources of protein, and of concentrated food value, such as cereal, whole-grain or enriched bread, potatoes, ice cream, custards, cheese, milk, cream, eggs and fruit juices. Meat and leafy green and yellow vegetables should be included as soon as tolerated. In-between feedings, such as high-calorie beverages that furnish energy and protein and additional fluids, are recommended. Examples are hot chocolate and malted milk with whipped cream, eggnogs and fruit juices with added sugar or Polycose. The average high-calorie diet contains approximately 3000 kcal. However, it may be necessary to provide as many as 5000 kcal. if the patient is large, growing or very restless and if there is great toxic destruction along with high temperature.

To increase the daily protein and energy intake in 500 kcal. steps, the plan in Table 27–9 is suggested. For example, the normal general hospital diet for an individual is calculated to be approximately 2000 kcal. If a diet of 2500 kcal. is desired, a step-up of 500 kcal. is added; or if 3000 kcal. are desired, then two such supplements are added. The choice of food for the addition of calories will be governed by the preference and tolerance of the patient. When the appetite is very poor, small meals and a concentrated supplement are tolerated best, since patients are often overwhelmed by the quantity of food served on the high-calorie, high-nutrient diets.

The Catabolic Response to Stress

Physiological stress can be due to many factors, including injury, starvation, surgery, burns, infections, flare-ups of chronic disease, extreme heat and extreme cold. There are many variables involved that relate to nutrition, such as the severity of the injury, the previous state of nutrition of the individual and the nutrients consumed following stress.

The acute *catabolic phase* is characterized by a *sympathetic nervous reaction*. The sympathetic activity causes release of glucagon by the pancreas and of glucocorticoid and epinephrine by the adrenals, as diagrammed in Figure 34–5. These substances inhibit the release of insulin and antagonize its actions. The net effect of this response is a reduced concentration of serum insulin, hyperglycemia and a resistance to insulin by the peripheral tissues, causing a pseudo-diabetic state. This explains why diabetics who normally are in good control become hyperglycemic during an infection and require more insulin. The lack of insulin in response to glucose and the tissue resistance to insulin action prevent muscle tissue from utilizing glucose, and a local fuel deficit develops. To satisfy its requirements for energy, skeletal muscle oxidizes the branched-chain amino acids (leucine, isoleucine and valine) from its own tissues. As this protein is mobilized for energy, the excess NH_3 that results from the oxidation is attached to pyruvate and carried back to the liver as the amino acid alanine. Alanine stimulates the pancreas to secrete glucagon, which induces gluconeogenesis and ureagenesis in the liver and clears the blood of alanine, glycerol and lactate. The basal level of insulin initially has an antilipolytic effect, so that the body does not adapt by oxidizing fatty acids and ketones for energy.

Sympathetic nervous activity also stimulates

Table 35–3. INCREASED PROTEIN CONTENT OF THE DAILY MEAL PLAN*†

DAILY MEAL PLAN *To increase the protein content of the day's meals from 100 gm. to 125 or 150, use the allowances of dried milk solids indicated in columns 2 and 3.*	PROTEIN CONTENT IN GRAMS		
	100 gm. (approx.)[a]	*125 gm. (approx.)*[b]	*150 gm. (approx.)*[c]
BREAKFAST			
Fruit juice, citrus, ½ cup	0.5	0.5	0.5
Cereal, enriched, ½ cup, cooked or prepared, with	2.5	2.5	2.5
½ cup whole milk	4.2	4.2	4.2
Plus 2 tbsp. dried non-fat milk solids	–	6.0	6.0
Egg, 1	6.5	6.5	6.5
Bread (white, enriched or whole-wheat), 1 slice	2.5	2.5	2.5
Butter or enriched margarine (as desired)			
Whole milk, 1 cup	8.5	8.5	8.5
LUNCH			
Meat, poultry, fish, 2 oz. cooked; or cheese	15.2	15.2	15.2
Salad, ½ cup (with dressing)	0.5	0.5	0.5
Cooked vegetable, green or yellow, ½ cup	2.0	2.0	2.0
Bread (white, enriched or whole-wheat), 1 slice	2.5	2.5	2.5
Butter or enriched margarine (as desired)			
Simple dessert,[d] fruit	0.5	0.5	0.5
Whole milk, 1 cup	8.5	8.5	8.5
Plus 2 tbsp. dried non-fat milk solids	–	6.0	6.0
MIDAFTERNOON SNACK			
Whole milk, 1 cup	–	8.5	8.5
Plus 2 tbsp. dried non-fat milk solids	–	–	6.0
Graham crackers, 2	–	–	2.5
DINNER			
Meat, poultry, fish (liver once a week); or cheese:			
4 oz. raw weight; 3 oz. cooked	22.8	22.8	22.8
Cooked vegetable, ½ cup	2.0	2.0	2.0
Potato	2.0	2.0	2.0
Plus 2 tbsp. dried non-fat milk solids	–	6.0	6.0
Bread (white, enriched or whole-wheat), 1 slice	2.5	2.5	2.5
Butter or enriched margarine (as desired)			
Simple dessert,[d] pudding	4.5	4.5	4.5
Plus 2 tbsp. dried non-fat milk solids	–	–	6.0
Whole milk, 1 cup	8.5	8.5	8.5
EVENING SNACK			
Whole milk, 1 cup	8.5	8.5	8.5
Plus 2 tbsp. dried non-fat milk solids	–	–	6.0
Total Gm. Protein	104.7	131.2	151.7

*Source of calculations: Turner, D. F.: Handbook of Diet Therapy, 5th ed. Chicago, University of Chicago Press, 1970. If additional calories are needed to maintain body weight, concentrated foods such as sugar, jelly, sauces and salad dressings may be added.

†To make these meal plans low in sodium, omit all salt in cooking and at the table, omit the cheese, substitute unsalted butter or fortified margarine and replace all or part of the whole milk and dried non-fat milk solids with low sodium milk, available in fresh fluid and canned forms and in powdered whole milk (Lonalac, Mead Johnson) and powdered skim milk (Cellu, Chicago Dietetic Supply House).

[a] 2400 kcal.
[b] 2700 kcal.
[c] 3000 kcal.
[d] Desserts: custards, puddings, plain ice cream, fruit.

the release of mineralocorticoids from the adrenal gland. These cause fluid and sodium retention and potassium excretion.

Protein catabolism during this phase does not take place solely to meet energy requirements. The amino acids mobilized from the skeletal muscles are also used by the liver to synthesize the proteins needed during stress: immunoglobulins, leukocytes and lymphocytes to fight infection, hemoglobin or albumin to replace blood loss, collagen to begin tissue healing and the enzymes necessary to make all of these proteins.

Table 35–4. CATABOLIC RESPONSE TO STRESS

IMMEDIATE RESPONSE	ADAPTIVE RESPONSE
Ventromedial hypothalamic activity ↑	VMH activity ↓
Sympathetic activity ↑	Sympathetic activity more specific
Epinephrine release ↑	Serum glucagon ↑
Serum glucagon ↑	Glucocorticoids normal
Glucocorticoid release ↑	Serum insulin in response to glucose challenge ↓
Serum insulin in response to glucose challenge ↓	Growth hormone normal
Peripheral tissue resistance to insulin	
Growth hormone ↑	
	These changes, after a few days of constant stress, result in:
These nervous and hormonal changes result in:	Serum glucose ↓
Hyperglycemia	Plasma fatty acids ↑
Inability of skeletal muscle to utilize glucose even though hyperglycemia is present	Ketonemia
	Ketonuria
Breakdown of skeletal muscle protein	Less breakdown of skeletal muscle protein
Ileus	Return of appetite
Anorexia	Urinary nitrogen excretion ↓
Urinary nitrogen excretion ↑	Mineralocorticoids normal; diuresis ensues
Mineralocorticoid release ↑, causing fluid and sodium retention and potassium excretion	

The net effect of the catabolic stress response as summarized in Table 35–4 is a hormonal environment that protects and defends the body at the expense of skeletal muscle. It is a beneficial response to stress that includes negative nitrogen balance as a necessary side effect. During this catabolic response, which lasts five to eight days, there is loss of nitrogen, sulfur, phosphorus, potassium, magnesium, zinc and creatine.

If stress continues, the body's sympathetic activity should also continue. If the sympathetic response stops when the body is still under stress, it indicates that the stress is overpowering the body, and this is a bad prognostic sign.

Assuming that the stress continues and that the body can maintain its sympathetic response and overcome the stress, the body will adapt somewhat to prolonged stress and enter an *adaptive catabolic phase* as outlined in Table 35–4. At this point, nutritional support should definitely be started either enterally or parenterally if it has not already begun.

The prominent feature of this stage is that the body uses a smaller amount of skeletal protein for its energy needs and adapts to using fatty acids and ketone bodies for energy, so that the nitrogen balance is not quite as negative. The blood glucose level is lower, and this is the clinical sign that the body has entered the adaptive phase. Serum fatty acid concentrations are higher.

Nutritional intake in this adapted phase is more efficiently utilized because the levels of epinephrine and glucocorticoids do not antagonize the action of insulin. Energy and protein given at this time can be used more efficiently.

Sudden development of hyperglycemia means that the stress has increased, usually owing to infection, and that the patient has again entered a catabolic stress response phase, with increased sympathetic activity and insulin resistance.

As the stress is relieved through treatment or by its own natural course, the sympathetic response decreases and the parasympathetic activity increases. The patient begins to feel hungry, a sign that he is feeling better. Nutritional care should be aimed at putting the patient into anabolism and restoring the tissue protein lost during stress.

Nutritional Care

Since the body does not adapt to its starvation fat economy unless the stress, trauma or infection is alleviated, the primary emphasis of nutritional care should be removal of the stress (draining the abscess, covering the burns, treating the infection, and so on). However, if the stress cannot be removed, nutritional support should be started. If support is not provided and the patient continues to use lean body mass for necessary protein synthesis, the consequences are severe. Eventually protein synthesis declines, and weakness, loss of immunocompetence, hypoalbuminemia, failure of wound healing, further infection, decubitus ulcers from skin breakdown, respiratory insufficiency from respiratory muscle weakness, and eventually multiple organ failure and death result.

The turn to anabolism should be promoted by offering food and nutrients as soon as the patient's blood glucose level begins to fall and gastrointestinal function returns. The patient should not be without nutritional support longer than five days following physiological trauma.[8]

The nutrients should be provided in the correct form and by the most efficient route—enteral or parenteral. During convalescence, the amounts of nutrients should be high in order to promote anabolism. The energy intake should be balanced with the protein intake for the most efficient utilization of protein.

If the goal of nutritional therapy is reached, the patient will achieve positive nitrogen balance. Another way to evaluate the nutritional care is to use the nutritional index as presented in Chapter 19. A daily comparison of the patient's *actual intake* with his *determined requirements* for protein and energy will give an index, either positive or negative, as to whether the nutritional care is meeting his requirements.

ENERGY. The energy requirement should be determined first and depends on the increase in metabolic expenditure caused by the patient's clinical situation. Rutten and coworkers have defined degrees of increased metabolic expenditure as classified in Table 35–5 by measuring the daily urinary urea nitrogen loss.[22] Appearance of 5 to 10 gm. of urea nitrogen in the urine in 24 hours means the energy requirement is 0 to 10 per cent above the basal requirement, while 10 to 15 gm. of urinary urea nitrogen in 24 hours indicates a 20 to 50 per cent increase. Patients with urinary urea nitrogen losses of more than 15 gm. in 24 hours have energy requirements 50 to 75 per cent above the basal need. The increase in energy and protein requirements is directly related to the output of urinary urea nitrogen (N) and the N output of other sites such as draining wounds or burns.

A more accurate method is to use indirect calorimetry to actually measure the basal metabolic rate (BMR) or resting metabolic rate (RMR) and the energy expenditure. Equipment to measure the patient's oxygen consumption and CO_2 production can be taken right to the bedside. From these measurements, energy consumption can be calculated as explained in Chapter 1.

Using several patients with mild to moderate degrees of catabolism, it was determined that calories provided at a level of 54 per cent above basal need, or 1.54 × BEE (basal energy expenditure), would provide enough energy to prevent breakdown of body tissues and promote anabolism and the repair of the body tissues in most patients. Burned or other severely traumatized patients will require more than this. For most patients, provision of calories to equal 1.54 × BEE gives about 40 to 45 kcal. per kg. ideal body weight (IBW), and this amount will put patients into anabolism and rehabilitate them. A level of 1.22 × BEE, or about 30 to 35 kcal. per kg. IBW, will maintain most patients and prevent negative nitrogen balance if they are already rehabilitated.[3] Most surgical patients have a resting energy expenditure of about 20 per cent above their basal expenditure.

PROTEIN. The optimal protein intake for depleted, stressed adults is 16 per cent of total energy. This level, in the presence of 40 to 45 kcal. per kg., promotes positive nitrogen balance and the restoration of lean body mass or of protein reserves.[4, 14a] A few calculations show that if 16 per cent of the total energy intake comes from protein, then the nitrogen to kcalorie ratio is 1 gm.:150 kcal. Therefore, the nitrogen requirement in grams can be determined from the en-

Table 35–5. CLASSIFICATION OF CATABOLISM*†

CLINICAL SITUATION	DEGREE OF CATABOLISM	UREA = N (gm./day)	INCREASE OF RESTING METABOLIC RATE OVER BMR (%)	TOTAL ENERGY REQUIREMENT[a] (kcal.)
Person in bed	1° (Normal)	<5	None	1800
Uncomplicated surgery	2° (Mild)	5–10	0–20	1800–2200
Multiple fractures or trauma	3° (Moderate)	10–15	20–50	2200–2700
Acute major infections or major burns	4° (Severe)	>15	50–125	2700–4000 or more

* Adapted from: Rutten, P., et al.: Determination of optimal hyperalimentation infusion rate. J. Surg. Res., *18*:477, 1975.

† Classification of patients according to the following: (1) obligate nitrogen loss (N obg.) expressed in gm. urea-N per 24 hr.; (2) energy expenditure expressed as per cent increase of the resting metabolic expenditure over calculated basal energy expenditure.

[a] This total resting metabolic requirement includes the amount needed for activity, about 20 per cent, since these patients usually are not active, and 10 per cent for specific dynamic action (SDA). This is a rough estimate for a 70-kg. man and depends on the patient's size.

ergy requirement by dividing the kcal. required by 150. The protein requirement can be determined by dividing the kcal. by 24.

Example: Ms. L's basal energy requirements = 1400 kcal. She has had a long bout with ulcerative colitis, followed by surgery with a resulting ileostomy.

Urinary urea N/24 hr. = 15 gm.

Her energy requirements = 54% over basal = 1400 + 756 = 2156 kcal.

Her protein requirements = 16% of kcal. = 2156 × 0.16 = 345 kcal.

Protein requirements in gm. = 345 kcal. ÷ 4 kcal./gm. protein = 86 gm. protein

Her requirements calculated using the nitrogen:calorie ratio of 1:150 or the N:Protein ratio of 24:

2156 kcal. ÷ 150 kcal./gm. N = 14.37 gm. N
2156 kcal. ÷ 24 kcal./gm. pro = 90 gm. protein
This is very close to the 86 gm. determined by the first method.

14.37 gm. N × 6.25 gm. pro/gm. N = 90 gm. protein, also very close to the 86 gm. determined by the first method.

Initial weight gain when the stressed patient switches from negative to positive nitrogen balance is really a reflection of body water retention. Following the initial gain, weight gain is minimal in spite of the continued positive nitrogen balance, because spontaneous diuresis keeps body water level down. Restoration of lean tissue and fat usually occurs at the rate of 250 gm. or ½ lb. per day with optimal nutritional support. Rates greater than this reflect an undesirable water retention.

VITAMINS AND MINERALS. Vitamins should be given at high levels, and a supplement is probably justified. Mineral intake will depend on the patient's prior nutritional status and mineral losses during stress.

Nutritional Support

ENTERAL FEEDING

The preferable and most palatable method for providing nutrition to meet the increased demands of the catabolic patient and of the patient who has come through a catabolic period is through abundant, nutritious and frequent meals and supplements given orally. Table 35–3 gives the amounts of foods needed to provide protein intakes of 100, 130 and 150 gm. and energy intakes of 2400, 2700 and 3000 kcal.

Nutritional Supplements

When a sufficient quantity of food is not eaten at meals, calorie and protein concentrates can be administered as between-meal drinks. As Table 35–8 shows, some nutritional supplements are adequate in all nutrients and provide complete nutrition, while others do not. Some supplements are concentrated with additional vitamins and minerals provided, while others are just commonly used foods. For example, powdered dried skim milk contains approximately 40 per cent protein of high biological value and provides 1.5 gm. of protein and 15 kcal. per tablespoon. Eight oz. of whole milk provides 160 kcal. and 8 gm. of protein. Although milk is an inexpensive and convenient protein supplement, many patients may not tolerate it because of a lactose intolerance, either primary (many non-Caucasians) or secondary to gastrointestinal disease. Milk is used frequently for liquid feedings because it is one of the few liquid forms of a complete protein. Casein and lactalbumin can be added to dried skim milk powder to increase its protein content at low cost. However, there are many formulas available that are not milk-based or are lactose-free and are suitable as nutritional supplements or for complete nutritional support.

Other forms of concentrated protein that can be used are powdered whole eggs and powdered dried egg albumin. The choice of a nutritional supplement will depend on the cost, availability, use and palatability of the product, staff available to prepare the supplement and the shelf-life of the supplement and on the patient's disease, extent of hypermetabolism and nutritional requirements. The composition and indications for use of available nutritional supplements are given in Table 35–8.

Complete Nutrition Formulas

Liquid feedings that meet all of the nutritional requirements are used in the nutritional care of patients unable to take solid food because of dysphagia, gastrointestinal obstruction or oral surgery. These patients need to have their food dispersed in water. Table 35–6 outlines the situations that may require the use of complete or supplemental liquid feeding. Ideally these feedings are given orally, but usually part or all of the intake must be given enterally by tube.

TUBE FEEDINGS. Because of gastrointestinal surgery, unconsciousness or esophageal obstruction that prevents oral intake, some patients require liquid feeding through a tube. Other patients cannot meet their nutritional requirements through oral intake alone and require additional nourishment through a tube.

The compositions of some commercial formulas that are suitable for tube feedings are given in Table 35–7. Commercial products save time in preparation, are less likely to be contaminated and are of a known composition, but they are not quite as flexible in meeting patient needs as

Table 35–6. SITUATIONS REQUIRING ARTIFICIAL FEEDING TECHNIQUES

PHYSIOLOGICAL PROBLEM	RECOMMENDED FEEDING	CLINICAL SITUATION OR DISORDER

Inability to ingest food	Liquid feedings: whole food or milk-based formula
	Route of administration:
	  Tube
	    nasogastric
	    gastrostomy
	    jejunostomy
	  Oral
		Carcinoma of esophagus or stomach
		Dental or oral surgery
		Inflammatory disease of esophagus
		Coma

Inability to digest food	Predigested or chemically defined diet
	  Amino acids and peptides
	  Glucose and dextrins
	  Minerals and vitamins
	Route of administration:
	  Oral
	  Tube
		Pancreatitis
		Enzyme deficiency
		Biliary tract disease

Decreased ability to absorb food	Chemically defined diet
	  Route of administration:
	    Oral
	    Tube
		Radiation therapy
		Sprue
		Inflammatory bowel disease
		Short bowel syndrome

Inability to absorb food	Peripheral vein nutritional support Total parenteral nutrition	

Inability to handle colonic residue	Chemically defined diet
	  Route of administration:
	    Oral
	    Tube
	Peripheral vein nutritional support
	Total parenteral nutrition
		Inflammatory bowel disease
		Presurgical preparation
		Ileostomy, colostomy
		Draining fistula

Inability to meet nutritional requirements fully with normal foods	Liquid feeding
	  Oral supplement
	  Tube feeding
	Peripheral vein nutritional support
	
	Central vein nutritional supplementation
		Major surgery
		Burns
		Trauma
		Extended fever
		Anorexia of chronic illness
		Anorexia nervosa

tube feedings prepared especially for the individual. These individualized feedings can be prepared by mixing modular components together. These modules are described in Table 35–8.

Feedings may be made from a mixture of the foods served in the adequate normal diet, finely homogenized in a mechanical blender and strained to ensure passage through the tube, or food combinations planned to meet specific therapeutic needs may be used. Formulas made from whole foods have the advantage of including trace minerals and vitamins that are naturally present in whole foods but may not be added to a chemically defined formula diet. Table 35–9 gives a typical formula made from whole foods. The disadvantages of the use of such a formula are the labor time required for its preparation and its thick consistency, which requires a larger feeding tube for its administration.

COMPOSITION. When evaluating a feeding formula it is useful to look at its osmolality, caloric concentration and protein, carbohydrate, fat, vitamin and mineral composition.

Osmolality. Osmolality is a measure of the osmotically active particles per kg. of the solvent in which the particles are dispersed, which in this case is water. Osmolality is expressed as milliosmoles of solute per kg. of solvent or mOsm./kg. *Osmolarity* is expressed as mOsm. per liter of the entire solution. The osmolality of normal body fluids is about 275 to 298 mOsm./kg. Solutions taken into the body that have an osmolality greater than this are hyperosmolar and cause water to be drawn into those areas where the hyperosmolar solutions are. Most tube feedings are hyperosmolar, and they will cause water to be drawn into the gastrointestinal tract if given too rapidly. Administration of the feeding slowly in the beginning

Table 35–7. COMPOSITION OF SELECTED COMMERCIAL FORMULAS

A. BLENDERIZED TUBE FEEDINGS

	COMPLEAT B (Doyle)	COMPLEAT MODIFIED (Doyle)	VITANEED (Organon)
Form	Liquid	Liquid	Liquid
Kcal/ml.	1.07	1.07	1.0
Protein % of calories	16	16	14
Carbohydrate % of calories	48	54	50
Fat % of calories	36	30	36
Protein gm./l.	43	43	35
Carbohydrate gm./l.	128	140	125
Fat gm./l.	43	37	40
Cal.:N	156	156	179
Sodium mEq./l.	56	30	22
Potassium mEq./l.	36	36	32
Osmolality mOsm./kg.	405	300	375
Volume to meet 100% of RDA for vitamins and minerals (ml.)	1500	1500	2000
Protein source	Beef, purée, non-fat dry milk	Beef, casein	Beef, sodium and calcium caseinate
Carbohydrate source	Hydrolyzed cereal solids, puréed foods, maltodextrin, non-fat dry milk	Hydrolyzed cereal solids, puréed vegetables	Maltodextrin, puréed fruits and vegetables
Fat source	Corn oil	Corn oil	Soy oil

B. WHOLE PROTEIN FORMULAS—LACTOSE-FREE

	ENSURE (Ross)	ISOCAL (Mead-Johnson)	NUTRI-AID (McGaw)	OSMOLITE (Ross)	PORTAGEN (Mead-Johnson)
Form	Liquid[a]	Liquid	Liquid	Liquid	Powder
kcal./ml.	1.06	1.06	1.06	1.06	1
Protein % of calories	14	13	15	14	14
Carbohydrate % of calories	55	50	53	55	45
Fat % of calories	31	37	32	31	41
Protein gm./l.	37	34	39	37	35
Carbohydrate gm./l.	148	132	142	148	117
Fat gm./l.	37	44	37	38	48
Cal.:N	179	195	169	179	179
Sodium mEq./l.	37	23	31	24	21
Potassium mEq./l.	40	34	31	26	33
Osmolality mOsm./kg.	450	300	350	300	158
Volume to meet 100% of RDA for vitamins and minerals (ml.)	1887	1887	1887	1887	1920[b]
Protein source	Sodium and calcium caseinate, soy protein isolate	Sodium and calcium caseinate, soy protein isolate	Sodium and potassium caseinate	Sodium and calcium caseinate, soy protein isolate	Sodium caseinate
Carbohydrate source	Hydrolyzed corn starch, sucrose	Maltodextrin	Corn syrup solids, sucrose	Hydrolyzed corn starch	Corn syrup solids, sucrose
Fat source	Corn oil	MCT, soy oil	Corn oil	MCT, corn oil, soy oil	MCT, corn oil

[a] Vanilla flavored.
[b] Except for folic acid and biotin.

Table continued on the following page

Table 35–7.   COMPOSITION OF SELECTED COMMERCIAL FORMULAS (*Continued*)
B. WHOLE PROTEIN FORMULAS—LACTOSE-FREE

	RENU (Organon)	SUSTACAL (Mead-Johnson)	TRAVASORB WHOLE PROTEIN LIQUID (Travenol)	TRAVASORB MCT (Travenol)
Form	Liquid	Liquid	Liquid	Powder
Kcal./ml.	1	1	1.06	1
Protein % of calories	14	24	14	20
Carbohydrate % of calories	50	55	55	50
Fat % of calories	36	21	31	30
Protein gm./l.	35	61	37	49
Carbohydrate gm./l.	125	140	144	123
Fat gm./l.	40	23	37	33
Cal.:N	179	103	179	128
Sodium mEq./l.	22	40	32	15
Potassium mEq./l.	32	53	33	47
Osmolality mOsm./kg.	300	625[c]	488	312
Volume to meet 100% of RDA for vitamins and minerals (ml.)	2000	1065	1887	2000
Protein source	Sodium and calcium caseinate	Sodium and calcium caseinate, soy protein isolate	Sodium and calcium caseinate, soy protein isolate	Lactalbumin, potassium caseinate
Carbohydrate source	Maltodextrin sucrose	Corn syrup, sucrose	Corn syrup solids, sucrose	Corn syrup solids
Fat source	Soy oil, soy lecithin, mono- and diglycerides	Soy oil	Corn oil, soy oil	MCT, sunflower oil

[c]Vanilla and eggnog flavor.

C. WHOLE PROTEIN FORMULAS—MILK-BASED

	MERITENE (Doyle)	SUSTACAL (Mead-Johnson)	SUSTAGEN (Mead-Johnson)
Form	Liquid	Powder[d]	Powder
Kcal./ml.	0.96	1.35	1.7
Protein % of calories	24	24	24
Carbohydrate % of calories	46	54	68
Fat % of calories	30	22	8
Protein gm./l.	58	82	113
Carbohydrate gm./l.	110	182	317
Fat gm./l.	32	33	17
Cal.:N	104	103	94
Sodium mEq./l.	38	53.8	55
Potassium mEq./l.	41	86	87
Osmolality mOsm./kg.	505	899	1100
Volume to meet 100% of RDA for vitamins and minerals (ml.)	1250	800	946
Protein source	Skim milk, sodium caseinate	Non-fat dry milk	Non-fat milk, powdered whole milk, sodium caseinate
Carbohydrate source	Corn syrup solids, sucrose	Corn syrup solids, sucrose	Corn syrup solids
Fat source	Corn oil	Milk fat (added with whole milk)	Milk fat

[d] With added whole milk, vanilla flavored.

Table 35–7.   COMPOSITION OF SELECTED COMMERCIAL FORMULAS (*Continued*)

D. WHOLE PROTEIN FORMULAS—HIGH-CALORIE LACTOSE-FREE

	ENSURE PLUS (*Ross*)	ISOCAL HCN (*Mead-Johnson*)	MAGNACAL (*Organon*)	SUSTACAL HC (*Mead-Johnson*)
Form	Liquid[a]	Liquid	Liquid	Liquid
Kcal./ml.	1.5	2	2	1.5
Protein % of calories	15	15	14	16
Carbohydrate % of calories	53	45	50	50
Fat % of calories	32	40	36	34
Protein gm./l.	55	75	70	61
Carbohydrate gm./l.	196	225	250	190
Fat gm./l.	53	91	80	58
Cal.:N	170	167	179	154
Sodium mEq./l.	50	35	44	36
Potassium mEq./l.	60	36	32	38
Osmolality mOsm./kg.	600	690	590	650
Volume to meet 100% of RDA for vitamins and minerals (ml.)	1600	1500	1000	1183
Protein source	Sodium and calcium caseinate, soy protein isolate	Sodium and calcium caseinate	Sodium and calcium caseinate	Sodium and calcium caseinate
Carbohydrate source	Hydrolyzed corn starch, sucrose	Corn syrup	Maltodextrin, sucrose	Corn syrup solids, sucrose
Fat source	Corn oil	MCT, soybean oil	Soy oil, soy lecithin, mono- and diglycerides	Soybean oil

[a] Vanilla flavored.

E. DEFINED FORMULA DIETS

	CRITICARE HN (*Mead-Johnson*)	ISOTEIN HN (*Doyle*)	PRECISION ISOTONIC (*Doyle*)	PRECISION HIGH NITROGEN (*Doyle*)	PRECISION LR (*Doyle*)
Form	Liquid	Powder	Powder	Powder	Powder
Kcal./ml.	1.06	1.2	1.0	1.05	1.1
Protein % of calories	14	23	12	17	10
Carbohydrate % of calories	83	52	60	82	89
Fat % of calories	3	25	28	1	1
Protein gm./l.	38	68	30	44	26
Carbohydrate gm./l.	222	156	150	216	246
Fat gm./l.	30	34	31	1.3	1.6
Cal.:N	174	110	208	149	264
Sodium mEq./l.	27	30	35	43	30
Potassium mEq./l.	34	22	26	23	23
Osmolality mOsm./kg.	650	300	300	525[e]	510[f]
Volume to meet 100% of RDA for vitamins and minerals (ml.)	1892	1770	1500	2857	1727
Protein source	Hydrolyzed casein	Lactalbumin, sodium caseinate	Egg white solids, sodium caseinate	Egg white solids	Egg white solids
Carbohydrate source	Maltodextrin, corn starch	Maltodextrin, fructose	Maltodextrin, sucrose	Maltodextrin, sucrose	Maltodextrin, sucrose
Fat source	Safflower oil	Soybean oil, MCT	Soybean oil	Soybean oil, MCT	Soybean oil, MCT

[e] Citrus fruit flavored.
[f] Orange flavored.

Table continued on the following page

Table 35–7.　COMPOSITION OF SELECTED COMMERCIAL FORMULAS (*Continued*)

E. DEFINED FORMULA DIETS

	TRAVASORB STD. (*Travenol*)	TRAVASORB HN (*Travenol*)	VITAL HN (*Ross*)	VIVONEX STD. (*Norwich-Eaton*)	VIVONEX HIGH NITROGEN (*Norwich-Eaton*)
Form	Powder	Powder	Powder	Powder	Powder
Kcal./ml. (mixed per directions)	1.0	1.0	1.0	1.0	1.0
Protein % of calories	12	18	17	8.2	18
Carbohydrate % of calories	76	70	74	90.5	81
Fat % of calories	12	12	9	1.3	1
Protein gm./l.	30	45	42	21	46
Carbohydrate gm./l.	190	175	188	231	210
Fat gm./l.	13.4	13.4	10.8	1.5	0.87
Cal.:N	208	139	150	298	136
Sodium mEq./l.	40	40	17	20	23
Potassium mEq./l.	30	30	30	30	30
Osmolality mOsm./kg.	560[g]	560	460	550	810
Volume to meet 100% of RDA for vitamins and minerals (ml.)	2000	2000	1500	1800	3000
Protein source	Hydrolyzed lactalbumin	Hydrolyzed lactalbumin	Hydrolyzed whey, meat and soy protein, free amino acids	Free L-amino acids	Free L-amino acids
Carbohydrate source	Glucose oligosaccharides	Glucose oligosaccharides	Hydrolyzed cornstarch, sucrose	Glucose oligosaccharides	Glucose oligosaccharides
Fat source	MCT, sunflower oil	MCT, sunflower oil	MCT, safflower oil	Safflower oil	Safflower oil

[g] Unflavored.

F. SPECIALLY DEFINED FORMULA DIETS

	AMIN-AID (*McGaw*)	HEPATIC-AID (*McGaw*)	TRAUM-AID HN (*McGaw*)	TRAVASORB HEPATIC (*Travenol*)	TRAVASORB RENAL (*Travenol*)
Form	Powder	Powder	Powder	Powder	Powder
Kcal./ml. (mixed per directions)	1.96	1.6	1.0	1.1	1.35
Protein % of calories	4	10	17	11	7
Carbohydrate % of calories	75	70	72	77	81
Fat % of calories	21	20	11	12	12
Protein gm./l.	19.3	42.6	43.4	29	23
Carbohydrate gm./l.	373	290.6	180	209	271
Fat gm./l.	47	36	12	14	18
Cal.:N	635	235	145	237	367
Sodium mEq./l.	15	15	23	19	Electrolyte-free
Potassium mEq./l.	6	6	21	29	Electrolyte-free
Osmolality mOsm./kg.	1095	1158	800	690	590
Volume to meet 100% of RDA for vitamins and minerals (ml.)	Incomplete	Incomplete	3000	2100	Incomplete
Protein source	Crystalline amino acids	Crystalline amino acids	Amino acids	Crystalline L-amino acids	Crystalline L-amino acids
Composition of protein source	Essential amino acids plus histidine	High in branched chain amino acids and arginine, low in aromatic amino acids and methionine	High in branched chain amino acids	High in branched chain amino acids	Essential amino acids plus histidine, arginine and non-essential amino acids
Carbohydrate source	Maltodextrin, sucrose	Maltodextrin, sucrose	Maltodextrin, sucrose	Glucose, oligosaccharides, sucrose	Glucose, oligosaccharides, sucrose
Fat source	Soybean oil, lecithin, mono- and diglycerides	Soybean oil, lecithin, mono- and diglycerides	Soybean oil, MCT, lecithin, mono- and diglycerides	MCT, sunflower oil	MCT, sunflower oil
Use	Renal failure	Liver disease	Catabolic state	Liver disease	Renal failure

Table 35–8. MODULAR COMPONENTS FOR ENTERAL FEEDING

PROTEIN

	CASEC (Mead-Johnson)	GEVRAL (Lederle)	PRO-MIX (Nubro)	PROPAC (Organon)
Form	Powder	Powder	Powder	Powder
Kcal./100 gm.	370	367	360	400
Protein % of calories	95	66	90	77
Carbohydrate % of calories	—	29	10	5
Fat % of calories	5	5	—	0.18
Protein gm./100 gm.	88	60	80	77
Carbohydrate gm./100 gm.		27	8	5
Fat gm./100 gm.	2	2	—	8.2
Cal.:N				
Sodium mEq./100 gm.	6.52	1.5	7	10
Potassium mEq./100 gm.	N.A.	1.3	41	13
Osmolality mOsm./kg.		VARIES WITH DILUTION		
Added vitamins and minerals	No	Yes	No	No
Protein source	Calcium caseinate from skim milk	Calcium caseinate	Whey protein	Whey protein
Carbohydrate source	—	Sucrose	—	Lactose
Fat source	—	—	—	Lecithin

CARBOHYDRATE

	CAL PLUS (Henkel)	MODUCAL (Mead-Johnson)	POLYCOSE (Ross)	SUMACAL (Organon)
Form	Powder	Powder	Powder	Powder
Kcal./100 gm.	400	380	380	380
Protein % of calories	—	—	—	—
Carbohydrate % of calories	90	95	94	95
Fat % of calories	—	—	—	—
Protein gm./100 gm.	—	—	—	—
Carbohydrate gm./100 gm.	90	95	94	95
Fat gm./100 gm.	—	—	—	—
Cal.:N	—	—	—	—
Sodium mEq./100 gm.	5	3	5	4.3
Potassium mEq./100 gm.	<0.2	0.13	1	≤1
Osmolality mOsm./kg.		VARIES WITH DILUTION		
Added vitaimins and minerals	No	No	No	No
Protein source	—	—	—	—
Carbohydrate source	Glucose polymers of hydrolyzed starch	Maltodextrin (hydrolyzed cornstarch)	Glucose polymers from hydrolyzed cornstarch	Maltodextrin (hydrolyzed cornstarch)
Fat source	—	—	—	—

CARBOHYDRATE

	HYCAL (Beecham)	MODUCAL (Mead-Johnson)	POLYCOSE (Ross)	KARO SYRUP (Best Foods)
Form	Liquid	Liquid	Liquid	Liquid
Kcal./ml.	2.5	2	2	4
Protein % of calories	—	—	—	—
Carbohydrate % of calories	100	100	100	100
Fat % of calories	—	—	—	—
Protein gm./100 ml.	—	—	—	—
Carbohydrate gm./100 ml.	60	50	50	104
Fat gm./100 ml.	—	—	—	—
Kcal:N	—	—	—	—
Sodium mEq./100 ml.	.71	1.5	2.5	6.9
Potassium mEq./100 ml.	<.02	0.06	0.05	0.14
Osmolality mOsm./kg.	2780	725	850	
Added vitamins and minerals	No	No	No	No
Protein source	—	—	—	—
Carbohydrate source	Dextrose	Maltodextrin (hydrolyzed cornstarch)	Glucose polymers from hydrolyzed cornstarch	Corn syrup
Fat source	—	—	—	—

Table continued on the following page

Table 35–8. MODULAR COMPONENTS FOR ENTERAL FEEDING (*Continued*)

FAT

	MCT (*Mead-Johnson*)	MICROLIPID (*Organon*)	VEGETABLE OIL[a]	LIPOMUL (*Upjohn*)
	Liquid	Liquid	Liquid	Liquid
Kcal./ml.	7.6	4.5	8.0	8.0
Protein % of calories	—	—	—	—
Carbohydrate % of calories	—	—	—	—
Fat % of calories	100	100	100	100
Protein gm./100 ml.	—	—	—	—
Carbohydrate gm./100 ml.	—	—	—	—
Fat gm./100 ml.	—	—	—	—
Cal:N	—	—	—	—
Sodium mEq./l.	—		—	—
Potassium mEq./l.	—	—	—	—
Osmolality mOsm./kg.	—	80	—	—
Added vitamins and minerals	No	No	No	No
Protein source	—	—	—	—
Carbohydrate source	—	—	—	—
Fat source	MCT from coconut oil	50% fat emulsion derived from safflower oil	Hydrogenated soybean oil, polyglycerides	Corn Oil

[a] Wesson brand

MIXED

	CITROTEIN (*Doyle*)	CONTROLYTE (*Doyle*)	CARNATION INSTANT BREAKFAST (*Carnation*)	NON-FAT DRY MILK	LONALAC (*Mead-Johnson*)
Form	Powder	Powder	Powder	Powder	Powder
Kcal./100 gm.	369	504	464	360	500
Protein % of calories	25	—	21	40	21
Carbohydrate % of calories	73	57	78	58	30
Fat % of calories	2	43	1	2	49
Protein gm./100 gm.	23	0.04	25	36	27
Carbohydrate gm./100 gm.	68	72	82	52	38
Fat gm./100 gm.	0.9	24	3.6	0.9	28
Cal:N					
Sodium mEq./100 gm.	<0.01	0.2	20[b]	23	0.86
Potassium mEq./100 gm.	<0.01	0.1		46	0.24
Osmolality mOsm./kg.	495[c]	598			
Added vitamins and minerals	Yes	No	Yes	No	Yes
Protein source	Egg white solids		Non-fat dry milk, calcium and sodium caseinate soy protein, egg yolk[d]	Non-fat dry milk	Casein
Carbohydrate source	Sucrose, maltodextrin	Polysaccharides from corn starch hydrolysate	Sucrose, lactose	Lactose	Lactose
Fat source	Soybean oil, mono- and diglycerides	Soybean oil	Corn syrup		Coconut oil

[b] Orange flavor.

[c] Chocolate flavor.

[d] Individual flavors vary.

Table 35-9. STANDARD BLENDED TUBE FEEDING USING WHOLE FOODS

(1 Liter)

FOOD	AMOUNT
Strained meat	1 jar (100 gm.) Select a variety.
Egg[a]	1 (50 gm. frozen egg or 30 gm. powdered egg)
Applesauce	2/3 cup (200 gm.)
Strained mixed vegetable	1 jar (200 gm.)
Instant mashed potato	2 tbsp. (50 gm.)
Powdered skim milk	1 cup (60 gm.)
Vegetable oil	1 tbsp. (15 gm.)
Orange juice (or vitamin C supplement)	1/2 cup (100 gm.)
Water	1 1/2 cups (400 cc.)

INGREDIENT	AMOUNT (gm.)	KCAL.	PRO. (gm.)	FAT (gm.)	CHO (gm.)	VIT. A (I.U.)	VIT. C (mg.)	NIACIN (mg.)	RIBO-FLAVIN (µg)	THIA-MIN (mg.)	CA (mg.)	P (mg.)	FE (mg.)	NA[b] (mg.)	K[b] (mg.)
Strained meat	100	97	14.5	4.3	–	–	4	3.7	151	0.01	8	81	1.6	192	234
Egg	50	78	6.0	5.5	–	570	–	–	140	0.05	26	50	1.1	59	62
Applesauce	200	182	0.4	0.2	48	80	2	–	20	0.04	8	10	1.5	4	130
Strained vegetable	200	82	2.8	0.2	17	7134	3	1.0	54	0.08	30	56	1.6	504	244
Instant mashed potato	50	182	3.6	0.3	42	–	32	5.4	30	0.11	17	86	0.8	40	800
Powdered skim milk	60	215	21.4	0.4	31	18	4	0.5	1060	0.2	777	603	0.4	315	1034
Vegetable oil	15	126	–	14.0	–	–	–	–	–	–	–	–	–	–	–
Orange juice	100	45	0.7	0.1	11	200	45	0.3	10	0.9	9	16	0.1	1	186
Total		1007	49.4	25.0	149	8002	90	10.9	1465	1.39	875	902	7.1	1115	2690

From Manual of Clinical Dietetics. Researched and Approved by Chicago Dietetic Association and South Suburban Dietetic Association of Chicago. 2nd ed. Philadelphia, W. B. Saunders Company, 1981.

[a]The use of fresh raw eggs should be discouraged because of salmonella hazard. Use cooked egg custard (1/2 cup), salmonella-free frozen or powdered eggs or canned baby egg yolks.

[b]Various degrees of sodium restriction are achieved by using low-sodium vegetables, meat and milk. Potassium restriction is achieved by reducing or omitting the orange juice and mashed potato.

with gradual increases in the amount will usually allow tolerance in most patients. Diluting the formula initially with gradual concentration to the normal concentration will also enhance tolerance. See Table 35–7 for the osmolality of feeding formulas.

Calories. Feedings usually provide 1 kcal./ml. when mixed full strength according to directions. Some high calorie formulas contain up to 2 kcal./ml. These calorically dense formulas are useful for patients with increased energy requirements who also have fluid restrictions or decreased ability to handle large volumes of liquid. However, they may not provide enough water, so the patient's hydration must be monitored. Other formulas have a lower concentration of calories. See Tables 35–7 and 35–8 for the energy content of formulas.

Protein. The protein content of formulas varies from 4 to 24 per cent of the calories. Stated another way, the Calorie:nitrogen ratio or the number of kcalories provided per gram of nitrogen can range from 100 to 300 kcal, or more per gram of nitrogen. Protein may be provided by a complete protein or may be partially hydrolyzed into peptide fragments or into the individual amino acids for easier digestion. The protein source can be casein (milk protein), puréed beef, egg albumin, skim milk powder, soy protein, hydrolyzed casein, hydrolyzed soy or amino acids. Formulas that contain the whole protein are much more palatable than those containing hydrolyzed protein or amino acids, and they are also cheaper. Many formulas are milk-based and have casein as the primary protein source because it is complete and easily digested and will make a solution of low viscosity. The hydrolyzed form of casein is a good source of peptides for a patient with protein maldigestion or malabsorption who needs a somewhat digested form of protein. The protein in formulas is also being modified to better meet the needs of patients with particular problems. For example, because of knowledge about changes in amino acid metabolism during trauma, formulas designed for these patients are higher in branched chain amino acids. See Table 35–7 for the listing of specially defined formulas.

Fat. The fat in most commercial formulas is corn, soy or safflower oil, and the amount may range from 1 to 43 per cent of the calories. A few products contain medium chain triglycerides (MCT) and thus are easier to absorb, and these should be used in cases of fat malabsorption. Alternatively, a fat-free formula can be used, with small amounts of fat (10 gm. per liter) added each day in order to increase the fat intake gradually. When limiting the fat in enteral feeding it is important to remain aware of essential fatty acid requirements (1 to 2 per cent of total energy intake) and to provide for these. Fat added to a feeding is important because it increases the calories yet does not increase the osmolality of the formula. It also gives the patient a feeling of satiety.

Carbohydrate. The many possible sources of carbohydrate in a liquid feeding range from puréed fruits and vegetables to corn syrup solids, maltodextrin, glucose, fructose, sucrose and lactose. The carbohydrate source greatly affects the palatability of the formula, and the amount of carbohydrate affects its osmolality. See Table 35–7 for the carbohydrate sources of common formulas.

Because many patients requiring liquid enteral feeding are lactase deficient because of disease or stress, many formulas eliminate lactose as a carbohydrate source.

Vitamins and Minerals. Most commercially available liquid diets are fortified with vitamins and minerals to meet the Recommended Dietary Allowances when a certain volume is taken, as Table 35–7 indicates. However, the allowances are designed for healthy people and are only guidelines to the vitamin and mineral needs of the ill person. Home-prepared or institutionally prepared formulas should have vitamins and minerals added, since some of these formulas may not be adequate depending on the choice of foods used in the feeding. The use of a multivitamin and mineral supplement is advised.

Additional vitamins would have to be added in cases of vitamin deficiency or excessively high requirements. For some patients, electrolytes may also need to be added to replace losses.

DEFINED FORMULA DIETS. These formulas are designed for easy digestion and absorption, and they leave minimal residue in the bowel. Stool passage is markedly reduced or stopped with the use of these formulas. These diets do contain known quantities of purified substances, but the substances are not truly elements, and the name "elemental diet," although widely used, is erroneous. It is true, however, that the protein and carbohydrate used in these diets are in simpler forms than those found in normal diets and in tube feedings formulated from whole foods. The carbohydrate is present in the form of glucose or dextrins (disaccharides and oligosaccharides). The protein in the form of amino acids or peptides, both of which have been found to be equally well absorbed.[17] There is very little fat, or else it is present in the form of MCT or is partially digested into mono- or diglycerides. (See Table 35-7C.) Because nutrients are present in simple forms, little digestion is required, and these formulas are especially suited for cases of steatorrhea and malabsorption caused by disease, short bowel syndrome, radiation therapy or antibiotic damage to the intestinal tract. Patients with as little as 100 cm. of remaining jejunum can be maintained with defined formulas because the nutrients are so easily absorbed. These formulas can also be made using modular components as listed in Table 35–8. All of the products are supplemented with vitamins and minerals to meet the RDA.

These products can be taken orally, although they are better tolerated when given through a tube. Because they are not viscous they can be given through a small-bore feeding tube, which makes feeding more comfortable for the patient. They are somewhat unpalatable when taken by mouth because of the peptides and amino acids. However, if they are to be taken orally, they should be offered to the patient well chilled, "on the rocks," masked with flavor supplements, and with a positive attitude.

High-nitrogen defined formula diets that contain more protein are available for severely traumatized, burned or very depleted patients who require a higher percentage of calories from protein. These have Calorie:nitrogen ratios of 100 to 150. See Table 35–10. for factors to consider when choosing a feeding formula.

ADMINISTRATION. The method and route of administration of a tube feeding as well as the condition of the patient will determine the type of formula to be used and how it will be tolerated by the patient. The route may be by nasogastric, esophagostomy, gastrostomy or jejunostomy tube. A smaller tube (number 8 French) is more comfortable for a nasopharyngeal feeding and many formulas will pass through this size tube especially if a pump is also used. A larger tube (number 16) would be required for administration of a blenderized tube feeding. However, the larger the feeding tube the greater the discomfort for the patient, and this should be a factor in considering the choice of formula and route of administration.

Continuous drip or pump administration of the feeding is probably the most common method of administration. If bolus feeding is used,

Table 35–10. FACTORS TO CONSIDER WHEN SELECTING A FEEDING FORMULA

Form of protein, fat and carbohydrate in the formula as related to patient's absorptive capacity (e.g., peptides vs. whole protein).

Type of carbohydrate (e.g., lactose) used.

Sodium and potassium content, particularly when contemplating use for patients with compromised hepatic, renal or cardiac function.

Recommended uses of the formula.

Caloric and protein density (i.e., kcal./ml., gm. protein/ml. and Cal:N ratio) when contemplating use for a debilitated patient.

---

200 to 350 ml. should be given in not less than 10 to 15 minutes, and this should be mixed with or followed by one half that amount of water. The additional water after feeding is important to prevent hypertonic dehydration from solute overload. The water is also used for careful rinsing of the tube, since the protein in the feeding tends to coagulate when it comes in contact with gastric HCl.

In the first few days, the feeding should be diluted to at least half strength, and not more than 40 to 60 ml. per hour should be given. This enables the patient to develop tolerance gradually to the osmolality of the formula. Many formulas are isoosmolar, but some are hyperosmolar (greater than 350 mOsm./kg.). This gradual administration is especially important with defined formula diets, which have osmolalities of 500 mOsm./kg. or more per kg. when the formula is taken at full strength. In these cases, it is wise to dilute the formula even further and start with one-quarter strength and then gradually increase to full strength and the required volume within four to five days. The gastrointestinal tract can adapt to accommodate a hyperosmolar formula when the formula is given in a way that increases the osmolality slowly. Initially, cramping and diarrhea may occur as the hyperosmolar formula draws water into the intestinal tract. Debilitated patients, those with gastrointestinal disorders, those being fed by gastrostomy and jejunostomy tubes and those whose gastrointestinal tracts have been without food for a long period of time are more likely to be intolerant of the hyperosmolar formula and to require special attention. *Remember: when a patient is not taking a formula full strength or is not taking the recommended amount, neither his energy needs nor his needs for vitamins and minerals are being met, and a supplement will be necessary.* Review Table 35–7 for the amount of formula needed to provide the RDA for vitamins and minerals.

The nurse should record the *actual* formula intake of the patient, any incidents of vomiting or diarrhea and any signs of hypertonic dehydration or inadequate feeding. Assessment of hydration is particularly important in comatose, weak, very ill or frightened patients who are unable to communicate their feelings of thirst. Patients with tracheostomies who are unable to express their thirst are typical of those who may become dehydrated from a tube feeding. Renal or cardiovascular disease that causes malfunction of a patient's water elimination and retention mechanism is also likely to cause dehydration. The amount of water given to a tube-fed patient should be increased if insensible water loss is great owing to fever, perspiration or fistula drainage or if the formula is high in protein or electrolytes. Hypernatremia, dehydration and azotemia have been reported in tube-fed patients. See Table 35–11 for a list of factors that should be monitored routinely for the tube-fed patient.

The feeding should be administered to the patient only when he is standing, sitting or lying in bed on his back with his head and thorax elevated at least 30 degrees from the horizontal. He should be in these positions during feeding and for at least one hour after feeding. This prevents possible aspiration of the formula into the lungs. The tube should be properly positioned in the stomach and not in the duodenum or jejunum, unless it is supposed to be there. The patient's stomach contents should be suctioned out before a new feeding is administered to make sure that there is only minimal residue from the previous feeding. Excessive residue may indicate an obstruction or digestive problem that should be resolved before the feeding is continued.

Diarrhea and cramping may be reduced by giving the tube feeding after it has reached room temperature or by warming it in hot water. Unused formula should be kept refrigerated and should not be used after 24 hours. If diarrhea continues even after dilution of the formula, it may be due to a lactose intolerance, either transitory or permanent, and a lactose-free formula listed in Table 35–7 should be tried. The addition of applesauce or pectin or the use of Probana, all good sources of pectin, may help to bring the diarrhea under control. Kaopectate or Lomotil (antidiarrheal agents) can be added to the feeding just before administration. After the patient has become stabilized on the tube feeding, constipation may develop because of the low fiber content of the formula and the large amounts of milk used. Methylcellulose and other forms of fiber can be added to the formula. However, these supplements increase the viscosity of the tube feeding, so that it may not go through the tube. If the constipation is still not resolved, stool softeners or cathartics may then be necessary.

Table 35–11. FACTORS TO MONITOR IN ROUTINE MANAGEMENT OF TUBE-FED PATIENTS

Weight (at least three times per week)
Signs of edema
Signs of dehydration
Fluid intake and output records
Records of calorie, protein, fat, carbohydrate, mineral and vitamin intakes
Blood urea nitrogen (BUN) level
Urine glucose concentration
Serum glucose concentration
Serum electrolyte concentrations

The goal of tube feeding is to put the patient into positive nitrogen balance or at least into nitrogen balance. If this is not achieved, a common reason is that the patient is not getting *enough* support either through lack of knowledge on the part of the medical staff or because the patient is not getting all of the nutritional support ordered. This may be due to intolerance or resistance on the part of the patient or inattention on the part of the hospital staff. Daily use of the nutritional index as discussed in Chapter 19, particularly for protein and energy, is also a valuable guide.

Patients who are being tube-fed need a great deal of encouragement to help them adjust to the situation. When administering the nourishment, the nurse can be of great assistance in establishing pleasant associations with the feedings.

PARENTERAL FEEDING

Maintenance of fluid balance and prophylaxis against nutritional depletion should be started during the first 24 hours after major surgery, trauma, burns or infection. Kidney function and excessive or abnormal loss of fluid or electrolytes should be monitored and intake adjusted accordingly. Sodium and water have a tendency to be retained following surgery or trauma, and excessive sodium chloride should be avoided during the first 48 hours. There is also an increase in potassium and nitrogen excretion in the urine in the first 24 to 48 hours, and if the patient is unable to take fluid orally in 24 hours, potassium should be added to the basic intravenous fluid.

Peripheral Parenteral Nutrition (PPN)

The usual regimen of fluid therapy is administration of a 5 per cent glucose solution intravenously, which gives the patient 50 gm. of glucose per liter, or about 100 to 150 gm. of glucose per day, or 400 to 600 kcal. This clinical practice is based on Gamble's observation that he could reduce ketosis and conserve water and salt in starving men by providing 100 gm. of carbohydrate daily.[10] This is true; however, it was also assumed that ketosis, known to be harmful to the diabetic patient, is also detrimental to the normal human being, which is not necessarily so. It is now known that, besides preventing ketosis and some protein breakdown, the administration of glucose during fasting prevents the body from adapting to conserve its body protein. As was mentioned in the discussion of starvation, the adaptation of the body that allows fat mobilization and decreased use of body protein for energy is dependent upon a drop in the level of serum insulin. A constant infusion of glucose as D_5W (5 per cent dextrose in water) stimulates the pancreas to release insulin, and the body is never allowed to adapt to starvation with a protective ketosis. The long-term effects of ketosis are unknown. The normal body has a feedback mechanism that stimulates the release of insulin and prevents ketonemia from becoming excessive.

Several researchers have shown that nitrogen balance improves even more when amino acids are given (either alone or in combination with glucose or fat) than when 5 per cent glucose is given by itself.[6, 12, 14] Second, it seems that the protein loss during stress is even less if the patient is given amino acids alone, without glucose or fat. Blackburn and others have been able to maintain nitrogen balance in patients by providing 30 to 60 gm. of amino acids daily via a peripheral vein.[5, 11, 14]

Amino acids instead of glucose can be given intravenously in a peripheral vein when it is known that the patient will be unable to eat for a few days during the catabolic phase. In these first few days, when the patient is hyper-catabolic, the amino acids will be converted to glucose and used for energy, and they seem to help spare body protein. The amino acids, usually given at about 1 to 1.5 gm. per kg. ideal body weight (IBW), maintain visceral protein mass (organ and serum proteins). The precise mechanism by which this occurs is still unclear. Researchers postulate that a hypoinsulinemia develops that allows endogenous fat mobilization. The insulin level would be high enough to allow the utilization of protein but not high enough to inhibit lipolysis. Dispensable fat stores, rather than expensive protein and lean body mass, are used for energy. However, this therapy is controversial and critics state that, for the patient who cannot eat for two to three days, the amount of protein saved by administration of amino acids (about 1 lb. or 0.5 kg.), is not worth the expense of giving the amino acids.

These solutions may be prepared as 500 ml. of 3 to 8.5 per cent amino acids added to 500 ml. of sterile water, normal saline or 5 or 10 per cent dextrose. Electrolytes and vitamins should also be added.

For the routine postoperative "clean" surgical patient, who will only be unable to eat for two to three days, 5 per cent glucose given intravenously is still the preferred therapy. However, for the patient who must be without oral intake longer than this and who has adequate fat stores, intravenous administration of isotonic amino acids might be considered. This procedure avoids the risk associated with insertion of the TPN catheter into the superior vena cava.

This form of parenteral nutrition is not a long-term therapy for the debilitated patient who has no fat stores. Patients who are unable to eat for more than five days require more aggressive parenteral alimentation.

More aggressive PPN would also include fat as a 10 per cent fat emulsion as well as glucose and amino acids. This would increase the caloric concentration over that of just 3 to 8.5 per cent amino acids or 5 per cent glucose but would not increase the osmolality. This type of nutritional support is useful to supplement enteral intake or in an interim period when the patient is changing from TPN to enteral intake or oral intake. The use of fat emulsion–amino acids–glucose in PPN can also lead to positive nitrogen balance and weight gain.

Total Parenteral Nutrition (TPN)

This method of feeding has also been called *intravenous hyperalimentation* because energy in excess of the normal requirements can be provided by it. For many patients, however, it is not hyperalimentation but merely normal alimentation—the maintenance of nutritional status or achievement of ideal body weight after being underweight. By providing all nutrients intravenously, positive nitrogen balance can be attained and sustained for a prolonged period of time without the use of the gastrointestinal tract.

INDICATIONS FOR USE. This method of feeding is used for individuals who are debilitated and malnourished, with a weight loss of 10 per cent of body weight or more, and who are unable to obtain adequate nutrition enterally or by peripheral intravenous feedings. A functioning gastrointestinal tract is always used in preference to intravenous nutrition if the patient can obtain an adequate intake by this route.

Patients with short bowel syndrome, bowel obstruction, inflammatory bowel disease or hypermetabolic states in which the gastrointestinal tract is completely or partially unusable, benefit from this form of nutritional support. It is useful for patients with cancer who are malnourished but who still have a chance of responding to oncological treatment if they can be nutritionally rehabilitated. TPN may meet the needs of burned patients who have great energy and protein needs but unusable gastrointestinal tracts because of multiple surgeries. It is also useful in the treatment of neonatal abnormalities (as discussed in Chapter 37), extreme cachexia, anorexia, pulmonary diseases in which aspiration of food is a danger and in acute hepatic and renal failure, when the composition of the amino acid intake must be manipulated. (See Chapters 24 and 30.) Table 35–6 summarizes those situations in which TPN is appropriate. Unlike the usual parenteral administration of glucose, which at most provides 600 kcal. per day, total parenteral nutrition can supply enough calories for anabolism—up to 5000 kcal. or more per day if necessary. This is possible because the concentrated solution is administered through a catheter inserted into the superior vena cava, where the hypertonic solution can be rapidly diluted by the large volume of blood. If such a concentrated solution were given in a peripheral vein, phlebitis would develop in four to eight hours.

NUTRIENT REQUIREMENTS AND COMPOSITION OF FORMULA. The body is less effective in using energy and nutrients provided by vein, so a greater amount must be given to keep the patient in positive nitrogen balance.

The composition of a typical TPN solution is shown in Table 35–12. It is a concentrated liquid that, at the usual strength, provides 1 kcal. per ml. or 1000 kcal. per liter of solution and about 42 gm. of protein per liter. The Calorie:nitrogen ratio of the solution is usually about 150:1, appropriate for protein synthesis and anabolism; however, there is great flexibility in designing the formula depending upon what is needed by the patient.

Protein. Protein is provided by crystalline amino acids or protein hydrolysates, although the crystalline amino acids are preferable because more of their protein is available for use and the amino acid composition of the formula can be manipulated to meet the patient's needs. Standard parenteral solutions contain 3.5 to 10 per cent protein with 5.6 to 16 gm. of nitrogen per liter in a Calorie:nitrogen ratio of 120 to 180:1. Commonly used solutions are Freamine Travasol and Aminosyn. Since the usual TPN solution contains 25 to 42 gm. of protein per liter, most patients require at least 2 to 3 liters per day in order to meet their protein requirements of 1 to 1.5 gm. of protein per kg. IBW per day. However, this depends on individual needs and should be individually determined. Infants usually require at least 2.0 gm. of protein per kg. IBW. Requirements for neonates are discussed in Chapter 37.

Carbohydrate. The carbohydrate in a TPN formula is usually a 50 per cent solution of glucose, which has a much higher osmolality than the usual 5 per cent glucose solution administered in peripheral intravenous therapy. The amount of glucose is usually 500 ml. in each liter of TPN solution. This provides 250 gm. of glucose or 850 kcal. per liter of TPN solution (250 gm. of glucose $\times$ 3.4 kcal. per gm. of glucose= 850 kcal.). To this is added the calories provided by the protein in the mixture (42.5 gm. of protein $\times$ 4 kcal. per gm. of protein = 170

kcal.), so that the final solution contains 1020 kcal. per liter, or about 1 kcal. per ml. Some patients require more concentrated carbohydrate energy sources because of large energy requirements or fluid restrictions. D_{70} (350 gm. of glucose per 500 ml.) is available. However, it has been reported that high glucose loads can increase minute ventilation, carbon dioxide production, the respiratory quotient (RQ) and oxygen consumption. Lipid does not have the same effect and has been shown to be useful in patients with impaired ventilatory function.

Fat. Patients usually also receive lipid as a separate additional energy source. Fat in a form suitable for intravenous use is available as Intralipid or Lyposyn. The addition of fat can increase the caloric concentration of the TPN fluid considerably. Lipid solutions are now available in 10 or 20 per cent concentrations if volume of intake is a problem for the patient. The 10 per cent solutions provide 1.1 kcal./ml. and the 20 per cent solutions 2.2 kcal./ml. Up to two thirds of the daily energy requirement can be provided as fat; however, it appears that fat has less nitrogen-sparing effect than glucose.

The addition of small amounts of lipid also prevents essential fatty acid (EFA) deficiency, which has been reported in babies and severely depleted adults receiving TPN.[9] The signs of EFA deficiency are: light, flaky and perhaps reddened skin lesions that appear on the scalp, arms and legs; thrombocytopenia; increased hemolysis; impaired wound healing; and growth retardation in the case of infants. (See Chapter 3 for further discussion.) To cure or prevent the deficiency state, lipid can be given in the TPN fluid 2 to 3 times per week. If lipid cannot be added to the TPN solution and cannot be taken orally, some success in relieving essential fatty acid deficiency may be achieved by rubbing sunflower seed oil or another highly polyunsaturated oil into the skin.[20]

Electrolytes. Electrolytes must be added to the solution to promote efficient tissue weight gain. Potassium is especially important because as the patient enters anabolism, glucose and potassium move into the cells, and the potassium requirement may be increased. Sodium and chloride are also important.

Phosphate is important because, in the presence of high-energy feedings, dangerous hypophosphatemia can develop. Calcium is necessary to balance the phosphate infusion. Table 35–12 gives the suggested electrolyte and major mineral concentrations during parenteral nutrition.

Vitamins. The precise vitamin requirements for patients receiving TPN are still not known. In the past usual multiple vitamin intravenous formulations based on oral dosage recommendations have been added to the TPN solution.

Table 35–12. ELECTROLYTE AND MINERAL REQUIREMENTS DURING PARENTERAL NUTRITION

(Normal Range of Daily Requirements)

Sodium	60 to 150 mEq. as sodium chloride and sodium lactate.
Potassium	70 to 150 mEq. as potassium chloride and potassium phosphate.
Chloride	Equal to Na to prevent acid-base disturbances.
Calcium	0.2 to 0.3 mEq./kg./day added as calcium gluconate.
Magnesium	0.35 to 0.45 mEq./kg./day added as magnesium sulfate. Give more if increased losses are present.
Phosphorous	7 to 10 mmoles per 1000 kcal., extremely variable—adjust to keep serum concentrations normal
*Zinc	2.5 to 4 mg. per day added as zinc sulfate. Additional 2.0 mg. for adult in acute metabolic state. 12.2 mg./l. of small bowel fluid lost; 17.1 mg./kg. of stool or ileostomy output
*Chromium	10 to 15 mg. per day added as chromic chloride 20 μg. in adult with intestinal losses
*Copper	0.5 to 1.5 mg./day added as copper sulfate
*Manganese	2 to 10 mg./day
Selenium	10 μg./day

* These are available in a single formulation in the amounts recommended by the AMA[†] and can be given as a single addition to the parenteral nutrition solution.

[†] AMA Dept. of Foods and Nutrition Guidelines for essential trace element preparations for parenteral use. A statement by an Expert Panel. JAMA, *241*:2051, 1979

Adapted from Grant J. P.: Handbook of Total Parenteral Nutrition. Philadelphia, W. B. Saunders Company, 1980.

However, active research in this area and study of patients on TPN for several years is rapidly adding to the knowledge in this area. New preparations are being formulated with the TPN patient in mind. As more knowledge is gained, these formulations will change. Table 35–13 presents the most recent recommendations for vitamins for children and adults on TPN. However, it is important to note that these are recommended guidelines for parenteral administration of vitamins for patients in non-stressed normal metabolic states.[1, 18] Additional unresolved problems are effects of nutritional composition of parenteral solutions on the patient's requirements for specific vitamins and the effects of infection and other disease states on requirements. For these reasons, the recommendations in Table 35–13 are just guidelines and are not meant to be all inclusive for all patients. Several others have proposed different regimens.[13, 19, 21] For example the need for vitamin C is higher in patients with burns or severe trauma than the 100 mg. recommended in Table 35–13.[25]

Products formulated for use with TPN, such as MVI–12, contain the usual multiple vitamin preparation with the addition of biotin, folic acid and vitamin B_{12}. They still may not be adequate for all patients. It may be preferable to give vitamin combinations to better meet the individual patient's needs. To prevent excessive excretion of the water-soluble vitamins, the daily dosage of the multiple vitamin preparation should be administered over several hours as part of the intravenous (IV) feeding schedule.

The requirements for fat-soluble vitamins by patients on TPN are not so clearly understood. Normal serum vitamin A levels can be maintained in patients receiving TPN using 1500 to 2000 I.U. per day, less than the RDA. However, in the case of vitamin E it is controversial. Although the recommendation in Table 35–13 is 10 I.U. (0.67 mg d,1-alpha-tocopherol), it appears that amounts greater than this are needed. Greig suggests that as much as 50 mg d,1-alpha-tocopherol may be needed.[13] However, much of this will be provided by the fat in the solution if it provides 50 per cent or more of the non-protein calories. In addition, the inclusion of this polyunsaturated fat in the TPN solution increases the requirement for vitamin E.

Vitamin K, normally provided by gut bacteria, should be adequate for the TPN patient. However, if there are changes in the gut flora due to antibiotic administration or the TPN feeding, additional vitamin K may be necessary. Ten mg. of Synkavite (water-soluble form) weekly in the TPN solution is adequate.

The need for vitamin D in TPN is not well established, even though 200 I.U. is the stated recommendation. In fact, a syndrome of skeletal calcium loss with a histological picture of increased bone osteoid, but with reduced calcification of the new osteoid, has been reported to be aggravated by giving vitamin D, at levels of 250 I.U. per day.[24] At present much more work needs to be done in this area. Greig and colleagues suggest that 100 I.U. of vitamin D once weekly is appropriate.[13]

Trace Minerals. Exact trace mineral needs during TPN are also not clarified, but it is well appreciated that there is a need for these nutrients. This has been demonstrated for several elements through study of patients for whom TPN is the sole source of nutrition for months or years.[15] At least one pharmaceutical company has formulated a trace mineral preparation containing zinc, copper, chromium and manganese that can be added to the TPN solution. Other formulations containing single minerals such as selenium and molybdenum are also available. In administering trace elements intravenously special care must be taken to avoid toxic complications and to consider the amounts of these elements that are already present in the parenteral nutrition solutions.

ADMINISTRATION. Insertion of the TPN catheter into the superior vena cava is a surgical technique performed under sterile conditions

Table 35–13. RECOMMENDATIONS FOR VITAMIN INTAKES FOR PATIENTS RECEIVING PARENTERAL NUTRITION

FORMULATIONS FOR INFANTS AND CHILDREN UNDER 11 YEARS[a]

VITAMINS	RDA			AAP[b] MINIMUM/ 100 KCAL ORALLY	SUGGESTED FORMATIONS	
	Range-infants per body wt 0.0–0.5 and 0.5–1.0 yr	Mean-infant	Range-children under 11 yrs		Multivitamin[c] for intravenous use for under 11 yrs	Water-soluble vitamins for intramuscular use
A (retinol), IU	233–222	227.0	2,000–3,300	250.0	2,300.0[d]	
D, IU	66–44	55.0	400	40.0	400.0[e]	
E (α tocopherol), IU	0.66–0.55	0.6	7–10	0.3	7.0	
K_1 (phylloquinone), mg					0.2	
Ascorbic acid, mg	6–4	5.0	40	8.0	80.0	80.0
Folacin, μg	8–6	7.0	100–300	4.0	140.0	140.0
Niacin, mg	0.9–0.8	0.85	9–16	0.25	17.0	17.0
Riboflavin, mg	0.07	0.07	0.8–1.2	0.06	1.4	1.4
Thiamin, mg	0.055–0.05	0.053	0.7–1.2	0.025	1.2	1.2
B_6 (pyridoxine), mg	0.05–0.04	0.045	0.6–1.2	0.035	1.0	1.0
B_{12} (cyanocobalamin), μg	0.04–0.03	0.035	1–2	0.15	1.0	1.0
Pantothenic acid, mg				0.3	5.0[f]	5.0
Biotin, μg					20.0[f]	20.0

CHILDREN AGE 11 YEARS AND ABOVE, AND ADULTS[a]

Ranges do not include requirements for pregnancy or lactation.

VITAMINS	RDA ADULT RANGE	MULTIVITAMIN FORMULATION FOR INTRAVENOUS USE	WATER-SOLUBLE VITAMIN FORMULATION FOR INTRAMUSCULAR USE
A, IU	4,000–5,000[g]	3,300	
D, IU	400	200	
E, IU	12–15	10.0	
Ascorbic acid, mg	45	100.0	100.0
Folacin, μg	400	400.0	400.0
Niacin, mg	12–20	40.0	40.0
Riboflavin, mg	1.1–1.8	3.6	3.6
Thiamin, mg	1.0–1.5	3.0	3.0
B_6 (pyridoxine), mg	1.6–2.0	4.0	4.0
B_{12} (cyanocobalamin), μg	3	5.0	5.0
Pantothenic acid,	5–10[h]	15.0	15.0
Biotin, μg	150–300[h]	60.0	60.0

[a] Adapted from Guidelines for Multivitamin Preparations for Parenteral Use, AMA, 1975.
[b] American Academy of Pediatrics.
[c] May be provided in appropriate salt or ester form in equivalent potency.
[d] 700 μg of retinol.
[e] As ergocalciferol or cholecalciferol.
[f] RDA not established; amount = 20 times the amount in 100 kcal. human milk.
[g] Assumes 50% intake as carotene, which is less available than vitamin A.
[h] RDA not established, amount considered adequate in usual dietary intake.

From Multivitamin preparations for parenteral use. A statement by the Nutrition Advisory Group. J. Parent. Ent. Nutr., 3:258, 1979. Copyright American Society for Parenteral and Enteral Nutrition, 428 E. Preston St., Baltimore, Md., 21202.

with a draped field. The patient is given local anesthesia. Once placement of the tube in the inferior vena cava has been confirmed, administration of TPN can begin. Because the TPN solution is hyperosmolar and a very concentrated source of glucose, it must be administered slowly at first. Usually, 1 liter is given in 24 hours using a constant drip infusion maintained by gravity or a pump. Blood glucose, urine glucose and electrolyte levels are watched closely. The rate of administration is gradually increased, usually over four to five days, until the patient is receiving the full requirement.

Monitoring of the blood glucose and urine glucose concentrations, urinary output, blood urea nitrogen (BUN) level and electrolyte levels show that the patient is stable and the insulin response is sufficient. Insulin may need to be added if the insulin response is not sufficient. Table 35–14 lists the clinical factors that should be monitored in the patient receiving TPN. Four liters per day of TPN is the maximum that most

Table 35–14. VARIABLES TO BE MONITORED DURING TOTAL PARENTERAL NUTRITION

VARIABLES TO BE MONITORED	SUGGESTED FREQUENCY*	
	Initial Period	Later Period
Growth Variables		
Weight	Daily	Daily
Length (infants only)	Weekly	Weekly
Head circumference (infants only)	Weekly	Weekly
Metabolic Variables		
Blood		
Serum electrolytes (Na^+, K^+, Cl^-)	Daily	3/week
Blood urea nitrogen	3/week	
Plasma total calcium and inorganic phosphorus	3/week	2/week
Blood glucose	Daily	3/week
Plasma transaminases	3/week	2/week
Plasma total protein and fractions	2/week	Weekly
Blood acid-base status	Daily	3/week
Hemoglobin	Weekly	Weekly
Prothrombin time	Weekly	Weekly
Ammonia	2/week	Weekly
Magnesium	2/week	Weekly
Zinc	Weekly	Weekly
Copper	Weekly	Weekly
Urine		
Glucose	4–6/day	2/day
Specific gravity or osmolarity	2–4/day	Daily
Urinary urea nitrogen	Weekly	Weekly
General Measurements		
Volume of infusate	Daily	Daily
Oral intake (if any)	Daily	Daily
Urinary output	Daily	Daily
Prevention and Detection of Infection		
Clinical observations (activity, temperature, etc.)	Daily	Daily
WBC[†] count and differential	As indicated	As indicated
Cultures	As indicated	As indicated

Sources: Winters, R. W., and Wilmore, D. W.: Evaluation of the patient. In White, P. L., Nagy, M. E., and Fletcher, D. C. (eds.): Total Parenteral Nutrition. Acton, Mass., Publishing Sciences Group, Inc., 1974; Grant, J. P.: Handbook of Total Parenteral Nutrition. Philadelphia, W. B. Saunders Company, 1980.

* *Initial period* refers to that period in which a full glucose intake is being achieved; *later period* implies that the patient has achieved a steady metabolic state. In the presence of metabolic instability, the more intensive monitoring outlined under *initial period* should be followed.

† WBC = white blood cells.

patients can tolerate. Patients requiring more than 3000 kcal. per day will probably require the addition of some lipid to the solution to increase its caloric concentration.

The solution should be administered at a steady rate. If the administration falls behind, the administration rate should be corrected. Do not attempt to "catch up," because an excessive glucose load will result. When hyperalimentation is no longer needed, it is important to decrease the amount infused gradually to prevent hypoglycemic shock. Oral intake should also be well established and should increase as the TPN decreases.

Some patients receiving TPN still feel hungry and, if possible, they can take some food orally. If complete bowel rest is required, however, the patient should not be given anything, not even water, by mouth but can only suck on ice chips.

TPN should be given in amounts to allow a daily weight gain of 1/4 to 1/2 lb. (0.1 to 0.2 kg.). This seems to be the limit for the amount of body tissue that can be synthesized in 24 hours. A weight gain greater than this indicates fluid retention. This is commonly seen initially in malnourished patients who are given TPN with non-protein calories as glucose only. It is not seen with systems that use lipid.[13] Once ideal weight is achieved, the TPN intake should be adjusted to maintain it.

CARE OF THE TPN CATHETER SITE. Care of the catheter site requires special attention because it is an easy entrance for microorganisms into a major vein. The dressings around the site and the tubing from the catheter to the TPN bottle should be changed two to three times per week. The area around the catheter insertion site should be cleansed with an antiseptic during each dressing change, and antibiotic ointment should be applied to the catheter site. The area is then covered with sterile dressings. The TPN catheter should not be used for any procedures other than TPN administration. The catheter is not removed until it is no longer needed or until there is indication of an infection at the catheter tip where it enters the vein (usually evidenced by a fever). With proper care, infectious complications of subclavian vein catheters should be infrequent.

EXERCISE. Skeletal muscle protein synthesis is enhanced if the muscles are exercised. For example, in states of protein depletion the heart muscle is spared until the end, apparently because it receives constant exercise. Exercise and physical therapy are very useful for the patient who is being nutritionally rehabilitated. They are an important part of the total therapy and allow efficient use to be made of the nutritional support being provided to the patient.

CYCLIC PARENTERAL NUTRITION. In cyclic parenteral nutrition the patient is fed amino acids and glucose parenterally for 10 to 16 hours and amino acids or amino acids and fat, either orally or parenterally, or nothing for the remainder of the 24-hour period.[16] This technique is valuable when (1) oral intake is not adequate to meet the patient's nutritional needs but total parenteral support is not necessary, (2) the patient is ambulatory or at home and does not want the encumbering I.V. bottle during the day or (3) essential fatty acid deficiency must be prevented.

It is postulated that cyclic parenteral nutrition with the withholding of glucose for 8 to 10 hours follows the body's normal intake of nutrients more closely, so that for a period of every day, usually at night during sleep, there is no nutritional intake. Serum insulin is reduced, which allows lipolysis to take place for a period of time. Cyclic parenteral nutrition prevents essential fatty acid deficiency because, during the period without hyperalimentation, the person uses some fatty acids from fat stored for energy and thus receives linoleic acid. Fatty livers do not develop and those already induced by continuous TPN resolve. A lower caloric intake is required to maintain nitrogen balance because some of the patient's fat stores are used.

PARENTERAL NUTRITION AT HOME. The patient who will never recover gastrointestinal tract function but who is free of disease can be maintained indefinitely with TPN. Patients have been kept alive and have returned to normal lives and work using this method. Such a person usually receives infusions for five to seven nights per week while sleeping, depending upon the requirements needed to maintain weight. The infusion is gradually decreased in the last few hours in order to prevent hypoglycemia in the non-alimentary period. The long-term effects of self-administered TPN will become better understood now that there is a sufficient number of patients that long-term term studies can be done.

Success with home parenteral nutrition requires an intensive training program to give patients and their families specialized skills for self-administration of parenteral fluids. There must also be supportive, available and frequent follow-up of these patients. There are also private companies that will deliver equipment and supplies to the home, maintain inventory and directly bill the patient or the insurance company.

COMPLICATIONS. Although TPN appears to be the answer to many clinical nutritional problems, it is not without risk. Some of the complications are listed in Table 35–15. The risk to the patient should always be balanced against the

Table 35–15. POTENTIAL COMPLICATIONS OF HYPERALIMENTATION

SUBCLAVIAN CATHETERIZATION
  Pneumothorax
  Hemothorax
  Hydrothorax
  Tension pneumothorax
  Subcutaneous emphysema
  Brachial plexus injury
  Subclavian artery injury
  Subclavian hematoma
  Central vein thrombophlebitis
  Arteriovenous fistula
  Thoracic duct injury
  Hydromediastinum
  Air embolism
  Catheter embolism
  Catheter misplacement
  Cardiac perforation; tamponade
  Endocarditis

INFECTION AND SEPSIS
  Catheter entrance site
      Contamination during insertion
      Long-term catheter placement
  Catheter seeding from blood-borne or distant infection
  Solution contamination

METABOLIC COMPLICATIONS
  Dehydration from osmotic diuresis
  Hyperosmolar, nonketotic, hyperglycemic coma
  Rebound hypoglycemia on sudden cessation of
      treatment
  Hypomagnesemia
  Hypocalcemia
  Hyperphosphatemia and hypophosphatemia
  Hyperchloremic metabolic acidosis
  Azotemia
  Hyperammonemia
  Electrolyte imbalance
  Trace mineral deficiencies

benefit of TPN, and risks and benefits of enteral nutrition. Patients receiving TPN or enteral nutrition should always be monitored closely.

Problems and Suggested Topics for Discussion

1. Describe what is happening metabolically in a healthy person who is fasting. Talk with a healthy person who has fasted and try to find out how he felt during the first two days of the fast and after about one week of fasting.
2. Give reasons for emphasis on (a) adequate protein therapy, (b) adequate fluid therapy, (c) adequate electrolyte therapy and (d) adequate calorie therapy in a patient with an infection.
3. Describe the catabolic stress response. How does it protect the body during stress?
4. Become familiar with the various types of tube feedings used for patients. What do they contain? When are they appropriate to use?
5. Talk with a patient who is receiving a defined formula diet. What is his or her reaction to it? How much is he or she taking? Does the patient need this form of therapy?
6. Under what conditions would intravenous hyperalimentation be indicated?

Cited References

1. American Medical Association, Nutrition Advisory Group: Statement on Guidelines for Multivitamin Preparations for Parenteral Use. Chicago, A.M.A., 1975.
2. Bistrian, B.R., Blackburn, G.L., and Scrimshaw, N.S.: Effect of mild infectious illness on nitrogen metabolism in patients on a modified fast. Am. J. Clin. Nutr., 28:1044, 1975.
3. Blackburn, G.L., and Bistrian, B.R.: Nutritional care of the injured or septic patient. Surg. Clin. North Am., 56:1195, 1976.
4. Blackburn, G.L., and Bistrian, B.R.: Protein-calorie curative therapy. In Schneider, H.: Nutritional Support in Medical Practice. New York, Harper & Row, 1976.
5. Blackburn, G.L., et al.: Peripheral intravenous feeding with isotonic amino acid solutions. Am. J. Surg., 125:447, 1973.
6. Blackburn, G.L., et al.: Protein-sparing therapy during periods of starvation with sepsis or trauma. Ann. Surg., 177:588, 1973.
7. DuBois, E.F., and Chambers, W.H.: Calories in medical practice. Handbook of Nutrition. Chicago, American Medical Association, 1943, pp. 55–70.
8. Dudrick, S.J., et al.: Total Parenteral Nutrition (videotape). Network for Continuing Medical Education, Houston, Texas, 1976.
9. Fleming, C.R., Smith, L.M., and Hodges, R.E.: Essential fatty acid deficiency in adults receiving total parenteral nutrition. Am. J. Clin. Nutr., 29:976, 1976.
10. Gamble, J.L.: Physiological information gained from studies on the life raft ration. Harvey Lect., 42:247, 1947.
11. Gazzaniga, A.B., et al.: Endogenous caloric sources and nitrogen balance. Arch. Surg., 111:1357, 1976.
12. Greenberg, G.R., et al.: Protein-sparing therapy in postoperative patients. N. Engl. J. Med., 294:1411, 1975.
13. Greig, P.D., Baker, J.P., and Jeejeebhoy, K.N.: Metabolic effects of total parenteral nutrition. Ann. Rev. Nutr., 2:179, 1982.
14. Hoover, H.C., et al.: Nitrogen-sparing intravenous fluids in postoperative patients. N. Engl. J. Med., 293:172, 1975.
14a. Hopkins, B.S., Bistrian, B.R., and Blackburn, G.L.: Protein-calorie management in the hospitalized patient. In Schneider, sin, D.B. (eds.): Nutritional Support in Medical Practice. 2nd ed. New York, Harper & Row, 1983.
15. Jeejeebhoy, K.N., et al.: Chromium deficiency, glucose intolerance, and neuropathy reversed by chromium supplementation in a patient receiving long-term parenteral nutrition. Am. J. Clin. Nutr., 30:531, 1977.
16. Maini, B., et al.: Cyclic hyperalimentation: an optimal technique for preservation of visceral protein. J. Surg. Res., 20:515, 1976.
17. Matthews, D.M., and Adibi, S.A.: Peptide absorption. Gastroenterology, 71:151, 1976.
18. Multivitamin preparations for parenteral use. A statement by the Nutrition Advisory Group. JPEN, 3:258, 1979.
19. Nicholalds, G.E., et al.: Vitamin requirements in patients receiving total parenteral nutrition. Arch. Surg., 112:1061, 1977.
20. Press, M., Hartop, P.J., and Prottey, C.: Correction of essential fatty acid deficiency in man by cutaneous application of sunflower seed oil. Lancet, 1:597, 1974.
21. Robinson, L.A., Mabry, C.D., and Wright, B.T.: Vitamin requirements in parenteral nutrition: a dilemma. JPEN, 6:76, 1982.
22. Rutten, P., et al.: Determination of optimal hyperalimentation infusion rate. J. Surg. Res., 18:477, 1975.
23. Scrimshaw, N.S.: Malnutrition and infection. Borden's Review, 26(2), 1965.
24. Shike, M., et al.: A possible role of vitamin D in the genesis of parenteral nutrition–induced metabolic bone disease. Ann. Intern. Med., 95:560, 1981.
25. Vallance, B.D.: Vitamin C, disease and surgical trauma. Br. Med. J., 2:955, 1979.

Additional References

AMA Dept. of Foods and Nutrition: "Guidelines for essential trace element preparations for parenteral use. A statement by an Expert Panel. JAMA, 241:2051, 1979.

Askanazi, J., et al.: Nutrition and the respiratory system. Crit. Care Med. 10:163, 1982.

Barron, J.: Tube feeding with liquified natural foods. Henry Ford Hospital Med. J., Vol. 1, June 1953.

Border, J.R., et al.: Multiple systems organ failure: muscle fuel deficit with visceral protein malnutrition. Surg. Clin. North Am., 56:1147, 1976.

Broviac, J.W., and Scribner, B.H.: Prolonged parenteral nutrition in the home. Surg. Gynecol. Obstet., 139:24, 1974.

Cahill, G.F.: Starvation in man. N. Engl. J. Med., 282:668, 1970.

Clowes, G.H.A. (ed.): Response to infection and injury. II. Metabolism. Surg. Clin. North Am., 56(5), 1976.

Del Rio, D., Williams, K., and Esveldt, B.: The Handbook of Enteral Nutrition. El Segundo, Cal., Medical Specifics Publishing, 1982.

Dudrick, S.J., et al.: Can intravenous feeding as the sole means of nutrition support growth in the child and restore weight loss in the adult? Ann. Surg., 169:974, 1969.

Dudrick, S.J., et al.: Long-term total parenteral nutrition and growth, development, and positive nitrogen balance. Surgery, 64:134, 1968.

Felig, P.: Intravenous nutrition: fact and fancy. N. Engl. J. Med., 294:1455, 1976.

Flatt, J.P., and Blackburn, G.L.: The metabolic fuel regulatory system: implications for protein-sparing therapies during caloric deprivation and disease. Am. J. Clin. Nutr., 27:175, 1974.

Gault, A.M., et al.: Hypernatremia, azotemia and dehydration due to high protein tube feeding. Ann. Intern. Med., 68:778, 1968.

Gordon, J.E.: Synergism of malnutrition and infectious disease. In Beaton, G.H., and Bengoa, J.M. (eds.): Nutrition in Preventive Medicine. Geneva, Switzerland, WHO, 1976, pp. 193–209.

Gormican, A.: Tube feeding. An overview. Dietetic Currents, 2(2), 1975.

Grant, J.P.: Handbook of Total Parenteral Nutrition. Philadelphia, W.B. Saunders Company, 1980.

Howard, L., et al.: Water soluble vitamin requirements in home parenteral nutrition patients. Am. J. Clin. Nutr., 37: 421, 1983.

Jeejeebhoy, K.N., et al.: Total parenteral nutrition at home: studies in patients surviving 4 months to 5 years. Gastroenterology, 71:943, 1976.

Jeejeebhoy, K.N. (ed.): Total Parenteral Nutrition in the Hospital and at Home. Boca Raton, Fla., CRC Press, 1983.

Kishi, H., Nishii, S., and Ono, T.: Thiamine and pyridoxine requirements during intravenous hyperalimentation. Am. J. Clin. Nutr., 32:332, 1979.

Kubo, W., et al.: Fluid and electrolyte problems of tube-fed patients. Am. J. Nurs., 76:912, 1976.

Lowry, F.L., et al.: Parenteral vitamin requirements during intravenous feeding. Am. J. Clin. Nutr., 31:2149, 1978.

McFarlane, H.: Nutrition and immunity. In Present Knowledge in Nutrition. 4th ed. New York, The Nutrition Foundation, Inc., 1976.

Mecray, P., Jr.: Nutrition and wound healing. Am. J. Clin. Nutr., 3:461, 1955.

Mullen, J.I., Crosby, L.O., and Rombeau, J.L. (eds.): Symposium on surgical nutrition. Surg. Clin. N. Am., 61(3), 1981.

Nutritional products. In Boyd, J.R. (ed.): Facts and Comparisons. Philadelphia, J.B. Lippincott & Company, 1982, pp. 1–60.

Riella, M.C., et al.: Essential fatty acid deficiency in human adults during total parenteral nutrition. Ann. Intern. Med., 83:786, 1975.

Rudman, D., et al.: Elemental balances during intravenous hyperalimentation of underweight adult subjects. J. Clin. Invest., 55:94, 1975.

Scribner, B.H., et al.: Long-term parenteral nutrition. JAMA, 212:457, 1970.

Shils, M.E.: A program for total parenteral nutrition at home. Am. J. Clin. Nutr., 28:1429, 1975.

Sieberman, H., and Eisenberg, D.: Parenteral Nutrition for the Hospitalized Patient. Norwalk, Conn., Appleton-Century-Crofts, 1982.

Skillman, J.J., et al.: Improved albumin synthesis in post-operative patients by amino acid infusion. N. Engl. J. Med., 295:1037, 1976.

Smith, J.L., and Heymsfield, S.B.: Enteral nutrition support: formula preparation from modular ingredients. JPEN, 7:280, 1983.

Stinnett, D. (ed.): Nutrition and the Immune Response. Boca Raton, Fla., CRC Press, 1983.

Stromberg, P., et al.: Vitamin status during total parenteral nutrition. JPEN, 5:295, 1981.

Walike, B.C., and Walike, J.W.: Lactose content of tube feeding diets as a cause of diarrhea. Laryngoscope, 83:1109, 1973.

NEOPLASTIC DISEASE

Nutrition, Diet and Cancer

DORICE M. CZAJKA-NARINS, PH.D. • CARRIE L. CHENEY, M.S.,
R.D. • SAUNDRA N. AKER, R.D.

Concepts of Neoplastic Disease

Definitions

The term *tumor* was applied to all masses before the nature of various types of lesions was understood. Eventually, swellings due to known causes, especially those due to infection, were excluded, and use of the term tumor was limited to those masses of unknown cause that apparently arose by unrestrained growth of the individual's own cells. *Cancer* is the general term for a malignant tumor that can exist in any tissue or organ. Cancers can differ greatly in appearance and growth patterns. *Neoplasia* means a purposeless, uncontrolled, progressive multiplication of cells. The neoplasm competes with normal cells for energy and nutritional substrates and is to a degree autonomous.

There are a few other words used to describe changes in cells that should be mentioned. *Dysplasia*, an alteration in adult cells characterized by variation in size, shape and organism, and *metaplasia*, a change in adult tissue to a type that is not normal for that tissue, are conditions in which it seems highly likely that normal controls over growth and development may be lacking. Dysplasia, in common medical usage, is the term applied to epithelial cells that have responded to chronic irritation and inflammation by undergoing irregularly atypical proliferative changes. In both the cervix and respiratory tract dysplasia is strongly implicated as the cause of cancer.

Classification

Tumors can be classified on the basis of the cell of origin and their behavior—benign, intermediate or malignant. A *benign* tumor is circumscribed, usually well encapsulated, and affects the host either by pressure atrophy or by obstruction. A *malignant* tumor, or cancer, invades surrounding tissue and releases cells that are carried to other parts of the body to set up secondary growth, or metastases. In tissue culture, cancer cells fail to adhere to each other or other support as do normal cells, and this may account in part for their ability to migrate. Malignant tumors produce a number of effects on the host, including mechanical pressure and obstruction, destruction of tissue, hemorrhage, infection, anemia, cachexia, hormonal abnormalities and other changes, such as muscle weakness, which cannot be explained. Tumors with patterns of behavior that do not fall into either category are classified as *intermediate* tumors. Intermediate tumors are locally invasive but do not metastasize.

The tissue of origin rather than the organ containing the tumor, determines the behavior of the tumor. Lipomas are therefore tumors arising from fatty tissue and fibromas arise from fibrocytes. The suffix -oma is used to denote the lesion. The prefix refers to the cell of origin, which is determined histologically. Clinically grading or staging a cancer is useful to indicate the extent and spread in an individual patient. No system is completely satisfactory. Most divide neoplasms into grades I, II, III and IV, with the higher numbers indicating more malignant tumors.

General Characteristics

Cancer cells tend to be large and have large nuclei with an irregular outline. There is often more than one nucleus. Mitotic cells are more frequent in tumor cells than in normal cells. In general most cancers grow more rapidly than benign tumors and the more anaplastic the cancer, the more numerous the mitoses and the more rapid the growth. Figure 36–1 shows the growth of a mass in terms of doubling time and number of cells. For Burkitt's lymphoma the doubling time may be five days or less. For other cancers the generation time may be as long as months. Chromosomal abnormalities are more common than originally thought and are not random, but affect specific loci. Cancers of blood cells involve translocation of chromosomal segments, whereas solid tumors usually involve deletions. Malignant tumors are surrounded by lymphocytes and evoke a substantial inflammatory response. These lymphocytes are T cells attacking the immunologically different non-host cancer. Patients receiving steroids, radiation or other drugs to suppress their immune response have an unusually high rate of new cancers.

Mode of Action

Mutagenesis is a heritable change in the cell produced by alteration of DNA. Most errors in DNA replication are corrected by the body's repair mechanisms. Virtually all carcinogens are mutagens, but not all mutagens are carcinogens. Carcinogenesis also involves a heritable change in DNA.

There are two types of mutagens: direct-acting mutagens and promutagens. *Direct-acting mutagens* do not require metabolic activation or transformation to manifest their mutagenic potential as do *promutagens*. Either type may be ingested with foods. Mutagens occur in foods naturally or as a result of processing. There are four categories of naturally occurring mutagens: those in edible plants, such as flavonoids; those produced by fungi, such as aflatoxin B_1; those produced by cooking, such as compounds in the charred parts of protein foods, and those formed by interactions of the food, such as when nitrites are added to food containing amines resulting in the formation of nitrosamines. Mutagens occurring in foods as a result of industrial processing can be removed, but naturally occurring mutagens are more difficult to remove.

Tumorigenesis or carcinogenesis is a two-stage process, involving initiation and promotion. In the *initiation* stage there is a transformation of the cell produced by interaction of chemicals, radiation or viruses with cellular DNA. This transformation occurs rapidly, but the resultant cell remains dormant for a variable period until activated by a promoting agent. Initiation of carcinogenesis may be irreversible. During the *promotion* stage, initiated cells multiply to form a discrete tumor. The effect of diet and nutrition on both the initiation and promotion stages of tumor development is currently the subject of intense scrutiny.

Nutrients or dietary compounds may inhibit mutagens or carcinogens by preventing them from reaching their target sites, by altering cell membrane permeability or by altering transport. Nutrients or dietary compounds may permit carcinogenesis by making conditions in the cell suitable. For example, localized deficiency of folate may increase the likelihood of chromosomal breakage at fragile points.

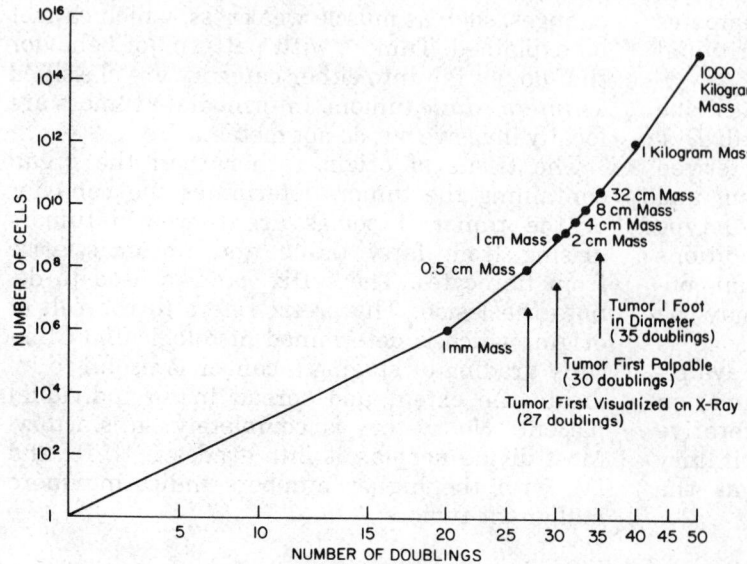

Figure 36–1. This graph shows the number of cells, the number of doublings, and the size of the mass. A tumor may be first visible only after 25 or more doublings. Growth from the point of first visibility becomes exponential. (From Thorn, G. W., et al. (eds.): Harrison's Principles of Internal Medicine. 8th ed. New York, McGraw-Hill, 1976.)

Our knowledge of nutrition related to cancer, although limited, is in two general areas: (1) nutrition in the etiology of cancer and (2) the role of nutrition in patients who have cancer. The second area can be subdivided into (a) the nutritional effects of cancer, (b) the nutritional problems resulting from cancer treatment and (c) the nutritional care for patients with cancer.

Nutrition in the Etiology of Cancer

If the estimate that 80 to 90 per cent of cancer is related to environmental factors is correct, then the majority of human cancer may be potentially preventable. An example of the influence of environmental factors is the observation that migrants from one culture to another show a shift in cancer pattern from that of the old habitat to that of the new one. For example, mortality from breast and colon cancer is low in Japan and mortality from stomach cancer is high, and the reverse is seen in the United States. After two or three generations, the pattern shifts in Japanese immigrants to that of the United States, coinciding with a change in dietary pattern of increased energy and fat. Puerto Ricans migrating to the mainland U.S. exhibit the same trend. If environmental factors can be specifically defined and this knowledge applied, the potential ramifications for treatment and prevention of cancer are tremendous.

One in five deaths in the United States is from cancer. Cancer kills more children aged 3 to 14 years than any other disease. In 1982, cancer was diagnosed in 835,000 people and 430,000 people died of cancer, one every 73 seconds. Figure 36–2 shows the 1982 estimates for cancer incidence and cancer deaths by site and sex. Statistically 7 of every 100 women will suffer from breast cancer, the leading cause of cancer in the United States. In men, lung cancer is the leading cause of death. The death rate for women from lung cancer has increased in recent years.

There are several points to remember when evaluating the role of diet in the etiology of cancer. First, diet alters immune response and an altered immune response may affect the ability of the body to inhibit cancer. Energy, protein, iron, zinc, vitamin A and several other nutrients play important roles in the maintenance of the immune system. Deficiencies of these nutrients may inhibit the immune response, which may in turn inhibit the initial responses against carcinogenesis. The role of specific nutrients in the immune response is discussed in Chapter 35. Second, there are interrelationships between diet and hormones that may lead to the development or enhancement of certain of the endocrine-dependent cancers, such as cancer of the ovary, prostate, breast, thyroid and uterine endometrium. Third, when one major component of the diet is altered, other changes take place simultaneously. For example, as the amount of animal protein is decreased, the amount of animal fat will also be decreased. These changes make interpretation of the data difficult. Fourth, many tumors have a long latency period, and diet at the time of initiation or promotion, not at the time of diagnosis, may be the important factor. Finally, different nutrients affect cancer differently, and one nutrient can have different effects on different types of cancer. Unfortunately, this area is just beginning to

1982 ESTIMATES

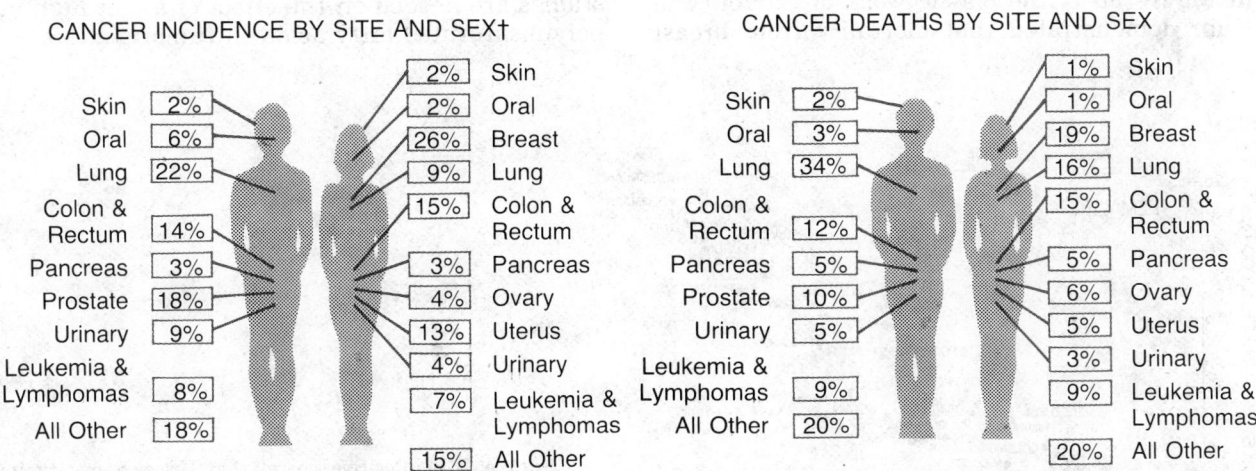

†Excluding non-melanoma skin cancer and carcinoma in situ.

Figure 36–2. Cancer incidence and deaths by site and sex. (From Cancer Facts and Figures, 1982. American Cancer Society, 1981.)

be explored, and the available data frequently appear to conflict.

Energy

In animal studies chronic restriction of food inhibits the growth of most experimentally induced tumors and the occurrence of many spontaneous tumors.[96] However, hepatic tumors are stimulated by such restriction, while adrenal adenomas are unaffected. How does energy restriction inhibit tumor growth? According to one theory, mitotic activity is inhibited by the limited amount of carbohydrate and carbohydrate intermediates available for energy production. Other theories postulate that changes in hormones produced by energy restriction inhibit tumorigenesis by a complex but unknown mechanism.

Energy excess is more difficult to relate to cancer incidence. Part of the difficulty arises from the use of body weight when the correlation really should be made to total body fat and percentage body fat. Obesity has frequently, but not always, been reported as a risk for endometrial cancer.[13, 97] The relationship may be due to differences in estrogen metabolism in obese and thin women.[64] Obese women convert a larger percentage of androstenedione to estrone than do thin women. Studies using rats also demonstrate that the incidence of various types of tumors is consistently greater in heavier animals.

Lipid

Extensive epidemiological data show a positive correlation between the amount of fat in the diet and the incidence of some neoplasms. High-fat Western diets are associated with intestinal cancer in both males and females and with cancer of the breast in females. As shown in Figure 36–3, the classic work of Carroll and Khor demonstrated that mortality from breast cancer varies geographically by per capita dietary fat consumption.[15] In the past many investigators failed to distinguish between animal fat and vegetable fat or between saturated fat and unsaturated fat or to discuss the trans fatty acid component. More recent studies include this information and should shortly provide enough data to clarify the relationship.

Concomitant with changes in the amount of fat in the diet are changes in the character of the feces, metabolic products and transit time. Fecal constituents have been analyzed to determine if the correlation of lipid content to cancer is better than that of fat. Within a geographic area, populations with different levels of fat intake excreted different levels of fecal bile acids.[74] Studies with animals confirmed that animals consuming a high-fat diet excreted more total bile acids. Whether the amount of total bile acids in the intestinal tract influences the incidence of cancer is still not clear.

Some of the effects of a high-fat diet may be due to alterations in these other variables. The relatively low lipid content and high fiber content of the typical Seventh Day Adventist (vegetarian) diet have been suggested to account for the relatively low incidence of certain types of cancer in this group. On the other hand, populations such as Indians and Eskimos, who consume large amounts of fat with or without fiber intake, are not usually prone to colonic cancer.

Tumor growth appears to be affected by the type of lipid as well as by the amount of lipid ingested. In animals consuming a low-fat diet of polyunsaturated fats, tumorigenesis is enhanced. When the total fat intake is increased, the effect of fat unsaturation becomes less. In humans the data are even less clear. Still other data suggest a possible role for trans fatty acids in tumorigenesis.[36] Obviously, more controlled studies are needed on the effect of a diet high in polyunsaturated fatty acids on tumorigenesis.

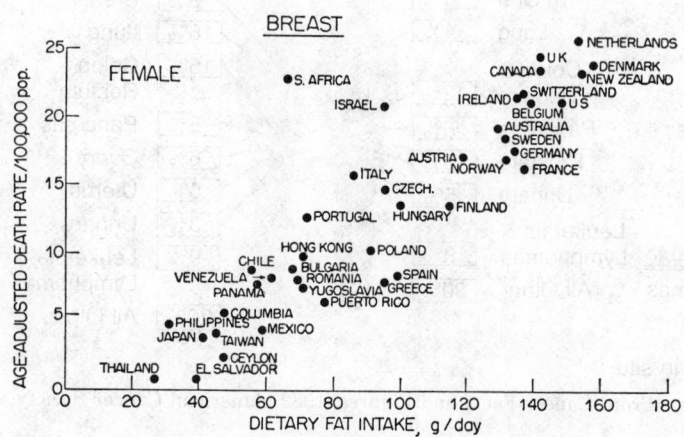

Figure 36–3. Positive correlation between per capita consumption of dietary fat and age-related mortality from cancer of the breast. (From: Carroll, K. K., and Khor, H. T.: Dietary fat in relation to tumorigenesis. Prog. Biochem. Pharmacol., *10*:308, 1975.)

The mechanism by which a high fat intake may facilitate tumor development may be hormonal. Certain hormone-dependent mammary tumors in rats require estrogen and prolactin for continued growth. In addition, a high fat intake raises the concentration of serum prolactin and thus might promote tumor growth. However, studies of plasma concentration of prolactin in women of various ethnic backgrounds suggest that elevation *per se* does not increase the risk of breast cancer in humans.[49] Hormones appear to make the cell susceptible to the carcinogenic event by their preparative and permissive properties.

Protein

Mortality from lymphoma and the consumption of animal protein, particularly beef protein, are positively correlated.[23] Understanding the role of protein in tumor development is complicated by the fact that most diets high in protein are also high in meat, which raises the fat content and lowers the fiber content of the diet. Epidemiological data indicate that those countries in which the intake of animal protein is increasing are also experiencing a concurrent rise in mortality from colonic cancer. However, the interaction between meat intake, fat intake and the incidence of colonic cancer is not at all clear.

The effect of protein on experimental carcinogenesis depends on the tissue of origin and the type and malignancy of the tumor, as well as on the type of protein and the caloric adequacy of the diet. Certain amino acid deficiencies inhibit some but not all tumors. Plasma amino acid concentrations and urinary amino acid excretion are altered in some patients with cancer, but the significance of these changes is not known.

Although the role of immunity in tumorigenesis is still questionable, the mechanism by which energy and protein affect the growth of tumors may involve cell-mediated immunity. Cell-mediated immunity is depressed when protein and energy intake are severely inadequate. Since cell-mediated immunity may be a defense against cancer, factors that alter cellular immunity could affect tumorigenesis. The effects of endocrine function (enhancement of tumorigenesis) seem to be in opposition to those of cell-mediated immunity (depression of tumorigenesis).

Vitamins

Deficiencies of some vitamins enhance tumor growth; deficiencies of other vitamins suppress it. Conversely, excesses of some vitamins enhance tumor growth, while excesses of others are inhibitory. The relationships are complex, knowledge of them is sparse, and many more studies are needed.

VITAMIN A. Epidemiological data suggest that relatively low dietary intakes of vitamin A are correlated with high incidence of cancer of the stomach, nasopharynx and lung when a correction is made for smoking habits. Plasma vitamin A and beta-carotene levels, indicators of the nutritional status of the vitamin in an individual, are low in patients with tumors of the alimentary tract.[8] However, these changes may be related to the presence of the tumor rather than being a cause of increased growth of the tumor.

Under certain conditions, retinol, retinoic acid, esters or ethers of retinol, and synthetic analogues of retinoic acid retard or inhibit tumor development. Studies in animals suggest that retinoic acid exerts its effect during promotion by a mechanism not yet identified. Theories state that vitamin A may stimulate the immune system, inhibit the binding of the carcinogen to DNA or control premalignant epithelial cell differentiation. Foods containing retinoids (forms of vitamin A) have some protective effect in preventing chemical carcinogenesis in epithelial tissues. Vitamin A deficiency in animals enhances their susceptibility to the chemical induction of some tumors. Since natural retinoids in the large doses required to produce this protective effect are also toxic and are largely deposited in the liver where they would have limited usefulness, the clinical application seems remote. Synthetic analogs of the vitamin have been used.

The positive results of initial, limited clinical trials suggest that retinoids can be combined with full dose chemotherapy. Beta-trans-retinoic acid delivered locally has resulted in reversal of pre-cancerous lesions of the cervix and 13-cis-retinoic acid has resulted in modest positive responses in patients with melanomas or tumors involving head, neck and lung.[67] Further testing will be required before these compounds are used routinely.

VITAMIN C. Ascorbic acid may also influence tumorigenesis. In one study 92 per cent of patients with malignant disease had leukocyte ascorbic acid levels less than the lower limit of normal range, and 60 per cent had very low levels.[58] Physical signs compatible with subclinical scurvy were seen in some patients with the lowest levels. Another study of cancer patients confirmed the low leukocyte ascorbic acid levels, and further, found that patients with bone metastases had lower vitamin C values than patients without bone metastases,[5] even though both groups were receiving vitamin supplements. These and other data suggest that large doses of vitamin C may retard collagen breakdown and, possibly, metastases.

There is a paucity of human epidemiological data regarding ascorbic acid and carcinogenesis. However, from available data, increased consumption of fruits and vegetables that contain substantial amounts of the vitamin are associated with lower risk for gastric and esophageal cancer. These studies provide mostly indirect evidence regarding a potential role of vitamin C in carcinogenesis. Addition of ascorbic acid to the medium of cells in culture has prevented chemically induced transformation in some cases and resulted in reversion of transformed cells in others. Laboratory studies suggest nitrosamine formation from nitrite can be prevented by ascorbic acid.

The best study negating the effects of supplemental ascorbic acid in patients with advanced cancer is a double-blind study conducted at the Mayo Clinic. The groups were well matched for age, sex, site of tumor, performance score, tumor grade and previous chemotherapy. No differences were found in survival, subjective improvement of symptoms, performance status, appetite or weight gain between those who recieved ascorbic acid and those who did not.[21]

VITAMIN E. There are no epidemiological reports on vitamin E intake and the risk of cancer. In mice, vitamin E has been shown to inhibit sarcoma cells from developing into tumors.[59] The amount of vitamin E needed depends on the amount of polyunsaturated fatty acids in the diet and the number of cancer cells present. Vitamin E may function by strengthening the antigenicity of cells, thereby exposing them to recognition and attack by the immune system. Vitamin E, like ascorbic acid, prevents the formation of nitrosamines in animals, but what role this may play in human cancer is not known. Finally vitamin E, as an antioxidant, may play a role in decreasing carcinogen-induced chromosomal breakage. The data are insufficient to draw any firm conclusions. Research presently underway should be most useful in clarifying the picture.

FOLIC ACID. Folic acid deficiency renders an individual more susceptible to environmental carcinogens. Folate deficiency increases the likelihood of breakage of chromosomes at fragile sites. Folate deficiency can be produced by a dietary lack or secondary to deficiencies of vitamin B_{12} or lipotropes such as methionine or choline. If the cell is incapable of synthesizing building blocks of DNA, it may fail to differentiate and replicate normally.

Folic acid therapy has recently been shown to improve mild to moderate dysplasia of the uterine cervix in a double-blind study. The authors of the study suggest that either a reversible, localized derangement of folate metabolism is misdiagnosed as cervical dysplasia or that the derangement is part of the dysplasia process and can be reversed by folate supplementation.[14]

Minerals

Industrial exposure to arsenic, cadmium, chromium and nickel results in increased incidence of various types of cancer in humans. Chromium and nickel salts are probably the most active carcinogens. Several other minerals produce tumors in animals, but have not been clearly identified as carcinogens in man.

There is a paucity of studies relating dietary minerals to carcinogenesis. Only two, selenium and iron, have been studied to any extent. High selenium in the soil is associated with a lower incidence of cancer of the colon, rectum and breast. Low selenium in the soil is associated with a higher incidence of cancer.[79] An antitumorigenic effect has also been demonstrated in animals, but the relevance of this for humans is not clear. Selenium may act as an antioxidant and work with other antioxidants such as vitamin E.

Animal experiments suggest that iron deficiency may increase susceptibility to some chemically induced tumors. Since iron sufficiency is required for optimal immune function[57] this could be the mechanism. Epidemiological evidence suggests a relationship to gastric cancer. High dietary zinc is associated with an increased incidence of cancer of the breast and stomach. Iodine deficiency and excess may increase the risk of thyroid carcinoma. The limited optimal range of intake of trace minerals makes their roles in carcinogenesis difficult to ascertain.

Fiber

In recent years much attention has been focused on the possible protective role of fiber in the prevention of cancer of the large bowel (colon and rectum). This interest has stemmed from the observation that the incidence of colonic cancer is lower among black Africans, who consume a diet high in unabsorbable fiber, than among Western populations who consume a diet low in fiber. As was mentioned earlier, no single component of the diet can change independently of other components. Consequently, dietary fiber intake affects meat, fat and refined carbohydrate intakes. The quantity of dietary fiber affects intestinal microflora, bile salt metabolism, transit time and fecal bulk, any or all of which may be involved in bowel carcinogenesis. There are other components of foods rich in fiber that may also affect carcinogenesis, but these are not well defined at present.

Higher numbers of certain anaerobes and lower counts of *Streptococcus* and other aerobic microorganisms were found in fecal specimens of individuals consuming a high-fat, high-meat diet or a high-beef diet. Other investigators found no significant differences, however. In addition to the variation in the number and types of microorganisms found in some individuals, there are differences in the metabolism of the microorganism of people following various dietary regimens. There also are variations in persons who have cancer compared with those who do not have cancer.

The results of a large collaborative study of diet, bowel function, fecal characteristics and large bowel cancer have recently been published.[52] Thirty men in each of four study areas varying in cancer incidence were studied extensively. Data from this and other studies[22, 48, 53] support the hypothesis that dietary fat promotes large bowel cancer by increasing bile acid output and that dietary fiber may reduce the risk by increasing fecal bulk thereby decreasing the concentration of carcinogens or cocarcinogens in contact with the colonic mucosa.

Alcohol

Several epidemiological studies suggest that alcohol plays a causative role in carcinogenesis. Alcohol could play a role in carcinogenesis either directly as a cell toxin or as a vehicle for cocarcinogens or indirectly by depressing the immune response or altering metabolism of vitamins. Well-controlled studies do not support a role for alcohol as a directly causative factor in carcinogenesis, but support the role of alcohol as an enhancer or promoter of tumorigenesis. Excessive alcohol intake appears to be most critical when the individual smokes.

Nitrates, Nitrites, Nitrosamines

Nitrates and nitrites have received a great deal of attention because of the relationship these compounds have with nitrosamines, which are potent carcinogens in various species. Nitrate can be readily reduced to nitrite, which in turn can interact with dietary substrates such as amines to produce N-nitroso compounds or nitrosamines. This conversion, known as N-nitrosation, has been demonstrated in the human stomach and colon, as well as in the bladder and saliva. It is not known, however, whether this mechanism is a cause of any human cancer.

Nitrates are present in a variety of foods, the main dietary sources being vegetables and drinking water. Meats that have been cured with nitrate are also contributors. The average person in the U.S. obtains 1.1 μg. of nitrosamines daily from food and if a smoker 17 μg. from each pack of cigarettes.[12] The use of nitrogen fertilizers has increased the nitrate levels of water in several areas and epidemiological studies have demonstrated an association between gastric cancer and fertilizer use. However, a relationship between cancer and nitrate levels of water supplies has not been consistently observed. Likewise, studies of the dietary habits of gastric cancer patients as compared with controls have not consistently identified a food item that is associated with increased risk, although food items have been linked with lower gastric cancer risk. These foods are in general rich in ascorbic acid, which has been shown to inhibit nitrosamine formation. A negative association between stomach cancer and ascorbic acid intake has been found, which lends further support to the hypothesis that stomach cancer is caused by endogenous formation of nitrosamine and that vitamin C may be protective.[56] The N-nitrosation reaction is also inhibited by tocopherol, although the significance of this is not known. At present, the evidence regarding dietary nitrate ingestion and human cancer is suggestive, but a conclusion must await further research.

Artificial Sweeteners

The use of artificial sweeteners has been investigated primarily in relation to bladder cancer, largely because of experimental evidence that large doses of *saccharin* produce tumors of the urinary tract and promote the action of carcinogens in the bladder of rats. In humans, several epidemiological studies suggest that the use of artificial sweeteners does not increase the risk of bladder cancer. It should be recognized, however, that detection of a weak carcinogenic effect is difficult and that there may be an effect of heavy use in certain individuals.[69]

On the other hand, the artificial sweetener *cyclamate* has been removed from the market because of toxic effects of its principal metabolite. These effects include chromosomal abnormalities and testicular atrophy in animals and dermatitis and convulsions in humans.[72]

Aspartame has not been seen to be carcinogenic in experimental studies; epidemiological data await its widespread use since it has been approved.

Other Additives

Butylated hydroxytoluene (BHT) and *butylated hydroxyanisole (BHA)* are antioxidants widely used as preservatives. Studies have suggested a tumor-promoting effect of BHT, but no such activity has been seen with BHA. On the other hand, BHT has been shown also to inhibit carcinogenesis under certain conditions.[83]

Method of Food Preparation

The mode of cooking may be associated with human cancers. Several investigators have found mutagenic activity in foods subjected to charcoal broiling and frying. Furthermore, mutagenic activity has been demonstrated in the urine of human subjects after eating fried meats.[3] Smoked foods are contaminated by carcinogenic polycyclic aromatic hydrocarbons. Accordingly, epidemiological studies have indicated an association between the increased incidence of cancer of the intestine and the frequent consumption of smoked foods.[39]

Coffee

There is little evidence linking coffee intake with increased cancer risk. According to laboratory studies, the caffeine component of coffee does not appear to be carcinogenic. A number of studies investigating the association between coffee drinking and bladder cancer show slightly increased risks and are not consistent between men and women. Results from a large international collaborative case-control study indicate that coffee drinking confers little or no risk of bladder cancer.[70] Recent reports suggest an association of coffee drinking with the occurrence of pancreatic cancer, although the evidence is limited and not conclusive.[62, 65] A large prospective cohort study of over 16,000 men and women in Norway found no increased rate of cancer of any site with coffee drinking.[51] The associations observed in this study are in the opposite direction; i.e., coffee appears to reduce the risk of certain cancers and of cancer over all. More research is needed, with an emphasis on distinguishing between types of processed coffees, such as freeze-dried and instant coffees.

DIETARY GUIDELINES FOR CANCER PREVENTION

Foods contain both promoters and inhibitors of carcinogenesis. The study of the effects of each component of foods on carcinogenesis may not provide the complete answer. The answer may be less clear-cut, because the overall effect of the diet may result from a particular balance of promoters and inhibitors. The balance may not be definable for all individuals under all circumstances. This does not mean that nothing can be done, but rather that practical advice may have to be more general.

The Committee on Diet, Nutrition and Cancer of the National Research Council has formulated interim dietary guidelines consistent with good nutritional practice that are *likely* to reduce the risk of cancer.[18] They are summarized in Table 36–1. To obtain maximal benefit all must be applied together with reduction in cigarette smoking. Since the data base is incomplete and there is a great deal of active research currently underway, the National Cancer Institute will review the guidelines at least every five years.

The interim guidelines may never be more specific, but if they are followed, the overall effect will be a decrease in cancer incidence.

Nutritional Effects of Cancer

The adverse nutritional effects of cancer can be severe, and may be compounded by the effects of the therapeutic regimens and the psychological impact of cancer. Often the result is a profound state of depletion. Since the increased morbidity and mortality of malnourished patients is well known, the incentive to prevent or reverse these effects is evident.

Cachexia

Malnutrition is a major cause of morbidity and mortality in cancer patients, in whom it is usually seen as a syndrome known as *cancer cachexia*. A number of factors predispose the patient to the development of cachexia; however, the malignancy itself is responsible for initiating the syndrome and its reversal is achieved only by control of the disease.[88] Cancer cachexia presents clinically with anorexia, weight loss, anemia, diminished reflexes, asthenia and emaciation. Although there are similarities in the cachexia of cancer patients and non-cancer patients, there is evidence that cancer cachexia

---

Table 36–1. NATIONAL RESEARCH COUNCIL INTERIM DIETARY GUIDELINES FOR CANCER PREVENTION

1. Decrease fat intake from 40 to 30% of calories.
2. Increase intake of fruits, vegetables and whole grains.
3. Minimize consumption of food preserved by salt curing, salt pickling or smoking.
4. Minimize contamination of foods with carcinogens from any source.
5. If alcoholic beverages are consumed, consumption should be moderate.
6. Decrease cigarette smoking*

* In the report, the NRC Committee recommends that alcohol consumption be reduced particularly by cigarette smokers. The authors believe cigarette smoking is a prime risk factor and should be severely reduced or stopped.

From: Committee on Diet, Nutrition and Cancer, National Research Council: Diet, Nutrition and Cancer. Washington, D.C., National Academy of Sciences, 1982.

is a complex metabolic problem unique to malignant disease and involves aberrations in substrate metabolism, water, electrolyte and acid-base balances, vitamin metabolism, enzyme systems, and immune and endocrine functions.

ENERGY METABOLISM. Weight loss results from a negative energy balance, although the nature of the negative balance is unclear. Is the wasting due to a reduction in energy intake or an increase in expenditure? There is experimental and clinical evidence that both mechanisms occur.

Energy intake has been repeatedly shown to be voluntarily reduced in tumor-bearing animals. Similar reductions have been reported in patients with various malignancies and stages of disease. However, the severity of the weight loss does not directly correlate with nutrient consumption; decreased intake cannot entirely explain the progressive weight loss.[88]

The normal response to decreased food intake, or semistarvation, is lowered basal metabolic rate (BMR). However, patients with cancer and tumor-bearing animals exhibit the opposite response. Significantly increased BMR and total energy expenditure have been seen in cancer patients as compared with age, sex, and activity-matched controls.[78] The mechanism for this increase is unknown; it does not appear to be a result of tumor growth alone, but of host metabolic alterations as well. One half of the resting energy expenditure has been estimated to be due to protein turnover.[98] Rates of protein synthesis and degradation may be changed in patients with cancer.[55, 63] These alterations, particularly those increasing the rates of synthesis, may account for the increase in energy expenditure. More research is needed to clarify the mechanisms involved.

SUBSTRATE METABOLISM. Energy metabolism is intimately related to carbohydrate, protein and lipid metabolism, all of which are altered by tumor growth. The tumor is a glucose drain, exerting a consistent demand for glucose on the host.[80] The neoplastic cell exhibits a characteristically high rate of anaerobic metabolism yielding lactate as the end product. This expanded lactic acid pool requires an increased rate of host gluconeogenesis via the Cori cycle which is significantly increased in cachectic cancer patients.[77] The high rate of gluconeogenesis may be largely responsible for promoting weight loss and is thought to be, in part, a manifestation of the noted relative resistance to endogenous and exogenous insulin.[50] Impaired glucose tolerance is also widely seen.

Alterations are seen in protein metabolism and appear to be directed toward providing adequate amino acids for tumor growth.[55] Most notable is the loss of skeletal muscle protein, which is due to both a decrease in the rate of synthesis and an increase in the rate of degradation of muscle protein.[41] Likewise, the rate of serum albumin synthesis diminishes and in some cases the rate of its degradation increases, accounting in part for the hypoalbuminemia characteristic of cachectic cancer patients. Negative nitrogen balance is frequently seen, and evidence suggests that the tumor retains nitrogen at the expense of host tissues.[9]

Also evident in patients with advanced cancer is the production of novel proteins and peptides, which are distinct from normal plasma and urine constituents. These are thought to be produced by the tumor, although it may be that the tumor induces the host to produce them.[88] The significance of these novel proteins is not clear.

Lipid metabolism is altered, as evidenced by inappropriate mobilization of free fatty acids from adipose tissues and subsequent depletion of total body fat. Disorders may also be seen as decreased lipid clearance from serum and elevated plasma free fatty acid levels. The mechanisms are not known, although insulin and other hormones (norepinephrine, ACTH, glucagon) have been implicated.[77] Supporting evidence suggests that the tumor produces lipolytic substances directly responsible for increased fat mobilization.[61]

Other Metabolic Abnormalities

Fluid and electrolyte imbalances are seen in patients with advanced cancer, the most frequent being hyponatremia. Hypoalbuminemia and hypocalcemia are also often seen. Severe imbalances in fluid and electrolyte status may be present in patients with cancers that promote excessive diarrhea or vomiting, and similar consequences result from hormone-secreting tumors that impair renal function.

Recent radioisotope tracer studies have shown advanced cancer patients to be overhydrated.[17, 95] Since body weight is widely used as an index of nutritional status, this overhydration may be misleading. Therefore, other indices of nutritional status should be used in conjunction with body weight.

Vitamin and mineral metabolism is altered in malignant disease, although much remains to be discovered. Serum levels of ascorbic acid, thiamin, folate, vitamin A, iron and zinc are often depressed, while serum copper is increased.[29, 42] The significance of these changes remains speculative; however, supplemental therapy may be useful for relieving symptoms.

The activities of several enzyme systems are affected, as are certain endocrine functions, and the nature of the alterations varies by tumor type. Host immunological function is impaired, apparently the result of both the neoplasm and the progressive malnutrition.

In addition to the cancer-induced metabolic effects, the mass of the tumor may anatomically alter the normal physiology of specific organ systems. This may be expected to disturb normal function and affect nutritional status accordingly.

Sensory Changes

Alterations in taste and smell sensations are common and contribute to the anorexia frequently seen in cancer patients. The recognition threshold for sweet is increased and for bitter is often lowered, while thresholds for sour and salt tend to increase, although there is considerable variation among reported studies.[25, 91] The sensation abnormalities do not consistently correlate with the extent of tumor involvement, tumor response to therapy, and food preferences and intake. Lowered taste threshold for bitter may lead to total meat aversion.

Nutritional Effects of Cancer Therapy

Antitumor therapy may involve chemotherapy, radiation or surgery or be a multimodal combination of these. Certain hematological malignancies are treated by bone marrow transplantation. Each of these therapeutic programs contributes to the nutritional alterations of the cancer patient by reducing food intake, decreasing absorption or altering metabolism.

Chemotherapy

The action of the chemotherapeutic agents is not limited to malignant tissue but affects normal cells as well. As a result, evidence of major organ toxicities are seen and dietary intake and nutritional status are adversely affected. Food intake is inhibited by the mucositis, (Figure 36–4), cheilosis, glossitis, stomatitis and esophagitis caused by many drugs. Table 36–2 summarizes the side effects of many drugs. Nausea and vomiting occur with almost all antineoplastic drugs. Taste abnormalities frequently result, leading to anorexia and *oligophagy* (eating few foods). Diarrhea may be induced or there may be constipation or *adynamic ileus* (inhibition of bowel motility). Symptoms of gastrointestinal toxicity are usually not long-lasting; however, some combination chemotherapeutic programs have severe and prolonged gastrointestinal effects.[30, 33] Some of the agents, especially corticosteroids, cause tissue breakdown and promote excessive urinary loss of protein, potassium and calcium. The intestinal mucosa and digestive

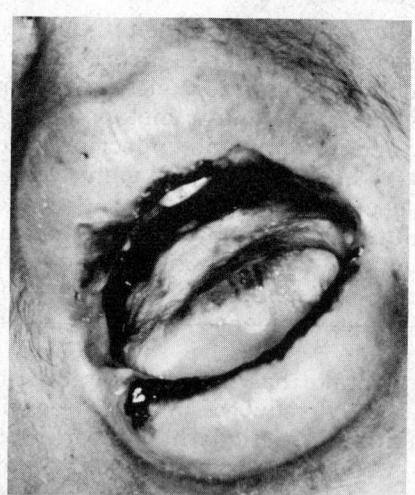

Figure 36–4. Severe oral mucositis following marrow transplantation. Patient has also had high dose cyclophosphamide and whole body radiation. (From Peterson, D. E., and Sonis, S. T. (eds.): Oral Complications of Cancer Therapy. The Hague, Martinus Nijhoff Publishing, 1983, p. 128.)

processes are affected, altering digestion and absorption to some degree. Protein, energy and vitamin metabolism may be altered, although the consequences of this are not known. Total lymphocyte count is depressed and does not accu-

Table 36–2. CHEMOTHERAPEUTIC AGENTS USED IN ONCOLOGY THAT MAY CAUSE NUTRITIONALLY LIMITING GASTROINTESTINAL TOXICITY

Anorexia, nausea, vomiting	Adriamycin
	5-Azacytidine
	cis-Diamminedichloroplatinum
	Cyclophosphamide
	Nitrogen mustard
	Procarbazine
Mucositis	Actinomycin D
	Adriamycin
	Bleomycin
	Daunomycin
	5-Fluorouracil
	Methotrexate
	Vinblastine
Diarrhea	Actinomycin D
	5-Azacytidine
	5-Fluorouracil
	Methotrexate
Constipation, adynamic ileus	Vinblastine
	Vincristine
Organ damage	
Liver	Asparaginase
	Azaserine
	Methotrexate
	6-Mercaptopurine
	Mithramycin
Pancreas	Asparaginase

From Donaldson, S.S.: Effects of therapy on nutritional status of the pediatric cancer patient. Cancer Res. *42*:(Suppl.), 729s, 1982. for page 744 rately reflect nutritional status when antineoplastic agents are administered.[84]

Radiation Therapy

The effects of radiation vary according to the region irradiated. Radiation to the head and neck causes a variety of food ingestion problems, including sore throat, mucositis, *xerostomia* (mouth dryness), severe dental and gum destruction, and altered taste and smell. Anorexia is common and weight loss is a major problem. Radiation to the thorax induces esophagitis with accompanying dysphagia. Esophageal stricture leading to obstruction can occur. Radiation to the abdomen may produce acute gastritis or enteritis with nausea, vomiting, diarrhea and anorexia; severe gastrointestinal damage is accompanied by malabsorption of glucose, lactose, fats and electrolytes. Radiation enteritis can develop into a chronic form, with symptoms of ulceration or obstruction intensifying the risk of malnutrition. Total body irradiation may cause all of the above acute symptoms to some degree. As with chemotherapy, radiation depresses immune function, thereby limiting the applicability of this as a nutritional assessment indicator.

Radiochemotherapy

The use of radiation concurrently with chemotherapy is preferred therapy for a number of malignant diseases. Although the information is limited, the deleterious nutrition effects of the radiation therapy are probably enhanced by its combination with antitumor drugs. In some cases the toxic effects are simply additive; however, in others the effects are much greater in severity than the sum of the individual effects.[33]

Surgery

The nutritional consequences of surgery depend upon the locale and the extensiveness of the procedure. Surgical resection of the oral cavity and pharynx interferes with the mechanics of food ingestion and may necessitate prolonged dependency on tube feedings. Esophageal resection often results in varying degrees of fat malabsorption, possibly due to disruption of the vagus nerve, with attendant steatorrhea and diarrhea. Resection of the stomach by partial or total gastrectomy may limit total energy intake owing to postoperative symptoms of the dumping syndrome. Absorption of fat, iron, vitamin B_{12} and calcium may be impaired, evidenced clinically by steatorrhea and anemia. Absorption of vitamins A, B and D may also be less efficient. Resection of the duodenum affects pancreatic and biliary secretion, with malabsorption of various nutrients. Compensatory changes in the ileum of patients who have had jejunal resection allow near normal absorption, although the efficiency is decreased. Resection of the ileum may cause vitamin B_{12} and bile salt malabsorption. Massive small bowel resection presents more serious nutritional problems, dependent upon the compensatory function of the remaining segments. Gastric hypersecretion may result from massive resection, intensifying the already present diarrhea.[60] Radical colonic surgery promotes water and electrolyte loss. Partial or total resection of the pancreas produces insufficiency or loss of pancreatic enzymes and insulin, resulting in malabsorption of fat, protein, and complex carbohydrates as well as the metabolic effects of insulin deficiency. Nutritional effects of surgery are discussed further in Chapter 34. Articles by Brennan[10] and Lawrence[60] discuss further the effects of cancer surgery on nutrition.

Marrow Transplantation

Marrow transplantation is performed for the treatment of certain hematological malignancies, such as leukemia and lymphoma and occasionally solid tumors. The preparative regimen includes cytotoxic chemotherapy and total body irradiation to suppress immunological reactivity and eradicate malignant cells. This is followed by intravenous infusion of bone marrow from a suitable donor.[89] Acute toxic reactions such as nausea, vomiting and diarrhea diminish 24 to 48 hours after administration of cytotoxic therapy and irradiation. Delayed effects during the first month to two months post-transplant include mucositis, stomatitis, esophagitis, salivary and taste alterations and gut damage. Patients typically have little or no oral intake during the first 30 days post-transplant and must be supported by parenteral nutrition.

Graft-versus-host disease (GVHD) is a major complication in which donor marrow cells react against the tissues of the "foreign" host. The functions of several target organs (skin, liver, gut, lymphoid cells) are disrupted and susceptibility to infection is increased.[90] GVHD of the intestinal tract is usually manifested within the first 70 days post-transplant[40] and may be resolved or may go on to a chronic form requiring long-term treatment and dietary management. Liver GVHD, evidenced by icterus and abnormal liver function tests, frequently accompanies gastrointestinal GVHD and further complicates nutritional management.

Hepatic veno-occlusive disease (VOD) is characterized by chemotherapy-induced damage to the hepatic venules. It can develop one to three weeks post-transplant, resulting in symptoms of hepatomegaly, ascites, jaundice and encephalopathy and presents a difficult clinical nutritional management situation.[82] The side effects of cancer therapy that may cause nutritional problems are summarized in Table 36–3.

Nutritional Care of the Patient with Cancer

A common secondary diagnosis in patients with advanced neoplastic disease is protein-energy malnutrition. Severe protein-energy malnutrition has been associated with decreased survival, reduced tolerance to therapy, and increased postoperative morbidity.[38, 47, 92] Even small amounts of weight loss prior to therapy (less than 5 per cent of body weight) may worsen prognosis significantly.[27] Because of this, the importance of early nutritional assessment and intervention as a preventive measure seems clear. The unclear issue, however, is the efficacy of nutritional repletion of already malnourished patients. Nutritional repletion is usually achieved by aggressive modes of support via enteral intubation or parenteral hyperalimentation. The beneficial effects of such support on tolerance to chemotherapy and radiation therapy, postsurgical complications and response to therapy have not been positively demonstrated. Improvements in nutritional support and neoplastic therapy are required to clarify the issue.[11, 20] Of concern also is the possibility that nutritional support will preferentially benefit the tumor. In tumor-bearing animals, nutritional repletion stimulates tumor growth while improving host nutritional status. This has not been observed in cancer patients, although further study is warranted. Thus, the controversy regarding the merits of nutritional support for cancer patients remains. Nevertheless, the adverse effects of malnutrition are clear. Nutritional support does serve as prevention and therapy for malnutrition, and in this function plays an important role in care of the cancer patient.

Goals of Care

The overall goals of the nutritional care of the cancer patient are to (1) prevent or correct nutritional deficiencies and (2) minimize weight loss.[87] The emphasis is on prevention. Unfortunately, nutritional consultation is often considered only after the patient becomes severely depleted. The health care plan should include initial assessment to determine the risk of nutritional depletion. This can be accomplished preferably at the first admission, and those at risk can effectively be identified and supportive care planned. The nutritional assessment should include: (1) medical, social and nutritional history, (2) anthropometric data, (3) nutrient and drug interactions, (4) biochemical measurements and (5) oral intake or dietary analysis. Routine periodic nutritional assessment at each clinic follow-up or at least monthly should be done. Nutritional assessment is discussed in Chapter 9 and suggestions for screening evaluation procedures and forms are given by Shils.[81] Nutritional care planning is discussed in Chapter 19.

Strategies for modifying nutrient intake will depend upon the specific feeding problem and the extent of depletion. The oral route is the preferred mode of feeding but may be resisted by the patient suffering from anorexia, nausea, altered taste sensations and dysphagia. Eating is encouraged by modifying the food and its presentation. Those patients experiencing altered taste acuity may benefit from increased use of sugar flavorings and seasonings in food preparation. Meat aversion requires emphasis of alternate sources of protein. Dysphagia due to lesions in the oral and esophageal tissues can be

Table 36–3. POTENTIAL SIDE EFFECTS OF CANCER THERAPY THAT MAY CAUSE NUTRITIONAL PROBLEMS

RADIATION TREATMENT

Nausea, vomiting and general loss of appetite
Taste and smell changes
Dental problems
Mucositis and xerostomia (mouth dryness)
Esophageal stricture from radiation to thorax
Diarrhea; malabsorption resulting from bowel damage
Depressed immune function

SURGICAL TREATMENT

Dependence on tube feeding as a result of resection of oropharyngeal area
Malabsorption resulting from resection of segments of gastrointestinal tract
Dumping syndrome resulting from gastrectomy
Hypoglycemia resulting from gastrectomy
Altered water and electrolyte balance resulting from ileostomy and colostomy
Diabetes mellitus resulting from pancreatectomy

CHEMOTHERAPY TREATMENT

Taste abnormalities
Mucositis, cheilosis, glossitis, stomatitis and esophagitis
Diarrhea and malabsorption from gastrointestinal toxicity
Nausea, anorexia and vomiting
Anemias
Depressed immune function

MARROW TRANSPLANTATION

Mucositis, stomatitis and esophagitis
Taste and salivary changes
Gastrointestinal damage
Graft versus host disease leading to disruption of skin, liver and gastrointestinal cells
Hepatic veno-occlusive disease causing severe liver dysfunction and metabolic problems

lessened with foods that are soft and liquid and at moderate or room temperature. Topical anesthetic solutions applied orally prior to eating are beneficial. Artificial saliva preparations and saliva stimulants are useful in cases of diminished salivation, as are foods with high moisture content. Patients with intestinal damage may require dietary modifications in lactose, fat and fiber content as well as texture. Commercial nutritional supplements can be useful in many dietary plans. Guidelines for oral feedings are presented in Table 36–4.

Timing of Food Presentation

The timing of food presentation deserves consideration. Cancer patients complain of decreased ability to eat as the day progresses, the morning being best for eating. This symptom may be due to sluggish digestion and gastric emptying as a result of decreased produc-

tion of digestive secretions, gastrointestinal mucosal atrophy, and gastric muscle atrophy.[25] Frequent small feedings with particular emphasis on the morning feedings would be beneficial.

The timing of meals or snacks relative to gastrointestinal (GI) toxic therapy may have a bearing on subsequent learned food aversions. *Learned food aversions* are developed by associating specific foods with unpleasant symptoms such as nausea and vomiting. Children introduced to a new food prior to GI toxic chemotherapy were less likely than similarly treated children not given the new food to choose that food after therapy.[6] The new food is paired with the unpleasant effects of therapy. Similar results were seen in adult cancer patients.[7] The effect may not be limited to new food items but also involve foods in the patient's usual diet eaten prior to treatment. Radiation-induced taste aversions have been demonstrated in animals, although it is not known whether this occurs in humans.[85]

TABLE 36–4. GUIDELINES FOR ORAL FEEDING DURING ANTITUMOR THERAPY

PROBLEM	DIET	SUPPLEMENTS AND AIDS	POORLY TOLERATED FOODS
Treatment phase: Acute GI toxicity	Clear liquid: cold liquids	None	Milk, milk products; hot soups; cereals; sandwiches
Post-treatment phase: Stomatitis, esophagitis	Liquid to soft: broth-based soups, fruit-ades, carbonated beverages, frozen grapes, melons, alter texture, temperature	Glucose polymers, mild-flavored supplements, topical anesthetics, frequent oral hygiene, frequent normal saline rinses	Juices, esp. citrus; milk, milk products; crisp or raw foods; meats; bread products; granular-textured foods
Viscous mucus production	Liquid: tea with lemon, juices, fruit-ades, popsicles, carbonated beverages, lemon-flavored liquids	Glucose polymers, artificial saliva, frequent normal saline rinses	Milk, milk products; gelatin; viscous liquids
Decreased salivation	Regular, high-moisture: gravies, sauces, casseroles, chicken, fish, beverages with foods, citric acid–containing foods	Milk- soy- or albumin-based supplements; artificial saliva; glucose polymers; saliva stimulants; sugarless lemon drops, gum; frequent normal saline rinses	Dry foods; bread products; meats
Hypogeusia	Regular, strongly flavored: highly spiced foods, emphasis on texture, aroma	Flavored supplements, frequent normal saline rinses	Bland foods
Dysgeusia	Regular, cold foods: milk, milk products; modify sweet, salt flavors; emphasis on experimentation	Fruit-flavored supplements	Red meats; chocolate; coffee
Steatorrhea, diarrhea	Liquid to soft, high-protein, high-calorie: modify lactose, fat, fiber content	Lactose-free, low-osmolality supplements; glucose polymers; lactose enzyme preparations; medium-chain triglycerides	Raw fruits; vegetables; milk, milk products; highly spiced foods

Developed by Carrie L. Cheney, M.S., R.D., and Saundra N. Aker, R.D., Fred Hutchinson Cancer Research Center, Seattle.

Accommodating Taste Changes

The patient should be the guide for which foods will be eaten and how well they are seasoned. Cold food, such as sandwiches, cottage cheese and salad plates, is frequently better accepted.[16, 43, 87] Aromas from hot foods sometimes aggravate nausea. Lemons and dill pickles are requested frequently by children and appear to curb nausea.[43] Popsicles are sometimes accepted when patients cannot tolerate other food.

Enteral Tube Feeding

Efforts to encourage oral intake sometimes fail or are inappropriate and more aggressive feeding methods are required. If the gut is functional, enteral tube feeding is utilized. The nasogastric route is most often used, although tubes may be inserted elsewhere in the intestinal tract as necessary. The selection of the enteral solution is determined by several factors, including the functional capacity of the gut, the intubation site, the patient's metabolic status, and the cost and convenience considerations, especially if used at home. Table 35–7 describes available enteral preparations. Blenderized formulas (Table 35–9) may be used with large-diameter tubes and have the advantage of lower cost, but are not suitable for the more common small-diameter feeding tubes. Commercial milk-based or soy-based formulas serve most needs. Defined formula diets can be utilized in patients with decreased digestive capacity. Patients with radiation enteritis or existing malnutrition may have multiple malabsorption problems and benefit from soy-based (lactose-free), low-residue and low-fat formulas.[28]

Parenteral Nutrition

If the gastrointestinal tract is not functioning, intravenous alimentation, or parenteral nutrition (PN), must be considered. This mode of feeding involves the administration of concentrated nutrient solutions via infusion into a larger-diameter vein, usually the subclavian vein. Parenteral nutritional support may be partial, to supplement a limited oral intake, or it may be the only source of nutrient intake, in which case it is referred to as *total parenteral nutrition* (TPN).

The ideal parenteral nutrient solution for cancer patients has not been determined. Energy and protein are usually given as glucose and a mixture of amino acids. Intravenous fat may be given to prevent essential fatty acid deficiency and as a concentrated source of calories. Electrolytes are added to the solution, as are certain trace metals and vitamins. Details regarding the nutrient composition and administration are given in Chapter 35.

Mullen[71] reviewed the frequency and severity of complications of PN in the cancer patient relative to those in the non-cancer patient and concluded that PN is equally safe for both. Complications of PN are occasionally seen, including catheter-related infections, venous thrombosis, and fluid overload. Mild to moderate elevations in tests of liver function have been reported in association with the use of TPN in cancer patients,[94] as has lactic acidosis.[66] Intense monitoring and specialized care are required. The use of PN on an outpatient basis is successful in selected cases if the patient and family are cooperative and instructed in its use. Parenteral nutrition at home is discussed on page 732.

Patient Cooperation

Regardless of which mode of feeding is utilized, nutritional goals should be specified. These should be achievable and limited in scope to encourage patient cooperation. The goals should be directed toward a visible means of feedback, such as body weight or some other meaningful index. Of primary importance in the success of any nutritional care plan is patient education. Instruction of the patient and family members regarding problems to be expected and their possible solutions should be initiated early in the course of cancer therapy and be ongoing in conjunction with follow-up nutritional assessment.

THE PEDIATRIC PATIENT WITH CANCER

Like the adult cancer patient, the child with cancer can suffer adverse nutritional consequences as a result of both the malignancy and the treatment. Overt malnutrition has been found in a high percentage of children at the time of diagnosis, indicating the substantial metabolic and symptomatic effects of the tumor.[31] The effects of antitumor therapy are similar to those described previously for cancer patients in general. Treatment commonly is multimodal and the complications of radiation may be enhanced by combination with chemotherapy. In addition, the nutrient requirements per kg of body weight of a child are greater. Thus, the child with cancer is at high risk for protein-energy malnutrition, and its impact is reflected in tolerance to treatment, incidence of complications, response to therapy, and survival.[76]

The psychological impacts of fear, unpleasant hospital routines, unfamiliar foods, learned food aversions, and pain require creative efforts to minimize their effects. Emphasis is placed on individual needs and making eating a pleasant experience. Nutritional supplements given orally can be useful, although their acceptance is often a problem and the child should be offered a selection from which to choose. As feeding by nasogastric tube is not usually an acceptable alternative in young children, efforts to encourage eating by serving familiar foods and encouraging parental involvement are vital.

If these efforts are not successful, or if the gastrointestinal tract is not functioning adequately, parenteral nutrition is an alternative. Parenteral nutrition is also indicated for children who present at the beginning of therapy in a malnourished state.[34, 76] Additionally, prophylactic use of PN and bowel rest for patients at risk for enteritis (those receiving abdominal or pelvic irradiation) might minimize intestinal trauma.[19] The efficacy of its routine use in all children at risk, however, has not been supported.[31] The use of PN in children is described in Chapter 35.

The nutritional requirements for the pediatric cancer patient are similar to those of normal growing children with the addition of a requirement for stress due to therapy and the tumor. DeWys[26] has estimated the "stress allowance" to be an additional 20 per cent of both protein and energy.

The long-term nutritional effects of cancer and its treatment in children are not well documented. Deficiencies in energy and protein can be expected to adversely affect growth, although the impact may be temporary and compensation may occur after cessation of successful tumor therapy. A survey of children with acute lymphocytic leukemia reported a delay in linear growth rate during the period of treatment followed by resumption of normal or even accelerated growth after completion of therapy.[93] On the other hand, the treatment may have effects on growth independent of nutritional deprivation. Pastore and coworkers[73] observed a high frequency of neurological and musculoskeletal sequelae after therapy in infancy. In older children kyphoscoliosis was a common late effect of radiotherapy for cancer. With the increase in survival rates for several childhood cancers, further studies of the long-term effects are needed.

THE TERMINAL CANCER PATIENT

The use of aggressive nutritional support techniques can prolong life, an unquestionable benefit for many patients undergoing therapy. It is of questionable benefit, however, for the patient for whom antitumor therapy has failed and who has no meaningful expectations of positive outcome. An extension of life in the case of the terminal cancer patient usually represents an extension of suffering and financial burden. More appropriate are suggestions for oral feedings as tolerated and the provision of emotional support. The pleasurable aspects of eating should be emphasized, without concern for quantity or nutrient content.

NUTRITIONAL CONSIDERATIONS FOR PATIENTS WITH SPECIFIC CANCERS

The nutritional impact of the disease and the therapy for most types of cancers is generally nonspecific and affects intake, absorption and metabolism. The intervention strategies to avoid or correct malnutrition will be determined by the number, type and severity of the complications of treatment. Malignancies of certain organs, however, do have specific nutritional considerations.

Oral Cavity, Pharynx, and Esophagus

The patient with cancer of the oral cavity, pharynx or esophagus may present with existing nutritional problems at the time of diagnosis, due to eating problems caused by the tumor mass, obstruction, oral infection and ulceration, or coexisting alcoholism frequently associated with these tumors.[35] This is compounded by the treatment, which commonly involves surgical resection and regional irradiation and may include chemotherapy. Chewing, swallowing, salivation and taste acuity are affected. Extensive dental decay, osteoradionecrosis and infections may occur. Chemotherapy, if given, can be expected to also produce nausea, vomiting and anorexia. Resection of the esophagus can result in fat malabsorption with varying degrees of steatorrhea.[60]

Initially, some form of nutritional support must be provided. Tube feedings are generally utilized if the remainder of the gastrointestinal tract is functional. The extent of the resection may require long-term feeding by tube if the ability to eat cannot be regained. If oral feeding is possible postsurgically, general dietary recommendations would include liquid or soft-textured moist foods for easy mastication and swallowing, and small, frequent meals of relatively high caloric density. The use of complex carbohydrates is preferred rather than the more cariogenic simple carbohydrates and simple sugars. Liquid nutritional supplements can be useful. Periodic application of an artificial saliva solution is also helpful, as is the frequent consumption of fluids to aid the dry mouth. Use of medium-chain triglycerides in food preparation can benefit the patient suffering from persistent steatorrhea.

A treatment regimen has been developed that significantly reduces morbidity from the therapeutic irradiation of the jaws.[75] During the pre-irradiation period, the patient's oropharyngeal area is evaluated by radiographic and oral examination, and then non-salvageable teeth are extracted and an aggressive oral hygiene regimen is begun. This includes daily home fluoride treatments. During the irradiation or chemotherapy period, the patient has daily prophylaxis with fluoride gel and continues with good brushing and flossing. Mucositis is improved with normal saline rinses and topical anesthetics as pain relievers. After radiation therapy, the regimen includes examination of the mouth and neck for detection of recurrent or new neoplastic disease, fluoridation prophylaxis, restoration procedures as needed and reinforcement of oral hygiene procedures. Medications are given to control infections, which are most commonly fungal. Fungal infections, besides causing inflammation and pain, also cause a metallic taste in the mouth and cause spicy foods to burn. This further compromises the patient's desire to eat.

Stomach

Malignant neoplasms of the stomach can lead to malnutrition by excessive blood and protein losses or, more commonly, by obstruction and mechanical interference with food intake. The majority of cancers of the stomach are treated by surgical resection; thus, the nutritional considerations are similar to those encountered in partial or total gastrectomy as discussed in Chapter 34. Surprisingly few of these patients have severe nutritional problems.[60]

Small Intestine and Colon

The nutritional problems seen at the time of diagnosis of intestinal tumors are due to progressive obstruction and are manifested by nausea, vomiting and fluid, electrolyte and protein losses. These may be compounded by a malabsorption syndrome similar to that seen in celiac disease or malabsorption due to bacterial overgrowth or simple food deprivation. The patients are often so depleted that nutritional repletion is necessary prior to cancer treatment. The nature of the malabsorption will dictate the mode of repletion, as discussed on page 451. A defined formula diet could be considered, although parenteral nutrition may be indicated.

As with gastric cancer, treatment of these cancers utilizes surgical resection. The nutritional consequences are related to the extent of the resection and the dietary management is similar to that described for the specific segment involved and is discussed in Chapter 34.

Radiation therapy may be given and radiation enteritis can be expected to occur to some degree. A defined formula diet can be useful in reducing symptoms of enteritis and maintaining nutritional status during radiotherapy,[33] although oral administration may meet with poor patient compliance. There is evidence that the use of a diet that is gluten-free, milk-free, low-fat and low-residue is beneficial both therapeutically and prophylactically for severe acute or chronic radiation-induced enteritis in children.[32] This dietary regimen should be initiated as a continuous drip tube feeding and slowly progressed to fractionated feedings supplemented by normal foods as intestinal repair is confirmed. The use of this dietary regimen in adults deserves consideration.

Pancreas

Surgical resection for carcinoma of the pancreas results in a decrease or loss of pancreatic enzymes and their replacement is difficult. Malnutrition from the resulting malabsorption of fat, protein and complex carbohydrates is common. Insulin deficiency or loss further complicates the clinical management. Nutritional care will depend upon remaining pancreatic function and is discussed on page 696.

Liver

Nutritional consequences of uncomplicated major hepatic resection are surprisingly minor. Levels of albumin and coagulation factors in the blood are decreased postoperatively, but rapidly return to normal as hepatic regeneration occurs. Hepatic regeneration is encouraged by adequate protein feeding.

MALIGNANCY TREATED BY MARROW TRANSPLANTATION

The marrow transplantation procedure presents severe nutritional consequences as previously described and requires prompt, aggressive nutritional intervention. A detailed review of the nutritional management of the marrow recipient is provided by Cunningham and colleagues.[24]

During the preparatory phase, the patient suffers nausea, vomiting and diarrhea caused by the chemoradiation conditioning therapy. Antiemetics may be helpful, but food intake is minimal. Cold, clear liquids and ices are given as tolerated. Use of low-lactose or soy milk products may help to lessen the diarrhea.

After marrow transplantation, the delayed-onset complications include varying degrees of mucositis, xerostomia, and dysgeusia. Topical anesthetics applied to the oral mucosa before eating help; bland liquids and soft solids are better tolerated. Salivary stimulants and substitutes are beneficial for temporary relief of dry mouth; liquids and foods with sauces and gravies are suggested. Changes in taste acuity persist 30 to 50 days post-transplant.[4] Strong flavored or spicy foods are better accepted, providing mucositis is not present. Nausea, vomiting and diarrhea may occur with administration of antibiotics and compound the existing complications.

As oral intake is virtually nil for an extended period of time and the function of the gastrointestinal tract is compromised, parenteral nutrition must be instituted. Parenteral nutrition is begun after the final dose of chemotherapy prior to marrow transplant. The adequacy of nutritional support is determined on a daily basis by monitoring serum electrolyte and glucose levels and by frequent nitrogen balance determinations; long-term adequacy is indicated by monthly anthropometic assessment. The administration of optimal levels of PN is complicated by its frequent interruption for the infusion of antibiotics, blood products and drugs, necessitating more concentrated nutrient solutions and increased flow rates.[2]

Additionally, two conditions can present particular challenges for nutritional care: gastrointestinal graft-versus-host disease (GVHD) and hepatic veno-occlusive disease (VOD), both of which are discussed on page 745. The symptoms of gastrointestinal GVHD are severe. The volumes of secretory diarrhea often exceed 3 liters per day and total gut rest is indicated until diarrhea is reduced to less than 500 ml. per day. Initial oral feedings begin with beverages that are iso-osmotic, low-fat and lactose-free because of the loss of intestinal enzymes due to intestinal villi and mucosa alterations. As those are tolerated, solids of the same nature are introduced individually. Dietary restrictions are progressively reduced as foods are gradually introduced in the absence of increasing symptoms. Readers are referred to Gauvreau and coworkers[40] for details.

The resulting symptoms of concern from VOD are fluid retention, with profound ascites in some cases, and encephalopathy. Fluid and protein restrictions are required; other modifications in nutritional support are frequently indicated. Nutritional and nursing care considerations are presented in depth by Ford and associates.[37]

PATIENT REHABILITATION

Concern for the patient with cancer should not stop when he or she is no longer acutely ill. It must continue until the patient has returned to a useful life. If at all possible, patients are encouraged to care for themselves and maintain their nutritional intake on their own. Many patients live at home or in temporary apartments during the later phases of treatment so that much of their food preparation is independent of the treatment center. A dietitian-nutritionist can be on hand in the clinic to guide selections, and patients could get together to encourage each other. Several books with high-calorie and high-protein recipes and suggestions for making foods palatable are listed at the end of this chapter and could be used by patients to help them maintain their dietary intake at home.

MISCONCEPTIONS IN NUTRITIONAL CARE

As can be anticipated from the obvious lack of knowledge about nutrition related to cancer, the area of nutritional care for cancer patients is fraught with mystique, misunderstanding and unsubstantiated claims. The most recent and most popularized example of this harmful situation is *Laetrile*.

The use of Laetrile for cancer has been reviewed by Jukes.[54] Laetrile, or more properly, *amygdalin*, is a cyanogenetic glycoside found in the seeds of apricots, peaches, plums, almonds and macadamia nuts. Upon hydrolysis, glucose and a mandelonitrile are produced. The mandelonitrile decomposes into benzaldehyde and cyanide, either spontaneously or by the action of an enzyme. Laetrile is not a vitamin but has been identified mistakenly as vitamin B_{17} by some people in order to avoid the federal requirements concerning food additives. Legislation has been passed in some states to make Laetrile legal to use. In controlled studies, Laetrile has been shown to have no effect on tumor growth.[68] In the popular literature, cases of improvement of patients who take the drug daily—frequently after having other forms of treatment—have been reported. Unfortunately, the popular literature never describes the patients who died or who did not improve as a result of taking this drug. The controversy over Laetrile illustrates that victims of incurable diseases are often susceptible to manipulation and exploitation by quacks.[44]

A related example is *pangamic acid,* called "vitamin B_{15}" by the same promoters who advanced Laetrile. Since there is no standard of identity for this product, pangamic acid could contain calcium gluconate, calcium chloride, glycine, dimethylglycine or diisopropylamine dichloroacetate in variable amounts.[45] It has no known nutritional worth and no vitamin properties. There is no proof that it has any therapeutic benefit or is safe for human use, and it may be mutagenic.[46, 86]

Summary

The role of nutrition and diet in the etiology of cancer is just beginning to be elucidated. Much additional research is needed before definite suggestions to alter the diet of large segments of the population can be made. Our knowledge of the role of nutrition in the treatment of patients with cancer is somewhat better. Well-nourished patients can cope with the disease better than malnourished patients can. Aggressive, understanding support of the patient can aid substantially in improving his or her nutritional status before, during and after therapy.

Problems and Suggested Topics for Discussion

1. Discuss the role of energy intake in the etiology of cancer.
2. Explain the etiological role of fat in the development of cancer.
3. Discuss the metabolic effects that result from the presence of a tumor in the body.
4. Assess the nutritional status of a patient receiving cancer treatment. Does he or she exhibit any biochemical or clinical signs of malnutrition? Evaluate the dietary intake. Is it adequate? How does he or she try to maintain food intake? Will there need to be changes as the cancer treatment continues?
5. Interview a patient receiving chemotherapy or radiotherapy. Ask about any changes in taste perception he or she is experiencing. Have these changes affected dietary intake?
6. What changes in food selection would you recommend to a patient with stomatitis? with decreased salivation? with viscous mucus?
7. Explain the nutritional care for a marrow transplant patient with graft-versus-host disease.

Cited References

1. Aker, S.N.: Oral feedings in the cancer patient. Cancer, *43*:2103, 1979.
2. Aker, S.N., et al.: Nutritional support in marrow graft recipients with single versus double lumen right atrial catheters. Exp. Hematol., *10*:732, 1982.
3. Baker, R., et al.: Detection of mutagenic activity in human urine following fried pork or bacon meals. Cancer Letters, *16*:81, 1982.
4. Barale, K.V., Aker, S.N., and Martinsen, C.S.: Primary taste thresholds in children with leukemia undergoing marrow transplantation. JPEN, *6*:287, 1982.
5. Basu, T.K.: Significance of vitamins in cancer. Oncology, *33*:183, 1976.
6. Bernstein, I.: Learned taste aversions in children receiving chemotherapy. Science, *200*:1302, 1978.
7. Bernstein, I.L., and Berstein, I.D.: Learned food aversions and cancer anorexia. Cancer Treat. Rep. *65* (Suppl. 5):43, 1981.
8. Bjelke, E.: Dietary vitamin A and human lung cancer. Semin. Oncol., *3*:17, 1976.
9. Blackburn, G.L., et al.: The effect of cancer on nitrogen, electrolyte, and mineral metabolism. Cancer Res., *37*:2348, 1977.
10. Brennan, M.F.: Metabolic response to surgery in the cancer patient: consequences of aggressive multimodal therapy. Cancer, *43*:2053, 1979.
11. Brennan, M.F., and Copeland, E.M.: Panel report on nutritional support of patients with cancer. Am. J. Clin. Nutr., *34*:1199, 1981.
12. Bright-See, E.: The role of vitamins C and E in the prevention of carcinogenesis. Presented at the 2nd Bristol-Myers Symposium, Nutritional Factors in the Induction and Maintenance of Malignancy. Washington, D.C., Dec. 9–10, 1982.
13. Brown, R.: Clinical features associated with endometrial carcinoma. J. Obstet. Gynaecol., *81*:933, 1974.
14. Butterworth, C.E., et al.: Improvement in cervical dysplasia associated with folic acid therapy in users of oral contraceptives. Am. J. Clin. Nutr., *35*:73, 1982.
15. Carroll, K.K., and Khor, H.T.: Dietary fat in relation to tumorigenesis. Prog. Biochem. Pharmacol., *10*:308, 1975.
16. Carson, J.A.S., and Gormican, A.: Taste acuity and food attitudes of selected patients with cancer. J. Am. Diet. Assoc., *70*:361, 1977.
17. Cohn, S.E., et al.: Compartmental body composition of cancer patients by measurement of total body nitrogen, potassium, and water. Metabolism, *30*:222, 1981.
18. Committee on Diet, Nutrition and Cancer, National Research Council: Diet, Nutrition and Cancer. Washington, D.C., National Academy of Sciences, 1982.
19. Copeland, E.M., Daly, J.M., and Dudrick, S.J.: Intravenous hyperalimentation, bowel rest, and cancer. Critical Care Manag., *8*:21, 1980.
20. Copeland, E.M., et al.: Intravenous hyperalimentation as an adjunct to radiation therapy. Cancer, *39*:609, 1977.
21. Cregan, E.T., et al.: Failure of high dose vitamin C (ascorbic acid) therapy to benefit patients with advanced cancer. N. Engl. J. Med., *301*:678, 1979.
22. Crowther, J.S., et al.: Faecal steroids and bacteria and large bowel cancer in Hong Kong by socio-economic groups. Br. J. Cancer, *34*:191, 1976.
23. Cunningham, A.S.: Lymphomas and animal protein consumption. Lancet, *2*:1184, 1976.
24. Cunningham, B.A., et al.: Nutritional considerations during marrow transplantation. Nurs. Clin. N. Am., *18*:585, 1983.
25. DeWys, W.D.: Anorexia as a general effect of cancer. Cancer, *43*:2013, 1979.
26. DeWys, W.D.: Pathophysiology of cancer cachexia: current understanding and areas for future research. Cancer Res. (Suppl.) *42*:721, 1982.
27. DeWys, W.D., et al.: Prognostic effect of weight loss prior to chemotherapy in cancer patients. Am. J. Med., *60*:491, 1980.
28. DeWys, W.D., and Kubota, T.T.: Enteral and parenteral nutrition in the care of the cancer patient. JAMA, *256*:1725, 1981.
29. Dickerson, J.W.T.: Nutrition and the patient with cancer. Proc. Nutr. Soc., *40*:31, 1981.
30. Dionigi, R., and Campani, M.: Nutritional and immunological abnormalities in malignant disease. Acta. Chir. Scand. (Suppl.) *507*:435, 1981.
31. Donaldson, S.S.: Effects of therapy on nutritional status of the pediatric cancer patient. Cancer Res. (Suppl.) *42*:729s, 1982.
32. Donaldson, S.S., et al.: Radiation enteritis in children: a retrospective review, clinicopathologic correlation, and dietary management. Cancer, *35*:1167, 1975.
33. Donaldson, S.S., and Lenon, R.A.: Alterations of nutritional status: impact of chemotherapy and radiation therapy. Cancer, *43*:2036, 1979.
34. Donaldson, S.S., et al.: A prospective randomized clinical trial of total parenteral nutrition in children with cancer. Med. Pediatr. Oncol., *10*:129, 1982.

35. Dwyer, J.T.: Dietetic assessment of ambulatory cancer patients. Cancer, *43*:2077, 1979.

36. Enig, M.G., Munn, R.J., and Kenney, M.: Dietary fat and cancer trends—a critique. Fed. Proc., *27*:2215, 1978.

37. Ford, R., McClain, K., and Cunningham, B.A.: Veno-occlusive disease following marrow transplantation—a nursing perspective. Nurs. Clin. N. Am., *18*:563, 1983.

38. Freeman, M., et al.: Prognostic nutrition factors in lung cancer patients. JPEN, *6*:122, 1982.

39. Fritz, W., and Soos, K.: Smoked food and cancer. Bibl. Nutr. Dieta, *29*:57, 1980.

40. Gauvreau, J.M., et al.: Nutritional management of patients with intestinal graft-versus-host disease. J. Am. Dietet. Assoc., *79*:673, 1981.

41. Goodlad, G.A.J., and Clark, C.M.: Protein metabolism in the tumor-bearing host. Acta. Chir. Scand. (Suppl.) *498*:137, 1980.

42. Harris, B.A., and Probert, J.C.: Nutrition and metabolism in cancer patients: a review. N. Z. Med. J., *94*: 227, 1981.

43. Hepedus, S., and Pelman, M.: Dietetics in a cancer hospital. J. Am. Diet. Assoc., *67*:235, 1975.

44. Herbert, V.: Laetrile: the cult of cyanide. Promoting poison for profit. Am. J. Clin. Nutr., *32*:1121, 1979.

45. Herbert, V.: Pangamic acid ("vitamin B_{15}"), Am. J. Clin. Nutr., *32*:1534, 1979.

46. Herbert, V., Gardner, A. and Colman, N.: Evidence for possible lack of safety for human consumption of dichloroacetate, a "sister compound" and frequent ingredient of the non-vitamin "B_{15}" (pangamate). Clin. Res., *27*:5512, 1979.

47. Hickman, D.M., et al.: Serum albumin and body weight as predictors of postoperative course in colorectal cancer. JPEN, *4*:314, 1980.

48. Hill, M.J., and Aries, V.: Fecal steroid composition and its relationship to cancer of the large bowel. J. Pathol. *104*:129, 1971.

49. Hill, P., et al.: Prolactin levels in populations at risk for breast cancer. Cancer Res., *36*:4102, 1976.

50. Holroyde, C.P., et al.: Altered glucose metabolism in metastatic carcinoma. Cancer Res., *35*:3710, 1975.

51. Jacobsen, B.J., and Bjelke, E.: Coffee consumption and cancer: a prospective study. Presented at the 13th International Cancer Congress, Seattle, 1982.

52. Jensen, O.M., MacLennan, R., and Wahrendorf, J.: Diet, bowel function, fecal characteristics of large bowel cancer in Denmark and Finland. Nutr. Cancer, *4*:5, 1982.

53. Jensen, O.M., et al.: A comparative study of the diagnostic basis for cancer of the colon and cancer of the rectum in Denmark and Finland. Int. J. Epidemiol., *3*: 183, 1974.

54. Jukes, J.H.: Laetrile for cancer. JAMA, *236*:1284, 1976.

55. Kawamura, I., et al.: Altered amino acid kinetics in rats with progressive tumor growth. Cancer Res., *42*: 824, 1982.

56. Kolonel, L.N., et al.: Association of diet and place of birth with stomach cancer incidence in Hawaii Japanese and Caucasians. Am. J. Clin. Nutr. *34*:2478, 1981.

57. Krantman, N., et al.: Immune function in pure iron deficiency. Am. J. Dis. Child, *136*:840, 1982.

58. Krasner, N., and Dymock, I.W.: Ascorbic acid deficiency in malignant diseases: a clinical and biochemical study. Br. J. Cancer, *30*:142, 1974.

59. Kurek, M.P. and Corwin, L.M.: Vitamin E protection against tumor formation by transplanted murine sarcoma cells. Nutrition and Cancer, *4*:128, 1982.

60. Lawrence, W.: Effects of cancer on nutrition: impaired organ system effects. Cancer, *43*:2020, 1979.

61. Liebelt, R.A., Liebelt, A.G., and Johnston, H.M.: Lipid metabolism and food intake in experimentally obese mice bearing transplanted tumors. Proc. Soc. Exp. Biol. Med., *138*:482, 1971.

62. Lin, R.S., and Kessler, I.I.: A multifactorial model for pancreatic cancer in man: epidemiologic evidence. JAMA, *245*:147, 1981.

63. Lundholm, K., Karlbert, I., and Schersten, T.: Albumin and hepatic protein synthesis in patients with early cancer. Cancer, *46*:71, 1980.

64. MacDonald, P.C., et al.: Effect of obesity on conversion of plasma androstenedione to estrone in post menopausal women with and without endometrial cancer. Am. J. Obstet. Gynecol., *130*:448, 1978.

65. MacMahon, B., et al.: Coffee and cancer of the pancreas. N. Engl. J. Med., *304*:630, 1981.

66. Merritt, R.J., et al.: Lactic acidosis in pediatric patients with cancer receiving total parenteral nutrition. J. Pediatr. *99*:247, 1981.

67. Meyskens, F.L.: Vitamin A and its synthetic derivatives in the prevention and treatment of cancer. Presented at the 2nd Bristol-Myers Symposium, Nutritional Factors in the Induction and Maintenance of Malignancy. Washington, D.C., Dec. 9–10, 1982.

68. Moertel, C.G., et al.: A clinical trial of amygdalin (Laetrile) in the treatment of human cancer. N. Engl. J. Med., *306*:201, 1982.

69. Morrison, A.S., and Buring, J.E.: Artificial sweeteners and cancer of the lower urinary tract. N. Engl. J. Med., *302*:537, 1980.

70. Morrison, A.S., et al.: Coffee drinking and cancer of the lower urinary tract. J. Nat. Cancer Inst., *68*:91, 1982.

71. Mullen, J.L.: Complications of total parenteral nutrition in the cancer patient. Cancer Treat. Rep., *65* (Suppl. 5):107, 1981.

72. Newell, G.R.: Artificial sweeteners and cancer. In Newell, G.R., and Ellison, N.M. (eds.): Nutrition and Cancer: Etiology and Treatment. New York, Raven Press, 1981.

73. Pastore, G., et al.: Late effects of treatment of cancer in infancy. Med. Pediatr. Oncol., *10*:369, 1982.

74. Reddy, B.S., and Wydner, E.L.: Large bowel carcinogenesis: fecal constituents of populations with diverse incidence rates of colon cancer. J. Nat. Cancer Inst., *50*:1437, 1973.

75. Regezi, J.A., Courtnem, R.M., and Kerr, D.A.: Dental management of patients irradiated for oral cancer. Cancer, *38*:994, 1976.

76. Rickard, K.A., et al.: Supportive nutritional intervention in pediatric cancer. Cancer Res. *42* (Suppl.):766, 1982.

77. Schein, R.S., et al.: Cachexia of malignancy: potential role of insulin in nutritional management. Cancer, *43*: 2070, 1979.

78. Schersten, T., et al.: Energy metabolism in cancer. Acta Chir. Scand. *498* (Suppl.):130, 1980.

79. Shamberger, R.J. and Willis, C.E.: Selenium distribution and human cancer mortality. CRC Crit. Rev. Clin. Lab. Sci., *2*:211, 1971.

80. Shapot, V.S.: The interrelationships of disturbances in the tumor host homeostasis. Acta Chir. Scand. *498* (Suppl.):141, 1980.

81. Shils, M.E.: Principles of nutritional therapy. Cancer, *43*:2093, 1979.

82. Shulman, H.M., et al.: An analysis of hepatic veno-occlusive disease and centrilobular hepatic degeneration following bone marrow transplantation. Gastroenterology, *79*:1178, 1980.

83. Slaga, T.J., and Bracken, W.M.: The effects of antioxidants on skin tumor initiation and aryl hydrocarbon hydrolase. Cancer Res., *37*:3126, 1977.

84. Sloan, G.M., Maher, M., and Brennan, M.F.: Nutritional effects of surgery, radiation therapy, and adjuvant

chemotherapy for soft tissue sarcomas. Am. J. Clin. Nutr., *34*:1094, 1981.

85. Smith, J.C., and Blumsack, J.T.: Learned taste aversion as a factor in cancer therapy. Cancer Treat. Rep. *65* (Suppl. 5):37, 1981.

86. Stacpoole, P.W., Moore, G.W., and Kornhauser, D.M.: Toxicity of chronic dichloroacetate. N. Engl. J. Med., *300*:372, 1979.

87. Theologides, A.: Nutritional management of the patient with advanced cancer. Postgrad. Med., *61*:97, 1977.

88. Theologides, A.: Cancer cachexia. Cancer, *43*:2004, 1979.

89. Thomas, E.D.: Marrow transplantation for acute leukemia. Cancer, *42*:895, 1978.

90. Thomas, E.D.: Marrow transplantation for marrow failure for leukemia. Comprehensive Therapy, *6*:69, 1980.

91. Trant, A.S., Serin, J., and Douglass, H.O.: Is taste related to anorexia in cancer patients? Am. J. Clin. Nutr., *36*:45, 1982.

92. VanEys, J.: Effect of nutritional status on response to therapy. Cancer Res. *42* (Suppl.):747s, 1982.

93. Verzosa, M.S., et al.: Five years after central nervous system irradiation of children with leukemia. Int. J. Radiat. Oncol. Biol. Phys., *1*:209, 1976.

94. Wagman, L.D., Burt, M.E., and Brennan, M.F.: The impact of total parenteral nutrition on liver function tests in patients with cancer. Cancer, *49*:1249, 1980.

95. Watson, W.S., and Sammon, A.M.: Body composition in cachexia resulting from malignant and non-malignant diseases. Cancer, *46*:2041, 1980.

96. Weindruch, R., and Walford, R.L.: Dietary restrictions in mice beginning at 1 year of age: effect on life span and spontaneous cancer incidence. Science, *215*:1415, 1982.

97. Wynder, E.L., Escher, G.C., and Mantel, N.: An epidemiological investigation of cancer of the endometrium. Cancer, *19*:489, 1966.

98. Young, V.R.: Energy metabolism and requirements in the cancer patient. Cancer Res., *37*:2336, 1977.

Additional References

Arnott, M.S., van Eys, J., and Wang, Y.M. (eds.): Molecular interactions of nutrition and cancer, New York, Raven Press, 1982.

Bernstein, I.L.: Physiological and psychological mechanisms of cancer anorexia. Cancer Res. *42* (Suppl.):715s, 1982.

Brennan, M.F.: Total parenteral nutrition in the cancer patient. N. Engl. J. Med., *305*:375, 1981.

Dickerson, J.W.T.: The role of enteral nutrition in malignant disease. Acta Chir. Scan., *507* (Suppl.):422, 1981.

Fraser, P., et al.: Nitrate and human cancer: a review of the evidence. Int. J. Epidemiol., *9*:3, 1980.

Frytak, S., and Moertel, C.G.: Management of nausea and vomiting in the cancer patient. JAMA, *245*:393, 1981.

Kluthe, R., and Lohr, G.W. (eds.): Nutrition and metabolism in cancer. Stuttgart, Georg Thieme Verlag, 1981.

Lawson, D.H., et al.: Metabolic approaches to cancer cachexia. Ann. Rev. Nutr., *2*:277, 1982.

Mendeloff, A.: Appraisal of "Diet, Nutrition and Cancer." Am. J. Clin. Nutr. 37:495, 1983.

Neumann, C.G., et al.: Nutritional assessment of the child with cancer. Cancer Res. *42* (Suppl.):699s, 1982.

Peterson, D.E., and Sonis, S.T. (eds.): Oral Complications of Cancer Chemotherapy, The Hague, Martinus Nijhoff Publishing, 1983.

Robbins, S.L., and Cotran, R.S.: Pathologic Basis of Disease. 2nd ed. Philadelphia, W.B. Saunders Company, 1979.

Shils, M.E., and Hermann, M.G.: Unproved dietary claims in the treatment of patients with cancer. Bull. N.Y. Acad. Med., *58*:323, 1982.

Van Eys, J.: Nutrition and neoplasia. Nutr. Rev., *40*:353, 1982.

Van Eys, J., Seelig, M.S. and Nichols, B.D., Jr. (eds.): Nutrition and Cancer. New York, S.P. Medical and Scientific Books, 1979.

Wollard, J.J. (ed.): Nutritional Management of the Cancer Patient. New York, Raven Press, 1979.

Suggestions for Patient Education:

Aker, S., and Lenssen, P.: A Guide to Good Nutrition During and After Chemotherapy and Radiation. Seattle, Fred Hutchinson Cancer Research Center, 1982.

Fishman, J., and Anrod, B.: Something's Got to Taste Good. Kansas City, Andrews and McMeel, Inc., 1981.

Gauvreau, J.M.: GVHD—A Nutrition Handbook for Patients with Graft-Versus-Host Disease. Seattle, Fred Hutchinson Cancer Research Center, 1981.

DISEASES OF INFANCY AND CHILDHOOD

Nutritional Care of the Low-Birth-Weight Infant

MARY J. O'LEARY, M.S., R.D.

The management of low-birth-weight infants requiring intensive care has improved dramatically during the past decade. With new technologies, better understanding of pathophysiology and cooperative interactions to regionalize the delivery of perinatal care, a greater number of immature infants are surviving. Recent studies indicate that the majority of these infants have the potential to lead long and productive lives.[24] To achieve this outcome, a team approach is required to overcome a multitude of complex medical and surgical problems. Nutritional support is receiving increasing attention as one of the important components affecting clinical and developmental outcome for low-birth-weight infants. This chapter will discuss the nutritional care of low-birth-weight infants who are separated prematurely from the maternal-placental supply line, or who are not able to feed successfully because of medical problems.

Definitions

An infant who weighs less than 2500 gm. (5 1/2 lb.) at birth is classified as being of *low birth weight (LBW)*, while an infant weighing less than 1500 gm. (3 1/2 pounds) at birth is frequently referred to as being of *very low birth weight (VLBW)*. An infant may be of low birth weight owing to a shortened period of gestation, which means that he or she is *premature*, or because of a retarded rate of growth, which makes him or her *small for gestational age (SGA)*. The *full-term* infant is born between the 38th and 42nd week of gestation. A premature infant is

one born before 38 weeks gestation. Infants born before the 25th week rarely survive. Modern neonatal intensive care is not able to meet the metabolic and medical needs of most infants born before the third trimester of gestation.

The *gestational age* of the infant is determined primarily by clinical assessment. Clinical parameters fall into two groups: (1) a series of neurologic signs, dependent mainly on postures and tone and (2) a series of external characteristics that reflect the physical maturity of the infant.[12] Accurate assessment of gestational age is important in establishing nutritional goals for individual infants, and in differentiating the premature from the SGA infant.

An SGA infant is defined as one who weighs less than the 10th percentile of the standard weight for that gestational age. This is usually a valid test, although sometimes an infant can be recognized as SGA only when compared with normal siblings who presumably have the same genetic potential. An SGA infant whose intrauterine weight gain was poor, but whose linear and head growth are *appropriate for gestational age (AGA)* (i.e., between the 10th and 90th percentiles on the intrauterine growth grid), has experienced *asymmetrical* intrauterine growth retardation. An SGA infant whose length and occipital frontal circumference (OFC) are also below the 10th percentile of the standards is said to be *symmetrically* growth retarded. Symmetrical *intrauterine growth retardation (IUGR)* usually reflects early and prolonged intrauterine deficit, and is apparently more detrimental to later growth and development.[28] The infant whose birth weight is above the 90th percentile on the intrauterine weight gain grid is referred

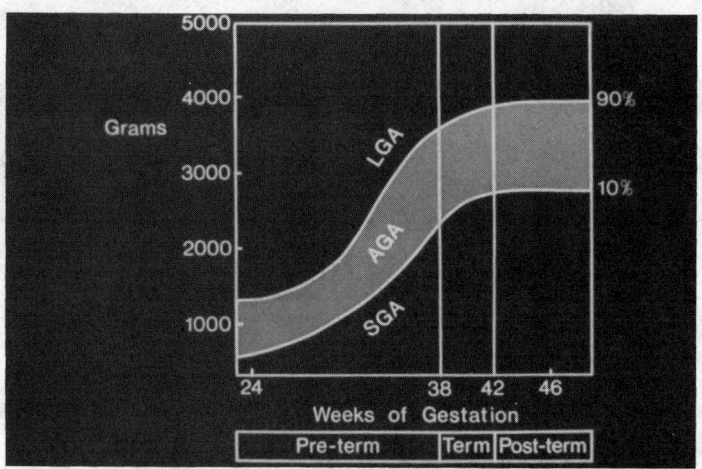

Figure 37–1. Classification of newborns based on maturity and intrauterine growth. SGA = small for gestational age; AGA = appropriate for gestational age; LGA = large for gestational age.

to as *large for gestational age (LGA)*. Figure 37–1 depicts the classification of newborns based on maturity and intrauterine growth.

Developmental Physiology

The premature or LBW infant has not had the chance to develop fully *in utero* and is physiologically different from the term infant weighing 2500 gm. or more, as Figure 37–2 shows. Consequently, some knowledge of relevant developmental physiology is prerequisite to understanding the nutritional requirements and methods of nutritional support for premature compared with full-term neonates.

Birth interrupts the influx of nutrients to the fetus and challenges the newborn with changes in source and type of nutrition. The healthy, full-term neonate generally adapts well to these changes and tolerates a wide variation in composition, quantity and frequency of feedings. The premature infant, however, is physiologically less well prepared to maintain homeostasis and more susceptible to feeding intolerance.

SMALLER METABOLIC RESERVES

Premature infants enter the world with smaller metabolic reserves than full-term babies. Because most of the infant's glycogen is stored in the fetal liver in the last four weeks of gestation, the glycogen reserve of the preterm infant is small and rapidly depleted. Fat stores are also limited, because most fetal fat is deposited during the last six weeks of pregnancy. In the premature infant weighing 1000 gm., fat contributes only 1 per cent of total body weight; in contrast, the body of the full-term infant (3500 gm.) is about 16 per cent fat.[55]

In general, the smallest infants have the smallest energy reserves of glycogen and fat. Tiny newborns become rapidly dependent on exogenous energy intake to meet their metabolic needs and support basic life functions. The 1000 gm. AGA premature infant, for example, has a glycogen and fat reserve equivalent to about 110 kcal./kg. of body weight. With basal metabolic needs of at least 50 kcal./kg./day, it is obvious that this baby will rapidly run out of fat and carbohydrate fuel unless adequate nutritional

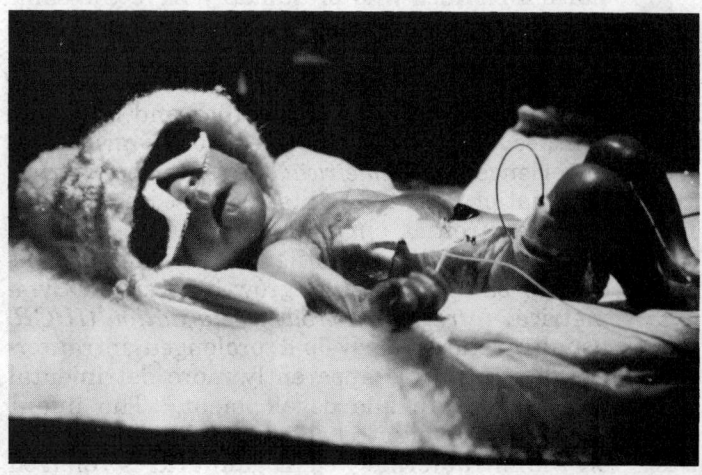

Figure 37–2. Briana on her second day of life, She was born prematurely at 26 weeks gestation, weighing 650 gm. (1½ lb.) Briana wears a little hat for warmth, and a mask to protect her eyes from the fluorescent radiation of the phototherapy lights used to treat hyperbilirubinemia.

support is established. Depletion time will vary between two and four days, depending upon the volume and concentration of parenteral dextrose that can be tolerated. Obviously, depletion time will be even shorter for premature babies weighing less than 1000 gm. at birth. Nutrient reserves are depleted most quickly by tiny infants suffering from intrauterine growth retardation.

It is often difficult, however, to provide adequate nutritional intake during the first several days of life because of immaturity of the organ systems and severe medical problems. When adequate dietary intake cannot be achieved and fat and glycogen reserves have been exhausted, the infant will begin to catabolize vital body protein tissue for energy. Heird and coworkers have theoretically estimated the survival time of starved and semistarved infants.[29] Their estimates, given in Table 37–1, assume depletion of all glycogen and fat, and about one third of body protein tissue at a rate of 50 kcal./kg./day with fluids as intravenous water (no exogenous calories) or 10 per cent dextrose solution. These projected survival times should, however, be interpreted with caution. It seems reasonable to question the quality of the survival that occurs at the expense of significant protein tissue catabolism. Furthermore, these may be unrealistically long periods of time, because the basal energy requirements upon which these figures are based do not allow for growth, biochemical maturation, activity or response to stress such as hypothermia or respiratory distress syndrome.

Although these data lack precision, they do serve to demonstrate the disadvantage of the small infant with respect to survival in the fasting state. The small premature baby is particularly vulnerable to undernutrition; inadequate intake for even a few days may adversely affect the infant's response to acute and chronic illness, recovery time and perhaps long-term outcome.

IMMATURE ORGAN SYSTEMS

Premature neonates, especially those of VLBW, suffer postnatal difficulties related to the immaturity of their organ systems. Developmental immaturity of the respiratory, cardiovascular and renal systems and of the mechanical and digestive function of the gastrointestinal tract must all be considered in the nutritional management of the premature infant.

The immaturity of the respiratory and cardiovascular systems can lead to hypoxia, respiratory acidosis, labored breathing and increased energy requirements. Because the renal system

Table 37–1. EXPECTED DURATION OF SURVIVAL OF INFANTS IN STARVATION (H_2O ONLY) AND SEMISTARVATION ($D_{10}W$)

BIRTH WEIGHT (GRAMS)	ESTIMATED SURVIVAL TIME (DAYS)	
	H_2O Only	$D_{10}W$
1000	4	11
2000	12	30
3500	32	80

Data from Heird, W. C., et al.: Intravenous alimentation in pediatric patients. J. Pediatr., *80*:351, 1972.

is immature, fluid balance is more difficult to manage. The renal solute load, or the amount of electrolytes and protein breakdown products excreted by the kidney, must be moderated according to the infant's fluid intake, extrarenal water losses and renal concentrating ability.

Mechanical immaturity of the digestive tract is reflected in poorly coordinated sucking and swallowing. The ability to swallow is well developed by mid-gestation; however, the ability to coordinate suck and swallow does not appear before about 34 weeks gestation. Esophageal motility is poor in LBW infants and the gastroesophageal sphincter is relatively incompetent, resulting in frequent regurgitation of food into the esophagus. Small gastric capacity, delayed gastric emptying time and poorly coordinated intestinal motility may be additional problems. The overall result of this mechanical immaturity is a tendency, most apparent in the smallest infants, toward frequent abdominal distention, gastric residuals and regurgitation, even in the absence of any recognized food intolerances or systemic illnesses.

In general, digestive function matures earlier in gestation than gastrointestinal mechanical activity. Based on studies of the intestinal mucosal content of disaccharidases, the capacity for carbohydrate digestion and absorption appears to be present by mid-gestation. An exception is lactase. Babies born prior to 28 to 34 weeks gestation have low intestinal lactase activity, although even the smallest infants usually tolerate lactose adequately.[39] Likewise, the ability to digest dietary protein does not seem to be impaired in the LBW infant. Gastric, pancreatic and intestinal enzymes responsible for protein hydrolysis are active by the third trimester, and the absorptive capacity for amino acids develops at the same time. Feeding studies corroborate the biochemical finding that neonates can digest and absorb an adequate quantity of dietary protein, although their digestive capacities are limited. In contrast, it has long been recognized that neonates, particularly premature infants and those who are SGA, are relatively inefficient in digestion and absorption of lipid. Low intraluminal concentrations of bile acids and lipases are primarily responsible, although the composition of the dietary fat may also play a role.

A more detailed discussion of the impact of digestive physiology on infant feeding follows in the section entitled Nutritional Requirements. Many LBW infants are initially unable to tolerate enteral feedings (via the gastrointestinal tract) and are temporarily supported by parenteral nutrition (via a blood vessel). However, the concepts of enteral nutrient requirements are better understood than those of parenteral nutrition, and are the focus of the following discussion. Refer to page 773 for discussion of specific information relating to nutrition that bypasses the physiological control mechanisms of the gastrointestinal tract.

Nutritional Requirements

The goals of nutritional management of LBW infants may be divided into three phases. Initial efforts to meet the infant's nutritional needs focus on the *maintenance of metabolic homeostasis.* Water and energy (glucose) must be provided almost immediately to replace ongoing losses, followed by electrolytes and calcium to meet metabolic requirements. This early postnatal phase is often one of crisis for the LBW infant, who suffers the stress of medical illness and the problems of extrauterine adaptation by immature organ systems. After this crisis period, which may last a few hours or even days, there is a *transition phase* during which a much greater variety of nutrients should be supplied. The addition of protein, essential fatty acids, vitamins and minerals should be considered at this time. As the infant's medical condition stabilizes, growth ensues, and the problems in maintaining homeostasis decrease. During this *growth phase*, the emphasis of nutritional management shifts to provide adequate quantities of all essential nutrients to support normal somatic growth and organ development.

The nutrient requirements of premature infants are apparently higher than those of full-term babies, because a greater portion of total nutrient intake is necessary for the synthesis of new tissue (i.e., growth). But precise nutrient requirements for premature babies have been difficult to establish because their optimal rate of postnatal growth is unknown. In recent years, the intrauterine growth rate has been suggested as a standard or objective.[37] Using this standard, the goal of nutritional management is postnatal resumption of the rate of fetal weight gain. Although perhaps a reasonable objective for some stable LBW babies, such rates of growth may be dangerous if overly aggressive efforts are made to provide fluid and nutrients.[34] Furthermore, weight gain alone is an insufficient measure of growth, since it may reflect water retention rather than tissue accretion. The quality of the weight that is gained is probably a more critical determinant of adequate nutrition for premature infants. Recently, investigators have begun to estimate the composition of the tissue that is accrued during growth.[54] The relationship of energy and other nutrients in the diet to new tissue composition has the potential to clarify precise nutrient requirements with appropriate empirical testing.

Essential nutrients should be supplied to LBW infants in quantities sufficient to maintain homeostasis without unnecessary weight loss or tissue catabolism, and yet not excessively to avoid potential toxicity and superfluous fat deposition. The exact quantities of nutrients required to meet these goals are still being defined. An approximation of the required amounts of protein and major minerals may be obtained by comparison with normal intrauterine accretion rates for these nutrients.[56] These estimates (called advisable intakes) provide temporary guides for nutritional management until more direct experimental data become available.

ENERGY

The energy requirement of premature babies varies with individual biological and environmental factors. Sinclair has estimated that 60 to 80 kcal./kg./day are required to meet maintenance energy needs, compared with 100 to 120 kcal./kg./day to provide adequate energy for growth as shown in Table 37–2. However, energy needs may be increased by stress and rapid growth, or decreased in a neutral thermal environment and when absorptive loss is eliminated with parenteral nutrition. To estimate the energy needs of individual infants, it is important to consider the dynamic biological and environmental factors that alter their needs. To evaluate the accuracy of the estimate, it is important to consider the infants' growth progress in relation to their average energy intakes. Some premature infants may require at least 120 to 150 kcal./kg./day to sustain an appropriate rate of growth, especially during their catch-up growth phase, which is discussed on page 776). To achieve these caloric intakes in babies with limited capacities to tolerate large fluid volumes, it is often necessary to concentrate the feedings to provide more than 20 kcal./oz. (i.e., more than 0.67 kcal./ml.).

Table 37–2. ENERGY REQUIREMENTS OF LOW-BIRTH-WEIGHT INFANTS

	KCAL./KG./DAY
Basal metabolic rate	50
Activity	15
Cold stress	10
Total Maintenance	75 (range 60–80)
Specific dynamic action	8
Fecal loss	12
Growth	25
Total Additional Requirements	45
Total Energy Needs for Growth	120 (range 100–120)

Adapted from Sinclair, J., et al.: Supportive management of the sick neonate: parenteral calories, water and electrolytes. Pediatr. Clin. N. Am., *17*:863, 1970.

PROTEIN

Although much attention has been directed toward determining the protein requirement of LBW infants, this is still a controversial subject. At the core of the controversy are basic questions relating to optimal postnatal growth and tissue composition changes of premature babies. Answers to these questions and data from direct clinical investigations are needed to establish precise protein requirements.

One approach to estimating the protein needs of preterm infants considers the intrauterine rate of protein accumulation to be the goal.[56] A reference fetus model is used to determine the amount of protein that would need to be ingested to match the quantity of protein that is deposited into newly formed fetal tissue.[57] In order to achieve these fetal accretion rates, additional protein must be supplied to compensate for intestinal losses and obligatory losses in urine and skin. Table 37–3 shows the advisable intakes for protein using this factorial method.

The advisable intakes derived by the factorial method are frequently cited as the goals for protein nurture of LBW babies. In stable infants who are growing rapidly, these protein intake levels of 3.5 to 4.0 gm./kg./day are apparently well tolerated. However, there are no clinical data to prove that these quantities of protein are necessary; indeed, such amounts may exceed the metabolic capacity of the very immature baby or may stress the sick infant.

Protein intakes greater than 4 gm./kg./day may be associated with both acute and long-term complications. Acute problems include fever, lethargy and various biochemical abnormalities, such as azotemia, hyperaminoacidemia and metabolic acidosis.[43, 45] Long-term complications (e.g., a higher incidence of strabismus and lower IQ scores) generally are thought to result from the biochemical abnormalities secondary to metabolic intolerance.[21] The upper limit for safe protein intake by growing LBW infants is about 4 gm./kg./day when fed by an enteral route.

Another approach to estimating the protein needs of preterm infants considers the effect that the quality or type of protein fed may have on the quantitative requirement. *Whey-predominant* proteins of high biological value for the preterm infant support sustained growth in quantities less than advisable intake estimates.[24] Low-birth-weight infants who ingest adequate calories and whey-predominant protein at 2.25 gm./kg./day show steady gains in weight and length,[43] although their rate of growth may be slower compared with intrauterine growth curves.[18] It can be argued that a slower rate of growth is normal for the preterm infant living in an extrauterine environment.

Breast-milk protein is composed of 60 per cent whey and 40 per cent casein, whereas most standard infant formulas are predominantly casein, usually 82 per cent casein and 18 per cent whey. Some commercial formula products contain additional demineralized whey protein (beta-lactoglobulin) resulting in a 60:40 whey:casein ratio. These whey-predominant feedings are the preferred choice for LBW infants because of improved metabolic tolerance.

Several studies have shown that premature infants tolerate whey better than casein.[20, 43–45] Premature babies fed casein-predominant formulas are more likely to develop metabolic acidosis and hyperammonemia. Plasma amino acid profiles may also be abnormal; plasma concentrations of tyrosine and phenylalanine, for example, are far higher than standard values. Although worrisome, these abnormal plasma aminograms are of unknown clinical significance.

Whey protein is also more soluble than casein in gastric acid secretions, and may be more easily digested by the premature infant. Unlike casein, whey protein does not form a curd. Avoiding gastric curd formation probably averts the potential for *lactobezoar* development.[49] A lactobezoar is a concretion in the stomach formed from milk products which provokes feeding intolerance and gastric upset in affected infants.

In addition, immature babies are deficient in certain enzymes necessary for protein metabolism. As a result, they are less able to catabolize the amino acid loads of casein-predominant proteins or to synthesize other amino acids, rendering them essential for premature infants. Whey-predominant proteins more adequately provide the amino acids essential for premature babies —histidine, cystine, tyrosine and possibly taurine—as well as the amino acids required by mature individuals.

Table 37-3. ESTIMATED REQUIREMENTS AND ADVISABLE INTAKES FOR PROTEIN AS DERIVED BY THE FACTORIAL METHOD

BODY WEIGHT OF INFANT	TISSUE INCREMENT (gm. per day)	DERMAL LOSS (gm. per day)	URINE LOSS (gm. per day)	INTESTINAL ABSORPTION (% intake)	ESTIMATED REQUIREMENT (gm. per day)	ADVISABLE INTAKE		
						(gm. per day)	(gm. per kg.)*	(gm. per 100 kcal.)†
800–1200 gm.	2.32	0.17	0.68	87†	3.64	4.0	4.0	3.1
1200–1800 gm.	3.01	0.25	0.90	87	4.78	5.2	3.5	2.7

* Assuming body weight of 1000 and 1500 gm., respectively, for the 800–1200 and 1200–1800 gm. infants.
† Assuming energy intake of 130 kcal./kg./day.
Adapted from Ziegler, E. E., Biga, R. L., and Fomon, S. J.: Nutritional requirements of the premature infant. In Suskind, R. M. (ed.): Textbook of Pediatric Nutrition. New York, Raven Press, 1981, p. 32.

An example of this is found in the essential amino acids *cystine* and *methionine*. The premature infant has a limited ability to convert methionine to cystine as a result of a lack of activity of the enzyme cystathionase. Whey protein contains more cystine and less methionine than does casein and may be more suitable for the immature baby during the first weeks of life. *Taurine*, an amino sulfonic acid, may provide another example of the preference by premature infants for whey proteins. Human milk is a rich source of taurine, whereas commercial cow's milk formulas contain only small amounts. Taurine may be important for the functioning of several developing organ systems, including the brain, retina, heart and liver. Although rapidly growing premature babies develop low plasma and urine concentrations of taurine without a dietary supply, no adverse clinical signs or symptoms have been identified in human infants fed commercial formulas lacking taurine.[46] Further study is required to determine whether premature infants have a dietary requirement for taurine.

In addition to the amount and type of protein, the distribution of protein calories (relative to carbohydrate and fat) affects the protein requirement. It is desirable that protein compose 7 to 16 per cent of total calories. Less than 7 per cent may be growth-limiting; more than 16 per cent may be toxic with consequent azotemia and acidosis.

FAT

The growing LBW infant needs an adequate amount of well-absorbed dietary fat to help meet the high energy needs of growth, to provide essential fatty acids, and to assist absorption of other important nutrients such as the fat-soluble vitamins and calcium. Neonates, particularly premature infants and those who are SGA are, however, relatively inefficient in digestion and absorption of lipid.

Fat digestion and absorption are primarily determined by the intraluminal concentration of lipases and bile acids, and by the composition of the dietary fat. Immature infants have low levels of the pancreatic enzyme lipase and consequently digest fat poorly. Physiologically, lingual lipases and gastric lipolysis may be important in neonates in view of inefficient duodenal lipid digestion.[26, 27] In addition to low lipase concentrations, premature infants have an intraluminal concentration of bile acids that is below the critical micellar concentration, and is therefore insufficient to solubilize most lipids for absorption. The combination of low lipase activity and a reduced bile acid pool in the duodenal lumen prevents complete hydrolysis and solubilization of lipids, resulting in a predictable decrease in lipolysis and transport of free fatty acids across the mucosal barrier.

In addition, the composition of dietary lipid has been shown to influence the level of absorption and retention of fat. Vegetable oils containing *polyunsaturated fatty acids (PUFA)* are absorbed more efficiently by LBW infants than saturated animal fats. Furthermore, medium chain fatty acids (8 to 12 carbon atoms) are absorbed and transported more readily than long chain fatty acids (12 carbon atoms or more). Unlike long chain fats, *medium chain triglycerides (MCT)* require few or no bile salts for digestion and absorption. When MCT is added to vegetable oils, there is improved fat absorption in LBW infants, resulting in alleviation of steatorrhea, increased weight gain, enhanced calcium absorption, and improved nitrogen retention.[53]

Dietary fat is also a source of *linoleic acid*, an essential long chain PUFA. The Committee on Nutrition of the American Academy of Pediatrics recommends that at least 3 per cent of the total calories for premature babies be provided in the form of linoleic acid.[2] Although arachidonic acid also has an important physiological role, linoleic acid is readily converted to arachidonic acid *in vivo* and is therefore the primary nutrient necessary for the prevention of essential fatty acid deficiency, as discussed on page 43. Vegetable oils and human milk fat do contain linoleic acid; MCT does not.

Adequate intake of essential fatty acids is important; however, an excessively high intake of PUFA may result in adverse effects. Because the fatty acid composition of the red blood cell membrane is primarily determined by the fatty acid composition of the diet, infants fed large amounts of PUFA have increased erythrocyte susceptibility to oxidative destruction. It is recommended that commercial formulas fed to LBW infants not contain more than about 12 per cent linoleic acid to prevent hemolytic anemia, which is discussed on page 765.

The percentage of total calories as fat relative to carbohydrate and protein is another important consideration. It is desirable that fat compose 30 to 55 per cent of total calories; fat intake greater than 60 per cent of calories may lead to ketosis. Furthermore, a diet high in fat and low in protein may yield more fat deposition than is desirable for the growing LBW infant.

CARBOHYDRATE

Carbohydrate is an important source of energy for biological reactions. There is a metabolic requirement for glucose at all times; however, there is no specific dietary requirement for carbohydrate because glucose can be manufactured in the body. Enzymes for endogenous production of glucose from carbohydrate, protein and fat are present in LBW infants.

Human milk and standard infant formulas contain approximately 40 per cent of the total calories as carbohydrate. An appropriate intake of carbohydrate is desirable; 35 to 65 per cent of total calories as carbohydrate is the recommended range. Too little carbohydrate may lead to hypoglycemia, while too much carbohydrate may provoke an osmotic diuresis or loose stools.

Lactose is the predominant carbohydrate in almost all mammalian milks, and may be important to the neonate in glucose homeostasis. Even though there is concern that the premature infant's ability to digest lactose may be marginal, in practice this is an infrequent problem, as already mentioned.[39] *Sucrose* is another disaccharide commonly found in commercial infant formula products. Because sucrase activity is present at 70 per cent of newborn levels early in the third trimester, sucrose is well tolerated by most premature infants. Both sucrase and lactase are sensitive to changes in the intestinal milieu, however, and babies afflicted by diarrhea, antibiotic therapy or undernutrition may develop a temporary intolerance to lactose and sucrose.

Glucose polymers are an increasingly common carbohydrate in the diets of LBW infants. The polymers, composed mainly of chains of five to nine glucose units linked together, are used to achieve the iso-osmolality of certain specialized formulas. Few data are available concerning the metabolism of glucose polymers in premature infants, although the polymers appear to be well digested and utilized.[10]

VITAMINS AND MINERALS

Premature infants require all of the vitamins and minerals essential for full-term infants; however, LBW babies have increased requirements for several of these because of poor body stores and physiological immaturity.

Calcium, Phosphorus and Vitamin D

Adequate intakes of calcium, phosphorus and vitamin D are required for optimal bone mineralization by growing premature infants. Because two thirds of the calcium and phosphorus content of the body of the full-term newborn is accumulated via active transport mechanisms during the last trimester of pregnancy, the infant born prematurely is deprived of this important intrauterine mineral deposition. During the final weeks of gestation, the fetus lays down approximately 120 to 150 mg. of calcium per kg.

per day in the form of new bone.[57] Table 37–4 compares the advisable intakes for calcium and phosphorus (based on intrauterine accretion rates) with the amounts contained in human milk, standard infant formulas, and specialized premature infant formula products. It is apparent that human milk and standard infant formulas do not provide enough calcium and phosphorus to meet normal fetal accretion rates. Since intestinal calcium absorption of standard formulas appears to be as low as 30 to 60 per cent of intake levels, the amount of calcium retained by the premature infant may only be 20 to 25 per cent of that which would have been received *in utero*. Indeed, several reports have documented *osteopenia* characterized by demineralization of bones in premature infants fed human milk or standard infant formulas.[22, 52] Premature infants fed milks low in calcium and phosphorus require supplementation, as discussed on page 769.

The etiology of osteopenia (i.e., rickets of prematurity) has been ascribed to a deficiency of calcium, phosphorus and vitamin D. The current state of knowledge is incomplete regarding the pathophysiology of the disease, and the relationship among hormones and mineral intakes in LBW infants is poorly understood. It is clear, however, that the intakes of calcium and phosphorus from human milk and standard infant formulas are far below fetal accumulation rates. It is also clear that calcium and phosphorus supplementation results in greater mineral retention as well as better bone mineralization.[11] Also, rickets associated with human milk feedings resolves solely with the provision of supplemental calcium and phosphorus.[22] Thus, regardless of the vitamin D requirement of the LBW infant, many of the current bone mineralization problems result from inadequate intakes of calcium and phosphorus. Specialized premature formulas now being marketed for LBW infants have a higher calcium and phosphorus content precisely for this reason. Premature infants fed these high-mineral formulas achieve bone mineralization comparable to that observed during intrauterine growth.[50] Consequently, no additional calcium and phosphorus supplementation is needed by LBW infants fed specialized premature formulas.

While delayed bone mineralization in LBW infants is primarily related to inadequate intakes of calcium and phosphorus, the role of vitamin D metabolites in the regulation of calcium and phosphorus absorption, and their effects on skeletal development should not be ignored. The premature infant probably has a higher vitamin D requirement than the full-term baby because of smaller vitamin D stores, a more rapid rate of growth, and immature bio-

Table 37-4. ADVISABLE INTAKES FOR CALCIUM, PHOSPHORUS, PROTEIN, SODIUM AND VITAMIN D COMPARED WITH SELECTED FEEDINGS

	ADVISABLE INTAKE		HUMAN MILK		STANDARD	PREMATURE		
	1 kg. Body Wt.	1.5 kg. Body Wt.	Preterm	Mature	Enfamil Similac SMA	Enfamil Premature	Premie SMA	Similac Special Care
Calcium (mg./100 kcal.)	160	140	40	43	66–78	117	92	178
Phosphorus (mg./100 kcal.)	108	95	18	20	49–66	58	49	89
Protein (gm./100 kcal.)	3.1	2.7	2.3 (range 0.9–2.8)*	1.5	2.2	3.0	2.5	2.7
Sodium (mEq./100 kcal.)	2.7	2.3	1.5 (range 1.9–2.3)	0.8	1.0–1.8	1.7	1.7	1.9
Caloric density (kcal./dl.)			73	67	81	81	81	81
Vitamin D (I.U./day)	600	600	?	4†	70–75†	75†	76†	180†

* Lemons, J. A., et al: Differences in the composition of preterm and term human milk during early lactation. Pediatr. Res., 16:113, 1982.
† At 120 kcal./kg./day for an infant weighing 1 kg.
Adapted from Brady, M. S., et al: Formulas and human milk for premature infants: a review and update. J. Am. Diet. Assoc., 81:547, 1982.

transformation of vitamin D to metabolically active forms.[7] Compared with term infants, those born prematurely appear to require higher amounts of vitamin D (as D_3) in order to maintain plasma $25\text{-}OHD_3$ levels in a normal range, possibly owing to inefficient metabolism or rapid turnover of metabolites.

Rickets has been described in VLBW infants (<1500 grams) fed standard formulas containing the amount of vitamin D required by full-term infants (i.e., 400 I.U./liter).[36] Because small infants consume small daily volumes of milk (often as little as 150 ml./kg./day), their actual vitamin D intake may be only a fraction of that ingested by full-term infants. A daily supplement of 400 I.U. of vitamin D has been reported to cure rickets in some of these VLBW infants;[36] other reports suggest that a daily dose of 400 I.U. vitamin D may not protect adequately against rickets.[7] Although the available data are insufficient for establishing a precise requirement for vitamin D for premature infants, an advisable intake of 600 I.U. per day has been tentatively proposed.[56] As Table 37–4 indicates, vitamin D intake is below this recommended level for human milk, standard formulas and specialized premature formulas, particularly when the small volume ingested is considered. Supplementation is generally recommended; in practice, an additional 400 to 600 I.U. of vitamin D per day is usually given as part of a multivitamin supplement.

Iron

Low-birth-weight infants are known to be at risk for developing iron deficiency anemia because of reduced iron stores associated with premature birth. Although these stores are sufficient to permit expansion of the premature infant's blood volume to nearly twice its initial size (i.e., until birth weight has doubled), they drop rapidly after about two months of age as active erythropoiesis resumes. Iron deficiency anemia may develop by three months postnatal age if iron supplementation is not provided. In contrast, full-term infants do not typically deplete their proportionately larger iron stores until after four to six months of life.

Recommendations for LBW infants call for supplementation of the diet with elemental iron at a dose of no more than 2 mg./kg./day, no later than two months postnatal age.[1] Specialized premature formulas contain low levels of iron (less than 0.5 mg./kg./day when providing 120 kcal./kg./day), and therefore need to be supplemented before the infant is about two months old. Similarly, the iron content of human milk does not meet the requirements of the premature, despite the enhanced absorption of iron

from human milk. For infants receiving human milk or premature formula, oral ferrous sulfate drops are an effective supplement. Larger premature infants (weighing 2 kg. or more) who are fed standard formula fortified with iron receive 1.8 to 2.0 mg. of elemental iron per 120 kcal. and do not require additional supplementation.

Iron intake in conjunction with vitamin E deficiency can lead to hemolytic anemia, as discussed in the following section. Because LBW infants are at risk for vitamin E deficiency, it is important that vitamin E intake recommendations be met if iron supplements are introduced in the immediate neonatal period (i.e., first 28 days of life). Furthermore, iron excess may theoretically decrease host resistance to infection through saturation and inactivation of the antibacterial, iron-binding proteins in serum and milk.[3] Since iron stores are ample for the first two months, the above considerations make it reasonable to consider withholding supplemental iron from LBW infants initially; however, supplements begun at about two to three weeks postnatal age have been shown to be both safe and effective.[38] Therefore, the recommended age for initiation of iron supplementation in LBW infants ranges from as early as two weeks to as late as two months postnatal age.

Vitamin E

Low-birth-weight infants may require more vitamin E than full-term infants. This has been assumed to be a result of poor absorption of the vitamin in the face of low body stores. Impaired absorption of vitamin E by premature infants was described in the early 1970's;[40] however, fat blends in current premature formulas are markedly improved, resulting in better absorption of both fat and vitamin E. In spite of this, the premature infant is born with poor vitamin E stores relative to the full-term baby. When supplemented with 30 I.U. of vitamin E per day, most premature infants show plasma tocopherol levels within the desired range. By comparison, unsupplemented infants are more apt to demonstrate biochemical signs of vitamin E deficiency, such as lower hemoglobin concentrations, higher reticulocyte counts, and more fragile red cells in weak solutions of hydrogen peroxide. The advisable intake of vitamin E in LBW infants is 30 I.U. per day.[56]

An important function of vitamin E is its protection of biological membranes against oxidative breakdown of lipids. Requirements for vitamin E increase when the level of PUFA in the diet is high. The PUFA gradually produce a change in the composition of the fatty acids in cellular and intracellular membranes. The membranes then become more susceptible to oxidative damage, which increases the requirement for the antioxidant effect of vitamin E. Because iron is a biological oxidant, a diet high in either iron or PUFA increases the risks of vitamin E deficiency. A premature infant suffering from vitamin E deficiency may experience oxidative destruction of red blood cells or *hemolytic anemia.*

Several studies in the early 1970's indicated that premature infants were at high risk for developing hemolytic anemia.[40] However, the formula products used in these studies were high in PUFA and iron, and contained fat blends that resulted in poor absorption of vitamin E. The combination of high PUFA content and high levels of the oxidant iron in the face of vitamin E deficiency resulted in red blood cell hemolysis by membrane destruction. Since that time, the composition of premature formulas has been favorably changed to correct these problems. Therefore, hemolytic anemia associated with vitamin E deficiency is rarely a problem today when careful attention is paid to the composition of the diet.

Since the dietary requirement for vitamin E depends upon the PUFA content of the diet, the recommended intake of vitamin E is commonly expressed as a ratio of vitamin E to PUFA. The Committee on Nutrition of the American Academy of Pediatrics recommends that milk fed to premature infants provide at least 0.6 mg. of d-alpha-tocopherol per gm. of PUFA.[2] Both human milk and the new premature formulas have E:PUFA ratios well above the minimum recommended by the American Academy of Pediatrics.

The use of pharmacological doses of vitamin E for the prevention of diseases related to oxygen toxicity is an area of much speculation. Pharmacological doses of parenteral vitamin E protect against oxygen-induced retinopathy in kittens, an animal model of the acute proliferative phase of human *retrolental fibroplasia (RLF).*[42] Preliminary clinical data also suggest that vitamin E deficiency may play a role in the development of RLF,[31] but the evidence is insufficient to draw conclusions at this time. A beneficial effect of high doses of vitamin E for the prevention of pulmonary oxygen toxicity in infants at risk for developing *bronchopulmonary dysplasia (BPD)* has also been suggested.[15] A subsequent study, however, could not demonstrate such an effect.[16] The appropriate use of pharmocological doses of vitamin E in preterm infants has not been documented as yet, and must be weighed in terms of potential benefit and possible toxicity. Thus, while available facts reinforce the need to provide supplemental vitamin E to LBW infants in quantities sufficient to produce normal blood levels (30 I.U. per day), the routine use of higher doses (100 I.U. or more per day) to produce greater than normal blood levels of vitamin E should be regarded with caution.

Folic Acid

Premature infants seem to have higher folic acid needs than infants born at term. Although serum folate levels are high at birth, they decrease dramatically soon thereafter. This may be a reflection of the high utilization of folic acid by the premature infant for DNA and tissue synthesis. Because the premature baby grows at a more rapid rate than the term infant, he or she may have a higher intrinsic need for folic acid.

A mild form of folic acid deficiency manifested by low serum folate concentrations and hypersegmentation of neutrophils is not unusual in premature infants. Megaloblastic anemia is much less commonly observed. A daily supplement of 50 to 70 μg. is effective in preventing neutrophil hypersegmentation and low serum folate concentrations.[51] Ziegler and associates recommend an intake of 60 μg. per day.[56]

Sodium

Low-birth-weight infants, especially those who are most premature, are prone to hyponatremia in the neonatal period. Up to 30 per cent of infants weighing less than 1300 gm. at birth may be hyponatremic during the first weeks of life.[47] These babies may experience excessive urinary sodium losses owing to renal immaturity. Furthermore, their sodium needs are high related to their rapid rate of growth. Dietary intake may be poor, especially for those infants who consume small volumes of milk.

Daily sodium intakes of 3 to 6 mEq. or more per kg. may be required by some infants to avoid hyponatremia and to correct associated growth failure.[17] The American Academy of Pediatrics does not recommend routine sodium supplementation of low-sodium milks.[2] However, it is important to consider the possibility that hyponatremia may occur and to monitor infants by frequent assessment of serum and/or urinary sodium concentrations.

Enteral Nutrition

Enteral alimentation is preferred for LBW infants because this approach is more physiologic and associated with fewer known complications than parenteral alimentation. However, the decision to initiate enteral feeding is often difficult and involves consideration of the degree of prematurity, history of perinatal insults, current medical condition, functioning of the gastrointestinal tract and several other individualized concerns. Because of the complexity of these factors, the choice of optimal feeding method must be personalized for each LBW infant, and altered according to the variable course of each baby.

METHODS OF FEEDING

Once the decision to feed enterally has been made, one must select the optimal enteral feeding technique. Infants may be fed either by gavage (tube) or nipple.

Oral gastric gavage feeding is often chosen for infants unable to suck because of immaturity or insults to the central nervous system. Infants of less than 32 to 34 weeks gestational age, regardless of birth weight, may be expected to have poorly coordinated sucking and swallowing activity related to their developmental immaturity, and are consequently unable to nipple-feed. Using the oral gastric gavage method, a soft feeding tube is inserted through the mouth and into the baby's stomach. The major risks of this technique include aspiration and gastric distention. Experience and proper positioning of the infant can minimize the danger of aspiration from regurgitation of stomach contents. Gastric distention and vagal nerve stimulation with resultant bradycardia are potential problems when oral gastric gavage feedings are delivered on an *intermittent bolus* schedule, with tube placement every two hours, for example. Elimination of the distention and vagal bradycardia may occasionally require the use of an indwelling tube for *continuous gastric gavage* feedings, instead of the preferred intermittent technique. *Nasal gastric gavage* is sometimes better tolerated than oral tube feeding. But because newborns are obligate nose breathers, this technique may compromise the nasal airway in LBW infants with associated deterioration in respiratory function.

Transpyloric gavage feeding is occasionally indicated for LBW infants. The goal of this method is to circumvent the often slow gastropyloric motility of the immature infant by passing the feeding tube through the stomach and pylorus and locating its tip within the duodenum or jejunum. Advantages to transpyloric feeding include the elimination of the pylorus as a barrier for adequate propulsion of milk, and a reduced chance of aspiration. But there are several disadvantages as well. Transpyloric feedings have been associated with decreased fat absorption, diarrhea, dumping syndrome, alteration of the intestinal microflora, contamination of the feeding system, intestinal perforation, and bilious fluid in the stomach.[48] Transpyloric tubes also require considerable expertise in their placement, and x-rays to determine the location of the catheter tip. Because of the problems inherent in using this technique, transpyloric feeding is probably not indicated for routine use in LBW infants. In certain critically ill infants, however, it may represent the best compromise between the benefits and risks of available alternatives.

Nipple-feeding may be attempted in infants whose gestational age is greater than 32 to 34 weeks. The ability to nipple-feed is usually indicated by evidence of an established sucking reflex and sucking motion. Because sucking requires considerable effort by the infant, any stress from other causes such as hypothermia or hypoxemia will diminish sucking ability. Nipple-feeding, therefore, should be offered only when the infant is free of stress and has sufficient maturity and strength for a sustained sucking effort. A soft, "premie" nipple may facilitate early nippling attempts; when a gestational age of 35 weeks is reached, a regular nipple is usually tolerated.

VOLUME OF FEEDING

The appropriate amount of milk to be fed to LBW infants depends upon their estimated stomach capacity. The undistended stomach volume varies with the size of the infant, and may be as small as 2 to 3 ml. in the 800 gm. newborn, or about 40 ml. in the 4000 gm. newborn. Although gastric capacity increases with postnatal age, individual infants vary in their ability to tolerate enteral volumes and should be monitored by regular measurement of gastric residuals. Exceeding the gastric capacity of the small baby may result in feeding intolerance and potentially serious morbidity. An example of a feeding schedule for LBW infants is shown in Table 37–5.

TOLERANCE OF FEEDINGS

All LBW babies receiving enteral nutrition should be consistently monitored for signs of feeding intolerance. *Vomiting* of feedings usually signals the inability of the infant to retain that amount of milk. When not associated with other signs of a systemic illness, vomiting may indicate a too rapid increase in feeding volumes or excessive volume for the infant's size and maturity. A reduction in volume may be all that is needed. If this does not eliminate vomiting, or if signs of a systemic illness coexist, feedings may need to be interrupted until the infant's condition has normalized.

Table 37-5. ENTERAL FEEDING SCHEDULE FOR LOW-BIRTH-WEIGHT INFANTS

	UP TO 1000 GM.		1001–1500 GM.		1501–2000 GM.		MORE THAN 2000 GM.	
	Amount	Frequency	Amount	Frequency	Amount	Frequency	Amount	Frequency
First feeding	Sterile water 1 ml.	1 hr.	2–3 ml.	2 hr.	4–5 ml.	2 hr.	10 ml.	3 hr.
Subsequent feedings (12–72 hr)	Human milk or formula Gradually increase by 0.5–1.0 ml. to maximum 3–5 ml.	2 hr.	Gradually increase by 1.0 ml. to maximum 7–10 ml.	2 hr.	Gradually increase by 2.0 ml. maximum 12–15	2–3 hr.	Gradually increase by 5.0 ml. to maximum 20 ml.	3 hr.
Final feeding schedule	Human milk or formula 6–12 ml.	2 hr.	18–28 ml.	3 hr.	28–37 ml.	3 hr.	37–50 ml.	3–4 hr.
Total volume (mg./kg./day)	120–150		150		150		150	

Adapted from Avery, G. B., and Fletcher, A. B.: Nutrition. In Avery, G. B. (ed.): Neonatology: Pathophysiology and Management of the Newborn. Philadelphia, J. B. Lippincott Company, 1981, p. 1025.

Abdominal distention may be caused by feeding of excessive volumes, organic obstruction, excessive swallowing of air, resuscitation or sepsis (i.e., systemic infection). Observation of the infant for abdominal distention should be a routine practice for the nurse caring for the infant. Intermittent measurement of abdominal circumference will aid in the early detection of distention. This symptom often indicates the need for interruption of feeding until the cause of the distention is determined and the abdomen is once more soft and flat.

Gastric residuals are measured by aspiration of the stomach contents, and should be routinely checked prior to each bolus gavage feeding and intermittently in all continuous drip feedings. Whether or not a residual is significant depends in part on its volume in relation to the total volume of the feeding; a residual whose volume is more than 20 per cent of the total feeding might be a sign of feeding intolerance. When interpreting the significance of a gastric residual, however, it is important to consider that residual in light of other concurrent signs of feeding intolerance and the pattern of residuals established for that infant. Gastric residuals that are bloody or bilious are more alarming than those that appear to be undigested milk.

The *frequency and consistency of bowel movements* require constant attention when feeding LBW infants. Furthermore, routine testing of stools for reducing substances is a useful procedure that promptly detects incomplete absorption of sugars by the intestine. Although the presence of gross blood can be detected by simple inspection, occult blood is not always visible, and should be investigated by a specific assay to detect small amounts of blood in the stool.

No one method of feeding is without hazards for LBW infants, and unless close attention is paid to symptoms indicative of poor feeding tolerance, serious complications may ensue. Certain diseases can be recognized clinically by determination of signs of feeding intolerance. Necrotizing enterocolitis is a serious and potentially fatal disease which is associated with such signs as abdominal distention and tenderness and abnormal gastric residuals.

NECROTIZING ENTEROCOLITIS

Several authors have suggested that aggressive enteral feeding in the early days of life may be an etiological factor in the development of *necrotizing enterocolitis (NEC)*. Necrotizing enterocolitis is a disease of complex multifactorial pathogenesis related to hypoxia with a consequent decrease in gut perfusion, bowel ischemia and mucosal damage. Early enteral feedings in susceptible infants, especially when volumes are rapidly increased and hypertonic formulas are fed, may predispose to NEC by contributing to mucosal damage.[14] When bacteria invade the damaged mucosa of an infant's intestine, necrosis and tissue death may result. Feedings may provide substrate for intestinal bacterial growth.

Although enteral feeding may play a part in the pathogenesis of NEC, evidence concerning the role of feeding is primarily circumstantial, particularly as the disease has been reported in a number of infants before enteral feeding was begun.[33] Other factors associated with the development of NEC include generalized asphyxia at birth or, in the neonate, arterial hypoxemia from respiratory disease, gut ischemia secondary to a patent ductus arteriosus or to congenital heart disease, and ischemia secondary to umbilical catheterization.[14] Enteral feeding is not singularly responsible for the pathogenesis of NEC; however, a conservative approach to enteral feeding may be warranted in LBW infants, particularly when other risk factors for the development of the disease are present.

COMPOSITION OF FEEDINGS—HUMAN MILK

Human milk is the reference standard for most commercial infant formulas, as human milk uniquely satisfies the nutritional requirements of the full-term baby. The nutritional adequacy of breast milk for small premature infants is, however, a controversial subject. There is a lack of adequate data concerning the composition of human milk, a lack of agreement regarding optimal growth and protein requirements of LBW babies, and some difficulty in performing and interpreting clinical nutritional studies of premature infants. Mature human milk contains less protein than the new formulas for premature babies listed in Table 37–4 and generally does not support growth of LBW infants at the intrauterine rate.[18] But growth does occur and is accompanied by fewer metabolic side effects than are seen with some high-protein formulas.[20, 43–45] Furthermore, no long-term developmental or intellectual sequelae have been attributed to feeding human milk to LBW infants. Whether failure to achieve intrauterine rates of growth is harmful is an unanswered question.

New investigations offer intriguing evidence that the composition of milk from mothers delivering prematurely differs from that of term mothers during the early weeks of lactation. As Table 37–4 indicates, it is higher in protein, sodium and chloride, and perhaps iron and magnesium, and theoretically may be more suitable for the preterm infant than mature human milk.[23, 35] In addition, the energy content of preterm human milk may be higher than that of more mature milk (i.e., 22 kcal./oz. compared with 20 kcal./oz.). The rate of growth of preterm infants fed their own mother's milk is more rapid than that of preterm infants fed human milk donated by mothers at a mature stage of lactation.[24] Other nutritional advantages in feeding human milk to preterm infants include its easily digested fat, low renal solute load, and desirable protein composition (i.e., whey-predominant protein with higher amounts of cystine and taurine).

A significant nutritional disadvantage for preterm infants exists with respect to the concentrations of calcium and phosphorus at all stages of human lactation. Human milk does not meet the calcium and phosphorus needs for normal bone mineralization for infants born prematurely.[22] Supplementation is recommended for rapidly growing LBW infants fed predominantly human milk. A new, powdered human milk fortifier (Mead Johnson) containing calcium and phosphorus (as well as protein, carbohydrate and certain other minerals) may be a useful supplement for preterm infants.

Nutritional considerations are not, however, the only basis on which to judge the adequacy of human milk for LBW infants. Providing breast milk to the premature infant can be a very positive experience for a mother, and often promotes maternal involvement and interaction. In addition, human colostrum and milk contain numerous factors that impart immunological and antimicrobial benefit to the infant. These agents may provide protection from infection for the developing gut mucosa, and provide possible prophylaxis against NEC. Although there is as yet no clinical evidence that human milk prevents NEC, there is a widespread clinical impression that NEC is less common in LBW infants fed human milk. There is also experimental evidence in a rat model that human milk macrophages protect against the development of NEC following an anoxic insult to the gut.[8]

After consideration of the nutritional, immunological and other risks and benefits related to the feeding of human milk to LBW infants, most authorities agree that it is the feeding of choice. Preterm mother's milk for her own infant is preferred owing to its favorable nutrient concentration and smaller logistical problems in collection and handling.

Since most preterm infants are neither strong nor mature enough to suckle at their mother's breast in the neonatal period, mothers usually express their milk for a considerable period of time before nursing can be established. Several factors relating to the technique of expression, storage and transport of milk must be considered in order to assure that the breast milk provided is appropriate for feeding. Because of the ready access of most medications to human milk and the risk of transmission of infection, both mothers and milk should be carefully screened as summarized in Table 11–11.

COMPOSITION OF FEEDINGS— FORMULAS

New formula preparations have been developed to meet the unique nutrient and physiological needs of growing LBW infants. The quantity and quality of nutrients contained in these products promote growth at intrauterine rates. When fed to *stable* premature infants who are growing rapidly, these specialized formulas are usually tolerated without metabolic consequences. Studies of stable babies weighing 1200 gm. or more indicate that these formulas are safe and promote weight gain, fat absorption, nitrogen retention and bone mineralization.[50] When fed to VLBW babies who are *stressed* and have not yet sustained a steady weight gain, premature formulas should be used cautiously. Because weight gain frequently does not occur in these small babies until after the first couple of weeks of life, premature formulas may be introduced by diluting with water to half strength (12 kcal./oz.) and fed in very small quantities. There is no proven advantage to prolonged dilute feedings; therefore, concentration may be increased to 24 kcal./oz. during the first 12 to 48 hours of enteral feeding, with a subsequent, gradual increase in volume over several days. The concentration of the premature formulas to 24 kcal./oz. at full strength more easily meets the LBW infants' energy needs in the face of fluid tolerance limitations.

These new premature formulas differ in many aspects from standard cow's milk–based formulas. Table 37–6 summarizes these differences and identifies some of the advantages of feeding premature formulas to LBW infants. Refer to Table 37–7 for a summary of the composition of human milk and that of premature and standard infant formulas.

SELECTION OF FEEDINGS

Choice of an optimal feeding for a LBW infant is complicated by the fact that no ideal feeding exists. The extrauterine environment represents an abrupt change for the preterm infant, and most of these babies require a period of adjustment before tolerance to any enteral feeding can be established.

There may be some advantage in feeding sterile water as the first feeding after birth, since

Table 37-6. COMPARISON OF PREMATURE VERSUS STANDARD FORMULAS FOR FEEDING LOW-BIRTH-WEIGHT INFANTS

PREMATURE FORMULAS*	STANDARD FORMULAS†
Designed, tested in preterm infants	Designed, tested in full-term infants
Energy: 24 kcal./oz.	20 kcal./oz.
Protein: whey-casein; 60:40	Whey-casein; 18:82‡
Fat: Part MCT; part long chain fats	100% long chain fats
Carbohydrate: part glucose polymers; part lactose	100% lactose
Calcium & phosphorus: fortified to meet needs of premature	Not fortified to meet needs of premature
Iron: not fortified	Available with or without added iron
Iso-osmolar (300 mOsm./kg. H_2O)	Iso-osmolar

* Enfamil Premature (Mead Johnson), Premie SMA (Wyeth Laboratories) and Similac Special Care (Ross Laboratories).

† Similac (Ross Laboratories).

‡ SMA (Wyeth Laboratories) contains whey-casein; 60:40. New *humanized standard* formulas with similar whey-predominant protein are also available, such as Enfamil (with Whey) (Mead Johnson) and Similac with Whey (Ross Laboratories). However, these standard products are not designed to meet the other unique nutrient and physiological needs of low-birth-weight infants.

animal evidence indicates that pulmonary damage from aspiration of water is less than that from either 5 per cent glucose in water or milk.[41] Following the first feeding, human milk or formula of the desired strength may be used in slowly increasing amounts.

During the initial period of feeding, premature infants are often still adjusting to enteral nutrition and may be experiencing concurrent stress, weight loss and diuresis. The primary goal of enteral feeding during this initial period is to facilitate *tolerance* to the milk provided. Aggressive nutritional support from the onset of enteral feeding often meets with failure, as babies appear unable to assimilate a large volume and concentration of nutrients until adjustment has been established. Supplementation of enteral feedings with parenteral fluids is often required until adequate oral volume is tolerated.

Selection of a milk with the characteristics listed in Table 37-8 may facilitate tolerance to enteral feedings during this initial period of adjustment. Feedings that meet these criteria include (1) human milk, (2) premature formula, or (3) a low-protein, low-mineral formula such as Similac PM 60/40 (Ross Laboratories).

When preterm mother's milk for her own infant is available, it is the feeding of choice. Premature formulas were designed for growing LBW infants and should be used with caution during the initial period of enteral feeding. The low renal solute load of such formulas as

Similac PM 60/40 may be of initial advantage to the stressed, immature infant experiencing obligatory water loss. However, the low protein and mineral concentrations in this formula are likely to be disadvantages for the stable infant once growth is established.

After the initial period of adjustment, the goal of enteral feeding changes to provide *complete nutrition* to promote growth and rapid organ development. All essential nutrients should be provided in quantities that support sustained growth in all parameters. For this effect, the following feeding choices are appropriate: (1) human milk, (2) premature formula or (3) standard infant formula.

Human milk continues to be the feeding of choice for the rapidly growing LBW infant. If fluid limitations exist, the volume of human milk ingested may be less than that needed to support adequate growth, and a powdered human milk fortifier (Mead Johnson), or a formula supplement (24 kcal./oz. or more) may be desirable until fluid intake can be liberalized.

In general, infants weighing less than about 2 kg. require special attention with respect to their nutritional needs and level of maturity. When human milk is not available, premature formulas are the usual choice for infants weighing less than 2 kg.; standard formulas are more appropriate for larger babies. The decision to change from premature to standard formula will vary in timing depending on such factors as the infant's growth history, energy requirements, volume limitations and discharge plans.

DIETARY MANIPULATIONS

It is occasionally desirable to increase the energy content of the formulas fed to small infants to more than 24 kcal./oz. This may be appropriate when the infant is not growing at a desirable rate and is already ingesting a maximum volume of fluid. One approach to providing hypercaloric formulas is to subtract water, thereby concentrating all nutrients, including energy. Concentrated infant formulas with energy contents of 24 kcal./oz. or greater are available to hospitals as ready-to-feed nursettes. When using such concentrated formulas, however, it is important to consider the infant's fluid intake and fluid losses in relation to the renal solute load of the concentrated feeding, to ensure that positive water balance is maintained.[9]

Another approach to increasing the energy content of formulas employs the use of caloric supplements such as MCT oil (Mead Johnson) and glucose polymers as Polycose (Ross Laboratories). These supplements increase the caloric density without marked alterations in solute load or osmolality; however, they do alter the

Table 37–7. COMPOSITION OF HUMAN MILK, PREMATURE FORMULAS, AND STANDARD FORMULAS

	CALORIC DENSITY	PROTEIN Whey/casein	PROTEIN % TOTAL CALORIES	CARBOHYDRATE	CARBOHYDRATE % TOTAL CALORIES	FAT	FAT % TOTAL CALORIES	Ca (mg./L)	P (mg./L)	RENAL (mOsm./L.)	GI (mOsm./kg. H_2O)
Human Milk											
Mature	20 kcal./oz. (0.67 kcal./ml.)		7	Lactose	38	Human milk fat	55	340	169	75	300
Premature	22 kcal./oz. (0.73 kcal./ml.)	60:40		Lactose		Human milk fat		293	134		300
Standard Formula											
Similac	20 kcal./oz.	18:82	9	Lactose	43	Coconut & soy oils	48	510 520	390 438	110–120	285
Humanized Standard Formulas											
SMA	20 kcal./oz.	60:40	9	Lactose	41–43	Corn, coconut, and/or soy, saf-oleo oils	48–51	420	310	105	250
Similac PM 60/40	20 kcal./oz.	60:40	9	Lactose	41			400	200	92	260
Enfamil	20 kcal./oz.	60:40	9	Lactose	41			460	345	97	285
Similac with whey	20 kcal./oz.	60:40	9	Lactose	43			400	300	104	300
Premature Formulas											
Similac Special Care	24 kcal./oz. (0.81 kcal./ml.)	60:40	11	Lactose/glucose polymers 50:50	42	MCT/corn/coconut 50:30:20	47	1440	702	208	300
Enfamil Premature	24 kcal./oz.	60:40	12	Lactose 40:60	42	40:40:20	44	940	470	220	300
Premie SMA	24 kcal./oz.	60:40	10	Lactose 50:50	42	Coconut/safflower/oleo/soy/ MCT 27:25:20:18:10	48	750	400	175	300

Table 37–8. CRITERIA THAT PROMOTE TOLERANCE TO INITIAL ENTERAL FEEDINGS

1. Nutrient composition that is readily digestible and absorable
2. Whey-casein protein 60:40
3. Low renal solute load
4. Iso-osmolality (300 mOsm./kg. H_2O)

relative distribution of total calories from protein, carbohydrate and fat. Because adding even small amounts of MCT oil and/or Polycose adversely dilutes the percentage of protein calories while altering the percentage of calories from fat and carbohydrate, adding these supplements to human milk or standard 20 kcal./oz. formula is not advised. Table 37–9 shows the potential dilutional effects of MCT oil and Polycose.

When a high-energy formula is appropriate, first add MCT oil to a 24 kcal./oz. base (either full-strength premature formula or a concentrated standard formula), to a maximum of 60 per cent of total calories as fat, and a minimum of 7 per cent of total calories as protein. If more energy is needed for sustained growth, Polycose may then be added. The guidelines in Table 37–10 are recommended for use of MCT oil and Polycose in LBW infants.

VITAMIN AND MINERAL SUPPLEMENTATION

The vitamin and mineral requirements of preterm infants are not precisely known. Estimates of advisable intakes take into account intrauterine accretion rates, full-term infants' needs and the unique physiological demands of LBW infants. Although these advisable intakes

Table 37–9. POTENTIAL ADVERSE EFFECTS OF MCT OIL (MCT) AND POLYCOSE (PC) SUPPLEMENTS IN HUMAN MILK AND STANDARD 20 KCAL./OZ. FORMULA

	DISTRIBUTION OF CALORIES (%)		
	Protein	*Carbohydrate*	*Fat*
Human Milk			
(150 ml./day)	7	38	55
+0.4 ml. MCT/oz.	5 (low)	33 (low)	63 (high)
+1.5 ml. PC/oz.	3–4 (low)	38	60 (high)
Standard Formula*			
(150 ml./day)	9	42	49
+0.4 ml. MCT/oz.	7	35 (low)	57
+1.5 ml. PC/oz.	6 (low)	43	50

* Standard formula as Similac (20 kcal./oz.).
From O'Leary, M. J.: Neonatal nutrition. In Hodson, W. A., and Truog, W. E. (eds.): Critical Care of the Newborn. Philadelphia, W. B. Saunders Company, 1983, p. 45.

Table 37–10. RECOMMENDATIONS FOR USE OF MCT OIL AND POLYCOSE BY LOW-BIRTH-WEIGHT INFANTS

1. To a 24 kcal./oz. formula base,
   Add: 0.4 ml. MCT oil*/oz. formula = 27 kcal./oz. formula
2. Then add: 1.5 ml. liquid Polycose[†]/oz. formula = 30 kcal./oz. formula
3. Increase volume of feeding as tolerated and wean off MCT oil and Polycose

* MCT oil (Mead Johnson).
[†] Polycose (Ross Laboratories).

lack precision, they do serve as guidelines until more precise empirical data are available. Ziegler and associates have reported advisable intakes for vitamins and minerals by preterm infants.[56] Table 37–11 compares the vitamin recommendations for preterm versus full-term babies.

Although human milk contains a full complement of vitamins, and premature formulas have been fortified to better meet the needs of the LBW infant, most tiny babies consume such small volumes of milk that a multivitamin supplement is usually recommended. The type, quantity and frequency of supplementation varies with individual body weight and predominant feeding, as Table 37–12 indicates.

Oral vitamin and mineral supplementation should be delayed until the infant has tolerated full-strength formula or breast milk for at least 48 hours at a volume sufficient to provide calo-

Table 37–11. ADVISABLE INTAKES OF VITAMINS FOR PRETERM COMPARED WITH FULL-TERM INFANTS

VITAMINS	PRETERM*	FULL-TERM[†] (0–12 mo.)
Vitamin A (I.U.)	500	500
Vitamin D (I.U.)	600	400
Vitamin E (I.U.)	30	4
Vitamin K (μg.)	15	15
Vitamin C (mg.)	60	20
Thiamin (mg.)	0.2	0.2
Riboflavin (mg.)	0.4	0.4
Niacin (mg.)	5	5
B_6 (mg.)	0.4	1.5
B_{12} (μg.)	1.5	—
Folic acid (μg.)	60	50
Pantothenic acid (mg.)	2	—
Biotin (μg.)	12	—

* Data from Ziegler, E. E., Biga, R. L., and Fomon, S. J.: Nutritional requirements of the premature infant. In Suskind, R. M. (ed.): Textbook of Pediatric Nutrition. New York, Raven Press, 1981, p. 36.
[†] Data from Anderson, T. A., and Fomon, S. J.: Vitamins. In Fomon, S. J. (ed.): Infant Nutrition. Philadelphia, W. B. Saunders Company, 1974, p. 212.

Table 37–12. SUGGESTED SCHEDULE FOR VITAMIN/MINERAL SUPPLEMENTATION FOR LBW INFANTS BASED ON BODY WEIGHT AND PREDOMINANT FEEDING

| | HUMAN MILK | PREMATURE FORMULA | | STANDARD, AND HUMANIZED STANDARD FORMULAS |
		Similac Special Care (Ross)	Premature Enfamil With Whey (Mead Johnson)	Similac, Similac With Whey, Enfamil, SMA
< 2000 Gram Infant:				
Premature vitamin compound* 0.6 ml. t.i.d.	yes	yes	yes	yes
Calcium (as gluceptate) 1.5 ml. = 27 mg. Ca	yes	no	no	yes
Phosphorus (as potassium phosphate) 0.2 ml. = 18 mg. P	yes	no	no	yes
Iron 2 mg./kg./day	*Prematures*: yes, when 1) body weight has doubled and/or 2) infant is 2 weeks to 2 months of age			No, if receiving formula with iron
> 2000 Gram Infant:				
Polyvisol 1.0 ml./day†	no	(these formulas are not usually fed to infants > 2000 grams body weight)		yes
Vitamin D (as D₃) 400 I.U./day	yes			no
Iron 1 mg./kg./day (full-term)	*Full-term*: yes, by 4 months of age			No, if receiving formula with iron

* Special vitamin preparation prepared by hospital pharmacy (based on Ziegler's advisable intakes for prematures[56]).

† Infants who weigh > 2500 grams and ingest about 0.5 liter per day receive 0.5 ml. per day.

Adapted from O'Leary, M.J.: Neonatal nutrition. In Hodson, W.A., and Truog, W.E. (eds.): Critical Care of the Newborn. Philadelphia, W.B. Saunders Company, 1983, p. 39.

ries for maintenance and growth. Because common liquid vitamin preparations have very high osmolalities, it is suggested that the supplements be administered in divided doses, and mixed with the iso-osmolar milk before feeding. This minimizes the adverse side effects of vitamin supplementation such as increased gastric residuals and regurgitation.

Parenteral Nutrition

Many critically ill LBW infants are unable to tolerate enteral nutrition in the first several days or even weeks of life. These sick premature babies are likely to develop protein-energy malnutrition unless adequate parenteral nutrition can be established.

Parenteral fluids are delivered either by lines placed in peripheral blood vessels or via central vascular catheters. The peripheral route is preferred for infants requiring parenteral support for a relatively brief period of time, usually less than two weeks, or for those infants needing supplemental fluids until adequate enteral intake is achieved. For the VLBW infant with limited peripheral vein access and prolonged parenteral nutrition need, and for neonates that require fluid restriction (e.g., those with congenital heart defects), central vascular delivery may be warranted. Although central and peripheral hyperalimentation can be life-saving or life-sustaining for many infants, both routes are associated with the metabolic and catheter-related complications listed in Table 37–13. When these risks are weighed against the nutritional benefits, most experts believe that there is no justification for the *routine* use of parenteral alimentation in LBW infants.

Formulations that may be given intravenously include glucose and amino acid solutions (with added electrolytes, vitamins and minerals) and lipid emulsions. Table 37–14 shows the typical nutrient composition of peripheral and central vein infusates.

Table 37–13.   METABOLIC AND CATHETER-
RELATED COMPLICATIONS OF PARENTERAL
NUTRITION

METABOLIC

Disorders Related to Metabolic Capacity of Infant

  Electrolyte and mineral imbalances
  Glucose
    Hyperglycemia
    Hypoglycemia
  Protein
    Azotemia
    Hyperammonemia
    Hyperaminoacidemia
    Metabolic Acidosis
  Fat
    Essential fatty acid deficiency
    Hyperlipidemia
  Vitamin excess or deficiency
  Trace element excess or deficiency

Hepatic Disorders

CATHETER-RELATED

Disorders Related to Catheter Site

  Malposition
  Pneumothorax

Disorders Related to Use of Catheter

  Sepsis
  Thrombosis
  Catheter dislodgement
  Perforation and/or infiltration leaks

Adapted from Heird, W.C.: Total parenteral nutrition. In Lebenthal, E. (ed.): Textbook of Gastroenterology and Nutrition in Infancy. New York, Raven Press, 1981, p. 662.

GLUCOSE

Glucose is usually the principal energy source. However, VLBW babies exhibit a significant degree of glucose intolerance in the early neonatal period. Hyperglycemia has been observed in more than 80 per cent of infants who weigh less than 1100 gm. at birth; this limits the amount of glucose that may be provided.[13] Furthermore, extremely premature infants may not tolerate a sudden increase in glucose load of more than 2 to 3 mg./kg./minute without becoming hyperglycemic and glycosuric. Such infants are at risk of becoming dehydrated from the osmotic diuresis that accompanies the glycosuria. Gradual increase in the amount of glucose infused may avert this problem. In addition to hyperglycemia, the infant already tolerating a high glucose load may suffer hypoglycemic episodes if the infusion is abruptly decreased or interrupted.

AMINO ACIDS

Protein hydrolysates of fibrin and casein were the first protein solutions available for intravenous use, but have now largely been replaced by crystalline amino acid solutions. Numerous in-vestigators have established that positive nitrogen balance and somatic growth occur when amino acid solutions are administered with adequate energy intake. An amino acid intake of 2.5 mg./kg./day results in nitrogen retention comparable to that observed in enterally fed, normal infants.[30] Provision of protein in excess of actual parenteral requirements is discouraged as the additional protein offers no apparent advantage and greatly increases the incidence of metabolic abnormalities. In practice, VLBW infants are usually given a small amount of amino acids initially (e.g., 1.0 gm./kg./day); the amount is gradually increased to 2.5 gm./kg./day according to individual infant tolerance.

The metabolic consequences of infusing amino acid mixtures into neonates are summarized in Table 37–13. It is important to note that the currently available amino acid solutions, such as Aminosyn (Abbott Laboratories), Freamine (American McGaw) and Travasol (Travenol Laboratories), were not designed to meet the particular needs of the immature infant, and may provoke imbalances in plasma amino acid levels. Although the significance of these abnormal plasma aminograms is unknown, there is concern for potential neurotoxic and developmental consequences. Amino acid solutions are currently being reformulated to contain an amino acid profile more like that of human milk; it is hoped that these future products will better meet the essential amino acid needs of the LBW infant without untoward metabolic effects.

LIPID

The availability of intravenous fat emulsions for use in LBW infants has added a new dimension to the nutritional support of these tiny babies. It is now feasible to deliver adequate calories for growth by peripheral vein, and to provide linoleic acid in sufficient quantity to prevent essential fatty acid deficiency. Biochemical evidence of essential fatty acid deficiency has been demonstrated by the end of the first week of life in the VLBW infant fed parenterally without fat.[19]

The rapidity with which the intravenously infused fat is metabolized is inversely related to gestational age, and is further decreased in infants who are SGA or acutely ill (e.g., those with sepsis or severe respiratory distress syndrome). In the presence of inadequate metabolism, hyperlipidemia characterized by high levels of plasma free fatty acids, triglycerides and cholesterol may occur and potentially serious complications may result (e.g., free fatty acids may displace bilirubin from albumin binding sites and potentiate kernicterus). Other conse-

Table 37–14.   COMPOSITION OF PERIPHERAL AND CENTRAL VEIN HYPERALIMENTATION FLUIDS

Component	DAILY AMOUNT (PER KG.)	
	Peripheral Vein	Central Vein
Glucose	10–15 gm.	20–30 gm.
Crystalline amino acids	1.0–2.5 gm.	2.5 gm.
Lipid	0.5–3.0 gm.	0.5–3 gm.
Electrolytes and minerals		
Sodium (as chloride)	3–4 mEq.	3–4 mEq.
Potassium (as phosphate and chloride)	2–4 mEq.	2–4 mEq.
Calcium (as gluconate)	1–4 mEq.	1–4 mEq.
Magnesium (as sulfate)	0.25 mEq.	0.25 mEq.
Phosphorus (as potassium phosphate)	1.36 mmole	1.36 mmole
Zinc (as sulfate)	150–300 μg.	150–300 μg.
Copper (as sulfate)	20–40 μg.	20–40 μg.
Vitamins: multivitamin preparation*	5 ml./day	5 ml./day
Volume	150 ml.	120 ml.

  * MVI Pediatric (U.S.V. Pharmaceutical Corporation) plus vitamin K, 1 mg. i.m., every 2 weeks.

  Adapted from Heird, W.C.: Total parenteral nutrition. In Lebenthal, E. (ed.): Textbook of Gastroenterology and Nutrition in Infancy. New York, Raven Press, 1981, p. 663.

quences of as yet undetermined significance include diminished pulmonary diffusion capacity, decreased arterial oxygen tension, pulmonary arterial and capillary lipid deposition, altered fatty acid composition of body tissue, and possibly impaired neutrophil function. Considering the various risks, it is suggested that fat emulsions, for example, Intralipid (Cutter Laboratories) and Liposyn (Abbott Laboratories), should not contribute more than 40 per cent of total calories or a maximum dose of 3.0 gm./kg./day. Essential fatty acid needs can be met by administration of as little as 0.5 to 1.0 gm./kg./day.[4]

VITAMINS AND MINERALS

The fat-soluble vitamins are generally added to parenteral fluids in amounts that match the recommended dietary allowances (RDA); vitamin C and the B vitamins are added to provide two to three times the RDA.[6] When this has been done, no vitamin deficiencies have been observed with the possible exception of biotin, which is not present in a commonly used parenteral vitamin preparation, MVI (U.S.V. Pharmaceutical Corporation). In addition, vitamin B_{12}, folate and vitamin K must be added separately to the solution or given intramuscularly if MVI is the sole multiple vitamin source. There is, however a new preparation (MVI Pediatric, U.S.V. Pharmaceutical Corporation) that contains biotin, folic acid and vitamin B_{12}, and is currently a preferred multivitamin infusion. Trace elements must also be provided to prevent deficiency in LBW infants receiving total parenteral nutrition.[5] Premature infants may be at risk for developing osteopenia and rickets when the duration of total parenteral nutrition is prolonged; the mineralization status of these infants should be monitored.[32]

Successful parenteral nutrition, whether infused by central or peripheral vein, is not easy to achieve. Adequate monitoring to detect metabolic and catheter-related complications is necessary; a schedule is suggested in Table 37–15.

Growth and Nutritional Assessment

All neonates typically lose some weight after birth. This is particularly true for LBW infants, who are born with more extracellular water than full-term infants and benefit from some degree of fluid loss. However, postnatal weight loss should not be excessive. Very-low-birth-weight infants who lose more than about 15 per cent of their birth weight can be expected to suffer from dehydration due to inadequate fluid intake or tissue wasting due to poor energy intake. Birth weight should be regained by the first or second week of life.

Weight is presently the most useful anthropometric determinant of nutritional status in the neonatal period. During this first month of life, the growth grid of Dancis and associates shown in Figure 37–3 is commonly used to assess weight progress. This grid has the advantages of depicting *daily* weight changes and *actual* growth curves; however, the chart is based on a small sample size and data that are now nearly 40 years old. The Dancis curves should not,

Table 37-15. SUGGESTED MONITORING SCHEDULE DURING PARENTERAL NUTRITION

VARIABLE	SUGGESTED FREQUENCY (PER WEEK)	
	*Initial Period**	*Later Period†*
Growth		
Weight	7	7
Length	1	1
Head circumference	1	1
Metabolic		
Blood or plasma		
Glucose	as indicated	as indicated
Na, K, Cl	3-4	1
Ca, Mg, P	2	1
Acid-base status	3-4	1
Urea nitrogen	2	1
Albumin	1	1
Liver function studies	1	1
Lipids	as indicated	as indicated
Hemoglobin	2	2
Urinary glucose	2-6/day	2/day
Prevention and Detection of Infection		
Clinical observation (activity, temperature, etc.)	daily	daily
WBC count and differential	as indicated	as indicated
Cultures	as indicated	as indicated

* *Initial* period is the time during which a full energy intake is being achieved.

† *Later* period implies that the infant has achieved a metabolic steady state. In the presence of metabolic instability, the more intensive monitoring outlined under the intial period should be followed.

Adapted from Heird, W.C.: Total parenteral nutrition. In Lebenthal, E. (ed.): Textbook of Gastroenterology and Nutrition in Infancy. New York, Raven Press, 1981, p. 669.

therefore, be interpreted to represent optimal growth, particularly for VLBW infants in modern neonatal intensive care units.

Intrauterine growth curves have also been developed using birth weight data of infants born at successive weeks of gestation, as shown in Figure 37-4. These curves do not depict the initial period of postnatal weight loss and are probably unrealistic goals for VLBW infants in the neonatal period. Once the infant's condition stabilizes and full nutrient intake is possible, the infant is often able to grow at a rate that parallels these curves (i.e., gain of 20 to 30 gm. per day).

Although weight is the only convenient and reliable anthropometric parameter by which to assess nutritional status during the early neonatal period, serial measurements of length and head circumference should be taken once the infant is stable. Growth curves such as those shown in Figure 37-5 are useful to evaluate the adequacy of growth in all parameters. Measurements of skinfold thickness or laboratory indicators of positive growth are still largely experimental for use in assessment of LBW infants.

During the first year of life, the healthy premature infant who is AGA grows at the same rate as the full-term infant of the same *post-conceptional* age. Growth progress is comparable as long as the premature infant's age is *corrected* for prematurity. For example, at 3 months postnatal age, the growth parameters of a premature infant born at 32 weeks gestation can be compared with those of a 1-month-old baby born at term. After discharge from a neonatal intensive care nursery, the standard growth grids from the National Center for Health Statistics shown in Appendices 15 to 18 can be used to evaluate growth of a premature infant, provided corrected age is used until at least 1 year of age.

Infants who have suffered severe medical stress or undernutrition in the early postnatal period and infants who are SGA often require a period of *catch-up growth* in order to fulfill their genetic potential. High energy intakes with appropriate concentrations of essential nutrients are frequently needed to potentiate catch-up growth. The catch-up period is characterized by the acceleration of the rate of growth in all parameters; once the infant has caught up, the rate of growth should slow to follow the normal channel for that child.

Monitoring of nutritional status by evaluation of anthropometric data is one of the few means

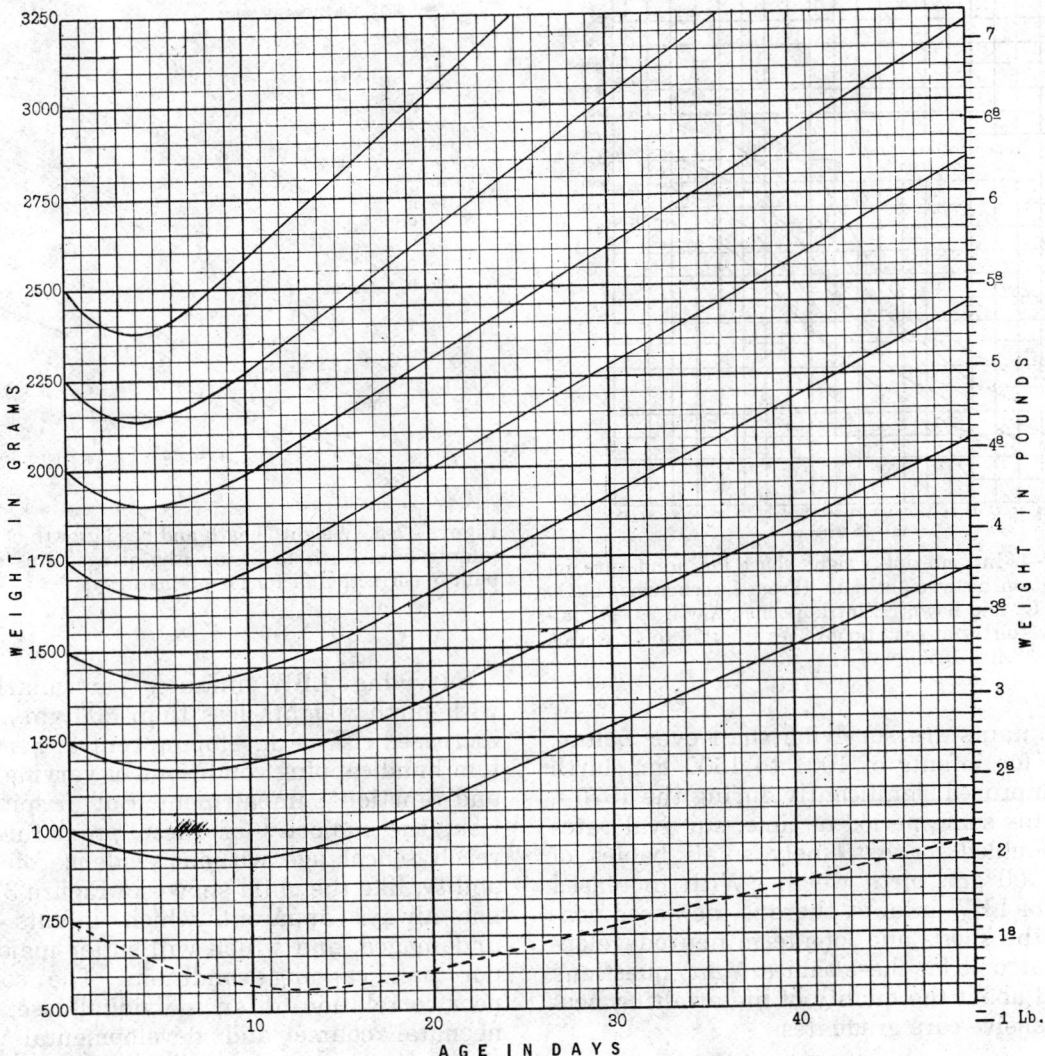

Figure 37–3. Weight chart for premature infants based on actual growth data. (From Dancis, J., O'Connell, J., and Holt, L.: A grid for recording the weight of premature infants. J. Pediatr., *33*:570, 1948.)

of assessment currently available. Nutritional care of LBW infants will take a giant step forward when optimal postnatal changes in tissue composition of premature infants are defined and non-invasive techniques developed to measure those changes. Until then, growth assessment and daily evaluation of nutrient intake and feeding tolerance are the best indicators of nutritional health. Certain biochemical parameters have been suggested as indices of nutritional status, such as serum albumin and total protein concentrations, but these are of limited usefulness, especially during the acute phase of the infant's hospitalization.

The development of practical guidelines for the nutritional management of LBW infants is complicated by the need to individualize the goals for each infant, and to vary them as the infant's medical condition changes. However,

the guidelines in Table 37–16 help to promote the nutritional support of small babies, especially when serious medical problems divert the focus of care away from nutritional needs. These guidelines are suggested, recognizing that they represent minimal rather than optimal needs. Low-birth-weight infants who are clinically stable will meet these nutritional recommendations sooner than infants who are ill.

NEURODEVELOPMENTAL OUTCOME

From the preceding discussion, it is apparent that it is possible to meet the metabolic and nutritional needs of premature and LBW infants in a manner sufficient to sustain life and to promote growth and development. With adequate nutritional support and recent advances in neonatal intensive care technology, more tiny, im-

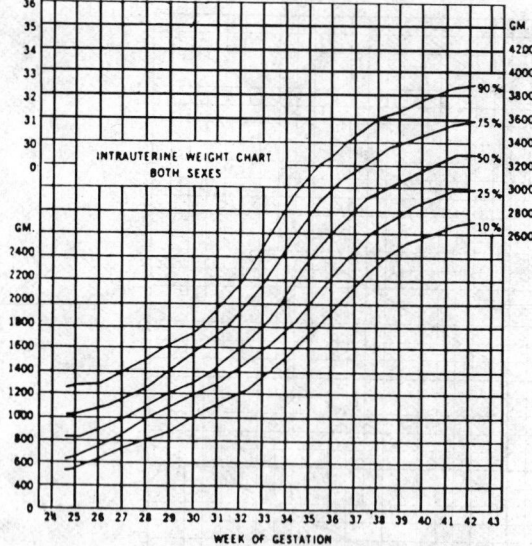

Figure 37–4. Intrauterine weight chart for premature infants based on birthweight data. (From Lubchencho, L. O., Hansman, C., and Boyd, E.: Intrauterine growth as estimated from live births at gestational ages from 26 to 42 weeks. Pediatrics, 37:403, 1966).

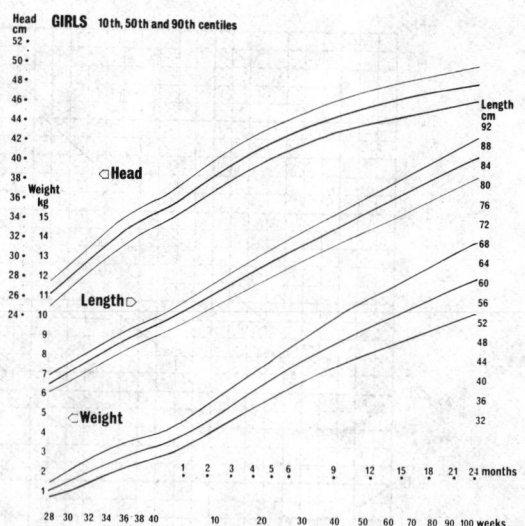

Figure 37–5. Weight, length and head growth of premature infants from birth to 24 months of age. This grid has a built-in correction factor for prematurity.

mature infants are surviving than ever before. Survival for infants of 1001 to 1500 gm. birth weight improved significantly during the 1970's. During this same period of time, survival rates nearly doubled for extremely small babies of 501 to 1000 gm. birth weight. With increased survival of LBW infants, there is increased concern for the short- and long-term neurodevelopmental outcome for these babies. Many questions are asked about the quality of life awaiting neonatal intensive care graduates.

Surviving LBW infants, particularly those with birth weights less than 800 gm., have an increased risk of developing central nervous system handicapping conditions of varying severity and functional impairment. But in spite of this risk, the majority of these premature babies reach school age without evidence of any disability, like the child shown in Figure 37–6. It is not always apparent which infants will be undamaged, and which will suffer major or minor handicapping conditions. The sometimes poor correlation, in an individual case, between neonatal course and developmental outcome

Table 37–16. ASSESSMENT GUIDELINES

3–5 DAYS OF AGE

If total energy intake is less than 60 kcal./kg./day parenterally or 80 kcal./kg./day enterally, consider these options:
1. If there are still no enteral feedings, consider:
   a. Peripheral vein alimentation fluids (glucose, electrolytes, amino acids, vitamins, and minerals), if further enteral limitation of short duration (1–2 weeks) is anticipated.
   b. Central vein alimentation fluids, if expect prolonged enteral limitation, or if poor peripheral vessel access. (Certain surgical or GI problems may require central hyperalimentation beginning earlier.)
2. If there is poor tolerance of enteral feedings, consider:
   a. Change in method or frequency of feeding.
   b. Change in type or concentration of feeding.

7 DAYS OF AGE

Consider introduction of intravenous fat emulsion to meet essential fatty acid needs of parenterally fed infants.

10 DAYS OF AGE

If there is no actual weight gain, or if energy intake is less than 80 kcal./kg./day (parenterally) or 100 kcal./kg./day (enterally), consider options to increase caloric intake (e.g., increase volume and/or concentration of feeding).

14 DAYS OF AGE

Total energy intake should meet infant's needs for sustained growth, i.e., 90–120 kcal./kg./day. *Note*: higher energy intakes may be needed by infants with elevated needs (e.g., SGA infant or infant with chronic lung disease).

Adapted from O'Leary, M.J.: Neonatal nutrition. In Hodson, W.A., and Truog, W.E. (eds.): Critical Care of the Newborn. Philadelphia, W.B. Saunders Co., 1983, p. 34.

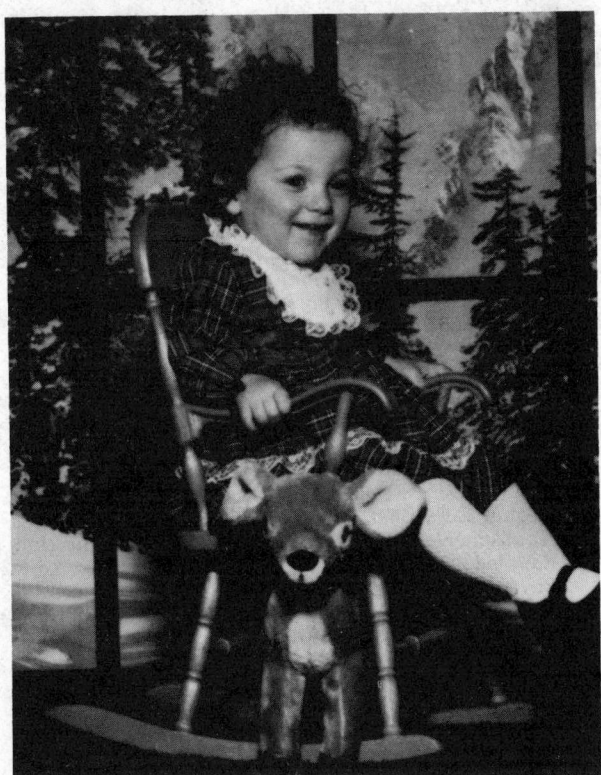

Figure 37–6. This photo shows the same Briana as in Figure 37–2, at a healthy 2½ years of age.

makes neonatal survival decisions extremely difficult. All premature and LBW infants merit personalized and sensitive screening and assessment, with intervention strategies employed as appropriate.

Conclusion

Although there are many means of providing nutrients to LBW infants, each has its benefits and limitations. Because of the complexities involved in the neonatal intensive care setting, a team including a skilled dietitian is necessary to promote optimal nutrition and to minimize undue delays and oversights of nutritional care. The dietitian may also function within a regionalized perinatal care system to provide consultation and guidance to community hospitals concerning the unique nutritional problems of premature infants.

Cited References

1. American Academy of Pediatrics, Committee on Nutrition: Iron supplementation for infants. Pediatrics, *58*:765, 1976.
2. American Academy of Pediatrics, Committee on Nutrition: Nutritional needs of low-birth-weight infants. Pediatrics, *60*:519, 1977.
3. American Academy of Pediatrics, Committee on Nutrition: Relationship between iron status and incidence of infection in infancy. Pediatrics, *62*:246, 1978.
4. American Academy of Pediatrics, Committee on Nutrition: Use of intravenous fat emulsions in pediatric practice. Pediatrics, *68*:738, 1981.
5. American Medical Association, Department of Foods and Nutrition: Guidelines for essential trace element preparations for parenteral use. J.A.M.A., *241*:2051, 1979.
6. American Medical Association, Department of Foods and Nutrition: Multivitamin preparations for parenteral use. JPEN, *3*:258, 1979.
7. Atkinson, S.A.: Calcium and phosphorus requirements of low-birth-weight infants: a nutritional and endocrinological perspective. Nutr. Rev., *41*:69, 1983.
8. Barlow, B., et al.: An experimental study of acute neonatal enterocolitis: the importance of breast milk. J. Pediatr. Surg., *9*:587, 1974.
9. Bergman, K.E., Ziegler, E.E., and Fomon, S.J.: Water and renal solute load. In Fomon, S.J. (ed.): Infant Nutrition. Philadelphia, W.B. Saunders Company 1974, p. 245.
10. Cicco, R., et al.: Glucose polymers tolerance in premature infants. Pediatrics, *67*:498, 1981.
11. Day, G.M., et al.: Growth and mineral metabolism in very-low-birth-weight infants: II. Effects of calcium supplementation on growth and divalent cations. Pediatr. Res. *9*:568, 1975.
12. Dubowitz, L.M.S., et al.: Clinical assessment of gestational age in the newborn infant. J. Pediatr., *77*:1, 1970.
13. Dweck, H.S., and Cassay, G.: Glucose intolerance in infants of very-low-birth-weight. I. Incidence of hyperglycemia in infants of birth weights 1,100 grams or less. Pediatrics, *53*:198, 1974.
14. Egan, E.A.: Neonatal necrotizing enterocolitis. In Lebenthal, E. (ed.): Textbook of Gastroenterology and Nutrition in Infancy. New York, Raven Press, 1981, p. 979.
15. Ehrenkranz, R.A., Ablow, R.C., and Warshaw, J.B.: Prevention of bronchopulmonary dysplasia with vitamin E administration during the acute stage of respiratory distress syndrome. J. Pediatr. *95*:873, 1979.
16. Ehrenkranz, R.A., et al.: Amelioration of broncho-pulmonary dysplasia after vitamin E administration. N. Engl. J. Med., *299*:564, 1978.
17. Engelke, S.C., et al.: Sodium balance in very-low-birth-weight infants. J. Pediatr., *93*:837, 1978.
18. Fomon, S.J., and Ziegler, E.E.: Protein intake of premature infants: interpretation of data. J. Pediatr., *90*:504, 1977.
19. Friedman, Z., et al.: Rapid onset of essential fatty acid deficiency in the newborn. Pediatrics, *58*:640, 1976.
20. Gaull, G.E., et al.: Milk protein quantity and quality in low-birth-weight infants: III. Effects on sulfur amino acids in plasma and urine. J. Pediatr., *90*:348, 1977.
21. Goldman, H.J., et al.: Late effects of early dietary protein intake on low-birth-weight infants. J. Pediatr., *85*:764, 1974.
22. Greer, F.R., Steichen, J.J., and Tsang, R.C.: Calcium and phosphate supplements in breast milk–related rickets. Am. J. Dis. Child., *136*:581, 1982.
23. Gross, S.J., et al.: Nutritional composition of milk products by mothers delivering preterms. J. Pediatr., *96*:641, 1980.
24. Gross, S.J., et al.: Growth and biochemical response of premature infants fed human milk or modified infant formula. N. Engl. J. Med., *308*:237, 1983.
25. Hack, M., Fanaroff, A.A., and Merkatz, I.R.: The low-birth-weight infant—evolution of a changing outlook. N. Engl. J. Med. *301*:1163, 1979.

26. Hamosh, M., and Scow, R.O.: Lingual lipase and its role in the digestion of dietary fat. J. Clin. Invest., *52*: 88, 1973.

27. Hamosh, M., et al.: Fat digestion in the stomach of premature infants. J. Pediatr., *93*:674, 1978.

28. Harvey, D., et al.: Abilities of children who were small for gestational age babies. Pediatrics, *69*:296, 1982.

29. Heird, W.C., et al.: Intravenous alimentation in pediatric patients. J. Pediatr., *80*:351, 1972.

30. Heird, W.C.: Total parenteral nutrition. In Lebenthal, E. (ed.): Textbook of Gastroenterology and Nutrition in Infancy. New York, Raven Press, 1981, p. 659.

31. Johnson, L., Schaffer, D., and Boggs, T.R., Jr.: The premature infant, vitamin E deficiency and retrolental fibroplasia. Am. J. Clin. Nutr., *27*:1158, 1974.

32. Kine, C.L., et al.: Rickets in premature infants receiving parenteral nutrition: a case report and review of the literature. J. Parent. Ent. Nutr., *6*:152, 1982.

33. Krouskop, R.W., Brown, E.G., and Sweet, A.Y.: The relationship of feeding to necrotizing enterocolitis. Pediatr. Res., *8*:109, 1974.

34. Lemons, J.A., et al: Considerations in feeding the very-low-birth-weight infant. Perinatol./Neonatol., May/June, 1982.

35. Lemons, J.A., et al.: Differences in the composition of preterm and term human milk during early lactation. Pediatr. Res., *16*:113, 1982.

36. Lewin, P.K., et al.: Iatrogenic rickets in very-low-birth-weight infants. J. Pediatr., *78*:207, 1971.

37. Lubchencho, L.O., Hansman, C., and Boyd, E.: Intrauterine growth in length and head circumference as estimated from live births at gestational ages from 26 to 42 weeks. Pediatrics, *37*:403, 1966.

38. Lundstrom, U., Siimes, M.A., and Dallman, P.R.: At what age does iron supplementation become necessary in low-birth-weight infants? J. Pediatr., *91*:878, 1977.

39. MacLean, W.C., and Fink, B.B.: Lactose malabsorption by premature infants: magnitude and clinical significance. J. Pediatr., *97*:383, 1980.

40. Melhorn, D.K., and Gross, S.: Vitamin E–dependent anemia in the premature infant: I. Effects of large doses of medicinal iron. J. Pediatr., *79*:569, 1971.

41. Olson, M.: The benign effects on rabbit's lungs of the aspiration of water compared with 5% glucose or milk. Pediatrics, *46*:538, 1970.

42. Phelps, D.L., and Rosenbaum, A.L.: The role of tocopherol in oxygen-induced retinopathy: kitten model. Pediatrics, *59*:998, 1977.

43. Raiha, N.C.R., et al.: Milk protein quantity and quality in low-birth-weight infants. I. Metabolic responses and effects on growth. Pediatrics, *57*:659, 1976.

44. Rassin, D.K., et al.: Milk protein quantity and quality in low-birth-weight infants. II. Effects of selected aliphatic amino acids in plasma and urine. Pediatrics, *59*: 407, 1977.

45. Rassin, D.K., et al.: Milk protein quantity and quality in low-birth-weight infants. IV. Effects on tyrosine and phenylalanine in plasma and urine. J. Pediatr., *90*: 356, 1977.

46. Rassin, D.K., Raiha, N.C.R., and Gaull, G.E.: Protein and taurine nutrition in infants. In Lebenthal, E. (ed.): Textbook of Gastroenterology and Nutrition in Infancy. New York, Raven Press, 1981, p. 397.

47. Roy, R.N., et al.: Late hyponatremia in very-low-birth-weight infants. (<1.3 kg). Pediatr. Res., *10*:526, 1976.

48. Schriener, R.L.: Continuous and bolus feeding techniques in the low-birth-weight infant: benefits and complications. In Report of 79th Ross Conference on Pediatric Research: Feeding the Neonate Weighing Less than 1,500 Grams—Nutrition and Beyond. Columbus, Ohio, Ross Laboratories, 1979, p. 78.

49. Schriener, R.L., et al.: Lack of occurrence of lacto-bezoars with predominantly whey protein formulas. Am. J. Dis. Child., *136*:437, 1982.

50. Shenai, J.P., Reynolds, J.W., and Babson, S.G.: Nutritional balance studies in very-low-birth-weight infants: enhanced nutrient retention rates by an experimental formula. Pediatrics, *66*:233, 1980.

51. Shojania, A.M., and Gross, S.: Folic acid deficiency and prematurity. J. Pediatr., *64*:323, 1964.

52. Steichen, J.J., Gratton, T.L., and Tsang, R.C.: Osteopenia of prematurity: The cause and possible treatment. J. Pediatr., *96*:528, 1980.

53. Tantibhedhyangkul, P., and Hashim, S.A.: Medium chain triglyceride feeding in premature infants: effects on fat and nitrogen absorption. Pediatrics, *55*:359, 1975.

54. Weil, W.J., Jr.: Energy balance in low-birth-weight infants. J. Pediatr., *99*:737, 1981.

55. Widdowson, E.M.: Growth and composition of the fetus and newborn. In Assali, N.S. (ed.): Biology of Gestation. Vol. II. New York, Academic Press, Inc., 1968, p. 1.

56. Ziegler, E.E., Biga, R.L., and Fomon, S.J.: Nutritional requirements of the premature infant. In Suskind, R.M. (ed.): Textbook of Pediatric Nutrition. New York, Raven Press, 1981, p. 29.

57. Ziegler, E.E. et al.: Body composition of the reference fetus. Growth, *40*:329, 1976.

Additional References

American Academy of Pediatrics, Committee on Nutrition: Calcium requirements in infancy and childhood. Pediatrics, *62*:826, 1978.

Bell, E.F., and Filer, L.J.: The role of vitamin E in the nutrition of premature infants. Am. J. Clin. Nutr., *34*:414, 1981.

Bell, E.F., and Oh, W.: Nutritional care. In Goldsmith, J.P., and Karotkin, E.H. (eds.): Assisted Ventilation of the Neonate. Philadelphia, W.B. Saunders Company, 1981, p. 281.

Benda, G.I.M.: Modes of feeding low-birth-weight infants. Semin. Perinatol., *3*:407, 1979.

Bennett, F.C.: Neurodevelopmental outcome of premature/low-birth-weight infants. In Kelley, V.C. (ed.): Practice of Pediatrics. Philadelphia, J.B. Lippincott Company, 1983.

Bose, C.L., et al.: Relactation by mothers of sick and premature infants. Pediatrics, *67*:565, 1981.

Brady, M.S., Gresham, E.L., and Rickard, K.: Nutritional care of the low-birth-weight infant requiring intensive care. Perinatal Press, *2*:125, 1978.

Brady, M.S., et al.: Formulas and human milk for premature infants: a review and update. J. Am. Diet. Assoc., *81*: 547, 1982.

Brandt, I.: Growth dynamics of low-birth-weight infants with emphasis on the perinatal period. In Falkner, F., and Tanner, J.M.: Human Growth—Postnatal Growth. New York, Plenum Press, 1978.

Chessey, P., et al.: Quality of growth in premature infants fed their own mother's milk. J. Pediatr., *102*:107, 1983.

Dobbing, J.: The later growth of the brain and its vulnerability. Pediatrics, *53*:2, 1974.

Dallman, P.R., Siimes, M.A., and Stekel, A.: Iron deficiency in infancy and childhood. Am. J. Clin. Nutr. *33*:86, 1980.

Ghadimi, H.: Total Parenteral Nutrition: Premises and Promises. New York, John Wiley & Sons, 1975, p. 407.

Harkavey, K.L.: Water and electrolyte requirements of the very-low-birth-weight infant. Perinatal Press, *6*:47, 1982.

Kerner, J.A., and Sunshine, P.: Parenteral alimentation. Semin. Perinatol., *3*:417, 1979.

Kessler, D.L.: Nutrition for the low-birth-weight infant. In Kelley, V.C. (ed.): Practice of Pediatrics. Hagerstown, Md., Harper & Row Publishers, Inc., 1979.

Klaus, M.H., and Fanaroff, A.A.: Care of the High Risk Neonate. Philadelphia, W.B. Saunders Company, 1979.

Lebenthal, E. (ed.): Textbook of Gastroenterology and Nutrition in Infancy. Vol. I & II. New York, Raven Press, 1981.

Lebenthal, E., Lee, P.C., and Heitlinger, L.A.: Impact of development of the gastrointestinal tract on infant feeding. J. Pediatr., 102:1, 1983.

Lowen, L.: Breastfeeding: when your baby is premature. Mothering, Winter:68, 1982.

Marks, K.H., et al.: Head growth in sick premature infants—a longitudinal study. J. Pediatr., 94:282, 1979.

National Research Council, Committee on Nutrition of the Mother and Preschool Child: Nutrition Services in Perinatal Care. Washington, D.C., National Academy Press, 1981.

Paneth, N., et al.: Newborn intensive care and neonatal mortality in low-birth-weight infants: A population study. N. Engl. J. Med. 307:149, 1982.

Prader, A.: Catch-up growth. Postgrad. Med. J., 54 (Suppl. 1):133, 1978.

Reichman, B.L., et al.: Partition of energy metabolism and energy cost of growth in the very-low-birth-weight infant. Pediatrics., 69:446, 1982.

Rickard, K., et al.: Nutritional outcome of 207 very-low-birth-weight infants in an intensive care unit. J. Am. Diet. Assoc., 81:674, 1982.

Ronnholm, K.A.R., Sipila, I., and Siimes, M.A.: Human milk protein supplementation for the prevention of hypoproteinemia without metabolic imbalance in breast milk–fed, very-low-birth-weight infants. J. Pediatr., 101:243, 1982.

Tsang, R.C., Steichen, J.J., and Chan, G.M.: Neonatal hypocalcemia: mechanism of occurrence and management. Crit. Care Med., 5:56, 1977.

Williams, F.H., and Pittard, W.B.: Human milk banking: practical concerns for feeding premature infants. J. Am. Diet. Assoc., 79:565, 1981.

Wilson, J.T.: Drugs in Breast Milk. New York, Adis Press, 1981.

CHAPTER 38

Nutritional Care in Diseases of Infancy and Childhood

The nutritional needs of a child who is ill are the same as or greater than those of a well child of the same age and development. Special consideration should be given to children who are receiving therapeutic regimens, to help them meet their nutritional needs for normal growth and development as well as their particular therapeutic requirements. Maintaining optimal nutritional status of the sick child plays an important part in the control of the disease and the rate of recovery.

A child's and family's response to illness and hospitalization may lead to undesirable changes in the child's eating behavior. Usually this is not a serious problem, and when feeling better the child will return to regular eating habits. Food must be served attractively and taste good to the sick child. At this time a child's desire for particular foods should be catered to as much as possible. Sometimes parents, particularly mothers, become demanding with regard to the child's food in an attempt to overcome feelings of helplessness and to do something for the child. In this situation, parents have a right to be demanding, and their demands should be met whenever possible.

If the child's appetite is poor, small meals served more frequently may be helpful, and ingenuity in meal planning and meal preparation may stimulate the appetite. Participation by the nurse in mealtime activities, as illustrated in Figure 38–1, encourages the child to eat.

Frequently a hospitalized child, such as a newly diagnosed diabetic child, must learn to eat in a new way. Education of the child and the family can begin in the hospital at mealtime if the child feels up to it. Children are usually interested in learning and desire to participate in activities such as learning to identify foods and even to prepare them to fit their new diets, as shown in Figure 38–2. Children usually can identify the foods that they believe to be good and those that they usually ingest. The nurse or dietitian accepts the child's suggestions and reinforces those that are appropriate. Using this approach the nurse or dietitian learns about the child's normal habits and the changes that may be necessary later.

Because emotional factors are involved with the child being separated from home, school, friends and perhaps family and the trauma of medical or surgical treatments, it is often difficult to alter food habits or introduce new foods. Any required education about dietary changes should always be followed up by counseling visits with the child and his parents after the child has returned home.

This chapter considers aspects of various dis-

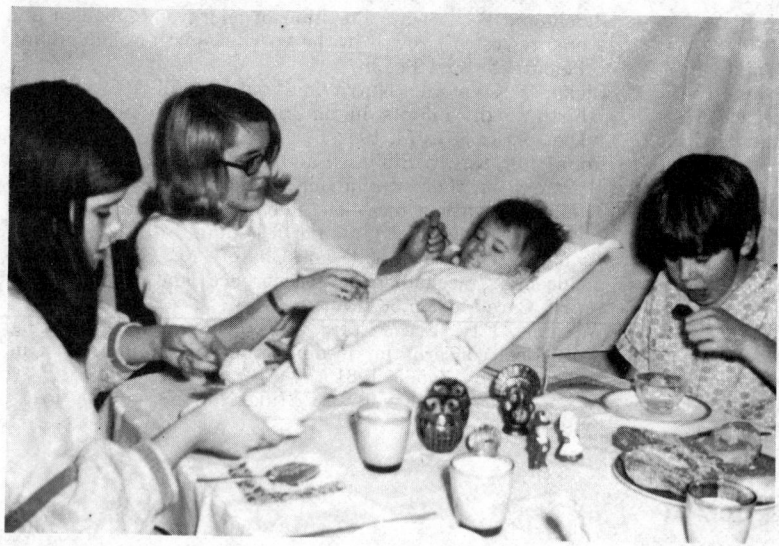

Figure 38-1. These children are obviously enjoying their breakfast under the supervision of an understanding nurse.

eases that relate specifically to children. Many other disorders also affect children, and the chapters throughout Part 2 of this volume on nutritional care in specific diseases should be consulted for information on care of children as well as adults.

Acute Infections

Children suffering from acute infections of short duration, such as the common cold, measles, pneumonia or chickenpox, usually have re-

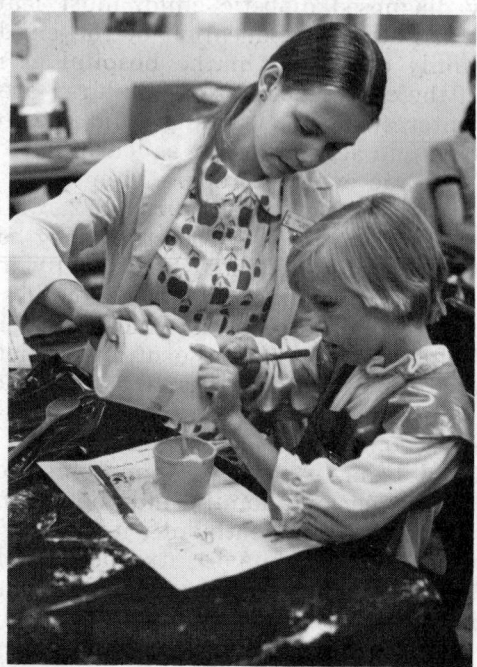

Figure 38-2. Dietitian helping a hospitalized child learn to prepare meals for her new diet. (Courtesy of Lutheran General Hospital, Des Plaines, Illinois.)

duced appetites. While it is not essential to insist that the nutritional requirements be met for the few days of the infection and fever, ketosis must be guarded against. (Consult Chapter 35 for discussions of the effect of infection on protein status and the requirements for energy and protein during this time.) During the first day or two of the illness, it is advisable to serve either small amounts of food or none at all, but fluids are supplied in quantities to meet the child's need. The infant's formula may be diluted with water, and when the fever subsides, the regular feeding formula is resumed in order to supply the required calories as soon as possible. The liquid diet prescribed for children includes fruit juices, soups, broth and milk as tolerated. As the fever subsides, the appetite usually improves, and the food intake can be increased accordingly. During convalescence, foods rich in protein, vitamins and minerals are advisable, and gradually the child can begin to consume his normal diet.

Chronic Infections

It is essential that adequate nutrition be maintained in children who have infections of long duration, such as rheumatic fever and tuberculosis. Chronic infections can be very debilitating if the child remains in negative nitrogen balance with tissue protein breakdown day after day, as discussed in Chapter 35.

Regurgitation and Vomiting

Regurgitation, or spitting up, is common in infants who take too much milk or swallow air. Burping should be practiced to give the baby a chance during each nursing to get rid of swallowed air.

Vomiting is a symptom of many disturbances that may or may not be serious. In a baby, vomiting of a whole feeding or a large portion of it is often an early sign of infectious disease. However, it may also be caused by indigestion, fatigue, overexcitement or a serious problem such as pyloric stenosis. A child who has eaten a meal while overtired, overexcited, angry or frightened many be unable to digest food well, and vomiting is nature's way of removing the undigested material. Such vomiting is not serious. Sometimes the condition results from an imbalance of food constituents in the formula, particularly from too much fat, which delays normal emptying of the stomach.

Persistent vomiting, especially when accompanied by diarrhea, will cause an imbalance of electrolytes and create a serious condition that demands immediate attention. The cause should be determined and feedings and fluids adjusted accordingly. In gastrointestinal upset it is useful to avoid lactose during the first two to three days. The reason for this is that the activity of the intestinal enzyme lactase is one of the first to be lost in gastrointestinal distress.

Diarrhea

Occasional diarrhea is common in infancy and childhood. The most frequent causes are contamination or spoilage of food, too much carbohydrate (sugar) or fat in the formula, irritants such as cathartics, allergic reactions to specific foods, and viral or bacterial infection. Diarrheal diseases are among the most common infections of children in the United States.

In the developing countries acute diarrheal diseases are commonly associated with the weaning period. Some are identified with a specific organism but the majority are not. The condition is listed among the first five causes of high infant mortality and, in many countries, ranks first in children under the age of two. Supplementary foods of low nutritive value, prepared under unsanitary conditions, are usually started during the latter part of the first year, and diarrhea follows.

The result of diarrhea is dehydration, which can lead to death unless corrected. Death from acute diarrheal disease can almost always be prevented with correction of intestinal fluid losses.

Nutritional Care

Nutritional care is directed toward rehydration by replacement of fluids and electrolytes lost in stool. For oral replacement glucose-elec-

Table 38–1. COMPOSITION OF ORAL REHYDRATION FORMULA—WHO RECOMMENDATION

Glucose (gm./100 ml.)	2.0
Sodium (mEq./l.)	90
Potassium (mEq./l.)	20
Bicarbonate (mEq./l.)	30
Osmolarity (mOsm./l.)	330

trolyte solutions have been found to be most effective. Various mixtures of glucose, electrolytes and water for rehydration fluids have been proposed, and there is still no agreement on the ideal solution for infants and children. What is apparent is that a wide variety of fluids are used as oral rehydration fluids to treat primarily mildly dehydrated youngsters, all with seeming effectiveness.[19,37] The World Health Organization has recommended a formula as shown in Table 38–1. Added to this should also be supplemental water and continued breast-feeding if possible.[28] Solutions with sodium contents of 50 mEq./l. or 90 mEq./l. are both effective and safe for rehydration.[35] A bottled preparation such as Lytren (Mead Johnson) or Pedialyte (Ross) or a home-prepared glucose-salt solution as described in Table 38–2 can be given orally. Recently there has been much scientific discussion regarding the effectiveness of oral rehydration in infantile diarrheal disease, and the consensus is that it can be just as effective as parenteral rehydration and much cheaper.[35] For the severely dehydrated child, parenteral fluid administration may be required.[29]

Usually feedings are withheld until the diarrhea subsides. However, a recent study showed that children given puréed foods (rice, banana, applesauce) after eight hours, regardless of whether the diarrhea had stopped, did just as well as children not allowed to eat.[35]

When feedings are resumed, the diet is built up gradually, starting with a lactose-free formula such as Prosobee, with addition of puréed or mashed fruits and vegetables. Pectin, apple or banana flakes may be given, since these substances have antidiarrheal properties. Cereals,

Table 38–2. GLUCOSE-SALT SOLUTION FOR REHYDRATION FOLLOWING ACUTE DIARRHEA

To 1 liter of water add:
- 3.5 gm. sodium chloride
- 2.5 gm. sodium bicarbonate
- 1.5 gm. potassium chloride
- 20.0 gm. glucose

The solution should be made up fresh every 24 hours.

From: The rehydration treatment of acute diarrhea with inexpensive oral fluids. Clin. Pediatr., *15*:1095, 1976.

breads and meats can be added next, with lactose-containing foods (such as milk or yogurt) being last. Finally, the normal or regular diet for the age and development of the child is resumed. As the condition improves, regular formula or whole milk can be used. An infant formula such as Pregestimil, Nutramigen or Portagen, in which the nutrients are present in an easily absorbable form, may be necessary in some instances. For further discussion of nutritional care for patients with diarrhea, see Chapter 23.

Constipation and Colic

Constipation is a fairly common disturbance of infancy and childhood. As a rule the bottle-fed baby has fewer stools than the breast-fed baby. Human milk is higher in carbohydrate (lactose) than cow's milk and tends to cause the baby to have more stools. Feces that are hard and expelled with difficulty should be reported to the physician. Sometimes constipation alternates with the uncontrolled passage of loose stools. This can become a distressing situation for older children and their families. It is also a more serious condition and may be indicative of Hirschsprung's disease or other intestinal disorder.

Treatment varies with the cause, as discussed in Chapter 23. In the case of the formula-fed infant, the amount of sugar can be increased or the type of sugar used in the formula can be changed. The breast-fed infant may have a supplementary bottle of fruit juice added to the feeding schedule. In infants receiving supplementary foods or for young children, the diet may include fruit juice (prune, orange), vegetable juice (tomato), fruit purées or fruits (prunes, apricots, applesauce, figs), vegetable purées or vegetables and whole-grain cereals, which may be added to or increased in the diet, depending upon the age of the child. For older children the suggestions outlined in Chapter 23 are appropriate.

Pyloric Stenosis

Pyloric stenosis of infancy is not uncommon. The condition is serious and, unless recognized and treated in the early stages, has a high rate of mortality. It is usually diagnosed during the first two months of life.

Mild cases are often treated successfully with medical management. Babies are usually fed at intervals of four hours. If vomiting occurs and a large part of the feeding is lost, the infant should be refed because refeedings are often retained. The nutritional status of the infant is usually poor because of nausea and limited food intake. Experience has demonstrated that artificially fed infants frequently show improvement when given thick cereal feedings every four hours. Some formula-fed babies show improvement when fed human milk.

Some severely affected infants may require parenteral hyperalimentation to correct dehydration, acid-base imbalance and malnutrition from the excessive vomiting. After rehydration and some improvement, surgery is generally advised.

Peptic Ulcers

Peptic ulcers occur more frequently in infants and children than was believed formerly. The majority of cases reported are diagnosed only when complications appear, and most cases occur with no obvious cause. The stress-inducing factors of modern urban society could be one cause of the increase in the occurrence of peptic ulcers at an early age, according to a survey of hospital and medical case records of children under 16 years of age.[31] Peptic ulceration in infants and children was also found to be associated with steroid therapy or a serious underlying illness.[42] Children's symptoms are closely allied to those of adult patients; i.e., they have pain in the upper abdomen, more marked when the stomach is empty, that is relieved by food or antacid medication. Chapter 22 discusses the nutritional care for peptic ulcers.

Ulcerative Colitis

Ulcerative colitis frequently appears in the pediatric age group. Although chronic ulcerative colitis is basically the same at all ages, the disease is usually more severe and treatment is less satisfactory in children than in adults. Because of its chronic, regressive nature, its occurrence at a time of active growth and its severe associated complications, the disease requires careful evaluation and active medical treatment, with early surgical intervention when indicated.

The psychological and social problems that can develop when this disease occurs in children also require empathy and attention from the medical staff. These patients are usually underweight and under emotional stress. Parents of these children may be overprotective or overaggressive in forcing them to compete beyond their desire or ability. A flareup of ulcerative colitis may occur after failure to meet a challenge or after an outburst of emotion or a severe stress. However, the belief that emotional factors *cause* ulcerative colitis is questionable.

Care should be aimed at helping the child obtain sufficient energy and an adequate intake of essential nutrients to provide for growth and development and to maintain good nutritional status. This is discussed in detail in Chapter 23.

Malabsorption

As noted earlier, in malabsorption the products of digestion available to the body are blocked because the absorbing surface of the small intestine is greatly reduced or malfunctioning. The microvilli are fewer and misshapen. The structural polarity of the epithelial cells is lost, and the intracellular enzymes that are responsible for the metabolism of epithelial cells are destroyed. With too few villi and microvilli, fat and fatty substances such as cholesterol and the lipid-soluble vitamins (A, D, E and K) are poorly absorbed and steatorrhea exists. A study of several children with malabsorption due to celiac disease, lymphangiectasia, abetalipoproteinemia, cystic fibrosis and obstructive jaundice showed that they all had deficient levels of serum vitamin E.[27] In addition, unabsorbed fats can combine with minerals, particularly with calcium and trace minerals, to form "soaps," which further prevent their absorption.

In some disorders there can also be malabsorption of protein and carbohydrate. The result is that the energy and nutrients of ingested food are not absorbed, and one of the early signs in the child is growth failure.

The primary focus of care is on determining the cause of the malabsorption. Once that is determined, nutritional care can be most effective. Complete nutritional care for malabsorption syndromes is discussed in Chapter 23. In in-fants, a defined formula such as Pregestimil or Nutramigen is often useful.

Cystic Fibrosis

Cystic fibrosis, a multisystem disorder affecting the exocrine glands, is the most common lethal genetic disease of Caucasians and in the U.S. and is the most common cause of life-threatening pulmonary disease in youth. Cystic fibrosis used to be a disease limited to infants and children, but the current median age of survival is approaching 20 years.

The major clinical manifestations are chronic pulmonary disease, pancreatic exocrine insufficiency and abnormally high sweat electrolyte levels, although there may also be involvement of other organs. Diagnosis is made when the chloride concentration in sweat is found to be greater than 60 mEq./l. Progressive pulmonary infections cause most of the morbidity and almost all of the mortality of this disease.

With an increasingly optimistic prognosis for longevity in cystic fibrosis patients, yet persistent incidence of growth impairment, renewed attention to details of optimal nutrition are merited.

Symptoms

The child with untreated cystic fibrosis will usually be malnourished, with bulky, foul-smelling stools (steatorrhea) and growth failure as shown in Figure 38–3. There will usually be pulmonary involvement such as chronic cough, asthma-like symptoms, recurrent pneumonia, nasal polyps and chronic sinusitis. Typically the child with cystic fibrosis has a ravenous appetite. Manifestations of the disease may develop before the child is born, with intestinal obstruction occurring in the neonatal period because of *meconium ileus*. On the other hand, the person

Figure 38–3. Three-month-old child with cystic fibrosis of the pancreas. He had loose stools, failed to gain weight and was fretful and irritable but had a good appetite. Although the muscles were well developed, there was a complete absence of subcutaneous fat. The abdomen was prominent. No enzymes were found in the duodenal juice. He was first given skim milk, banana powder, dried milk protein and large doses of vitamin A. Later he was given 1 gm. of powdered pancreatin before each feeding of evaporated milk formula. He improved rapidly and at three years, after being maintained on a high-calorie, low-fat diet and pancreatin, appeared to be relatively normal (From Andersen, D. H.: J. Pediatr., *15*:10, 1939.)

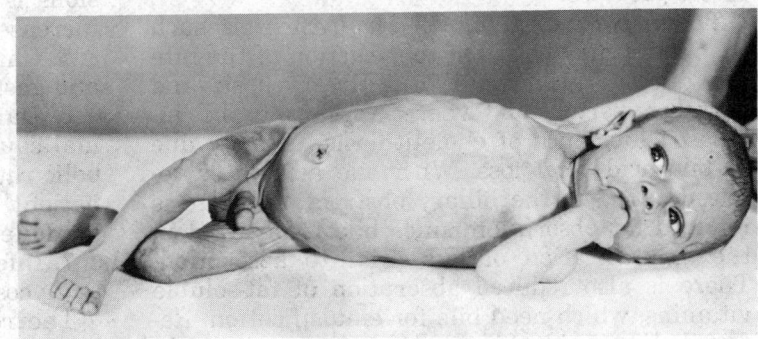

may remain asymptomatic through childhood and adolescence and develop his or her first pulmonary symptoms as an adult.

Some patients over 15 to 20 years of age seem to do better than younger patients, perhaps because survival to this age usually depends on a relatively mild degree of pulmonary involvement. Patients also appear to need less dietary attention with advancing age. However, others with severe involvement may have decreased pulmonary function, more frequent infections, and body deformity with age.

Gastrointestinal Involvement

Pancreatic involvement, causing reduced secretion of bicarbonate and the enzymes amylase, lipase and trypsin, causes steatorrhea and malabsorption. If 5 to 15 per cent of pancreatic enzyme activity is preserved, fecal fat, nitrogen, and bile loss are not present and there are no symptoms of malabsorption. Recent evidence suggests that cystic fibrosis patients with "normal" pancreatic function might have a milder form of the disease than those who present with steatorrhea and clinical malabsorption.

Pancreatic islet cells may eventually become abnormal with the development of glucose intolerance. Glucose intolerance or hyperglycemia is present in the majority of cystic fibrosis patients, but only 2.5 per cent of those with glucose intolerance require additional insulin.

Because of *intestinal mucus involvement*, the intestinal enzymes on the surface of the villi may not function properly even though an intestinal biopsy is normal. This may lead to a malabsorption of disaccharides. This usually is not a clinical problem. Deficient activity of the enzyme lactase causes most of the clinical problems that do occur, and dietary lactose omission should be considered if all other measures to control malabsorption are not effective.

The development of viscous intestinal mucus may cause a thick mass leading to ileus, intussusception (prolapse of the intestine into another part of the intestine), fecal impaction or rectal prolapse.

The *hepatic and biliary involvement* is such that there may be mucus obstruction of the biliary ducts, which may result in cirrhosis and portal hypertension. There appears to be increased incidence of cholelithiasis, possibly due to bile acid fecal loss. With bile acid pools reduced owing to the biliary obstruction, there is reduced fat absorption, since bile is involved in the emulsification of fats prior to absorption. There is also reduced absorption of fat-soluble vitamins, which need bile for emulsification. Reduced bile acids may also affect the reabsorption of B_{12} in the ileum. Sometimes bile salts

are added to the treatment regimens for patients not nutritionally well controlled with enzymes alone.

Sweat Gland Involvement

The sweat glands produce an abnormal excretion with high sodium, potassium, and chloride concentrations. This can lead to massive salt depletion and even cardiovascular collapse under some conditions, such as with heavy physical exercise in hot, humid climates.

Nutritional Care

The nutritional status of cystic fibrosis patients is of utmost importance because malnutrition means not only reduced height and weight, little subcutaneous fat, poor growth and delayed puberty, but also diminished resistance to pulmonary infections and diminished lung function.

Cystic fibrosis patients tend to fall into three categories: (1) those who have a good appetite, metabolize nutrients well, and achieve weight gain and growth; (2) those who have a good appetite but are unable to metabolize nutrients adequately or meet their increased energy demands, and hence do *not* thrive and show signs of nutritional deficiency; and (3) those who have a poor appetite, do not eat well, and consequently do *not* gain or grow well. This last group is the greatest nutritional challenge.

ENERGY. It is difficult for people with cystic fibrosis to meet their energy needs for the following reasons:

1. Some energy is "wasted" because of malabsorption.

2. Extra energy is required for the labored breathing, and the amount depends on the individual.

3. Fatigue from breathing can lead to anorexia and disinterest in food, especially during illness.

4. Chest physical therapy (PT) can cause postprandial vomiting. When the child or adolescent is ill, the number and length of chest PT sessions is usually increased, and this can lead to increased fatigue and anorexia.

5. Chronic coughing can also lead to vomiting and gastroesophageal reflux with loss of intake.

6. During fever each 1°C. elevation above normal causes a 7 per cent increase in basal metabolic rate (BMR). Even though it is not high, the patient with CF may have a persistent low-grade fever.

7. Infection is a physiological stress that leads to glycosuria and the loss of additional energy.

The recommendation for energy intake is at least 150 per cent of the RDA for sex and age. However, the Cystic Fibrosis Foundation and others recommend about 150 kcal./kg. per day, depending upon the age and requirements of the child. Since the energy requirements seem to be so individualized depending upon the extent of pancreatic insufficiency and pulmonary disease, it is probably best to individualize the intake in order to maintain growth and weight at least above the 25th percentile of weight for height (see Appendices 16, 18, 20 and 22).

Adeniyi-Jones showed that ten children with cystic fibrosis had higher basal energy expenditures (BEE) than normal adolescents.[1] Suskind showed that the BEE of children 8 to 14 years old was 30 per cent higher than that of controls.[41]

Even though there are reports that children with CF have voracious appetites, a study by Bell showed that, in fact, adolescents with CF had intakes (based upon food records kept for 28 days) that were close to the RDA and between 99 and 117 per cent of the intakes for normal adolescents of the same age.[2] In other words, they were not meeting their tremendous energy requirements or in some cases even the RDA for normal children of their age.

The energy loss from malabsorption can be as much as 16 per cent in some patients. This points to the need for aggressive counseling regarding the necessity for eating large amounts of food very often and that many times hunger cannot be the guide for energy intake.

FAT. Without lipase, fat is poorly digested and absorbed. This accounts for the greatest energy loss. In some patients, 50 per cent of the ingested fat is found in the stools, but more commonly 10 to 35 per cent of the ingested fat is not absorbed. Normal intestinal loss is less than 5 gm. of fat in 72 hours. In one study mean values of absorption of total intake of energy, fat and nitrogen were 86.7, 60.5 and 81.3 per cent, respectively.[36] MCT oil may be recommended as an energy supplement because it may be absorbed a little better than long chain triglyceride. However, its absorption is better in the presence of the enzyme lipase, so its use in children with CF should be coupled with pancreatic enzyme replacement. Generally, fat does not need to be severely restricted except in children who suffer from recurrent rectal prolapse.

PROTEIN. Without trypsin there is poor digestion and absorption of protein. Artificial diets have been tried in the hope that more elemental forms of protein and amino acids would be better absorbed and result in better weight gain. Some of these studies have shown improved weight gain, whereas others have not. However, most nutritionists working with CF patients have concluded that the unpleasant taste and inconvenience of defined formula diets make their use not worthwhile. In addition, essential fatty acid deficiency may develop with their use.

CARBOHYDRATE. As previously mentioned, omission of lactose from the diet may be tried as a means of treating malabsorption due to lactase deficiency in CF patients. Otherwise, carbohydrate should not be restricted but rather encouraged as a source of extra energy.

VITAMINS AND MINERALS. Because fat-soluble vitamins are poorly absorbed, they should be taken as additional supplements in water-soluble form. Additional amounts of water-soluble vitamins and minerals are also given as recommended in Table 38–3.

PANCREATIC ENZYMES. Pancreatin in 1943 became the first pancreatic enzyme supplement used. Fat absorption improved from 46 to 67 per cent with 5 mg. of pancreatin per meal. Nitrogen retention was also increased considerably. Patients with 10 per cent or more residual pancreatic function appear to tolerate a normal diet without enzyme supplements. Viokase and Cotazyme are newer preparations that contain lipase, amylase and trypsin. The newest forms of enzymes are Pancrease and Cotazyme-S, which are the enzymes in enteric-coated spherules so that their contents are released upon contact with the alkaline pH of the duodenum. This prevents inactivation of the pancreatic enzyme contents by acidic gastric contents. However, the duodenal contents are more acidic in cystic fibrosis patients with pancreatic insufficiency because of the lower bicarbonate output of the pancreas, so that these enzymes may not be totally released. Nevertheless, they appear to be much more clinically effective than previous forms. Capsules can be opened and the spherules sprinkled on a child's food when the child is too young to take capsules.

Pancrease is as effective as Viokase and Cotazym at substantially lower daily doses. Pancrease is taken in amounts of about two capsules with meals and one capsule with snacks, whereas six to ten capsules with meals and three to five capsules with snacks may be needed with Viokase or Cotazym.

During therapy with Pancrease, fat absorption reaches 95 per cent and nitrogen absorption 85 per cent. However, even at the highest dose complete absorption is not achieved. Enzymes affect but *do not resolve* the problem.

Constipation is frequently a problem and can be solved by reducing the dosage of pancreatic enzymes. A mild laxative may also be necessary.

Optimal dosage of enzyme therapy is an educated guess and varies with the individual. Because the activity of the enzymes is dependent upon the environment in the duodenum, increased amounts of pancreatic enzymes do not always yield the anticipated results.

Table 38–3. SUMMARY OF NUTRITIONAL CARE FOR PATIENTS WITH CYSTIC FIBROSIS

NUTRIENT	COMMENTS	RECOMMENDED SUPPLEMENTS
Energy	Energy intake great enough to promote growth and weight gain. Growth curve should be at or above 25th percentile weight for height.	Enough to maintain growth. Much higher than that recommended for normal children of same age. Infants (up to 1 yr.) — 150–200 kcal./kg./day Children (1–9 yr.) — 130–180 kcal./kg./day Males (9–18 yr.) — 100–130 kcal./kg./day Females (9–18 yr.) — 100–130 kcal./kg./day Adult requirements may be higher as patient's pulmonary condition worsens.
Protein	Protein can be lost in stool owing to lack of enzyme trypsin for digestion.	2–4 times the RDA for age. 12–15% of total energy intake.
Carbohydrate	Carbohydrate supplements (Polycose) may be useful.	As necessary to meet energy requirements. Best digested of 3 energy-producing nutrients.
Fat	Fat also lost in stool owing to lack of enzyme lipase. Intake varies with degree of fat tolerance.	Rigid restriction of fat should be avoided. MCT better digested and absorbed and may be useful in order to keep energy intake high.
Essential fatty acids (EFA)		Safflower oil or some source of polyunsaturated oil at 1 ml./kg./day.

Fat-soluble vitamins
  Vitamin A
  Vitamin D
  Vitamin E
		5000–10,000 I.U./day. Provided in water-miscible form.
		RDA + 400–800 I.U./day. Exposure to sunlight.
		Alpha-tocopherol acetate 100 I.U./day for infants, 200 I.U./day for older children and adults. Provided in water-miscible form.

Vitamin K	Especially important in infants, patients with hemoptysis or cirrhosis, patients to have surgery, and those on long-term antibiotic therapy.	50–100 μg./day orally or one 5 mg. tablet every 3rd day or 0.5–1.0 mg. parenterally once a month.
Water-soluble vitamins Vitamin B_{12}		RDA + 0.1 μg./day. With deficiency 100 μg. every other day I.M. for one month. Supplements to provide the RDA for age.
Riboflavin	Requirement increased with antibiotic administration.	5–10 times the RDA.
Minerals Sodium chloride	Intake depends upon use of "fast foods" and salty items in the diet. Infants may require supplements because salt omitted from baby foods.	500 to 1000 mg. per day extra during hot weather and heavy physical exercise.
Zinc	This amount supplied in a multiple vitamin/mineral supplement.	RDA for age.
Iron	Provided in multiple vitamin with iron or multiple vitamin/mineral supplement.	RDA for age.
Selenium		Not routinely recommended. 0.01–0.2 mg. elemental selenium per day (Na_2SeO_3) depending on age for those who wish to supplement. See ESADDI.*
Copper		Not routinely recommended. 0.5–3.0 mg./day elemental Cu for those who wish to supplement. See ESADDI.*
Pancreatic enzymes	Given with meals and snacks. Enteric-coated more efficacious than powders.	Dosage and timing sufficient to eliminate steatorrhea yet avoid constipation.

* ESADDI: Estimated Safe and Adequate Daily Dietary Intakes. From Food and Nutrition Board, National Research Council: Recommended Dietary Allowances. 9th ed. Washington, D.C., National Academy of Sciences, 1980.

Nutritional Status of Cystic Fibrosis Patients

GROWTH. Growth retardation is common, and CF patients who are tall for their age or obese are rare. Catch-up growth in newly diagnosed and treated infants with CF has been well documented, however.[14]

The more severe the pulmonary involvement, the greater the weight and height retardation. Severity of pulmonary insufficiency correlates better with the growth curve than does malabsorption.[39] Delayed bone age, puberty and onset of menarche are not unusual.

VITAMIN DEFICIENCIES. Fat-soluble vitamins are poorly absorbed because of poor fat absorption, although this is corrected significantly with enteric-coated enzymes. Vitamin A, carotene, retinol-binding protein and prealbumin are low in patients with untreated cystic fibrosis.

Deficiencies of all the fat-soluble vitamins have been reported, but it is important to consider the type of pancreatic enzymes the affected patients were taking, since the new enteric-coated enzymes are so much more effective. However, because malabsorption is not completely resolved with enzyme replacement, it is important that individuals with CF be given vitamin supplements as stated in Table 38–3. Gross clinical signs of vitamin deficiency are rare today in well-managed patients with CF.

TRACE MINERAL DEFICIENCIES. There are few studies of the trace mineral status and requirements of individuals with CF. The minerals that have been studied are calcium, copper, zinc, selenium and iron. Plasma copper and ceruloplasmin have shown some changes (both elevated), but the significance of this is not known. Increases in plasma copper seemed to parallel the clinical deterioration.[38]

Some children with cystic fibrosis have been reported to have low plasma zinc levels.[18, 21] Zinc deficiency is closely linked to vitamin A in two ways: first, it results in a decrease in retinol dehydrogenase, which converts retinol to retinal for night vision; second, it is necessary for the production of retinol-binding protein (RBP), which is essential in mobilization of vitamin A from the liver. However, in children with cystic fibrosis the low plasma vitamin A and RBP levels did not improve following zinc supplementation.

The recommendations for mineral supplementation of patients with CF as shown in Table 38–3 are based on very limited data.

ESSENTIAL FATTY ACIDS. Abnormal fatty acid composition can be found in the blood and tissue lipids of 85 to 90 per cent of CF patients. At least one study showed that linoleic acid supplementation had a positive effect on pulmonary function studies in CF patients.[6] It has been suggested that linoleic acid plays a role in the manifestation of this disease because linoleic acid is important in the control of prostaglandin biosynthesis, and some prostaglandins are associated with bronchoconstriction and pulmonary vasoconstriction. No conclusions can be made at present. In fact, it is not even clear whether essential fatty acid biochemical deficiency seen in CF patients is secondary to their disease or a primary derangement of the disease. Much more work needs to be done in this area.

Emotional Adjustment

Because cystic fibrosis is such a debilitating disease, with a prognosis for a short life span, it is important for health professionals to be aware of the emotional and psychological adjustment of the patient. One study showed that at first glance adolescents with cystic fibrosis appeared to function adequately on a daily basis. However, four sources of psychological stress were identified: altered physical appearance causing distorted body images and denial of sexuality, strained interpersonal relationships, conflicts in upbringing, and increased awareness of the future and of death.[4] These issues should be dealt with by a team approach of clinicians working with cystic fibrosis patients. Help for patients and families can be obtained from The Cystic Fibrosis Foundation, 600 Executive Blvd., Rockville, Md. 20852.

Protein-Energy Malnutrition (PEM)

Malnutrition is usually thought of in reference to children. Malnourished children do not get adequate energy and nutrients, either because they do not ingest sufficient food to supply their needs or because they have faulty digestion, absorption or assimilation. Protein-energy malnutrition in preschool children is probably the most common and important current nutritional problem in the world.

Over half the world's population is the victim of hunger or inadequate nutrition in one form or another, and the principal victims are infants and children. Millions die in their early years because they do not get adequate food.

Nutritional Care

Mild cases of protein-energy malnutrition (PEM) can be treated on an outpatient basis with an adequate diet, education in the home for the mothers and others who care for the child, and treatment of the usually coexistent infections. Treatment of severe PEM such as the case shown in Figure 38–4 requires hospitalization.

Initially, fluid and electrolyte imbalances are corrected and treatment of the usual concomitant infections is started. Later the objective of treatment is to raise the level of the child's nutritional status as rapidly as possible. Diluted infant formula is generally used at first, followed by undiluted formula and eventually concentrated formula if necessary to meet energy requirements and if tolerated. Patients may have to be tube-fed in the beginning, but as they become rehydrated and gain strength, their appetites will return and they can take nourishment by themselves.

Depending upon their clinical condition and tolerance, patients by the end of the first week of rehabilitation should receive energy at a level of 125 to 150 kcal./kg./day and protein at 3 to 5 gm./kg./day. Formulas may need to be concentrated to 1 kcal./ml. To reach this concentra-

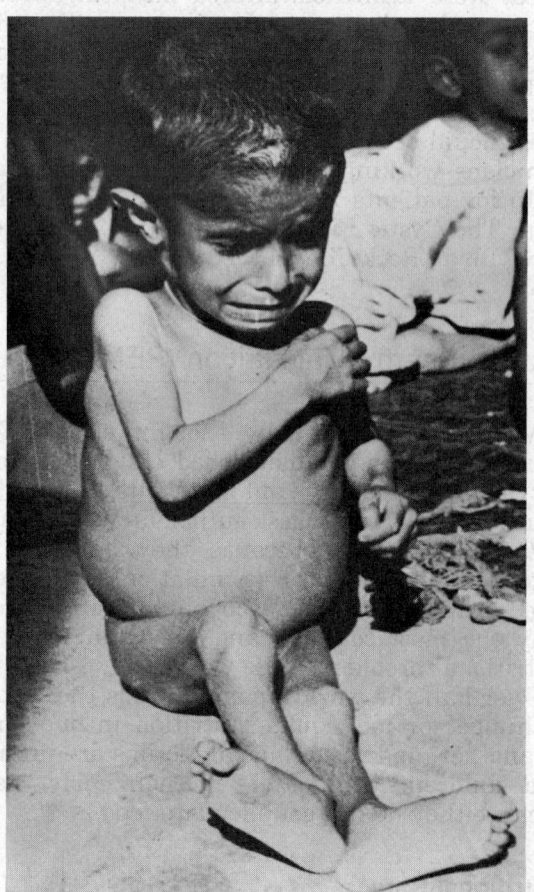

Figure 38–4. An Iranian girl admitted in an advanced stage of malnutrition to a foundling home in Teheran. After 12 months of treatment she became a normal, lively child. (Courtesy FAO.)

tion, the standard commercially prepared liquid formula concentrate (133 kcal./dl.) is mixed with only half the usual required amount of water to give a 100 kcal./dl. formula instead of the usual 67 kcal./dl. This caloric concentration should be reached gradually over a period of four to five days. Diarrhea is commonly present in patients with PEM but should not be a reason to stop the feeding. It will probably resolve itself as the nutritional status improves. Some children may not tolerate lactose, in which case milk and other lactose-containing foods will aggravate diarrhea. Other high-protein liquids and foods such as a chemically defined liquid diet or lactose-free formula (Prosobee or Neo-Mull-Soy) can be used. Solid foods are added when improvement is noted and appetite increases. Foods are added as tolerated, with emphasis on energy and protein. Frequent small feedings are tolerated better than the customary three daily meals, because they prevent overloading of the gastrointestinal tract and the development of hypothermia and hypoglycemia.

The goal of nutritional rehabilitation is the most rapid weight gain and catch-up growth possible. In catch-up growth during recovery from PEM it is not uncommon to see rates of weight gain 20 times that of normal children of the same age. This can occur especially in children receiving 200 kcal./kg./day.

Supplementary vitamins are given as indicated. Vitamin A is required to prevent ocular lesions that can occur when children who also have an unsuspected vitamin A deficiency are rehabilitated. DeMaeyer recommends an initial intramuscular injection of 100,000 I.U. of a water-miscible preparation. This should be followed by a daily oral supplement (water-miscible or oil-soluble) of 10,000 I.U. until the child is taking adequate amounts of vitamin A in the diet.[12]

Potassium should be supplied daily during the first two weeks of therapy in the form of 1 to 2 gm. of potassium chloride. This is necessary because of the increased potassium uptake that occurs during this period of rapid protein synthesis.

Magnesium (250 mg. to 1 gm. daily, depending on the child's weight) may also be required and is given intramuscularly until the child is able to take it orally.

The continuation of an adequate diet to correct deficiencies is the objective of complete nutritional care. This means that there must be follow-up and that attention must be paid to the home environment to which the child will return when he or she leaves the hospital. There should also be attention to mental stimulation of the child both in the hospital during rehabilitation and at home. These are difficult tasks that require governmental support and the attention of educators and health workers in the community.

Vitamin Deficiency Diseases

Vitamin deficiency diseases are discussed in Chapter 6. However, hemolytic anemia of the premature infant related to vitamin E is discussed in Chapter 37.

Diabetes Mellitus

The etiology of diabetes in children is not clear, but it is thought to be a genetic predisposition aggravated by environmental factors, as discussed in Chapter 25. It is almost always insulin-dependent, and good nutritional care is very important to maintain blood glucose control and proper growth in the child. The majority of children are undernourished when the disease is first recognized, and the onset of symptoms is relatively sudden.

Insulin Therapy

The basics of insulin therapy, diet management, home glucose monitoring and exercise are discussed in Chapter 25. Only comments particular to the management of children are mentioned here.

Sometime after beginning insulin therapy, some juvenile patients appear to have a remission and do not need as much or, in rare cases, any insulin. This *"honeymoon period"* may last for months or years, but it is *always temporary*, and the child and parents should be so informed. This temporary remission is not well understood, but it appears to be a "last ditch" effort by the pancreas to secrete insulin and control the level of blood glucose.

This phenomenon has been the focus of much study, and there is some indication that the length of this period correlates with the length of time that elapsed before diagnosis and treatment of the child.[20] Those children diagnosed and treated early, before or soon after the onset of overt diabetes, may have lower insulin requirements and a longer period of partial remission. Those children diagnosed and treated when they were in severe acidosis appear to have higher insulin requirements and shorter partial remission. However, these findings are still controversial.

After this "honeymoon period," insulin requirements increase and then remain fairly stable, except during periods of increased growth rate, when they will increase. Requirements also increase after a hypoglycemic attack because the body develops a transitory insulin resistance as a protective mechanism. Insulin resistance and increased insulin requirements also occur during an infection.

As the child reaches adulthood and energy requirements lessen, it is important to reduce insulin dosage and energy intake accordingly.

Nutritional Care

The diabetic child's diet follows the same general pattern as that suggested for the adult (Chapter 25). However, a child's energy and protein requirements per kilogram of body weight are higher, to allow for proper growth and development. Recommended allowances for energy, protein, vitamins and minerals for normal children as listed in Table 10-1 should be used as the starting point for designing the diet for the diabetic child. Chapters 12, 13 and 14 provide further discussion of the nutritional needs of infants, children and adolescents.

Controversy exists regarding the necessity for strict supervision of the food intake. However, most authorities believe that there is a close relationship between the control of diabetes and the development of complications. Consequently, it is advocated that food intake, exercise and insulin distribution be adjusted to avoid insulin reactions and, insofar as practical, to avoid glycosuria.

The diet is adjusted to provide 15 to 20 per cent of the calories from protein, 25 to 35 per cent from fat and 50 to 60 per cent from carbohydrate. The distribution of the carbohydrates and calories throughout the day must be relatively uniform to maintain a high degree of control and prevent dangerous hypoglycemia.

Nutritional Counseling

The interpretation of diets for diabetic children should be particularly liberal, especially if the child and family are conscientious about glucose monitoring. If favorite party dishes are planned occasionally, the child may cooperate more cheerfully and adhere more closely to the established regimen. The many emotional conflicts of childhood and adolescence must be considered in the treatment of the diabetic child and require sympathetic understanding and tact. Some of these problems and ways to deal with them are reviewed by Lum.[22] Planning the diabetic eating plan around the usual dietary pattern of the family helps the child to accept it. The child need not appear to be different from other members of the family at the table and can learn to eat at regular intervals and to live a normal life.

Children are apt students and learn quickly how to plan their own diets once they have accepted their disease and are ready to learn. When possible, it is advisable to give diabetic children the responsibility for planning their own diets from the family meals. They are then able to plan their eating to include those foods that will be eaten outside the home. They will appreciate and accept the obligation of the task.

It is highly important that the diabetic child and the parents be clearly informed concerning the disease and the later complications that inevitably develop to some degree. While there is no known cure at this time, the condition need not interfere with a happy, well-adjusted life, provided the diabetic receives adequate treatment and education to control the disorder.

Hyperthyroidism (Graves' Disease)

A discussion of hyperthyroidism appears in Chapter 26 and will not be repeated here. The treatment for children follows the same general principles outlined for the adult; however, attention is directed to the need for additional energy and protein so the child can meet the requirements for growth and development.

Hypothyroidism (Cretinism and Juvenile Myxedema)

Hypothyroidism that develops in fetal life or early infancy, is referred to as *cretinism* (Fig. 38–5). The main cause of cretinism is insufficient thyroid hormone in the newborn, either because (1) the structure is defective or (2) the iodine intake of the mother has been inadequate. In this country, even in the "goiter belts," the latter is seldom encountered. Distribution of foods that contain iodine and the use of iodized table salt have minimized the danger. In certain areas such as Ecuador, however, the prevalence of endemic goiter as a result of iodine deficiency among school children is high.

Hypothyroidism acquired in childhood is known as *juvenile myxedema*. It usually is suspected in an older child who begins to lag or drop behind in school, loses interest, tires easily and has definitely delayed growth and development.

Treatment

Thyroid hormone supplementation is the main therapy. Without this therapeutic management the course is regressive, and the physical and mental growth of the child are stunted.

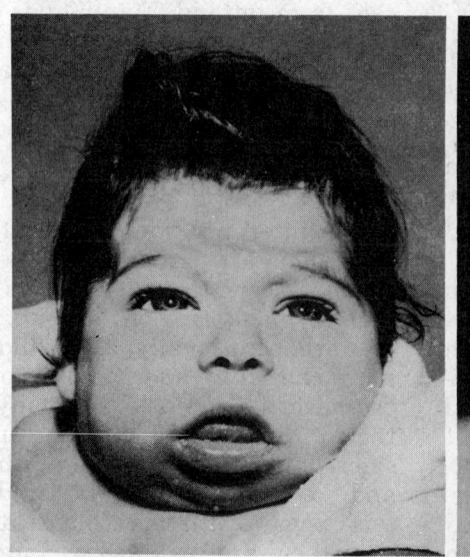
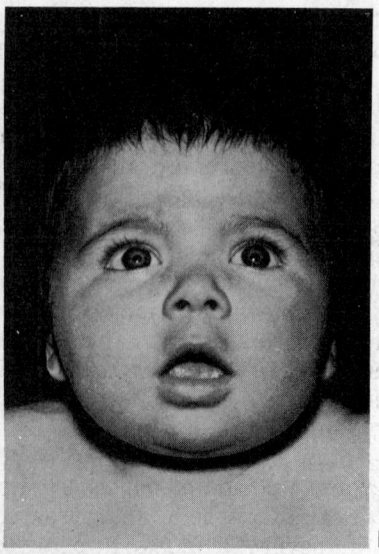

Figure 38–5. Cretinism. Congenitally hypothyroid infant at six months of age. Infant fed poorly in neonatal period and was constipated, had persistent nasal discharge and large tongue, was very lethargic and had no social smile and no head control. *A*, Note puffy face, dull expression, hirsute forehead. Serum cholesterol 172 mg. per 100 ml., alkaline phosphatase 4.8 Bodansky units, negligible uptake to radioiodine. Osseous development that of newborn. *B*, Four months after treatment with U.S.P. thyroid. Note decreased puffiness of face, decreased hirsutism of forehead and alert appearance. (From Behrman, R. E., and Vaughan, V. C.: Nelson Textbook of Pediatrics, 12th ed., Philadelphia, W. B. Saunders Co., 1983.)

When medication is instituted during the first two years, the results are sometimes excellent, although a certain number of children remain slightly subnormal for their age. Signs of improvement may be noted within a few weeks or months, and the dosage is regulated by checking the patient's response to thyroid extract. As a rule, this form of therapy is continued throughout life.

As in all patients who lack thyroid, there is a tendency toward overweight. The tissues are not firm but flabby, mottled and cool to the touch. The amount of calories in the customary diet is reduced in order to lose and then maintain weight at the desired level. See Chapter 26 for additional discussion of hypothyroidism.

Overweight

Overnutrition in infants, children and adolescents in this country is a matter of medical and public health concern. The child whose weight for height is above the 90th percentile as determined by using Appendices 16, 18, 20 and 22 should warrant further evaluation and possible treatment.

Factors in the etiology of obesity development are thoroughly discussed in Chapter 27. Heredity may be one of the factors that lead to overweight, but frequently there are also environmental factors leading to overfeeding and underexercising in overweight children. Even with a genetic tendency toward obesity, a person's diet can be changed and an exercise program can be started in order to prevent expression of the tendency or at least to attenuate its expression. If obesity is prevalent among family members, the entire family needs to review their dietary and exercise patterns and change them.

Mild overweight between the ages of 8 and 14 often occurs because of a spurt in body weight gain prior to a rapid gain in height and is simply a brief stage of development. The weight will usually adjust itself automatically through normal appetite and activity, providing there is no abnormality.

Frequently, food is the center of interest at social gatherings. Children, and especially teenagers, meet at favorite places for a soft drink, sandwich, pizza or other snack, and although Type A school lunches provide a well-balanced meal, there is the ever-present distraction on school grounds of vending machines that make high-calorie, low-nutrition foods such as soda pop, candy and pastries easily available. The energy equivalent of these extra snacks may well exceed energy expenditure and can result in weight gain.

Besides the fact that their social world revolves around food, another frequent reason for obesity development, especially for teenagers, is low activity. Obese adolescents, in general, are less active than non-obese youngsters of the same age group. Bullen and associates[5] compared the activity of obese and non-obese adolescent girls engaged in sports at summer camp by using motion picture sampling. The striking degree of inactivity of the obese girls appears to be a significant factor in their overweight conditions. Obesity in adolescence is discussed in Chapter 14. Obesity and other eating disorders in adolescence have been extensively reviewed by Rees.[30]

Nutritional Care

Unless a child is grossly obese, vigorous reducing is generally not advised. Weight maintenance is the preferable approach with the child "growing into" the present weight. It is important that linear growth and development continue at the same rate. The child's customary food pattern and eating habits are evaluated, and the child is encouraged to become interested in making the necessary changes to improve his or her diet.

For a child less than about five years of age, the family will need to take almost complete responsibility for the behavioral and environmental changes. However, the older child should be allowed to take as much responsibility as possible for weight management. Frequently it is more difficult for the parents to give up responsibility for and "control" of the child's diet than it is for the child to take control. It is important to remind parents, however, to set consistent limits, with consequences for the child if they are exceeded.

After deciding appropriate behavioral changes with the child and family, monitoring the ability to make those changes is important. This can be done with a star or point system in which the child receives a point for making a behavior change each day. The points are earned and lead to rewards which are motivators for the child. It is important that parents follow through with providing the rewards. See Chapter 27 for the principles involved in the dietary treatment of obesity.

Emotional and Social Factors

Understanding a child's weight problem—the reasons for the overweight—is more important than formulating the correct diet for losing weight. Diets should be avoided and rather the reasons for the child's overeating and underactivity must be identified. It is thought that the obese child cannot accurately recognize hunger and mistakes feelings of guilt, anger or frustration for it. The comfort gained from a full stomach allays the other feelings but reinforces the obesity and the social ostracism felt by the obese child. This leads to depression and then eating to relieve depression, and the vicious circle continues.

Adolescents especially have many physiological and psychological characteristics[17] that must be taken into account, for at this age there is great self-awareness, as discussed in Chapter 14. While girls are sometimes more concerned about their weight than boys are, the markedly obese adolescent of either sex is usually self-conscious and unhappy. Teenagers are great imitators, and here the dietitian-nutritionist or nurse can be of invaluable help by setting a good example for weight control. Adolescents appreciate any interest and understanding about their weight problems. Time spent in counseling is usually rewarding. Acceptance by their peers is vital, because children seek group approval. The feeling that they will be more popular after a reduction in weight such as that shown in Figure 38–6 is a strong motivation for changing

food habits, but they need tremendous amounts of support. Individualized treatment is the cornerstone of management.

Group discussions with other overweight adolescents may be useful in helping the obese teenager get involved in new activities, participate in enjoyable sports and get some regular form of exercise. Discussion of common problems is helpful. The focus should be on the learning of new attitudes and behaviors that promote weight loss instead of weight gain.

Family interaction around food, weight and dieting must be assessed. Frequently the overeating, underexercising obese child becomes the focus of parental attention so that parents do not have to focus on their poor interaction. The child can become a buffer, and maintaining overweight or an eating disorder as a center for this diverted attention may act to maintain family function. The "function" is really malfunction, and until this can be changed, successful weight reduction and weight maintenance in the child or young adolescent is very difficult. Minuchin discusses characteristics of families with children who have eating disorders.[26] Also see Chapter 14 and the section on eating disorders in Chapter 32.

Cooperation of parents and other members of the family is necessary to prevent frustration. Overall adolescent adjustment problems require evaluation to make sure the pressures of obesity are not increased by an impossible regimen.

It is easier to prevent obesity than to treat it, and most of the attention should be directed toward that goal. Prevention and even reduction of obesity have been demonstrated through school programs where the activity of the children was significantly increased through daily structured exercise. It is important that health professionals and parents encourage and set good examples for regular energy-requiring activity. Obesity is a public health problem that can be solved only through learning on the part of individuals to avoid unwanted weight gain at any time in life.

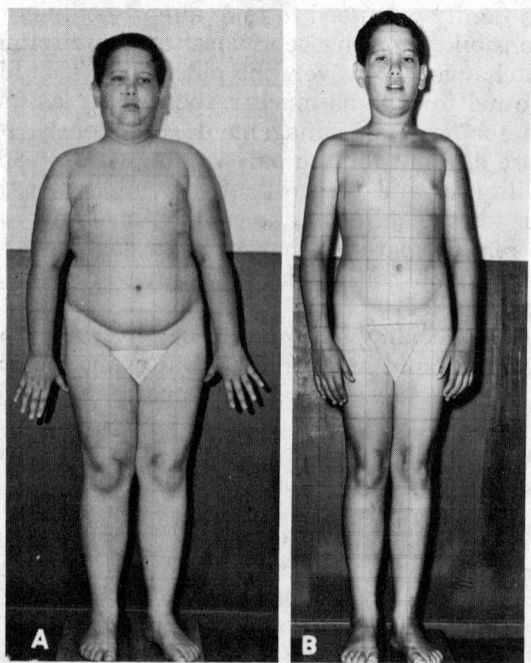

Figure 38–6. Obesity. Before and after 10 months' treatment for obesity in an 11-year-old boy. Weight loss was 42½ lb. However, since there was a growth of 1½ inches during this period, the effective weight loss is calculated to be 49½ lb. The change in facial expression is as dramatic as the weight loss, a frequent observation in such cases. (Courtesy of Dr. R. H. Hoffman.)

Underweight

Although slimness in itself does not indicate malnutrition, if a child is below the 10th percentile for weight for height (Appendices 16, 18, 20 and 22) or if the rate of weight gain is slowing down, this should warrant a more complete assessment of additional anthropometric data as discussed in Chapter 9 and a physical examination. If no disease can be demonstrated, further evaluation of the family, school and home situation is also important. There may be psychosocial reasons why the child is not eating enough. Disorganized family eating patterns may be responsible.

In some instances, a scanty breakfast or no breakfast starts the child's day, while in others essential foods are omitted without suitable substitutes. Some children become tea or coffee addicts at an early age. Many resort to nibbling, which spoils the appetite for regular meals. Some children become so engrossed with the business of play that they eat too rapidly. Adolescents of both sexes are often figure-conscious and skip some nutritious foods in an attempt to keep slim.

The nervous, irritable child with a finicky appetite should receive attractive meals served at regular hours. Nutritious snacks at midmorning and midafternoon may prove beneficial. A diet high in all the vitamins, especially the B-complex group, usually stimulates the appetite.

The avoidance of fatigue by restricting activity and encouraging additional rest is advised for some children. For others who are kept indoors and have limited activity, plenty of fresh air and sunshine may stimulate the appetite. Underweight is further discussed in Chapter 27.

Hypertension

There is increasing evidence that childhood may be an appropriate time to initiate strategies to prevent hypertension, especially in children with a family history of essential hypertension.[15] As in adults, obesity is the main environmental factor contributing to hypertension development in children, and weight management should be the primary focus of nutritional care. Sodium intake should also be addressed, as discussed in Chapter 28.

Congenital Heart Disease

Congenital anomalies of the heart make up 12 per cent of all congenital anomalies. Although most infants with congenital heart anomalies are appropriate size at birth, growth retardation becomes apparent early. This growth retardation can be due to chronic hypoxia, but inadequate nutrition can also be present. One factor that can lead to inadequate nutrition is decreased food intake. Chronic labored respiration and rapid fatigue while feeding can reduce the amount the infant will consume. Such infants also may refuse to nurse or may vomit or spit out food given to them, a tendency that for some unknown reason is resolved by reparative surgery.[13]

Besides decreased food intake in the child with severe heart disease, gastrointestinal absorption is less efficient, which can further prevent the meeting of nutritional requirements. Furthermore, these patients are hypermetabolic and have increased energy requirements. Other factors that can lead to failure to thrive are congestive heart failure and the increased susceptibility to infections that accompanies congenital heart disease. All these factors act to deter the growth and development of children with severe heart disease, and by nine months of age most have fallen below the 5th percentile for length and weight.[32]

Since surgical correction of the congenital defect is usually attempted when the child is 12 to 15 months of age, it is important that he or she be in the best possible nutritional condition. This requires early initiation of nutritional care.

Nutritional Care

ENERGY. Most of these infants require more than the usual amount of energy for an infant the same age. Their requirement is usually about 120 to 135 kcal./kg./day, and some infants may need as much as 150 to 175 kcal./kg./day to gain weight and grow.

FORMULA. Because of their increased energy needs and their inability to take more than a small volume of food at one time (many under one year of age can take only 450 ml. per day), these infants should be given calorically dense formulas. Formulas can be concentrated by mixing them with less water so that they provide up to 24 kcal./oz. (9 per cent protein) without jeopardizing the fluid status of the infant. Carbohydrate and fat can be added to a standard premature infant formula (80 kcal./dl. or 24 kcal./oz.) so that it will contain 100 kcal./dl. (30 kcal./oz.). This manipulation can be done using standard formula (67 kcal./dl. or 20 kcal./oz.), but the protein content may be diluted so much that the infant will not get enough for growth, particularly if he or she can take only a small volume of formula. The formula should not contain butterfat (evaporated milk formula) because of its poor digestibility. The infant will excrete butterfat in the stool, and thus the energy intake will be decreased.

It is preferable to use proprietary formula with vegetable oil and to raise the caloric density of the formula by adding vegetable oil. Karo syrup or a carbohydrate supplement (Polycose) can also be used to increase the caloric density of the formula. See Table 38–4 for the methods for increasing the energy concentration of formulas.

Table 38–4.　METHODS FOR INCREASING THE ENERGY CONCENTRATION
OF FORMULAS

	KCAL./OZ.	% CHO	% PRO	% FAT
13　oz. regular formula concentrate 13　oz. water	20	42	9	49
13　oz. regular formula concentrate 11　oz. water	22	42	9	49
13　oz. concentrate 9　oz. water	24	42	9	49
13　oz. concentrate 9　oz. water 1　tsp. light Karo syrup (5 ml.) ½　tsp. vegetable oil (2.5 ml.)	26	42	8	50
13　oz. concentrate 9　oz. water 2　tsp. light Karo syrup (10 ml.) 1　tsp. vegetable oil (5 ml.)	28	42	8	50
13　oz. concentrate 9　oz. water 1　tbsp. light Karo syrup (15 ml.) 1½　tsp. vegetable oil (7.5 ml.)	30	43	7	50

Later, when the child takes semisolids that are sources of carbohydrate and fat, the carbohydrate and fat added to the formula can be omitted, but the formula should be mixed with a smaller amount of water so that it is still a concentrated source of protein. The commercially prepared concentrated liquid (133 kcal./dl.) can be mixed with half the usual amount of water to give a formula with a caloric concentration of 100 kcal./dl. instead of the usual 67 kcal./dl.

Whenever infants are taking a concentrated food, their fluid balance should be watched closely because of the increased renal solute load presented by the formula and the possibility of excessive renal water loss and dehydration. Careful attention is required to balance the child's water needs and the decreased volume of intake with the increased calorie and protein requirements.

SODIUM. Sodium balance is important because excess sodium can precipitate congestive heart failure or disrupt the water balance. Eight mEq. of sodium per day is advised for adequate growth, although the estimated requirement is 2.1 to 2.6 mEq. per day. Standard formulas are usually given, and low-sodium formulas are needed only during periods of severe cardiac failure or excessive sodium retention. Commercial baby foods are appropriate because salt is no longer added to these products. Homemade baby foods prepared without added salt would also be appropriate. Strained fruits would appear to be a good choice for first baby foods because they are low in sodium.

POTASSIUM. Diuretics are used to control congestive heart failure, and if used regularly may cause hypokalemia, digitalis toxicity and impaired renal concentrating ability. Potassium replacements may be necessary.

VITAMINS AND MINERALS. Supplements of vitamins and iron should be given because of possible inadequate intake and inefficient gastrointestinal absorption. For example, an increased prevalence of biochemical riboflavin deficiency has been seen in these children,[40] and folic acid deficiency is frequent. [33] Calcium supplements such as Neo-Calglucon are also given because of poor absorption of calcium. Table 38–5 presents the amounts of calcium, folic acid and sodium in 450 ml. of several infant formulas. This amount is the maximum intake for many infants who have a severe heart problem. Note that the amounts received from this volume of formula are low compared with the estimated requirements and advisable intakes stated by Fomon.[16] Supplementation is therefore necessary.

Nutritional Counseling

The parents must understand the special nutritional needs of their infant in order for the child to grow properly. This may require exten-

Table 38–5. ADEQUACY OF SELECTED VITAMINS AND MINERALS IN 450 ML. OF SEVERAL INFANT FORMULAS

FORMULA (20 kcal./oz.)	CALCIUM (mg./450 ml.)	FOLIC ACID (µg./450 ml.)	SODIUM (mEq./450 ml.)	
Enfamil	260	47	5	
Isomil	315	45	5.8	
PM 60/40	158	22.5	3	
Prosobee	351	45	8	
SMA	179	23	3	

	0–4 MONTHS	4–12 MONTHS	0–12 MONTHS	0–4 MONTHS	4–12 MONTHS
[a]Estimated requirement	388	289	<50	2.5	2.1
[a]Advisable intake	450	350	50	8	6

From Rickard, K., Brady, M. S., and Gresham, E. L.: Nutritional management of the chronically ill child. Pediatr. Clin. North Am., *24*:157, 1977.

[a] Estimated requirements and advisable intakes during infancy are those suggested by Fomon and associates.[16]

sive counseling. A mother may equate weight gain with edema, which she knows is deleterious to her infant's health, and thus feed the child less than he or she needs in order to avoid weight gain. Parents may associate atherosclerotic heart disease with their child's condition and inappropriately modify the diet to lower cholesterol and fat by using skim milk or by omitting all types of fat from the child's diet, with the result that the child's energy intake is reduced.

When these infants grow older they are frequently the center of the family's attention and can become very manipulative. It is important that the parents receive adequate counseling and support in their attempts to provide the proper nutritional care.

The children should be followed closely, with regular measurement of growth, serum albumin and urine osmolarity. The urine osmolarity should be maintained below 400 mOsm. per liter. In addition, the osmolarity of the formula can be measured to determine if it is being prepared with the proper dilution. Parents should be instructed carefully in formula preparation and the accurate recording of the infant's fluid intake. They should observe the frequency of urination (number of wet diapers) and the color of the urine.

When the rate of weight gain is less than the 25th percentile for normal infants, modification of the formula is necessary. If the urine osmolarity is 300 mOsm. per liter or less, the concentration of the formula can be increased by adding less water to the commercially prepared concentrated liquid. However, if the urine osmolarity is greater than 300 mOsm. per liter and

the child is not growing, then the concentration of the formula should be increased by adding more carbohydrate and fat without significantly increasing the renal solute load. If an infant still does not grow properly, a fat absorption test should be made to determine if malabsorption exists. If it does, using a formula in which medium chain triglycerides (MCT) supply the fat or using MCT oil in the diet may be helpful.

After successful surgical repair of the anomaly, the child typically feels better and begins to gain weight. This may partially be due to increased intestinal absorption caused by increased splanchnic blood flow.[25] The absorption rate from the intestine is directly affected by the amount of blood flowing through the intestinal wall.

Anemia

Nutritional or iron deficiency anemia is the most common form of anemia in infancy and childhood. It affects individuals of all ages, but particularly women and infants, and occurs most frequently among infants 6 to 24 months old. Most of the babies involved received a poor supply of iron from an anemic mother or had fetal blood loss.

Evidence has accumulated to indicate that sensitivity to cow's milk may cause occult loss of significant quantities of blood into the gastrointestinal tracts of some children with hypochromic microcytic anemia. Furthermore, cow's milk is almost devoid of iron, and the anemic infant is not likely to improve unless a supplementary source of iron is given. In the rapidly growing infant, lack of iron in a milk diet unsupplemented by other foodstuffs is usually the cause of iron deficiency anemia.

Breast-fed infants rarely become anemic as long as they are nursing, possibly because the iron in breast milk is present in a more easily absorbed form than the iron in cow's milk or cow's milk formula. Other factors in human milk may also be responsible, as discussed in Chapter 12.

Introduction of iron-rich supplementary foods, such as infant cereal, egg yolk, strained beef and liver, certain fruits and green vegetables, when the infant is five or six months old is helpful. Continuing the child on an iron-fortified formula or on an older infant formula such as Advance (Ross), which contains iron, during the entire first year of life may help to prevent iron deficiency anemia. (See Appendix Table 11 for iron-rich foods.) The iron content of some baby foods and formulas is given in Table 38–6. See Table 10–1 for the recommended allowances for iron at different ages.

Factors that promote the absorption of iron from the diet are discussed in Chapters 7 and 29. Iron deficiency in the premature infant and appropriate supplementation are discussed in Chapter 37.

Lowered blood hemoglobin levels are not uncommon among adolescents who consume less iron than is recommended. Iron deficiency anemia is frequently seen in girls at puberty.

Growth requires additional iron, and it is easy to understand how some adolescent males, undergoing tremendous growth, could become anemic. Girls frequently become anemic when they diet to remain slim at the peak of their adolescent growth spurt and when they also begin to menstruate. Complete discussion of the anemias and the nutritional care for them appears in Chapter 29.

Lead Poisoning

Children with *pica*, an abnormal craving for non-food substances, are particularly prone to chronic lead poisoning, or *plumbism*. The non-food substances they eat are frequently sources of lead, the most common being chips of lead-based paint. Pica may result from nutritional deficiencies or from emotional disorders. Thorough discussions of pica have been presented.[3,9] A recent report revealed that the prevalence of elevated lead levels in children age 6 months to 5 years is higher (4 per cent) than previously believed. It is much higher in black children (12.2 per cent) than in white children.[24]

Most of the paint currently used on children's furniture and toys is free from lead; however, lead-based paints may still be found in many older houses and apartments and on homemade toys and furniture. Infants and young children may chew their cribs, toys or window sills and eat the sweet-tasting chips (Fig. 38–7). A chip of

Table 38–6. IRON CONTENT OF SELECTED FOODS FED TO INFANTS IN THE UNITED STATES

FOOD	ELEMENTAL IRON	
	(mg./100 gm. of food)	(mg./100 kcal.)
Milk or formula		
Human milk[a]	0.05	0.07
Cow's milk[a]	0.05	0.07
Iron-fortified formula	0.9–1.3	1.2–1.8
Formula unfortified with iron	<0.05	<0.05
Infant cereals		
Iron-fortified (dry) mixed with milk[b]	4.2	7–14
Wet-packed cereal-fruit	3.3	1.3–7.5
Strained and junior foods		
Meats		
Liver and a few others	4–6	4–6
Most meats	1–2	1–2
Egg yolks	2–3	1.0–1.5
"Dinners"		
High meat	<1	<1
Vegetable-meat	<0.5	<0.5
Vegetables[c]	<0.5	<0.5
Fruits[c]	<0.5	<0.5

From Fomon, S. J.: Infant Nutrition, 2nd ed. Philadelphia, W. B. Saunders Co., 1974, p. 314.
[a] Data reviewed by Underwood (1971).
[b] Assuming that one part by weight of dry cereal is mixed with six parts of milk.
[c] A few varieties of vegetables and fruits provide 1 to 2 mg. of iron/100 gm. (1 to 3 mg./100 kcal.).

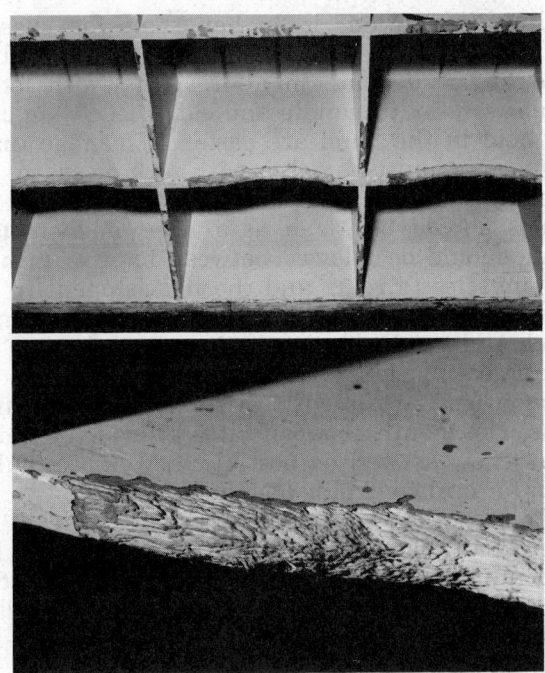

Figure 38–7. A bookself with the paint chewed off by an infant. (From Bicknell, D. J.: Pica, A Childhood Symptom. London, Butterworth and Co., Ltd., 1975, p. 133.)

paint the size of a penny can contain 50 to 100 μg. of lead. Repeated ingestion of this amount daily for a three-month period could easily occur and could result in clinical symptoms. This would mean a daily ingestion of 100 times the adult tolerable intake.[8] Other potential sources of lead are slightly acidic beverages, such as fruit juices, stored in earthenware pitchers painted with lead-based glaze; food canned in lead-soldered containers; food from crops fertilized with sewage sludge; air polluted with automotive emissions from automobiles using leaded gasoline or from industrial smokestacks; and dirt in city yards or parks that may be eaten by young children.

When an excess amount of lead enters the body, lead poisoning may follow. The normal blood lead level is less than 40 μg./dl. Children with blood levels of 60 to 80 μg./dl. usually have symptoms of vomiting, irritability, loss of weight, weakness, headache, abdominal pain, insomnia and anorexia. These early symptoms after six to eight weeks of lead ingestion are not specific, and the child may be incorrectly diagnosed and treated unless the nurse and physician are alert to the possibility of lead poisoning in the community. With blood lead levels greater than 80 μg./dl., children exhibit more severe symptoms such as anemia, acute renal tubular injury, peripheral neuritis, muscular incoordination, joint pains and encephalopathy. Eventual-

ly death will result. Sometimes chronic nephritis without the acute encephalopathy results from long-term chronic lead poisoning.

Treatment

Since the tubular injury to the kidneys results in *Fanconi syndrome*—increased urinary loss of amino acids, glucose and phosphate—the first step in treating severe acute lead poisoning is to restore fluid and electrolyte balance, with particular concern to correcting the hypophosphatemia. After fluid and electrolyte balance is restored in the acute phase, the child is started on a regimen of chelating agents, which pick up lead from the tissues and allow its removal by the kidney and liver. A common chelating agent is *ethylenediaminetetraacetic acid (EDTA)*, which is given intramuscularly along with *British Anti-Lewisite (BAL)* for five days, usually while the child is hospitalized. *Penicillamine* can be used for less severe cases or as follow-up therapy. During chelation therapy it is important for the nurse to maintain the child's fluid intake to allow maximal excretion of the lead. At least 200 ml. of some fluid should be given each hour. Most of the body's burden of lead will have been deposited in the long bones as "lead lines," and some will never be drawn out. However, in the bones it is relatively harmless.

The number of cases of lead toxicity drastically increases during the summer months. Although this observation cannot be explained, it may be that exposure to sunlight during these months and the consequent formation by the skin of vitamin D causes an increased absorption of lead from the gut.[7] Vitamin D appears to enhance lead absorption, and calcium seems to compete with it. Therefore, a diet high in calcium is indicated. Zinc and iron in the diet also seem to have a protective effect against lead absorption.[23]

Prognosis

Children with confirmed lead poisoning often have severe neurological and psychological sequelae even after treatment. It has been shown that children with elevated lead levels during the first three years of life had abnormalities of IQ, fine motor coordination and behavior when they were tested at ages seven and eight.[11] Others report that subclinical lead poisoning may lead to a hyperkinetic behavioral pattern, including hyperactivity, impulsiveness and short attention span.[10] Because there seems to be lasting brain damage in 25 per cent of those children who are successfully treated and not reexposed to lead, it is important to prevent the disease, and treated children should have their blood lead levels tested periodically thereafter, and their environments should be tested for lead.

Dental Caries

A youngster has a good chance of developing good teeth if his mother was properly nourished and received adequate calcium and vitamins during the pregnancy. Proper nourishment with adequate calcium and vitamin D during the child's early years rates next in importance. Further, prevention of dental caries can be aided by regular brushing of the teeth and by avoidance of sticky foods and sweets, such as cola drinks, candy and sugar. Nutritional care to prevent dental caries and periodontal disease is discussed in Chapter 33.

Cerebral Palsy

Cerebral palsy, a disturbance of muscular action caused by damage to portions of the brain, is a real challenge to health professionals helping the child who is handicapped since birth to make use of his potential abilities. Difficulty in sucking and swallowing causes feeding problems. The spasticity of the muscles often makes eating and drinking difficult. Observations of cerebral palsy children in a residential school suggest that the extent of "mouth area" involvement is closely associated with poor food intake and, correspondingly, with the general growth curve.[34] The many problems of these individuals—food lost through dribbling due to poor function of mouth, tongue or throat and tiring easily while eating—may contribute to inadequate food intake and poor growth. The nurse can not only feed these children but can aid in teaching them to feed themselves. Dishes that will not tip over and easy-to-handle cups, glasses and silver should be given to cerebral palsy patients, and a great deal of patience should be exercised in helping them to use them.

Nutritional Care

Many of these children are underweight and require increased energy intake to meet the added expenditure of energy produced by the nature of the disease. However, energy requirements for some spastic patients may be lower than for normal children. Obesity has been observed in some of these children, especially when they reach the early teens. The calorie requirement for athetoid children, with their in-voluntary motion, is higher than for spastic patients who expend less energy. The diet should be adequate in all respects, with foods that are easy to handle and eat. Foods than can be held in the hand are easier to manage than those that must be eaten with fork or spoon. In feeding these patients, small amounts of food or fluids should be given at a time, and enough time should be allowed between bites or drinks for muscles to relax and the nourishment to be swallowed. It is helpful for the child's trunk, neck and head to be well supported when he or she is eating. It is also helpful for the nurse or person feeding the child to support the jaw and close the mouth between bites so that the child may chew as well as possible. Sensory stimulation for oral control is also helpful.

Each patient will have specific problems of eating, and the success in resolving them will be determined by the child's ability and mental capacity as well as the support that the family, school personnel and other caretakers receive in carrying through with recommendations.

Problems and Suggested Topics for Discussion

1. Observe the eating habits of the children in your hospital. What considerations should be observed in feeding the sick child?
2. Why is diarrhea so prevalent in the less-developed countries? What is being done to improve the situation?
3. If possible, observe an infant who is suffering from pyloric stenosis. Follow the eating program and evaluate food intake for a day or two. Compare the diet with the accepted nutritional standard allowances for the same age. Observe if any vomiting occurs and estimate the food lost.
4. Interview a child with cystic fibrosis and talk with the family. Evaluate the child's typical intake. How many kcal./kg. are being received? Evaluate growth. Are there enzyme supplements? What is the status of lung disease?
5. Plan a diet with a child who has diabetes. Determine what the child needs to know about food and meal planning. Involve the child in developing an eating plan on the basis of family meals.
6. Take a dietary history from an obese adolescent. Be sure to ask about physical activity. Why is he or she overweight? What emotional or social factors are involved? Talk with the teenager about ways to increase activity and reduce food intake.
7. Plan a diet for a child who is 12 years old and 10 lb. underweight.
8. Describe the nutritional problems of an infant with severe congenital heart disease. Design an appropriate diet and counsel the mother about this.
9. In what periods of life does iron deficiency anemia usually occur? What can be done to prevent its occurrence?
10. Talk with a mother whose child has an elevated blood lead level in order to learn about the child's environment. What are the potential sources of lead? Are there any dietary changes that you would recommend?
11. How can the nurse help a cerebral palsy patient with self-feeding?

Cited References

1. Adeniyi-Jones, S.K., et al.: Growth, energy metabolism and T$_3$ levels in malnutrition in cystic fibrosis. Cystic Fibrosis Club Abstracts, Atlanta, 1979.
2. Bell, L., et al.: Nutrient intakes of adolescents with cystic fibrosis. J. Canad. Diet. Assoc., 42:62, 1981.
3. Bicknell, D.J.: Pica, A Childhood Symptom. London, Butterworth and Co., Ltd., 1975.
4. Boyle, I.R., et al.: Emotional adjustment of adolescents and young adults with cystic fibrosis. J. Pediatr., 88:318, 1976.
5. Bullen, B.A., et al.: Physical activity of obese and nonobese adolescent girls appraised by motion picture sampling. Am. J. Clin. Nutr., 14:211, 1964.
6. Chase, H.P., Cotton, E.K., and Elliott, R.B.: Intravenous linoleic acid supplementation in children with cystic fibrosis. Pediatrics, 64:207, 1979.
7. Chisholm, J.J.: Disturbances in the biosynthesis of heme in lead intoxication. J. Pediatr., 64:174, 1964.
8. Chisholm, J.J.: Lead poisoning. Sci. Am., 224:15, 1971.
9. Danford, D.E.: Pica and nutrition. Ann. Rev. Nutr., 2:303, 1982.
10. David, O.J., et al.: Lead and hyperactivity. Behavioral response to chelation: a pilot study. Am. J. Psychol., 133:1155, 1976.
11. de la Burdé, B., and Choate, M.S.: Early asymptomatic lead exposure and development at school age. J. Pediatr., 87:638, 1975.
12. DeMaeyer, E.M.: Protein-energy malnutrition. In Beaton, G.H., and Bengoa, J.M. (eds): Nutrition in Preventive Medicine. Geneva, World Health Organization, 1976, p. 40.
13. Dobell, A.R.C., et al.: Severe feeding difficulty in infants with increased pulmonary flow. J. Thorac. Cardiovasc. Surg., 72:303, 1976.
14. Ellis, C.E., and Hill, E.: Growth, intelligence and school performances in children with cystic fibrosis who have an episode of malnutrition in infancy. J. Pediatr., 87:565, 1975.
15. Ellison, R.C., Newburger, J.W., and Gross, D.M.: Pediatric aspects of essential hypertension. J. Am. Diet. Assoc., 80:21, 1982.
16. Fomon, S.J.: Infant Nutrition. 2nd ed. Philadelphia, W. B. Saunders Company, 1974, pp. 212, 269.
17. Gallagher, J.R.: Weight control in adolescence. J. Am. Diet. Assoc., 40:519, 1962.
18. Halsted, J.A., and Smith, J.C., Jr.: Plasma zinc in health and disease. Lancet, 1:322, 1970.
19. Hirschhorn, N.: The treatment of acute diarrhea in children. An historical and physiological perspective. Am. J. Clin. Nutr., 33:637, 1980.
20. Jackson, R.L., et al.: The Child with Diabetes. Columbia, Mo., University of Missouri, 1973, pp. 18–19.
21. Jacob, R.L., et al.: Zinc status and vitamin A transport in cystic fibrosis. Am. J. Clin. Nutr., 31:638, 1978.
22. Lum, B.O.: Preventing ketoacidosis in the child with juvenile-onset diabetes mellitus. J. Am. Diet. Assoc., 69:157, 1976.
23. Mahaffey, K.R.: Nutritional factors in lead poisoning. Nutr. Rev., 39:353, 1981.
24. Mahaffey, K.R., et al.: National estimates of blood lead levels: United States 1976–1980. Association with selected demographic and socioeconomic factors. N. Engl. J. Med., 307:573, 1982.
25. Markiewicz, A., Wajczuk, D., and Iljin, W.: Xylose absorption before and after surgical correction of atrial septal defect (ASD) and ventricular septal defect (VSD). Eur. J. Pediatr., 124:57, 1976.
26. Minuchin, S., Rosman, B.L., and Baker, L.: Psychosomatic Families. Anorexia Nervosa in Context. Cambridge, Mass., Harvard University Press, 1978.
27. Muller, D.P.R., Harries, J.T., and Lloyd, J.K.: The relative importance of the factors involved in the absorption of vitamin E in children. Gut, 15:966, 1974.

28. Nalin, D.R., et al.: Oral rehydration and maintenance of children with rotavirus and bacterial diarrheas. Bull. WHO, 57:453, 1979.
29. Pierce, N.F., and Hirschhorn, N.: Oral fluid—a simple weapon against dehydration in diarrhea: how it works and how to use it. WHO Chron., 31:87, 1977.
30. Rees, J.M.: Eating disorders. In Mahan, L.K., and Rees, J.M.: Nutrition in Adolescence. St. Louis, C.V. Mosby Company, 1984.
31. Review: Are peptic ulcers on the increase in children? Food and Nutrition News, 42(2), 1970.
32. Rickard, K., Brady, M.S., and Gresham, E.L.; Nutritional management of the chronically ill child. Congenital heart disease and myelomeningocele. Pediatr. Clin. North Am., 24:157, 1977.
33. Rook, G.D., et al.: Folic acid deficiency in infants and children with heart disease. Br. Heart J., 35:87, 1973.
34. Ruby, D.O., and Matheny, W.D.: Comments on growth of cerebral palsied children. J. Am. Diet. Assoc., 40:525, 1962.
35. Santosham, M., et al.: Oral rehydration therapy of infantile diarrhea. A controlled study of well-nourished children hospitalized in the United States and Panama. N. Engl. J. Med., 306:1070, 1982.
36. Shwachman, H.: Nutritional considerations in the treatment of children with cystic fibrosis. In Suskind, R.E. (ed.): Textbook of Pediatric Nutrition. New York, Raven Press, 1981.
37. Snyder, J.D.: From Pedialyte to popsicles: a look at oral rehydration therapy used in the United States and Canada. Am. J. Clin. Nutr., 35:157, 1982.
38. Solomons, N.W., et al.: Some biochemical indices of nutrition in treated cystic fibrosis patients. Am. J. Clin. Nutr., 34:462, 1981.
39. Sproul, A., and Huang, N.: Growth patterns in children with cystic fibrosis. J. Pediatr., 65:664, 1964.
40. Steir, M., Lopez, R., and Cooperman, J.M.: Riboflavin deficiency in infants and children with heart disease. Am. Heart J., 92:139, 1976.
41. Suskind, R.M.: Nutritional Support of the Child With Cystic Fibrosis. Abstract. Annual Meeting, American Dietetic Association, San Antonio, Texas, October, 1982.
42. Thomson, N.B., Jr., and Jewett, T.C.: Peptic ulcers in infancy and childhood. JAMA, 189:539, 1964.

Additional References

Accuado, P.J. (ed.): Failure to Thrive in Infancy and Early Childhood: A Multidisciplinary Team Approach. Baltimore, University Park Press, 1982.

Boyle, I.R., et al.: Emotional adjustment of adolescents and young adults with cystic fibrosis. J. Pediatr., 88:318, 1979.

Chase, H.P., Long, M.A., and Lavin, M.H.: Cystic fibrosis and malnutrition. J. Pediatr., 95:337, 1979.

Collip, P.J. (ed.): Childhood Obesity. Acton, Mass., Publishing Sciences Group, Inc., 1975.

Committee on Toxicology, Assembly of Life Sciences, National Research Council: Recommendations for the prevention of lead poisoning in children. Nutr. Rev., 34:321, 1976.

Davis, P.B., and di Sant'Agnese, P.: A review—cystic fibrosis at forty—quo vadis? Pediatr. Res., 14:83, 1980.

Effect of lactose on intestinal absorption of lead. Nutr. Rev., 40:116, 1982.

Fajans, S.S., et al.: The various faces of diabetes in the young. Arch. Intern. Med., 136:194, 1976.

Finberg, L.: The role of oral electrolyte-glucose solutions in hydration for children—international and domestic aspects. J. Pediatr., 96:51, 1980.

Green, V.A., Wise, G.W., and Callenbach, J.: Lead poisoning. Clin. Toxicol., 9:33, 1976.

Hammond, M.I., et al.: A nutritional study of cerebral palsied children. J. Am. Diet. Assoc., *49*:196, 1966.

Hirschhorn, N.: Oral rehydration therapy for diarrhea in children—a basic primer. Nutr. Rev., *40*:97, 1982.

Huse, D.M., et al.: Infants with congenital heart disease. Food intake, body weight and energy metabolism. Am. J. Dis. Child., *129*:65, 1975.

Lloyd-Still, J.D., Johnson, S., and Holman, R.T.: Essential fatty acid status in cystic fibrosis and the effects of safflower oil supplementation. Am. J. Clin. Nutr., *34*:1, 1981.

Mahaffey, K.R.: Relations between quantities of lead ingested and health effects of lead in humans. Pediatrics, *59*:448, 1977.

McCollum, A.T.: The Chronically Ill Child: A Guide for Parents and Professionals. New Haven, Yale University Press, 1981.

Pollack, M.M., et al.: Malnutrition in critically ill infants and children. JPEN, *6*:20, 1982.

Queen, P.M., et al.: Nutritional assessment of pediatric patients. Nutr. Support Services, *3*(5):23, 1983.

Rayner, P.H.W.: Diet for diabetic children: a change in emphasis. Arch. Dis. Child., *57*:487, 1982.

Shwachman, H.: Cystic fibrosis. In Kendig, E.L., and Chernick, V. (eds.): Disorders of the Respiratory Tract in Children. 4th ed. Philadelphia, W.B. Saunders Company, 1983.

Sperling, M.A.: Diabetes mellitus. In Behrman, R.E., and Vaughan, V.C., III (eds.): Nelson Textbook of Pediatrics. 12th ed. Philadelphia, W.B. Saunders Company, 1983.

Strangway, A., et al.: Diet and growth in congenital heart disease. Pediatrics, *57*:75, 1976.

Wilson, J.F., et al.: Milk-induced gastrointestinal bleeding in infants with hypochromic microcytic anemia. JAMA, *189*:568, 1964.

CHAPTER 39

Nutritional Care for Children with Metabolic Disorders

CRISTINE M. TRAHMS, M.S., R.D.

Metabolic disorders are inherited traits that cause disease when the normal metabolism of a compound is impaired because of the absence or reduced activity of a specific enzyme or cofactor. Most metabolic disorders are inherited as autosomal recessive conditions with each parent being a carrier for the gene in question. This chapter will focus on metabolic disorders that affect protein and carbohydrate metabolism and the attendant nutritional therapy. (For further reading, Ampola[4] provides a catalogue of the currently known metabolic disorders and the basics of therapy.)

It is important to remember that not all biochemical "disorders" are diseases; some may, in fact, be normal variations that are benign and do not require treatment. For example, a biochemical difference for which treatment is controversial is histidinemia.[38] Many questions related to diagnosis and treatment still need to be answered for many of the metabolic disorders.

Most inherited metabolic disorders are associated with severe clinical manifestations, often appearing soon after birth. Mental retardation and severe neurological involvement may be the result of delayed diagnosis and treatment. Prenatal diagnosis is available for many metabolic disorders, but unfortunately, it usually requires the identification of a family at risk, which can be done only after the birth of an affected child.

Goals of Nutritional Care

In many cases, nutritional treatment is available to modify the effect of the disorder by "working around" the missing or inactive enzyme. Nutritional treatments can be viewed in major categories based on the model in Figure 39–1.

The goals of nutritional therapy are to (1) maintain biochemical equilibrium for the specific pathway, (2) provide adequate nutrients to support normal growth and development and (3) provide support for social and emotional development.

An effective nutritional treatment program meets more than the obvious nutritional needs.

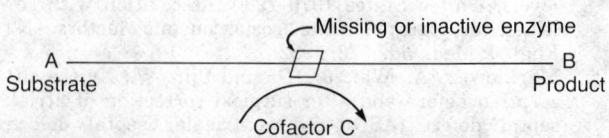

Figure 39–1. Nutritional treatment can be used to: (1) restrict the amount of substrate (A) available; (2) supplement the amount of product (B); (3) supplement the cofactor (C); or (4) combine two or all three of these approaches.

Families and children need information and skills that enable them to adhere to their regimen. These tools for compliance consist of factual information on the disease and its outcome, genetic counseling, and nutrition education regarding management of feeding behaviors and appropriate food choices. Although biochemical control is essential, nutritional counseling and support are needed to enable patients to achieve that goal.

Amino Acid Disorders and Their Management

Nutritional therapy for amino acid disorders most frequently consists of substrate restriction, which involves limiting a dietary essential amino acid to the minimum requirement while providing adequate energy and nutrients to promote normal growth and development. In many disorders, an inadequate intake of an essential amino acid can be as detrimental as an excess of that amino acid,[17] and dietary supplementation is the second most common type of nutritional therapy for amino acid disorders.

Requirements for individual amino acids are difficult to determine, as normal growth and development can be achieved over a wide range of intake. The data of Holt and Snyderman[20, 21] are often used as the basis for amino acid requirements (Table 39-1) and the prescription for nutritional therapy. This type of nutritional therapy requires careful and frequent monitoring of the child to ensure the adequacy of the prescription. Although nitrogen studies would be the most precise, weight gain in infants is a sensitive and easily monitored index of well-being and nutritional adequacy.

HYPERPHENYLALANINEMIAS

Of the amino acid disorders listed in Table 39-2, the hyperphenylalaninemias are the most frequent. They provide a reasonable model for detailed discussion because (1) they are relatively frequent and the majority of newborns are screened for these disorders; (2) they have a predictable course, that is, the greatest available documentation of "natural" and "intervention" history; (3) nutritional therapy is "successful"; (4) the effects of various therapies, positive or negative, have been observed over time; and (5) the effect on the next generation can be observed.

Of the hyperphenylalaninemias, "classic" phenylketonuria or PKU is the most common. In PKU, phenylalanine is not metabolized to tyrosine because of a deficiency or inactivity of phenylalanine hydroxylase, as shown in Figure 39-2. Nutritional treatment involves restriction of the substrate (phenylalanine) and supplementation of the product (tyrosine). Approximately 97 per cent of the cases have this deficiency; the remainder have a defect in associated pathways, either in activity of dihydropteridine reductase or in the synthesis of biopterin. These rare types have been labeled "malignant PKU" because the low-phenylalanine diet does not prevent neurological deterioration.[14, 15]

Diagnosis and Outcome

Currently, most states have newborn screening programs for PKU and other disorders. The Guthrie bacterial inhibition assay is the most frequently used screening test. It is recommended by the American Academy of Pediatrics that newborns with a positive screening test be tested again by both qualitative and quantitative methods.[31]

The criteria for the diagnosis of phenylketonuria are blood levels of phenylalanine consistently above 16 to 20 mg./dl. and tyrosine less than about 3 mg./dl. and the presence of phenylpyruvic acid and o-hydroxyphenylacetic acid in the urine.[22] Confirmation of the diagnosis of PKU requires quantitative elevations of phenylalanine compounds in both blood and urine. Frequently, a 72-hour phenylalanine challenge diet is administered at the end of the first year of life to reconfirm the diagnosis.[32]

Outcome, that is, IQ attainment or intellectual functioning, depends upon the age at diagnosis and start of nutritional therapy, biochemical control over time, and the ability of the family to comply with the regimen. The age at diagnosis and start of nutritional therapy depend on an effective screening program and an organized follow-up program, since infants with PKU do not manifest any clinical signs of abnormality in the immediate postnatal period. The advantage of rigorous nutritional therapy is proven by a comparison of children with PKU who were treated and those who were not. Individuals who have not received diet therapy are severely retarded (mean IQ about 40), whereas children treated since birth have IQ's in the normal range of intellectual functioning.[12, 13, 40]

Nutritional Care for Infants and Children

FORMULA. The restricted phenylalanine diet consists primarily of a formula with a reduced phenylalanine content (Fig. 39-3). The most commonly used formulas are Lofenalac for in-

Text continued on page 808

Table 39–1. APPROXIMATE DAILY REQUIREMENTS FOR SELECTED NUTRIENTS AND AMINO ACIDS IN INFANCY AND CHILDHOOD[a]

AMINO ACID	UNIT	0 to 2 mo.	2 to 5 mo.	6 to 12 mo.	1 to 2 yr.	2 to 3 yr.	3 to 4 yr.	4 to 6 yr.	6 to 8 yr.	8 to 10 yr.
Phenylalanine										
Infants	mg./kg.	47–90	47–90	25–47	—	—	—	—	—	—
Children	mg./day	—	—	—	200–500[b]	200–500[b]	200–500[b]	200–500[b]	200–500[b]	200–500[b]
Histidine	mg./kg.	16–34	16–34	16–34	—	—	—	—	—	—
Tyrosine[c]	mg./kg.	60–80	60–80	40–60	25–85	25–85	25–85	8–50	8–50	25
Leucine										
Infants	mg./kg.	76–150	76–150	76–150	—	—	—	—	—	—
Children	mg./day	—	—	—	1000	1000	1000	1000	1000	1000
Isoleucine										
Infants	mg./kg.	79–110	79–110	50–75	—	—	—	—	—	—
Children	mg./day	—	—	—	1000	1000	1000	1000	1000	1000
Valine										
Infants	mg./kg.	65–105	65–105	50–80	—	—	—	—	—	—
Children	mg./day	—	—	—	400–600	400–600	400–600	400–600	400–600	400–600
Methionine[d]										
Infants	mg./kg.	20–45	20–45	20–45	—	—	—	—	—	—
Children	mg./day	—	—	—	400–800	400–800	400–800	400–800	400–800	400–800
Cyst(e)ine[e]										
Infants	mg./kg.	15–50	15–50	15–50	—	—	—	—	—	—
Children	mg./day	—	—	—	400–800	400–800	400–800	400–800	400–800	400–800
Lysine										
Infants	mg./kg.	90–120	90–120	90–120	—	—	—	—	—	—
Children	mg./day	—	—	—	1200–1600	1200–1600	1200–1600	1200–1600	1200–1600	1200–1600

	Units									
Threonine										
Infants	mg./kg.	45–87	45–87	45–87	—	—	—	—	—	—
Children	mg./day	—	—	—	800–1000	800–1000	800–1000	800–1000	800–1000	800–1000
Tryptophan										
Infants	mg./kg.	13–22	13–22	13–22	—	—	—	—	—	—
Children	mg./day	—	—	—	60–120	60–120	60–120	60–120	60–120	60–120
Energy[f]										
Infants	kcal./kg.	120	110	100	—	—	—	—	—	—
Children	kcal./day	—	—	—	1100	1250	1400	1600	2000	2200
Water										
Infants	ml./kg.	100	110	100	—	—	—	—	—	—
Children	ml./day	—	—	—	1100	1250	1400	1600	2000	2200
Carbohydrate[g]	gm.					kcal. × 0.50	→	→	→	→
Protein										
Infants	gm./kg.	1.8–2.2	1.8–2.0	1.8	—	—	—	—	—	—
Children	gm./day	—	—	—	25	25	30	30	35	40
Fat[h]	gm.					kcal. × 0.35	→	→	→	→

[a] Compiled from amino acid data of Holt and Snyderman. There is limited information on amino acid requirements of infants and children at different ages; the figures given here are in excess of minimum requirements. Consequently, this table should be used only as a guide and should not be regarded as an authoritative statement to which individual patients must conform.

[b] More phenylalanine (> 800 mg) is required in the absence of tyrosine.

[c] Total phenylalanine plus tyrosine should be considered in the prescription since most phenylalanine is converted to tyrosine.

[d] More methionine is required in the absence of cyst(e)ine.

[e] More cyst(e)ine is required in the presence of a blocked trans-sulfuration outflow pathway for methionine metabolism.

[f] The energy requirement is increased when a protein is provided as a mixture of the corresponding free L-amino acids.

[g] Minimum fraction is 50% of total calories; optimum value given.

[h] Minimum fraction is 4% of total calories, optimum value given.

Adapted from Committee on Nutrition, American Academy of Pediatrics: Special diets for infants with inborn errors of metabolism. Pediatrics, *57*:783, 1976.

Table 39–2. SOME AMINO ACID DISORDERS THAT RESPOND TO DIETARY TREATMENT

DISORDER	ENZYME DEFECT	INCIDENCE	CLINICAL/ BIOCHEMICAL FEATURES	DIETARY TREATMENT
Hyperphenylalaninemias				
"Classic" phenylketonuria	Phenylalanine hydroxylase	1:15,000	Blood Phe >20 mg./dl. ↑ Phenylketones in urine Progressive severe MR, prevented by early treatment	↓ Phe, ↑ tyrosine diet to maintain serum Phe at 2–10 mg./dl.
"Atypical" phenylketonuria	Phenylalanine hydroxylase	?1:13,000	Blood Phe >12 mg./dl. ↑ Phe in urine MR less severe than in classic PKU	↓ Phe diet (less restrictive than for classic disease)
Hyperphenylalaninemia, benign	Phenylalanine hydroxylase	?1:19,000	Blood Phe <10 mg./dl. ?No effect	?Not necessary
Neonatal hyperphenylalaninemia	Phenylalanine hydroxylase Not inherited		Apparently benign	Not necessary
Offspring of maternal phenylketonuria	None	—	Fetal brain damage	None
Dihydropteridine reductase deficiency	Dihydropteridine reductase	Rare	Blood Phe <20 mg./dl. Irritability, dev. delay, seizures	None 5-hydroxytryptophan, L-3,4-dihydroxyphenylalanine carbidopa may help
Tyrosinemias				
Hereditary tyrosinemia	?	Rare	Vomiting, acidosis, diarrhea, FTT, hepatomegaly, rickets, often fatal ↑ Blood/urine tyrosine, methionine,↑ urine parahydroxy derivatives of tyrosine	? ↓ Tyrosine, ↓ Phe diet, vitamin D for rickets
Hypertyrosinemia	Cytosol tyrosine aminotransferase	Rare	Keratosis, MR, corneal dystrophy ↑ Blood/urine tyrosine ↑ Urine parahydroxy derivatives of tyrosine	↓ Tyrosine, ↓ Phe diet
Transient neonatal tyrosinemia	?Para-hydroxyphenyl-pyruvic acid oxidase (appears slowly after birth) Not inherited	?	Initial lethargy ?Long-term effects ↑ Blood/urine tyrosine	Vitamin C 100 mg./day ?↓ Protein intake until tyrosine cleared
Maple Syrup Urine Diseases				
Classic MSUD	Keto acid decarboxylase <5% activity	1:225,000	Early onset, convulsions, acidosis, severe MR, often death Plasma leucine, isoleucine, valine levels 10× normal	Low leucine, isoleucine, valine diet
Intermediate MSUD	Keto acid decarboxylase 25% activity	?1:600,000	Later onset, moderate MR Plasma leucine, isoleucine and valine levels 5–15× normal	As above
Intermittent MSUD	Keto acid decarboxylase 10–20% activity between episodes	Rare	Intermittent symptoms, can cause death, some MR Plasma leucine, isoleucine and valine levels 10× normal during episodes	As above
Thiamin-responsive MSUD		Rare	Mild MR Plasma leucine, isoleucine and valine levels 3× normal	Thiamin 100 mg./day Diet as above
Other Amino Acid Disorders				
Homocystinuria	Cystathionine synthase	1:300,000	Arterial and venous thromboses, bony abnormalities, dislocated lens, fair hair and skin, mild to moderate MR ↑ Methionine, ↑ homocystine	Trial of 500 mg. of vitamin B$_6$ per day for 1 mo. (if normal folate levels) ?Low-protein, low-methionine diet with added L-cystine

Table 39–2.   SOME AMINO ACID DISORDERS THAT RESPOND TO DIETARY TREATMENT (*Continued*)

DISORDER	ENZYME DEFECT	INCIDENCE	CLINICAL/ BIOCHEMICAL FEATURES	DIETARY TREATMENT
			dislocated lens, fair hair and skin, mild to moderate MR ↑ Methionine, ↑ homocystine	Trial of 500 mg. of vitamin B_6 per day for 1 mo. (if normal folate levels) ?Low-protein, low-methionine diet with added L-cystine
Hyperlysinuria	Lysine ketoglutarate reductase, saccharopine oxidoreductase, saccharopine dehydrogenase	Rare	Probably benign ↑ Blood/urine lysine	Does not require dietary treatment
Histidinemia	Histidinase	1:18,000	Benign ↑ Blood/urine histidine	Does not require dietary treatment
Urea Cycle Disorders				
Carbamyl phosphate synthetase deficiency	Carbamyl phosphate synthetase	Rare	Vomiting, seizures, coma → death Survivors usually have MR ↑ Plasma ammonia, glutamine	Long-term treatment: Low-protein diet as tolerated and sodium benzoate Acute treatment: hemodialysis or peritoneal dialysis with calories and fluids
Ornithine transcarbamylase deficiency	Ornithine transcarbamylase (X-linked)	Rare	Vomiting, seizures coma → death as newborn usual in males Plasma ammonia, glutamine, glutamic acid, alanine	?Low-protein diet and sodium benzoate
Citrullinemia	Argininosuccinic acid synthetase	Rare	Neonatal: vomiting, seizures, coma → death Infantile: vomiting, seizures, progressive dev. delay ↑ Plasma citrulline, ammonia, alanine	Low-protein diet, arginine supplements Sodium benzoate
Argininosuccinic aciduria	Argininosuccinic acid lyase	Rare	Neonatal: hypotonia, seizures Subacute: vomiting, FTT, progressive dev. delay ↑ Plasma argininosuccinic acid, citrulline, ammonia	Neonatal: low-protein diet, though often untreatable Subacute: low-protein diet, arginine supplement, dialysis for crisis Sodium benzoate
Argininemia	Arginase	Rare	Periodic vomiting, seizures, coma Progressive spastic diplegia and dev. delay ↑ Arginine, ↑ ammonia with protein intake	?Low-protein diet
Organic Acidemias				
Methylmalonic acidemia	Methylmalonyl CoA mutase or coenzyme B_{12}	Rare	Metabolic acidosis Vomiting, seizures, coma, often death Progressive dev. delay in survivors ↑ Organic acids, ammonia	Long-term: ↑ kcal., ↓ protein diet, B_{12} supplements Acute: IV fluid, bicarbonate
Propionic acidemia	Propionyl CoA carboxylase	Rare	Metabolic acidosis, ↑ ammonia,↑ propionic acid in blood, ↑ methylcitric acid in urine	Long-term: ↑ kcal., ↓ protein diet Acute: IV fluid, bicarbonate
Carbohydrate Disorders				
Galactosemia	Galactose-1-phosphate uridyl transferase	1:65,000	Vomiting, hepatomegaly, hypoglycemia, FTT, cataracts, MR, often early sepsis ↑ Urine/blood galactose	Galactose- and lactose-free diet
Galactokinase deficiency	Galactokinase	1:40,000	Cataracts ↑ Blood/urine galactose after lactose feeding	As above

Table continued on the following page

Table 39–2. SOME AMINO ACID DISORDERS THAT RESPOND TO DIETARY TREATMENT *(Continued)*

DISORDER	ENZYME DEFECT	INCIDENCE	CLINICAL/ BIOCHEMICAL FEATURES	DIETARY TREATMENT
Hereditary fructose intolerance	Fructose-1-phosphate aldolase	Rare	Vomiting, hepatomegaly, hypoglycemia, FTT, renal tubular defects after fructose introduction ↑ Blood/urine fructose after fructose feeds	Fructose-, sucrose- and sorbitol-free diet
Fructose 1,6-diphosphate deficiency	Fructose 1,6-diphosphate	Rare	Hypoglycemia, hepatomegaly, hypotonia, metabolic acidosis → fructose introduction No ↑ fructose in blood or urine	As above
Other Disorders				
Gyrate atrophy of the choroid and retina	Ornithine keto acid transferase	Rare	Progressive gyrate atrophy of choroid and retina with cataracts May also have FTT, hepatic cirrhosis, seizures, MR ↑ Blood/urine ornithine ↓ Blood lysine	?Low-protein diet (low ornithine) with lysine supplements
Cystinuria	Defective proximal renal tubular transport of cystine and dibasic amino acids	1:13,000	Urinary tract calculi ↑ Cystine, ornithine, lysine, and arginine in urine	↑ Fluid intake Bicarbonate to alkalinize urine

MR, mental retardation; FTT, failure to thrive; Phe, phenylalanine; dev., developmental.

fants and Phenyl-free for children and adolescents. *Lofenalac* is a protein hydrolysate with about 95 per cent of the phenylalanine removed, and *Phenyl-free* is completely free of phenylalanine. The formulas described in Table 39–3 provide a major portion of the daily protein and energy needs for the affected infants and children.

The formula is supplemented with evaporated milk or regular infant formula during infancy and early childhood to provide high biological value protein, non-essential amino acids, and phenylalanine to meet the requirements of the growing child. The Lofenalac and milk mixture should provide 90 per cent of the protein and 80 per cent of the energy needed by infants and toddlers.[2] A method for calculating Lofenalac intake is shown in Table 39–4. It must be stressed that formula calculations should provide adequate but not excessive energy intake for in-

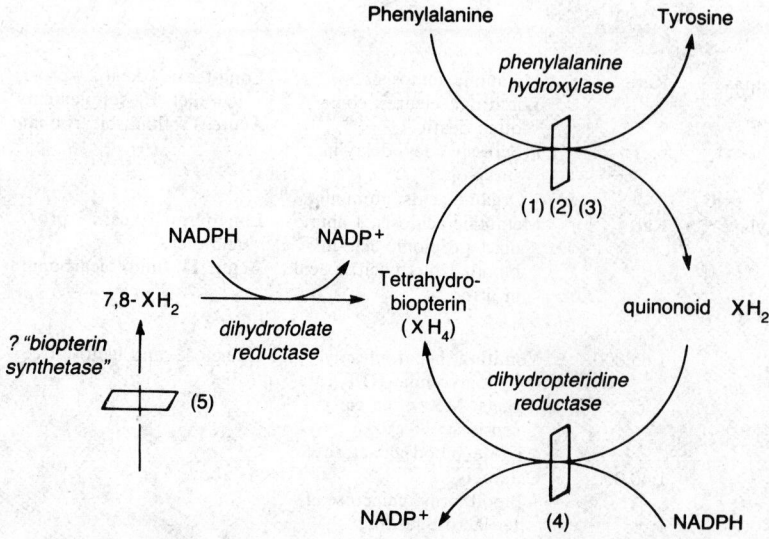

Figure 39–2. Hyperphenylalaninemias: (1) "classic" phenylketonuria, (2) "atypical" phenylketonuria, (3) benign hyperphenylalaninemia, (4) dihydropteridine reductase deficiency, and (5) "biopterin synthetase" deficiency.

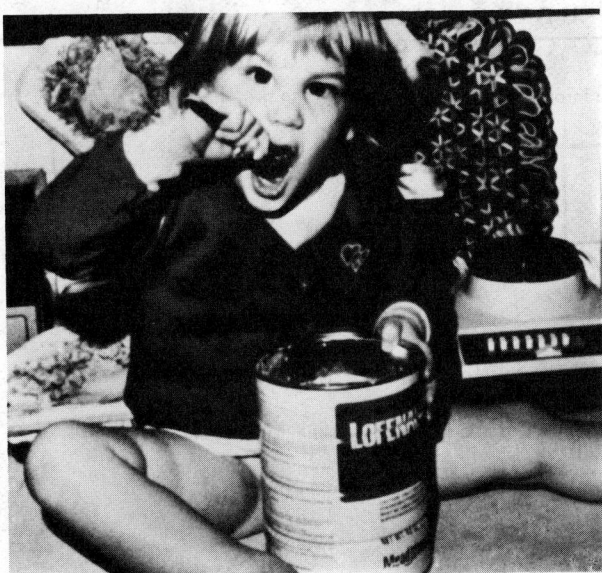

Figure. 39–3. Obviously this youngster enjoys her Lofenalac. Families must respond positively to the low-phenylalanine formula to encourage to child's compliance with the restricted diet.

Table 39–3. PRODUCTS FOR THE MANAGEMENT OF DIETS FOR INBORN ERRORS OF METABOLISM

DISORDER	PRODUCT	FORMULATED FOR: Infant	Child
PKU	Lofenalac*	X	
	Phenyl-free*		X
	PKU 1[†]	X	
	PKU 2[†]		X
Tyrosinemia	3200AB*	X	X
	TYR 1[†]	X	
	TYR 2[†]		X
MSUD and branched chain amino acid disorders	MSUD Diet Powder*	X	X
	MSUD 1[†]	X	
	MSUD 2[†]		X
Homocystinuria	3200K*	X	X
	HOM 1[†]	X	
	HOM 2[†]		X
Organic acid disorders	OS 1[†]	X	
	OS 2[†]		X
	80056*	X	X

* Formulas produced by Mead Johnson & Co., Evansville, Ind., 47221, are primarily a mix of amino acids and hydrolyzed protein; corn syrup solids and modified tapioca starch to provide carbohydrate; and corn oil to provide fat plus vitamin and mineral supplements. 80056 is similar in composition but is protein-free. There is some variation in ingredients and supplementation levels among products, so each intake must be monitored carefully to meet individual needs according to age and metabolic needs.

† Formulas produced by Milupa Corp., Darien, Conn., 06820, are amino acid, vitamin and mineral mixes which contain no fat and small amounts of carbohydrate from sucrose. Generally, they are supplemented with vegetable oil and a carbohydrate source such as corn syrup to meet individual energy needs. It is necessary to carefully monitor the osmolarity of these formula mixtures for the young infant.

fants and provide appropriate fluid to maintain hydration.

BLOOD PHENYLALANINE CONTROL. The blood phenylalanine level must be checked frequently to maintain it within the range of 2 to 10 mg./dl. Phenylalanine-containing foods are offered as tolerated as long as the blood phenylalanine level remains in the range of good control. The child's rate of growth and mental development must be carefully monitored. Effective management requires a cohesive team of child, parents, nutritionist, pediatrician, psychologist, nurse and social worker working together to achieve and maintain biochemial control and provide an atmosphere for normal mental and emotional development.

Elevations in blood phenylalanine level are generally caused by (1) intake of too much phenylalanine (that in excess of the amount required for growth accumulates in the blood); (2) intake of too little energy (a deficient calorie intake promotes tissue catabolism to meet energy needs and thus an accumulation of phenylalanine in the blood); and (3) illness (during infection, tissue catabolism causes release of amino acids into the blood). During illness some would recommend that phenylalanine intake be limited to half the usual amount to avoid prolonged high blood levels. In general, the anorexia of illness limits phenylalanine intake, and the essential concept is to maintain the intake of formula as much as possible to intervene in tissue catabolism by providing at least some, if not all, of the prescribed protein and energy. Although oc-

casionally it may be necessary to offer only clear liquids during an illness, the low-phenylalanine formula should be reintroduced as soon as it is feasible.

LOW-PHENYLALANINE FOODS. Foods of moderate or low phenylalanine content are used as a supplement to the formula mixture. These foods are offered at the same ages as they are usually offered to children who do not have PKU to support developmental readiness and also to meet energy needs. Puréed foods from a spoon might be introduced at five to six months, finger foods at seven to eight months, and the cup at eight to nine months of age, using the same timing and progression of texture as recommended in Tables 12–9 and 12–10 for children on free-choice food patterns. Table 39–5 lists phenylalanine values for selected foods. More complete lists of phenylalanine content of foods can be obtained from the sources listed at the end of this chapter.

Low-protein pastas, breads and baked goods made from wheat starch add variety to the food pattern and allow children to eat some foods "to appetite." Sources for low-protein products are

Table 39–4. GUIDELINES FOR PKU DIET CALCULATIONS

Case Study

M.S. is a six-month-old infant with phenylketonuria. The information provided in Tables 39–1 and 39–5, can be utilized in planning a diet for this child.

BASELINE DATA

Age	6 months
Sex	Male
Weight (kg.)	7.7
Weight percentile	50th
Height (cm.)	67.8
Height percentile	50th
Head circumference (cm.)	43.3
General health	Good
Activity	Very active

STEP 1. Calculate the child's requirement for phenylalanine, protein and kilocalories using Table 39–1.

    A. Phenylalanine

        7.7 kg. body weight × 60* mg. phenylalanine/kg./day = 462 mg. phenylalanine/day

    B. Protein

        7.7 kg. body weight × 3.3 gm. protein/kg./day = 25.4 gm. protein/day

    C. Kilocalories

        7.7 kg. body weight × 115 kcal./kg./day = 885 kcal./day

STEP 2. Determine the amount of Lofenalac required per day. This information is determined from the infant's or child's protein requirement.

    25.4 gm. protein/day × 90% of protein from Lofenalac = 22.9 gm. protein ÷ 1.5 gm. protein/ms.† Lofenalac = 15 ms., which is equal to 150 gm. of Lofenalac per day.

STEP 3. Determine the amount of evaporated milk to be included in the diet. 2 to 2½ oz. of evaporated milk is recommended for an infant 4 to 6 months of age.

STEP 4. Determine the amount of water to mix with the Lofenalac. The fluid consistency of the formula varies according to the infant's age and fluid requirements. For an infant consuming a formula of 20 kcal./oz., 1 level 8-oz. measuring cup of Lofenalac is mixed with 1 qt. of water.

    To prepare formula for the infant described in the case study, mix 15 ms. (150 gm.) of Lofenalac and 2½ oz. (75 ml.) of evaporated milk with 4 oz. of water to prevent lumps from forming. Then add water to make a total of 32 oz. of formula. This provides 4 bottles of 8 oz. each.

STEP 5. Determine the amounts of phenylalanine, protein and kilocalories in the Lofenalac and evaporated milk.

	Phenylalanine (mg.)	Protein (gm.)	Kcal.
Lofenalac, 15 ms.	120	22.5	681
Evaporated milk, 2½ oz.	265	5.5	97
Total	385	28.0	778

STEP 6. Determine the amount of phenylalanine, protein and kilocalories‡ to be obtained from foods other than the formula.

    Total phenylalanine = 462 mg./day
    Phenylalanine in formula = 385 mg./day
    Phenylalanine from other foods = 77 mg./day

Total protein	25.4 gm./day
Protein in formula	28.0 gm./day
Protein from other foods	1.0–2.0 gm./day
Total kcalories	885 kcal./day
Kcalories in formula	778 kcal./day
Kcalories from other foods	107 kcal./day

STEP 7. Determine the amount of foods other than formula to be included in the dietary plan. Use exchange lists in Table 39–5.

	Phenylalanine (mg.)	Protein (gm.)	Kcal.
Baby rice cereal	18	0.4	18
Applesauce, 6 Tbsp.	8	0.2	72
Green beans, strained, 2 Tbsp.	18	0.4	8
Banana, mashed, 50 gm.	22	0.6	44
Carrots, strained, 3 Tbsp.	9	0.3	12
Total	75	1.9	154

Table 39–4.   GUIDELINES FOR PKU DIET CALCULATIONS (*Continued*)

Step 8.   Determine the actual amounts of phenylalanine, protein and kcal. per kg. of body weight by dividing the body weight (in kg.) into the total available nutrients:

Phenylalanine (mg.)
    460 mg. phenylalanine ÷ 7.7 kg. body weight = 60 mg. phenylalanine/kg./day
Protein
    29.9 gm. protein ÷ 7.7 kg. body weight = 3.9 gm. protein/kg./day
Kilocalories
    932 kcal. ÷ 7.7 kg. body weight = 121 kcal./kg./day

* 60 mg. phenylalanine/kg./day is chosen as a moderate phenylalanine intake. The prescription for phenylalanine must be adapted to individual needs as judged by growth and blood levels.
† ms. = measure, 1 ms. of Lofenalac = 1 packed tablespoon.
‡ Total energy intake must be adjusted to meet individual needs and an excess must be avoided.

given at the end of the chapter. In addition, cookbooks providing recipes low in phenylalanine content are listed. In many cases, parents have created recipes or adapted family favorites to meet the needs of their children. These recipes enable the children to have a variety of textures and food choices and to participate in family meals. Families are also able to meet the energy and phenylalanine needs of their children without resorting to excessive intakes of sugars and concentrated sweets.

Phenyl-free is generally introduced between three and six years of age. Generally, the criteria for introduction are that the child accept the food pattern and formula well and that the child reliably consume a wide variety of foods from the low-phenylalanine food lists. Phenyl-free provides a greater flexibility in food choices and menu planning for children and families, which is particularly important as the child enters school or other group settings. Most children and families who are not compliant on a food pattern including Lofenalac are unlikely to be compliant with a different formula. The use of Phenyl-free generally allows a slight liberalization in low-protein food choices. The comparison of a food pattern using Phenyl-free with a regular food pattern of a child is shown in Table 39–6.

The necessity of continuing the restricted phenylalanine diet beyond age four to six years is a consideration in the management of children with phenylketonuria. Progressively decreasing IQ's, learning difficulties, poor attention span and behavioral difficulties have been reported in some of the children who have discontinued the dietary regimen.[10,23,34] Even though others have reported no difficulties,[24] the cur-

Table 39–5.   FOOD EXCHANGE LISTS FOR PHENYLALANINE- OR TYROSINE-RESTRICTED DIET

VEGETABLES

Contain per serving an average of 15 mg. phenylalanine, 10 mg. tyrosine, 0.5 gm. protein and 10 kcal. Protein averages 2.8% phenylalanine and 2% tyrosine.

	PHENYLALANINE (mg.)	TYROSINE (mg.)	PROTEIN (gm.)	ENERGY (kcal.)
Asparagus, raw, 1½ spears (25 gm.)	14	11	0.5	6
Asparagus, canned, green, 1½ spears (28 gm.)	17	12	0.6	5
Beans, snap, green, 4 T. (31 gm.)	11	15	0.4	8
Beets, solids, ¼ c. (42 gm.)	7	14	0.4	15
Cabbage, raw, ⅓ c. (33 gm.)	16	10	0.5	8
Cabbage, cooked, 5 T. (50 gm.)	12	11	0.5	10
Carrots, raw, 1 small (50 gm.)	15	13	0.5	21
Carrots, cooked, ⅔ c. (100 gm.)	18	8	0.5	30
Cauliflower, cooked, 3 T. (25 gm.)	18	8	0.6	5
Cucumber, raw, ½ med. (50 gm.)	12	–	0.5	8
Eggplant, cooked, 2 T. (25 gm.)	11	10	0.2	5
Lettuce, (25 gm.)	17	9	0.3	5
Okra, cooked, 2 pods	18	7	0.5	7
Tomato, raw, ½ small (50 gm.)	16	7	0.6	11
Tomato, canned, ¼ c. (50 gm.)	14	6	0.5	10
Tomato juice, canned, ¼ c. (50 gm.)	13	6	0.4	10
Turnip root, white raw, 6 T. (50 gm.)	9	7	0.4	15
Turnip root, cooked, ⅔ c. (100 gm.)	14	12	0.8	23

Table continued on the following page

Table 39–5. FOOD EXCHANGE LISTS FOR PHENYLALANINE- OR TYROSINE-RESTRICTED DIET
(*Continued*)

GERBER'S STRAINED AND JUNIOR VEGETABLES

	PHENYLALANINE (mg.)	TYROSINE (mg.)	PROTEIN (gm.)	ENERGY (kcal.)
Amounts in 1 T.				
Beets	2	7	0.2	5
Carrots	3	2	0.1	4
Green beans	9	4	0.2	4
Sweet potatoes	10	5	0.2	10

FRUITS

Contain per serving an average of 10 mg. phenylalanine, 5 mg. tyrosine, 0.4 gm. protein and 55 kcal. Protein averages 2.2% phenylalanine and 1.4% tyrosine.

	PHENYLALANINE (mg.)	TYROSINE (mg.)	PROTEIN (gm.)	ENERGY (kcal.)
Apple, raw, 1 small (100 gm.)	10	6	0.4	58
Applesauce, ⅔ c. (200 gm.)	10	6	0.4	182
Apple juice, 1½ c.	10	6	0.4	174
Apricots, raw, 1½ med. (50 gm.)	6	5	0.4	25
Apricots, canned, 1½ halves (50 gm.)	10	6	0.3	43
Avocado, 2 T. (20 gm.)	9	6	0.3	33
Banana, ¼ small (25 gm.)	11	7	0.3	22
Dates, dried, 1 date (10 gm.)	7	2	0.3	27
Orange, ⅓ small (33 gm.)	10	5	0.3	16
Orange juice, frozen, 3 T. (1½ oz.)	10	5	0.3	22
Peaches, raw, ½ med. (50 gm.)	9	10	0.4	19
Peaches, canned, 2 med. halves (100 gm.)	9	10	0.4	78
Strawberries, raw, 3 large (25 gm.)	6	7	0.2	9

GERBER'S STRAINED AND JUNIOR FRUITS

	PHENYLALANINE (mg.)	TYROSINE (mg.)	PROTEIN (gm.)	ENERGY (kcal.)
Apple juice (3 oz.)	<3	2	0.1	49
Orange juice (3 oz.)	<3	8	0.5	50
Per Tablespoon				
Applesauce	1.4	0.4	0.03	12
Applesauce & apricots	1.5	0.6	0.04	12
Apricots with tapioca	1.2	1.1	0.06	11
Bananas with tapioca	2.0	1.6	0.07	13
Peaches	3.1	2.1	0.09	12
Pears	1.5	0.9	0.06	10

BREAD AND CEREAL

Contain per serving an average of 18 mg. phenylalanine, 12 mg. tyrosine, 0.4 gm. protein and 15 kcal. Protein averages 4.6% phenylalanine and 3.2% tyrosine.

	PHENYLALANINE (mg.)	TYROSINE (mg.)	PROTEIN (gm.)	ENERGY (kcal.)
Dry Cereals				
Cheerios, 2 T.	22	14	0.4	12
Cornflakes, 3 T.	17	15	0.4	18
Rice Flakes, 3 T.	19	13	0.4	23
Rice Krispies, 4 T.	19	14	0.4	27
Rice, Puffed, 8 T.	19	14	0.4	26
Kix, 4T.	20	14	0.4	28
Hot Cereals				
Cream of Wheat, cooked, 1 T.	13	9	0.3	8
Farina, cooked, 2 T.	22	15	0.5	18
Grits, cooked, 2 T.	18	14	0.4	15
Malt-O-Meal, cooked, 1 T.	13	9	0.3	8

Table 39–5.   FOOD EXCHANGE LISTS FOR PHENYLALANINE- OR TYROSINE-RESTRICTED DIET
(Continued)

Miscellaneous				
Corn, canned, 1 T.	14	10	0.3	9
Macaroni, cooked, tender, 1 T.	16	10	0.3	9
Potatoes, boiled, ¼ med. (25 gm.)	21	13	0.5	16
Rice, brown, cooked, 1 T.	12	9	0.2	11
Rice, white, parboiled, cooked, 2 T.	20	14	0.4	20
Yams, cooked, 1 T.	16	6	0.4	17
Special Products				
Aproten*				
Anellini, uncooked, ¾ c. (100 gm.)	12	12	0.5	340
Rigatini, uncooked, 1½ c. (100 gm.)	12	12	0.5	340
Paygel Low Protein Bread, 1 slice (32 gm.)	7	5	0.3	83
Rusks, 1 slice (11.5 gm.)	4	3	0.1	48
Tagliatelle, uncooked, 1¼ c. (100 gm.)	12	12	0.5	340

GERBER'S BABY CEREALS (dry)	PHENYLALANINE *(mg.)*	TYROSINE *(mg.)*	PROTEIN *(gm.)*	ENERGY *(kcal.)*
Per Tablespoon				
Oatmeal cereal	18	18	0.4	9
Rice cereal	9	6	0.2	9

FATS

Contain per serving an average of 4 mg. phenylalanine, 6 mg. tyrosine, 0.1 gm. protein and 90 kcal. Protein averages 4.9% phenylalanine and 5.1% tyrosine.

	PHENYLALANINE *(mg.)*	TYROSINE *(mg.)*	PROTEIN *(gm.)*	ENERGY *(kcal.)*
Butter, 2 tsp.	4	5	0.1	72
Cream, heavy (40% fat), 1 tsp. (5 gm.)	5	5	0.1	17
Italian dressing, 3 T. (14 gm.)	4	4	0.1	231
Margarine, 1 T. (14 gm.)	5	5	0.1	100
Mayonnaise, 1 T. (14 gm.)	5	5	0.1	101
Tartar sauce, ½ T. (10 gm.)	4	4	0.1	47
Thousand Island dressing, 1 T. (14 gm.)	4	4	0.1	57

FREE FOODS

These foods contain little or no protein and may be used as desired in the diet as long as appetite is not depressed by their use and the child is not overweight.

	ENERGY *(kcal.)*
Candies:	
Butterscotch, 1 piece	20
Cream mints, 1 piece	7
Fondant, patties or mint, 1 piece	40
Gum drops, 1 large	35
Hard candy, 2 pieces	39
Jelly beans, 10	110
Lollipops, 1 med. (2¼″ diameter)	108
Corn syrup, 1 T.	58
Danish dessert, ½ c.	123
Fruit ices, ½ c.	69
Kool-Aid, ½ c.	53
Maple syrup, 1 T.	50
Molasses, 1 T.	46
Popsicle, 1 twin bar	95
Prono,* ⅓ c.	55
Start, liquid, ½ c.	60
Sugar, granulated, 1 T.	43
Tang, liquid, ½ c.	59

Adapted from Acosta, P., and Elsas, L.: Dietary Management of Inherited Metabolic Disease: Phenylketonuria, Galactosemia, Tyrosinemia, Maple Syrup Urine Disease. Atlanta, Ga., ACELMU Publishers, 1976.

* Available from Henkel Corporation, Special Dietary Foods, 4620 W. 77th Street, Minneapolis, Minnesota, 55435.

Table 39–6. COMPARISON OF MENUS FOR CHILDREN
WITH AND THOSE WITHOUT PKU

	PKU Menu	Phe (mg)*	Regular Menu	Phe (mg)*
Breakfast	Phenyl-free	0	Milk	450
	Rice Krispies		Rice Krispies	
	Orange juice		Orange juice	
Lunch	Jelly sandwich with	18	Jelly sandwich with	260
	low-protein bread		white bread	
	Banana		Banana	
	Carrot and celery		Carrot and celery	
	sticks		sticks	
	Low-protein choco-	4	Chocolate chip	60
	late chip cookies		cookies	
	Juice		Juice	
Snack	Phenyl-free	0	Milk	450
	Orange		Orange	
	Potato chips		Potato chips	
	(small bag)			
Dinner	Phenyl-free	0	Milk	450
	Salad		Salad	
	Low protein spa-	8	Spaghetti with	240
	ghetti with toma-		meatballs	600
	to sauce			
	Baskin-Robbins			
	fruit ice	10	Ice cream	120
Estimated intake		400		2900

* Phenylalanine values provided only for those foods that differ between the two patterns.

rent recommendation from most treatment centers is that the restricted phenylalanine diet be continued into the foreseeable future.[33]

EDUCATION ON DIET MANAGEMENT. The energy needs and amino acid requirements of these children do not differ appreciably from children in general.[1, 3] Normal growth can be expected.[19] However, parents may tend to offer excessive energy as sweets because they feel that the child is being deprived of food experiences. It is imperative that health care providers stress to parents that children with PKU are *well* children who must make careful food choices for themselves as opposed to chronically ill children who require food indulgences. Appropriate clinical interaction with the family will provide them with the information and skills to differentiate between food behaviors normal to the age and developmental level of the child and those related specifically to PKU. To avoid power struggles and conflicts over food, it is advisable to involve the child in choosing appropriate foods at an early age. Two- and three-year-old children can master the concept of appropriate choices when foods are categorized as *YES* foods and *NO* foods. The concept of an appropriate quantity of a food can be introduced to a three- or four-year-old as "how many" by counting crackers or raisins, and then as "how much" by weighing or measuring foods such as cereal or fruit.[18] The child then moves to more complex tasks such as formula and food preparation.

Planning meals such as breakfast or a packed lunch is the next logical step in self-management. Responsibility for planning a full day's menus by calculating the phenylalanine in portions of food and compiling the daily phenylalanine total is the ultimate goal.

PSYCHOSOCIAL DEVELOPMENT. The necessity for maintaining a carefully controlled food intake may encourage parents to overprotect their children and perhaps restrict their social activities. The children, in turn, may react against their parents and their nutritional therapy. Thus, continuation of nutritional therapy beyond early childhood requires that children become knowledgeable about and responsible for management of their own food choices (Fig. 39–4). It also becomes the responsibility of the health care team to work with families and children to provide them with strategies that enable children and adolescents to participate in social and school activities, interact with peers, and progress through the usual developmental stages with self-confidence and self-esteem.

Children require parental and professional support in assuming responsibility for their food management. Self-management of food choices avoids the risk of the child using dietary noncompliance as a wedge against parental restrictions. Normal intellectual development is a laudable goal of management of PKU, but to be entirely successful, the children with PKU need to concomitantly develop self-assurance and a

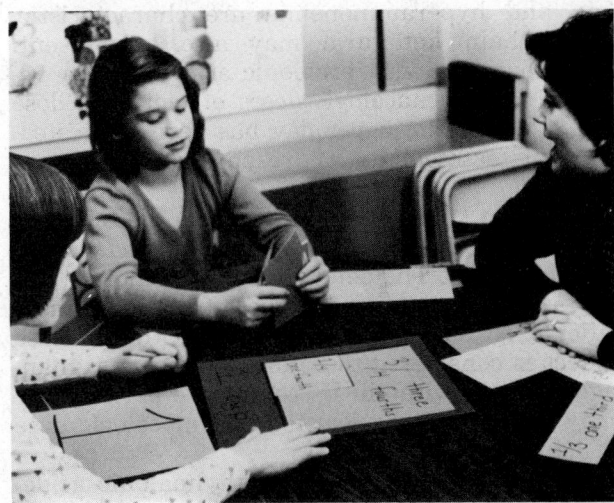

Figure 39–4. Older children learning to mange their own low-phenylalanine diets by calculating their intakes and by sharing with peers.

Table 39–7. CHILDREN OF MOTHERS WITH CLASSIC PKU*	
Mentally retarded	92%
Microcephalic	73%
Low birth weight	40%
Congenital heart disease	12%

* Blood phenylalanine concentration > 20 mg./dl.

From Lenke, R. R., and Levy, H. L.: Maternal phenylketonuria and hyperphenylalaninemia: an international survey of the outcome of treated and untreated pregnancies. N. Engl. J. Med. 303:1202, 1980.

strong self-image. This can, in part, be achieved by fostering self-management, independence, and a "normal" lifestyle for these children.

Nutritional Care in Maternal Phenylketonuria

A pregnant woman with elevated blood phenylalanine levels endangers her fetus because of the amplified transport of amino acids across the placenta. The fetus is exposed to about twice the phenylalanine level of maternal blood. Babies whose mothers have elevated blood phenylalanine levels have an increased occurrence of cardiac defects, retarded growth, microcephaly and mental retardation, as listed in Table 39–7. It appears that the higher the mother's blood phenylalanine level is, the more severe will be the effect on the fetus.[28] It appears that the fetus is at risk for being damaged with only minor elevations in maternal blood phenylalanine levels.

The management of nutritional therapy during pregnancy for a woman with hyperphenylalaninemia is complex. The changing physiology of pregnancy and concomitant changing nutritional needs are difficult to monitor with the precision required to maintain appropriately low blood phenylalanine levels. Even with meticulous attention to phenylalanine intake, blood phenylalanine levels and the nutritional requirements of pregnancy, a woman cannot be assured of a normal infant. Pre-pregnancy management of blood phenylalanine levels may decrease the risk to the fetus, but again success cannot be assured. When pre-pregnancy management is not possible, the restricted phenylalanine diet should be started as soon as possible after conception.[27, 29, 35] The risks of abnormal development of the fetus even with dietary management are an important consideration for young women with PKU who are considering pregnancy.

Nutritional management during pregnancy is difficult even for those women who have consistently been on a low-phenylalanine diet since infancy. Women who have been off the diet generally find reinstitution of formula consumption and limitation of food choices to be a difficult if not an overwhelming task. Compliance with nutritional therapy during pregnancy for even the well-motivated woman requires family and professional support as well as frequent monitoring of biochemical and nutritional aspects of both pregnancy and phenylketonuria.

Nutritional Care for Older Retarded Individuals

Adults with phenylketonuria most likely have some neurological damage and mental retardation due to delayed diagnosis and treatment, although with improved treatment the proportion of adults so affected will decline in the future. Frequently, hyperactivity and self-abuse are major concerns before the institution of a low-phenylalanine diet to modify behavior is considered. Results are inconsistent, as little, if any, intellectual or behavioral improvement has been observed.[30] However, it has been recommended that for the older patient who is difficult to manage, a trial of the low-phenylalanine diet be tried. If successful, continued diet therapy may aid in management.

TYROSINEMIA

Tyrosinemia is a poorly understood syndrome in which deficiency of para-hydroxyphenylpyruvic acid oxidase has been described. However, this deficiency may not be the primary cause of the syndrome. Plasma tyrosine concentration is high, as is methionine. It is unclear what causes the severe liver damge.

Nutritional therapy for tyrosinemia is controversial. Some patients have benefited from a low-tyrosine, low-phenylalanine diet supplemented with vitamin D. Methionine restriction has also been suggested for these patients.

ORGANIC ACID DISORDERS

In the past ten years, organic acid disorders have been more frequently identified than previously. It is assumed that this is largely a function of more effective diagnosis rather than an increase in incidence. Defects in the metabolism of propionic and methylmalonic acid, though rare, are the most common of the organic acid disorders.

Propionic acidemia is a defect of propionyl CoA carboxylase in the pathway of propionyl CoA to methylmalonyl CoA, as illustrated in Figure 39–5. The clinical course can be varied but is generally marked by vomiting, lethargy, hypotonia, dehydration, seizures and coma. Survivors often have permanent neurological damage. Metabolic acidosis with a marked anion gap and hyperammonemia are characteristic. Long chain ketonuria may also be present. Some patients with propionic acidemia may respond to pharmacologic doses of biotin. A dose of 10 mg. of biotin per day has been suggested. Careful assessment of responsiveness is required.[41]

At least five separate enzyme deficiencies have been identified that result in *methylmalonic acidemia*. The defect of methylmalonyl CoA mutase apoenzyme is the most frequently identified (Fig. 39–5). The patient with this mutase defect is considered to be more difficult to manage than the vitamin B_{12} responsive patient who may respond to a suggested pharmacologic dose of 1 to 2 mg. per day.[39]

The clinical features of methylmalonic acidemia are similar to those of propionic acidemia. Acidosis is common and diagnosis is documented by large amounts of methylmalonic acid in blood and urine. Other findings include hypoglycemia, ketonuria, and elevation of plasma ammonia and lactate. There is also a need to rule out frank vitamin B_{12} deficiency, as vitamin B_{12} yields two cofactors that are required to convert methylmalonate to succinate and homocysteine to methionine.

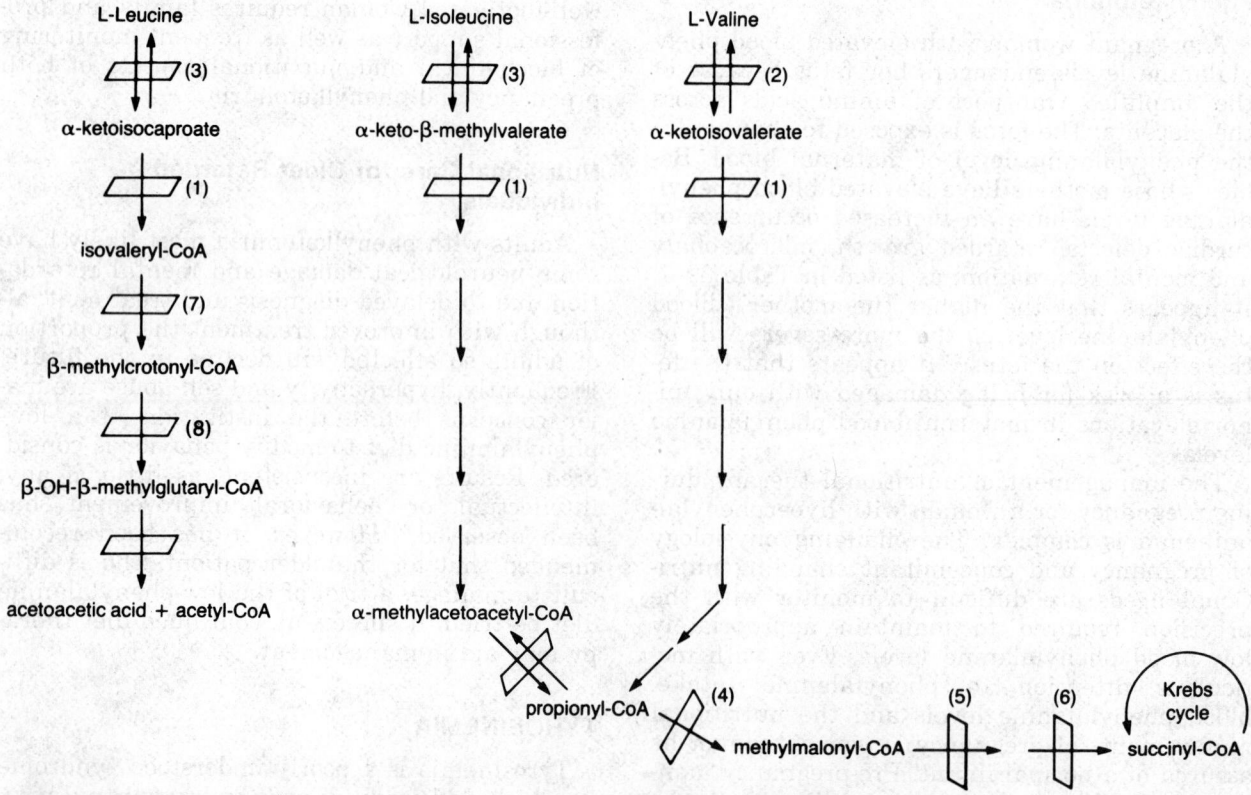

Figure 39–5. Organic acidemias and MSUD: (1) branched-chain ketoacid decarboxylase (MSUD), (2) valine aminotransferase, (3) leucine-isoleucine aminotransferase, (4) propionyl CoA carboxylase (propionic acidemia), (5) methylmalonyl CoA racemase (methylmalonic aciduria), (6) methylmalonyl CoA mutase (methylmalonic aciduria), (7) isovaleryl CoA dehydrogenase (isovaleric acidemia), and (8) beta-methylcroteryl CoA carboxylase (biotin-responsive multiple carboxylase deficiency).

The goals of management of acute episodes of propionic acidemia and methylmalonic acidemia are to provide and maintain normal nutrient intake and to restore and maintain biochemical balance. It is important to prevent tissue catabolism by maintaining energy intake and to prevent dehydration by maintaining fluid intake. Electrolyte imbalances are corrected by the ususal methods, and abnormal metabolites are removed by urinary excretion promoted by a large fluid intake.

Relapses of metabolic acidoses may result from excessive protein intake, infection, or unidentified reasons. Parents become skilled at identifying early signs of illness. Treatment for these episodes must be rapid.

Long-term nutritional therapy includes an appropriate balance of essential nutrients and a protein intake restricted to 1.0 to 1.5 gm./kg./day. Response to protein intake is variable, as some patients require little or no protein restriction and can be self-regulated, while some may need severely restricted protein intakes. In conjunction with dilute standard infant formula, 80056 (Mead Johnson) is frequently used to ensure an adequate intake of vitamins, minerals, and energy. An adequate fluid intake is required to influence blood ammonia levels. Information on long-term prognosis is very limited.

UREA CYCLE DEFECTS

Defects in the urea cycle have also been more frequently identified in the past several years. All defects in the urea cycle result in an ammonia accumulation in the blood. The clinical signs of elevated ammonia are vomiting and lethargy, which may progress to seizures, coma and ultimately death. In infants the adverse effects of elevated ammonia levels are rapid and devastating. In older children, symptoms of elevated ammonia may be preceded by hyperactivity and irritability. The severity and variation of the clinical course of all of the urea cycle defects may be related to the degree of residual enzyme activity.

Most common urea cycle defects are discussed in a progression that proceeds around the urea cycle as shown in Figure 39–6.

Ornithine transcarbamylase deficiency (OTC deficiency) is an X-linked recessive disorder with a block in the conversion of ornithine and carbamyl phosphate to citrulline. OTC deficiency is identified by hyperammonemia, increased urinary orotic acid, and normal levels of citrulline, argininosuccinic acid and arginine.[8] OTC deficiency is usually lethal in males, whereas heterozygous females with various degrees of enzyme activity may not demonstrate symptoms of this defect until stressed by infection or by a significant increase in the protein content of the diet. The usual treatment is a moderately low protein diet (about 2 gm./kg./day).

Citrullinemia is the deficiency of argininosuccinic acid synthetase in the metabolism of citrulline to argininosuccinic acid. Citrullinemia is identified by markedly elevated citrulline in the urine and blood. Argininosuccinic acid synthetase activity is absent or decreased in cultured skin fibroblasts. Symptoms may be present in the neonatal period or gradually develop in early infancy. These symptoms are poor feeding and recurrent vomiting which, without immediate treatment, progress to seizures, neurological abnormalities and coma.

Argininosuccinic aciduria (ASA) is the deficiency of argininosuccinate lyase in the metabolism of argininosuccinic acid to arginine. ASA is identified by the presence of argininosuccinic acid in urine and blood. Citrulline may be mod-

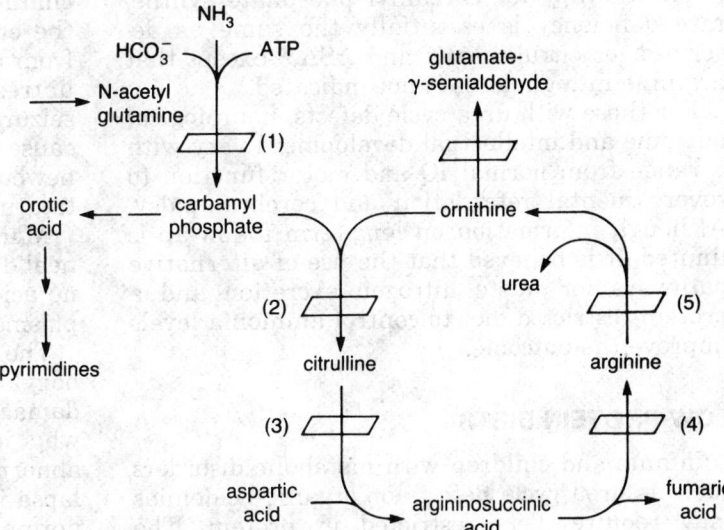

Figure 39–6. Urea cycle disorders: (1) carbamyl phosphate synthetase (CPS deficiency), (2) ornithine carbamyl transferase (OTC deficiency), (3) argininosuccinic acid synthetase (citrullinemia), (4) argininosuccinic acid lyase (argininosuccinic aciduria) and (5) arginase (arginemia).

erately elevated in blood and urine. Argininosuccinate lyase activity is absent or decreased in cultured fibroblasts or red blood cells.

Citrullinemia and ASA have essentially the same clinical presentation, and the aim of therapy for both of these defects is to prevent or decrease hyperammonemia and the detrimental neurological consequences associated with the high amino acid levels. Acute episodes of illness are managed by discontinuation of protein intake and the administration of intravenous fluids and glucose to correct the dehydration and provide energy. If hyperammonemia is severe, peritoneal dialysis, hemodialysis or exchange transfusion may be required. Intravenous arginine and sodium benzoate have also been beneficial in reducing the hyperammonemia.

Long-term therapy consists of a restricted protein diet at 1.0 to 2.0 gm./kg./day, depending on individual tolerance. The diet should be supplemented with L-arginine (1 gm./day for infants, 2 gm./day for older children) to prevent arginine deficiency and to assist in waste nitrogen excretion.[9] Sodium benzoate at 0.25 gm./kg./day is frequently prescribed to aid in ammonia excretion. Keto analogues of essential amino acids have also been tried but are reported to be no more effective than a low-protein diet plus arginine.[6, 7] Because of the effect of infection and illness on the urea cycle, infections should be treated aggressively.

Carbamyl phosphate synthetase deficiency (CPS deficiency) is manifested in a very similar manner with hyperammonemic episodes. The onset is usually in the early neonatal period with vomiting, irritability, hypothermia, respiratory distress, altered muscle tone, lethargy and often coma. Specific laboratory findings usually include elevated plasma glutamine and normal or low orotic acid in urine.

The therapy for carbamyl phosphate synthetase deficiency is essentially the same as described for citrullinemia and ASA,[37] except that arginine in high doses is not indicated.

For those with urea cycle defects, neurological outcome and intellectual development vary with a range from normal IQ and motor function to severe mental retardation and cerebral palsy. Although information on long-term follow-up is limited, it is believed that the use of alternative pathways for waste nitrogen excretion and a protein-restricted diet to control ammonia levels improve the outcome.

LOW-PROTEIN DIETS

Infants and children with metabolic disorders such as urea cycle defects or organic acidemias may require diets restricted in protein. The most usual restrictions are for 1.0, 1.5, and 2.0 gm. of protein per kg. body weight. The appropriate prescription for protein level is based on the individual tolerance of the infant or child. Clearly, the infant or child should be fed the highest level of protein that can be tolerated to ensure adequate growth and a margin of nutritional safety.

In general, low-protein or restricted-protein diets can be formulated from readily available infant and toddler foods. Infant formula can be diluted so that it meets the prescribed protein level. The resulting energy deficit is made up by supplementing carbohydrate and fat. The supplement can be 80056 (Mead Johnson), a protein-free carbohydrate, fat, vitamin and mineral supplement; Polycose (Ross), a protein- and fat-free formulation of glucose polymers; corn oil; or MCT oil. The appropriate choice depends on the level of restriction, age, and condition of the child. Formulas should be at 20 kcal./oz. and energy at least 100 kcal./kg. Usual recommendations for vitamins and minerals are appropriate.

Diet plans are given for 1.0, 1.5, and 2.0 gm./kg. protein levels for a theoretical infant (3 kg.) and toddler (11 kg.) in Table 39–8. These example diet plans illustrate the wide variety of foods that may be offered.

MAPLE SYRUP URINE DISEASE

Classical *maple syrup urine disease* (MSUD) or *branched chain ketoaciduria* results from a defect in decarboxylation that affects the metabolism of leucine, isoleucine and valine (Figure 39–5). This rare autosomal recessive metabolic defect is estimated to occur in 1 in 225,000 newborns. Infants appear normal at birth but by four or five days of age demonstrate poor feeding, vomiting, lethargy and periodic hypertonia. A characteristic sweet, malty odor appears toward the end of the first week of life and is present from urine and perspiration. If this condition is untreated, acidosis, neurological deterioration, seizures and coma proceed to eventual death. Because of the rapid onset of symptoms, results of newborn screening are often too late to initiate treatment before symptoms appear.

Management of acute disease requires peritoneal dialysis and hydration. Branched chain amino acids (BCAA) are gradually introduced when plasma leucine levels are decreased to 1 mM.[11]

The precise mechanism of the complete decarboxylase reaction and the resulting neurological damage are not known. Neither is it understood why leucine metabolism is significantly more abnormal than the other two BCAA. Clinical relapse is most often related to the degree of abnormality of the leucine level,[36] and these

Table 39–8.   SAMPLE LOW-PROTEIN DIET PLANS

1.0 GM. PROTEIN PER KG. BODY WEIGHT FOOD PATTERN

Infant (Newborn, Weight = 3 kg.)

AMOUNT	COMPONENT	PROTEIN (gm.)	ENERGY (kcal.)
6½ oz. (or 3 tbsp. + ¾ tsp. Powder)	Similac with Fe*	3.0	130
4 tbsp. (40 gm.)	80056†	0.0	196
	Water to total 16½ oz.		
	Total:	3.0	326

Toddler (18 mo. old, 11 kg.)

AMOUNT	COMPONENT	PROTEIN (gm.)	ENERGY (kcal.)
18 oz. (or 9 tbsp. Powder)	Similac with Fe*	8.4	360
8.5 tbsp. (85 gm.)	80056	0.0	417
	Water to 36 oz.		
¼ small	Banana	0.3	22
2 tbsp.	Rice Krispies	0.25	15
8 oz.	Apple juice	0.25	168
1	Saltine with ½ tsp. margarine	0.3	20
3 tbsp.	Vegetarian vegetable soup (condensed)	0.3	12
2 tbsp.	Green beans with ½ tsp. margarine	0.3	10
1	Ritz cracker	0.2	15
4 tbsp.	Applesauce	0.1	46
2	Peach halves	0.4	78
1½ tbsp.	Rice, white	0.25	15
	Total:	11.05	1178

1.5 GM. PROTEIN PER KG. BODY WEIGHT FOOD PATTERN

Infant (Newborn, Weight = 3 kg.)

AMOUNT	COMPONENT	PROTEIN (gm.)	ENERGY (kcal.)
10 oz. (or 5 tbsp. Powder)	Similac with Fe*	4.6	200
3 tbsp. (30 gm.)	80056	0.0	147
	Total:	4.6	347

Toddler (18 mo. old, 11 kg.)

AMOUNT	COMPONENT	PROTEIN (gm.)	ENERGY (kcal.)
25 oz. (or 12½ tbsp. Powder)	Similac with Fe*	11.6	500
5 tbsp.	80056	0.0	245
	Water to 37 oz.		
½ small	Banana	0.6	44
4 tbsp.	Rice Krispies	0.5	30
8 oz.	Apple juice	0.25	168
1	Saltine	0.25	20
3 tbsp.	Tomato soup (condensed)	0.4	16
2 tbsp.	Green beans	0.3	10
2	Ritz crackers	0.4	15
4 tbsp.	Applesauce	0.1	46
3 tbsp.	Rice	0.5	29
⅓ cup	Carrots	0.5	16
2	Peach halves	0.4	78
6 oz.	Apple juice	0.1	126
1	Graham cracker	0.6	21
	Total:	16.4	1364

Table continued on the following page

Table 39–8. SAMPLE LOW-PROTEIN DIET PLANS(*Continued*)

2.0 GM. PROTEIN PER KG. BODY WEIGHT FOOD PATTERN

Infant (Newborn, Weight = 3 kg.)

AMOUNT	COMPONENT	PROTEIN (gm.)	ENERGY (kcal.)
13 oz. or (6½ tbsp. Powder)	Similac with Fe*	6.0	260
1½ tbsp. (15 gm.)	80056	0.0	74
	Water to 17 oz.		
	Total:	6.0	334

Toddler (18 mo. old, 11 kg.)

AMOUNT	COMPONENT	PROTEIN (gm.)	ENERGY (kcal.)
33 oz. (or 1 cup + ½ tbsp. Powder)	Similac with Fe*	15.3	660
—	80056	—	—
	No additional water		
½ small	Banana	0.6	44
4 tbsp.	Oatmeal	1.2	40
8 oz.	Apple juice	0.25	168
2	Saltines	0.5	40
3 tbsp.	Tomato soup (condensed)	0.4	16
2 tbsp.	Green beans	0.3	10
½ slice	White bread with jam	1.0	30
4 tbsp.	Applesauce	0.1	46
3 tbsp.	Macaroni	0.9	40
⅓ cup	Carrots	0.5	16
2	Peach halves	0.4	78
1	Graham cracker	0.6	21
	Total:	22.1	1209

* Similac = 0.465 gm. protein/oz. and 20 kcal./oz., either ready-to-feed or diluted according to manufacturer's instructions.

† 80056 = 0 gm. protein/tbsp. and 49 kcal./tbsp.

Specific formula products are mentioned as an example only. Low protein bread and pasta may be offered to provide additional food experiences and energy to satisfy individual appetites.

relapses are frequently related to infection. Acute infections are a medical emergency and most children who have died despite being on therapy have done so during an episode of infection. If the plasma leucine level rises to over 20 mg./dl., BCAA should immediately be removed from the diet and intravenous therapy started.

Nutritional Care

Nutritional therapy requires very careful monitoring of blood levels, especially leucine, and growth and general nutritional adequacy. Several formulas such as MSUD diet powder and MSUD 1 and MSUD 2 are now available to provide a reasonable amino acid and vitamin mixture. These generally are supplemented with a small quantity of infant formula or cow's milk to provide the BCAA needed to support growth and development. Lists of the leucine values of foods have been developed and are given in Table 39–9.

Recent reports have indicated that early intervention and meticulous biochemical control can provide a more hopeful prognosis than previously realized. Reasonable growth and intellectual development in the normal to low normal range have been described in a series of four patients, the oldest aged nine years.[11] It is recommended that plasma leucine levels be maintained between 2 and 5 mg./dl. Levels above 10 mg./dl. are associated with alpha-ketoacidemia and neurological symptoms.

Disorders of Carbohydrate Metabolism

A second category of inborn errors of metabolism is the carbohydrate disorders. These disorders are rare. Nutritional intervention appears to be effective.

GALACTOSEMIA

Galactosemia, a high level of plasma galactose combined with galactosuria, is found in two metabolic disorders that are both of autosomal

Table 39–9. FOOD EXCHANGE LISTS FOR DIETS RESTRICTED IN ISOLEUCINE, LEUCINE AND VALINE

VEGETABLES

Contain per serving an average of 23 mg. isoleucine, 30 mg. leucine, 27 mg. valine, 0.7 gm. protein and 15 kcal. Protein is 3.48% isoleucine, 4.55% leucine and 4.09% valine.

	ILEU. (mg.)	LEU. (mg.)	VAL. (mg.)	PRO. (gm.)	ENERGY (kcal.)
Asparagus, raw, 1½–2 spears (33 gm.)	18	32	26	0.7	9
Asparagus, canned, green, 2 med. spears (38 gm.)	26	32	35	0.7	7
Beans, green, raw, cooked in small amount of water, ¼ c. (31 gm.)	22	29	24	0.5	8
Beans, green, canned, drained solids ¼ c. (31 gm.)	20	26	21	0.4	8
Beans, yellow wax, canned, drained solids ¼ c. (50 gm.)	32	40	33	0.7	12
Beets, canned, drained, ½ c. (100 gm.)	29	28	25	0.8	31
Beet greens, cooked, 2 T. (25 gm.)	18	27	21	0.2	4
Brussels sprouts, cooked, drained, 1 sprout (17 gm.)	29	31	31	0.7	6
Cabbage, raw, ½ c. shredded (50 gm.)	26	26	20	0.6	12
Cabbage, cooked in small amount of water, 5 T. (50 gm.)	22	22	16	0.6	10
Carrots, raw, ½ large (50 gm.)	16	25	25	0.55	21
Carrots, canned, drained solids, ½ c.	24	34	30	0.64	24
Chard, frozen cooked, 3 T. (33 gm.)	26	32	23	0.8	8
Collards, frozen cooked, 1½ T. (18 gm.)	16	30	27	0.6	6
Cucumber, not pared, 1 med. (100 gm.)	18	26	20	0.1	16
Eggplant, cooked, drained, ¼ c. (50 gm.)	26	31	30	0.5	10
Kale, frozen cooked, 2 T. (17 gm.)	17	32	24	0.5	5
Lettuce, raw, (25 gm.)	12	21	18	0.3	4
Mustard greens, frozen cooked, ¼ c. (50 gm.)	36	30	52	1.1	10
Okra, cooked, 2 pods (25 gm.)	21	31	28	0.55	10
Onion, raw, 6 T. chopped (60 gm.)	18	30	40	1.2	24
Potato, boiled in skin, ⅓ med. (33 gm.)	31	35	37	0.7	25
Spinach, frozen cooked, 1 T. (12 gm.)	17	28	20	0.4	3
Squash, summer, cooked, drained, ½ c. (100 gm.)	29	41	33	0.9	14
Squash, winter, boiled, 3 T. (50 gm.)	17	25	20	0.55	19
Sweet potato, baked, ¼ small (25 gm.)	25	30	39	0.52	35
Tomato, raw, 1 small (100 gm.)	32	45	31	1.1	22
Tomato, canned, 6 T. (75 gm.)	22	31	21	0.75	16
Tomato juice, canned, ½ c. (100 gm.)	26	37	25	0.9	19
Turnip greens, cooked in small amount of water (12 gm.)	14	27	19	0.37	4

GERBER'S STRAINED AND JUNIOR VEGETABLES

	ILEU. (mg.)	LEU. (mg.)	VAL. (mg.)	PRO. (gm.)	ENERGY (kcal.)
Amounts in 1 T. (14 gm.)					
Beets	6.7	6.6	5.9	0.19	5.4
Carrots	3.7	5.3	4.7	0.1	4.3
Green beans	8.1	10.7	8.9	0.19	4.1
Squash	3.6	5.1	4.1	0.11	3.9
Sweet potatoes	9.6	11.6	15	0.2	9.9

FRUITS

Contain per serving an average of 15 mg. isoleucine, 25 mg. leucine, 25 mg. valine, 0.6 gm. protein and 90 kcal. Protein is 2.85% isoleucine, 4.35% leucine and 3.73% valine.

	ILEU. (mg.)	LEU. (mg.)	VAL. (mg.)	PRO. (gm.)	ENERGY (kcal.)
Apple, raw, 1 small 2″ diam. (100 gm.)	13	23	15	0.4	58
Applesauce, canned, sweetened, ⅔ c. (200 gm.)	13	23	15	0.4	182
Apple juice, 1½ c.	13	23	15	0.4	174
Apricot, raw, 2–3 med. (100 gm.)	14	23	19	0.8	51
Apricot, canned, sweetened, 4 med. halves (133 gm.)	14	23	19	0.8	115
Apricots, dried, 3 halves (18 gm.)	14	23	19	0.8	52
Avocado, 3½ T. (33 gm.)	16	25	21	0.5	56
Banana, ½ small (50 gm.)	16	26	22	0.6	42

Table continued on the following page

Table 39–9. FOOD EXCHANGE LISTS FOR DIETS RESTRICTED IN ISOLEUCINE, LEUCINE AND VALINE (*Continued*)

Dates, domestic natural, 2 med. pitted (20 gm.)	15	15	19	0.4	55
Figs, raw, 1 large (50 gm.)	18	26	23	0.6	40
Orange, raw, 1 small 2½" diam. (100 gm.)	23	22	31	0.8	49
Orange juice, canned, ⅖ c. (100 gm.)	23	22	31	0.8	48
Peach, raw, 1 med. (100 gm.)	13	29	30	0.8	38
Peaches, canned, 4 med. halves & 4 T. syrup (200 gm.)	13	29	30	0.8	156
Peach nectar, canned, 1½ c. (370 gm.)	13	29	30	0.8	178
Pear, canned in syrup, 6 small halves & 6 T. syrup (300 gm.)	17	26	22	0.6	226
Pear, raw, ½ pear (100 gm.)	20	30	26	0.7	61
Pineapple, raw, 1½ c. diced (200 gm.)	23	35	30	0.8	104
Pineapple juice, 1 c. (240 gm.)	23	35	30	0.8	128
Pumpkin, canned, 3⅓ T. (50 gm.)	19	26	19	0.5	17
Strawberries, fresh, 7½ large (75 gm.)	14	32	17	0.6	28
Strawberries, frozen, & sugar, ½ c. (128 gm.)	14	32	17	0.6	140

GERBER'S STRAINED AND JUNIOR FRUITS

	ILEU. (mg.)	LEU. (mg.)	VAL. (mg.)	PRO. (gm.)	ENERGY (kcal.)
Apple juice (3 oz.)	3	6	4	0.1	49
Orange juice (3 oz.)	14	14	19	0.5	50
Amounts in 1 T. (14 gm.)					
Applesauce	<1	1.7	1.1	0.03	11.6
Apricots with tapioca	<1	1.7	1.3	0.06	11.4
Peaches	1.4	3.1	3.1	0.09	11.7
Pears	1.6	2.4	2.1	0.06	9.9
Pears & pineapple	1.6	2.4	2.1	0.06	10.1

BREAD AND CEREAL

Contain per serving an average of 15 mg. isoleucine, 35 mg. leucine, 20 mg. valine, 0.4 gm. protein and 20 kcal. Protein is 3.83% isoleucine, 8.08% leucine and 5.12% valine.

	ILEU. (mg.)	LEU. (mg.)	VAL. (mg.)	PRO. (gm.)	ENERGY (kcal.)
Ready to Serve					
Bran, All, Kellogg's, 1 T. (3.5 gm.)	13	26	19	0.4	12
Bran Flakes, 40%, 2 T. (4.7 gm.)	16	32	24	0.5	17
Bran, Raisin, Kellogg's, 2 T. (5 gm.)	15	30	22	0.4	18
Cheerios, 2 T. (3 gm.)	17	33	23	0.4	13
Cornflakes, 2 T. (3 gm.)	10	34	12	0.3	12
Rice Krispies, 4 T. (¼ c.) (7 gm.)	18	35	24	0.4	27
Rice, puffed, 8 T. (½ c.) (6 gm.)	18	35	24	0.4	25
Cooked					
Farina, cooked, 2 T.	23	33	21	0.5	18
Rice, brown, cooked, 2 T.	16	30	24	0.4	17
Rice, white, cooked, 2 T.	17	30	25	0.4	17
Special Low Protein Products*†					
Aproten Macaroni Products					
Anellini, uncooked, ¾ c. (100 gm.)	13	26	15	0.5	340
Rigatini, uncooked, 1½ c. (100 gm.)	13	26	15	0.5	340
Tagliatelle, uncooked, 1¼ c. (100 gm.)	13	26	15	0.5	340
Paygel Low Protein Bread, 1 slice (32 gm.)				0.3	83
Aproten Rusks, 1 slice (11.5 gm.)	4	6	4	0.1	48

GERBER'S DRY CEREALS	ILEU. (mg.)	LEU. (mg.)	VAL. (mg.)	PRO. (gm.)	ENERGY (kcal.)
Amounts in 1 T. (2.4 gm.)					
Oatmeal	14	6	20	0.359	9
Rice	6	12	10	0.159	9

Table 39–9. FOOD EXCHANGE LISTS FOR DIETS RESTRICTED IN ISOLEUCINE, LEUCINE AND VALINE (*Continued*)

FATS

Contain per serving an average of 7 mg. isoleucine, 10 mg. leucine, 8 mg. valine, 0.1 gm. protein and 70 kcal. Protein averages 5.83% isoleucine, 8.33% leucine and 6.67% valine.

Butter, 1 T. (14 gm.)	6	10	7	0.1	100
Cream, whipping (40%), 1 tsp. (5 gm.)	6	10	7	0.1	17
Coffee Rich, liquid, 1 T. (14 gm.)	8	11	8	0.1	24
French dressing, 2 T. (28 gm.)	6	7	7	0.2	114
Margarine, 2 tsp. (10 gm.)	5	7	5	0.1	72
Mayonnaise, 1 T. (14 gm.)	10	13	11	0.15	101
Tartar sauce, ½ T. (10 gm.)	7	9	7	0.1	47
Thousand Island dressing, 1 T. (14 gm.)	7	10	8	0.11	70

Adapted from Acosta, P., and Elsas, L.: Dietary Management of Inherited Metabolic Disease: Phenylketonuria, Galactosemia, Tyrosinemia, Maple Syrup Urine Disease. Atlanta, Ga., ACELMU Publishers, 1976.

* Manufactured by Henkel Corporation, Special Dietary Foods, 4620 W. 77th Street, Minneapolis, Minnesota, 55435.

† Not calculated in mean figures for amino acid content of Bread and Cereal list.

recessive inheritance. The disorders are *galactokinase deficiency* and *galactose-1-phosphate uridyl transferase deficiency*, which is also called *classic galactosemia.*

Galactosemia results from a disturbance in the conversion of galactose to glucose because of the absence of one of the enzyme activities as shown in Figure 39–7. The deficiencies cause an accumulation of galactose, or galactose and galactose-1-phosphate in body tissues. It is believed that galactose-1-phosphate in intercellular fluids causes the cellular disturbances in classic galactosemia.

If an infant has no galactose-1-phosphate uridyl transferase activity, illness generally occurs within the first two weeks of life. Symptoms are vomiting, diarrhea, lethargy, failure to thrive, jaundice, hepatomegaly and cataracts. Infants with galactosemia may be hypoglycemic and are prone to infection from gram-negative organisms. If the condition is not treated, death

is frequently caused by septicemia. If diagnosis and therapy are delayed, mental retardation can result.

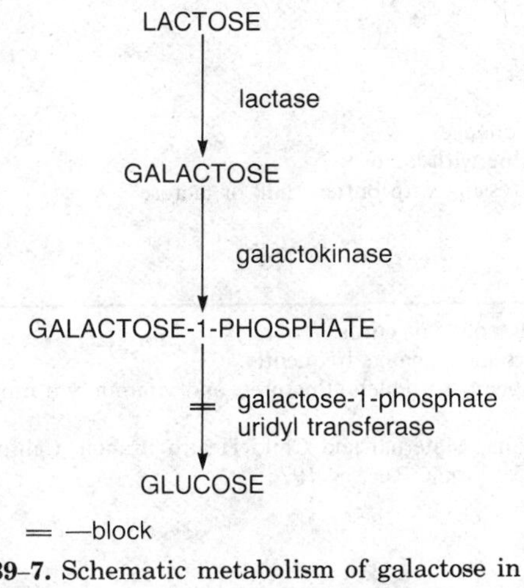

Diagnosis of transferase deficiency is accomplished in a stepwise fashion. First, sick newborns are screened for reducing sugars that are not glucose, which are shown to be present if Benedict's test is positive and the glucose paper strip test is negative. Then the Beutler test for transferase enzyme activity is done and confirmation of diagnosis by specific enzyme tests is completed.

Treatment for galactosemia is galactose restriction. If all galactose is omitted from the food intake, the galactose required for production of galactolipids and cerebrosides is produced by an alternative pathway. Galactose restriction mandates that all milk and milk products be strictly avoided as lactose divides into galactose and glucose. In addition, organ meats such as liver, pancreas and brain and monosodium glutamate must be eliminated because they contain galactose. The galactose-restricted food pattern must be maintained throughout life.

Effective galactose restriction makes it essential to read labels on all food products carefully. Milk is added to many products, and the tablet form of medications often has lactose in the coating. Table 39–10 presents a galactose-free diet.

With early diagnosis and treatment, physical progress should be good with resolution of physical problems, sometimes even of cataracts.[26] Mental development is generally slightly less than expected; patients often have an IQ of 85 to 100, and visual-perceptual difficulties are common.[16]

A few treated women with galactosemia have become pregnant and given birth to healthy ba-

LACTOSE

↓ lactase

GALACTOSE

↓ galactokinase

GALACTOSE-1-PHOSPHATE

⫧ galactose-1-phosphate
uridyl transferase

↓

GLUCOSE

= —block

Figure 39–7. Schematic metabolism of galactose in galactosemia.

Table 39–10. FOOD LIST FOR GALACTOSE-FREE DIET

FOODS ALLOWED	FOODS NOT ALLOWED
MILK AND MILK SUBSTITUTES	
Isomil	Breast milk
Neo-Mull-Soy	All forms of animal milk
Nutramigen	Imitation or filled milk
Prosobee	Cream
Soyalac	Cottage cheese
Meat-base formula	Hard cheeses
	Yogurt
	Ice cream, ice milk, sherbet
FRUITS	
All fresh, frozen, canned or dried, except those listed in column two	Fruits processed with unsafe ingredients*
	Diabetic or dietetic fruits processed with unsafe ingredients
VEGETABLES	
All fresh, frozen, canned or dried, except those listed in column two	Vegetables processed with unsafe ingredients, seasoned with butter or margarine, breaded or creamed
	Instant mashed potatoes containing lactose or other unsafe ingredients
	Commercially packaged fried potatoes containing lactose or other unsafe ingredients
MEAT, POULTRY, FISH, EGGS AND NUTS	
Plain beef, lamb, veal, pork, ham	Creamed, buttered or breaded meat, fish, eggs or poultry
Plain fish, turkey, chicken, game, fowl	Frankfurters, cold cuts or liver sausage made with milk, lactose or unsafe ingredients
Kosher frankfurters	
Eggs prepared without milk, cream, butter or margarine	Organ meats: liver, brains, sweetbreads, kidneys, pancreas, heart
Nut butters (peanut butter)	
Nuts	
BREADS AND CEREALS	
Cooked and dry cereals without milk or lactose added	Cereals, bread, or crackers that have milk, milk products, or lactose added
Bread or crackers without milk or lactose added (saltines, graham crackers, water breads, hard rolls). Contact bakery if not sure. Read all labels.	Dry cereals
	Cream of wheat or rice
Macaroni, spaghetti, noodles, rice	Pancakes, waffles, French toast
Tortilla, flour, and corn	Zwieback
	Crackers made with butter or margarine
	Prepared muffin or biscuit mixes
FATS	
All vegetable oils (soybean, corn, olive, cottonseed, safflower, peanut)	Butter
	Cream
All shortening, lard, margarines containing safe ingredients	Cream cheese
	Margarine with lactose
Bacon	Salad dressing with butter, milk or lactose
Mayonnaise	
Olives	
Salad dressings with safe ingredients	

* Unsafe ingredients are milk, lactose, galactose, casein, whey, dry milk solids or curds.
Labels should be regularly and carefully checked, as formulations of products change frequently.
Lactose is often used as a pharmaceutical bulking agent, filler, or excipient, so tablets, tinctures, and vitamin and mineral mixtures should be carefully evaluated.
From Parents' Guide to the Galactose-Restricted Diet, Davis, California, Maternal and Child Health Branch, California Department of Health Services, Department of Nutrition, University of California. Revised 1976.

bies, though ovarian failure is now a commonly recognized problem in adolescent females affected with galactosemia.[25]

Galactokinase deficiency also requires the same restricted galactose regimen as galactosemia. Cataracts form, but the other sequelae of galactosemia have not been described in galactokinase deficiency. Other disorders of carbohydrate metabolism (except diabetes mellitus, which is discussed in Chapter 25) are exceedingly rare.

FRUCTOSE INTOLERANCE

Hereditary fructose intolerance and *fructose 1,6-diphosphatase deficiency* manifest as clinical features only after introduction of fructose. The former manifests as vomiting, hepatomegaly, severe hypoglycemia and renal tubular defects. Diagnosis is made by elevated urinary and blood levels of fructose after fructose feedings. The latter is manifested by hypoglycemia, episodic hepatomegaly, hypotonia, and metabolic acidosis. In both cases, diagnosis is confirmed by enzyme assay and treatment is a diet free of fructose, sucrose and sorbitol, as presented in Table 39–11.[5, 42]

OTHER DISORDERS

Table 39–2 outlines additional disorders and the enzymatic defects, outstanding clinical and biochemical features and current dietary treatment.

Summary

There are a relatively large number of rare metabolic disorders that theoretically respond to dietary manipulation. Though the specific adjustments may differ, the general principles of nutritional management are similar. The primary goal is to maintain biochemical balance. That goal can be achieved only by providing the patient and family with long-term clinical and psychological support. Implementation of the principles of treatment is a difficult task. An experienced and understanding health care team, particularly a pediatrician, nutritionist and psychologist, will be able to encourage and assist families as they learn to adjust to the necessary therapeutic restrictions. An organized nutrition education program will provide patients with the information and skills required to manage their own regimen successfully.

Problems and Suggested Topics for Discussion

1. Describe the problems that may be encountered in providing nutritional counseling to parents of children with inborn errors of metabolism.
2. Discuss the nutritional management goals for a child with phenylketonuria.
3. A child with galactosemia is admitted to the outpatient clinic. What information should be obtained before a proper diet can be planned?
4. Write a day's menu for a 9-month-old infant with citrullinemia.
5. Write a day's menu for a 12-month-old infant with maple syrup urine disease.

Table 39–11. FOODS THAT MUST BE ELIMINATED IN A FRUCTOSE- AND SUCROSE-FREE DIET*

Milk	Infant formulas containing fructose or sucrose; sweetened condensed milk, commercial chocolate milk, milk drinks with added sugar, ice cream or sherbet
Meats	Meats processed in sugar brine, such as ham, bacon and luncheon meat; commercially prepared infant meat and vegetable dinners to which sucrose may be added; some processed cheese spreads
Fats	Mayonnaise, salad dressings, peanut butter
Cereals	Sugar-coated cereals, defatted wheat germ, rice bran
Desserts	Cookies, cakes and other desserts made with sugar, sweet or chocolate milk, syrup or molasses
Potatoes	Sweet potatoes; regular white cooking potatoes may provide a significant source of fructose, depending upon harvesting, storage and cooking techniques
Vegetables	All vegetables and vegetable juices are eliminated*
Fruits	All fruits and fruit juices should be eliminated
Miscellaneous	Granulated, powdered and brown sugars; sugar substitutes containing sorbital; milk and sweet chocolate; honey, jelly, syrup, molasses, sorghum; peanuts and other nuts; coconut and coconut milk, preserves made with corn syrup or invert sugar

* The first foods to add back to increase fructose and sucrose intake in order to determine tolerance are all vegetables *except*: broccoli, cucumber, peas, rhubarb, beets, carrots, parsnips, pumpkins, rutabagas, winter squash, turnips, corn, hominy and dry beans.

Adapted from Francis, D. E. M.: Diets for Sick Children. 3rd ed. Oxford, Blackwell Scientific Publications, 1974.

Sources of Low-Protein Foods

Source	Products
Henkel Corporation 4620 W. 77th Street Minneapolis, Minn. 55435	Low-protein pastas Low-protein rusks Wheat starch Prono (Gelled Dessert Mix) Porridge
Chicago Dietetic Supply, Inc. 1750 W. Van Buren Street Chicago, Ill. 60612	Cellu wheat starch Low-protein pastas, baking mix, and bread
Ener-G Foods, Inc. 6901 Fox Ave. S. P.O. Box 24723 Seattle, Wash. 98124	Jolly Joan low-protein bread and mix Egg replacer Low-protein pastas and cookies

Kingsmill Foods Co. Ltd.
1399 Kennedy Road, Unit 17
Scarborough, Ontario
Canada M1P 2L6

Unimix low-protein bread and mix

Low-protein pastas and cookies

Guides for Parents

Acosta, P.B., et al.: A Parent's Guide to the Child with Maple Syrup Urine Disease. Florida State University, Center for Family Services, 103 Sandels Building, Tallahassee, Fla. 32306, 1980.

Acosta, P.B., et al.: Parents' Guide to the Child with PKU. Florida State University, Center for Family Services, 103 Sandels Building, Tallahassee, Fla. 32306, 1980.

Lo-Pro Diet Guide. 2nd ed. Metabolism Office, James Whitcomb Riley Hospital for Children, Rm. A-36, 1100 W. Michigan St., Indianapolis, Ind. 46223, 1982.

Read, E., et al.: The PKU Cookbook. Program in Dietetics, Emory University, 2040 Ridgewood Drive N.E., Atlanta, Ga. 30322, 1976.

Schuett, V.E.: Low Protein Cookery for Phenylketonuria. University of Wisconsin Press, Box 1379, Madison, Wis. 53701, 1977.

Schuett, V.E.: Low Protein Food List: For Phenylketonuria and Metabolic Diseases Requiring a Low Protein Diet. The Waisman Center, University of Wisconsin, 1500 Highland Avenue, Madison, Wis. 53706, 1981.

Taylor, M., and Schuett, V.E.: You and PKU. Waisman Center on Mental Retardation and Human Development, 1500 Highland Avenue, Madison, Wis. 53706, 1978.

Materials for Health Care Professionals

Acosta, P.B., and Elsas, L.J.: Dietary Management of Inherited Metabolic Disease: Phenylketonuria, Galactosemia, Tyrosemia, Homocystinuria, Maple Syrup Urine Disease. ACELMU Publishers, 1939 Westminister Way, Atlanta, Ga. 30307, 1976.

Acosta, P.B., and Wenz, E.: Diet Management of PKU for Infants and Preschool Children. DHEW Publication No. (HSA) 78–5209, 1978.

Bell, L.: Arginine Equivalency System. Clinical Investigation Unit, Nutrition Division, The Hospital for Sick Children, 555 University Avenue, Toronto, Ontario, Canada, M5X 1G8, 1980.

Bell, L.: H.S.C. Equivalency System for Dietary Treatment of Maple Syrup Urine Disease. Clinical Investigation Unit, Nutrition Division, The Hospital for Sick Children, 555 University Avenue, Toronto, Ontario, Canada, M5X 1G8, 1979.

Bell, L.: Low Protein Equivalency System. Clinical Investigation Unit, Nutrition Division, The Hospital for Sick Children, 555 University Avenue, Toronto, Ontario, Canada, M5X 1G8, 1981.

Bell, L.: The Phenylalanine Content of Foods. Clinical Investigation Unit, Nutrition Division, The Hospital for Sick Children, 555 University Avenue, Toronto, Ontario, Canada, M5X 1G8, 1980.

Henderson, R.A., et al.: PKU and the Schools: Information for Teachers, Administrators, and Other School Personnel. DHEW Publication No. (HSA) 80–5233, 1980.

Holtzman, N.A.: Newborn Screening for Genetic Metabolic Diseases: Progress, Principles and Recommendations. DHEW Publication No. (HSA) 77–5207, 1977.

Management of Newborn Infants with Phenylketonuria. DHEW Publication No. (HSA) 70–5211, 1979.

PKU: Phenylketonuria: A Guide to Dietary Management, Mead Johnson & Co., Evansville, Ind. 47721, 1981.

Products for Dietary Management of Inborn Errors of Metabolism and Other Special Feeding Problems. Mead Johnson & Co., Evansville, Ind. 47721, 1979, Revised 1981.

Schuett, V.E., and Gurda, R.F.: Treatment Programs for PKU in the United States: A Survey. DHEW Publication No. (HSA) 77–5207, 1977.

Cited References

1. Acosta, P.B., et al.: Intakes of one to six year old children with phenylketonuria (PKU) undergoing therapy. Am. J. Clin. Nutr., *38*:694, 1983.
2. Acosta, P.B., and Wenz, E.: Diet Management of PKU for infants and preschool children. DHEW Publication No. (HSA) 77–5209. Washington, D.C., U.S. Department of Health, Education and Welfare, 1977.
3. Acosta, P.B., Wenz, E., and Williamson, M.: Nutrient intake of treated infants with phenylketonuria. Am. J. Clin. Nutr., *30*:198, 1977.
4. Ampola, M.G.: Metabolic Disease in Pediatric Practice. Boston, Little, Brown & Co., 1982.
5. Baerlocher, K., et al.: Hereditary fructose intolerance in early childhood: a major diagnostic challenge. Helv. Paediat. Acta., *33*:465, 1978.
6. Batshaw, M.L., et al.: Treatment of inborn errors of urea synthesis: activation of alternative pathways of waste nitrogen synthesis and excretion. N. Engl. J. Med., *306*:1387, 1982.
7. Batshaw, M.L., Thomas, G.H., and Brusilow, S.W.: New approaches to diagnosis and treatment of inborn errors of urea synthesis. Pediatrics, *68*:290, 1981.
8. Brubakk, A.M., et al.: Successful treatment of severe OTC deficiency. J. Pediatr., *100*:929, 1982.
9. Brusilow, S.W., and Batshaw, M.L.: Arginine therapy of arginine-succinase deficiency. Lancet, *1*:124, 1979.
10. Cabalska, B., et al.: Termination of dietary treatment in phenylketonuria. Eur. J. Pediatr., *126*:253, 1977.
11. Clow, C.L., Reade, T.M., and Scriver, C.R.: Outcome of early and long-term management of classical maple syrup urine disease. Pediatrics, *68*:856, 1981.
12. Dobson, J.C., et al.: Intellectual performance of 36 phenylketonuria patients and their non-affected siblings. Pediatrics, *58*:53, 1976.
13. Dobson, J.C., et al.: Intellectual assessment of 111 4-year-old children with phenylketonuria. Pediatrics, *60*:885, 1977.
14. Editorial: New varieties of PKU. Lancet, *1*:304, 1979.
15. Editorial: Early diagnosis of hyperphenylalaninemia due to tetrahydrobiopterin deficiency (malignant hyperphenylalaninemia). J. Pediatr., *96*:854, 1980.
16. Fischler, K., et al.: Developmental aspects of galactosemia from infancy to childhood. Clin. Pediatr., *19*:38, 1980.
17. Hanley, W.B., et al.: Malnutrition with early treatment of phenylketonuria. Pediatr. Res., *4*:318, 1970.
18. Heffernan, J.F., and Trahms, C.M.: A model preschool for patients with phenylketonuria. J. Am. Diet Assoc., *79*:306, 1981.
19. Holm, V.A., et al.: Physical growth in phenylketonuria. II. Growth of treated children in the PKU collabortive study from birth to 4 years of age. Pediatrics, *63*:700, 1979.
20. Holt, L.E., and Snyderman, S.E.: The amino acid requirements of infants. JAMA, *175*:100, 1961.
21. Holt, L.E., and Snyderman, S.E.: The amino acid requirements of children. In Nyhan W.L. (ed.): Amino Acid Metabolism and Genetic Variation. New York, McGraw-Hill, 1967, pp. 381–390.
22. Koch, R., et al.: An approach to management of phenylketonuria. J. Pediatr., *76*:815, 1970.
23. Koch, R., et al.: Preliminary report on the effects of diet discontinuation on PKU. J. Pediatr., *100*:870, 1982.
24. Koff, E., et al.: Intelligence and phenylketonuria: effects of diet termination. J. Pediatr., *94*:534, 1979.

25. Komrower, G.M.: Inborn errors of metabolism. Ped. Rev., *2*:175, 1980.
26. Komrower, G.M., and Lee, D.H.: Long-term follow-up of galactosemia. Arch. Dis. Child., *45*:367, 1970.
27. Komrower, G.M., et al.: Management of maternal phenylketonuria: an emerging clinical problem. Brit. Med. J., *1*:1383, 1979.
28. Lenke, R.R., and Levy, H.L.: Maternal phenylketonuria and hyperphenylalaninemia: an international survey of the outcome of untreated and treated pregnancies. N. Engl. J. Med., *303*:1202, 1980.
29. Lenke, R.R., and Levy, H.L.: Maternal phenylketonuria: results of dietary therapy. Am. J. Obstet. Gynecol., *142*:548, 1982.
30. Levy, H.L.: Treatment of phenylketonuria. Prog. Clin. Biol. Res., *34*:171, 1979.
31. New issues in newborn screening for phenylketonuria and hypothyroidism: a commentary from the Committee on Genetics of the American Academy of Pediatrics. Pediatrics, *69*:104, 1982.
32. O'Flynn, M.E., et al.: The diagnosis of phenylketonuria: A report from the collaborative study of children treated for phenylketonuria. Amer. J. Dis. Child., *134*:769, 1980.
33. Schuett, V.E., Gurda, R.F., and Brown, E.S.: Diet discontinuation policies and practices of PKU clinics in the U.S. Publ. Health Rep., *70*:498, 1980.
34. Smith, I., et al.: Effect of stopping low-phenylalanine diet on intellectual progress of children with phenylketonuria. Brit. Med. J., *2*:723, 1978.
35. Smith, I., et al.: Fetal damage despite low-phenylalanine diet after conception in a phenylketonuric woman. Lancet, *1*:17, 1979.
36. Snyderman, S.: Medical and nutritional aspects of maple syrup urine disease. In Koch, R., Shaw, K.N.F., and Durkin, F. (eds.): Maple Syrup Urine Disease Symposium. DHEW Publication No. (HSA) 79–5294. Washington, D.C., U.S. Department of Health, Education and Welfare, 1979.
37. Snyderman, S.E.: Clinical aspects of disorders of the urea cycle. Pediatrics, *68*:284, 1981.
38. Snyderman, S.E., et al.: The nutritional therapy of histidinemia. J. Pediatr., *95*:712, 1979.
39. Walsher, M., and Stewart, P.M.: Organic acidemia and hyperammonaemia: review. J. Inher. Metab. Dis., *4*: 177, 1981.
40. Williamson, M.L., et al.: Correlates of intelligence tests results in treated phenylketonuric children. Pediatrics, *68*:161, 1981.
41. Wolf, B., et al.: Propionic acidemia: a clinical update. J. Pediatr., *99*:835, 1981.
42. Yudkoff, M., et al.: Errors of carbohydrate metabolism in infants and children, a survey. Clin. Pediatr., *17*: 810, 1978.

Additional References

Bell L., et al.: Dietary management of maple-syrup urine disease: extension of equivalency systems. J. Am. Diet. Assoc., *74*:357, 1979.
Bell, L., et al.: Dietary treatment of hyperornithinemia in gyrate atrophy. J. Am. Diet. Assoc., *79*:139, 1981.
DiGeorge, A., et al.: Prospective study of maple-syrup-urine disease for the first four days of life. N. Engl. J. Med., *307*: 1492, 1982.
Koch, R., and Friedman, E.G.: Accuracy of newborn screening programs for phenylketonuria. J. Pediatr., *98*:267, 1981.
Koch, R., Shaw, K.N.F., and Durkin, F. (eds.): Maple Syrup Urine Disease Symposium. DHEW Publication No. (HSA) 79–5294. Washington, D.C., U.S. Department of Health, Education and Welfare, 1979.
Levy, H.L., et al.: Maternal PKU: Proceedings of a Conference. DHHS Publication No. (HSA) 81–5299. Office of Maternal and Child Health. Rockville, Md., U.S. Department of Health and Human Services, 1981.
Levy, H.L., and Hammersen, G.: Newborn screening for galactosemia and other galactose metabolic defects. J. Pediatr., *92*:871, 1978.
Naylor, E.M., and Guthrie, R.: Newborn screening for maple-syrup urine disease. Pediatr., *61*:262, 1978.
Stanbury, J.B., et al. (eds.): The Metabolic Basis of Inherited Disease. New York, McGraw-Hill, 1982.

PART

3

FOODS

In this chapter, the four groups of foods (milk and milk products, meats and meat alternates, fruits and vegetables, and grains and cereals) will be discussed. The nutrient contributions, role in the diet, and techniques for shopping will be presented for each group.

Milk Group

The use of milk from cattle goes back to antiquity. It is mentioned in the Bible at least 50 times, and there is evidence of the common use of milk, cheese and butter in Egyptian, Greek and Roman civilizations. A 5000-year-old frieze, unearthed in the Euphrates valley, portrays men seated on low stools milking cows. Marco Polo reported in the 13th century that the Asians used dairy products.

RECOMMENDED DAILY INTAKE. The following amounts of milk are recommended every day: Children under 9 years of age should drink 2 to 3 cups. Children 9 to 12 years old should have 3 or more cups. Teenagers should receive 4 or more cups, and the adult requirement is 2 or more cups daily.

Calcium Equivalents

On the basis of calcium content, cheese and ice cream can replace the milk recommended daily. On the basis of the calcium they provide, the following are alternates for 1 cup of milk:

1$1/3$ oz. Cheddar, American or Swiss cheese
16 oz. cream cheese
1$1/3$ cups cottage cheese
1$2/3$ cups ice cream
3 cups milk sherbet
1 cup baked custard
1 cup non-fat milk
1 cup buttermilk
$1/2$ cup undiluted evaporated milk
$1/4$ cup dried non-fat milk powder
$1/4$ cup dried whole milk powder

MILK BEVERAGES

The most common use of milk is as a drink. It is also the basic ingredient in making many good-tasting, nutritious beverages. Cow's milk is most generally used, although milk from other animals such as goats is consumed in some countries where cows are scarce. Milk is available in whole, skim, evaporated, condensed, dried whole and dried skim (non-fat solids) forms.

COMPOSITION OF MILK. Milk contains high-quality protein (mainly casein with small amounts of lactalbumin and lactoglobulin), fat (cream), carbohydrate (lactose or milk sugar), the minerals calcium and phosphorus and the vitamins riboflavin, niacin, vitamin A and (when the milk is fortified) vitamin D.

The composition of milk varies to some degree with the breed of cattle, the season of the year and the feed given to the animal. However, milk purchased in the market is a mixture from different breeds and maintains a fairly constant average composition. Local and state regulations set the required butterfat and solids contents. The average composition of cow's milk is given on page 274.

NUTRITIONAL VALUE AND DIGESTIBILITY. The value of milk in the diet for all age levels has been repeatedly emphasized throughout this text. It furnishes about a hundred nutrients but is outstanding in importance for calcium, riboflavin, protein, vitamin D (when fortified) and phosphorus. Three-fourths of the calcium, nearly one-half of the riboflavin and one-fourth of the protein in the country's food supply come from milk. If milk is omitted or sparingly used in the diet, it is difficult to meet the requirement for calcium and riboflavin.

A pint of milk in the diet for an adult yields approximately 320 kcal. If energy intake must be kept down, skim milk can be used to supply all the nutients in whole milk except fat and vitamin A. (Fortified skim milk provides vitamin A and usually vitamin D.) One pint of skim milk has 180 kcal. If energy is to be increased in the diet, ingredients such as cocoa, chocolate, ice cream and malted milk can be added to milk. For example, one pint of malted milk beverage contains approximately 560 kcal. Energy values of various milk products are listed in Table 40–1.

The protein in milk, casein, is of high quality. It contains all the amino acids needed for body building and tissue repair. The carbohydrate is in the form of lactose, a disaccharide that is not as sweet as cane sugar. Lactose does not ferment readily and does not cause gastric disturbances, as do some sugars. However, some people do not digest lactose because of a defi-

Table 40–1.   APPROXIMATE NUMBER OF CALORIES IN MILK AND MILK PRODUCTS

MILK PRODUCT	QUANTITY	KCAL.
Fresh fluid whole milk	1 cup (½ pt.)	160
Fresh fluid skim milk	1 cup	90
Buttermilk (non-fat)	1 cup	90
Half-and-half	1 cup	325
Chocolate-flavored milk drink	1 cup	190
Cocoa	1 cup	235
Malted milk beverage	1 cup	280
Evaporated milk, diluted with equal amount of water	1 cup	173
Non-fat dry milk	4 tblsp. (¼ cup)	63
Ice cream	1 slice (⅛ of qt. brick)	145
Ice milk	½ cup	143
Cheddar cheese	1-in. cube	70
Cottage cheese, creamed	½ cup	120
Cottage cheese, uncreamed	½ cup	98

ciency of the enzyme lactase, and this can lead to gastrointestinal disturbances, as discussed on page 458.

The minerals found in milk, calcium and phosphorus, are essential for the structure of bones and teeth for individuals of all ages, especially infants and children.

Milk is a dependable source of vitamin A, thiamin, niacin and riboflavin. Some vitamin C is present but not in adequate quantities. Natural milk does not contain adequate vitamin D to prevent rickets and produce normal growth and tooth development, but it is especially adaptable for fortification with this vitamin. Nearly all homogenized milk, skim milk and non-fat dry milk available today is fortified with vitamin D. The fat (cream) in milk is in an emulsified form that contains vitamin A and is easily digested and well tolerated.

MILK IN THE DAILY DIET. In the amounts recommended, milk contributes significant amounts of protein to the diet. The mineral and vitamin contributions of milk are equally important.

Adults often feel that milk is not a necessary food for them, but as a source of calcium and vitamin D it appears to be extremely important in delaying osteoporosis. The objections that it is fattening or not liked can be overcome by encouraging the use of skim milk in reducing diets and incorporating milk in dishes that the person especially enjoys if milk is not liked as a beverage. Milk can be taken in the form of cheese or used in creamed soups, creamed dishes, baked products, vegetables, milk desserts and in beverages made with milk.

MAKING MILK SAFE. Most milk is pasteurized. *Pasteurized* milk has been heated to destroy pathogenic bacteria and then cooled rapidly, making it safe to drink. In addition to being pasteurized, milk may also be *homogenized*, a process that reduces the size of the

cream particles. As a result, the cream does not rise to the top of the milk but stays suspended. *Certified* milk is not pasteurized but must meet standards of cleanliness. Federal, state and local public health service legislation protects the public milk supply.

A new technique has been developed for processing milk, aseptic vacuum packing. The milk so processed is referred to as *ultra high temperature (UHT)* milk, and its advantage is its extremely long shelf life. During processing, it is heated to a very high temperature, which kills all bacteria without changing the nutritional value or taste, and then it is vacuum packed in a sterile container. Without refrigeration it can keep for a fairly long time, and with normal refrigeration it will stay fresh for many weeks and even months.

BUYER'S INFORMATION. Fresh whole or skim milk is purchased pasteurized. If the milk is "raw" it should be home-pasteurized before being consumed. Evaporated milk is purchased either in tall cans (14½ oz. by weight or 12 fluid oz.) containing 1⅔ cups or in small "baby" cans (6 oz. by weight or 5⅓ fluid oz.) containing ⅔ of a cup. Dried milk is sold in powdered form and packaged in cartons of different sizes. Dry milk costs less than other milk and can be used in place of other milk.

FILLED DAIRY PRODUCTS

Filled dairy products are often promoted as beverage alternatives to milk. These products usually have an inconsistent nutritional profile and their nutritional value is not the same as milk. Filled dairy products have about one third less calcium, half as much protein, and more sodium than real cow's milk. The fat is usually coconut oil, which is more saturated than milk fat, and instead of lactose the sugars are glucose and maltose, which have greater cariogenic properties. Many trace minerals present in milk are not present in filled dairy products.

COCOA AND CHOCOLATE

Dried cocoa beans or seeds are imported from Central and South America. Chocolate has a higher fat content, while cocoa has cornstarch incorporated into the defatted powdered form. *Theobromine*, a substance similar to caffeine, is the stimulant substance present in cocoa and chocolate.

MALTED MILK

The malted milk added to flavor a beverage is a dried and condensed mixture of milk, malt and wheat (which has had the fiber eliminated). *Malt* is defined as germinated grain, usually sprouted barley, in which the enzyme diastase has changed the starch molecules to maltose. The nutritive value of a malted milk beverage is high. Malted milk is higher in protein, calories, thiamin and vitamin A and has seven times as much iron as whole milk. There is 0.7 mg. of iron in one cup of malted milk, making it a fair source of that mineral. Sometimes ice cream is whipped into the beverage or added as a float.

WHITE SAUCE

White sauce is useful for making a number of cream-style dishes and for adding milk to the diet. Thin white sauce is blended with puréed or strained vegetables to make creamed soups; a medium white sauce is blended with meat, fish, fowl or eggs and vegetables to make creamed dishes; a thick white sauce is used as the base for soufflés and a very thick white sauce is blended with other ingredients to make croquettes. To make a white sauce, milk or some other liquid is thickened with flour or another cereal product to the desired consistency.

CREAM SOUPS

Cream soups are blends of vegetable purées or mixtures of chopped, diced or minced vegetables and meat, fish or poultry in a white sauce base.

MILK IN SIMPLE DESSERTS

Desserts bring milk to the table in simple and easy-to-digest ways. Milk sherbets, ice cream, custards (baked or soft) and puddings (bread, cornstarch, Junket, rice and Bavarian cream) belong on the list.

CHEESE

Dishes prepared with milk, eggs and cheese are sometimes called meat alternates. They can be interchanged in the menu with meat dishes because of the similarity of their nutrients, particularly animal, or complete, proteins.

BUYER'S INFORMATION. Cheeses are classified into categories of soft, semihard and hard cheeses. Cottage cheese, cream cheese and Neufchatel are unripened soft cheeses. Camembert and Brie are soft cheeses that are ripened by molds; Limburger and Liederkranz are soft cheeses ripened by bacteria. Gorgonzola, Roquefort, bleu and Stilton are semihard cheeses ripened by molds, and brick and Muenster are semihard cheeses ripened by bacteria. Among the hard cheeses without air or "gas" holes are Cheddar, Edam and Gouda, and those with holes include Swiss, Gruyère and Parmesan. Skim milk is the basis for longhorn and cottage cheese, while Cheddar is made from whole milk. A combination of milk and cream is blended into cream cheese. The domestic cheeses are usually less expensive than the imported varieties. See Table 40–2 for information about various cheeses and their uses.

COMPOSITION. Cheese of the Cheddar type contains about 25 per cent protein, 32 per cent fat, 2 per cent lactose (milk sugar), minerals (especially calcium and phosphorus), vitamins (especially vitamin A and riboflavin) and 40 per cent water. It retains most of the calcium, phosphorus and iron of milk. Except for cottage cheese, it is high in fat and, consequently, a rich source of vitamin A, containing approximately 1700 I.U. per ounce. There is considerable variation in water and fat content, depending upon whether it is made from whole or skim milk. Cottage cheese is lower in fat, with about 4.2 per cent fat if creamed and 0.3 per cent fat if uncreamed. Other low-fat cheeses are designated by asterisks in Table 40–2.

NUTRITIVE VALUE. Cheese is not equal in food value to the milk from which it is made, since some of the protein (lactalbumin), lactose, certain mineral salts (some calcium) and a portion of the vitamins are separated out and left in the whey. The milk from which cheese is made is usually not vitamin D fortified, so *cheese is not a good source of vitamin D*. The casein of milk is the main constituent of cheese. It is a high biological value protein with a high calcium content, making it a valuable food.

In general, it takes about one half pound of Cheddar cheese to give the same amount of protein as a pound of meat containing a moderate amount of bone and fat. Cottage cheese is less concentrated than Cheddar cheese, with about four fifths as much protein per pound. Cream cheese is almost entirely fat and should not be considered a protein source.

The *sodium content* of milk and milk products is fairly high, and processed cheeses have the highest sodium content. (Sodium is added in

Table 40–2.   GUIDE TO NATURAL CHEESES

KIND	CHARACTERISTICS	USES
American	See Cheddar.	See Cheddar.
Bel Paese (Bel Pah-A-say)	Mild, sweet flavor; light, creamy yellow interior; slate gray surface; soft to medium firm, creamy texture.	Appetizers, sandwiches, desserts and snacks.
Bleu	Tangy, piquant flavor; semisoft, pasty, sometimes crumbly texture; white interior marbled or streaked with blue veins of mold; resembles Roquefort.	Appetizers, salads and salad dressings, desserts and snacks.
Brick	Mild to moderately sharp flavor; semisoft to medium firm, elastic texture; creamy white to yellow interior; brownish exterior.	Appetizers, sandwiches, desserts and snacks.
Brie (Bree)	Mild to pungent flavor; soft, smooth texture; creamy yellow interior; edible thin brown and white crust.	Appetizers, sandwiches, desserts and snacks.
Caciocavallo (Ca-cheo-ca-VAL-lo)	Piquant, somewhat salty flavor—similar to Provolone, but not smoked; smooth, very firm texture; light or white interior; clay or tan colored surface.	Snacks and desserts. Suitable for grating and cooking when fully cured.
Camembert (KAM-em-bear)	Distinctive mild to tangy flavor; soft, smooth texture—almost fluid when fully ripened; creamy yellow interior; edible thin white or gray-white crust.	Appetizers, desserts and snacks.
Cheddar (often called American)	Mild to very sharp flavor; smooth texture, firm to crumbly; light cream to orange color.	Appetizers, main dishes, sauces, soups, sandwiches, salads, desserts and snacks.
Colby	Mild to mellow flavor, similar to Cheddar; softer body and more open texture than Cheddar; light cream to orange.	Sandwiches and snacks.
Cottage*	Mild, slightly acid flavor; soft, open texture with tender curds of varying size; white to creamy white.	Appetizers, salads, used in some cheesecakes.
Cream	Delicate, slightly acid flavor; soft, smooth texture; white.	Appetizers, salads, sandwiches, desserts and snacks.
Edam	Mellow, nutlike, sometimes salty flavor; rather firm, rubbery texture; creamy yellow or medium yellow-orange interior; surface coated with red wax; usually shaped like a flattened ball.	Appetizers, salads, sandwiches, sauces, desserts and snacks.
Gjetost* (YET-ost)	Sweetish, caramel flavor; firm, buttery consistency; golden brown.	Desserts and snacks.
Gorgonzola (Gor-gon-ZO-la)	Tangy, rich, spicy flavor; semisoft, pasty, sometimes crumbly texture; creamy white interior, mottled or streaked with blue-green veins of mold; clay colored surface.	Appetizers, salads, desserts and snacks.
Gouda (GOO-da)	Mellow, nutlike, often slightly acid flavor; semisoft to firm, smooth texture, often containing small holes; creamy yellow or medium yellow-orange interior; usually has red wax coating; usually shaped like a flattened ball.	Appetizers, salads, sandwiches, sauces, desserts and snacks.
Gruyère (Grew-YARE)	Nutlike, salty flavor, similar to Swiss but sharper; firm, smooth texture with small holes or eyes; light yellow.	Appetizers, desserts and snacks.
Liederkranz (LEE-der-krontz)	Robust flavor, similar to very mild Limburger; soft, smooth texture; creamy yellow interior; russet surface.	Appetizers, desserts and snacks.
Limburger	Highly pungent, very strong flavor and aroma; soft, smooth texture that usually contains small irregular openings; creamy white interior; reddish yellow surface.	Appetizers, desserts and snacks.
Mozzarella (also called Scamorza) (Mottza-REL-la)	Delicate, mild flavor; slightly firm, plastic texture; creamy white.	Main dishes such as pizza or lasagna; sandwiches and snacks.
Muenster (MUN-stir)	Mild to mellow flavor; semisoft texture with numerous small openings; creamy white interior; yellowish tan surface.	Appetizers, sandwiches, desserts and snacks.
Mysost (MEWS-ost)	Sweetish, caramel flavor; firm, buttery consistency; light brown.	Desserts and snacks.
Neufchatel (New-sha-TEL)	Mild, acid flavor; soft, smooth texture similar to cream cheese but lower in fat; white.	Salads, sandwiches, desserts and snacks.
Parmesan	Sharp, distinctive flavor; very hard, granular texture; yellowish white.	Grated for seasoning.
Port du Salut (Pore du sa-LOO)	Mellow to robust flavor similar to Gouda; semisoft, smooth elastic texture; creamy white or yellow.	Appetizers, desserts and snacks.
Provolone (Pro-vo-LO-na)	Mellow to sharp flavor, smoky and salty; firm, smooth texture; cuts without crumbling; light creamy yellow; light brown or golden yellow surface.	Appetizers, main dishes, sandwiches, desserts and snacks.
Ricotta (Ri-COT-ah)*	Mild, sweet, nutlike flavor; soft, moist texture with loose curds (fresh ricotta) or dry and suitable for grating; white.	Salads, main dishes such as lasagna and ravioli, and desserts.

Table continued on the following page

Table 40–2 GUIDE TO NATURAL CHEESES (*Continued*)

KIND	CHARACTERISTICS	USES
Romano	Very sharp, piquant flavor; very hard, granular texture; yellowish-white interior; greenish-black surface.	Seasoning and general table use; when cured one year it is suitable for grating.
Roquefort	Sharp, peppery, piquant flavor; semisoft, pasty, sometimes crumbly texture; white interior streaked with blue-green veins of mold.	Appetizers, salads and salad dressings, desserts and snacks.
Sap Sago*	Sharp, pungent, cloverlike flavor; very hard texture suitable for grating; light green or sage green.	Grated for seasoning.
Stilton	Piquant flavor, milder than Gorgonzola or Roquefort; open, flaky texture; creamy white interior streaked with blue-green veins of mold; wrinkled, melon-like rind.	Appetizers, salads, desserts and snacks.
Swiss (also called Emmentaler)	Mild, sweet, nutlike flavor; firm, smooth, elastic body with large round eyes; light yellow.	Sandwiches, salads and snacks.

From U.S. Department of Agriculture: Cheese in Family Meals: A Guide for Consumers. Home and Garden Bulletin No. 112. Washington, D.C., U.S. Government Printing Office, 1966.
*Low in fat—appropriate for low-fat diets.

processing.) For example, the sodium content of a 1-oz. slice of Cheddar cheese is 168 mg., while that of the same size slice of processed American cheese is 307 mg.

DIGESTIBILITY. Cheese is easily digested, being rich in easily assimilated fat and in protein of high biological value. In "ripened" cheese, the protein has been partially digested by bacterial action and made more soluble in the process.

YOGURT

Yogurt is a fermented milk product made from whole, low-fat or skim milk. The bacteria usually used are *Lactobacillus bulgaricus, Streptococcus thermophilus* and possibly *Lactobacillus acidophilus*. Yogurt contains all the food value of the milk from which it was made. The curd is made by the bacteria clotting the milk. There is no evidence to justify the idea that the bacteria in yogurt are needed to maintain healthy gastrointestinal tract flora.

Yogurt is not exceptionally low in calories unless it is made from skim milk and is unsweetened. One cup of this kind of yogurt would contain 90 to 100 kcal. and 8 gm. of protein, a very low kcal.:protein ratio. Sweetened, one cup of yogurt can contain as much as 260 kcal. and still only 8 gm. of protein.

Meat Group

Two or more servings from this group are suggested daily. These may consist of meats (beef, veal, pork, lamb), poultry, fish or eggs. Dry beans, dry peas and nuts may be used as alternates.

MEAT

Meat is a popular, high-quality protein food that satisfies the appetites and tastes of many people. Roasts, steaks and chops are the most popular cuts of meat, and the increased demand seems to put such cuts of meat in the highest price range. With the exception of the organ meats, which are much richer in nutrients, most of the parts of the animal are equally nutritious, although the muscular sections are tougher because of the muscle cells and connective tissue. Therefore, different methods of cooking are employed: dry heat for tender roasts, steaks and chops and moist heat for the tougher cuts.

Beef is the most popular meat eaten in this country, and there is a wide range of cuts, as shown in Figure 40–1, and quality.

KINDS OF MEAT. The kinds of meat are *beef* from cattle, *veal* from calves, *pork* from swine and *lamb* (young) and *mutton* (mature) from sheep.

A cut of meat from the market includes muscle tissue, connective tissue, fat and bone. Edible glands and organs, such as liver, heart, kidney, brains, sweetbreads and tongue are classified as glandular, organ, or *variety* meats.

NUTRITIVE VALUE. Meat is classified as a protein food with a variable amount of fat. A study by Leverton and Odell[2] of the nutritive value of cooked beef, lamb, veal and pork was made to serve as a guide in the planning and calculation of diets. It was suggested that extremely lean portions average 32 per cent protein and 8 per cent fat and that lean-plus-marble portions contain 28 per cent protein and 16 per cent fat. These figures are of special value in planning a diet of limited fat content.

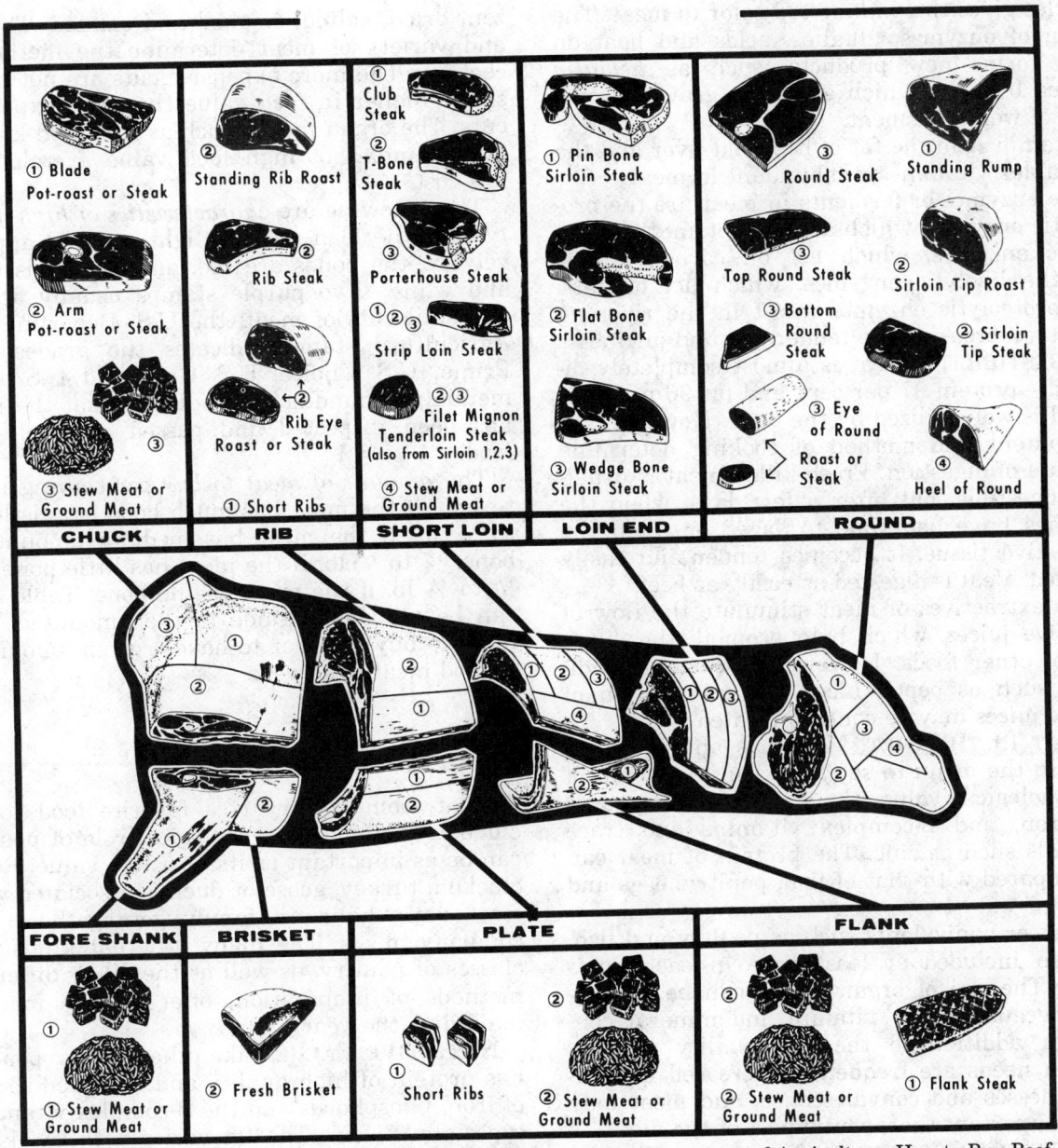

Figure 40–1. Beef chart. (From Consumer and Marketing Service, U.S. Department of Agriculture: How to Buy Beef Roasts. Home and Garden Bulletin No. 146. Washington D.C., U.S. Government Printing Office, 1968.)

Yellow connective tissue consists chiefly of the protein *elastin*, and cooking does not make it tender. White connective tissue consists chiefly of the protein *collagen*, and cooking does make it tender and soft.

The age of the animal, the amount and character of connective tissue and the deposits of fat are factors that influence the tenderness of meat. Most meat in this country is produced to contain large amounts of marbling, which Americans seem to like. However, efforts are being made to develop feeding methods that will produce meat with a lower fat content or with fat that has a greater concentration of unsatu-

rated fatty acids. This is a result of the increasing knowledge that relates a high fat intake, especially of saturated fats, to the incidence of atherosclerosis.

Meat is considered a rich source of the minerals iron and phosphorus and contains a variable amount of calcium. *Glycogen* is the type of carbohydrate found in meat. It changes to lactic acid, the non-nitrogenous extractive. The nitrogenous extractives give meat its distinctive flavor. They are the end products of protein metabolism and include such examples as creatine, creatinine, purines and other products.

The hemoglobin present in the tissues and

muscles gives the pink or red color to meat. The action of enzymes, alkalies, acids and heat on meat forms new products, such as *hematin* formed by heat, which gives the grayish-brown color of well-done meat.

Vitamin A in the fat of beef and liver and the B-complex vitamins are abundant in meat.

The enzymes or ferments in meat are the proteolytic enzymes, which act on protein, the amylolytic enzymes, which act on carbohydrates, and the lipolytic enzymes, which act on fats. The proteolytic enzymes assist in the ripening process, increasing the tenderness and juiciness.

DIGESTIBILITY. Meat is almost completely digested—protein 97 per cent and fat 96 per cent —and is well utilized by the body. However, the fat content and method of cooking determine the rate of digestion. Fresh-killed meat is usually indigestible, but after a few days, when the enzymes have had time to "age" or ripen the connective tissue, it becomes tender and easily digested. Veal is digested as easily as beef.

The extractives of meat stimulate the flow of digestive juices, which help promote the digestion of other foods. However, in certain conditions, such as peptic ulcer, the stimulation of gastric juices may be contraindicated.

MEAT IN THE DIET. Meat has an important place in the menu to supply essential protein of high biological value, the minerals phosphorus and iron, and B-complex vitamins and trace minerals such as zinc. The protein of meat can be compared with that of fish, poultry, eggs and milk.

Meat, or equivalents such as poultry and fish, is often included at least once in each day's menu. The use of organ meats can be encouraged because of the vitamin and mineral content in addition to the high-quality protein. Protein needs are frequently increased in various illnesses and convalescence, and meat may be an important therapeutic part of the diet.

EFFECT OF COOKING ON NUTRITIVE VALUE. Meat is cooked to destroy microorganisms and tenderize connective tissue. Since meat is usually eaten in cooked form, it has been necessary to determine the vitamin content of cooked meat. Studies have shown that if meat is properly cooked and all the drippings are used, 30 per cent of the thiamin, 5 per cent of the riboflavin and 5 per cent of the niacin are lost. Excessive heat destroys many nutrients in meat. Roasting and frying, for example, require high temperatures, but the damage to the heat-labile substances is counteracted somewhat by the retention of juices.

BUYER'S INFORMATION. Meat is sold cut into the standardized pieces for roasts, steaks, chops, stews and other meat dishes. It is sold fresh, frozen, dried, salted, smoked and canned. The cut and variety of meat determine the method of cookery. The more expensive cuts are not necessarily higher in food value than less expensive cuts. The organ meats, such as liver and kidney, are examples of high food value at relatively low cost.

The following are *characteristics of high-quality beef*: the lean meat is light red and appears velvety, the bones are red, and the fat is flaky and white. Two purple stamps usually appear on retail cuts of meat: the U.S. Department of Agriculture stamp indicates the grades U.S. Prime, U.S. Choice, U.S. Good and U.S. Commercial; a round stamp indicates that the meat has been inspected and passed as wholesome food.

The *amount of meat to buy* per serving is: ½ to 1 lb. if the meat has much bone or gristle, ⅓ to ½ lb. if the meat has medium amounts of bone, ¼ to ⅓ lb. if the meat has little bone and ⅕ to ¼ lb. if the meat has no bone. Table 40–3 can be used as a guide to the amount of raw meat to buy in order to have a given amount of cooked meat to serve.

POULTRY

Meat from poultry is a favorite food to include in diets. The psychological role of poultry can be as important as its nutritive value. Roast chicken, turkey, goose or duck is associated with feast days, holidays, family get-togethers and company meals. The many different kinds and classes of poultry, as well as the many different methods of preparation, offer variety for the main dish the year round.

NUTRITIVE VALUE. Like other meats, poultry has protein of high quality and is a good source of iron, phosphorus and the B-complex vitamins, especially niacin. The fat varies with the kind, age and quality of the bird. In addition, the dark meat is slightly higher in fat content than the white meat, while the white meat contains more niacin.

Poultry, as a rule, is lower in fat than beef is. For instance, 3 oz. of a lean beef cut such as flank steak has about 6 gm. of fat, while the same amount of chicken without the skin (which contains most of the fat) contains about 3 gm. of fat.

DIGESTIBILITY. The high coefficient of digestibility, as well as rapidity and ease of digestion, makes poultry a valuable addition to the menu. Since the white meat contains a little less connective tissue and fat than the dark meat, it is slightly easier to digest. Duck and goose are comparatively high in fat. Broilers and fryers,

Table 40–3.   YIELD OF COOKED MEAT PER POUND OF RAW MEAT

MEATS AS PURCHASED	MEAT AFTER COOKING (Less Drippings)	
	PARTS WEIGHED	APPROXIMATE WEIGHT OF COOKED PARTS PER LB. OF RAW MEAT (oz.)
Chops or steaks for broiling or frying		
With bone and relatively large amount of fat, such as pork or lamb chops, beef rib, sirloin or porterhouse steaks	Lean, bone and fat	10–12
	Lean and fat	7–10
	Lean only	5–7
Without bone and with very little fat, such as round of beef, veal steaks	Lean and fat	12–13
	Lean only	9–12
Ground meat for broiling or frying, such as beef, lamb or pork patties	Patties	9–13
Roasts for oven cooking (no liquid added)		
With bone and relatively large amount of fat, such as beef rib, loin, chuck; lamb shoulder, leg; pork, fresh or cured	Lean, bone and fat	10–12
	Lean and fat	8–10
	Lean only	6–9
Without bone	Lean and fat	10–12
	Lean only	7–10
Cuts for pot-roasting, simmering, braising, stewing		
With bone and relatively large amount of fat, such as beef chuck, pork shoulder	Lean, bone and fat	10–11
	Lean and fat	8–9
	Lean only	6–8
Without bone and with relatively small amount of fat, such as trimmed beef; veal	Lean with adhering fat	9–11

From Nutritive Value of Foods. Home and Garden Bulletin No. 72. Washington, D.C., U.S. Department of Agriculture, 1970.

being younger, have less fat than the older roasters and stewing birds. Turkey can be classed with the latter group.

BUYER'S INFORMATION. Many factors should be considered when buying poultry.

Kinds of Poultry. Chicken, turkey, duck and goose are the kinds of poultry most commonly eaten and, of these, chicken is by far the most plentiful and popular. Less common and more expensive birds enjoyed are Cornish game hen, guinea hen and squab (pigeon).

Class. Poultry classes within each kind are based on age, weight and sex and therefore are related to tenderness and suitable methods of cooking. A plump young chicken (usually 9 to 12 weeks of age), selected for broiling, weighs not over 2½ lb. The weight of a frying chicken averages 2½ lb to 3½ lb., and a roasting chicken (usually 3 to 5 months of age) averages 3 to 6 lb. Capons (castrated male birds), deluxe in quality, are usually under 8 months of age and weigh 6 to 9 lb., ready-to-cook weight. They are exceptionally meaty, and the flesh is juicy, tender, and unusually fine in flavor. A capon is usually roasted. Fowls or stewing chickens are mature birds (usually more than 10 months of age) and their weights are variable.

Turkeys are classed as fryers or roasters. Ducks weigh 4 lb. or under for the small size and 5 lb. or more for the large size. Ducks are usually marketed young as ducklings. Geese weigh 8 lb. or under for the small size and 10 lb. or more for the large size. Squabs and guineas are sold in some markets.

Style of Processing. Most poultry is currently marketed ready-to-cook (whole or parts), although live and dressed birds are still available in some markets. Dressed and ready-to-cook poultry is sold fresh-chilled, cold storage or quick-frozen. Cold storage poultry is kept in refrigerated storage for a minimum of 60 days. Dressed poultry indicates that the bird has been bled and the feathers removed, but the head, feet and internal organs remain. The ready-to-cook (eviscerated) poultry has been bled, feathers removed and picked and internal organs, head, feet and oil sac removed. The meat of chicken and turkey is sold frozen or canned.

Government Standards. Some poultry is labeled to show government inspection and grading, some to show inspection only, and some is neither graded nor inspected. The bird that carries an official grade mark has been examined for quality and then assigned a U.S. Grade A, B or C, according to Government standards. The inspection mark refers to the bird's wholesomeness or fitness for food.

The *best quality* poultry show these characteristics: full-fleshed and meaty breast and legs, well-distributed fat, and skin with few blemishes and pinfeathers. Young chickens and turkeys have smooth, tender skin, soft, tender meat and a flexible breastbone. An older chicken or turkey, suitable for stewing or braising, has coarser skin and a firm breastbone.

The *number of servings* obtained from poultry is dependent upon the kind, weight, age, sex, grade and method of cooking. Ready-to-cook weight of poultry to buy per serving is: ¼ to ½ chicken for broiling, about ½ lb. of chicken for frying, roasting and stewing, about 1 lb. of duck, about ⅔ lb. of goose and about ¾ lb. of turkey.

FISH

Fish is a high-quality protein food classified into categories of fresh-water fish (caught in fresh-water lakes, rivers and streams), salt-water fish and shellfish.

COMPOSITION. Fish and shellfish contain about 19 per cent protein that is similar in amino acid composition to that found in muscle meats. The fat content varies from 1 to 20 per cent, depending upon the species and the season of the year. In general, this is a lower fat content than beef. (See Appendix Table 1.)

NUTRITIVE VALUE. Fish contains protein of high biological value, essential minerals, vitamins and fats. In general, the nutritive value of fish is similar to that of beef, except that shellfish and salt-water fish are rich in iodine and fluorine, plus appreciable amounts of cobalt, and for that reason make a valuable contribution to the diet. Fish is also a satisfactory source of magnesium, phosphorus, iron and copper. The iron content of fish is lower than that found in meat, but calcium is about equal. Shellfish generally have a higher calcium and iodine content than fish. Herring and oysters are exceptionally high in zinc.

A serving of fatty fish, such as salmon or mackerel, will supply about 10 per cent of the daily allowance of vitamin A and all of the vitamin D. The natural oil found in canned fish should be used, since it too is a valuable source of these vitamins. An average serving of either fatty or lean fish will supply about 10 per cent of the thiamin, 15 per cent of the riboflavin and 50 per cent of the niacin required daily.

Fish and shellfish have high levels of polyunsaturated fatty acids, especially ω-3 fatty acids, which, as discussed on page 565, tend to lower blood cholesterol. This makes their use in certain dietary regimens desirable. However, the cholesterol content of fish muscle is similar to that of meat and poultry (50 to 70 mg. cholesterol per 100 gm. tissue). Shellfish are low in fat but relatively rich in cholesterol. (See Appendix Table 5.)

DIGESTIBILITY. Fish and shellfish are excellent sources of easily digestible protein of high nutritional value. Tests have shown that from 85 to 95 per cent of the protein is assimilable. Some individuals are very allergic to shellfish and occasionally to other fish.

BUYER'S INFORMATION. Fish is sold fresh, frozen, salted, dried and canned.

Certain varieties of fresh fish are more economical when plentiful during specific seasons of the year. Signs of freshness to be looked for in buying whole fresh fish are: eyes are bright, clear and bulging; gills are reddish-pink and free from slime; scales are tight to the skin, bright and shiny; flesh is firm and elastic; and odor is fresh. Fresh fish are marketed (1) whole or round (internal organs, scales, head, tail and fins must be removed at home before cooking), (2) drawn (whole or round fish sold after internal organs are removed), (3) dressed or pan dressed (whole or round fish sold after internal organs and scales are removed), (4) as steaks, which are cross-section slices of the larger dressed fish and are ready to cook as purchased and (5) as fillets, which are the meaty sides of the fish, cut lengthwise away from the bone. These require no preparation for cooking, and there is no waste. Here are the suggested amounts to buy per serving: 1 lb. whole or round fish, ½ lb. large dressed fish and ⅓ lb. steaks and fillets.

Smoked, dried and salted fish are sold either whole (such as herring or small whitefish) or in slices (such as codfish).

Frozen fish consist of steaks and fillets that are quick-frozen and packaged.

Canned fish include tuna, salmon, sardines and other varieties. Some manufacturers can fish with less oil or in water for the dietetic market.

The popular varieties of shellfish include oysters, clams, shrimp, crabs and lobsters.

EGGS

COMPOSITION. The average hen's egg, without shell, weighs 50 gm. The fat and protein are about equally divided, with 13 per cent protein and 12 per cent fat. The egg yolk contains half of the protein and all of the fat, minerals (except sulfur) and vitamins (except riboflavin). The egg white contains the other half of the protein and riboflavin and part of the sulfur. One egg yields an *average* of 80 kcal., of which

64 are from the yolk and only 16 from the white.

NUTRITIVE VALUE. Eggs are a good source of complete, high-quality protein, easily assimilated unsaturated fats, iron, copper, phosphorus, vitamin A, riboflavin, vitamin B_{12}, vitamin D, pantothenic acid and thiamin. All the nutritive substances, minerals and vitamins necessary for the development of the chick are furnished by the egg and can be compared in food value with milk and meat. The yolk contains most of the mineral and vitamin activity of whole egg. Eggs lack vitamin C and are a poor source of niacin. Egg protein contains somewhat higher amounts of the sulfur amino acids (methionine and cystine) than does meat. Egg yolk is high in cholesterol; the average egg yolk contains 275 mg.

The color of the shell depends upon the breed of the fowl and does not affect the nutritive value of the egg or the flavor. Neither is it a guide to yolk color. The color of the egg yolk may vary from light to deep yellow. Yolk color is influenced by heredity and diet but does not necessarily affect flavor and nutritive value. The food ration of the hen tends to affect the flavor of the egg and color of the yolk and to influence the vitamin content, especially vitamin A.

Cholesterol-free egg products have been developed for use by those who have been advised to reduce their cholesterol intake. These egg substitutes have no cholesterol, but their sodium content is often higher than that of regular eggs.

There is no evidence to say that fertile eggs have more nutritional value than infertile eggs. That the hormones in fertile eggs are needed by human beings is a fallacy.

EGGS IN THE DAILY DIET. Eggs may be served in innumerable ways for breakfast and as a main dish for luncheon or dinner, or they can be combined with other foods in the preparation of beverages, bread, cake, desserts, salads, salad dressings, sandwiches, sauces, vegetables and countless other dishes.

Fresh eggs are served poached, coddled, scrambled, baked, in omelets and in custards. Cold storage eggs are used in cooking and baking in which the flavor of the ingredients helps to mask the taste of "held" eggs. Frozen eggs and dried or dehydrated eggs can also be used in baked goods.

Eggs are useful in cooking and baking. When air is whipped into whole egg, egg yolk or egg white, the role of leavening agent comes into play. Eggs are used to thicken liquids (custards), to bind ingredients (sauces), to clarify (consommé) and to act as an emulsifying agent (mayonnaise).

DIGESTIBILITY. Eggs are easily digested and almost completely utilized. The fat in the yolk is of superior quality and is in a finely emulsified form similar to that of milk. Methods of cooking eggs affect their digestibility to some degree but do not affect their total utilization.

BUYER'S INFORMATION. Large and medium-size eggs are the most common sizes on the market. Small (pullet) eggs are usually more plentiful in the late summer and fall months. The size does not affect the quality but does affect price. Weight for weight, the nutritive value is the same for small and large eggs of equal quality.

The retail grades for shell eggs are: U.S. Grades AA, A, B and C. Factors that determine the grade are (1) cleanliness and soundness of shell, (2) size of the air cell and (3) condition of the yolk and white, which are judged by candling. Retail cartons of officially graded eggs carry a certificate stating grade, size and the date of grading.

MEAT ALTERNATES

When meat is limited, other foods—macaroni, noodles, spaghetti, rice or legumes (dried peas, beans, lentils)—can be combined with it. This is known as mutual supplementation. Meat loaf, extended with dried milk, oats, wheat germ and grated carrots and bound with egg, is an excellent source of protein. Dried skim milk, split peas or beans flavored with ham bone (or any kind of bone) furnish protein as desirable as that in expensive lamb chops. One half cup of cooked dried peas or beans furnishes about the same amount of protein as 1 oz. of meat.

At a time when famine and malnutrition exist among one eighth of the population of the world, finding less expensive ways of obtaining protein than from animals becomes very important. Grain-fed beef, so popular in the United States, is by far the most expensive form of edible protein, not only in terms of money but in terms of the amounts of protein and energy needed to raise the animal, as Figure 40–2 shows.

Nuts

Nuts are defined as a dry fruit consisting of a kernel in a shell. Since they are generally high in protein and fat, they are sometimes used as meat alternates or extenders. The nuts most commonly used are peanuts (and peanut butter), almonds, filberts, chestnuts, walnuts, cashews and Brazil nuts.

COMPOSITION. Except for the chestnut, which is high in carbohydrate and low in protein and fat, nuts are generally high in fat and protein, as shown in Table 40–4.

NUTRITIVE VALUE AND DIGESTIBILITY. Although the protein of nuts is not equal in quali-

LIVESTOCK PROTEIN CONVERSION EFFICIENCY

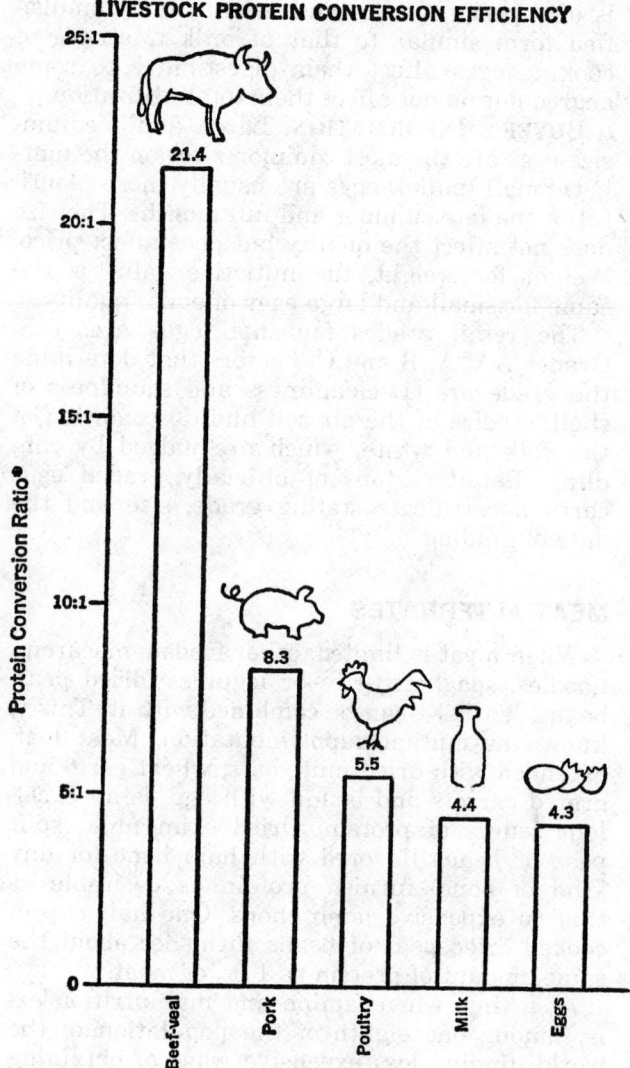

Figure 40–2. Livestock protein conversion efficiency. *Protein Conversion ratio is the number of lb. of protein fed to livestock in order to produce 1 lb. of protein for human consumption. (From Lappé, F. M.: Diet for a Small Planet. New York, Ballantine, 1971, p.7.)

ty to that of milk, eggs, cheese, meat, fish and poultry, it is of good quality and makes a valuable contribution to the diet. Nuts are a good source of the B-complex vitamins thiamin, riboflavin and niacin and of the minerals iron, copper, phosphorus and manganese. They also contain varying amounts of calcium, depending upon the variety. Since nuts are high in fat (except chestnuts), they are digested slowly. Chopped nuts and nut spreads, such as peanut butter, are more easily utilized.

USE IN THE DIET. Nuts are used as good sources of protein and as meat alternates and extenders, such as in stuffing for poultry, nut loaf, stuffed peppers, potato cakes, fritters and croquettes. In whole or chopped form they are also used as an ingredient in cakes, cookies, pies and various dessert dishes and are also used as a spread for sandwiches in the form of nut butters.

Legumes

Dry beans, peas and lentils are nutritious, low-cost foods that can be used in combination with other foods to provide good quality protein, as indicated in Figure 10–2 and Table 10–10. There are many varieties of legumes, including lima beans, split peas, lentils, red kidney beans, pinto beans, black-eyed peas, chickpeas and many others.

NUTRITIVE VALUE. Legumes supply important quantities of protein, iron, thiamin, riboflavin and trace minerals and are low in fat. One cup of cooked legumes supplies about 290 kcal., 31 per cent of the protein, 42 per cent of the iron, 26 per cent of the thiamin and 13 per cent of the riboflavin needed by an adult male.

BUYER'S INFORMATION. Beans, peas and lentils should have a bright, uniform color, be free of visible defects and be of uniform size. They

Table 40–4.   AVERAGE COMPOSITION OF COMMON NUTS

KIND	WATER (%)	PROTEIN (%)	FAT (%)	CHO (%)	KCAL. (per 100 gm.)
Almonds, dried	5	19	54	20	598
Brazil nuts	5	14	67	11	654
Butternuts	4	24	61	8	629
Cashew nuts	5	17	46	29	561
Chestnuts, fresh	53	3	2	42	194
Chestnuts, dried	8	7	4	79	377
Filberts (hazelnuts)	6	13	62	17	634
Hickory nuts	3	13	69	13	673
Peanuts, roasted	2	26	49	21	582
Pecans	3	9	71	15	687
Pistachio nuts	5	19	54	19	594
Walnuts, black	3	21	59	15	628
Walnuts, English	4	15	64	16	651

should be kept tightly covered in a cool, dry place. To compare the relative cost of legumes, nuts, peanut butter and meat, quotations of prices can be obtained from a retail store, but they should be evaluated in terms of grams of protein provided. This is easier now that nutritional labeling of food products is available. As discussed in Chapter 4, when a person is consuming most of his protein intake in the form of incomplete proteins, he may require more than the RDA of 0.8 gm. per kg. body weight.

Vegetable and Fruit Group

Four or more servings from the vegetable and fruit group are recommended daily. These should include citrus fruit or another fruit or vegetable rich in ascorbic acid, a dark green or deep yellow vegetable or vitamin A-rich vegetable (at least every other day) and other vegetables and fruits, including potatoes.

VEGETABLES

Vegetables play an important part in the diet. Yellow vegetables provide vitamin A and green vegetables furnish iron and vitamin A, while all of the vegetables are good sources of minerals, vitamins, and fiber.

Appetizing and palatable vegetables depend upon the selection of quality produce and the careful adherence to proper food preparation techniques. Overcooked, woody-textured and soggy vegetables are not appetizing and are usually refused. Rapid transportation facilities and the canning and freezing processes have largely eliminated the regional and seasonal factors in availability. Sources of supply vary with the changing seasons and with crop development in many divergent producing areas. Vegetables are usually lowest in price in any given market

area when the local supply is most abundant. Scarcity or abundance of a commodity regulates the price more often than any other factor. Many families obtain fresh vegetables from a garden planted in the back yard, and in some areas apartment dwellers can rent space in vacant lots for raising vegetables. Home food freezers and refrigerators with enough space for storing frozen foods have changed buying habits. However, the fresh vegetable flavor remains the criterion for judging both frozen and canned vegetables.

CLASSIFICATION BY NUTRITIVE VALUE. Vegetables may be classified according to the part of the plant used for food and according to nutritive value. Vegetables and parts of vegetables vary in nutritive value.

Green Leafy Vegetables. Lettuce, romaine, chicory, escarole, endive, cabbage, collards, Chinese cabbage and all greens are examples. They are most valuable for minerals, vitamins and cellulose; they are important sources of the minerals calcium and iron and of the vitamins A, K and riboflavin, and they are valuable sources of ascorbic acid. The young, tender growing leaves contain more ascorbic acid than the mature plants. The green outer leaves of lettuce and cabbage are much richer in vitamin A, calcium and iron than the white inner leaves. The thinner and greener the leaf, the richer it is in nutritive value. Green leafy vegetables are generally low in calories.

Flowering Vegetables. Broccoli and cauliflower are the two most commonly used flowering vegetables. Broccoli, being greener, rates higher in nutritive value than cauliflower and is a good source of iron, phosphorus, vitamin A, ascorbic acid and riboflavin. Cauliflower is also a good source of ascorbic acid. One half cup of cooked cauliflower contains about 70 mg. The outer leaves of cauliflower and broccoli are much higher in nutritive value than the flower buds and should be cooked or used in salads.

Seed Vegetables. Peas, beans and lentils are classified as seed vegetables or legumes. The more mature legumes provide protein (incomplete) and are frequently supplemented with complete protein foods, such as milk, eggs, meat, cheese, or other incomplete or complementary proteins, such as wheat, rice or corn, as summarized in Figure 10–2. They may be used as a main dish and are valuable for phosphorus, iron, zinc and thiamin. The fiber in soybeans appears to have unique serum cholesterol –lowering qualities. (see page 566).

Root Vegetables. Carrots, beets, turnips and white and sweet potatoes are examples of root vegetables, of which the yellow and orange varieties are rich sources of carotene. The deeper the yellow color, the greater the content of *carotene*, the precursor of vitamin A. Root vegetables in general are good sources of thiamin. White potatoes (modified underground stems) contain some ascorbic acid, and although they are not a rich source, when properly prepared and used in quantity they can add significantly to the total day's allowance.

Stem or Stalk Vegetables. Celery and asparagus are examples of stem vegetables. They contain minerals and vitamins in proportion to the green color, similar to that found in green leafy vegetables. Asparagus is a particularly good source of folic acid.

Fruit Vegetables. The tomato and pepper are the outstanding vegetables that are the fruit of the plant. Both are rich in ascorbic acid. Other fruit vegetables are cucumbers, squash, pumpkin and eggplant. Deeper green or yellow color indicates greater carotene content.

Bulb Vegetables. The onion is the outstanding example of a bulb vegetable and is a fair source of ascorbic acid.

COMPOSITION OF VEGETABLES. In general, the fresh raw product contains more vitamins and minerals than the processed product. In the raw state, vegetables are also an excellent source of dietary fiber. All vegetables have a high water content and vary in composition, even within one variety, depending upon the species, conditions of growth and method of cooking. Vegetables are composed chiefly of carbohydrates. The carbohydrate content, in general, ranges from 3 per cent—as found in the leafy and stem vegetables—to 27 per cent in sweet potatoes. The root and seed vegetables are among the richest in carbohydrate content. With the exception of legumes, vegetables contain very little protein, averaging from 1 to 3 per cent. There is little or no fat in vegetables. As discussed in Chapter 17, no evidence exists that organically grown vegetables are any richer in nutrients than traditionally grown vegetables, although they will have less pesticide residue.

DIGESTIBILITY. The great value of fresh vegetables in keeping the digestive tract functioning normally has been mentioned previously. The bulky, fibrous foods, in contrast with highly refined, concentrated foods, are essential for good digestion and elimination. Adequate bulk makes laxatives generally unnecessary.

There are some conditions, such as diarrhea, peptic ulcers and ulcerative colitis (Chapters 22 and 23), in which the use of bulky vegetables and roughage may be restricted or must be avoided. Furthermore, in conditions such as gallbladder (Chapter 24) and cardiac disease (Chapter 28) certain vegetables, commonly termed "gas-forming," may cause distress and must be used with discretion. However, the normal individual can digest vegetables with ease.

BUYER'S INFORMATION. Supply, demand and distribution are factors that influence the price of produce. Although practice is the best teacher in the selection of fresh vegetables, here are some suggested criteria for judging:

Selecting the fresh and avoiding the shriveled, wilted or decayed is the best rule to follow. Freshness, state of ripeness, firmness, lack of blemishes and no sign of spoilage are some of the guiding factors. Best quality and price are available at the peak of the season.

CANNED VEGETABLES. Commercially canned vegetables offer a large variety of products to choose from the year round, helping to keep the food budget down when certain vegetables are out of season. They are cooked and ready to eat, thus saving time and assuring no waste. The vegetables used for canning are especially grown for that purpose, picked at just the right point of maturity, vacuum sealed and subjected to pressure heat in the briefest possible time after harvesting. The process used in industrial canning does not affect the food value of carbohydrate, protein and fat, and most of the vitamin and mineral nutritive values are retained. Quality canned vegetables are preferable for plain-cooked dishes, salads or serving "as is." Second quality may do for combination dishes such as stews, casseroles or soups or when wholeness or color is not so important.

For those who count calories, limit sodium or potassium intake or are diabetic, there is an increasing number of dietetic-pack canned vegetables.

FROZEN VEGETABLES. Frozen vegetables are becoming increasingly popular and are available all year. They are ready to cook and therefore save labor and time in preparation. The nutritive value is usually equal to that of the fresh product. The best of the crop is harvested at the peak of quality and rapidly frozen within a few hours. Only solid-frozen packages should be selected, never those that are soft and starting to thaw. Refreezing after thawing lowers quality.

DRIED VEGETABLES. Besides fresh, frozen and canned, vegetables are also available in dried or dehydrated form. Legumes are the most popular dried foods and are used as supplementary protein foods. Other dried foods such as soups and seasonings (onion, garlic, parsley) are also available. They take little storage space and have a definite place in the menu.

MAINTAINING NUTRITIONAL VALUE DURING PREPARATION. Cook vegetables quickly (just until tender) in a minimum amount of water (just enough to prevent scorching) in a covered pan and serve immediately. In this respect, steaming and pressure cooking have advantages over boiling. The iron content of broccoli, for example, diminishes 50 per cent after 20 minutes of boiling. Adding bicarbonate of soda to the water softens the fiber and retains the color of green vegetables but encourages mineral and vitamin loss. Vegetables deteriorate quickly in vitamin value if exposed to air while cooking or if cooked too long. The nutritional content also suffers when vegetables are allowed to stand in the open or are warmed over. This is especially true of the ascorbic acid content of vegetables. Gordon and Noble[1] analyzed ascorbic acid values following three methods of cooking vegetables: in a pressure saucepan, in a "waterless" saucepan, and covered with boiling water. The percentage retention of ascorbic acid was highest with the pressure saucepan. The "waterless" saucepan ranked second (except for broccoli and Brussels sprouts).

Use the liquid remaining from cooked and canned vegetables to flavor soups, sauces and gravies.

Cook potatoes without peeling to retain more nutrients.

Peel or scrape any vegetables sparingly. The dark outer leaves of cabbage, head lettuce and other greens are rich in iron, calcium and vitamins.

FRUIT

Modern methods of transportation and refrigeration make it possible to have fresh fruits all year. Consumption of citrus fruits has increased greatly in the last century. Even so, clinical studies reveal that many children and adults do not get enough ascorbic acid, often because they lack knowledge about its sources and nutritive value rather than because of cost or availability.

COMPOSITION. Fruits provide energy value (through the carbohydrate content), protective vitamins and minerals and cellulose. They contain very little protein and are practically fat-free. Two exceptions to the fat rule are avocados and olives, both of which contain appreciable amounts of fat. Fruits vary widely in their carbohydrate content. The caloric value of fresh and reconstituted dried fruit is comparatively low. Dried fruit, as such, and fruits canned or frozen with sugar have increased calories, depending upon the ingredients used in processing.

NUTRITIVE VALUE. All fresh fruits contribute some ascorbic acid, but the citrus fruits are outstanding as a source of this vitamin. For example, one medium-size orange will furnish the normal adult daily requirement. Strawberries and cantaloupe are good sources, while apples and peaches are fair sources. However, a fair source can be taken in sufficient quantity to contribute substantially to the diet.

Most fruits also supply varying amounts of vitamin A and the B-complex vitamins. The yellow fruits, such as peaches, cantaloupe and apricots, are good sources of vitamin A, whereas plums and dried fruits (those not treated with sulfur dioxide) are the best sources of thiamin.

Fruits contribute appreciable amounts of the minerals iron and calcium. Among the fruits richest in iron are dried fruits of all kinds, apricots, peaches, bananas, grapes and berries. Calcium is found in small amounts in the citrus fruits (the whole fruit contains double the amount contained in an equal amount of the juice), strawberries and dried figs. Sodium, magnesium and potassium, which account for the alkaline ash of fruits when metabolized by the body, are also present in varying amounts in most fruits. Fruits are therefore an important part of the alkaline ash diets used in treating conditions such as certain types of kidney stones and kidney diseases, as discussed in Chapter 30.

Careful preparation, storage and service are essential procedures to retain the maximum value of vitamins and minerals. There is some loss of nutritive value in the process of cooking, drying or canning, but losses are not so great as at one time supposed. The frozen fruits compare favorably in vitamin content with fresh ones. Bruising, cutting and allowing fruit and fruit juice to be exposed to the air cause considerable loss of ascorbic acid.

DIGESTIBILITY. Ripe fruits are easily digested, because the sugar content (glucose and fructose) is in readily absorbable form. Emphasis should be on *ripeness*, since the sugar in green fruits is not fully developed and is therefore difficult to digest. For example, bananas are high in starch when green but when ripe the starch changes to thoroughly digestible sugars. In some conditions, fruits are tolerated better if cooked.

Fruits, like vegetables, contain indigestible cellulose that furnishes bulk necessary for good elimination and intestinal health. Of course, in certain conditions cellulose is to be avoided, as discussed in Chapters 22 and 23. Prunes and figs are especially valuable as mild laxatives.

BUYER'S INFORMATION. In selecting fresh

fruits, those with no disfigurements or just a few removable blemishes should be picked, while shriveled, wilted and decayed fruit should be rejected.

Bananas are usually purchased by the hand (5 or 6 bananas attached to stem) and by weight, and the color indicates degree of ripeness. The skin of a fully ripened banana shows brown flecks and no green tips.

Among the citrus fruits, the markings on the peel or the color of the peel does not influence the quality. Those with smooth thin skins usually indicate a high juice content. Those that are heavy for size are preferred.

MAINTAINING NUTRITIONAL VALUE DURING PREPARATION. To conserve nutrients, fruits should be peeled thinly. Juice should be extracted from fruit just before serving. Fruit juice should not be allowed to stand long after extraction or after opening the can. If juices (fresh or canned) are stored in the refrigerator, they should be put in covered containers to reduce oxidation and loss of vitamin C. Fresh fruit should be chilled before extraction of the juice.

Bread and Cereal Group

Cereal derives its name from the mythological Roman goddess of grains and harvest, Ceres, and furnishes the bulk of the world's food supply. Cereal grains are the source of many food items that are included in normal and modified diet plans. Examples are bread, crackers, cooked cereals, ready-to-eat cereals, macaroni, spaghetti, noodles, rice and barley.

CEREALS AND FLOUR

COMPOSITION. Cereal grains furnish an average of 75 per cent carbohydrate, 10 to 15 per cent protein and 2 per cent fat. A cereal grain consists of three parts: the inner germ, the protective endosperm and the outer bran layer, as shown in Figure 2–7. The *germ* is the heart or embryo of the grain, which sprouts when the seed is planted. It is one of the best sources of thiamin and vitamin E, and it contains protein of high quality, other B-complex vitamins, fat, minerals (especially iron) and carbohydrate. The *endosperm* makes up by far the largest part of the grain, or approximately 85 per cent, and is chiefly carbohydrate, with some protein in the form of gluten. The *bran*, or outer layer, is chiefly cellulose plus the B-complex vitamins and minerals, especially iron.

NUTRITIVE VALUE. In Chapter 2 the nutritive value of carbohydrates from grain sources is discussed. Cereal and cereal products furnish ap-

proximately 50 per cent of the calories for the people of the world. Whole-grain cereals, or those enriched with vitamins and minerals to whole-grain value, provide significant amounts or iron, thiamin, riboflavin and niacin.

The protein of the germ is a complete protein, but since this is the portion of the grain that spoils first, it is removed in the refining process. The protein in the endosperm is not of such high quality but contributes significantly to the total daily protein requirement. For example, when milk is used with or added to cereals and cereal products such as breakfast cereal and in bread-making, the endosperm proteins complement the protein amino acids in milk and become important and economical sources of protein.

The vitamin and mineral content of cereal grain products depends upon the amount of germ, endosperm and bran present. Whole grains include all three parts, while highly refined cereal grain products contain only the endosperm. Enriched and restored cereal products and flours have had returned some of the vitamins and minerals that were removed during the milling process, namely thiamin, riboflavin, niacin and iron. Table 40–5 reviews the enrichment requirements for flour and cereal grain foods in the United States.

BUYER'S INFORMATION. There are four different types of wheat flour. (1) Whole-wheat flour, graham flour and entire wheat flour are synonymous. (2) Flour, white flour, wheat flour and plain flour are synonymous terms, and the flour may be either bleached or unbleached. (3) Self-rising flour contains the correct proportions of leavening agent and salt. (4) Enriched flour is white flour with added vitamins and minerals.

CLASSIFICATION OF FLOURS. Flours are identified by the following classification: (1) Macaroni flours are made from durum wheats, high in protein content. (2) Bread flours are milled from blends of hard spring and hard winter wheats, bleached or unbleached. (3) General purpose or all-purpose family flours are milled from hard wheats (northern areas) and soft wheats (southern areas). (4) Pastry flours are milled usually from soft wheats. (5) Cake flours are milled from soft wheats. Other types of flour are buckwheat flour, corn flour (a byproduct of making corn meal), cottonseed flour, lima bean flour, peanut flour, potato flour, soy flour (full-fat and low-fat), rice flour and rye flour.

CEREAL GRAIN PRODUCTS. A variety of products are manufactured and processed from cereal grains. Corn meal, cornstarch and hominy (pearl, lye, granulated and grits) are processed from corn. Oatmeal or rolled oats, both regular and quick-cooking, are processed from oats. The varieties of rice include coated (white) or

Table 40-5. STANDARDS FOR ENRICHMENT OF CEREAL PRODUCTS

Minimum and Maximum Amounts of Required and Optimal Nutrients Specified for Foods Labeled "Enriched"[1]

| CEREAL PRODUCT | REQUIRED NUTRIENTS | | | | | | | | | | | OPTIONAL NUTRIENTS | | | |
	THIAMIN Min. (mg.)	THIAMIN Max. (mg.)	RIBOFLAVIN Min. (mg.)	RIBOFLAVIN Max. (mg.)	NIACIN Min. (mg.)	NIACIN Max. (mg.)	IRON Min. (mg.)	IRON Max. (mg.)	CALCIUM Min. (mg.)	CALCIUM Max. (mg.)	CALCIUM Min. (mg.)	CALCIUM Max. (mg.)	VITAMIN D Min. (I.U.)	VITAMIN D Max. (I.U.)
Per Lb. of Product														
Bread, rolls and buns, white	1.1	1.8	0.7	1.6	10.0	15.0	8.0	12.5	–	–	300	800	150	750
Cornmeal; corn grits	2.0	3.0	1.2	1.8	16.0	24.0	13.0	26.0	–	–	500	750	250	1000
Cornmeal, self-rising	2.0	3.0	1.2	1.8	16.0	24.0	13.0	26.0	–	–	500	1750	250	1000
Farina	2.0	2.5	1.2	1.5	16.0	20.0	13.0	(2)	–	–	500	(2)	250	(2)
Flour, white	2.0	2.5	1.2	1.5	16.0	20.0	13.0	16.5	–	–	500[3]	625[3]	250	1000
Flour, self-rising	2.0	2.5	1.2	1.5	16.0	20.0	13.0	16.5	500	1500	–	–	250	1000
Macaroni products; noodle products	4.0	5.0	1.7	2.2	27.0	34.0	13.0	16.5	–	–	500	625	250	1000
Rice, milled	2.0	4.0	1.2[4]	2.4[4]	16.0	32.0	13.0	26.0	–	–	500	1000	250	1000
Per 100 Gm. of Product														
Bread, rolls and buns, white	0.24	0.40	0.15	0.35	2.20	3.31	1.76	2.76	–	–	66	176	33	165
Cornmeal; corn grits	0.44	0.66	0.26	0.40	3.53	5.29	2.87	5.73	–	–	110	165	55	220
Cornmeal, self-rising	0.44	0.66	0.26	0.40	3.53	5.29	2.87	5.73	–	386	–	–	55	220
Farina	0.44	0.55	0.26	0.33	3.53	4.41	2.87	(2)	–	–	110	(2)	55	(2)
Flour, white	0.44	0.55	0.26	0.33	3.53	4.41	2.87	3.64	–	–	110[3]	138	55	220
Flour, self-rising	0.44	0.55	0.26	0.33	3.53	4.41	2.87	3.64	110	331	–	–	55	220
Macaroni products; noodle products	0.88	1.10	0.37	0.48	5.95	7.50	2.87	3.64	–	–	110	138	55	220
Rice, milled	0.44	0.88	0.26[4]	0.53[4]	3.53	7.05	2.87	5.73	–	–	110	220	55	220

*Information here, except for rice and self-rising cornmeal, from: Federal Register, Dec. 20, 1955. Information for rice and self-rising cornmeal from: Federal Register, Aug. 27, 1957 and Aug. 10, 1961 respectively. Standards became effective for latter on Jan. 27, 1962.

[1]Standards for enrichment provide for inclusion of calcium and vitamin D within stated limits as optional ingredients for products here, except self-rising cornmeal and self-rising flour; for these items calcium is required as indicated.

[2]No maximum level established.

[3]When acidified with monocalcium phosphate at specified range of 0.25 to 0.75 per cent of the finished product, calcium levels may range from 680 to 1165 mg. per lb. (150 to 257 mg. per 100 gm.).

[4]Requirement for riboflavin stayed pending further hearings.

uncoated (brown), long-, medium- and short-grain, rice bran, rice polish and wild rice. Soy grits are obtained from the soybean plant. Tapioca is available in pearl and quickcooking varieties. Crushed wheat, cracked wheat, farina, macaroni and noodle products are processed from wheat.

Seasonings

Seasoning is frequently termed the soul of cooking. The greater the skill in the art of seasoning, the better the cook. While seasonings do not add food value to the diet, they often make a dish that has been unacceptable a desirable food. The main purpose in seasoning foods is to make the product more palatable. Seasonings can do this in several ways: (1) by intensifying the basic flavor of a food, (2) by blending flavors into a more pleasing composite flavor or (3) by changing a flavor or combination of basic flavors to something quite different. Use imagination when adding that extra salt and pepper to cooked vegetables. Experiment by adding garlic or onion salt or herbs to a favorite dish. Sodium-restricted diets can be made palatable by using allowed spices, herbs and other seasonings. In general, seasonings include condiments, spices, herbs and other flavorings. It is difficult to be specific about what should be grouped under each term. They all overlap and can be grouped together roughly as "seasoning."

CONDIMENTS

Salt (sodium chloride) is by far the most commonly used seasoning and is also an essential body mineral. When used in moderation, it gives zest to and brings out the natural flavor of otherwise tasteless food. However, care should be taken not to use excess amounts that mask the natural food flavor and blunt the appetite.

Pepper ranks next to salt as the most common seasoning. It comes in two forms, white and black. Both come from the dried berries of the same tropical vine. The difference is in processing. For white pepper, the outer dark surface of the tiny berries is rubbed off and only the inside is used. White pepper is chiefly valued for its light hue. In creamy sauces, pale soups and other light-colored dishes it leaves none of the dark specks that black pepper does. It is also somewhat less pungent than black pepper.

Cayenne pepper and *paprika* are members of the pepper family. Cayenne is a pungent chili pepper used in sauces, meat and egg dishes and seafood. Paprika is a mild member of the pepper family, usually sprinkled on and used to add color and flavor to canapes, gravies, salad dressings, certain vegetables, fish and meats.

SPICES

Among the more common spices used to add flavor are cinnamon, ginger, cloves, allspice (resembles a blend of cinnamon, nutmeg and cloves), mace (flavor similar to nutmeg) and aniseed (licorice-like flavor). Table 40–6 lists the more common spices with their sources and uses.

Some spices in large amounts have been found to have pharmacological properties. Nutmeg, for instance, in doses of 1 to 2 tbsp. within 3 to 6 hours, will cause thirst, tachycardia, cutaneous flushing, hallucinations and a feeling of unreality. It has been used for this purpose by prison inmates, among others.

MONOSODIUM GLUTAMATE

Monosodium glutamate (MSG) intensifies taste rather than adding any of its own. It is a fine white powder derived from vegetable protein. Oriental cultures have used it for centuries; in fact, it is sometimes called "Chinese powder." Some people have an adverse reaction to monosodium glutamate and may experience headache, dizziness, a burning sensation in the extremities and chest pain after eating a Chinese meal, since MSG is used so much in this kind of cooking. This is called "Chinese restaurant syndrome."

HERBS

Herbs are different from spices in that spices are plant products, whereas herbs are the nonwoody plants themselves. Herbs do wonders for flavoring and seasoning foods. Go slowly at first and use only a small amount. For best results, use one teaspoonful of fresh herbs or a quarter teaspoonful of the dried varieties.

Oregano, imported from Italy and Mexico, is good in or on green salads, tomatoes, cheese dishes, lasagna, omelets, spaghetti sauces, lamb, pork, beef, beef soup, stews and meat balls.

Marjoram is of the mint family, comes from France and Chile and should be used sparingly in or on vegetables such as carrots, greens, asparagus, lima beans and squash. It can also be used in cheese, egg and chicken dishes, roast lamb, meat pies, hash, stews, stuffings, fish and vegetable sauces.

Tarragon is a leaf with anise flavor and is good added to steaks, chops, chicken, fish, vinegar, French dressing, green salad, duckling, egg dishes, sauces, tomato dishes and vegetables such as beets, greens, peas and mushrooms.

Table 40–6. SPICES—SOURCES AND USES

NAME	DESCRIPTION AND SOURCE	USES
Allspice	Dried berry of the pimento tree, grown in West Indies. Named allspice because flavor resembled blend of cinnamon, nutmeg and cloves.	Whole: for pickling, spicing meats, seasoning gravies and boiling fish. Ground: for boiled foods, cakes, puddings and relishes.
Caraway seed	Dried seeds of plant grown in Northern Europe, notably Holland.	In rye bread, sauerkraut, new cabbage and on pork, liver and kidney before cooking. In cream and other mild cheeses.
Cayenne	Ground small hot red pepper. Grown in Africa.	With meats, fish, sauces and egg dishes.
Celery seed	Small dried ripe seed-like fruit of celery. Grown in many countries, including France, India, Holland and the United States.	For fish, potato salad, tomato dishes and tomato soup. Used in pickling and salad dressing. Excellent for Irish stews. Gives variety to hamburgers.
Chili powder (blend)	Ground chili peppers (grown in Mexico, California, Carolinas and Louisiana) and blended spices. Two varieties: mild or hot.	For such Mexican dishes as *chili con carne*. Good in shellfish and oyster cocktail sauces; for boiled and scrambled eggs, gravy and stew seasoning, canned corn.
Cinnamon	Dried aromatic bark of cinnamon tree. Major source, Sri Lanka (Ceylon).	Whole pieces of bark: in pickling, preserving and stewed fruits. Ground: in baked goods and to season mincemeat.
Cloves	Nail-shaped flower bud of the clove tree. Imported from Indonesia, the Malagasy Republic and Zanzibar.	Whole: for roast ham garnish, pickling, preserving, spiced syrups and drinks. Ground: for baked goods, puddings and stews.
Curry powder (blend)	Blend of many spices, originating in India.	For curried meat, fish, eggs and chicken, curry sauce, French dressing, scalloped tomatoes and clam and fish chowder.
Ginger	Root stalk of plant grown mainly in Jamaica, West Africa, India and the Orient.	Ground: in cakes, puddings, pumpkin pie and cookies. Whole *fresh* root is used in many oriental dishes. Many canned fruits benefit by a dash of ginger, especially canned pears. Used in preserved, candied (or crystallized) and dried forms.
Mace	Part of nutmeg between shell and outer husk, orange-red in color; flavor resembles nutmeg. From Indonesia and the West Indies.	Blades used in pickling, preserving and fish sauces. Used ground in pound cake, doughnuts, yellow dishes, chocolate dishes and oyster stew. Use sparingly.
Mustard	Seed of mustard plant grown in England and other areas.	Dry ground mustard used as flavoring for sauces and gravy. Prepared mustard (blended with other spices and vinegar) used in salad dressing, with ham, frankfurters and cheese.
Nutmeg	Kernel of a fruit of that name, grown in Indonesia and the West Indies.	Whole: to be grated as needed. Ground: used in baked goods, sauces and puddings. Good sprinkled over certain vegetables, such as cauliflower. Merges well with spinach. Topping for eggnog and custards. Favorite spice for doughnuts.
Paprika	Ground sweet red pepper grown chiefly in Spain and Hungary.	For color and mild flavor in, and sprinkled on, fish, shellfish and salad dressing. Used lavishly as a garnish, also served with sweet corn on the cob. Mixed with butter to make paprika butter.
Pepper	Most generally used of all spices. A small round berry picked before ripe; grows on a climbing vine. Grown in Indonesia and India. White pepper is the mature berry with hull removed.	Whole (black and white): used in pickling, soups and meats. Ground (black and white): used in meat sauces, gravies, vegetables and egg dishes.
Poppy seed	Tiny seeds of poppy plant imported from Holland. About 900,000 seeds to the pound.	Whole: as topping for breads, rolls and cookies. Oil used in salad dressings and margarine.

Adapted from U.S. Department of the Navy publication, Navsanda, P-277.

Dill is good added to potato dishes (salad or boiled), cream or cottage cheese mixtures (canapés), fish, fish sauces, gravies, pickles, cucumbers, lamb, vegetable salads, spaghetti and tomato dishes.

Basil is an herb from west Europe that is good cooked with or sprinkled on tomato dishes especially, and on eggplant, salads, green beans, peas, potatoes, squash, meats (especially ham and lamb chops), stew, sausage, eggs, poultry, sauces, salad dressings, soups and spaghetti.

Thyme is especially good in stews, chowders, and stuffings and on tomatoes, eggplant, carrots, peas, fish and cheese dishes, breads, veal and pork. *Sage* is less subtle and may be substituted for thyme.

Fresh Plant Flavorings

For fresh flavoring, onions, garlic, parsley, shallots, mint, sage, dill and chives are among the more staple and commonly used plants.

DESSERT FLAVORINGS

Flavorings are most often thought of in connection with desserts, cakes, cookies or foods that are enhanced by the addition of extracts to lend a pleasing flavor. Vanilla, almond and fruit extracts are the ones most frequently used. Do not limit the use to one or two flavors. Try new ones or combine flavors such as vanilla and almond or lemon and orange. Coffee and chocolate are also used as flavorings. Flavorings can be purchased in artificial or natural form, and this is always noted on the label.

BUYING AND STORAGE INFORMATION

When buying a spice or an herb, make a note of the purchase date on the label and six months later discard the product if it has not been used. By that time it will have lost its true bouquet and taste. Buy in small amounts. Keep away from heat (do not put a spice shelf over a stove), because heat promotes drying and staleness. So does air; hence, a tightly covered container is a must. Shaker tops are approved as long as the openings are closed after the spice has been used. Prepared mustard and horseradish best retain flavor if refrigerated.

No matter what precautions are taken, spices start to lose savor (through evaporation of volatile oils) as soon as they are ground.

Cited References

1. Gordon, J., and Noble, I.: "Waterless" vs. boiling water cooking of vegetables. J. Am. Diet. Assoc., *44*:378, 1964.
2. Leverton, R.M., and Odell, G.V.: The Nutritive Value of Meat. Miscellaneous Publication MP–49, Stillwater, Oklahoma, Oklahoma Agricultural Experimental Station, Oklahoma State University, 1959.

APPENDIX

Appendix Table 1. NUTRITIVE VALUES OF THE EDIBLE PART OF FOODS

(Dashes (—) denote lack of reliable data for a constituent believed to be present in measurable amount)

Item No. (A)	Foods, approximate measures, units, and weight (edible part unless footnotes indicate otherwise) (B)		Grams	Water (C) Percent	Food energy (D) Calories	Protein (E) Grams	Fat (F) Grams	Fatty Acids Saturated (total) (G) Grams	Unsaturated Oleic (H) Grams	Unsaturated Linoleic (I) Grams	Carbohydrate (J) Grams	Calcium (K) Milligrams	Phosphorus (L) Milligrams	Iron (M) Milligrams	Potassium (N) Milligrams	Vitamin A value (O) International units	Thiamin (P) Milligrams	Riboflavin (Q) Milligrams	Niacin (R) Milligrams	Ascorbic acid (S) Milligrams
	DAIRY PRODUCTS (CHEESE, CREAM, IMITATION CREAM, MILK; RELATED PRODUCTS)																			
	Butter. See Fats, oils; related products, items 103-108.																			
	Cheese:																			
	Natural:																			
1	Blue	1 oz	28	42	100	6	8	5.3	1.9	0.2	1	150	110	0.1	73	200	0.01	0.11	0.3	0
2	Camembert (3 wedges per 4-oz container)	1 wedge	38	52	115	8	9	5.8	2.2	.2	Trace	147	132	.1	71	350	.01	.19	.2	0
	Cheddar:																			
3	Cut pieces	1 oz	28	37	115	7	9	6.1	2.1	.2	Trace	204	145	.2	28	300	.01	.11	Trace	0
4		1 cu in	17.2	37	70	4	6	3.7	1.3	.1	Trace	124	88	.1	17	180	Trace	.06	Trace	0
5	Shredded	1 cup	113	37	455	28	37	24.2	8.5	.7	1	815	579	.8	111	1,200	.03	.42	.1	0
	Cottage (curd not pressed down):																			
	Creamed (cottage cheese, 4% fat):																			
6	Large curd	1 cup	225	79	235	28	10	6.4	2.4	.2	6	135	297	.3	190	370	.05	.37	.3	Trace
7	Small curd	1 cup	210	79	220	26	9	6.0	2.2	.2	6	126	277	.3	177	340	.04	.34	.3	Trace
8	Low fat (2%)	1 cup	226	79	205	31	4	2.8	1.0	.1	8	155	340	.4	217	160	.05	.42	.3	Trace
9	Low fat (1%)	1 cup	226	82	165	28	2	1.5	.5	.1	6	138	302	.3	193	80	.05	.37	.3	Trace
10	Uncreamed (cottage cheese dry curd, less than 1/2% fat)	1 cup	145	80	125	25	1	.4	.1	Trace	3	46	151	.3	47	40	.04	.21	.2	0
11	Cream	1 oz	28	54	100	2	10	6.2	2.4	.2	1	23	30	.3	34	400	Trace	.06	Trace	0
	Mozzarella, made with—																			
12	Whole milk	1 oz	28	48	90	6	7	4.4	1.7	.2	1	163	117	.1	21	260	Trace	.08	Trace	0
13	Part skim milk	1 oz	28	49	80	8	5	3.1	1.2	.1	1	207	149	.1	27	180	.01	.10	Trace	0
	Parmesan, grated:																			
14	Cup, not pressed down	1 cup	100	18	455	42	30	19.1	7.7	.3	4	1,376	807	1.0	107	700	.05	.39	.3	0
15	Tablespoon	1 tbsp	5	18	25	2	2	1.0	.4	Trace	Trace	69	40	Trace	5	40	Trace	.02	Trace	0
16	Ounce	1 oz	28	18	130	12	9	5.4	2.2	.3	1	390	229	.3	30	200	.01	.11	.1	0
17	Provolone	1 oz	28	41	100	7	8	4.8	1.7	.1	1	214	141	.1	39	230	.01	.09	Trace	0
	Ricotta, made with—																			
18	Whole milk	1 cup	246	72	430	28	32	20.4	7.1	.7	7	509	389	.9	257	1,210	.03	.48	.3	0
19	Part skim milk	1 cup	246	74	340	28	19	12.1	4.7	.5	13	669	449	1.1	308	1,060	.05	.46	.2	0
20	Romano	1 oz	28	31	110	9	8	—	—	—	1	302	215	—	—	160	—	.11	Trace	0
21	Swiss	1 oz	28	37	105	8	8	5.0	1.7	.2	1	272	171	Trace	31	240	.01	.10	Trace	0
	Pasteurized process cheese:																			
22	American	1 oz	28	39	105	6	9	5.6	2.1	.2	Trace	174	211	.1	46	340	.01	.10	Trace	0
23	Swiss	1 oz	28	42	95	7	7	4.5	1.7	.1	1	219	216	.2	61	230	Trace	.08	Trace	0
24	Pasteurized process cheese food, American.	1 oz	28	43	95	6	7	4.4	1.7	.1	2	163	130	.2	79	260	.01	.13	Trace	0
25	Pasteurized process cheese spread, American.	1 oz	28	48	80	5	6	3.8	1.5	.1	2	159	202	.1	69	220	.01	.12	Trace	0
	Cream, sweet:																			
26	Half-and-half (cream and milk)	1 cup	242	81	315	7	28	17.3	7.0	.6	10	254	230	.2	314	260	.08	.36	.2	2
27		1 tbsp	15	81	20	Trace	2	1.1	.4	Trace	1	16	14	Trace	19	20	.01	.02	Trace	Trace
28	Light, coffee, or table	1 cup	240	74	470	6	46	28.8	11.7	1.0	9	231	192	.1	292	1,730	.08	.36	.1	2
29		1 tbsp	15	74	30	Trace	3	1.8	.7	.1	1	14	12	Trace	18	110	Trace	.02	Trace	Trace

(A)	(B)	(C)	(D)	(E)	(F)	(G)	(H)	(I)	(J)	(K)	(L)	(M)	(N)	(O)	(P)	(Q)	(R)	(S)
	Whipping, unwhipped (volume about double when whipped):																	
30	Light — 1 cup (239 g)	64	700	5	74	46.2	18.3	1.5	7	166	146	0.1	231	2,690	0.06	0.30	0.1	1
31	1 tbsp (15 g)	64	45	Trace	5	2.9	1.1	.1	Trace	10	9	Trace	15	170	Trace	.02	Trace	Trace
32	Heavy — 1 cup (238 g)	58	820	5	88	54.8	22.2	2.0	7	154	149	Trace	179	3,500	.05	.26	.1	Trace
33	1 tbsp (15 g)	58	80	Trace	6	3.5	1.4	.1	Trace	10	9	Trace	11	220	Trace	.02	Trace	0
34	Whipped topping, (pressurized) — 1 cup (60 g)	61	155	Trace	13	8.3	3.4	.3	7	61	54	.1	88	550	.02	.04	0	0
35	1 tbsp (3 g)	61	10	Trace	1	.4	.2	Trace	Trace	3	3	Trace	4	30	Trace	Trace	0	0
36	Cream, sour — 1 cup (230 g)	71	495	7	48	30.0	12.1	1.1	10	268	195	.1	331	1,820	.08	.34	.2	2
37	1 tbsp (12 g)	71	25	Trace	3	1.6	.6	.1	1	14	10	Trace	17	90	Trace	.02	Trace	Trace
	Cream products, imitation (made with vegetable fat): Sweet: Creamers:																	
38	Liquid (frozen) — 1 cup (245 g)	77	335	2	24	22.8	.3	Trace	28	23	157	.1	467	[1]220	0	0	0	0
39	1 tbsp (15 g)	77	20	Trace	1	1.4	Trace	Trace	2	1	10	Trace	29	[1]10	0	0	0	0
40	Powdered — 1 cup (94 g)	2	515	5	33	30.6	.9	Trace	52	21	397	.1	763	[1]190	0	[1].16	0	0
41	1 tsp (2 g)	2	10	Trace	1	.7	Trace	0	1	Trace	8	Trace	16	[1]Trace	0	[1]Trace	0	0
	Whipped topping:																	
42	Frozen — 1 cup (75 g)	50	240	1	19	16.3	1.0	.2	17	5	6	.1	14	[1]650	0	0	Trace	0
43	1 tbsp (4 g)	50	15	Trace	1	.9	.1	Trace	1	Trace	Trace	Trace	1	[1]30	0	0	0	0
44	Powdered, made with whole milk — 1 cup (80 g)	67	150	3	10	8.5	.6	.1	13	72	69	Trace	121	[1]290	.02	.09	Trace	1
45	1 tbsp (4 g)	67	10	Trace	Trace	.4	Trace	Trace	1	4	3	Trace	6	[1]10	Trace	Trace	0	Trace
46	Pressurized — 1 cup (70 g)	60	185	1	16	13.2	1.4	.2	11	4	13	Trace	13	[1]330	0	0	0	0
47	1 tbsp (4 g)	60	10	Trace	1	.8	.1	Trace	Trace	Trace	1	Trace	1	[1]20	0	0	0	0
48	Sour dressing (imitation sour cream) made with nonfat dry milk — 1 cup (235 g)	75	415	8	39	31.2	4.4	1.1	11	266	205	.1	380	[1]120	.09	.38	.2	2
49	1 tbsp (12 g)	75	20	Trace	2	1.6	.2	.1	1	14	10	Trace	19	[1]Trace	.01	.02	Trace	Trace
	Ice cream. See Milk desserts, frozen (items 75–80).																		
	Ice milk. See Milk desserts, frozen (items 81–83).																		
	Milk: Fluid:																		
50	Whole (3.3% fat) — 1 cup (244 g)	88	150	8	8	5.1	2.1	.2	11	291	228	.1	370	[2]310	.09	.40	.2	2
51	Lowfat (2%): No milk solids added — 1 cup (244 g)	89	120	8	5	2.9	1.2	.1	12	297	232	.1	377	500	.10	.40	.2	2
52	Milk solids added: Label claim less than 10 g of protein per cup — 1 cup (245 g)	89	125	9	5	2.9	1.2	.1	12	313	245	.1	397	500	.10	.42	.2	2
53	Label claim 10 or more grams of protein per cup (protein fortified) — 1 cup (246 g)	88	135	10	5	3.0	1.2	.1	14	352	276	.1	447	500	.11	.48	.2	3
54	Lowfat (1%): No milk solids added — 1 cup (244 g)	90	100	8	3	1.6	.7	.1	12	300	235	.1	381	500	.10	.41	.2	2
55	Milk solids added: Label claim less than 10 g of protein per cup — 1 cup (245 g)	90	105	9	2	1.5	.6	.1	12	313	245	.1	397	500	.10	.42	.2	2
56	Label claim 10 or more grams of protein per cup (protein fortified) — 1 cup (246 g)	89	120	10	3	1.8	.7	.1	14	349	273	.1	444	500	.11	.47	.2	3
57	Nonfat (skim): No milk solids added — 1 cup (245 g)	91	85	8	Trace	.3	.1	Trace	12	302	247	.1	406	500	.09	.34	.2	2

[1] Vitamin A value is largely from beta-carotene used for coloring. Riboflavin value for items 40–41 apply to products with added riboflavin.
[2] Applies to product without added vitamin A. With added vitamin A, value is 500 International Units (I.U.).

Table continued on the following page

From Nutritive Value of Foods. Home and Garden Bulletin Number 72. U.S. Department of Agriculture. Washington, D.C., U.S. Government Printing Office, 1981.

Appendix Table 1. NUTRITIVE VALUES OF THE EDIBLE PART OF FOODS (Continued)

(Dashes (—) denote lack of reliable data for a constituent believed to be present in measurable amount)

Item No. (A)	Foods, approximate measures, units, and weight (edible part unless footnotes indicate otherwise) (B)	Grams	Water (C) Percent	Food energy (D) Calories	Protein (E) Grams	Fat (F) Grams	Fatty Acids Saturated (total) (G) Grams	Unsaturated Oleic (H) Grams	Unsaturated Linoleic (I) Grams	Carbohydrate (J) Grams	Calcium (K) Milligrams	Phosphorus (L) Milligrams	Iron (M) Milligrams	Potassium (N) Milligrams	Vitamin A value (O) International units	Thiamin (P) Milligrams	Riboflavin (Q) Milligrams	Niacin (R) Milligrams	Ascorbic acid (S) Milligrams
	DAIRY PRODUCTS (CHEESE, CREAM, IMITATION CREAM, MILK; RELATED PRODUCTS)—Con.																		
	Milk—Continued																		
	Fluid—Continued																		
	Nonfat (skim)—Continued																		
	Milk solids added:																		
58	Label claim less than 10 g of protein per cup. — 1 cup	245	90	90	9	1	0.4	0.1	Trace	12	316	255	0.1	418	500	0.10	0.43	0.2	2
59	Label claim 10 or more grams of protein per cup (protein fortified). — 1 cup	246	89	100	10	1	.4	.1	Trace	14	352	275	.1	446	500	.11	.48	.2	3
	Buttermilk:																		
60	— 1 cup	245	90	100	8	2	1.3	.5	Trace	12	285	219	.1	371	380	.08	.38	.1	2
	Canned:																		
	Evaporated, unsweetened:																		
61	Whole milk — 1 cup	252	74	340	17	19	11.6	5.3	0.4	25	657	510	.5	764	[3]610	.12	.80	.5	5
62	Skim milk — 1 cup	255	79	200	19	1	.3	.1	Trace	29	738	497	.7	845	[4]1,000	.11	.79	.4	3
63	Sweetened, condensed — 1 cup	306	27	980	24	27	16.8	6.7	.7	166	868	775	.6	1,136	[3]1,000	.28	1.27	.6	8
	Dried:																		
64	Buttermilk — 1 cup	120	3	465	41	7	4.3	1.7	.2	59	1,421	1,119	.4	1,910	[3]260	.47	1.90	1.1	7
	Nonfat instant:																		
65	Envelope, net wt., 3.2 oz[5]	91	4	325	32	1	.4	.1	Trace	47	1,120	896	.3	1,552	[6]2,160	.38	1.59	.8	5
66	Cup[7] — 1 cup	68	4	245	24	Trace	.3	.1	Trace	35	837	670	.2	1,160	[6]1,610	.28	1.19	.6	4
	Milk beverages:																		
	Chocolate milk (commercial):																		
67	Regular — 1 cup	250	82	210	8	8	5.3	2.2	.2	26	280	251	.6	417	[3]300	.09	.41	.3	2
68	Lowfat (2%) — 1 cup	250	84	180	8	5	3.1	1.3	.1	26	284	254	.6	422	500	.10	.42	.3	2
69	Lowfat (1%) — 1 cup	250	85	160	8	3	1.5	.7	.1	26	287	257	.6	426	500	.10	.40	.2	2
70	Eggnog (commercial) — 1 cup	254	74	340	10	19	11.3	5.0	.6	34	330	278	.5	420	890	.09	.48	.3	4
	Malted milk, home-prepared with 1 cup of whole milk and 2 to 3 heaping tsp of malted milk powder (about 3/4 oz):																		
71	Chocolate — 1 cup of milk plus 3/4 oz of powder.	265	81	235	9	9	5.5	—	—	29	304	265	.5	500	330	.14	.43	.7	2
72	Natural — 1 cup of milk plus 3/4 oz of powder.	265	81	235	11	10	6.0	—	—	27	347	307	.3	529	380	.20	.54	1.3	2
	Shakes, thick:[8]																		
73	Chocolate, container, net wt., 10.6 oz. — 1 container	300	72	355	9	8	5.0	2.0	.2	63	396	378	.9	672	260	.14	.67	.4	0
74	Vanilla, container, net wt., 11 oz. — 1 container	313	74	350	12	9	5.9	2.4	.2	56	457	361	.3	572	360	.09	.61	.5	0
	Milk desserts, frozen:																		
	Ice cream:																		
	Regular (about 11% fat):																		
75	Hardened — 1/2 gal	1,064	61	2,155	38	115	71.3	28.8	2.6	254	1,406	1,075	1.0	2,052	4,340	.42	2.63	1.1	6
76	— 1 cup	133	61	270	5	14	8.9	3.6	.3	32	176	134	.1	257	540	.05	.33	.1	1
77	— 3-fl oz container	50	61	100	2	5	3.4	1.4	.1	12	66	51	Trace	96	200	.02	.12	.1	Trace
78	Soft serve (frozen custard) — 1 cup	173	60	375	7	23	13.5	5.9	.6	38	236	199	.4	338	790	.08	.45	.2	1
79	Rich (about 16% fat), hardened. — 1/2 gal	1,188	59	2,805	33	190	118.3	47.8	4.3	256	1,213	927	.8	1,771	7,200	.36	2.27	.9	5
80	— 1 cup	148	59	350	4	24	14.7	6.0	.5	32	151	115	.1	221	900	.04	.28	.1	1
	Ice milk:																		
81	Hardened (about 4.3% fat) — 1/2 gal	1,048	69	1,470	41	45	28.1	11.3	1.0	232	1,409	1,035	1.5	2,117	1,710	.61	2.78	.9	6
82	— 1 cup	131	69	185	5	6	3.5	1.4	.1	29	176	129	.1	265	210	.08	.35	.1	1

(A)	(B)		(grams)	(C)	(D)	(E)	(F)	(G)	(H)	(I)	(J)	(K)	(L)	(M)	(N)	(O)	(P)	(Q)	(R)	(S)
83	Soft serve (about 2.6% fat)	1 cup	175	70	225	8	5	2.9	1.2	0.1	38	274	202	0.3	412	180	0.12	0.54	0.2	31
84	Sherbet (about 2% fat)	1/2 gal	1,542	66	2,160	17	31	19.0	7.7	.7	469	827	594	2.5	1,585	1,480	.26	.71	1.0	31
85		1 cup	193	66	270	2	4	2.4	1.0	.1	59	103	198	.3	198	190	.03	.09	.1	4
	Milk desserts, other:																			
86	Custard, baked	1 cup	265	77	305	14	15	6.8	5.4	.7	29	297	310	1.1	387	930	.11	.50	.3	1
	Puddings:																				
	From home recipe:																				
	Starch base:																				
87	Chocolate	1 cup	260	66	385	8	12	7.6	3.3	.3	67	250	255	1.3	445	390	.05	.36	.3	1
88	Vanilla (blancmange)	1 cup	255	76	285	9	10	6.2	2.5	.2	41	298	232	Trace	352	410	.08	.41	.3	2
89	Tapioca cream	1 cup	165	72	220	8	8	4.1	2.5	.5	28	173	180	.7	223	480	.07	.30	.2	2
	From mix (chocolate) and milk:																				
90	Regular (cooked)	1 cup	260	70	320	9	8	4.3	2.6	.2	59	265	247	.8	354	340	.05	.39	.3	2
91	Instant	1 cup	260	69	325	8	7	3.6	2.2	.3	63	374	237	1.3	335	340	.08	.39	.3	2
	Yogurt:																				
	With added milk solids:																				
	Made with lowfat milk:																				
92	Fruit-flavored[9]	1 container, net wt., 8 oz	227	75	230	10	3	1.8	.6	.1	42	343	269	.2	439	[10]120	.08	.40	.2	1
93	Plain	1 container, net wt., 8 oz	227	85	145	12	4	2.3	.8	.1	16	415	326	.2	531	[10]150	.10	.49	.3	2
94	Made with nonfat milk	1 container, net wt., 8 oz	227	85	125	13	Trace	.3	.1	Trace	17	452	355	.2	579	[10]20	.11	.53	.3	2
	Without added milk solids:																				
95	Made with whole milk	1 container, net wt., 8 oz	227	88	140	8	7	4.8	1.7	.1	11	274	215	.1	351	280	.07	.32	.2	1
	EGGS																				
	Eggs, large (24 oz per dozen):																				
	Raw:																				
96	Whole, without shell	1 egg	50	75	80	6	6	1.7	2.0	.6	1	28	90	1.0	65	260	.04	.15	Trace	0
97	White	1 white	33	88	15	3	Trace	0	0	0	Trace	4	4	Trace	45	0	Trace	.09	Trace	0
98	Yolk	1 yolk	17	49	65	3	6	1.7	2.1	.6	Trace	26	86	.9	15	310	.04	.07	Trace	0
	Cooked:																				
99	Fried in butter	1 egg	46	72	85	5	6	2.4	2.2	.6	1	26	80	.9	58	290	.03	.13	Trace	0
100	Hard-cooked, shell removed	1 egg	50	75	80	6	6	1.7	2.0	.6	1	28	90	1.0	65	260	.04	.14	Trace	0
101	Poached	1 egg	50	74	80	6	6	1.7	2.0	.6	1	28	90	1.0	65	260	.04	.13	Trace	0
102	Scrambled (milk added) in butter. Also omelet.	1 egg	64	76	95	6	7	2.8	2.3	.6	1	47	97	.9	85	310	.04	.16	Trace	0
	FATS, OILS; RELATED PRODUCTS																				
	Butter:																				
	Regular (1 brick or 4 sticks per lb):																				
103	Stick (1/2 cup)	1 stick	113	16	815	1	92	57.3	23.1	2.1	Trace	27	26	.2	29	[11]3,470	.01	.04	Trace	0
104	Tablespoon (about 1/8 stick).	1 tbsp	14	16	100	Trace	12	7.2	2.9	.3	Trace	3	3	Trace	4	[11]430	Trace	Trace	Trace	0
105	Pat (1 in square, 1/3 in high; 90 per lb).	1 pat	5	16	35	Trace	4	2.5	1.0	.1	Trace	1	1	Trace	1	[11]150	Trace	Trace	Trace	0
	Whipped (6 sticks or two 8-oz containers per lb).																				
106	Stick (1/2 cup)	1 stick	76	16	540	1	61	38.2	15.4	1.4	Trace	18	17	.1	20	[11]2,310	Trace	.03	Trace	0
107	Tablespoon (about 1/8 stick).	1 tbsp	9	16	65	Trace	8	4.7	1.9	.2	Trace	2	2	Trace	2	[11]290	Trace	Trace	Trace	0
108	Pat (1 1/4 in square, 1/3 in high; 120 per lb).	1 pat	4	16	25	Trace	3	1.9	.8	.1	Trace	1	1	Trace	1	[11]120	0	Trace	Trace	0

[3] Applies to product without vitamin A added.
[4] Applies to product with added vitamin A. Without added vitamin A, value is 20 International Units (I.U.).
[5] Yields 1 qt of fluid milk when reconstituted according to package directions.
[6] Applies to product with added vitamin A.
[7] Weight applies to product with label claim of 1 1/3 cups equal 3.2 oz.
[8] Applies to products made from thick shake mixes and that do not contain added ice cream. Products made from milk shake mixes are higher in fat and usually contain added ice cream.
[9] Content of fat, vitamin A, and carbohydrate varies. Consult the label when precise values are needed for special diets.
[10] Applies to product made with milk containing no added vitamin A.
[11] Based on year-round average.

Table continued on the following page

Appendix Table 1. NUTRITIVE VALUES OF THE EDIBLE PART OF FOODS (Continued)

(Dashes (—) denote lack of reliable data for a constituent believed to be present in measurable amount)

NUTRIENTS IN INDICATED QUANTITY

Item No. (A)	Foods, approximate measures, units, and weight (edible part unless footnotes indicate otherwise) (B)	Grams	Water (C) Percent	Food energy (D) Calories	Protein (E) Grams	Fat (F) Grams	Fatty Acids Saturated (total) (G) Grams	Oleic (H) Grams	Linoleic Grams	Carbohydrate (I) Grams	Calcium (K) mg	Phosphorus (L) mg	Iron (M) mg	Potassium (N) mg	Vitamin A value (O) I.U.	Thiamin (P) mg	Riboflavin (Q) mg	Niacin (R) mg	Ascorbic acid (S) mg
	FATS, OILS; RELATED PRODUCTS—Con.																		
109	Fats, cooking (vegetable shortenings). 1 cup	200	0	1,770	0	200	48.8	88.2	48.4	0	0	0	0	0	—	0	0	0	0
110	Lard——— 1 tbsp	13	0	110	0	13	3.2	5.7	3.1	0	0	0	0	0	0	0	0	0	0
111	1 cup	205	0	1,850	0	205	81.0	83.8	20.5	0	0	0	0	0	0	0	0	0	0
112	1 tbsp	13	0	115	0	13	5.1	5.3	1.3	0	0	0	0	0	0	0	0	0	0
	Margarine: Regular (1 brick or 4 sticks per lb):																		
113	Stick (1/2 cup)——— 1 stick	113	16	815	1	92	16.7	42.9	24.9	Trace	27	26	.2	29	[1][2]3,750	.01	.04	Trace	0
114	Tablespoon (about 1/8 stick)— 1 tbsp	14	16	100	Trace	12	2.1	5.3	3.1	Trace	3	3	Trace	4	[1]2,470	Trace	Trace	Trace	0
115	Pat (1 in square, 1/3 in high; 90 per lb). 1 pat	5	16	35	Trace	4	.7	1.9	1.1	Trace	1	1	Trace	1	[1]2,170	Trace	Trace	Trace	0
116	Soft, two 8-oz containers per lb. 1 container	227	16	1,635	1	184	32.5	71.5	65.4	Trace	53	52	.4	59	[1][2]7,500	.01	.08	.1	0
117	1 tbsp	14	16	100	Trace	12	2.0	4.5	4.1	Trace	3	3	Trace	4	[1]2,470	Trace	Trace	Trace	0
	Whipped (6 sticks per lb):																		
118	Stick (1/2 cup)——— 1 stick	76	16	545	Trace	61	11.2	28.7	16.7	Trace	18	17	.1	20	[1][2]2,500	Trace	.03	Trace	0
119	Tablespoon (about 1/8 stick)— 1 tbsp	9	16	70	Trace	8	1.4	3.6	2.1	Trace	2	2	Trace	2	[1]2,310	Trace	Trace	Trace	0
	Oils, salad or cooking: Corn:																		
120	1 cup	218	0	1,925	0	218	27.7	53.6	125.1	0	0	0	0	0	—	0	0	0	0
121	1 tbsp	14	0	120	0	14	1.7	3.3	7.8	0	0	0	0	0	—	0	0	0	0
	Olive:																		
122	1 cup	216	0	1,910	0	216	30.7	154.4	17.7	0	0	0	0	0	—	0	0	0	0
123	1 tbsp	14	0	120	0	14	1.9	9.7	1.1	0	0	0	0	0	—	0	0	0	0
	Peanut:																		
124	1 cup	216	0	1,910	0	216	37.4	98.5	67.0	0	0	0	0	0	—	0	0	0	0
125	1 tbsp	14	0	120	0	14	2.3	6.2	4.2	0	0	0	0	0	—	0	0	0	0
	Safflower:																		
126	1 cup	218	0	1,925	0	218	20.5	25.9	159.8	0	0	0	0	0	—	0	0	0	0
127	1 tbsp	14	0	120	0	14	1.3	1.6	10.0	0	0	0	0	0	—	0	0	0	0
	Soybean oil, hydrogenated (partially hardened).																		
128	1 cup	218	0	1,925	0	218	31.8	93.1	75.6	0	0	0	0	0	—	0	0	0	0
	Soybean-cottonseed oil blend, hydrogenated.																		
129	1 tbsp	14	0	120	0	14	2.0	5.8	4.7	0	0	0	0	0	—	0	0	0	0
130	1 cup	218	0	1,925	0	218	38.2	63.0	99.6	0	0	0	0	0	—	0	0	0	0
131	1 tbsp	14	0	120	0	14	2.4	3.9	6.2	0	0	0	0	0	—	0	0	0	0
	Salad dressings: Commercial: Blue cheese:																		
132	Regular——— 1 tbsp	15	32	75	1	8	1.6	1.7	3.8	1	12	11	Trace	6	30	Trace	.02	Trace	Trace
133	Low calorie (5 Cal per tsp) 1 tbsp	16	84	10	Trace	1	.5	.3	Trace	1	10	8	Trace	5	30	Trace	.01	Trace	Trace
	French:																		
134	Regular——— 1 tbsp	16	39	65	Trace	6	1.1	1.3	3.2	3	2	2	.1	13	—	—	—	—	—
135	Low calorie (5 Cal per tsp) 1 tbsp	16	77	15	Trace	1	.1	.1	.4	2	2	2	.1	13	—	—	—	—	—
	Italian:																		
136	Regular——— 1 tbsp	15	28	85	Trace	9	1.6	1.9	4.7	1	2	1	Trace	2	Trace	Trace	Trace	Trace	—
137	Low calorie (2 Cal per tsp) 1 tbsp	15	90	10	Trace	1	.1	.1	.4	Trace	2	1	Trace	2	Trace	Trace	Trace	Trace	—
138	Mayonnaise——— 1 tbsp	14	15	100	Trace	11	2.0	2.4	5.6	Trace	3	4	.1	5	40	Trace	.01	Trace	—
	Mayonnaise type:																		
139	Regular——— 1 tbsp	15	41	65	Trace	6	1.1	1.4	3.2	2	2	4	Trace	1	30	Trace	Trace	Trace	—
140	Low calorie (8 Cal per tsp) 1 tbsp	16	81	20	Trace	2	.4	.4	1.0	2	3	4	Trace	1	40	Trace	Trace	Trace	Trace
141	Tartar sauce, regular——— 1 tbsp	14	34	75	Trace	8	1.5	1.8	4.1	1	3	4	.1	11	30	Trace	Trace	Trace	Trace
	Thousand Island:																		
142	Regular——— 1 tbsp	16	32	80	Trace	8	1.4	1.7	4.0	2	2	3	.1	18	50	Trace	Trace	Trace	Trace
143	Low calorie (10 Cal per tsp) 1 tbsp	15	68	25	Trace	2	.4	.4	1.0	2	2	3	.1	17	50	Trace	Trace	Trace	Trace
	From home recipe:																		
144	Cooked type[13]——— 1 tbsp	16	68	25	1	2	.5	.6	.3	2	14	15	.1	19	80	.01	.03	Trace	Trace

FISH, SHELLFISH, MEAT, POULTRY; RELATED PRODUCTS

(A)	(B)	(C)	(D)	(E)	(F)	(G)	(H)	(I)	(J)	(K)	(L)	(M)	(N)	(O)	(P)	(Q)	(R)	(S)
	Fish and shellfish:																	
145	Bluefish, baked with butter or margarine. — 3 oz (85 g)	68	135	22	4	—	—	—	0	25	244	0.6	—	40	0.09	0.08	1.6	—
	Clams:																	
146	Raw, meat only — 3 oz (85 g)	82	65	11	1	0.2	Trace	Trace	2	59	138	5.2	154	90	.08	.15	1.1	8
147	Canned, solids and liquid — 3 oz (85 g)	86	45	7	1	—	—	—	2	47	116	3.5	119	—	.01	.09	.9	—
148	Crabmeat (white or king), canned, not pressed down. — 1 cup (135 g)	77	135	24	3	.6	0.4	0.1	1	61	246	1.1	149	—	.11	.11	2.6	—
149	Fish sticks, breaded, cooked, frozen (stick, 4 by 1 by 1/2 in). — 1 fish stick or 1 oz (28 g)	66	50	5	3	—	—	—	2	3	47	.1	—	0	.01	.02	.5	—
150	Haddock, breaded, fried[14] — 3 oz (85 g)	66	140	17	5	1.4	2.2	1.2	5	34	210	1.0	296	—	.03	.06	2.7	2
151	Ocean perch, breaded, fried[14] — 1 fillet (85 g)	59	195	16	11	2.7	4.4	2.3	6	28	192	1.1	242	—	.10	.10	1.6	—
152	Oysters, raw, meat only (13–19 medium Selects). — 1 cup (240 g)	85	160	20	4	1.3	.2	.1	8	226	343	13.2	290	740	.34	.43	6.0	—
153	Salmon, pink, canned, solids and liquid. — 3 oz (85 g)	71	120	17	5	.9	.8	.1	0	[15]167	243	.7	307	60	.03	.16	6.8	—
154	Sardines, Atlantic, canned in oil, drained solids. — 3 oz (85 g)	62	175	20	9	3.0	2.5	.5	0	372	424	2.5	502	190	.02	.17	4.6	—
155	Scallops, frozen, breaded, fried, reheated. — 6 scallops (90 g)	60	175	16	8	—	—	—	9	—	—	—	—	—	—	—	—	—
156	Shad, baked with butter or margarine, bacon. — 3 oz (85 g)	64	170	20	10	—	—	—	0	20	266	.5	320	30	.11	.22	7.3	—
	Shrimp:																	
157	Canned meat — 3 oz (85 g)	70	100	21	1	.1	.1	Trace	1	98	224	2.6	104	50	.01	.03	1.5	—
158	French fried[16] — 3 oz (85 g)	57	190	17	9	2.3	3.7	2.0	9	61	162	1.7	195	70	.03	.07	2.3	—
159	Tuna, canned in oil, drained solids. — 3 oz (85 g)	61	170	24	7	1.7	1.7	.7	0	7	199	1.6	—	—	.04	.10	10.1	2
160	Tuna salad[17] — 1 cup (205 g)	70	350	30	22	4.3	6.3	6.7	7	41	291	2.7	—	590	.08	.23	10.3	—
	Meat and meat products:																	
161	Bacon, (20 slices per lb, raw), broiled or fried, crisp. — 2 slices (15 g)	8	85	4	8	2.5	3.7	.7	Trace	2	34	.5	35	0	.08	.05	.8	—
	Beef,[18] cooked:																	
	Cuts braised, simmered or pot roasted:																	
162	Lean and fat (piece, 2 1/2 by 2 1/2 by 3/4 in). — 3 oz (85 g)	53	245	23	16	6.8	6.5	.4	0	10	114	2.9	184	30	.04	.18	3.6	—
163	Lean only from item 162 — 2.5 oz (72 g)	62	140	22	5	2.1	1.8	.2	0	10	108	2.7	176	10	.04	.17	3.3	—
	Ground beef, broiled:																	
164	Lean with 10% fat — 3 oz or patty 3 by 5/8 in (85 g)	60	185	23	10	4.0	3.9	.3	0	10	196	3.0	261	20	.08	.20	5.1	—
165	Lean with 21% fat — 2.9 oz or patty 3 by 5/8 in (82 g)	54	235	20	17	7.0	6.7	.4	0	9	159	2.6	221	30	.07	.17	4.4	—
	Roast, oven cooked, no liquid added:																	
166	Relatively fat, such as rib: Lean and fat (2 pieces, 4 1/8 by 2 1/4 by 1/4 in). — 3 oz (85 g)	40	375	17	33	14.0	13.6	.8	0	8	158	2.2	189	70	.05	.13	3.1	—
167	Lean only from item 166 — 1.8 oz (51 g)	57	125	14	7	3.0	2.5	.3	0	6	131	1.8	161	10	.04	.11	2.6	—
168	Relatively lean, such as heel of round: Lean and fat (2 pieces, 4 1/8 by 2 1/4 by 1/4 in). — 3 oz (85 g)	62	165	25	7	2.8	2.7	.2	0	11	208	3.2	279	10	.06	.19	4.5	—

12 Based on average vitamin A content of fortified margarine. Federal specifications for fortified margarine require a minimum of 15,000 International Units (I.U.) of vitamin A per pound.
13 Fatty acid values apply to product made with regular-type margarine.
14 Dipped in egg, milk or water, and breadcrumbs; fried in vegetable shortening.
15 If bones are discarded, value for calcium will be greatly reduced.
16 Dipped in egg, breadcrumbs, and flour or batter.
17 Prepared with tuna, celery, salad dressing (mayonnaise type), pickle, onion, and egg.
18 Outer layer of fat on the cut was removed to within approximately 1/2 in of the lean. Deposits of fat within the cut were not removed.

Table continued on the following page

Appendix Table 1. NUTRITIVE VALUES OF THE EDIBLE PART OF FOODS (Continued)

(Dashes (—) denote lack of reliable data for a constituent believed to be present in measurable amount)

							Fatty Acids												
								Unsaturated											
Item No.	Foods, approximate measures, units, and weight (edible part unless footnotes indicate otherwise)		Water	Food energy	Protein	Fat	Saturated (total)	Oleic	Linoleic	Carbohydrate	Calcium	Phosphorus	Iron	Potassium	Vitamin A value	Thiamin	Riboflavin	Niacin	Ascorbic acid
(A)	(B)	Grams	Percent	Calories	Grams	Grams	Grams	Grams	Grams	Grams	Milligrams	Milligrams	Milligrams	Milligrams	International units	Milligrams	Milligrams	Milligrams	Milligrams
			(C)	(D)	(E)	(F)	(G)	(H)	(I)	(I)	(K)	(L)	(M)	(N)	(O)	(P)	(Q)	(R)	(S)
	FISH, SHELLFISH, MEAT, POULTRY; RELATED PRODUCTS—Con.																		
	Meat and meat products—Continued																		
	Beef,[18] cooked—Continued																		
	Roast, oven cooked, no liquid added—Continued																		
	Relatively lean such as heel of round—Continued																		
169	Lean only from item 168--- 2.8 oz	78	65	125	24	3	1.2	1.0	0.1	0	10	199	3.0	268	Trace	0.06	0.18	4.3	—
	Steak:																		
	Relatively fat—sirloin, broiled:																		
170	Lean and fat (piece, 2 1/2 by 2 1/2 by 3/4 in), 3 oz	85	44	330	20	27	11.3	11.1	.6	0	9	162	2.5	220	50	.05	.15	4.0	—
171	Lean only from item 170--- 2.0 oz	56	59	115	18	4	1.8	1.6	.2	0	7	146	2.2	202	10	.05	.14	3.6	—
	Relatively lean—round, braised:																		
172	Lean and fat (piece, 4 1/8 by 2 1/4 by 1/2 in), 3 oz	85	55	220	24	13	5.5	5.2	.4	0	10	213	3.0	272	20	.07	.19	4.8	—
173	Lean only from item 172--- 2.4 oz	68	61	130	21	4	1.7	1.5	.2	0	9	182	2.5	238	10	.05	.16	4.1	—
	Beef, canned:																		
174	Corned beef--- 3 oz	85	59	185	22	10	4.9	4.5	.2	0	17	90	3.7	440	—	.01	.20	2.9	—
175	Corned beef hash--- 1 cup	220	67	400	19	25	11.9	10.9	.5	24	29	147	4.4	142	—	.02	.20	4.6	—
176	Beef, dried, chipped--- 2 1/2-oz jar	71	48	145	24	4	2.1	2.0	.1	0	14	287	3.6	142	—	.05	.23	2.7	0
177	Beef and vegetable stew--- 1 cup	245	82	220	16	11	4.9	4.5	.2	15	29	184	2.9	613	2,400	.15	.17	4.7	17
178	Beef potpie (home recipe), baked[19] (piece, 1/3 of 9-in diam. pie). 1 piece	210	55	515	21	30	7.9	12.8	6.7	39	29	149	3.8	334	1,720	.30	.30	5.5	6
179	Chili con carne with beans, canned. 1 cup	255	72	340	19	16	7.5	6.8	.3	31	82	321	4.3	594	150	.08	.18	3.3	—
180	Chop suey with beef and pork (home recipe). 1 cup	250	75	300	26	17	8.5	6.2	.7	13	60	248	4.8	425	600	.28	.38	5.0	33
181	Heart, beef, lean, braised--- 3 oz	85	61	160	27	5	1.5	1.1	.6	1	5	154	5.0	197	20	.21	1.04	6.5	1
	Lamb, cooked:																		
	Chop, rib (cut 3 per lb with bone), broiled:																		
182	Lean and fat--- 3.1 oz	89	43	360	18	32	14.8	12.1	1.2	0	8	139	1.0	200	—	.11	.19	4.1	—
183	Lean only from item 182--- 2 oz	57	60	120	16	6	2.5	2.1	.2	0	6	121	1.1	174	—	.09	.15	3.4	—
	Leg, roasted:																		
184	Lean and fat (2 pieces, 4 1/8 by 2 1/4 by 1/4 in). 3 oz	85	54	235	22	16	7.3	6.0	.6	0	9	177	1.4	241	—	.13	.23	4.7	—
185	Lean only from item 184--- 2.5 oz	71	62	130	20	5	2.1	1.8	.2	0	9	169	1.4	227	—	.12	.21	4.4	—
	Shoulder, roasted:																		
186	Lean and fat (3 pieces, 2 1/2 by 2 1/2 by 1/4 in). 3 oz	85	50	285	18	23	10.8	8.8	.9	0	9	146	1.0	206	—	.11	.20	4.0	—
187	Lean only from item 186--- 2.3 oz	64	61	130	17	6	3.6	2.3	.2	0	8	140	1.0	193	—	.10	.18	3.7	—
188	Liver, beef, fried[20] (slice, 6 1/2 by 2 3/8 by 3/8 in).[22] 3 oz	85	56	195	22	9	2.5	3.5	.9	5	9	405	7.5	323	[2]145,390	.22	3.56	14.0	23
	Pork, cured, cooked:																		
189	Ham, light cure, lean and fat, roasted (2 pieces, 4 1/8 by 2 1/4 by 1/4 in).[22] 3 oz	85	54	245	18	19	6.8	7.9	1.7	0	8	146	2.2	199	0	.40	.15	3.1	—
	Luncheon meat:																		
190	Boiled ham, slice (8 per 8-oz pkg.). 1 oz	28	59	65	5	5	1.7	2.0	.4	0	3	47	.8	—	0	.12	.04	.7	—
191	Canned, spiced or unspiced: Slice, approx. 3 by 2 by 1/2 in. 1 slice	60	55	175	9	15	5.4	6.7	1.0	1	5	65	1.3	133	0	.19	.13	1.8	—

(A)	(B)	(C)	(D)	(E)	(F)	(G)	(H)	(I)	(J)	(K)	(L)	(M)	(N)	(O)	(P)	(Q)	(R)	(S)
	Pork, fresh,[18] cooked:																	
	Chop, loin (cut 3 per lb with bone), broiled:																	
192	Lean and fat — 2.7 oz (78)	42	305	19	25	8.9	10.4	2.2	0	9	209	2.7	216	0	0.75	0.22	4.5	—
193	Lean only from item 192 — 2 oz (56)	53	150	17	9	3.1	3.6	.8	0	7	181	2.2	192	0	.63	.18	3.8	—
	Roast, oven cooked, no liquid added:																	
194	Lean and fat (piece, 2 1/2 by 2 1/2 by 3/4 in) — 3 oz (85)	46	310	21	24	8.7	10.2	2.2	0	9	218	2.7	233	0	.78	.22	4.8	—
195	Lean only from item 194 — 2.4 oz (68)	55	175	20	10	3.5	4.1	.8	0	9	211	2.6	224	0	.73	.21	4.4	—
	Shoulder cut, simmered:																	
196	Lean and fat (3 pieces, 2 1/2 by 2 1/2 by 1/4 in) — 3 oz (85)	46	320	20	26	9.3	10.9	2.3	0	9	118	2.6	158	0	.46	.21	4.1	—
197	Lean only from item 196 — 2.2 oz (63)	60	135	18	6	2.2	2.6	.6	0	8	111	2.3	146	0	.42	.19	3.7	—
	Sausages (see also Luncheon meat (items 190-191)):																	
198	Bologna, slice (8 per 8-oz pkg.) — 1 slice (28)	56	85	3	8	3.0	3.4	.5	Trace	2	36	.5	65	—	.05	.06	.7	—
199	Braunschweiger, slice (6 per 6-oz pkg.) — 1 slice (28)	53	90	4	8	2.6	3.4	.8	1	3	69	1.7	—	1,850	.05	.41	2.3	—
200	Brown and serve (10-11 per 8-oz pkg.), browned — 1 link (17)	40	70	3	6	2.3	2.8	.7	Trace	—	—	—	—	—	—	—	—	—
201	Deviled ham, canned — 1 tbsp (13)	51	45	2	4	1.5	1.8	.4	0	1	12	.3	—	0	.02	.01	.2	—
202	Frankfurter (8 per 1-lb pkg.), cooked (reheated) — 1 frankfurter (56)	57	170	7	15	5.6	6.5	1.2	1	3	57	.8	—	—	.08	.11	1.4	—
203	Meat, potted (beef, chicken, turkey), canned — 1 tbsp (13)	61	30	2	2	—	—	—	0	—	—	—	—	—	Trace	.03	.2	—
204	Pork link (16 per 1-lb pkg.), cooked — 1 link (13)	35	60	2	6	2.1	2.4	.5	Trace	1	21	.3	35	0	.10	.04	.5	—
	Salami:																	
205	Dry type, slice (12 per 4-oz pkg.) — 1 slice (10)	30	45	2	4	1.6	1.6	.1	Trace	1	28	.4	—	—	.04	.03	.5	—
206	Cooked type, slice (8 per 8-oz pkg.) — 1 slice (28)	51	90	5	7	3.1	3.0	.2	Trace	3	57	.7	—	—	.07	.07	1.2	—
207	Vienna sausage (7 per 4-oz can) — 1 sausage (16)	63	40	2	3	1.2	1.4	.2	Trace	1	24	.3	—	—	.01	.02	.4	—
	Veal, medium fat, cooked, bone removed:																	
208	Cutlet (4 1/8 by 2 1/4 by 1/2 in), braised or broiled — 3 oz (85)	60	185	23	9	4.0	3.4	.4	0	9	196	2.7	258	—	.06	.21	4.6	—
209	Rib (2 pieces, 4 1/8 by 2 1/4 by 1/4 in), roasted — 3 oz (85)	55	230	23	14	6.1	5.1	.6	0	10	211	2.9	259	—	.11	.26	6.6	—
	Poultry and poultry products:																	
	Chicken, cooked:																	
210	Breast, fried,[23] bones removed, 1/2 breast (3.3 oz with bones) — 2.8 oz (79)	58	160	26	5	1.4	1.8	1.1	1	9	218	1.3	—	70	.04	.17	11.6	—
211	Drumstick, fried,[23] bones removed (2 oz with bones) — 1.3 oz (38)	55	90	12	4	1.1	1.3	.9	Trace	6	89	.9	—	50	.03	.15	2.7	—
212	Half broiler, broiled, bones removed (10.4 oz with bones) — 6.2 oz (176)	71	240	42	7	2.2	2.5	1.3	0	16	355	3.0	483	160	.09	.34	15.5	—
213	Chicken, canned, boneless — 3 oz (85)	65	170	18	10	3.2	3.8	2.0	0	18	210	1.3	117	200	.03	.11	3.7	3
214	Chicken a la king, cooked (home recipe) — 1 cup (245)	68	470	27	34	12.7	14.3	3.3	12	127	358	2.5	404	1,130	.10	.42	5.4	12
215	Chicken and noodles, cooked (home recipe) — 1 cup (240)	71	365	22	18	5.9	7.1	3.5	26	26	247	2.2	149	430	.05	.17	4.3	Trace

[18] Outer layer of fat on the cut was removed to within approximately 1/2 in of the lean. Deposits of fat within the cut were not removed.
[19] Crust made with vegetable shortening and enriched flour.
[20] Regular-type margarine used.
[21] Value varies widely.
[22] About one-fourth of the outer layer of fat on the cut was removed. Deposits of fat within the cut were not removed.
[23] Vegetable shortening used.

Table continued on the following page

Appendix Table 1. NUTRITIVE VALUES OF THE EDIBLE PART OF FOODS (*Continued*)

(Dashes (—) denote lack of reliable data for a constituent believed to be present in measurable amount)

Item No. (A)	Foods, approximate measures, units, and weight (edible part unless footnotes indicate otherwise) (B)	Grams	Water Percent (C)	Food energy Calories (D)	Protein Grams (E)	Fat Grams (F)	Saturated (total) Grams (G)	Oleic Grams (H)	Linoleic Grams (I)	Carbohydrate Grams (J)	Calcium Milligrams (K)	Phosphorus Milligrams (L)	Iron Milligrams (M)	Potassium Milligrams (N)	Vitamin A value International units (O)	Thiamin Milligrams (P)	Riboflavin Milligrams (Q)	Niacin Milligrams (R)	Ascorbic acid Milligrams (S)
	FISH, SHELLFISH, MEAT, POULTRY; RELATED PRODUCTS—Con.																		
	Poultry and poultry products—Continued																		
	Chicken chow mein:																		
216	Canned ------ 1 cup ------	250	89	95	7	Trace	—	—	—	18	45	35	1.3	418	150	0.05	0.10	1.0	13
217	From home recipe ------ 1 cup ------	250	78	255	31	10	2.4	3.4	3.1	10	58	293	2.5	473	280	.08	.23	4.3	10
218	Chicken potpie (home recipe), baked,[19] piece (1/3 or 9-in diam. pie). ------ 1 piece ------	232	57	545	23	31	11.3	10.9	5.6	42	70	232	3.0	343	3,090	.34	.31	5.5	5
	Turkey, roasted, flesh without skin:																		
	Dark meat, piece, 2 1/2 by 1 5/8 by 1/4 in.																		
219	4 pieces ------	85	61	175	26	7	2.1	1.5	1.5	0	—	—	2.0	338	—	.03	.20	3.6	—
	Light meat, piece, 4 by 2 by 1/4 in.																		
220	2 pieces ------	85	62	150	28	3	.9	.6	.7	0	—	—	1.0	349	—	.04	.12	9.4	—
	Light and dark meat:																		
	Chopped or diced:																		
221	1 cup ------	140	61	265	44	9	2.5	1.7	1.8	0	11	351	2.5	514	—	.07	.25	10.8	—
222	Pieces (1 slice white meat, 4 by 2 by 1/4 in with 2 slices dark meat, 2 1/2 by 1 5/8 by 1/4 in). ------ 3 pieces ------	85	61	160	27	5	1.5	1.0	1.1	0	7	213	1.5	312	—	.04	.15	6.5	—
	FRUITS AND FRUIT PRODUCTS																		
	Apples, raw, unpeeled, without cores:																		
223	2 3/4-in diam. (about 3 per lb with cores). ------ 1 apple ------	138	84	80	Trace	1	—	—	—	20	10	14	.4	152	120	.04	.03	.1	6
224	3 1/4 in diam. (about 2 per lb with cores). ------ 1 apple ------	212	84	125	Trace	1	—	—	—	31	15	21	.6	233	190	.06	.04	.2	8
225	Applejuice, bottled or canned[24] ------ 1 cup ------	248	88	120	Trace	Trace	—	—	—	30	15	22	1.5	250	—	.02	.05	.2	2[52]
	Applesauce, canned:																		
226	Sweetened ------ 1 cup ------	255	76	230	1	Trace	—	—	—	61	10	13	1.3	166	100	.05	.03	.1	3[53]
227	Unsweetened ------ 1 cup ------	244	89	100	Trace	Trace	—	—	—	26	10	12	1.2	190	100	.05	.02	.1	2[52]
	Apricots:																		
228	Raw, without pits (about 12 per lb with pits). ------ 3 apricots ------	107	85	55	1	Trace	—	—	—	14	18	25	.5	301	2,890	.03	.04	.6	11
229	Canned in heavy sirup (halves and sirup). ------ 1 cup ------	258	77	220	2	Trace	—	—	—	57	28	39	.8	604	4,490	.05	.05	1.0	10
	Dried:																		
230	Uncooked (28 large or 37 medium halves per cup). ------ 1 cup ------	130	25	340	7	1	—	—	—	86	87	140	7.2	1,273	14,170	.01	.21	4.3	16
231	Cooked, unsweetened, fruit and liquid. ------ 1 cup ------	250	76	215	4	1	—	—	—	54	55	88	4.5	795	7,500	.01	.13	2.5	8
232	Apricot nectar, canned ------ 1 cup ------	251	85	145	1	Trace	—	—	—	37	23	30	.5	379	2,380	.03	.03	.5	2[36]
	Avocados, raw, whole, without skins and seeds:																		
233	California, mid- and late-winter (with skin and seed, 3 1/8-in diam.; wt., 10 oz). ------ 1 avocado ------	216	74	370	5	37	5.5	22.0	3.7	13	22	91	1.3	1,303	630	.24	.43	3.5	30
234	Florida, late summer and fall (with skin and seed, 3 5/8-in diam.; wt., 1 lb). ------ 1 avocado ------	304	78	390	4	33	6.7	15.7	5.3	27	30	128	1.3	1,836	880	.33	.61	4.9	43
235	Banana without peel (about 2.6 per lb with peel). ------ 1 banana ------	119	76	100	1	Trace	—	—	—	26	10	31	.8	440	230	.06	.07	.8	12
236	Banana flakes ------ 1 tbsp ------	6	3	20	Trace	Trace	—	—	—	5	2	6	.2	92	50	.01	.01	.2	Trace

(A)	(B)	Measure	Grams	(C)	(D)	(E)	(F)	(G)	(H)	(I)	(J)	(K)	(L)	(M)	(N)	(O)	(P)	(Q)	(R)	(S)
237	Blackberries, raw	1 cup	144	85	85	2	1	—	—	—	19	46	27	1.3	245	290	0.04	0.06	0.6	30
238	Blueberries, raw	1 cup	145	83	90	1	1	—	—	—	22	22	19	1.5	117	150	.04	.09	.7	20
	Cantaloups. See Muskmelons (item 271).																			
	Cherries:																			
239	Sour (tart), red, pitted, canned, water pack.	1 cup	244	88	105	2	Trace	—	—	—	26	37	32	.7	317	1,660	.07	.05	.5	12
240	Sweet, raw, without pits and stems.	10 cherries	68	80	45	1	Trace	—	—	—	12	15	13	.3	129	70	.03	.04	.3	7
241	Cranberry juice cocktail, bottled, sweetened.	1 cup	253	83	165	Trace	Trace	—	—	—	42	13	8	.8	25	Trace	.03	.03	.1	[27]81
242	Cranberry sauce, sweetened, canned, strained.	1 cup	277	62	405	Trace	1	—	—	—	104	17	11	.6	83	60	.03	.03	.1	6
	Dates:																			
243	Whole, without pits	10 dates	80	23	220	2	Trace	—	—	—	58	47	50	2.4	518	40	.07	.08	1.8	0
244	Chopped	1 cup	178	23	490	4	1	—	—	—	130	105	112	5.3	1,153	90	.16	.18	3.9	0
245	Fruit cocktail, canned, in heavy sirup.	1 cup	255	80	195	1	Trace	—	—	—	50	23	31	1.0	411	360	.05	.03	1.0	5
	Grapefruit:																			
	Raw, medium, 3 3/4-in diam. (about 1 lb 1 oz):																			
246	Pink or red	1/2 grapefruit with peel[28]	241	89	50	1	Trace	—	—	—	13	20	20	.5	166	540	.05	.02	.2	44
247	White	1/2 grapefruit with peel[28]	241	89	45	1	Trace	—	—	—	12	19	19	.5	159	10	.05	.02	.2	44
248	Canned, sections with sirup	1 cup	254	81	180	2	Trace	—	—	—	45	33	36	.8	343	30	.08	.05	.5	76
	Grapefruit juice:																			
249	Raw, pink, red, or white	1 cup	246	90	95	1	Trace	—	—	—	23	22	37	.5	399	(29)	.10	.05	.5	93
	Canned, white:																			
250	Unsweetened	1 cup	247	89	100	1	Trace	—	—	—	24	20	35	1.0	400	20	.07	.05	.5	84
251	Sweetened	1 cup	250	86	135	1	Trace	—	—	—	32	20	35	1.0	405	30	.08	.05	.5	78
	Frozen, concentrate, unsweetened:																			
252	Undiluted, 6-fl oz can	1 can	207	62	300	4	1	—	—	—	72	70	124	.8	1,250	60	.29	.12	1.4	286
253	Diluted with 3 parts water by volume.	1 cup	247	89	100	1	Trace	—	—	—	24	25	42	.2	420	20	.10	.04	.5	96
254	Dehydrated crystals, prepared with water (1 lb yields about 1 gal).	1 cup	247	90	100	1	Trace	—	—	—	24	22	40	.2	412	20	.10	.05	.5	91
	Grapes, European type (adherent skin), raw:																			
255	Thompson Seedless	10 grapes	50	81	35	Trace	Trace	—	—	—	9	6	10	.2	87	50	.03	.02	.2	2
256	Tokay and Emperor, seeded types	10 grapes[30]	60	81	40	Trace	Trace	—	—	—	10	7	11	.2	99	60	.03	.02	.2	2
	Grapejuice:																			
257	Canned or bottled	1 cup	253	83	165	1	Trace	—	—	—	42	28	30	.8	293	—	.10	.05	.5	[25]Trace
	Frozen concentrate, sweetened:																			
258	Undiluted, 6-fl oz can	1 can	216	53	395	1	Trace	—	—	—	100	22	32	.9	255	40	.13	.22	1.5	[31]32
259	Diluted with 3 parts water by volume.	1 cup	250	86	135	1	Trace	—	—	—	33	8	10	.3	85	10	.05	.08	.5	[31]10
260	Grape drink, canned	1 cup	250	86	135	Trace	Trace	—	—	—	35	8	10	.3	88	—	[32].03	.03	.3	(32)
261	Lemon, raw, size 165, without peel and seeds (about 4 per lb with peels and seeds).	1 lemon	74	90	20	1	Trace	—	—	—	6	19	12	.4	102	10	.03	.01	.1	39
	Lemon juice:																			
262	Raw	1 cup	244	91	60	1	Trace	—	—	—	20	17	24	.5	344	50	.07	.02	.2	112
263	Canned, or bottled, unsweetened	1 cup	244	92	55	1	Trace	—	—	—	19	17	24	.5	344	50	.07	.02	.2	102
264	Frozen, single strength, unsweetened, 6-fl oz can.	1 can	183	92	40	1	Trace	—	—	—	13	13	16	.5	258	40	.05	.02	.2	81
	Lemonade concentrate, frozen:																			
265	Undiluted, 6-fl oz can	1 can	219	49	425	Trace	Trace	—	—	—	112	9	13	.4	153	40	.05	.06	.7	66
266	Diluted with 4 1/3 parts water by volume.	1 cup	248	89	105	Trace	Trace	—	—	—	28	2	3	.1	40	10	.01	.02	.2	17

[19] Crust made with vegetable shortening and enriched flour.
[24] Also applies to pasteurized apple cider.
[25] Applies to product without added ascorbic acid. For value of product with added ascorbic acid, refer to label.
[26] Based on product with label claim of 45% of U.S. RDA in 6 fl oz.
[27] Based on product with label claim of 100% of U.S. RDA in 6 fl oz.
[28] Weight includes peel and membranes between sections. Without these parts, the weight of the edible portion is 123 g for item 246 and 118 g for item 247.
[29] For white-fleshed varieties, value is about 20 International Units (I.U.) per cup; for red-fleshed varieties, 1,080 I.U.
[30] Weight includes seeds. Without seeds, weight of the edible portion is 57 g.
[31] Applies to product without added ascorbic acid. With added ascorbic acid, based on claim that 6 fl oz of reconstituted juice contain 45% or 50% of the U.S. RDA, value in milligrams is 108 or 120 for a 6-fl oz can (item 258), 36 or 40 for 1 cup of diluted juice (item 259).
[32] For products with added thiamin and riboflavin but without added ascorbic acid, values in milligrams would be 0.60 for thiamin, 0.80 for riboflavin, and trace for ascorbic acid. For products with only ascorbic acid added, value varies with the brand. Consult the label.

Table continued on the following page

Appendix Table 1. NUTRITIVE VALUES OF THE EDIBLE PART OF FOODS (Continued)

(Dashes (—) denote lack of reliable data for a constituent believed to be present in measurable amount)

Item No. (A)	Foods, approximate measures, units, and weight (edible part unless footnotes indicate otherwise) (B)	Grams	Water Percent (C)	Food energy Calories (D)	Protein Grams (E)	Fat Grams (F)	Saturated (total) Grams (G)	Unsaturated Oleic Grams (H)	Unsaturated Linoleic Grams (I)	Carbohydrate Grams (J)	Calcium Milligrams (K)	Phosphorus Milligrams (L)	Iron Milligrams (M)	Potassium Milligrams (N)	Vitamin A value International units (O)	Thiamin Milligrams (P)	Riboflavin Milligrams (Q)	Niacin Milligrams (R)	Ascorbic acid Milligrams (S)
	FRUITS AND FRUIT PRODUCTS—Con.																		
	Limeade concentrate, frozen:																		
267	Undiluted, 6-fl oz can — 1 can	218	50	410	Trace	Trace	—	—	—	108	11	13	0.2	129	Trace	0.02	0.02	0.2	26
268	Diluted with 4 1/3 parts water by volume. 1 cup	247	89	100	Trace	Trace	—	—	—	27	3	3	Trace	32	Trace	Trace	Trace	Trace	6
	Limejuice:																		
269	Raw — 1 cup	246	90	65	1	Trace	—	—	—	22	22	27	.5	256	20	.05	.02	.2	79
270	Canned, unsweetened — 1 cup	246	90	65	1	Trace	—	—	—	22	22	27	.5	256	20	.05	.02	.2	52
	Muskmelons, raw, with rind, without seed cavity:																		
271	Cantaloup, orange-fleshed (with rind and seed cavity, 5-in diam., 2 1/3 lb). 1/2 melon with rind[33]	477	91	80	2	Trace	—	—	—	20	38	44	1.1	682	9,240	.11	.08	1.6	90
272	Honeydew (with rind and seed cavity, 6 1/2-in diam., 5 1/4 lb). 1/10 melon with rind[33]	226	91	50	1	Trace	—	—	—	11	21	24	.6	374	60	.06	.04	.9	34
	Oranges, all commercial varieties, raw:																		
273	Whole, 2 5/8-in diam., without peel and seeds (about 2 1/2 per lb with peel and seeds). 1 orange	131	86	65	1	Trace	—	—	—	16	54	26	.5	263	260	.13	.05	.5	66
274	Sections without membranes — 1 cup	180	86	90	2	Trace	—	—	—	22	74	36	.7	360	360	.18	.07	.7	90
	Orange juice:																		
275	Raw, all varieties — 1 cup	248	88	110	2	Trace	—	—	—	26	27	42	.5	496	500	.22	.07	1.0	124
276	Canned, unsweetened — 1 cup	249	87	120	2	Trace	—	—	—	28	25	45	1.0	496	500	.17	.05	.7	100
	Frozen concentrate:																		
277	Undiluted, 6-fl oz can — 1 can	213	55	360	5	Trace	—	—	—	87	75	126	.9	1,500	1,620	.68	.11	2.8	360
278	Diluted with 3 parts water by volume. 1 cup	249	87	120	2	Trace	—	—	—	29	25	42	.2	503	540	.23	.03	.9	120
279	Dehydrated crystals, prepared with water (1 lb yields about 1 gal). 1 cup	248	88	115	1	Trace	—	—	—	27	25	40	.5	518	500	.20	.07	1.0	109
	Orange and grapefruit juice: Frozen concentrate:																		
280	Undiluted, 6-fl oz can — 1 can	210	59	330	4	1	—	—	—	78	61	99	.8	1,308	800	.48	.06	2.3	302
281	Diluted with 3 parts water by volume. 1 cup	248	88	110	1	Trace	—	—	—	26	20	32	.2	439	270	.15	.02	.7	102
282	Papayas, raw, 1/2-in cubes — 1 cup	140	89	55	1	Trace	—	—	—	14	28	22	.4	328	2,450	.06	.06	.4	78
	Peaches:																		
283	Raw: Whole, 2 1/2-in diam., peeled, pitted (about 4 per lb with peels and pits). 1 peach	100	89	40	1	Trace	—	—	—	10	9	19	.5	202	[34]1,330	.02	.05	1.0	7
284	Sliced — 1 cup	170	89	65	1	Trace	—	—	—	16	15	32	.9	343	[34]2,260	.03	.09	1.7	12
	Canned, yellow-fleshed, solids and liquid (halves or slices):																		
285	Sirup pack — 1 cup	256	79	200	1	Trace	—	—	—	51	10	31	.8	333	1,100	.03	.05	1.5	8
286	Water pack — 1 cup	244	91	75	1	Trace	—	—	—	20	10	32	.7	334	1,100	.02	.07	1.5	7
	Dried:																		
287	Uncooked — 1 cup	160	25	420	5	1	—	—	—	109	77	187	9.6	1,520	6,240	.02	.30	8.5	29
288	Cooked, unsweetened, halves and juice. 1 cup	250	77	205	3	1	—	—	—	54	38	93	4.8	743	3,050	.01	.15	3.8	5

NUTRIENTS IN INDICATED QUANTITY — Fatty Acids

(A)	(B)		(C)	(D)	(E)	(F)	(G)	(H)	(I)	(J)	(K)	(L)	(M)	(N)	(O)	(P)	(Q)	(R)	(S)
	Frozen, sliced, sweetened:																			
289	10-oz container	1 container	284	77	250	1	Trace	—	—	—	64	11	37	1.4	352	1,850	0.03	0.11	2.0	[35]116
290	Cup	1 cup	250	77	220	1	Trace	—	—	—	57	10	33	1.3	310	1,630	.03	.10	1.8	[35]103
	Pears:																			
291	Raw, with skin, cored: Bartlett, 2 1/2-in diam. (about 2 1/2 per lb with cores and stems)	1 pear	164	83	100	1	1	—	—	—	25	13	18	.5	213	30	.03	.07	.2	7
292	Bosc, 2 1/2-in diam. (about 3 per lb with cores and stems)	1 pear	141	83	85	1	1	—	—	—	22	11	16	.4	83	30	.03	.06	.1	6
293	D'Anjou, 3-in diam. (about 2 per lb with cores and stems)	1 pear	200	83	120	1	1	—	—	—	31	16	22	.6	260	40	.04	.08	.2	8
294	Canned, solids and liquid, sirup pack, heavy (halves or slices)	1 cup	255	80	195	1	1	—	—	—	50	13	18	.5	214	10	.03	.05	.3	3
	Pineapple:																			
295	Raw, diced	1 cup	155	85	80	1	Trace	—	—	—	21	26	12	.8	226	110	.14	.05	.3	26
	Canned, heavy sirup pack, solids and liquid:																			
296	Crushed, chunks, tidbits	1 cup	255	80	190	1	Trace	—	—	—	49	28	13	.8	245	130	.20	.05	.5	18
	Slices and liquid:																			
297	Large	1 slice; 2 1/4 tbsp liquid	105	80	80	Trace	Trace	—	—	—	20	12	5	.3	101	50	.08	.02	.2	7
298	Medium	1 slice; 1 1/4 tbsp liquid	58	80	45	Trace	Trace	—	—	—	11	6	3	.2	56	30	.05	.01	.1	4
299	Pineapple juice, unsweetened, canned	1 cup	250	86	140	1	Trace	—	—	—	34	38	23	.8	373	130	.13	.05	.5	[27]80
	Plums:																			
300	Raw, without pits: Japanese and hybrid (2 1/8-in diam., about 6 1/2 per lb with pits)	1 plum	66	87	30	Trace	Trace	—	—	—	8	8	12	.3	112	160	.02	.03	.3	4
301	Prune-type (1 1/2-in diam., about 15 per lb with pits)	1 plum	28	79	20	Trace	Trace	—	—	—	6	3	5	.1	48	80	.01	.01	.1	1
	Canned, heavy sirup pack (Italian prunes), with pits and liquid:																			
302	Cup[36]	1 cup[36]	272	77	215	1	Trace	—	—	—	56	23	26	2.3	367	3,130	.05	.05	1.0	5
303	Portion	3 plums; 2 3/4 tbsp liquid[36]	140	77	110	1	Trace	—	—	—	29	12	13	1.2	189	1,610	.03	.03	.5	3
	Prunes, dried, "softenized," with pits:																			
304	Uncooked	4 extra large or 5 large prunes[36]	49	28	110	1	Trace	—	—	—	29	22	34	1.7	298	690	.04	.07	.7	1
305	Cooked, unsweetened, all sizes, fruit and liquid	1 cup[36]	250	66	255	2	1	—	—	—	67	51	79	3.8	695	1,590	.07	.15	1.5	2
306	Prune juice, canned or bottled	1 cup	256	80	195	1	Trace	—	—	—	49	36	51	1.8	602	—	.03	.03	1.0	5
	Raisins, seedless:																			
307	Cup, not pressed down	1 cup	145	18	420	4	Trace	—	—	—	112	90	146	5.1	1,106	30	.16	.12	.7	1
308	Packet, 1/2 oz (1 1/2 tbsp)	1 packet	14	18	40	Trace	Trace	—	—	—	11	9	14	.5	107	Trace	.02	.01	.1	Trace
	Raspberries, red:																			
309	Raw, capped, whole	1 cup	123	84	70	1	1	—	—	—	17	27	27	1.1	207	160	.04	.11	1.1	31
310	Frozen, sweetened, 10-oz container	1 container	284	74	280	2	1	—	—	—	70	37	48	1.7	284	200	.06	.17	1.7	60
	Rhubarb, cooked, added sugar:																			
311	From raw	1 cup	270	63	380	1	Trace	—	—	—	97	211	41	1.6	548	220	.05	.14	.8	16
312	From frozen, sweetened	1 cup	270	63	385	1	Trace	—	—	—	93	211	32	1.9	475	190	.05	.11	.5	16

[27] Based on product with label claim of 100% of U.S. RDA in 6 fl oz.

[33] Weight includes rind. Without rind, the weight of the edible portion is 272 g for item 271 and 149 g for item 272.

[34] Represents yellow-fleshed varieties. For white-fleshed varieties, value is 50 International Units (I.U.) for 1 peach, 90 I.U. for 1 cup of slices.

[35] Value represents products with added ascorbic acid. For products without added ascorbic acid, value in milligrams is 116 for a 10-oz container, 103 for 1 cup.

[36] Weight includes pits. After removal of the pits, the weight of the edible portion is 258 g for item 302, 133 g for item 303, 43 g for item 304, and 213 g for item 305.

Table continued on the following page

Appendix Table 1. NUTRITIVE VALUES OF THE EDIBLE PART OF FOODS (Continued)

(Dashes (—) denote lack of reliable data for a constituent believed to be present in measurable amount)

Item No. (A)	Foods, approximate measures, units, and weight (edible part unless footnotes indicate otherwise) (B)	Grams	Water (C) Percent	Food energy (D) Calories	Protein (E) Grams	Fat (F) Grams	Fatty Acids Saturated (total) (G) Grams	Unsaturated Oleic (H) Grams	Linoleic (I) Grams	Carbohydrate (I) Grams	Calcium (K) Milligrams	Phosphorus (L) Milligrams	Iron (M) Milligrams	Potassium (N) Milligrams	Vitamin A value (O) International units	Thiamin (P) Milligrams	Riboflavin (Q) Milligrams	Niacin (R) Milligrams	Ascorbic acid (S) Milligrams
	FRUITS AND FRUIT PRODUCTS—Con.																		
	Strawberries:																		
313	Raw, whole berries, capped——— 1 cup	149	90	55	1	1	—	—	—	13	31	31	1.5	244	90	0.04	0.10	0.9	88
	Frozen, sweetened:																		
314	Sliced, 10-oz container——— 1 container	284	71	310	1	1	—	—	—	79	40	48	2.0	318	90	.06	.17	1.4	151
315	Whole, 1-lb container (about 1 3/4 cups)——— 1 container	454	76	415	2	1	—	—	—	107	59	73	2.7	472	140	.09	.27	2.3	249
316	Tangerine, raw, 2 3/8-in diam., size 176, without peel (about 4 per lb with peels and seeds)——— 1 tangerine	86	87	40	1	Trace	—	—	—	10	34	15	.3	108	360	.05	.02	.1	27
317	Tangerine juice, canned, sweetened——— 1 cup	249	87	125	1	Trace	—	—	—	30	44	35	.5	440	1,040	.15	.05	.2	54
318	Watermelon, raw, 4 by 8 in wedge with rind and seeds (1/16 of 32 2/3-lb melon, 10 by 16 in)——— 1 wedge with rind and seeds[37]	926	93	110	2	1	—	—	—	27	30	43	2.1	426	2,510	.13	.13	.9	30
	GRAIN PRODUCTS																		
	Bagel, 3-in diam.:																		
319	Egg——— 1 bagel	55	32	165	6	2	0.5	0.9	0.8	28	9	43	1.2	41	30	.14	.10	1.2	0
320	Water——— 1 bagel	55	29	165	6	1	.2	.4	.6	30	8	41	1.2	42	0	.15	.11	1.4	0
321	Barley, pearled, light, uncooked——— 1 cup	200	11	700	16	2	.3	.2	.8	158	32	378	4.0	320	0	.24	.10	6.2	0
	Biscuits, baking powder, 2-in diam. (enriched flour, vegetable shortening):																		
322	From home recipe——— 1 biscuit	28	27	105	2	5	1.2	2.0	1.2	13	34	49	.4	33	Trace	.08	.08	.7	Trace
323	From mix——— 1 biscuit	28	29	90	2	3	.6	1.1	.7	15	19	65	.6	32	Trace	.09	.08	.8	Trace
324	Breadcrumbs (enriched):[38] Dry, grated——— 1 cup	100	7	390	13	5	1.0	1.6	1.4	73	122	141	3.6	152	Trace	.35	.35	4.8	Trace
	Breads:																		
	Soft. See White bread (items 349-350).																		
325	Boston brown bread, canned, slice 3 1/4 by 1/2 in.[38]——— 1 slice	45	45	95	2	1	.1	.2	.2	21	41	72	.9	131	[39]0	.06	.04	.7	0
	Cracked-wheat bread (3/4 enriched wheat flour, 1/4 cracked wheat):[38]																		
326	Loaf, 1 lb——— 1 loaf	454	35	1,195	39	10	2.2	3.0	3.9	236	399	581	9.5	608	Trace	1.52	1.13	14.4	Trace
327	Slice (18 per loaf)——— 1 slice	25	35	65	2	1	.1	.2	.2	13	22	32	.5	34	Trace	.08	.06	.8	Trace
	French or vienna bread, enriched:[38]																		
328	Loaf, 1 lb——— 1 loaf	454	31	1,315	41	14	3.2	4.7	4.6	251	195	386	10.0	408	Trace	1.80	1.10	15.0	Trace
	Slice:																		
329	French (5 by 2 1/2 by 1 in)——— 1 slice	35	31	100	3	1	.2	.4	.4	19	15	30	.8	32	Trace	.14	.08	1.2	Trace
330	Vienna (4 3/4 by 4 by 1/2 in)——— 1 slice	25	31	75	2	1	.2	.3	.3	14	11	21	.6	23	Trace	.10	.06	.8	Trace
	Italian bread, enriched:																		
331	Loaf, 1 lb——— 1 loaf	454	32	1,250	41	4	.6	.3	1.5	256	77	349	10.0	336	0	1.80	1.10	15.0	0
332	Slice, 4 1/2 by 3 1/4 by 3/4 in——— 1 slice	30	32	85	3	Trace	Trace	Trace	.1	17	5	23	.7	22	0	.12	.07	1.0	0
	Raisin bread, enriched:[38]																		
333	Loaf, 1 lb——— 1 loaf	454	35	1,190	30	13	3.0	4.7	3.9	243	322	395	10.0	1,057	Trace	1.70	1.07	10.7	Trace
334	Slice (18 per loaf)——— 1 slice	25	35	65	2	1	.2	.3	.2	13	18	22	.6	58	Trace	.09	.06	.6	Trace

(A)	(B)		(C)	(D)	(E)	(F)	(G)	(H)	(I)	(J)	(K)	(L)	(M)	(N)	(O)	(P)	(Q)	(R)	(S)
	Rye Bread:																		
	American, light (2/3 enriched wheat flour, 1/3 rye flour):																		
335	Loaf, 1 lb	1 loaf	454	36	1,100	41	5	0.7	0.5	2.2	236	340	667	9.1	658	0	1.35	0.98	12.9	0
336	Slice (4 3/4 by 3 3/4 by 7/16 in)	1 slice	25	36	60	2	Trace	Trace	Trace	.1	13	19	37	.5	36	0	.07	.05	.7	0
	Pumpernickel (2/3 rye flour, 1/3 enriched wheat flour):																		
337	Loaf, 1 lb	1 loaf	454	34	1,115	41	5	.7	.5	2.4	241	381	1,039	11.8	2,059	0	1.30	.93	8.5	0
338	Slice (5 by 4 by 3/8 in)	1 slice	32	34	80	3	Trace	.1	Trace	.2	17	27	73	.8	145	0	.09	.07	.6	0
	White bread, enriched:[38]																		
	Soft-crumb type:																		
339	Loaf, 1 lb	1 loaf	454	36	1,225	39	15	3.4	5.3	4.6	229	381	440	11.3	476	Trace	1.80	1.10	15.0	Trace
340	Slice (18 per loaf)	1 slice	25	36	70	2	1	.2	.3	.3	13	21	24	.6	26	Trace	.10	.06	.8	Trace
341	Slice, toasted	1 slice	22	25	70	2	1	.2	.3	.3	13	21	24	.6	26	Trace	.08	.06	.8	Trace
342	Slice (22 per loaf)	1 slice	20	36	55	2	1	.2	.2	.2	10	17	19	.5	21	Trace	.08	.05	.7	Trace
343	Slice, toasted	1 slice	17	25	55	2	1	.2	.2	.2	10	17	19	.5	21	Trace	.06	.05	.7	Trace
344	Loaf, 1 1/2 lb	1 loaf	680	36	1,835	59	22	5.2	7.9	6.9	343	571	660	17.0	714	Trace	2.70	1.65	22.5	Trace
345	Slice (24 per loaf)	1 slice	28	36	75	2	1	.2	.3	.3	14	24	27	.7	29	Trace	.11	.07	.9	Trace
346	Slice, toasted	1 slice	24	25	75	2	1	.2	.3	.3	14	24	27	.7	29	Trace	.09	.07	.9	Trace
347	Slice (28 per loaf)	1 slice	24	36	65	2	1	.2	.3	.3	12	20	23	.6	25	Trace	.10	.06	.8	Trace
348	Slice, toasted	1 slice	21	25	65	2	1	.2	.3	.3	12	20	23	.6	25	Trace	.08	.06	.8	Trace
349	Cubes	1 cup	30	36	80	3	1	.2	.3	.3	15	25	29	.8	32	Trace	.12	.07	1.0	Trace
350	Crumbs	1 cup	45	36	120	4	1	.3	.5	.5	23	38	44	1.1	47	Trace	.18	.11	1.5	Trace
	Firm-crumb type:																		
351	Loaf, 1 lb	1 loaf	454	35	1,245	41	17	3.9	5.9	5.2	228	435	463	11.3	549	Trace	1.80	1.10	15.0	Trace
352	Slice (20 per loaf)	1 slice	23	35	65	2	1	.2	.3	.3	12	22	23	.6	28	Trace	.09	.06	.8	Trace
353	Slice, toasted	1 slice	20	24	65	2	1	.2	.3	.3	12	22	23	.6	28	Trace	.07	.06	.8	Trace
354	Loaf, 2 lb	1 loaf	907	35	2,495	82	34	7.7	11.8	10.4	455	871	925	22.7	1,097	Trace	3.60	2.20	30.0	Trace
355	Slice (34 per loaf)	1 slice	27	35	75	2	1	.2	.3	.3	14	26	28	.7	33	Trace	.11	.06	.9	Trace
356	Slice, toasted	1 slice	23	24	75	2	1	.2	.3	.3	14	26	28	.7	33	Trace	.09	.06	.9	Trace
	Whole-wheat bread:																		
	Soft-crumb type:[38]																		
357	Loaf, 1 lb	1 loaf	454	36	1,095	41	12	2.2	2.9	4.2	224	381	1,152	13.6	1,161	Trace	1.37	.45	12.7	Trace
358	Slice (16 per loaf)	1 slice	28	36	65	3	1	.2	.2	.2	14	24	71	.8	72	Trace	.09	.03	.8	Trace
359	Slice, toasted	1 slice	24	24	65	3	1	.1	.2	.2	14	24	71	.8	72	Trace	.07	.03	.8	Trace
	Firm-crumb type:[38]																		
360	Loaf, 1 lb	1 loaf	454	36	1,100	48	14	2.5	3.3	4.9	216	449	1,034	13.6	1,238	Trace	1.17	.54	12.7	Trace
361	Slice (18 per loaf)	1 slice	25	36	60	3	1	.1	.2	.3	12	25	57	.8	68	Trace	.06	.03	.7	Trace
362	Slice, toasted	1 slice	21	24	60	3	1	.1	.2	.3	12	25	57	.8	68	Trace	.05	.03	.7	Trace
	Breakfast cereals:																		
	Hot type, cooked:																		
	Corn (hominy) grits, degermed:																		
363	Enriched	1 cup	245	87	125	3	Trace	Trace	Trace	.1	27	2	25	.7	27	[40]Trace	.10	.07	1.0	0
364	Unenriched	1 cup	245	87	125	3	Trace	Trace	Trace	.1	27	2	25	.2	27	[40]Trace	.05	.02	.5	0
365	Farina, quick-cooking, enriched	1 cup	245	89	105	3	Trace	Trace	Trace	.1	22	147	[41]113	(42)	25	0	.12	.07	1.0	0
366	Oatmeal or rolled oats	1 cup	240	87	130	5	2	.4	.8	.9	23	22	137	1.4	146	0	.19	.05	.2	0
367	Wheat, rolled	1 cup	240	80	180	5	1	—	—	—	41	19	182	1.7	202	0	.17	.07	2.2	0
368	Wheat, whole-meal	1 cup	245	88	110	4	1	—	—	—	23	17	127	1.2	118	0	.15	.05	1.5	0
	Ready-to-eat:																		
369	Bran flakes (40% bran), added sugar, salt, iron, vitamins	1 cup	35	3	105	4	1	—	—	—	28	19	125	5.6	137	1,540	.46	.52	6.2	0
370	Bran flakes with raisins, added sugar, salt, iron, vitamins	1 cup	50	7	145	4	1	—	—	—	40	28	146	7.9	154	[43]2,200	(44)	(44)	(44)	0

[37] Weight includes rind and seeds. Without rind and seeds, weight of the edible portion is 426 g.
[38] Made with vegetable shortening.
[39] Applies to product made with white cornmeal. With yellow cornmeal, value is 30 International Units (I.U.).
[40] Applies to white varieties. For yellow varieties, value is 150 International Units (I.U.).
[41] Applies to products that do not contain di-sodium phosphate. If di-sodium phosphate is an ingredient, value is 162 mg.
[42] Value may range from less than 1 mg to about 8 mg depending on the brand. Consult the label.
[43] Applies to product with added nutrient. Without added nutrient, value is trace.
[44] Value varies with the brand. Consult the label.

Table continued on the following page

Appendix Table 1. NUTRITIVE VALUES OF THE EDIBLE PART OF FOODS (*Continued*)

(Dashes (—) denote lack of reliable data for a constituent believed to be present in measurable amount)

Item No. (A)	Foods, approximate measures, units, and weight (edible part unless footnotes indicate otherwise) (B)	Grams	Water (C) Percent	Food energy (D) Calories	Protein (E) Grams	Fat (F) Grams	Saturated (total) (G) Grams	Oleic (H) Grams	Linoleic (I) Grams	Carbohydrate (I) Grams	Calcium (K) Milligrams	Phosphorus (L) Milligrams	Iron (M) Milligrams	Potassium (N) Milligrams	Vitamin A value (O) International units	Thiamin (P) Milligrams	Riboflavin (Q) Milligrams	Niacin (R) Milligrams	Ascorbic acid (S) Milligrams
	GRAIN PRODUCTS—Con.																		
	Breakfast cereals—Continued																		
	Ready-to-eat—Continued																		
	Corn flakes:																		
371	Plain, added sugar, salt, iron, vitamins. 1 cup	25	4	95	2	Trace	—	—	—	21	[44]	9	[44]	30	[44]	[44]	[44]	[44]	[44]13
372	Sugar-coated, added salt, iron, vitamins. 1 cup	40	2	155	2	Trace	—	—	—	37	1	10	[44]	27	1,760	.53	.50	7.1	[44]21
373	Corn, oat flour, puffed, added sugar, salt, iron, vitamins. 1 cup	20	4	80	2	1	—	—	—	16	4	18	5.7	—	880	.26	.30	3.5	11
374	Corn, shredded, added sugar, salt, iron, thiamin, niacin. 1 cup	25	3	95	2	Trace	—	—	—	22	1	10	.6	—	0	.33	.05	4.4	13
375	Oats, puffed, added sugar, salt, minerals, vitamins. 1 cup	25	3	100	3	1	—	—	—	19	44	102	4.0	—	1,100	.33	.38	4.4	13
	Rice, puffed:																		
376	Plain, added iron, thiamin, niacin. 1 cup	15	4	60	1	Trace	—	—	—	13	3	14	.3	15	0	.07	.01	.7	0
377	Presweetened, added salt, iron, vitamins. 1 cup	28	3	115	1	0	—	—	—	26	3	14	[44]	43	[45]1,240	[44]	[44]	[44]	[45]15
378	Wheat flakes, added sugar, salt, iron, vitamins. 1 cup	30	4	105	3	Trace	—	—	—	24	12	83	4.8	81	1,320	.40	.45	5.3	16
	Wheat, puffed:																		
379	Plain, added iron, thiamin, niacin. 1 cup	15	3	55	2	Trace	—	—	—	12	4	48	.6	51	0	.08	.03	1.2	0
380	Presweetened, added salt, iron, vitamins. 1 cup	38	3	140	3	Trace	—	—	—	33	7	52	[44]	63	1,680	.50	.57	6.7	[44]20
381	Wheat, shredded, plain. 1 oblong biscuit or 1/2 cup spoon-size biscuits.	25	7	90	2	1	—	—	—	20	11	97	.9	87	0	.06	.03	1.1	0
382	Wheat germ, without salt and sugar, toasted. 1 tbsp	6	4	25	2	1	—	—	—	3	3	70	.5	57	10	.11	.05	.3	1
383	Buckwheat flour, light, sifted. 1 cup	98	12	340	6	1	0.2	0.4	0.4	78	11	86	1.0	314	0	.08	.04	.4	0
384	Bulgur, canned, seasoned. 1 cup	135	56	245	8	4	—	—	—	44	27	263	1.9	151	0	.08	.05	4.1	0
	Cake icings. See Sugars and Sweets (items 532–536).																		
	Cakes made from cake mixes with enriched flour:[6]																		
	Angelfood:																		
385	Whole cake (9 3/4-in diam. tube cake). 1 cake	635	34	1,645	36	1	—	—	—	377	603	756	2.5	381	0	.37	.95	3.6	0
386	Piece, 1/12 of cake. 1 piece	53	34	135	3	Trace	—	—	—	32	50	63	.2	32	0	.03	.08	.3	0
	Coffeecake:																		
387	Whole cake (7 3/4 by 5 5/8 by 1 1/4 in). 1 cake	430	30	1,385	27	41	11.7	16.3	8.8	225	262	748	6.9	469	690	.82	.91	7.7	1
388	Piece, 1/6 of cake. 1 piece	72	30	230	5	7	2.0	2.7	1.5	38	44	125	1.2	78	120	.14	.15	1.3	Trace
	Cupcakes, made with egg, milk, 2 1/2-in diam.:																		
389	Without icing. 1 cupcake	25	26	90	1	3	.8	1.2	.7	14	40	59	.3	21	40	.05	.05	.4	Trace
390	With chocolate icing. 1 cupcake	36	22	130	2	5	2.0	1.6	.6	21	47	71	.4	42	60	.05	.06	.4	Trace
	Devil's food with chocolate icing:																		
391	Whole, 2 layer cake (8- or 9-in diam.). 1 cake	1,107	24	3,755	49	136	50.0	44.9	17.0	645	653	1,162	16.6	1,439	1,660	1.06	1.65	10.1	1
392	Piece, 1/16 of cake. 1 piece	69	24	235	3	8	3.1	2.8	1.1	40	41	72	1.0	90	100	.07	.10	.6	Trace
393	Cupcake, 2 1/2-in diam. 1 cupcake	35	24	120	2	4	1.6	1.4	.5	20	21	37	.5	46	50	.03	.05	.3	Trace

(A)	(B)	(C)	(D)	(E)	(F)	(G)	(H)	(I)	(J)	(K)	(L)	(M)	(N)	(O)	(P)	(Q)	(R)	(S)
	Gingerbread:																	
394	Whole cake (8-in square)------	1 cake------	570	1,575	18	39	9.7	16.6	10.0	291	513	570	8.6	1,562	Trace	0.84	1.00	7.4	Trace
395	Piece, 1/9 of cake------	1 piece------	63	175	2	4	1.1	1.8	1.1	32	57	63	.9	173	Trace	.09	.11	.8	Trace
	White, 2 layer with chocolate icing:																	
396	Whole cake (8- or 9-in diam.)-	1 cake------	1,140	4,000	44	122	48.2	46.4	20.0	716	1,129	2,041	11.4	1,322	680	1.50	1.77	12.5	2
397	Piece, 1/16 of cake------	1 piece------	71	250	3	8	3.0	2.9	1.2	45	70	127	.7	82	40	.09	.11	.8	Trace
	Yellow, 2 layer with chocolate icing:																	
398	Whole cake (8- or 9-in diam.)-	1 cake------	1,108	3,735	45	125	47.8	47.8	20.3	638	1,008	2,017	12.2	1,208	1,550	1.24	1.67	10.6	2
399	Piece, 1/16 of cake------	1 piece------	69	235	3	8	3.0	3.0	1.3	40	63	126	.8	75	100	.08	.10	.7	Trace
	Cakes made from home recipes using enriched flour:[47]																	
	Boston cream pie with custard filling:[47]																	
400	Whole cake (8-in diam.)------	1 cake------	825	2,490	41	78	23.0	30.1	15.2	412	553	833	8.2	[48]734	1,730	1.04	1.27	9.6	2
401	Piece, 1/12 of cake------	1 piece------	69	210	3	6	1.9	2.5	1.3	34	46	70	.7	[48]61	140	.09	.11	.8	Trace
402	Fruitcake, dark: Loaf, 1-lb (7 1/2 by 2 by 1 1/2 in).	1 loaf------	454	1,720	22	69	14.4	33.5	14.8	271	327	513	11.8	2,250	540	.72	.73	4.9	2
403	Slice, 1/30 of loaf------	1 slice------	15	55	1	2	.5	1.1	.5	9	11	17	.4	74	20	.02	.02	.2	Trace
	Plain, sheet cake:																	
	Without icing:																	
404	Whole cake (9-in square)-----	1 cake------	777	2,830	35	108	29.5	44.4	23.9	434	497	793	8.5	[48]614	1,320	1.21	1.40	10.2	2
405	Piece, 1/9 of cake------	1 piece------	86	315	4	12	3.3	4.9	2.6	48	55	88	.9	[48]68	150	.13	.15	1.1	Trace
	With uncooked white icing:																	
406	Whole cake (9-in square)-----	1 cake------	1,096	4,020	37	129	42.2	49.5	24.4	694	548	822	8.2	[48]669	2,190	1.22	1.47	10.2	2
407	Piece, 1/9 of cake------	1 piece------	121	445	4	14	4.7	5.5	2.7	77	61	91	.8	[48]74	240	.14	.16	1.1	Trace
408	Pound:[49] Loaf, 8 1/2 by 3 1/2 by 3 1/4	1 loaf------	565	2,725	31	170	42.9	73.1	39.6	273	107	418	7.9	345	1,410	.90	.99	7.3	0
409	Slice, 1/17 of loaf------	1 slice------	33	160	2	10	2.5	4.3	2.3	16	6	24	.5	20	80	.05	.06	.4	0
	Spongecake:																	
410	Whole cake (9 3/4-in diam. tube cake).	1 cake------	790	2,345	60	45	13.1	15.8	5.7	427	237	885	13.4	687	3,560	1.10	1.64	7.4	2
411	Piece, 1/12 of cake------	1 piece------	66	195	5	4	1.1	1.3	.5	36	20	74	1.1	57	300	.09	.14	.6	Trace
	Cookies made with enriched flour:[50][51]																	
	Brownies with nuts:																	
	Home-prepared, 1 3/4 by 1 3/4 by 7/8 in:																	
412	From home recipe------	1 brownie------	20	95	1	6	1.5	3.0	1.2	10	8	30	.4	38	40	.04	.03	.2	Trace
413	From commercial recipe------	1 brownie------	20	85	1	4	.9	1.4	1.3	13	9	27	.4	34	20	.03	.02	.2	Trace
414	Frozen, with chocolate icing,[52] 1 1/2 by 1 3/4 by 7/8 in.	1 brownie------	25	105	1	5	2.0	2.2	.7	15	10	31	.4	44	50	.03	.03	.2	Trace
	Chocolate chip:																	
415	Commercial, 2 1/4-in diam., 3/8 in thick.	4 cookies------	42	200	2	9	2.8	2.9	2.2	29	16	48	1.0	56	50	.10	.17	.9	Trace
416	From home recipe, 2 1/3-in diam.	4 cookies------	40	205	2	12	3.5	4.5	2.9	24	14	40	.8	47	40	.06	.06	.5	Trace
417	Fig bars, square (1 5/8 by 1 5/8 by 3/8 in) or rectangular (1 1/2 by 1 3/4 by 1/2 in).	4 cookies------	56	200	2	3	.8	1.2	.7	42	44	34	1.0	111	60	.04	.14	.9	Trace
418	Gingersnaps, 2-in diam., 1/4 in thick.	4 cookies------	28	90	2	2	.7	1.0	.6	22	20	13	.7	129	20	.08	.06	.7	0
419	Macaroons, 2 3/4-in diam., 1/4 in thick.	2 cookies------	38	180	2	9	—	—	—	25	10	32	.3	176	0	.02	.06	.2	0
420	Oatmeal with raisins, 2 5/8-in diam., 1/4 in thick.	4 cookies------	52	235	3	8	2.0	3.3	2.0	38	11	53	1.4	192	30	.15	.10	1.0	Trace

[44]Value varies with the brand. Consult the label.
[45]Applies to product with added nutrient. Without added nutrient, value is trace.
[46]Excepting angelfood cake, cakes were made from mixes containing vegetable shortening; icings, with butter.
[47]Excepting spongecake, vegetable shortening used for cake portion; butter, for icing. If butter or margarine used for cake portion, vitamin A values would be higher.
[48]Applies to product made with a sodium aluminum-sulfate type baking powder. With a low-sodium type baking powder containing potassium, value would be about twice the amount shown.
[49]Equal weights of flour, sugar, eggs, and vegetable shortening.
[50]Products are commercial unless otherwise specified.
[51]Made with enriched flour and vegetable shortening except for macaroons which do not contain flour or shortening.
[52]Icing made with butter.

Table continued on the following page

Appendix Table 1. NUTRITIVE VALUES OF THE EDIBLE PART OF FOODS (Continued)

(Dashes (—) denote lack of reliable data for a constituent believed to be present in measurable amount)

Item No. (A)	Foods, approximate measures, units, and weight (edible part unless footnotes indicate otherwise) (B)	Grams	Water (C) Percent	Food energy (D) Calories	Protein (E) Grams	Fat (F) Grams	Fatty Acids Saturated (total) (G) Grams	Unsaturated Oleic (H) Grams	Unsaturated Linoleic (I) Grams	Carbohydrate (J) Grams	Calcium (K) Milligrams	Phosphorus (L) Milligrams	Iron (M) Milligrams	Potassium (N) Milligrams	Vitamin A value (O) International units	Thiamin (P) Milligrams	Riboflavin (Q) Milligrams	Niacin (R) Milligrams	Ascorbic acid (S) Milligrams
	GRAIN PRODUCTS—Con.																		
	Cookies made with enriched flour[50][51]—Continued																		
421	Plain, prepared from commercial chilled dough, 2 1/2-in diam., 1/4 in thick. 4 cookies	48	5	240	2	12	3.0	5.2	2.9	31	17	35	0.6	23	30	0.10	0.08	0.9	0
422	Sandwich type (chocolate or vanilla), 1 3/4-in diam., 3/8 in thick. 4 cookies	40	2	200	2	9	2.2	3.9	2.2	28	10	96	.7	15	0	.06	.10	.7	0
423	Vanilla wafers, 1 3/4-in diam., 1/4-in thick. 10 cookies	40	3	185	2	6	—	—	—	30	16	25	.6	29	50	.10	.09	.8	0
	Cornmeal:																		
424	Whole-ground, unbolted, dry form. 1 cup	122	12	435	11	5	.5	1.0	2.5	90	24	312	2.9	346	[53]620	.46	.13	2.4	0
425	Bolted (nearly whole-grain), dry form. 1 cup	122	12	440	11	4	.5	.9	2.1	91	21	272	2.2	303	[53]590	.37	.10	2.3	0
	Degermed, enriched:																		
426	Dry form 1 cup	138	12	500	11	2	.2	.4	.9	108	8	137	4.0	166	[53]610	.61	.36	4.8	0
427	Cooked 1 cup	240	88	120	3	Trace	Trace	.1	.2	26	2	34	1.0	38	[53]140	.14	.10	1.2	0
	Degermed, unenriched:																		
428	Dry form 1 cup	138	12	500	11	2	.2	.4	.9	108	8	137	1.5	166	[53]610	.19	.07	1.4	0
429	Cooked 1 cup	240	88	120	3	Trace	Trace	.1	.2	26	2	34	.5	38	[53]140	.05	.02	.2	0
	Crackers:[38]																		
430	Graham, plain, 2 1/2-in square 2 crackers	14	6	55	1	1	.3	.5	.3	10	6	21	.5	55	0	.02	.08	.5	0
431	Rye wafers, whole-grain, 1 7/8 by 3 1/2 in. 2 wafers	13	6	45	2	Trace	—	—	—	10	7	50	.5	78	0	.04	.03	.2	0
432	Saltines, made with enriched flour. 4 crackers or 1 packet	11	4	50	1	1	.3	.5	.4	8	2	10	.5	13	0	.05	.05	.4	0
	Danish pastry (enriched flour), plain without fruit or nuts:[54]																		
433	Packaged ring, 12 oz 1 ring	340	22	1,435	25	80	24.3	31.7	16.5	155	170	371	6.1	381	1,050	.97	1.01	8.6	Trace
434	Round piece, about 4 1/4-in diam. by 1 in. 1 pastry	65	22	275	5	15	4.7	6.1	3.2	30	33	71	1.2	73	200	.18	.19	1.7	Trace
435	Ounce 1 oz	28	22	120	2	7	2.0	2.7	1.4	13	14	31	.5	32	90	.08	.08	.7	Trace
	Doughnuts, made with enriched flour:[38]																		
436	Cake type, plain, 2 1/2-in diam., 1 in high. 1 doughnut	25	24	100	1	5	1.2	2.0	1.1	13	10	48	.4	23	20	.05	.05	.4	Trace
437	Yeast-leavened, glazed, 3 3/4-in diam., 1 1/4 in high. 1 doughnut	50	26	205	3	11	3.3	5.8	3.3	22	16	33	.6	34	25	.10	.10	.8	0
	Macaroni, enriched, cooked (cut lengths, elbows, shells):																		
	Firm stage (hot):																		
438	1 cup	130	64	190	7	1	—	—	—	39	14	85	1.4	103	0	.23	.13	1.8	0
	Tender stage:																		
439	Cold macaroni 1 cup	105	73	115	4	Trace	—	—	—	24	8	53	.9	64	0	.15	.08	1.2	0
440	Hot macaroni 1 cup	140	73	155	5	1	—	—	—	32	11	70	1.3	85	.0	.20	.11	1.5	0
	Macaroni (enriched) and cheese:																		
441	Canned[55] 1 cup	240	80	230	9	10	4.2	3.1	1.4	26	199	182	1.0	139	260	.12	.24	1.0	Trace
442	From home recipe (served hot)[56] 1 cup	200	58	430	17	22	8.9	8.8	2.9	40	362	322	1.8	240	860	.20	.40	1.8	Trace
	Muffins made with enriched flour:[38]																		
	From home recipe:																		
443	Blueberry, 2 3/8-in diam., 1 1/2 in high. 1 muffin	40	39	110	3	4	1.1	1.4	.7	17	34	53	.6	46	90	.09	.10	.7	Trace
444	Bran, 1 muffin	40	35	105	3	4	1.2	1.4	.8	17	57	162	1.5	172	90	.07	.10	1.7	Trace
445	Corn (enriched degermed cornmeal and flour), 2 3/8-in diam., 1 1/2 in high. 1 muffin	40	33	125	3	4	1.2	1.6	.9	19	42	68	.7	54	[57]120	.10	.10	.7	Trace

(A)	(B)		grams (C)	(C)	(D)	(E)	(F)	(G)	(H)	(I)	(I)	(K)	(L)	(M)	(N)	(O)	(P)	(Q)	(R)	(S)
446	Plain, 3-in diam., 1 1/2 in high.	1 muffin	40	38	120	3	4	1.0	1.7	1.0	17	42	60	0.6	50	40	0.09	0.12	0.9	Trace
447	From mix, egg, milk: Corn, 2 3/8-in diam., 1 1/2 in high.[58]	1 muffin	40	30	130	3	4	1.2	1.7	—	20	96	152	.6	44	100[57]	.08	.09	.7	Trace
448	Noodles (egg noodles), enriched, cooked.	1 cup	160	71	200	7	2	—	—	—	37	16	94	1.4	70	110	.22	.13	1.9	0
449	Noodles, chow mein, canned.	1 cup	45	1	220	6	11	—	—	—	26	—	—	—	—	—	—	—	—	—
450	Pancakes, (4-in diam.):[38] Buckwheat, made from mix (with buckwheat and enriched flours), egg and milk added.	1 cake	27	58	55	2	2	.8	.9	.4	6	59	91	.4	66	60	.04	.05	.2	Trace
451	Plain: Made from home recipe using enriched flour.	1 cake	27	50	60	2	2	.5	.8	.5	9	27	38	.4	33	30	.06	.07	.5	Trace
452	Made from mix with enriched flour, egg and milk added.	1 cake	27	51	60	2	2	.7	.7	.3	9	58	70	.3	42	70	.04	.06	.2	Trace
	Pies, piecrust made with enriched flour, vegetable shortening (9-in diam.):																			
	Apple:																			
453	Whole	1 pie	945	48	2,420	21	105	27.0	44.5	25.2	360	76	208	6.6	756	280	1.06	.79	9.3	9
454	Sector, 1/7 of pie	1 sector	135	48	345	3	15	3.9	6.4	3.6	51	11	30	.9	108	40	.15	.11	1.3	2
	Banana cream:																			
455	Whole	1 pie	910	54	2,010	41	85	26.7	33.2	16.2	279	601	746	7.3	1,847	2,280	.77	1.51	7.0	9
456	Sector, 1/7 of pie	1 sector	130	54	285	6	12	3.8	4.7	2.3	40	86	107	1.0	264	330	.11	.22	1.0	1
	Blueberry:																			
457	Whole	1 pie	945	51	2,285	23	102	24.8	43.7	25.1	330	104	217	9.5	614	280	1.03	.80	10.0	28
458	Sector, 1/7 of pie	1 sector	135	51	325	3	15	3.5	6.2	3.6	47	15	31	1.4	88	40	.15	.11	1.4	4
	Cherry:																			
459	Whole	1 pie	945	47	2,465	25	107	28.2	45.0	25.3	363	132	236	6.6	992	4,160	1.09	.84	9.8	Trace
460	Sector, 1/7 of pie	1 sector	135	47	350	4	15	4.0	6.4	3.6	52	19	34	.9	142	590	.16	.12	1.4	Trace
	Custard:																			
461	Whole	1 pie	910	58	1,985	56	101	33.9	38.5	17.5	213	874	1,028	8.2	1,247	2,090	.79	1.92	5.6	0
462	Sector, 1/7 of pie	1 sector	130	58	285	8	14	4.8	5.5	2.5	30	125	147	1.2	178	300	.11	.27	.8	0
	Lemon meringue:																			
463	Whole	1 pie	840	47	2,140	31	86	26.1	33.8	16.4	317	118	412	6.7	420	1,430	.61	.84	5.2	25
464	Sector, 1/7 of pie	1 sector	120	47	305	4	12	3.7	4.8	2.3	45	17	59	1.0	60	200	.09	.12	.7	4
	Mince:																			
465	Whole	1 pie	945	43	2,560	24	109	28.0	45.9	25.2	389	265	359	13.3	1,682	20	.96	.86	9.8	9
466	Sector, 1/7 of pie	1 sector	135	43	365	3	16	4.0	6.6	3.6	56	38	51	1.9	240	Trace	.14	.12	1.4	1
	Peach:																			
467	Whole	1 pie	945	48	2,410	24	101	24.8	43.7	25.1	361	95	274	8.5	1,408	6,900	1.04	.97	14.0	28
468	Sector, 1/7 of pie	1 sector	135	48	345	3	14	3.5	6.2	3.6	52	14	39	1.2	201	990	.15	.14	2.0	4
	Pecan:																			
469	Whole	1 pie	825	20	3,450	42	189	27.8	101.0	44.2	423	388	850	25.6	1,015	1,320	1.80	.95	6.9	Trace
470	Sector, 1/7 of pie	1 sector	118	20	495	6	27	4.0	14.4	6.3	61	55	122	3.7	145	190	.26	.14	1.0	Trace
	Pumpkin:																			
471	Whole	1 pie	910	59	1,920	36	102	37.4	37.5	16.6	223	464	628	7.3	1,456	22,480	.78	1.27	7.0	Trace
472	Sector, 1/7 of pie	1 sector	130	59	275	5	15	5.4	5.4	2.4	32	66	90	1.0	208	3,210	.11	.18	1.0	Trace
473	Piecrust (home recipe) made with enriched flour and vegetable shortening, baked.	1 pie shell, 9-in diam.	180	15	900	11	60	14.8	26.1	14.9	79	25	90	3.1	89	0	.47	.40	5.0	0
474	Piecrust mix with enriched flour and vegetable shortening, 10-oz pkg. prepared and baked.	Piecrust for 2-crust pie, 9-in diam.	320	19	1,485	20	93	22.7	39.7	23.4	141	131	272	6.1	179	0	1.07	.79	9.9	0

[38] Made with vegetable shortening.
[50] Products are commercial unless otherwise specified.
[51] Made with enriched flour and vegetable shortening except for macaroons which do not contain flour or shortening.
[53] Applies to yellow varieties; white varieties contain only a trace.
[54] Contains vegetable shortening and butter.
[55] Made with corn oil.
[56] Made with regular margarine.
[57] Applies to product made with yellow cornmeal.
[58] Made with enriched degermed cornmeal and enriched flour.

Table continued on the following page

Appendix Table 1. NUTRITIVE VALUES OF THE EDIBLE PART OF FOODS (Continued)

(Dashes (—) denote lack of reliable data for a constituent believed to be present in measurable amount)

NUTRIENTS IN INDICATED QUANTITY

Item No. (A)	Foods, approximate measures, units, and weight (edible part unless footnotes indicate otherwise) (B)		Grams	Water (C) Percent	Food energy (D) Calories	Protein (E) Grams	Fat (F) Grams	Saturated (total) (G) Grams	Unsaturated Oleic (H) Grams	Linoleic (I) Grams	Carbohydrate (J) Grams	Calcium (K) Milligrams	Phosphorus (L) Milligrams	Iron (M) Milligrams	Potassium (N) Milligrams	Vitamin A value (O) International units	Thiamin (P) Milligrams	Riboflavin (Q) Milligrams	Niacin (R) Milligrams	Ascorbic acid (S) Milligrams
	GRAIN PRODUCTS—Con.																			
475	Pizza (cheese) baked, 4 3/4-in sector; 1/8 of 12-in pie.[19]	1 sector	60	45	145	6	4	1.7	1.5	0.6	22	86	89	1.1	67	230	0.16	0.18	1.6	4
	Popcorn, popped:																			
476	Plain, large kernel	1 cup	6	4	25	1	Trace	—	.1	.2	5	1	17	.2	—	—	—	.01	.1	0
477	With oil (coconut) and salt added, large kernel.	1 cup	9	3	40	1	2	1.5	.2	.2	5	1	19	.2	—	—	—	.01	.2	0
478	Sugar coated	1 cup	35	4	135	2	1	.5	.2	.4	30	2	47	.5	—	—	—	.02	.4	0
	Pretzels, made with enriched flour:																			
479	Dutch, twisted, 2 3/4 by 2 5/8 in.	1 pretzel	16	5	60	2	1	—	—	—	12	4	21	.2	21	0	.05	.04	.7	0
480	Thin, twisted, 3 1/4 by 2 1/4 by 1/4 in.	10 pretzels	60	5	235	6	3	—	—	—	46	13	79	.9	78	0	.20	.15	2.5	0
481	Stick, 2 1/4 in long	10 pretzels	3	5	10	Trace	Trace	—	—	—	2	1	4	Trace	4	0	.01	.01	.1	0
	Rice, white, enriched: Instant, ready-to-serve, hot																			
482		1 cup	165	73	180	4	Trace	Trace	Trace	Trace	40	5	31	1.3	—	0	.21	(59)	1.7	0
	Long grain:																			
483	Raw	1 cup	185	12	670	12	1	.2	.2	.2	149	44	174	5.4	170	0	.81	.06	6.5	0
484	Cooked, served hot	1 cup	205	73	225	4	Trace	.1	.1	.1	50	21	57	1.8	57	0	.23	.02	2.1	0
	Parboiled:																			
485	Raw	1 cup	185	10	685	14	1	.2	.1	.2	150	111	370	5.4	278	0	.81	.07	6.5	0
486	Cooked, served hot	1 cup	175	73	185	4	Trace	.1	.1	.1	41	33	100	1.4	75	0	.19	.02	2.1	0
	Rolls, enriched:[38] Commercial:																			
487	Brown-and-serve (12 per 12-oz pkg.), browned.	1 roll	26	27	85	2	2	.4	.7	.5	14	20	23	.5	25	Trace	.10	.06	.9	Trace
488	Cloverleaf or pan, 2 1/2-in diam., 2 in high.	1 roll	28	31	85	2	2	.4	.6	.4	15	21	24	.5	27	Trace	.11	.07	.9	Trace
489	Frankfurter and hamburger (8 per 11 1/2-oz pkg.).	1 roll	40	31	120	3	2	.5	.8	.6	21	30	34	.8	38	Trace	.16	.10	1.3	Trace
490	Hard, 3 3/4-in diam., 2 in high.	1 roll	50	25	155	5	2	.4	.6	.5	30	24	46	1.2	49	Trace	.20	.12	1.7	Trace
491	Hoagie or submarine, 11 1/2 by 3 by 2 1/2 in.	1 roll	135	31	390	12	4	.9	1.4	1.4	75	58	115	3.0	122	Trace	.54	.32	4.5	Trace
	From home recipe:																			
492	Cloverleaf, 2 1/2-in diam., 2 in high.	1 roll	35	26	120	3	3	.8	1.1	.7	20	16	36	.7	41	30	.12	.12	1.2	Trace
	Spaghetti, enriched, cooked:																			
493	Firm stage, "al dente," served hot.	1 cup	130	64	190	7	1	—	—	—	39	14	85	1.4	103	0	.23	.13	1.8	0
494	Tender stage, served hot	1 cup	140	73	155	5	1	—	—	—	32	11	70	1.3	85	0	.20	.11	1.5	0
	Spaghetti (enriched) in tomato sauce with cheese:																			
495	From home recipe	1 cup	250	77	260	9	9	2.0	5.4	.7	37	80	135	2.3	408	1,080	.25	.18	2.3	13
496	Canned	1 cup	250	80	190	6	2	.5	.3	.4	39	40	88	2.8	303	930	.35	.28	4.5	10
	Spaghetti (enriched) with meat balls and tomato sauce:																			
497	From home recipe	1 cup	248	70	330	19	12	3.3	6.3	.9	39	124	236	3.7	665	1,590	.25	.30	4.0	22
498	Canned	1 cup	250	78	260	12	10	2.2	3.3	3.9	29	53	113	3.3	245	1,000	.15	.18	2.3	5
499	Toaster pastries	1 pastry	50	12	200	3	6	—	—	—	36	[60]54	[60]67	1.9	[60]74	500	.16	.17	2.1	([60])
	Waffles, made with enriched flour, 7-in diam.:[38]																			
500	From home recipe	1 waffle	75	41	210	7	7	2.3	2.8	1.4	28	85	130	1.3	109	250	.17	.23	1.4	Trace
501	From mix, egg and milk added	1 waffle	75	42	205	7	8	2.8	2.9	1.2	27	179	257	1.0	146	170	.14	.22	.9	Trace

LEGUMES (DRY), NUTS, SEEDS; RELATED PRODUCTS

(A)	(B)	(C)	(D)	(E)	(F)	(G)	(H)	(I)	(J)	(K)	(L)	(M)	(N)	(O)	(P)	(Q)	(R)	(S)
	Wheat flours:																	
	All-purpose or family flour, enriched:																	
502	Sifted, spooned——— 1 cup	12	420	12	1	0.2	0.1	0.5	88	18	100	3.3	109	0	0.74	0.46	6.1	0
503	Unsifted, spooned——— 1 cup	12	455	13	1	.2	.1	.5	95	20	109	3.6	119	0	.80	.50	6.6	0
504	Cake or pastry flour, enriched, sifted, spooned. 1 cup	12	350	7	1	.1	.1	.3	76	16	70	2.8	91	0	.61	.38	5.1	0
505	Self-rising, enriched, unsifted, spooned. 1 cup	12	440	12	1	.2	.1	.5	93	331	583	3.6	—	0	.80	.50	6.6	0
506	Whole-wheat, from hard wheats, stirred. 1 cup	12	400	16	2	.4	.2	1.0	85	49	446	4.0	444	0	.66	.14	5.2	0
	LEGUMES (DRY), NUTS, SEEDS; RELATED PRODUCTS																	
	Almonds, shelled:																	
507	Chopped (about 130 almonds)——— 1 cup	5	775	24	70	5.6	47.7	12.8	25	304	655	6.1	1,005	0	.31	1.20	4.6	Trace
508	Slivered, not pressed down (about 115 almonds). 1 cup	5	690	21	62	5.0	42.2	11.3	22	269	580	5.4	889	0	.28	1.06	4.0	Trace
	Beans, dry:																	
	Common varieties as Great Northern, navy, and others:																	
	Cooked, drained:																	
509	Great Northern——— 1 cup	69	210	14	1	—	—	—	38	90	266	4.9	749	0	.25	.13	1.3	0
510	Pea (navy)——— 1 cup	69	225	15	1	—	—	—	40	95	281	5.1	790	0	.27	.13	1.3	0
	Canned, solids and liquid:																	
	White with—																	
511	Frankfurters (sliced)——— 1 cup	71	365	19	18	2.4	2.8	.6	32	94	303	4.8	668	330	.13	.15	3.3	Trace
512	Pork and tomato sauce——— 1 cup	71	310	16	7	4.3	5.0	1.1	48	138	235	4.6	536	330	.20	.08	1.5	5
513	Pork and sweet sauce——— 1 cup	66	385	16	12				54	161	291	5.9	673		.15	.10	1.3	—
514	Red kidney——— 1 cup	76	230	15	1				42	74	278	4.6	—	10	.13	.10	1.5	—
515	Lima, cooked, drained——— 1 cup	64	260	16	1				49	55	293	5.9	1,163		.25	.11	1.3	—
516	Blackeye peas, dry, cooked (with residual cooking liquid). 1 cup	80	190	13	1				35	43	238	3.3	573	30	.40	.10	1.0	—
517	Brazil nuts, shelled (6-8 large kernels). 1 oz	5	185	4	19	4.8	6.2	7.1	3	53	196	1.0	203	Trace	.27	.03	.5	—
518	Cashew nuts, roasted in oil 1 cup	5	785	24	64	12.9	36.8	10.2	41	53	522	5.3	650	140	.60	.35	2.5	—
	Coconut meat, fresh:																	
519	Piece, about 2 by 2 by 1/2 in 1 piece	51	155	2	16	14.0	.9	.3	4	6	43	.8	115	0	.02	.01	.2	1
520	Shredded or grated, not pressed down. 1 cup	51	275	3	28	24.8	1.6	.5	8	10	76	1.4	205	0	.04	.02	.4	2
521	Filberts (hazelnuts), chopped (about 80 kernels). 1 cup	6	730	14	72	5.1	55.2	7.3	19	240	388	3.9	810	—	.53	—	1.0	Trace
522	Lentils, whole, cooked 1 cup	72	210	16	Trace	—	—	—	39	50	238	4.2	498	40	.14	.12	1.2	0
523	Peanuts, roasted in oil, salted (whole, halves, chopped). 1 cup	2	840	37	72	13.7	33.0	20.7	27	107	577	3.0	971	—	.46	.19	24.8	0
524	Peanut butter——— 1 tbsp	2	95	4	8	1.5	3.7	2.3	3	9	61	.3	100	—	.02	.02	2.4	0
525	Peas, split, dry, cooked——— 1 cup	70	230	16	1	—	—	—	42	22	178	3.4	592	80	.30	.18	1.8	—
526	Pecans, chopped or pieces (about 120 large halves). 1 cup	3	810	11	84	7.2	50.5	20.0	17	86	341	2.8	712	150	1.01	.15	1.1	2
527	Pumpkin and squash kernels, dry, hulled. 1 cup	4	775	41	65	11.8	23.5	27.5	21	71	1,602	15.7	1,386	100	.34	.27	3.4	—
528	Sunflower seeds, dry, hulled——— 1 cup	5	810	35	69	8.2	13.7	43.2	29	174	1,214	10.3	1,334	70	2.84	.33	7.8	—
	Walnuts:																	
	Black:																	
529	Chopped or broken kernels——— 1 cup	3	785	26	74	6.3	13.3	45.7	19	Trace	713	7.5	575	380	.28	.14	.9	—
530	Ground (finely), chopped——— 1 cup	3	500	16	47	4.0	8.5	29.2	12	Trace	456	4.8	368	240	.18	.09	.6	—
531	Persian or English, chopped (about 60 halves). 1 cup	4	780	18	77	8.4	11.8	42.2	19	119	456	3.7	540	40	.40	.16	1.1	2

19 Crust made with vegetable shortening and enriched flour.
38 Made with vegetable shortening.
59 Product may or may not be enriched with riboflavin. Consult the label.
60 Value varies with the brand. Consult the label.

Table continued on the following page

Appendix Table 1. NUTRITIVE VALUES OF THE EDIBLE PART OF FOODS (Continued)

(Dashes (—) denote lack of reliable data for a constituent believed to be present in measurable amount)

NUTRIENTS IN INDICATED QUANTITY

Item No. (A)	Foods, approximate measures, units, and weight (edible part unless footnotes indicate otherwise) (B)	Grams	Water (C) Percent	Food energy (D) Calories	Protein (E) Grams	Fat (F) Grams	Saturated (total) (G) Grams	Unsaturated Oleic (H) Grams	Linoleic (I) Grams	Carbohydrate (J) Grams	Calcium (K) Milligrams	Phosphorus (L) Milligrams	Iron (M) Milligrams	Potassium (N) Milligrams	Vitamin A value (O) International units	Thiamin (P) Milligrams	Riboflavin (Q) Milligrams	Niacin (R) Milligrams	Ascorbic acid (S) Milligrams
	SUGARS AND SWEETS																		
	Cake icings:																		
	Boiled, white:																		
532	Plain	94	18	295	1	0	0	0	0	75	2	2	Trace	17	0	Trace	0.03	Trace	0
533	With coconut	166	15	605	3	13	11.0	.9	Trace	124	10	50	0.8	277	0	0.02	.07	0.3	0
	Uncooked:																		
534	Chocolate made with milk and butter.	275	14	1,035	9	38	23.4	11.7	1.0	185	165	305	3.3	536	580	.06	.28	.6	1
535	Creamy fudge from mix and water.	245	15	830	7	16	5.1	6.7	3.1	183	96	218	2.7	238	Trace	.05	.20	.7	Trace
536	White	319	11	1,200	2	21	12.7	5.1	.5	260	48	38	Trace	57	860	Trace	.06	Trace	Trace
	Candy:																		
537	Caramels, plain or chocolate	28	8	115	1	3	1.6	1.1	.1	22	42	35	.4	54	Trace	.01	.05	.1	Trace
	Chocolate:																		
538	Milk, plain	28	1	145	2	9	5.5	3.0	.3	16	65	65	.3	109	80	.02	.10	.1	Trace
539	Semisweet, small pieces (60 per oz).	170	1	860	7	61	36.2	19.8	1.7	97	51	255	4.4	553	30	.02	.14	.9	0
540	Chocolate-coated peanuts	28	1	160	5	12	4.0	4.7	2.1	11	33	84	.4	143	Trace	.10	.05	2.1	Trace
541	Fondant, uncoated (mints, candy corn, other).	28	8	105	Trace	1	.1	.3	.1	25	4	2	.3	1	0	Trace	Trace	Trace	0
542	Fudge, chocolate, plain	28	8	115	1	3	1.3	1.4	.6	21	22	24	.3	42	Trace	.01	.03	.1	Trace
543	Gum drops	28	12	100	Trace	Trace	—	—	—	25	2	Trace	.1	1	0	0	Trace	Trace	0
544	Hard	28	1	110	0	Trace	—	—	—	28	6	2	.5	1	0	0	0	0	0
545	Marshmallows	28	17	90	1	Trace	—	—	—	23	5	2	.5	2	0	0	Trace	Trace	0
	Chocolate-flavored beverage powders (about 4 heaping tsp per oz):																		
546	With nonfat dry milk	28	2	100	5	1	.5	.3	Trace	20	167	155	.5	227	10	.04	.21	.2	1
547	Without milk	28	1	100	5	1	.4	.2	Trace	25	9	48	.6	142	—	.01	.03	.2	Trace
548	Honey, strained or extracted	21	17	65	Trace	0	0	0	0	17	1	1	.1	11	0	Trace	.01	.1	Trace
549	Jams and preserves	20	29	55	Trace	Trace	—	—	—	14	4	2	.2	18	Trace	Trace	.01	Trace	Trace
550	Jellies	14	29	40	Trace	Trace	—	—	—	10	3	1	.1	12	Trace	Trace	.01	Trace	Trace
551		18	29	50	Trace	Trace	—	—	—	13	4	1	.3	14	Trace	Trace	.01	Trace	1
552		14	29	40	Trace	Trace	—	—	—	10	3	1	.1	11	Trace	Trace	Trace	Trace	1
	Sirups:																		
	Chocolate-flavored sirup or topping:																		
553	Thin type	38	32	90	1	1	.5	.3	Trace	24	6	35	.6	106	Trace	.01	.03	.2	0
554	Fudge type	38	25	125	2	5	3.1	1.6	.1	20	48	60	.5	107	60	.02	.08	.2	Trace
	Molasses, cane:																		
555	Light (first extraction)	20	24	50	—	—	—	—	—	13	33	9	.9	183	—	.01	.01	Trace	—
556	Blackstrap (third extraction)	20	24	45	—	—	—	—	—	11	137	17	3.2	585	—	.02	.04	.4	—
557	Sorghum	21	23	55	—	—	—	—	—	14	35	5	2.6	1	—	—	.02	Trace	—
558	Table blends, chiefly corn, light and dark.	21	24	60	0	0	0	0	0	15	9	3	.8	1	0	0	0	0	0
	Sugars:																		
559	Brown, pressed down	220	2	820	0	0	0	0	0	212	187	42	7.5	757	0	.02	.07	.4	0
	White:																		
560	Granulated	200	1	770	0	0	0	0	0	199	0	0	.2	6	0	0	0	0	0
561	1 tbsp	12	1	45	0	0	0	0	0	12	0	0	Trace	Trace	0	0	0	0	0
562	1 packet	6	1	23	0	0	0	0	0	6	0	0	Trace	Trace	0	0	0	0	0
563	Powdered, sifted, spooned into cup.	100	1	385	0	0	0	0	0	100	0	0	.1	3	0	0	0	0	0

VEGETABLE AND VEGETABLE PRODUCTS

(A)	(B)	grams	(C)	(D)	(E)	(F)	(G)	(H)	(I)	(J)	(K)	(L)	(M)	(N)	(O)	(P)	(Q)	(R)	(S)
	Asparagus, green:																		
	Cooked, drained:																		
	Cuts and tips, 1 1/2- to 2-in lengths:																		
564	From raw -------- 1 cup	145	94	30	3	Trace	—	—	—	5	30	73	0.9	265	1,310	0.23	0.26	2.0	38
565	From frozen ------ 1 cup	180	93	40	6	Trace	—	—	—	6	40	115	2.2	396	1,530	.25	.23	1.8	41
	Spears, 1/2-in diam. at base:																		
566	From raw --------- 4 spears	60	94	10	1	Trace	—	—	—	2	13	30	.4	110	540	.10	.11	.8	16
567	From frozen ------ 4 spears	60	92	15	2	Trace	—	—	—	2	13	40	.7	143	470	.10	.08	.7	16
568	Canned, spears, 1/2-in diam. at base ---- 4 spears	80	93	15	2	Trace	—	—	—	3	15	42	1.5	133	640	.05	.08	.6	12
	Beans:																		
	Lima, immature seeds, frozen, cooked, drained:																		
569	Thick-seeded types (Fordhooks) -- 1 cup	170	74	170	10	Trace	—	—	—	32	34	153	2.9	724	390	.12	.09	1.7	29
570	Thin-seeded types (baby limas) -- 1 cup	180	69	210	13	Trace	—	—	—	40	63	227	4.7	709	400	.16	.09	2.2	22
	Snap:																		
	Green:																		
571	Cooked, drained: From raw (cuts and French style) ---- 1 cup	125	92	30	2	Trace	—	—	—	7	63	46	.8	189	680	.09	.11	.6	15
	From frozen:																		
572	Cuts ----- 1 cup	135	92	35	2	Trace	—	—	—	8	54	43	.9	205	780	.09	.12	.5	7
573	French style ---- 1 cup	130	92	35	2	Trace	—	—	—	8	49	39	1.2	177	690	.08	.10	.4	9
574	Canned, drained solids (cuts) --- 1 cup	135	92	30	2	Trace	—	—	—	7	61	34	2.0	128	630	.04	.07	.4	5
	Yellow or wax:																		
575	Cooked, drained: From raw (cuts and French style) -- 1 cup	125	93	30	2	Trace	—	—	—	6	63	46	.8	189	290	.09	.11	.6	16
576	From frozen (cuts) -- 1 cup	135	92	35	2	Trace	—	—	—	8	47	42	.9	221	140	.09	.11	.5	8
577	Canned, drained solids (cuts) -- 1 cup	135	92	30	2	Trace	—	—	—	7	61	34	2.0	128	140	.04	.07	.4	7
	Beans, mature. See Beans, dry (items 509-515) and Blackeye peas, dry (item 516).																		
	Bean sprouts (mung):																		
578	Raw ---- 1 cup	105	89	35	4	Trace	—	—	—	7	20	67	1.4	234	20	.14	.14	.8	20
579	Cooked, drained ---- 1 cup	125	91	35	4	Trace	—	—	—	7	21	60	1.1	195	30	.11	.13	.9	8
	Beets:																		
	Cooked, drained, peeled:																		
580	Whole beets, 2-in diam. -- 2 beets	100	91	30	1	Trace	—	—	—	7	14	23	.5	208	20	.03	.04	.3	6
581	Diced or sliced --- 1 cup	170	91	55	2	Trace	—	—	—	12	24	39	.9	354	30	.05	.07	.5	10
	Canned, drained solids:																		
582	Whole beets, small --- 1 cup	160	89	60	2	Trace	—	—	—	14	30	29	1.1	267	30	.02	.05	.2	5
583	Diced or sliced --- 1 cup	170	89	65	2	Trace	—	—	—	15	32	31	1.2	284	30	.02	.05	.2	5
584	Beet greens, leaves and stems, cooked, drained --- 1 cup	145	94	25	2	Trace	—	—	—	5	144	36	2.8	481	7,400	.10	.22	.4	22
	Blackeye peas, immature seeds, cooked and drained:																		
585	From raw --- 1 cup	165	72	180	13	1	—	—	—	30	40	241	3.5	625	580	.50	.18	2.3	28
586	From frozen --- 1 cup	170	66	220	15	1	—	—	—	40	43	286	4.8	573	290	.68	.19	2.4	15
	Broccoli, cooked, drained:																		
	From raw:																		
587	Stalk, medium size --- 1 stalk	180	91	45	6	1	—	—	—	8	158	112	1.4	481	4,500	.16	.36	1.4	162
588	Stalks cut into 1/2-in pieces -- 1 cup	155	91	40	5	Trace	—	—	—	7	136	96	1.2	414	3,880	.14	.31	1.2	140
	From frozen:																		
589	Stalk, 4 1/2 to 5 in long -- 1 stalk	30	91	10	1	Trace	—	—	—	1	12	17	.2	66	570	.02	.03	.2	22
590	Chopped --- 1 cup	185	92	50	5	1	—	—	—	9	100	104	1.3	392	4,810	.11	.22	.9	105
	Brussels sprouts, cooked, drained:																		
591	From raw, 7-8 sprouts (1 1/4- to 1 1/2-in diam.) -- 1 cup	155	88	55	7	1	—	—	—	10	50	112	1.7	423	810	.12	.22	1.2	135
592	From frozen -- 1 cup	155	89	50	5	Trace	—	—	—	10	33	95	1.2	457	880	.12	.16	.9	126

Table continued on the following page

Appendix Table 1. NUTRITIVE VALUES OF THE EDIBLE PART OF FOODS (*Continued*)

(Dashes (—) denote lack of reliable data for a constituent believed to be present in measurable amount)

Item No. (A)	Foods, approximate measures, units, and weight (edible part unless footnotes indicate otherwise) (B)		Grams	Water (C) Per cent	Food energy (D) Calories	Pro-tein (E) Grams	Fat (F) Grams	Fatty Acids Saturated (total) (G) Grams	Unsaturated Oleic (H) Grams	Linoleic (I) Grams	Carbo-hydrate (J) Grams	Calcium (K) Milligrams	Phos-phorus (L) Milligrams	Iron (M) Milligrams	Potas-sium (N) Milligrams	Vitamin A value (O) International units	Thiamin (P) Milligrams	Ribo-flavin (Q) Milligrams	Niacin (R) Milligrams	Ascorbic acid (S) Milligrams
	VEGETABLE AND VEGETABLE PRODUCTS—Con.																			
	Cabbage:																			
	Common varieties:																			
	Raw:																			
593	Coarsely shredded or sliced—	1 cup	70	92	15	1	Trace	—	—	—	4	34	20	0.3	163	90	0.04	0.04	0.2	33
594	Finely shredded or chopped—	1 cup	90	92	20	1	Trace	—	—	—	5	44	26	.4	210	120	.05	.05	.3	42
595	Cooked, drained—	1 cup	145	94	30	2	Trace	—	—	—	6	64	29	.4	236	190	.06	.06	.4	48
596	Red, raw, coarsely shredded or sliced.	1 cup	70	90	20	1	Trace	—	—	—	5	29	25	.6	188	30	.06	.04	.3	43
597	Savoy, raw, coarsely shredded or sliced.	1 cup	70	92	15	2	Trace	—	—	—	3	47	38	.6	188	140	.04	.06	.2	39
598	Cabbage, celery (also called pe-tsai or wongbok), raw, 1-in pieces.	1 cup	75	95	10	1	Trace	—	—	—	2	32	30	.5	190	110	.04	.03	.5	19
599	Cabbage, white mustard (also called bokchoy or pakchoy), cooked, drained.	1 cup	170	95	25	2	Trace	—	—	—	4	252	56	1.0	364	5,270	.07	.14	1.2	26
	Carrots:																			
	Raw, without crowns and tips, scraped:																			
600	Whole, 7 1/2 by 1 1/8 in, or strips, 2 1/2 to 3 in long.	1 carrot or 18 strips—	72	88	30	1	Trace	—	—	—	7	27	26	.5	246	7,930	.04	.04	.4	6
601	Grated—	1 cup	110	88	45	1	Trace	—	—	—	11	41	40	.8	375	12,100	.07	.06	.7	9
602	Cooked (crosswise cuts), drained	1 cup	155	91	50	1	Trace	—	—	—	11	51	48	.9	344	16,280	.08	.08	.8	9
	Canned:																			
603	Sliced, drained solids—	1 cup	155	91	45	1	Trace	—	—	—	10	47	34	1.1	186	23,250	.03	.05	.6	3
604	Strained or junior (baby food)	1 oz (1 3/4 to 2 tbsp)—	28	92	10	Trace	Trace	—	—	—	2	7	6	.1	51	3,690	.01	.01	.1	1
	Cauliflower:																			
605	Raw, chopped—	1 cup	115	91	31	3	Trace	—	—	—	6	29	64	1.3	339	70	.13	.12	.8	90
	Cooked, drained:																			
606	From raw (flower buds)—	1 cup	125	93	30	3	Trace	—	—	—	5	26	53	.9	258	80	.11	.10	.8	69
607	From frozen (flowerets)—	1 cup	180	94	30	3	Trace	—	—	—	6	31	68	.9	373	50	.07	.09	.7	74
	Celery, Pascal type, raw:																			
608	Stalk, large outer, 8 by 1 1/2 in, at root end.	1 stalk	40	94	5	Trace	Trace	—	—	—	2	16	11	.1	136	110	.01	.01	.1	4
609	Pieces, diced—	1 cup	120	94	20	1	Trace	—	—	—	5	47	34	.4	409	320	.04	.04	.4	11
	Collards, cooked, drained:																			
610	From raw (leaves without stems)—	1 cup	190	90	65	7	1	—	—	—	10	357	99	1.5	498	14,820	.21	.38	2.3	144
611	From frozen (chopped)—	1 cup	170	90	50	5	1	—	—	—	10	299	87	1.7	401	11,560	.10	.24	1.0	56
	Corn, sweet:																			
	Cooked, drained:																			
612	From raw, ear 5 by 1 3/4 in—	1 ear[61]—	140	74	70	2	1	—	—	—	16	2	69	.5	151	[62]310	.09	.08	1.1	7
	From frozen:																			
613	Ear, 5 in long—	1 ear[61]—	229	73	120	4	1	—	—	—	27	4	121	1.0	291	[62]440	.18	.10	2.1	9
614	Kernels—	1 cup	165	77	130	5	1	—	—	—	31	5	120	1.3	304	[62]580	.15	.10	2.5	8
	Canned:																			
615	Cream style—	1 cup	256	76	210	5	2	—	—	—	51	8	143	1.5	248	[62]840	.08	.13	2.6	13
	Whole kernel:																			
616	Vacuum pack—	1 cup	210	76	175	5	1	—	—	—	43	6	153	1.1	204	[62]740	.06	.13	2.3	11
617	Wet pack, drained solids—	1 cup	165	76	140	4	1	—	—	—	33	8	81	.8	160	[62]580	.05	.08	1.5	7
	Cowpeas. See Blackeye peas. (Items 585-586).																			
	Cucumber slices, 1/8 in thick (large, 2 1/8-in diam.; small, 1 3/4-in in diam.):																			
618	With peel—	6 large or 8 small slices	28	95	5	Trace	Trace	—	—	—	1	7	8	.3	45	70	.01	.01	.1	3

(A)	(B)			(C)	(D)	(E)	(F)	(G)	(H)	(I)	(J)	(K)	(L)	(M)	(N)	(O)	(P)	(Q)	(R)	(S)
619	Without peel	6 1/2 large or 9 small pieces	28	96	5	Trace	Trace	—	—	—	1	7	5	0.1	45	Trace	0.01	0.01	0.1	3
620	Dandelion greens, cooked, drained	1 cup	105	90	35	2	1	—	—	—	7	147	44	1.9	244	12,290	.14	.17	—	19
621	Endive, curly (including escarole), raw, small pieces	1 cup	50	93	10	1	Trace	—	—	—	2	41	27	.9	147	1,650	.04	.07	.3	5
622	Kale, cooked, drained: From raw (leaves without stems and midribs)	1 cup	110	88	45	5	1	—	—	—	7	206	64	1.8	243	9,130	.11	.20	1.8	102
623	From frozen (leaf style)	1 cup	130	91	40	4	1	—	—	—	7	157	62	1.3	251	10,660	.08	.20	.9	49
624	Lettuce, raw: Butterhead, as Boston types: Head, 5-in diam	1 head[6.3]	220	95	25	2	Trace	—	—	—	4	57	42	3.3	430	1,580	.10	.10	.5	13
625	Leaves	1 outer or 2 inner or 3 heart leaves	15	95	Trace	Trace	Trace	—	—	—	Trace	5	4	.3	40	150	.01	.01	Trace	1
626	Crisphead, as Iceberg: Head, 6-in diam	1 head[6.4]	567	96	70	5	1	—	—	—	16	108	118	2.7	943	1,780	.32	.32	1.6	32
627	Wedge, 1/4 of head	1 wedge	135	96	20	1	Trace	—	—	—	4	27	30	.7	236	450	.08	.08	.4	8
628	Pieces, chopped or shredded	1 cup	55	96	5	Trace	Trace	—	—	—	2	11	12	.3	96	180	.03	.03	.2	3
629	Looseleaf (bunching varieties including romaine or cos), chopped or shredded pieces	1 cup	55	94	10	1	Trace	—	—	—	2	37	14	.8	145	1,050	.03	.04	.2	10
630	Mushrooms, raw, sliced or chopped pieces	1 cup	70	90	20	2	Trace	—	—	—	3	4	81	.6	290	Trace	.07	.32	2.9	2
631	Mustard greens, without stems and midribs, cooked, drained	1 cup	140	93	30	3	Trace	—	—	—	6	193	45	2.5	308	8,120	.11	.20	.8	67
632	Okra pods, 3 by 5/8 in, cooked	10 pods	106	91	30	2	Trace	—	—	—	6	98	43	.5	184	520	.14	.19	1.0	21
633	Onions: Mature: Raw: Chopped	1 cup	170	89	65	3	Trace	—	—	—	15	46	61	.9	267	[6.5]Trace	.05	.07	.3	17
634	Sliced	1 cup	115	89	45	2	Trace	—	—	—	10	31	41	.6	181	[6.5]Trace	.03	.05	.2	12
635	Cooked (whole or sliced), drained	1 cup	210	92	60	3	Trace	—	—	—	14	50	61	.8	231	[6.5]Trace	.06	.06	.4	15
636	Young green, bulb (3/8 in diam.) and white portion of top	6 onions	30	88	15	Trace	Trace	—	—	—	3	12	12	.2	69	Trace	.02	.01	.1	8
637	Parsley, raw, chopped	1 tbsp	4	85	Trace	Trace	Trace	—	—	—	Trace	7	2	.2	25	300	Trace	.01	Trace	6
638	Parsnips, cooked (diced or 2-in lengths)	1 cup	155	82	100	2	1	—	—	—	23	70	96	.9	587	50	.11	.12	.2	16
639	Peas, green: Canned: Whole, drained solids	1 cup	170	77	150	8	1	—	—	—	29	44	129	3.2	163	1,170	.15	.10	1.4	14
640	Strained (baby food)	1 oz (1 3/4 to 2 tbsp)	28	86	15	1	Trace	—	—	—	3	3	18	.3	28	140	.02	.03	.3	3
641	Frozen, cooked, drained	1 cup	160	82	110	8	Trace	—	—	—	19	30	138	3.0	216	960	.43	.14	2.7	21
642	Peppers, hot, red, without seeds, dried (ground chili powder, added seasonings)	1 tsp	2	9	5	Trace	Trace	—	—	—	1	5	4	.3	20	1,300	Trace	.02	.2	Trace
643	Peppers, sweet (about 5 per lb, whole), stem and seeds removed: Raw	1 pod	74	93	15	1	Trace	—	—	—	4	7	16	.5	157	310	.06	.06	.4	94
644	Cooked, boiled, drained	1 pod	73	95	15	1	Trace	—	—	—	3	7	12	.4	109	310	.05	.05	.4	70
645	Potatoes, cooked: Baked, peeled after baking (about 2 per lb, raw)	1 potato	156	75	145	4	Trace	—	—	—	33	14	101	1.1	782	Trace	.15	.07	2.7	31
646	Boiled (about 3 per lb, raw): Peeled after boiling	1 potato	137	80	105	3	Trace	—	—	—	23	10	72	.8	556	Trace	.12	.05	2.0	22
647	Peeled before boiling	1 potato	135	83	90	3	Trace	—	—	—	20	8	57	.7	385	Trace	.12	.05	1.6	22
648	French-fried, strip, 2 to 3 1/2 in long: Prepared from raw	10 strips	50	45	135	2	7	1.7	1.2	3.3	18	8	56	.7	427	Trace	.07	.04	1.6	11
649	Frozen, oven heated	10 strips	50	53	110	2	4	1.1	.8	2.1	17	5	43	.9	326	Trace	.07	.01	1.3	11
650	Hashed brown, prepared from frozen	1 cup	155	56	345	3	18	4.6	3.2	9.0	45	28	78	1.9	439	Trace	.11	.03	1.6	12
651	Mashed, prepared from— Raw: Milk added	1 cup	210	83	135	4	2	.7	.4	Trace	27	50	103	.8	548	40	.17	.11	2.1	21

[6.1] Weight includes cob. Without cob, weight is 77 g for item 612, 126 g for item 613.
[6.2] Based on yellow varieties. For white varieties, value is trace.
[6.3] Weight includes refuse of outer leaves and core. Without these parts, weight is 163 g.
[6.4] Weight includes core. Without core, weight is 539 g.
[6.5] Value based on white-fleshed varieties. For yellow-fleshed varieties, value in International Units (I.U.) is 70 for item 633, 50 for item 634, and 80 for item 635.

Table continued on the following page

Appendix Table 1. NUTRITIVE VALUES OF THE EDIBLE PART OF FOODS (*Continued*)

(Dashes (—) denote lack of reliable data for a constituent believed to be present in measurable amount)

Item No. (A)	Foods, approximate measures, units, and weight (edible part unless footnotes indicate otherwise) (B)	Grams	Water (C) Per cent	Food energy (D) Calories	Protein (E) Grams	Fat (F) Grams	Fatty Acids Saturated (total) (G) Grams	Oleic (H) Grams	Linoleic (I) Grams	Carbohydrate (I) Grams	Calcium (K) Milligrams	Phosphorus (L) Milligrams	Iron (M) Milligrams	Potassium (N) Milligrams	Vitamin A value (O) International units	Thiamin (P) Milligrams	Riboflavin (Q) Milligrams	Niacin (R) Milligrams	Ascorbic acid (S) Milligrams
	VEGETABLE AND VEGETABLE PRODUCTS—Con.																		
	Potatoes, cooked—Continued																		
	Mashed, prepared from—Continued																		
	Raw—Continued																		
652	Milk and butter added-- 1 cup	210	80	195	4	9	5.6	2.3	0.2	26	50	101	0.8	525	360	0.17	0.11	2.1	19
653	Dehydrated flakes (without milk), water, milk, butter, and salt added. 1 cup	210	79	195	4	7	3.6	2.1	.2	30	65	99	.6	601	270	.08	.08	1.9	11
654	Potato chips, 1 3/4 by 2 1/2 in oval cross section. 10 chips	20	2	115	1	8	2.1	1.4	4.0	10	8	28	.4	226	Trace	.04	.01	1.0	3
655	Potato salad, made with cooked salad dressing. 1 cup	250	76	250	7	7	2.0	2.7	1.3	41	80	160	1.5	798	350	.20	.18	2.8	28
656	Pumpkin, canned-- 1 cup	245	90	80	2	1	—	—	—	19	61	64	1.0	588	15,680	.07	.12	1.5	12
657	Radishes, raw (prepackaged) stem ends, rootlets cut off. 4 radishes	18	95	5	Trace	Trace	—	—	—	1	5	6	.2	58	Trace	.01	.01	.1	5
658	Sauerkraut, canned, solids and liquid. 1 cup	235	93	40	2	Trace	—	—	—	9	85	42	1.2	329	120	.07	.09	.5	33
	Southern peas. See Blackeye peas (items 585-586).																		
	Spinach:																		
659	Raw, chopped-- 1 cup	55	91	15	2	Trace	—	—	—	2	51	28	1.7	259	4,460	.06	.11	.3	28
660	Cooked, drained: From raw-- 1 cup	180	92	40	5	1	—	—	—	6	167	68	4.0	583	14,580	.13	.25	.9	50
	From frozen:																		
661	Chopped-- 1 cup	205	92	45	6	1	—	—	—	8	232	90	4.3	683	16,200	.14	.31	.8	39
662	Leaf-- 1 cup	190	92	45	6	1	—	—	—	7	200	84	4.8	688	15,390	.15	.27	1.0	53
663	Canned, drained solids-- 1 cup	205	91	50	6	1	—	—	—	7	242	53	5.3	513	16,400	.04	.25	.6	29
	Squash, cooked:																		
664	Summer (all varieties), diced, drained. 1 cup	210	96	30	2	Trace	—	—	—	7	53	53	.8	296	820	.11	.17	1.7	21
665	Winter (all varieties), baked, mashed. 1 cup	205	81	130	4	1	—	—	—	32	57	98	1.6	945	8,610	.10	.27	1.4	27
	Sweetpotatoes:																		
	Cooked (raw, 5 by 2 in; about 2 1/2 per lb):																		
666	Baked in skin, peeled-- 1 potato	114	64	160	2	1	—	—	—	37	46	66	1.0	342	9,230	.10	.08	.8	25
667	Boiled in skin, peeled-- 1 potato	151	71	170	3	1	—	—	—	40	48	71	1.1	367	11,940	.14	.09	.9	26
668	Candied, 2 1/2 by 2-in piece-- 1 piece	105	60	175	1	3	2.0	.8	.1	36	39	45	.9	200	6,620	.06	.04	.4	11
	Canned:																		
669	Solid pack (mashed)-- 1 cup	255	72	275	5	1	—	—	—	63	64	105	2.0	510	19,890	.13	.10	1.5	36
670	Vacuum pack, piece 2 3/4 by 1 in. 1 piece	40	72	45	1	Trace	—	—	—	10	10	16	.3	80	3,120	.02	.02	.2	6
	Tomatoes:																		
671	Raw, 2 3/5-in diam. (3 per 12 oz pkg.). 1 tomato[66]	135	94	25	1	Trace	—	—	—	6	16	33	.6	300	1,110	.07	.05	.9	[6][7]28
672	Canned, solids and liquid-- 1 cup	241	94	50	2	Trace	—	—	—	10	[6]14	46	1.2	523	2,170	.12	.07	1.7	41
673	Tomato catsup-- 1 cup	273	69	290	5	1	—	—	—	69	60	137	2.2	991	3,820	.25	.19	4.4	41
674	1 tbsp	15	69	15	Trace	Trace	—	—	—	4	3	8	.1	54	210	.01	.01	.2	2
	Tomato juice, canned:																		
675	Cup-- 1 cup	243	94	45	2	Trace	—	—	—	10	17	44	2.2	552	1,940	.12	.07	1.9	39
676	Glass (6 fl oz)-- 1 glass	182	94	35	2	Trace	—	—	—	8	13	33	1.6	413	1,460	.09	.05	1.5	29
677	Turnips, cooked, diced-- 1 cup	155	94	35	1	Trace	—	—	—	8	54	37	.6	291	Trace	.06	.08	.5	34
	Turnip greens, cooked, drained:																		
678	From raw (leaves and stems)-- 1 cup	145	94	30	3	Trace	—	—	—	5	252	49	1.5	—	8,270	.15	.33	.7	68
679	From frozen (chopped)-- 1 cup	165	93	40	4	Trace	—	—	—	6	195	64	2.6	246	11,390	.08	.15	.7	31
680	Vegetables, mixed, frozen, cooked-- 1 cup	182	83	115	6	1	—	—	—	24	46	115	2.4	348	9,010	.22	.13	2.0	15

MISCELLANEOUS ITEMS

(A)	(B)		(C)	(D)	(E)	(F)	(G)	(H)	(I)	(J)	(K)	(L)	(M)	(N)	(O)	(P)	(Q)	(R)	(S)
	Baking powders for home use:																		
	Sodium aluminum sulfate:																		
681	With monocalcium phosphate monohydrate.	1 tsp	3.0	2	5	Trace	Trace	0	0	0	1	58	87	—	5	0	0	0	0	0
682	With monocalcium phosphate monohydrate, calcium sulfate.	1 tsp	2.9	1	5	Trace	Trace	0	0	0	1	183	45	—	—	0	0	0	0	0
683	Straight phosphate.	1 tsp	3.8	2	5	Trace	Trace	0	0	0	1	239	359	—	6	0	0	0	0	0
684	Low sodium.	1 tsp	4.3	2	5	Trace	Trace	0	0	0	2	207	314	—	471	0	0	0	0	0
685	Barbecue sauce.	1 cup	250	81	230	4	17	2.2	4.3	10.0	20	53	50	2.0	435	900	.03	.03	.8	13
686	Beverages, alcoholic: Beer.	12 fl oz	360	92	150	1	0	0	0	0	14	18	108	Trace	90	—	.01	.11	2.2	—
	Gin, rum, vodka, whisky:																		
687	80-proof.	1 1/2-fl oz jigger	42	67	95	—	—	—	—	—	Trace	—	—	—	1	—	—	—	—	—
688	86-proof.	1 1/2-fl oz jigger	42	64	105	—	—	—	—	—	Trace	—	—	—	1	—	—	—	—	—
689	90-proof.	1 1/2-fl oz jigger	42	62	110	—	—	—	—	—	Trace	—	—	—	1	—	—	—	—	—
	Wines:																			
690	Dessert.	3 1/2-fl oz glass	103	77	140	Trace	0	0	0	0	8	8	—	—	77	—	.01	.02	.2	—
691	Table.	3 1/2-fl oz glass	102	86	85	Trace	0	0	0	0	4	9	10	.4	94	—	Trace	.01	.1	—
	Beverages, carbonated, sweetened, nonalcoholic:																			
692	Carbonated water.	12 fl oz	366	92	115	0	0	0	0	0	29	—	—	—	—	0	0	0	0	0
693	Cola type.	12 fl oz	369	90	145	0	0	0	0	0	37	—	—	—	—	0	0	0	0	0
694	Fruit-flavored sodas and Tom Collins mixer.	12 fl oz	372	88	170	0	0	0	0	0	45	—	—	—	—	0	0	0	0	0
695	Ginger ale.	12 fl oz	366	92	115	0	0	0	0	0	29	—	—	0	0	0	0	0	0	0
696	Root beer.	12 fl oz	370	90	150	0	0	0	0	0	39	—	—	0	0	0	0	0	0	0
	Chili powder. See Peppers, hot, red (item 642).																			
	Chocolate:																			
697	Bitter or baking.	1 oz	28	2	145	3	15	8.9	4.9	.4	8	22	109	1.9	235	20	.01	.07	.4	0
	Semisweet, see Candy, chocolate (item 539).																			
	Gelatin, dry.																			
698		1 7-g envelope	7	13	25	6	Trace	0	0	0	0	—	—	—	—	0	0	0	0	0
699	Gelatin dessert prepared with gelatin dessert powder and water.	1 cup	240	84	140	4	0	0	0	0	34	—	—	—	—	0	0	0	0	0
700	Mustard, prepared, yellow.	1 tsp or individual serving pouch or cup.	5	80	5	Trace	Trace	—	—	—	Trace	4	4	.1	7	—	—	—	—	—
	Olives, pickled, canned:																			
701	Green.	4 medium or 3 extra large or 2 giant.[69]	16	78	15	Trace	2	.2	1.2	.1	Trace	8	2	.2	7	40	—	—	—	—
702	Ripe, Mission.	3 small or 2 large[69]	10	73	15	Trace	2	.2	1.2	.1	Trace	9	1	.1	2	10	Trace	Trace	—	—
	Pickles, cucumber:																			
703	Dill, medium, whole, 3 3/4 in long, 1 1/4-in diam.	1 pickle	65	93	5	Trace	Trace	—	—	—	1	17	14	.7	130	70	Trace	.01	Trace	4
704	Fresh-pack, slices 1 1/2-in diam., 1/4 in thick.	2 slices	15	79	10	Trace	Trace	—	—	—	3	5	4	.3	—	20	Trace	Trace	Trace	1
705	Sweet, gherkin, small, whole, about 2 1/2 in long, 3/4-in diam.	1 pickle	15	61	20	Trace	Trace	—	—	—	5	2	2	.2	—	10	Trace	Trace	Trace	1
706	Relish, finely chopped, sweet.	1 tbsp	15	63	20	Trace	Trace	—	—	—	5	3	2	.1	—	—	—	—	—	—
	Popcorn. See items 476-478.																			
707	Popsicle, 3-fl oz size.	1 popsicle	95	80	70	0	0	0	0	0	18	0	—	Trace	—	0	0	0	0	0

[66] Weight includes cores and stem ends. Without these parts, weight is 123 g.
[67] Based on year-round average. For tomatoes marketed from November through May, value is about 12 mg; from June through October, 32 mg.
[68] Applies to product without calcium salts added. Value for products with calcium salts added may be as much as 63 mg for whole tomatoes, 241 mg for cut forms.
[69] Weight includes pits. Without pits, weight is 13 g for item 701, 9 g for item 702.

Table continued on the following page

Appendix Table 1. NUTRITIVE VALUES OF THE EDIBLE PART OF FOODS (*Continued*)

(Dashes (—) denote lack of reliable data for a constituent believed to be present in measurable amount)

Item No. (A)	Foods, approximate measures, units, and weight (edible part unless footnotes indicate otherwise) (B)		Water (C)	Food energy (D)	Protein (E)	Fat (F)	Saturated (total) (G)	Oleic (H)	Linoleic (I)	Carbohydrate (J)	Calcium (K)	Phosphorus (L)	Iron (M)	Potassium (N)	Vitamin A value (O)	Thiamin (P)	Riboflavin (Q)	Niacin (R)	Ascorbic acid (S)
		Grams	Percent	Calories	Grams	Grams	Grams	Grams	Grams	Grams	Milligrams	Milligrams	Milligrams	Milligrams	International units	Milligrams	Milligrams	Milligrams	Milligrams
	MISCELLANEOUS ITEMS—Con.																		
	Soups:																		
	Canned, condensed:																		
	Prepared with equal volume of milk:																		
708	Cream of chicken------- 1 cup	245	85	180	7	10	4.2	3.6	1.3	15	172	152	0.5	260	610	0.05	0.27	0.7	2
709	Cream of mushroom------ 1 cup	245	83	215	7	14	5.4	2.9	4.6	16	191	169	.5	279	250	.05	.34	.7	1
710	Tomato------ 1 cup	250	84	175	7	7	3.4	1.7	1.0	23	168	155	.8	418	1,200	.10	.25	1.3	15
	Prepared with equal volume of water:																		
711	Bean with pork------ 1 cup	250	84	170	8	6	1.2	1.8	2.4	22	63	128	2.3	395	650	.13	.08	1.0	3
712	Beef broth, bouillon, consomme. 1 cup	240	96	30	5	0	0	0	0	3	Trace	31	.5	130	Trace	Trace	.02	1.2	—
713	Beef noodle------ 1 cup	240	93	65	4	3	.6	.7	.8	7	7	48	1.0	77	50	.05	.07	1.0	Trace
714	Clam chowder, Manhattan type (with tomatoes, without milk). 1 cup	245	92	80	2	3	.5	.4	1.3	12	34	47	1.0	184	880	.02	.02	1.0	Trace
715	Cream of chicken------ 1 cup	240	92	95	3	6	1.6	2.3	1.1	8	24	34	.5	79	410	.02	.05	.5	Trace
716	Cream of mushroom------ 1 cup	240	90	135	2	10	2.6	1.7	4.5	10	41	50	.5	98	70	.02	.12	.7	Trace
717	Minestrone------ 1 cup	245	90	105	5	3	.7	.9	1.3	14	37	59	1.0	314	2,350	.07	.05	1.0	—
718	Split pea------ 1 cup	245	85	145	9	3	1.1	1.2	.4	21	29	149	1.5	270	440	.25	.15	1.5	1
719	Tomato------ 1 cup	245	91	90	2	3	.5	.5	1.0	16	15	34	.7	230	1,000	.05	.05	1.2	12
720	Vegetable beef------ 1 cup	245	92	80	5	2	—	—	—	10	12	49	.7	162	2,700	.05	.05	1.0	—
721	Vegetarian------ 1 cup	245	92	80	2	2	—	—	—	13	20	39	1.0	172	2,940	.05	.05	1.0	—
	Dehydrated:																		
722	Bouillon cube, 1/2 in------ 1 cube	4	4	5	1	Trace	—	—	—	Trace	—	—	—	4	—	—	—	—	—
	Mixes:																		
	Unprepared:																		
723	Onion------ 1 1/2-oz pkg	43	3	150	6	5	1.1	2.3	1.0	23	42	49	.6	238	30	.05	.03	.3	6
	Prepared with water:																		
724	Chicken noodle------ 1 cup	240	95	55	2	1	—	—	—	8	7	19	.2	19	50	.07	.05	.5	Trace
725	Onion------ 1 cup	240	96	35	1	1	—	—	—	6	10	12	.2	58	Trace	Trace	Trace	Trace	2
726	Tomato vegetable with noodles. 1 cup	240	93	65	1	1	—	—	—	12	7	19	.2	29	480	.05	.02	.5	5
727	Vinegar, cider------ 1 tbsp	15	94	Trace	Trace	0	0	0	0	1	1	1	.1	15	—	—	—	—	—
728	White sauce, medium, with enriched flour. 1 cup	250	73	405	10	31	19.3	7.8	.8	22	288	233	.5	348	1,150	.12	.43	.7	2
	Yeast:																		
729	Baker's, dry, active------ 1 pkg	7	5	20	3	Trace	—	—	—	3	3	90	1.1	140	Trace	.16	.38	2.6	Trace
730	Brewer's, dry------ 1 tbsp	8	5	25	3	Trace	—	—	—	3	[70]17	140	1.4	152	Trace	1.25	.34	3.0	Trace

[70]Value may vary from 6 to 60 mg.

Appendix Table 2. ENERGY VALUES OF BEVERAGES AND SNACK FOODS

FOOD	WEIGHT (gm.)	APPROXIMATE MEASURE	KCALORIES	FOOD	WEIGHT (gm.)	APPROXIMATE MEASURE	KCALORIES
Beverages				Doughnut, cake type,			
Carbonated, cola type	369	1 bottle, 12 ounces	145	plain	32	1 average	125
Malted milk	235	1 regular (1 cup)	245	Doughnut, jelly	65	1 average	226
Chocolate milk				Doughnut, raised	30	1 average	120
(made with skim milk)	250	1 cup	190				
Cocoa	250	1 cup	245	**Fruits**			
soda, vanilla ice cream	242	1 regular	60	Apple	150	1 medium, 2½ in. diameter	70
				Banana	100	1 medium, 6 by 1½ in.	85
Beverages, alcoholic				Grapes, European type	160	1 cup	95
Beer	360	1 bottle, 12 ounces	150	Orange	180	1 medium, 2⅝ in.	65
Brandy	30	1 brandy glass	75			diameter	
Gin	43	1 jigger	107	Pear	182	1 medium, 3 by 2½ in.	100
Liqueurs (average)	20	1 cordial glass	165			diameter	
Martini		1 cocktail glass	145				
Manhattan		1 cocktail glass	165	**Miscellaneous**			
Rum	43	1 jigger	105	Hamburger and bun	96	1 average	334
Whiskey	43	1 jigger	107	Ice cream, vanilla	62	3-ounce container	95
Wine, port	100	1 wine glass	160	Sherbet	96	½ cup	130
Wine, sauterne	100	1 wine glass	85	Jams, jellies,			
				marmalades, preserves	21	1 tablespoon	55
Cake				Syrup, blended	21	1 tablespoon	60
Angel food	53	1 piece	135	Waffles	75	1 waffle, 4½ by 5½ by	210
Cupcake, chocolate, iced	36	1 cake, 2¾ in.	130			½ inch	
		diameter					
Fruit cake	30	1 piece, 2 by 2 by ½ in.	110	**Nuts**			
				Mixed, shelled	15	8 to 12	94
Candy and Popcorn				Peanut butter	16	1 tablespoon	95
Butterscotch	15	3 pieces	60	Peanuts, shelled,			
Candy bar, plain	28	1 bar	145	roasted	144	1 cup	840
Caramels	28	3 medium	115	**Pie**			
Choc. coated peanuts	28	1 ounce	160	Apple	135	4-inch sector	350
Fudge	28	1 piece	115	Cherry	135	4-inch sector	350
Peanut brittle	30	1 ounce	128	Custard	130	4-inch sector	285
Popcorn with oil added	9	1 cup	40	Lemon meringue	120	4-inch sector	305
				Mince	135	4-inch sector	365
Cheese				Pumpkin	130	4-inch sector	275
Camembert	38	1 wedge	115				
Cheddar	28	1 ounce	115	**Potato chips**			
Cream	28	1 ounce	106	Potato chips	20	10 chips, 2 inches in	115
Swiss (domestic)	28	1 ounce	100			diameter	
Cookies				**Sandwiches**			
Brownies, made with				Bacon, lettuce, tomato	148	1 sandwich	282
mix	20	1 piece	85	Egg salad	138	1 sandwich	279
Cookies, plain and		1 cooky, 3 in.		Ham	81	1 sandwich	281
assorted	25	diameter	120	Liverwurst	91	1 sandwich	251
				Peanut butter	83	1 sandwich	328
Crackers							
Cheese	18	5 crackers	86	**Soups, commercial canned**			
Graham	14	2 medium	55	Bean with pork	250	1 cup	170
Saltines	11	4 crackers	50	Beef noodle	250	1 cup	70
Rye	26	4 crackers	85	Chicken noodle	198	1 cup	51
				Cream (mushroom)	241	1 cup	215
Dessert type cream puff				Tomato	198	1 cup	73
and doughnuts				Vegetable with beef			
Cream puff – custard				broth	241	1 cup	80
filling	100	1 average	233				

Appendix Table 3. COMMON CARBOHYDRATES IN FOODS PER 100 GM. EDIBLE PORTION**

FOOD	MONO-SACCHARIDES		REDUC-ING SUGARS*	DISACCHARIDES			POLYSACCHARIDES					
	Fructose	Glucose		Lactose	Maltose	Sucrose	Cellulose	Dextrins	Hemi-cellulose	Pectin	Pento-sans	Starch
Fruits												
	gm.	*gm.*	*gm.*	*gm.*	*gm.*	*gm.*	*gm.*	*gm.*	*gm.*	*gm.*	*gm.*	*gm.*
Agave juice	17.0		19.0	†								
Apple	5.0	1.7	8.3			3.1	0.4		0.7	0.6		0.6
Apple juice			8.0			4.2						
Apricots	0.4	1.9				5.5	0.8		1.2	1.0		
Banana												
Yellow green			5.0			5.1						8.8
Yellow			8.4			8.9						1.9
Flecked	3.5	4.5				11.9						1.2
Powder			32.6			33.2		9.6				7.8
Blackberries	2.9	3.2				0.2						
Blueberry juice, commercial			9.6			0.2						
Boysenberries			5.3			1.1				0.3		
Breadfruit												
Hawaiian			1.8			7.7						
Samoan			4.9			9.7						
Cherries												
Eating	7.2	4.7	12.5			0.1				0.3		
Cooking	6.1	5.5	11.6			0.1						
Cranberries	0.7	2.7				0.1						
Currants												
Black	3.7	2.4				0.6						
Red	1.9	2.3				0.2						
White	2.6	3.0										
Dates												
Invert sugar, seedling type	23.9	24.9				0.3						
Deglet Noor			16.2			45.4						
Egyptian			35.8			48.5						
Figs, Kadota												3.0
Fresh	8.2	9.6				0.9						0.1
Dried	30.9	42.0				0.1						0.3
Gooseberries	4.1	4.4				0.7						
Grapes												
Black	7.3	8.2										
Concord	4.3	4.8	9.5			0.2						
Malaga			22.2			0.2						
White	8.0	8.1										
Grapefruit	1.2	2.0				2.9					1.3	
Guava			4.4			1.9						
Lemon												
Edible portion			1.3			0.2				3.0	0.7	
Whole	1.4	1.4				0.4						
Juice	0.9	0.5				0.1						
Peel			3.4			0.1						
Loganberries	1.3	1.9				0.2						
Loquat												
Champagne		12.0				0.8						
Thales		9.0				0.9						
Mango			3.4			11.6						0.3
Melon												
Cantaloupe	0.9	1.2	2.3			4.4				0.3		
Cassaba,												
Vine ripened			2.8			6.2						
Picked green			3.2			3.9						
Honeydew												
Vine ripened			3.3			7.4						
Picked green			3.6			3.3						
Yellow	1.5	2.1				1.4						
Mulberries	3.6	4.4										
Orange												
Valencia (Calif.)	2.3	2.4	4.7			4.2						
Composite values	1.8	2.5	5.0			4.6	0.3		0.3	1.3	0.3	
Juice												
Fresh	2.4	2.4	5.1			4.7						
Frozen, reconstituted			4.6			3.2						

**From: Hardinge, M. G., et al.: Carbohydrate in foods. J. Am. Diet. Assoc., *46*:197, 1965.

Appendix Table 3. COMMON CARBOHYDRATES IN FOODS PER 100 GM. EDIBLE PORTION
(Continued)

FOOD	MONO-SACCHARIDES Fructose	Glucose	REDUCING SUGARS*	DISACCHARIDES Lactose	Maltose	Sucrose	POLYSACCHARIDES Cellulose	Dextrins	Hemi-Cellulose	Pectin	Pentosans	Starch
	gm.	gm.	gm.	gm.	gm.	gm.	gm.	gm.	gm.	gm.	gm.	gm.
FRUITS, continued												
Palmyra palm, tender kernel	1.5	3.2				0.4						
Papaw (*Asimina triloba*) (North America)			5.9			2.7						
Papaya (*Carica papaya*) (tropics)			9.0			0.5						
Pashion fruit juice	3.6	3.6				3.8						1.8
Peaches	1.6	1.5	3.1			6.6		0.7		0.7		
Pears												
Anjou			7.6			1.9				0.7		
Bartlett	5.0	2.5	8.0			1.5				0.6		
Bosc	6.5	2.6				1.7				0.6		
Persimmon			17.7									
Pineapple												
Ripened on plant	1.4	2.3	4.2			7.9						
Picked green			1.3			2.4						
Plums												
Damson	3.4	5.2	8.4			1.0						
Green Gage	4.0	5.5				2.9						
Italian prunes			4.6			5.4				0.9		
Sweet	2.9	4.5	7.4			4.4		0.5		1.0	0.1	
Sour	1.3	3.5				1.5				1.0		
Pomegranate			12.0			0.6						
Prunes, uncooked	15.0	30.0	47.0			2.0	2.8		10.7	0.9	2.0	0.7
Raisins, Thompson seedless			70.0							1.0		
Raspberries	2.4	2.3	5.0			1.0				0.8		
Sapote	3.8	4.2		0.7								
Strawberries												
Ripe	2.3	2.6				1.4						
Medium ripe			3.8			0.3						
Tangerine			4.8			9.0						
Tomatoes	1.2	1.6	3.4				0.2		0.3	0.3		
Canned			3.0			0.3						
Seedless pulp			6.5			0.4	0.4			0.5		
Watermelon												
Flesh red and firm, ripe			3.8			4.0				0.1		
Red, mealy, overripe			3.0			4.9				0.1		
Vegetables												
Asparagus, raw			1.2						0.3			
Bamboo shoots			0.5			0.2	1.2					
Beans												
Lima												
Canned						1.4						
Fresh						1.4						
Snap, fresh			1.7			0.5	0.3		1.0	0.5	1.2	2.0
Beets, sugar						12.9	0.9		0.8			
Broccoli						0.9			0.9		0.9	1.3
Brussel Sprouts							1.1		1.5			
Cabbage, raw			3.4			0.3	0.8		1.0			
Carrots, raw			5.8			1.7	1.0		1.7	0.9		
Cauliflower		2.8				0.3	0.7		0.6			
Celery												
Fresh			0.3			0.3						
Hearts			1.7			0.2						
Corn												
Fresh		0.5				0.3	0.6	0.1	0.9		1.3	14.5
Bran									77.1		4.0	
Cucumber			2.5			0.1						
Eggplant			2.1			0.6			0.5			
Lettuce			1.4			0.2	0.4		0.6			
Licorice root	1.4					3.2						22.0
Mushrooms, fresh			0.1				0.9		0.7			2.5
Onions, raw			5.4			2.9			0.3	0.6		
Parsnips, fresh						3.5						7.0
Peas, green						5.5	1.1		2.2			4.1

Table continued on the following page

Appendix Table 3. COMMON CARBOHYDRATES IN FOODS PER 100 GM. EDIBLE PORTION
(*Continued*)

FOOD	MONO-SACCHARIDES		REDUC-ING SUGARS*	DISACCHARIDES			POLYSACCHARIDES					
	Fructose	Glucose		Lactose	Maltose	Sucrose	Cellulose	Dextrins	Hemi-Cellulose	Pectin	Pentosans	Starch
	gm.	gm.	gm.	gm.	gm.	gm.	gm.	gm.	gm.	gm.	gm.	gm.
VEGETABLES, continued												
Potatoes, white	0.1	0.1	0.8			0.1	0.4		0.3			17.0
Pumpkin			2.2			0.6			0.5			0.1
Radishes			3.1			0.3			0.3	0.4		
Rutabagas		5.0				1.3					0.8	
Spinach			0.2				0.4		0.8			
Squash												
Butternut	0.2	0.1				0.4						2.6
Blue Hubbard	1.2	1.1				0.4	0.7					4.8
Golden Crookneck			2.8			1.0						
Sweet potato												
Raw	0.3	0.4	0.8		1.6	4.1	0.6		1.4	2.2		16.5
Baked			14.5			7.2						4.0
Mature Dry Legumes												
Beans												
Mung												
Black gram						1.6						
Green gram						1.8						
Navy							3.1	3.7	6.4		8.2	35.2
Soy			1.6			7.2	2.6	1.4	6.6		4.0	1.9
Cow pea						1.5	5.4		4.8			
Garbanzo (chick peas)						2.4						
Garden pea (*Pisum sativum*)‡						6.7	5.0		5.1			38.0
Horse gram (*Dolichos biplorus*)						2.7						
Lentils						2.1						28.5
Pigeon pea (red gram)						1.6						
Soybean												
Flour						6.8						
Meal						6.8						
Milk and Milk Products												
Buttermilk												
Dry				39.9								
Fluid, genuine and cultured				5.0								
Casein		0.1		4.9								
Ice cream (14.5% cream)				3.6		16.6						
Milk												
Ass				6.0								
Cow				4.9								
Dried												
Skim				52.0								
Whole				38.1								
Fluid												
Skim				5.0								
Whole				4.9								
Sweetened, condensed				14.1		43.5						
Ewe				4.9								
Goat				4.7								
Human												
Colustrum				5.3								
Mature				6.9								
Whey				4.9								
Yogurt				3.8								
Nuts and Nut Products												
Almonds, blanched			0.2			2.3					2.1	
Chestnuts			2.2			3.6					1.2	18.0
Virginia			1.2			8.1		0.3			2.8	18.6
French			3.3			3.6					2.5	33.1
Coconut milk, ripe						2.6						
Copra meal, dried	1.2	1.2				14.3	15.6	0.6			2.2	0.9
Macadamia nut			0.3			5.5						

Appendix Table 3.   COMMON CARBOHYDRATES IN FOODS PER 100 GM. EDIBLE PORTION
(Continued)

FOOD	MONO-SACCHARIDES		REDUC-ING SUGARS*	DISACCHARIDES			POLYSACCHARIDES					
	Fructose	Glucose		Lactose	Maltose	Sucrose	Cellulose	Dextrins	Hemi-cellulose	Pectin	Pento-sans	Starch
Nuts and Nut Products, continued												
	gm.	gm.	gm.	gm.	gm.	gm.	gm.	gm.	gm.	gm.	gm.	gm.
Peanuts			0.2			4.5	2.4	2.5	3.8			4.0
Peanut butter			0.9									5.9
Pecans						1.1					0.2	
Cereals and Cereal Products												
Barley												
Grain, hulled							2.6		6.0		8.5	62.0
Flour						3.1					1.2	69.0
Corn, yellow							4.5		4.9		6.2	62.0
Flaxseed							1.8		5.2			
Millet grain									0.9		6.5	56.0
Oats, hulled											6.4	56.4
Rice												
Bran			1.4			10.6	11.4		7.0		7.4	
Brown, raw			0.1			0.8		2.1			2.1	69.7
Polished, raw		2.0	trace#			0.4	0.3	0.9			1.8	72.9
Polish			0.7								3.8	
Rye												
Grain							3.8		5.6		6.8	57.0
Flour											4.1	71.4
Sorghum grain											2.5	70.2
Soya-wheat (cereal)											3.3	46.4
Wheat												
Germ, defatted						8.3					6.2	
Grain		2.0				1.5	2.0	2.5	5.8		6.6	59.0
Flour, patent		2.0			0.1	0.2		5.5			2.1	68.8
Spices and Condiments												
Allspice (pimenta)			18.0			3.0						
Cassia			23.3									
Cinnamon			19.3									
Cloves			9.0									2.7
Nutmeg			17.2									14.6
Pepper, black			38.6									34.2
Sirups and Other Sweets												
Corn sirup		21.2			26.4			34.7				
High conversion		33.0			23.0			19.0				
Medium conversion		26.0			21.0			23.0				
Corn sugar		87.5			3.5			0.5				
Chocolate, sweet dry						56.4						
Golden sirup			37.5			31.0						
Honey	40.5	34.2				1.9		1.5				
Invert sugar			74.0			6.0						
Jellies, pectin						40-65						
Royal jelly	11.3	9.8				0.9						
Jellies, starch						25-60						7=12
Maple sirup			1.5			62.9						
Milk chocolate				8.1		43.0						
Molasses	8.0	8.8				53.6						
Blackstrap	6.8	6.8	26.9			36.9						
Sorghum sirup			27.0			36.0						
Miscellaneous												
Beer			1.5					2.8			0.3	
Cacao beans, raw, Arriba	0.6	0.5	1.1			1.9						
Carob bean												
Pod			11.2			23.2				1.4		
Pod and seeds			11.1			19.4						
Soy sauce	0.9											

°Mainly monosaccharides plus the disaccharides, maltose and lactose.
†Blanks indicate lack of acceptable data.
‡Also known as Alaska pea, field pea, and common pea.
#Trace = less than 0.05 gm.

Appendix Table 4. DIETARY FIBER AND CARBOHYDRATE
CONTENT OF FOODS PER 100 GM. EDIBLE PORTION

FOOD	CARBOHYDRATE			DIETARY FIBER (gm.)
	Total (gm.)	Sugar* (gm.)	Starch (gm.)	
Cereals and breads				
Arrowroot	94.0	Trace	94.0	—
Barley (pearl), raw	83.6	Trace	83.6	6.5
Barley, boiled	27.6	Trace	27.6	2.2
Bemax	44.7	16.0	28.7	—
Bran (wheat)	26.8	3.8	23.0	44.0
Corn flour	92.0	Trace	92.0	—
Custard powder	92.0	Trace	92.0	—
Flour (whole meal 100%)	65.8	2.3	63.5	9.6
Flour, brown (85%)	68.8	1.9	66.9	7.5
Flour, white (72%)	74.8	1.5	73.3	3.0
Flour, household, plain	80.1	1.7	78.4	3.4
Flour, self-rising	77.5	1.4	76.1	3.7
Patent (40%)	78.0	1.4	76.6	—
Macaroni, raw	79.2	Trace	79.2	—
Macaroni, boiled	25.2	Trace	25.2	—
Oatmeal, raw	72.8	Trace	7.28	7.0
Porridge	8.2	Trace	8.2	0.8
Rice, polished, raw	86.8	Trace	86.8	2.4
Rice, boiled	29.6	Trace	26.9	0.8
Rye flour (100%)	75.9	Trace	15.9	—
Sago, raw	94.0	Trace	94.0	—
Semolina, raw	77.5	Trace	77.5	—
Soya flour, full fat	23.5	11.2	12.3	11.9
Soya flour, low fat	28.2	13.4	14.8	14.3
Spaghetti, raw	84.0	2.7	81.3	—
Spaghetti, boiled	26.0	0.8	25.2	—
Spaghetti, canned, in tomato sauce	12.2	3.4	8.8	—
Tapioca, raw	95.0	Trace	95.0	—
Bread				
Whole meal	41.8	2.1	39.7	8.5
Brown	44.7	1.8	42.9	5.1
Hovis	45.1	2.4	42.7	4.6
White	49.7	1.8	47.9	2.7
White, fried	51.3	1.7	49.6	(2.2)†
Toasted	64.9	2.1	62.8	(2.8)
Dried crumbs	77.5	2.6	74.9	(3.4)
Currant	51.8	13.0	38.8	(1.7)
Malt	49.4	18.6	30.8	—
Soda	56.3	3.0	53.3	2.3
Rolls, brown, crusty	57.2	2.1	55.1	(5.9)
Rolls, brown, soft	47.9	1.9	46.0	(5.4)
Rolls, white, crusty	57.2	2.1	55.1	(3.1)
Rolls, white, soft	53.6	1.9	51.7	(2.9)
Rolls, starch reduced	45.7	1.6	44.1	(2.0)
Chapatis with fat	50.2	1.8	46.5	3.7
Chapatis without fat	43.7	1.6	42.1	(3.4)
Breakfast cereals				
All-Bran	43.0	15.4	27.6	26.7
Corn Flakes	85.1	7.4	77.7	11.0
Grape Nuts	75.9	9.5	66.4	7.0
Muesli	66.2	26.2	40.0	7.4
Puffed Wheat	68.5	1.5	67.0	15.4
Ready Brek	69.9	2.2	67.7	7.6
Rice Krispies	88.1	9.0	79.1	4.5
Shredded wheat	67.9	0.4	67.5	12.3
Special K	78.2	9.6	68.6	5.5
Sugar Puffs	84.5	56.5	28.0	6.1
Weeta Bix	70.3	6.1	66.5	12.7
Biscuits				
Chocolate, full coated	67.4	43.4	24.0	3.1
Cream crackers	68.3	Trace	68.3	(3.0)
Crisp bread, rye	70.6	3.2	67.4	11.7

Appendix Table 4.   DIETARY FIBER AND CARBOHYDRATE
CONTENT OF FOODS PER 100 GM. EDIBLE PORTION (*Continued*)

FOOD	CARBOHYDRATE Total (gm.)	Sugar* (gm.)	Starch (gm.)	DIETARY FIBER (gm.)
Biscuits (*Continued*)				
Crisp wheat, starch reduced	36.9	7.4	29.5	4.9
Digestive, plain	66.0	16.4	49.6	(5.5)
Digestive, chocolate	66.5	28.5	38.0	3.5
Ginger nuts	79.1	35.8	43.3	2.0
Homemade	65.5	26.8	38.7	1.7
Matzo	86.6	4.2	82.4	3.9
Oatcakes	63.0	3.1	59.9	4.0
Sandwich	69.2	30.2	39.0	1.2
Semisweet	74.8	22.3	52.5	2.3
Short-sweet	62.2	24.1	38.1	1.7
Shortbread	65.5	17.2	48.3	2.1
Wafers, filled	66.0	44.7	21.3	1.6
Water biscuits	75.8	2.3	73.5	(3.2)
Fruits				
Apples, just flesh	11.9	11.8	0.1	2.0
Apples, flesh, skin, core	9.2	9.1	0.1	1.5
Apples, cooking, raw	9.6	9.2	0.4	2.4
Apples, stewed, no sugar	8.2	7.9	0.3	2.1
Apples, stewed, with sugar	17.3	17.0	0.3	1.9
Apricots, fresh, raw	6.7	6.7	0	2.1
Apricots, stewed, no sugar	5.7	5.6	0	1.7
Apricots, stewed, with sugar	15.6	15.6	0	1.6
Apricots, dried, raw	43.4	43.4	0	24.0
Apricots, dried, stewed, without sugar	16.1	16.1	0	8.9
Apricots, dried, stewed, with sugar	19.9	19.9	0	8.5
Apricots, canned	27.7	27.7	0	1.3
Avocados	1.8	1.8	Trace	2.0
Bananas, raw	19.2	16.2	3.0	3.4
Blackberries, raw	6.4	6.4	0	7.3
Blackberries, stewed, no sugar	5.5	5.5	0	6.3
Blackberries, stewed, with sugar	14.8	14.8	0	5.7
Cherries, eating, raw	11.9	11.9	0	1.7
Cherries, cooking, raw	11.6	11.6	0	1.7
Cherries, stewed, no sugar	9.8	9.7	0	1.4
Cherries, stewed, with sugar	20.1	19.7	0	1.2
Cranberries, raw	3.5	3.5	0	4.2
Currants, black, raw	6.6	6.6	0	8.7
Currants, black, stewed, no sugar	5.6	5.6	0	7.4
Currants, black, stewed, with sugar	15.0	15.0	0	6.8
Currants, red, raw	4.4	4.4	0	8.2
Currants, red, stewed, no sugar	3.8	3.8	0	7.0
Currants, red, stewed, with sugar	13.3	13.3	0	6.4
Currants, white, raw	5.6	5.6	0	6.8
Currants, stewed, no sugar	4.8	4.8	0	5.8
Currants, stewed, with sugar	14.2	14.2	0	5.3

Table continued on the following page

Appendix Table 4. DIETARY FIBER AND CARBOHYDRATE
CONTENT OF FOODS PER 100 GM. EDIBLE PORTION (*Continued*)

| FOOD | CARBOHYDRATE | | | DIETARY FIBER (gm.) |
	Total (gm.)	Sugar* (gm.)	Starch (gm.)	
Fruits (*Continued*)				
Currants, dried	63.1	63.1	0	6.5
Dates, dried	63.9	63.9	0	8.7
Dates, dried, with pits	54.9	54.9	0	7.5
Figs, green, raw	9.5	9.5	0	2.5
Figs, dried, raw	52.9	52.9	0	18.5
Figs, stewed, no sugar	29.4	29.4	0	10.3
Figs, stewed, with sugar	34.3	34.3	0	9.7
Fruit pie filling, canned	25.1	23.2	1.9	(1.8)
Fruit salad, canned	25.0	25.0	0	1.1
Gooseberries, green, raw	3.4	3.4	0	3.2
Gooseberries, stewed, no sugar	2.9	2.9	0	2.7
Gooseberries, stewed, with sugar	12.5	12.5	0	2.5
Gooseberries, ripe, raw	9.2	9.2	0	3.5
Grapes, black, raw	15.5	15.5	0	0.4
Grapes, white, raw	16.1	16.1	0	0.9
Grapefruit, raw	5.3	5.3	0	0.6
Grapefruit, canned	15.5	15.5	0	0.4
Green gages	11.8	11.8	0	2.6
Green gages, stewed, no sugar	10.0	10.0	0	2.2
Green gages, stewed, with sugar	19.4	19.2	0	2.1
Guavas, canned	15.7	15.7	Trace	3.6
Lemons, whole	3.2	3.2	0	5.2
Lemon juice, fresh	1.6	1.6	0	0
Loganberries, raw	3.4	3.4	0	6.2
Loganberries, stewed, no sugar	3.1	3.1	0	5.7
Loganberries, stewed, with sugar	13.4	13.4	0	5.2
Loganberries, canned	26.2	26.2	0	3.3
Lychees, raw	16.0	16.0	0	(0.5)
Lychees, canned	17.7	17.7	0	0.4
Mandarin oranges, canned	14.2	14.2	0	0.3
Mangoes, raw	15.3	15.3	Trace	(1.5)
Mangoes, canned	20.3	20.2	0.1	1.0
Melons				
Cantaloupe, raw	5.3	5.3	0	1.0
Yellow honeydew, raw	5.0	5.0	0	0.9
Watermelon, raw	5.3	5.3	0	—
Mulberries, raw	8.1	8.1	0	1.7
Nectarines, raw	12.4	12.4	0	2.4
Olives, in brine	Trace	Trace	0	4.4
Oranges, raw	8.5	8.5	0	2.0
Orange juice, fresh	9.4	9.4	0	0
Passion fruit, raw	6.2	6.2	0	15.9
Pawpaw, canned	17.0	17.0	0	0.5
Peaches, fresh, raw	9.1	9.1	0	1.4
Peaches, dried, raw	53.0	53.0	0	14.3
Peaches, stewed, no sugar	19.6	19.6	0	5.3
Peaches, stewed, with sugar	23.3	23.3	0	5.1
Peaches, canned	22.9	22.9	0	1.0
Pears, eating	10.6	10.6	0	2.3
Pears, cooking, raw	9.3	9.3	Trace	2.9
Pears, stewed, no sugar	7.9	7.9	Trace	2.5
Pears, stewed, with sugar	17.1	17.1	Trace	2.3

Appendix Table 4.   DIETARY FIBER AND CARBOHYDRATE CONTENT OF FOODS PER 100 GM. EDIBLE PORTION (*Continued*)

FOOD	CARBOHYDRATE			DIETARY FIBER (gm.)
	Total (gm.)	Sugar* (gm.)	Starch (gm.)	
Fruits (*Continued*)				
Pears, canned	20.0	20.0	0	1.7
Pineapple, fresh	11.6	11.6	0	1.2
Pineapple, canned	20.2	20.2	0	0.9
Plums, Victoria dessert, raw	9.6	9.6	0	2.1
Plums, cooking, raw	6.2	6.2	0	2.5
Plums, stewed, no sugar	5.2	5.2	0	2.2
Plums, stewed, with sugar	15.3	15.1	0	1.9
Pomegranate juice	11.6	11.6	0	0
Prunes, dried, raw	40.3	40.3	0	16.1
Prunes, stewed, no sugar	20.4	20.4	0	8.1
Prunes, stewed, with sugar	26.5	26.5	0	7.7
Raisins, dried	64.4	64.4	0	6.8
Raspberries, raw	5.6	5.6	0	7.4
Raspberries, stewed, no sugar	5.9	5.9	0	7.8
Raspberries, stewed, with sugar	17.3	17.3	0	7.0
Raspberries, canned	22.5	22.5	0	(5.0)
Rhubarb, raw	1.0	1.0	0	2.6
Rhubarb, stewed, no sugar	0.9	0.9	0	2.4
Rhubarb, stewed, with sugar	11.4	11.4	0	2.2
Strawberries, raw	6.2	6.2	0	2.3
Strawberries, canned	21.1	21.1	0	1.0
Sultanas, dried	64.7	64.7	0	7.0
Tangerines, raw	8.0	8.0	0	1.9
Nuts				
Almonds	4.3	4.3	0	14.3
Barcelona nuts	5.2	3.4	1.8	10.3
Brazil nuts	4.1	1.7	2.4	9.0
Chestnuts	36.6	7.0	29.6	6.8
Cob or hazelnuts	6.8	4.7	2.1	6.1
Coconut, fresh	3.7	3.7	0	13.6
Coconut, milk	4.9	4.9	0	(Trace)
Coconut, desiccated	6.4	6.4	0	23.5
Peanuts, fresh	8.6	3.1	5.5	8.1
Peanuts, roasted, salted	8.6	3.1	5.5	8.1
Peanut butter, smooth	13.1	6.7	6.4	7.6
Walnuts	5.0	3.2	1.8	5.2
Vegetables				
Artichokes, globe, boiled	2.7	—	0	—
Asparagus, boiled	1.1	1.1	0	1.5
Aubergine, raw	3.1	2.9	0.2	2.5
Beans, French, boiled	1.1	0.8	0.3	3.2
Beans, runner, raw	3.9	2.8	1.1	2.9
Beans, broad, boiled	7.1	0.6	6.5	4.2
Beans, red kidney, raw	45.0	(3.0)	(42.0)	(25.0)
Bean sprouts, canned	0.8	0.4	0.4	3.0
Broccoli, tops, raw	2.5	2.5	Trace	3.6
Broccoli, boiled	1.6	1.5	0.1	4.1
Brussels sprouts, raw	2.7	2.6	0.1	4.2
Brussels sprouts, boiled	1.7	1.6	0.1	2.9
Cabbage, red, raw	3.5	3.5	Trace	3.4
Cabbage, white, raw	3.5	3.7	0.1	2.7
Carrots, old, raw	5.4	5.4	0	2.9

Table continued on the following page

Appendix Table 4.   DIETARY FIBER AND CARBOHYDRATE
CONTENT OF FOODS PER 100 GM. EDIBLE PORTION (*Continued*)

FOOD	CARBOHYDRATE			DIETARY FIBER (gm.)
	Total (gm.)	Sugar* (gm.)	Starch (gm.)	
Vegetables (*Continued*)				
Carrots, boiled	4.3	4.2	0.1	3.1
Carrots, young, boiled	4.5	4.4	0.1	3.0
Carrots, canned	4.4	4.4	Trace	3.7
Cauliflower, raw	1.5	1.5	Trace	2.1
Cauliflower, boiled	0.8	0.8	Trace	1.8
Celery, raw	1.3	1.2	0.1	1.8
Celery, boiled	0.7	0.7	0	2.2
Chicory, raw	1.5	—	0	—
Corn, sweet, on-the-cob, raw	23.7	1.7	22.0	3.7
Corn, sweet, on-the-cob, boiled	22.8	1.7	21.1	4.7
Corn, sweet, canned, kernels	16.1	8.9	7.2	5.7
Cucumber, raw	1.8	1.8	0	0.4
Endive, raw	1.0	1.0	0	2.2
Horseradish, raw	11.0	7.3	3.7	8.3
Leeks, raw	6.0	6.0	0	3.1
Leeks, boiled	4.6	4.6	0	3.9
Lentils, raw	53.2	2.4	50.8	11.7
Lentils, split, boiled	17.0	0.8	16.2	3.7
Lettuce, raw	1.2	1.2	Trace	1.5
Mushrooms, raw	0	0	0	2.5
Mustard and cress, raw	0.9	0.9	0	3.7
Okra, raw	2.3	2.3	Trace	(3.2)
Onions, raw	5.2	5.2	0	1.3
Onions, boiled	2.7	2.7	0	1.3
Parsley, raw	Trace	Trace	0	9.1
Parsnips, raw	11.3	8.8	2.5	4.0
Parsnips, boiled	13.5	2.7	10.8	2.5
Peas, fresh, raw	10.6	4.0	6.6	5.2
Peas, fresh, boiled	7.7	1.8	5.9	5.2
Peas, frozen, raw	7.2	4.1	3.4	7.8
Peas, frozen, boiled	4.3	1.0	3.3	12.0
Peas, canned, garden	7.0	3.6	3.4	6.3
Peas, processed	13.7	1.3	12.4	7.9
Peas, dried, raw	50.0	2.4	47.6	16.7
Peas, dried, boiled	19.1	0.9	18.2	4.8
Peas, split, dried, raw	56.6	1.9	54.7	11.9
Peas, split, dried, boiled	21.9	0.9	21.0	5.1
Peas, chick Bengal gram, raw	50.0	(10.0)	(40.0)	(15.0)
Peas, red pidgeon, raw	54.0	(9.0)	(45.0)	(15.0)
Peppers, green, raw	2.2	2.2	Trace	0.9
Peppers, green, boiled	1.8	1.7	0.1	0.9
Plantain, green, raw	28.3	0.8	27.5	(5.8)
Plantain, green, boiled	31.1	0.9	30.2	6.4
Potatoes, old, raw	20.8	0.5	20.3	2.1
Potatoes, boiled	19.7	0.4	19.3	1.0
Potatoes, mashed, with margarine and milk	18.0	0.6	17.4	0.9
Potatoes, baked	25.0	0.6	24.4	2.5
Potatoes, new, boiled	18.3	0.7	17.6	2.0
Potatoes, new, canned	12.6	0.4	12.2	2.5
Potatoes, instant powder	73.2	2.2	71.0	16.5
Potatoes, instant powder, made up	16.1	0.5	15.6	3.6
Potato chips	49.3	0.7	48.6	11.9
Pumpkin, raw	3.4	2.7	0.7	0.5
Radishes, raw	2.8	2.8	0	1.0
Spinach, boiled	1.4	1.2	0.2	6.3
Spring greens, boiled	0.9	0.9	0	3.8
Sweet potatoes, raw	21.5	(9.7)	(11.8)	(2.5)

Appendix Table 4. DIETARY FIBER AND CARBOHYDRATE
CONTENT OF FOODS PER 100 GM. EDIBLE PORTION (*Continued*)

FOOD	CARBOHYDRATE Total (gm.)	Sugar* (gm.)	Starch (gm.)	DIETARY FIBER (gm.)
Vegetables (*Continued*)				
Sweet potatoes, boiled	20.1	9.1	11.0	2.3
Tomatoes, raw	2.8	2.8	Trace	1.5
Tomatoes, canned	2.0	2.0	Trace	0.9
Turnips, raw	3.8	3.8	0	2.8
Turnips, boiled	2.8	2.3	0	2.2
Turnip tops, boiled	0.1	0	0.1	3.9
Watercress, raw	0.7	0.6	0.1	3.3
Yams, raw	32.4	1.0	31.4	(4.1)
Yams, boiled	29.8	0.2	29.6	3.9

Adapted from Floch, M.H.: Nutrition and Diet Therapy in Gastrointestinal Disease. New York, Plenum Medical Book Company, 1981. Data from Paul, A.A., and Southgate, D.A.T.: McCance and Widdowson's The Composition of Foods. 4th ed. New York, Elsevier/North Holland Biomedical Press, 1978.

* Sugar includes all free monosaccharides and disaccharides.

† Values in parentheses are taken from the literature.

Appendix Table 5. FATTY ACID AND CHOLESTEROL CONTENT OF FOODS

Food	Amount	Total Fat, g	Fatty Acids, g* Saturated	Polyunsaturated	Cholesterol, mg
Meat, lean (≤ 3 g fat/oz)	1 oz				
Beef		2.6	0.9	0.1	25
Lamb		2.9	1.2	0.1	28
Pork		2.8	0.8	0.3	25
Veal		3.1	1.3	0.2	28
Poultry (without skin)	1 oz				
Chicken					
Light		1	trace	trace	22
Dark		2.7	0.7	0.5	25
Turkey					
Light		0.7	trace	trace	22
Dark		1.5	0.4	0.3	28
Others: duck, goose, pheasant		2.3	0.5	0.2	25
Finfish	1 oz				
≤ 5% fat		0.5	trace	trace	18
Bass, cod, halibut, haddock, skipjack tuna, sole, red snapper, pike perch					
5–10% fat		2	trace	trace	18
Trout; drained anchovy, salmon, albacore, and sardines; mackerel; Atlantic herring					
≥ 12% fat		3.8	0.6	0.6	27
Pacific herring					

Table continued on the following page

Appendix Table 5. FATTY ACID AND CHOLESTEROL CONTENT OF FOODS (*Continued*)

Food	Amount	Total Fat, g	Fatty Acids, g*		Cholesterol, mg
			Saturated	Polyunsaturated	
Shellfish	1 oz				
< 2% fat		0.5	...	0.2	15
Abalone, clams, mussel, oysters, scallops					
Crab, lobster		0.5	...	0.2	26
Shrimp		0.4	...	0.2	42
Caviar		4.2	...	...	84
Organ meats	1 oz				
Heart		1.6	0.5	0.2	77
Liver					
Beef, veal		1.1	0.4	0.2	122
Chicken		1.2	0.5	0.3	208
Brains		2.4	0.6	0.3	560
Sweetbreads		6.5	2.7	0.3	130
Kidney		3.4	1.3	0.5	225
Tongue		4.7	1.6	0.6	25
Giblets		0.9	0.3	0.2	60
Gizzard		0.9	0.3	0.2	55
Meat, medium-fat (≤ 5 g fat/oz):	1 oz				
cooked, separable lean					
Beef		4.3	1.8	0.2	25
Pork		4	1.3	0.4	25
Meat, high-fat (≥ 10 g fat/oz)	1 oz				
Beef		9	3.7	0.3	26
Pork		8.6	3.3	1.0	25
Lamb (untrimmed)		8.2	3.8	0.5	27
Veal (untrimmed)		7	2.6	0.4	28
Cold cuts		7.6	2.7	0.9	25
Sausage		12.4	4.5	1.5	25
Bacon: cooked, 50% fat	1 slice	3.4	1.3	0.4	3
Dairy products					
Milk	1 cup				
Skim (< 1% fat)		0.2	0.1	...	4
Buttermilk		0.2	0.1	...	4
1%		2.4	1.4	trace	7
2%		4.8	2.9	0.2	14
Whole		8.4	5.3	0.3	32
Chocolate					
Skim		5.5	2.2	0.1	16
Whole		8.2	5.2	0.3	32
Yogurt	1 cup				
Part skim milk		2	1.3	0.1	11
Whole milk		8.2	5.3	2.4	32
Processed milk	1 oz				
Condensed		2.4	1.5	0.1	10
Evaporated		2.4	1.4	trace	9
Cottage cheese	1/4 cup (2 oz)				
1%		0.5	0.3	trace	2
2%		1	0.6	trace	3
Regular		2.3	1.4	0.7	7

Appendix Table 5.   FATTY ACID AND CHOLESTEROL CONTENT OF FOODS *(Continued)*

Food	Amount	Total Fat, g	Fatty Acids, g* Saturated	Fatty Acids, g* Polyunsaturated	Cholesterol, mg
Dairy products *(Continued)*					
Cheese	1 oz				
<1% fat		0.3	0.2	trace	2
Dietetic					
<10% fat		2.2	1.4	0.1	9
Imitation processed cheese spread					
<20% fat		4.6	2.9	0.1	18
Farmer, mozzarella (part skim), ricotta					
<30% fat		7.4	4.7	0.2	27
Pasteurized processed cheese foods and spreads, Bel Paese, Camembert, Edam, feta, Gouda, Limburger, mozzarella (low-moisture), Neufchâtel, Parmesan, Samsoe, Swiss					
>30% fat		9.2	5.6	0.3	29
Blue, brick, cheddar, colby, cream, Muenster, Port du Salut					
Polyunsaturated cheese		6.4	0.8	3.7	1
Cream	1 oz				
Half-and-half		3.3	2.0	0.9	12
Light (sweet or sour)		5.8	3.6	0.2	18
Heavy		10.6	6.6	0.4	38
Whipped (aerosol)		6.5	4.1	0.3	24
Dairy desserts	3 1/2 oz				
Ice milk		5.1	3.2	0.2	14
Ice cream					
Regular		10.6	6.6	0.4	40
Rich		16	10	0.6	57
Ice cream sandwich		8.2	4.7	0.5	40
Butterfat	1 tsp				
Butter		4	2.5	0.2	12
Butter oil		5	3.1	0.2	14
Eggs					
Whole	1				
Small (≤ 40 g)		4.5	1.4	0.5	192
Medium (≤ 44 g)		5	1.5	0.6	222
Large (≤ 50 g)		5.7	1.7	0.6	252
Extra large (≤ 57 g)		6.4	1.9	0.7	281
Yolk	100 g	33.5	10.1	3.8	1,480
Fats and oils					
Margarine	1 tsp				
Vegetable (P/S ratio†)					
>3: e.g., soft safflower		4	0.5	2.3	…
2.6–3: e.g., stick safflower		4	0.6	1.7	…
2–2.5: e.g., soft corn		4	0.7	1.8	…
1.6–1.9: e.g., stick corn		4	0.8	1.3	…
1–1.5: e.g., liquid soybean		4	0.9	1.3	…
0.5–0.9: e.g., partially hydrogenated oil		4	0.8	0.5	…
<0.5: e.g., hydrogenated oil		4	0.8	0.5	…

Table continued on the following page

Appendix Table 5. FATTY ACID AND CHOLESTEROL CONTENT OF FOODS (*Continued*)

Food	Amount	Total Fat, g	Fatty Acids, g*		Cholesterol, mg
			Saturated	Polyunsaturated	
Fats and oils (Continued)					
Vegetable-animal		4	1.7	0.3	4
Animal fats					
Beef	1 tsp				
Tallow		5	2.4	0.2	5
Lard		5	2	0.6	5
Chicken					
Fat	1 tsp	5	1.6	0.8	4
Skin, 35% fat	5 g	1.8	0.5	0.5	6
Salt pork, raw	1 oz	23.8	8.5	2.7	19
Mutton	5 g	5	2.2	0.4	4
Vegetable oils	1 tsp				
Safflower		5	0.5	3.7	...
Sunflower		5	0.5	3.2	...
Soybean					
Nonhydrogenated		5	0.8	2.9	
Part hydrogenated		5	0.7	2	...
Wheat germ		5	0.9	3	...
Corn		5	0.6	2.9	...
Sesame		5	0.8	2	...
Cottonseed		5	1.3	2.5	...
Peanut		5	0.9	1.2	...
Olive		5	0.7	0.4	...
Palm		5	2.4	0.5	...
Cocoa butter		5	3	0.2	...
Coconut		5	4.3	0.1	...
Soybean lecithin		5	0.8	2.4	...
Processed vegetable oils	1 tsp				
Oil blends					
90% sunflower and 10% cottonseed		5	0.6	3.1	...
90% soybean and 10% cottonseed		5	0.8	2.8	...
50% cottonseed and 50% soybean		5	1.2	2.7	...
10% olive and 90% other vegetable		5	0.7	1.8	...
Shortenings					
All-vegetable		5	1.6	1	...
Vegetable-animal		5	2.1	0.5	3
Dressings					
Mayonnaise		4	0.6	2.3	4
Mayonnaise-type		2.1	0.3	1.1	2.5
Salad					
All creamy: e.g., French, garlic		2	0.3	1.1	...
Creamy with egg or mayonnaise or both: e.g., tartar sauce, Thousand Island		2.5	0.4	1.3	3
Clear: e.g., French, Italian		3	0.5	1.7	...
Sandwich spread		2.5	0.3	1.5	2.6

Appendix Table 5. FATTY ACID AND CHOLESTEROL CONTENT OF FOODS (*Continued*)

Food	Amount	Total Fat, g	Fatty Acids, g*		Cholesterol, mg
			Saturated	Polyunsaturated	
Meat substitutes					
Meat loaf	1 oz	2.5	0.4	1.4	...
Sausage, piece					
Link	23 g	4.3	1	1.6	...
Patty	38 g	7.2	1.5	2.6	...
Ham, slice	1 oz	2.4	0.4	0.8	...
Frankfurter	1 oz	5.5	0.8	2.9	...
Textured vegetable protein	1 oz	2	0.3	1.1	...
Nuts	1/2 oz				
Peanuts					
Runner		7.6	1.3	2.1	...
Virginia		7.1	1.2	1.8	...
Spanish		7.4	1.4	2.4	...
Unspecified		7.3	1.3	2	...
Almonds		8.1	0.6	1.5	...
Brazil nuts		10.2	2.6	3.8	...
Cashews		6.8	1.4	1.1	...
Chestnuts		0.4	trace	0.2	...
Filberts		9.7	0.7	1	...
Macadamia nuts		11.3	1.5	0.2	...
Pecans		10.6	0.9	2.7	...
Pistachios		8.1	1.1	1.1	...
Walnuts					
English		9.6	1	6.1	...
Black		8.9	0.7	4.9	...
Peanut butter	2 tbsp				
Hydrogenated		14.4	2.9	4.2	...
Unhydrogenated		13.8	2.5	4.1	...
Avocado, 50 g	1/4	8.2	1.2	0.9	...
Coconut: shredded, sweetened	1 tbsp	5.3	4.7	1	...
Olives	1/2 oz				
Green		3.6	0.5	0.3	...
Black		3.9	0.5	0.3	...
Cereal products					
Bread, all varieties	1 slice	0.8	0.2	0.3	...
Bagel, small	1/2				
Plain		2	0.3	0.9	...
Egg		2	0.3	0.9	28
English muffin	1/2	0.9	0.2	trace	...
Roll	1	0.8	0.2	0.3	...
Bun, frankfurter or hamburger	1/2	1.5	0.6	0.2	...
Cereals					
Dry	3/4 cup	trace	trace	trace	...
Cooked	1/2 cup	trace	trace	trace	...
Pasta	1/2 cup				
Plain		trace	...	...	...
Egg		2	0.2	0.2	31
Wheat germ	1/4 cup	2.5	0.5	1.6	...

Table continued on the following page

Appendix Table 5. FATTY ACID AND CHOLESTEROL CONTENT OF FOODS (*Continued*)

Food	Amount	Total Fat, g	Fatty Acids, g* Saturated	Fatty Acids, g* Polyunsaturated	Cholesterol, mg
Cereal Products *(Continued)*					
Crackers	5				
Low-fat (< 12%)					
Saltines		<1	<0.7	0.2	. . .
High-fat (> 12%)					
Ritz		3.2	1.3	0.4	3
Prepared foods					
Biscuit	1 oz	2	‡	‡	. . .
Corn bread, small	1 oz	2.8	‡	‡	. . .
Muffin, small	1 oz	2.1	‡	‡	. . .
Potatoes, fried	1 oz	5	‡	‡	. . .
Potato chips	1 oz	11	‡	‡	. . .
Pancake, 4 in. round	1 oz	2	‡	‡	. . .
Waffle, 4 1/2 in. sq	1 1/2 oz	5	‡	‡	. . .

*Polyunsaturated fats include all unsaturated fats with two or more double bonds. Monounsaturated fats (one double bond) are not listed in the table because they do not affect serum lipids and are not used in calculating the ratio of polyunsaturated to saturated fat (P/S ratio).

†Check label for content of saturates, polyunsaturates, and cholesterol.

‡Fatty acid content depends on type of fat used in preparation.

From Mayo Clinic Diet Manual. A Handbook of Dietary Practices. 5th ed. Philadelphia, W. B. Saunders Company, 1981.

SELECTED BIBLIOGRAPHY

Comprehensive evaluation of fatty acids in foods (series), J. Am. Diet. Assoc.

I. Dairy products (Posati, L. P., Kinsella, J. E., and Watt, B. K.). 66:482–488, 1975.
II. Beef products (Anderson, B. A., Kinsella, J. E., and Watt, B. K.). 67:35–41, 1975.
III. Eggs and egg products (Posati, L. P., Kinsella, J. E., and Watt, B. K.). 67:111–115, 1975.
IV. Nuts, peanuts, and soups (Fristrom, G. A., Stewart, B. C., Weihrauch, J. L., and Posati, L. P.). 67:351–355, 1975.
V. Unhydrogenated fats and oils (Brignoli, C. A., Kinsella, J. E., and Weihrauch, J. L.). 68:224–229, 1976.
VI. Cereal products (Weihrauch, J. L., Kinsella, J. E., and Watt, B. K.). 68:335–340, 1976.
VII. Pork products (Anderson, B. A.). 69:44–49, 1976.
VIII. Finfish (Exler, J., and Weihrauch, J. L.). 69:243–248, 1976.
IX. Fowl (Fristrom, G. A., and Weihrauch, J. L.). 69:517–522, 1976.
X. Lamb and veal (Anderson, B. A., Fristrom, G. A., and Weihrauch, J. L.). 70:53–58, 1977.
XI. Leguminous seeds (Exler, J., Avena, R. M., and Weihrauch, J. L.). 71:412–415, 1977.
XII. Shellfish (Exler, J., and Weihrauch, J. L.). 71:518–521, 1977.

Adams, C. F.: Nutritive Value of American Foods in Common Units. Agriculture Handbook No. 456, Washington, D. C., United States Department of Agriculture, 1975.
Feeley, R. M., Criner, P. E., and Watt, B. K.: Cholesterol content of foods. J. Am. Diet. Assoc., 61:134–149, 1972.
Nazir, D. J., Moorecroft, B. J., and Mishkel, M. A.: Fatty acid composition of margarines. Am. J. Clin. Nutr., 29:331–339, 1976.

Appendix Table 6. AMINO ACID CONTENT OF FOODS PER 100 GM. EDIBLE PORTION*

ITEM, PROTEIN CONTENT, AND NITROGEN CONVERSION FACTOR	TRYPTO-PHAN	THREO-NINE	ISO-LEUCINE	LEUCINE	LYSINE	SULFUR CONTAINING			PHENYL-ALANINE	TYRO-SINE†	VALINE	ARGININE	HISTIDINE
						Meth-ionine†	Cystine†	Total					
	Gm.	Gm.	Gm.	Gm.	Gm.	Gm.	Gm.	Gm.	Gm.	Gm.	Gm.	Gm.	Gm.
Milk; Milk Products:													
Milk (Protein, N x 6.38):													
Cow:													
Fluid, whole and nonfat (3.5% protein)	0.049	0.161	0.223	0.344	0.272	0.086	0.031	0.117	0.170	0.178	0.240	0.128	0.092
Canned:													
Evaporated, unsweetened (7.0% protein)	.099	.323	.447	.688	.545	.171	.063	.234	.340	.357	.481	.256	.185
Condensed, sweetened (8.1% protein)	.114	.374	.518	.796	.631	.198	.072	.271	.393	.413	.557	.296	.214
Dried:													
Whole (25.8% protein)	.364	1.191	1.648	2.535	2.009	.632	.231	.863	1.251	1.316	1.774	.944	.680
Nonfat (35.6% protein)	.502	1.641	2.271	3.493	2.768	.870	.318	1.188	1.724	1.814	2.444	1.300	.937
Goat (3.3% protein)	.039	.217	.087	.278	.312	.065			.121	.071	.139	.174	.068
Human (1.4% protein)	.023	.062	.075	.124	.090	.028	.027	.055	.060		.086	.055	.030
Indian buffalo (4.2% protein)	.059	.212	.204	.420	.331	.112	.058	.170	.177		.255	.136	.086
Milk Products:													
Buttermilk (3.5% protein, N x 6.38)	.038	.165	.219	.348	.291	.082	.032	.114	.186	.137	.262	.168	.099
Casein (100.0% protein, N x 6.29)	1.335	4.277	6.550	10.048	8.013	3.084	.382	3.466	5.389	5.819	7.393	4.070	3.021
Cheese (protein, N x 6.38):													
Blue mold (21.5% protein)	.293	.799	1.449	2.096	1.577	.559	.121	.680	1.153	1.028	1.543	.785	.701
Camembert (17.5% protein)	.239	.650	1.179	1.706	1.284	.455	.099	.554	.938	.837	1.256	.639	.571
Cheddar (25.0% protein)	.341	.929	1.685	2.437	1.834	.650	.141	.791	1.340	1.195	1.794	.913	.815
Cheddar processed (23.2% protein)	.316	.862	1.563	2.262	1.702	.604	.131	.735	1.244	1.109	1.665	.847	.756
Cheese foods, cheddar (20.5% protein)	.280	.761	1.382	1.998	1.504	.533	.116	.649	1.099	.980	1.472	.749	.668
Cottage (17.0% protein)	.179	.794	.989	1.826	1.428	.469	.147	.616	.917	.917	.978	.802	.549
Cream cheese (9.0% protein)	.080	.408	.519	.923	.721	.229	.085	.314	.547	.408	.538	.313	.278
Limburger (21.2% protein)	.289	.788	1.429	2.067	1.555	.552	.120	.672	1.136	1.014	1.522	.774	.691
Parmesan (36.0% protein)	.491	1.337	2.426	3.510	2.641	.937	.203	1.140	1.930	1.721	2.584	1.315	1.174
Swiss (27.5% protein)	.375	1.021	1.853	2.681	2.017	.715	.155	.870	1.474	1.315	1.974	1.004	.896
Swiss processed (26.4% protein)	.360	.981	1.779	2.574	1.937	.687	.149	.836	1.415	1.262	1.895	.964	.861
Lactalbumin (100.0% protein, N x 6.49)	2.203	5.239	6.209	12.342	9.060	2.250	3.405	5.655	4.360	3.806	5.686	3.498	1.911
Whey (Protein, N x 6.49):													
Fluid (0.9% protein)	.010	.048	.052	.074	.055	.013	.018	.031	.023	.009	.045	.017	.011
Dried (12.7% protein)	.147	.677	.734	1.043	.769	.188	.250	.438	.323	.131	.640	.235	.159

* Adapted from the more comprehensive Table 2 complied by M.L. Orr and B.K. Watt in "Amino Acid Content of Foods." Home Economics Research Report No. 4. U.S. Department of Agriculture. Washington, D.C., U.S. Government Printing Office, 1968.

†All amino acids except those designated with † are essential to man. Histidine is essential for the human infant and may be essential for adults.

Table continued on the following page

Appendix Table 6. AMINO ACID CONTENT OF FOODS PER 100 GM. EDIBLE PORTION (*Continued*)

ITEM, PROTEIN CONTENT, AND NITROGEN CONVERSION FACTOR	TRYPTO-PHAN	THREO-NINE	ISO-LEUCINE	LEUCINE	LYSINE	SULFUR CONTAINING			PHENYL-ALANINE	TYRO-SINE	VALINE	ARGININE	HISTIDINE
						Meth-ionine	Cystine	Total					
	Gm.	Gm.	Gm.	Gm.	Gm.	Gm.	Gm.	Gm.	Gm.	Gm.	Gm.	Gm.	Gm.
Eggs, Chicken (Protein, N x 6.25):													
Fresh or stored:													
Whole (12.8% protein)	0.211	0.637	0.850	1.126	0.819	0.401	0.299	0.700	0.739	0.551	0.950	0.840	0.307
Whites (10.8% protein)	.164	.477	.698	.950	.648	.420	.263	.683	.689	.449	.842	.634	.233
Yolks (16.3% protein)	.235	.827	.996	1.372	1.074	.417	.274	.691	.717	.756	1.121	1.132	.368
Dried:													
Whole (46.8% protein)	.771	2.329	3.108	4.118	2.995	1.468	1.093	2.561	2.703	2.014	3.474	3.070	1.123
Whites (85.9% protein)	1.306	3.793	5.553	7.559	5.154	3.340	2.089	5.429	5.484	3.573	6.693	5.044	1.855
Yolks (31.2% protein)	.449	1.582	1.907	2.626	2.057	.799	.524	1.323	1.373	1.448	2.147	2.167	.704
Meat; Poultry; Fish and Shellfish; Their Products:													
Meat (Protein, N x 6.25):													
Beef carcass or side:													
Thin (18.8% protein)	.220	.830	.984	1.540	1.642	.466	.238	.704	.773	.638	1.044	1.212	.653
Medium fat (17.5% protein)	.204	.773	.916	1.434	1.529	.434	.221	.655	.720	.594	.972	1.128	.608
Fat (16.3% protein)	.190	.720	.853	1.335	1.424	.404	.206	.610	.670	.553	.905	1.051	.566
Very fat (13.7% protein)	.160	.605	.717	1.122	1.197	.340	.173	.513	.563	.465	.761	.883	.476
Medium fat, trimmed to retail basis (18.2% protein)	.213	.804	.952	1.491	1.590	.451	.230	.681	.748	.617	1.010	1.174	.632
Beef cuts, medium fat:													
Chuck (18.6% protein)	.217	.821	.973	1.524	1.625	.461	.235	.696	.765	.631	1.033	1.199	.646
Flank (19.9% protein)	.232	.879	1.041	1.630	1.738	.494	.252	.746	.818	.675	1.105	1.283	.691
Hamburger (16.0% protein)	.187	.707	.837	1.311	1.398	.397	.202	.599	.658	.543	.888	1.032	.556
Porterhouse (16.4% protein)	.192	.724	.858	1.343	1.433	.407	.207	.614	.674	.556	.911	1.057	.569
Rib roast (17.4% protein)	.203	.768	.910	1.425	1.520	.432	.220	.652	.715	.590	.966	1.122	.604
Round (19.5% protein)	.228	.861	1.020	1.597	1.704	.484	.246	.730	.802	.661	1.083	1.257	.677
Rump (16.2% protein)	.189	.715	.848	1.327	1.415	.402	.205	.607	.666	.550	.899	1.045	.562
Sirloin (17.3% protein)	.202	.764	.905	1.417	1.511	.429	.219	.648	.711	.587	.960	1.116	.601
Beef, canned (25.0% protein)	.292	1.104	1.308	2.048	2.184	.620	.316	.936	1.028	.848	1.388	1.612	.868
Beef, dried or chipped (34.3% protein)	.401	1.515	1.795	2.810	2.996	.851	.434	1.285	1.410	1.163	1.904	2.212	1.191
Lamb carcass or side:													
Thin (17.1% protein)	.222	.782	.886	1.324	1.384	.410	.224	.634	.695	.594	.843	1.114	.476
Medium fat (15.7% protein)	.203	.718	.814	1.216	1.271	.377	.206	.583	.638	.545	.774	1.022	.437
Fat (13.0% protein)	.168	.595	.674	1.007	1.052	.312	.171	.483	.528	.451	.641	.847	.362
Lamb cuts, medium fat:													
Leg (18.0% protein)	.233	.824	.933	1.394	1.457	.432	.236	.668	.732	.625	.887	1.172	.501
Rib (14.9% protein)	.193	.682	.772	1.154	1.206	.358	.195	.553	.606	.517	.734	.970	.415
Shoulder (15.6% protein)	.202	.714	.809	1.208	1.263	.374	.205	.579	.634	.542	.769	1.016	.434

Meat; Poultry; Fish and Shellfish; Their Products—Continued

Meat (Protein, N x 6.25)—Continued

	Gm.	Gm.	Gm.	Gm.	Gm.	Gm.	Gm.	Gm.	Gm.	Gm.	Gm.	Gm.	Gm.
Pork, packer's carcass or side:													
Thin (14.1% protein)	0.183	0.654	0.724	1.038	1.157	0.352	0.165	0.517	0.555	0.503	0.733	0.864	0.487
Medium fat (11.9% protein)	.154	.552	.611	.876	.977	.297	.139	.436	.468	.425	.619	.729	.411
Fat (9.8% protein)	.127	.455	.503	.721	.804	.245	.114	.359	.386	.350	.510	.601	.339
Pork cuts, medium fat, fresh:													
Ham (15.2% protein)	.197	.705	.781	1.119	1.248	.379	.178	.557	.598	.542	.790	.931	.525
Loin (16.4% protein)	.213	.761	.842	1.207	1.346	.409	.192	.601	.646	.585	.853	1.005	.567
Miscellaneous lean cuts (14.5% protein)	.188	.673	.745	1.067	1.190	.362	.169	.531	.571	.517	.754	.889	.501
Pork, cured:													
Bacon, medium fat (9.1% protein)	.095	.306	.399	.728	.587	.141	.106	.247	.434	.234	.434	.622	.246
Fat back or salt pork (3.9% protein)	.006	.141	.110	.367	.317	.055	.043	.098	.157	.052	.168	.379	.035
Ham (16.9% protein)	.162	.692	.841	1.306	1.420	.411	.273	.684	.646	.652	.879	1.068	.544
Luncheon meat:													
Boiled ham (22.8% protein)	.219	.934	1.135	1.762	1.915	.554	.368	.923	.872	.879	1.186	1.441	.733
Canned, spiced (14.9% protein)	.143	.610	.741	1.151	1.252	.362	.241	.603	.570	.575	.775	.942	.479
Rabbit, domesticated, flesh only (21.0% protein)		1.021	1.082	1.636	1.818	.541			.793		1.021	1.176	.474
Veal, carcass or side:													
Thin (19.7% protein)	.258	.854	1.040	1.444	1.645	.451	.233	.684	.801	.709	1.018	1.283	.634
Medium fat (19.1% protein)	.251	.828	1.008	1.400	1.595	.437	.226	.663	.776	.688	.987	1.244	.614
Fat (18.5% protein)	.243	.802	.977	1.356	1.545	.423	.219	.642	.752	.666	.956	1.205	.595
Veal cuts, medium fat:													
Round (19.5% protein)	.256	.846	1.030	1.429	1.629	.446	.231	.677	.792	.702	1.008	1.270	.627
Shoulder (19.4% protein)	.255	.841	1.024	1.422	1.620	.444	.230	.674	.788	.698	1.003	1.263	.624
Stew meat (18.3% protein)	.240	.793	.966	1.341	1.528	.419	.217	.636	.744	.659	.946	1.192	.589
Poultry (Protein, N x 6.25):													
Chicken, flesh only:													
Broilers or fryers (20.6% protein)	.250	.877	1.088	1.490	1.810	.537	.277	.814	.811	.725	1.012	1.302	.593
Hens (21.3% protein)	.259	.907	1.125	1.540	1.871	.556	.286	.842	.838	.750	1.046	1.346	.613
Ducks, domesticated, flesh only (21.4% protein)		.935	1.109	1.657	1.842	.531			.842		1.027	1.301	.486
Turkey, flesh only (24.0% protein)		1.014	1.260	1.836	2.173	.664	.330	.994	.960		1.187	1.513	.649
Fish and Shellfish (Protein, N x 6.25):													
Blue fish (20.5% protein)	.203	.889	1.040	1.548	1.797	.597	.276	.873	.761	.554	1.092	1.155	
Cod:													
Fresh (16.5% protein)	.164	.715	.837	1.246	1.447	.480	.222	.702	.612	.446	.879	.929	
Dried (81.8% protein)	.811	3.547	4.149	6.178	7.172	2.383	1.099	3.481	3.036	2.212	4.358	4.607	

Table continued on the following page

Appendix Table 6. AMINO ACID CONTENT OF FOODS PER 100 GM. EDIBLE PORTION (*Continued*)

ITEM, PROTEIN CONTENT, AND NITROGEN CONVERSION FACTOR	TRYPTO-PHAN	THREO-NINE	ISO-LEUCINE	LEUCINE	LYSINE	SULFUR CONTAINING			PHENYL-ALANINE	TYRO-SINE	VALINE	ARGININE	HISTIDINE
						Meth-ionine	Cystine	Total					
	Gm.	Gm.	Gm.	Gm.	Gm.	Gm.	Gm.	Gm.	Gm.	Gm.	Gm.	Gm.	Gm.
Meat; Poultry; Fish and Shellfish; Their Products—Continued													
Fish and Shellfish (Protein, N x 6.25)—Continued													
Croaker (17.8% protein)	0.177	0.772	0.903	1.344	1.561	0.518	0.239	0.757	0.661	0.481	0.948	1.002	——
Eel (18.6% protein)	.185	.806	.943	1.405	1.631	.542	.250	.792	.690	.503	.991	1.048	——
Flounder (14.9% protein)	.148	.646	.756	1.125	1.306	.434	.200	.634	.553	.403	.794	.839	——
Haddock (18.2% protein)	.181	.789	.923	1.374	1.596	.530	.245	.775	.676	.492	.970	1.025	——
Halibut (18.6% protein)	.185	.806	.943	1.405	1.631	.542	.250	.792	.690	.503	.991	1.048	——
Herring:													
Atlantic (18.3% protein)	.182	.793	.928	1.382	1.605	.533	.246	.779	.679	.495	.975	1.031	——
Lake (18.5% protein)	.184	.802	.938	1.397	1.622	.539	.249	.788	.687	.500	.986	1.042	——
Pacific (16.6% protein)	.165	.720	.842	1.254	1.455	.483	.223	.706	.616	.449	.884	.935	——
Mackerel:													
Raw, common Atlantic (18.7% protein)	.186	.811	.948	1.412	1.640	.545	.251	.796	.694	.506	.996	1.053	——
Canned, solids and liquid:													
Atlantic (19.3% protein)	.191	.837	.979	1.458	1.692	.562	.259	.821	.716	.522	1.028	1.087	——
Pacific (21.1% protein)	.209	.915	1.070	1.593	1.850	.614	.284	.898	.783	.571	1.124	1.188	——
Salmon:													
Raw, Pacific (Chinook or King) (17.4% protein)	.173	.754	.883	1.314	1.526	.507	.234	.741	.646	.470	.927	.980	——
Canned, solids and liquid (Sockeye or red) (20.2% protein)	.200	.876	1.025	1.526	1.771	.588	.271	.859	.750	.546	1.076	1.138	——
Sardines, canned, solids and liquid:													
Atlantic type (21.1% protein)	.209	.915	1.070	1.593	1.850	.614	.284	.898	.783	.571	1.124	1.188	——
Pacific type (17.7% protein)	.176	.767	.898	1.337	1.552	.515	.238	.753	.657	.479	.943	.997	——
Shrimp, canned, solids and liquid (18.7% protein)	.186	.811	.948	1.412	1.640	.545	.251	.796	.694	.506	.996	1.053	——
Products from Meat, Poultry, and Fish (Protein, N x 6.25):													
Brains (10.4% protein)	.138	.494	.504	.845	.760	.220	.145	.365	.506	.433	.536	.614	0.278
Chitterlings (8.6% protein)	.094	.398	.308	.457	.670	.193	.109	.302	.359	.228	.462	1.406	.169
Fish flour (76.0% protein)	.754	4.378	4.232	6.189	7.381	2.019			2.845		3.916	5.204	1.289
Gelatin (85.6% protein, N x 5.55)	.006	1.912	1.357	2.930	4.226	.787	.077	.864	2.036	.401	2.421	7.866	.771
Gizzard, chicken (23.1% protein)	.207	1.072	1.094	1.689	1.567	.554	.218	.772	.968	.680	1.116	1.741	.480
Heart:													
Beef or pork (16.9% protein)	.219	.776	.857	1.509	1.387	.403	.168	.571	.765	.627	.973	1.068	.433
Chicken (20.5% protein)	.266	.941	1.040	1.830	1.683	.489	.203	.692	.928	.761	1.181	1.296	.525

Products from Meat, Poultry, and Fish (Protein N x 6.25)—*Continued*

	Gm.	Gm.	Gm.	Gm.	Gm.	Gm.	Gm.	Gm.	Gm.	Gm.	Gm.	Gm.	Gm.
Kidney:													
Beef (15.0% protein)	0.221	0.665	0.730	1.301	1.087	0.307	0.182	0.489	0.706	0.557	0.876	0.934	0.377
Pork (16.3% protein)	.240	.722	.793	1.414	1.181	.334	.198	.532	.767	.605	.952	1.015	.409
Sheep (16.6% protein)	.244	.736	.807	1.440	1.203	.340	.202	.542	.781	.616	.969	1.033	.417
Liver:													
Beef or pork (19.7% protein)	.296	.936	1.031	1.819	1.475	.463	.243	.706	.993	.738	1.239	1.201	.523
Calf (19.0% protein)	.286	.903	.994	1.754	1.423	.447	.234	.681	.958	.711	1.195	1.158	.505
Chicken (22.1% protein)	.332	1.050	1.156	2.040	1.655	.520	.272	.792	1.114	.827	1.390	1.347	.587
Sheep or lamb (21.0% protein)	.316	.998	1.099	1.939	1.572	.494	.259	.753	1.058	.786	1.320	1.280	.558
Pancreas:													
Beef (13.5% protein)	.175	.626	.683	1.054	.996	.244			.562	.590	.724	.771	.266
Pork (14.5% protein)	.188	.673	.733	1.132	1.070	.262			.603	.633	.777	.828	.285
Pork and beef, canned (14.3% protein)	.151	.618	.730	1.190	1.345	.327	.261	.588	.579	.570	.810	1.050	.460
Potted meat (16.1% protein)	.149	.662	.641	1.203	1.061	.361			.641		.943	1.002	.322
Sausage:													
Bologna (14.8% protein)	.126	.606	.718	1.061	1.191	.313	.185	.498	.540	.481	.744	1.028	.398
Braunschweiger (15.4% protein)	.172	.668	.754	1.291	1.200	.320	.187	.507	.700	.471	.956	.954	.458
Frankfurters (14.2% protein)	.120	.582	.688	1.018	1.143	.300	.177	.477	.518	.461	.713	.986	.382
Head cheese (15.0% protein)	.079	.418	.509	.946	.907	.250	.209	.459	.569	.569	.617	1.075	.278
Liverwurst (16.7% protein)	.187	.724	.818	1.400	1.301	.347	.203	.550	.759	.510	1.037	1.034	.497
Pork, links or bulk, raw (10.8% protein)	.092	.442	.524	.774	.869	.228	.135	.363	.394	.351	.543	.750	.290
Pork, bulk, canned (15.4% protein)	.131	.631	.747	1.104	1.239	.325	.192	.517	.562	.500	.774	1.069	.414
Salami (23.9% protein)	.203	.979	1.159	1.713	1.923	.505	.298	.803	.872	.776	1.201	1.660	.642
Vienna sausage, canned (15.8% protein)	.134	.647	.766	1.133	1.272	.334	.197	.531	.576	.513	.794	1.097	.425
Tongue:													
Beef (16.4% protein)	.197	.708	.792	1.286	1.364	.357	.207	.564	.661	.548	.840	1.065	.412
Pork (16.8% protein)	.202	.726	.812	1.317	1.398	.366	.212	.578	.677	.562	.860	1.091	.422
Veal and pork loaf, canned (17.2% protein)	.198	.627	.859	1.236	1.258	.418	.209	.627	.619	.468	.958	.916	.388
Legumes (Dry Seed); Common Nuts; Other Nuts and Dry Seeds; Their Products:													
Legume Seeds and Their Products:													
Beans (Phaseolus vulgaris) (N x 6.25):													
Pinto and red Mexican (23.0% protein)	.213	.997	1.306	1.976	1.708	.232	.228	.460	1.270	.887	1.395	1.384	.655

Table continued on the following page

Appendix Table 6. AMINO ACID CONTENT OF FOODS PER 100 GM. EDIBLE PORTION (*Continued*)

ITEM, PROTEIN CONTENT, AND NITROGEN CONVERSION FACTOR	TRYPTO-PHAN	THREO-NINE	ISO-LEUCINE	LEUCINE	LYSINE	SULFUR CONTAINING — Meth-ionine	SULFUR CONTAINING — Cystine	SULFUR CONTAINING — Total	PHENYL-ALANINE	TYRO-SINE	VALINE	ARGININE	HISTIDINE
	Gm.	Gm.	Gm.	Gm.	Gm.	Gm.	Gm.	Gm.	Gm.	Gm.	Gm.	Gm.	Gm.
Legumes (Dry Seed); Common Nuts; Other Nuts and Dry Seeds; Their Products—Continued													
Legume Seeds and Their Products—Continued													
Beans (Phaseolus vulgaris) (N x 6.25)—Continued													
Red kidney:													
Raw (23.1% protein)	0.214	1.002	1.312	1.985	1.715	0.233	0.229	0.462	1.275	0.891	1.401	1.390	0.658
Canned, solids and liquid (5.7% protein)	.053	.247	.324	.490	.423	.057	.057	.114	.315	.220	.346	.343	.162
Other common beans including navy, peabean, white marrow:													
Raw (21.4% protein)	.199	.928	1.216	1.839	1.589	.216	.212	.428	1.181	.825	1.298	1.287	.609
Baked with pork, canned (5.8% protein)	.057	.274	.291	.486	.354	.059	.018	.077	.333	.165	.312	.251	.186
Black gram, raw (23.6% protein, N x 6.25)	.242	.801	1.390	2.062	1.510	.332	.287	.619	1.242	.551	1.450	1.552	.559
Broadbeans, raw (25.4% protein, N x 6.25)	.236	.829	1.593	2.211	1.426	.106	.179	.285	1.057	.687	1.276	1.780	.748
Chickpeas (20.8% protein, N x 6.25)	.170	.739	1.195	1.538	1.434	.276	.296	.572	1.012	.692	1.025	1.551	.559
Cowpeas (22.9% protein, N x 6.25)	.220	.901	1.110	1.715	1.491	.352	.297	.649	1.198	.678	1.293	1.473	.692
Dolichos, twinflower (21.6% protein, N x 6.25)	.221	.836	1.448	1.707	1.700	.294	.480	.774	1.486	.560	1.286	1.230	.650
Lentils, whole (25.0% protein, N x 6.25)	.216	.896	1.316	1.760	1.528	.180	.204	.384	1.104	.664	1.360	1.908	.548
Lima beans (20.7% protein, N x 6.25)	.195	.980	1.199	1.722	1.378	.331	.311	.642	1.222	.543	1.298	1.315	.669
Lupine (32.3% protein, N x 6.25)		1.101	1.618	1.964	1.447	.114			1.271		1.328	2.718	.811
Moth beans (24.4% protein, N x 6.25)	.164	.765	1.093	1.484	1.202	.191	.109	.300	1.003	1.245	.695	1.370	.722
Mung beans (24.4% protein, N x 6.25)	.180	.828	1.351	2.202	1.667	.265	.152	.417	1.167	.390	1.444		.543
Peanuts (26.9% protein, N x 5.46)	.340		1.266	1.872	1.099	.271	.463	.734	1.557	1.104	1.532	3.296	.749
Peanut flour (51.2% protein, N x 5.46)	.647	1.575	2.410	3.563	2.091	.516	.881	1.397	2.963	2.100	2.916	6.273	1.425
Peanut butter (26.1% protein, N x 5.46)	.330	.803	1.228	1.816	1.066	.263	.449	.712	1.510	1.071	1.487	3.198	.727
Peas (Pisum sativum) (N x 6.25):													
Entire seeds (23.8% protein)	.251	.918	1.340	1.969	1.744	.286	.308	.594	1.200	.960	1.333	2.102	.651
Split (24.5% protein)	.259	.945	1.380	2.027	1.795	.294	.318	.612	1.235	.988	1.372	2.164	.670
Pigeonpeas, without seed coat (21.9% protein, N x 6.25)	.119	.834	1.346	1.717	1.580	.256	.308	.564	1.875	.725	1.153	1.489	.617
Soybeans, whole (34.9% protein, N x 5.71)	.526	1.504	2.054	2.946	2.414	.513	.678	1.191	1.889	1.216	2.005	2.763	.911
Soybean flour, flakes, and grits (protein, N x 5.71):													
Low fat (44.7% protein)	.673	1.926	2.630	3.773	3.092	.658	.869	1.527	2.419	1.558	2.568	3.538	1.166
Medium fat (42.5% protein)	.640	1.831	2.501	3.588	2.940	.625	.826	1.451	2.300	1.481	2.441	3.364	1.109
Full fat (35.9% protein)	.541	1.547	2.112	3.030	2.483	.528	.698	1.226	1.943	1.251	2.062	2.842	.937
Soybean curd (7.0% protein, N x 5.71)						.081	.091	.172					
Soybean milk (3.4% protein, N x 5.71)	.051	.176	.175	.305	.269	.054	.071	.125	.195	.193	.186	.302	.121
Vetch (28.8% protein, N x 6.25)	.203	.899	2.198	2.290	1.898	.346	.336	.682	1.014	.369	1.442	2.249	.659

Table continued on the following page

Legumes (Dry Seed); Common Nuts; Other Nuts and Dry Seeds; Their Products:—Continued

Common Nuts and Their Products:

	Gm.	Gm.	Gm.	Gm.	Gm.	Gm.	Gm.	Gm.	Gm.	Gm.	Gm.	Gm.	Gm.
Almonds (18.6% protein, N x 5.18)	0.176	0.610	0.873	1.454	0.582	0.259	0.377	0.636	1.146	0.618	1.124	2.729	0.517
Brazil nuts (14.4% protein, N x 5.46)	.187	.422	.593	1.129	.443	.941	.504	1.445	.617	.483	.823	2.247	.367
Cashews (18.5% protein, N x 5.30)	.471	.737	1.222	1.522	.792	.353	.527	.880	.946	.712	1.592	2.098	.415
Coconut (3.4% protein, N x 5.30)	.033	.129	.180	.269	.152	.071	.062	.133	.174	.101	.212	.486	.069
Coconut meal (20.3% protein, N x 5.30)	.199	.770	1.076	1.605	.908	.421	.372	.793	1.038	.605	1.268	2.899	.414
Filberts (12.7% protein, N x 5.30)	.211	.415	.853	.939	.417	.139	.165	.304	.537	.434	.934	2.171	.288
Peanuts. See Legumes.													
Pecans (9.4% protein, N x 5.30)	.138	.389	.553	.773	.435	.153	.216	.369	.564	.316	.525	1.185	.273
Walnuts (English or Persian) (15.0% protein, N x 5.30)	.175	.589	.767	1.228	.441	.306	.320	.626	.767	.583	.974	2.287	.405

Other Nuts and Seeds and Their Products (Protein, N x 5.30):

	Gm.	Gm.	Gm.	Gm.	Gm.	Gm.	Gm.	Gm.	Gm.	Gm.	Gm.	Gm.	Gm.
Acorns (10.4% protein)	.126	.434	.561	.808	.636	.139	.184	.323	.473	—	.718	.722	.251
Amaranth (14.6% protein)	.149	.832	.882	1.209	1.074	.372	.521	.893	1.141	.617	.849	1.747	.441
Balsampear seed meal (41.9% protein)	.261	.373	.543	1.041	.418	.056	.142	—	2.609	.453	.927	5.914	.147
Breadnuttree, Ramon (9.6% protein)													
Chinese tallow tree-nut flour (57.6% protein)	.837	2.174	3.510	4.347	1.587	.924	.696	1.620	2.847	2.011	4.510	10.031	1.587
Chocolatetree, Nicaragua (38.5% protein)	.588	1.496	2.092	3.952	2.223	.276	—	—	2.630	—	2.404	4.220	.683
Cottonseed flour and meal (42.3% protein)	.591	1.764	1.884	2.945	2.139	.686	.814	1.500	2.610	1.365	2.458	5.603	1.325
Earpodtree, Guanacaste (34.1% protein)	.444	1.165	2.213	4.581	1.930	.360	—	—	1.325	—	1.570	2.857	1.004
Leadtree (24.1% protein)	.191	.828	1.651	1.787	1.164	.055	—	—	.855	—	.864	2.410	.564
Pumpkin seed (30.9% protein)	.560	.933	1.737	2.437	1.411	.577	.495	—	1.749	—	1.679	4.810	.711
Safflower seed meal (42.1% protein)	.675	1.462	1.914	2.740	1.525	.731	.857	—	2.605	—	2.446	4.623	.985
Sesame:													
Seed (19.3% protein)	.331	.707	.951	1.679	.583	.637	—	1.132	1.457	.951	.885	1.992	.441
Meal (33.4% protein)	.573	1.223	1.645	2.905	1.008	1.103	—	1.960	2.521	1.645	1.531	3.447	.763
Sunflower:													
Kernel (23.0% protein)	.343	.911	1.276	1.736	.868	.443	.464	.907	1.220	.647	1.354	2.370	.586
Meal (39.5% protein)	.589	1.565	2.191	2.981	1.491	.760	.797	1.557	2.094	1.110	2.325	4.069	1.006

Grains and Their Products:

	Gm.	Gm.	Gm.	Gm.	Gm.	Gm.	Gm.	Gm.	Gm.	Gm.	Gm.	Gm.	Gm.
Barley (12.8% protein, N x 5.83)	.160	.433	.545	.889	.433	.184	.257	.441	.661	.466	.643	.659	.239
Bread, white (4% nonfat dry milk, flour basis) (8.5% protein, N x 5.70)	.091	.282	.429	.668	.225	.142	.200	.342	.465	.243	.435	.340	.192

Appendix Table.6. AMINO ACID CONTENT OF FOODS PER 100 GM. EDIBLE PORTION (*Continued*)

ITEM, PROTEIN CONTENT, AND NITROGEN CONVERSION FACTOR	TRYPTO-PHAN	THREO-NINE	ISO-LEUCINE	LEUCINE	LYSINE	SULFUR CONTAINING			PHENYL-ALANINE	TYRO-SINE	VALINE	ARGININE	HISTIDINE
						Meth-ionine	Cystine	Total					
	Gm.	Gm.	Gm.	Gm.	Gm.	Gm.	Gm.	Gm.	Gm.	Gm.	Gm.	Gm.	Gm.
Grains and Their Products—Continued													
Buckwheat flour:													
Dark (11.7% protein, N x 6.25)	0.165	0.461	0.440	0.683	0.687	0.206	0.228	0.434	0.442	0.240	0.607	0.930	0.256
Light (6.4% protein, N x 6.25)	.090	.252	.241	.374	.376	.113	.125	.238	.242	.131	.332	.509	.140
Cañihua (14.7% protein, N x 6.25)	.118	.706	1.000	.851	.882	.263	.162	.425	.529	.294	.677	1.162	.367
Cereal combinations:													
Corn and soy grits (18.0% protein, N x 6.25)	.161	.792	.841	1.656	.772	.271	.311	.582	.832	.562	1.054	.982	.472
Infant food, precooked, mixed cereals with non-fat dry milk and yeast (19.4% protein, N x 6.25)	.118					.310	.137	.447	.543	.447		.447	.233
Oat-corn-rye mixture, puffed (14.5% protein, N x 5.83)	.172	.545	.841	1.368	.273	.388	.234	.622	.933	.622	.900	.776	.326
Corn, field (10.0% protein, N x 6.25)	.061	.398	.462	1.296	.343	.186	.130	.316	.454	.611	.510	.352	.206
Corn flour (7.8% protein, N x 6.25)	.047	.311	.361	1.011	.288	.145	.101	.246	.354	.477	.398	.275	.161
Corn grits (8.7% protein, N x 6.25)	.053	.347	.402	1.128	.225	.161	.113	.274	.395	.532	.444	.306	.180
Cornmeal:													
Whole ground (9.2% protein, N x 6.25)	.056	.367	.425	1.192	.251	.171	.119	.290	.418	.562	.470	.324	.190
Degermed (7.9% protein, N x 6.25)	.048	.315	.365	1.024	.265	.147	.102	.249	.359	.483	.403	.278	.163
Corn products:													
Flakes (8.1% protein, N x 6.25)	.052	.275	.306	1.047	.228	.135	.152	.287	.354	.283	.386	.231	.226
Germ (14.5% protein, N x 6.25)	.144	.622	.578	1.030	.791	.232	.130	.362	.483	.343	.789	1.134	.464
Gluten (10.0% protein, N x 6.25)	.059	.344	.443	1.563	.154	.282	.141	.423	.558	.582	.512	.322	.200
Hominy (8.7% protein, N x 6.25)	.084	.316	.349	.810	.179	.099			.333	.331	.398	.444	.203
Masa (2.8% protein, N x 6.25)	.010				.358	.108	.030	.138					
Pozol (5.9% protein, N x 6.25)	.042	.336	.304	.591	.103	.087			.254		.267	.197	.122
Tortilla (5.8% protein, N x 6.25)	.031	.235	.345	.939	.234	.111			.252		.304	.223	.128
Zein (16.1% protein, N x 6.25)	.010	.495	.822	3.184	.145	.281	.162	.443	1.664		.654	.286	.216
Job's tears (13.8% protein, N x 5.83)	.066	.620	1.065	3.506	.362	.459	.265	.724	.703	.981		.518	.317
Millets:													
Foxtail millet (9.7% protein, N x 5.83)	.103	.323	.790	1.737	.218	.291			.697		.717	.374	.218
Little millet (7.2% protein, N x 5.83)	.047	.262	.517	.841	.138	.178			.370		.471	.363	.147
Pearlmillet (11.4% protein, N x 5.83)	.248	.456	.635	1.746	.383	.270	.152	.422	.506		.682	.524	.240
Ragimillet (6.2% protein, N x 5.83)	.085	.270	.398	.620	.202	.270	.187	.457	.263		.473	.100	.079
Oatmeal and rolled oats (14.2% protein, N x 5.83)	.183	.470	.733	1.065	.521	.209	.309	.518	.758	.524	.845	.935	.261
Quinoa (11.0% protein, N x 6.25)	.120	.523	.722	.781	.729	.278	.107	.385	.394	.253	.447	.820	.297
Rice:													
Brown (7.5% protein, N x 5.95)	.081	.294	.352	.646	.296	.135	.102	.237	.377	.343	.524	.432	.126
White and converted (7.6% protein, N x 5.95)	.082	.298	.356	.655	.300	.137	.103	.240	.382	.347	.531	.438	.128

Grains and Their Products—Continued

	Gm.	Gm.	Gm.	Gm.	Gm.	Gm.	Gm.	Gm.	Gm.	Gm.	Gm.	Gm.	Gm.
Rice products:													
Flakes or puffed (5.9% protein, N x 5.95).....	0.046	—	—	—	0.056	—	0.044	—	0.286	0.124	—	0.137	0.137
Germ (14.2% protein, N x 5.95).....	.270	2.177	.630	.838	1.707	.420	.169	.589	.750	.929	.938	1.559	.430
Rye (12.1% protein, N x 5.83).....	.137	.448	.515	.813	.494	.191	.241	.432	.571	.390	.631	.591	.276
Rye flour:													
Light (9.4% protein, N x 5.83).....	.106	.348	.400	.632	.384	.148	.187	.335	.443	.303	.490	.459	.214
Medium (11.4% protein, N x 5.83).....	.129	.422	.485	.766	.465	.180	.227	.407	.538	.368	.594	.557	.260
Sorghum (11.0% protein, N x 6.25).....	.123	.394	.598	1.767	.299	.190	.183	.373	.547	.303	.628	.417	.211
Teosinte (22.0% protein, N x 6.25).....	.049				.348	.496							
Wheat, whole grain:													
Hard red spring (14.0% protein, N x 5.83).....	.173	.403	.607	.939	.384	.214	.307	.521	.691	.523	.648	.670	.286
Hard red winter (12.3% protein, N x 5.83).....	.152	.354	.534	.825	.338	.188	.270	.458	.608	.460	.570	.589	.251
Soft red winter (10.2% protein, N x 5.83).....	.126	.294	.443	.684	.280	.156	.224	.380	.504	.382	.472	.488	.208
White (9.4% protein, N x 5.83).....	.116	.271	.408	.630	.258	.143	.206	.349	.464	.351	.435	.450	.192
Durum (12.7% protein, N x 5.83).....	.157	.366	.551	.852	.348	.194	.279	.473	.627	.475	.588	.608	.259
Wheat flour:													
Whole grain (13.3% protein, N x 5.83).....	.164	.383	.577	.892	.365	.203	.292	.495	.657	.497	.616	.636	.271
Intermediate extraction (12.0% protein, N x 5.70).....		.392	.619	.924	.356	.198	.320	.518	.732	.335	.583	.549	.286
White (10.5% protein, N x 5.70).....	.129	.302	.483	.809	.239	.138	.210	.348	.577	.359	.453	.466	.210
Wheat products:													
Bran (12.0% protein, N x 6.31).....	.196	.342	.485	.717	.491	.145	.270	.415	.434	.259	.552	.742	.280
Burghul (12.4% protein, N x 5.83).....	.070				.430	.300	.319	.619	.579	.447		.424	.268
Farina (10.9% protein, N x 5.70).....	.124	.356	.496	.891	.199	.143	.184	.327	.478	.311	.572	.559	.231
Flakes (10.8% protein, N x 5.70).....	.121				.360	.127	.191	.318					
Germ (25.2% protein, N x 5.80).....	.265	1.343	1.177	1.708	1.534	.404	.287	.691	.908	.882	1.364	1.825	.687
Gluten, commercial (80.0% protein, N x 5.70).....	.856	2.119	3.677	5.993	1.530	1.389	1.726	3.115	4.351	2.596	3.789	3.481	1.825
Gluten flour (41.4% protein, N x 5.70).....	.443	1.097	1.903	3.101	.792	.719	.893	1.612	2.252	1.344	1.961	1.801	.944
Macaroni or spaghetti (12.8% protein, N x 5.70).....	.150	.499	.642	.849	.413	.193	.243	.436	.669	.422	.728	.582	.303
Noodles, contain egg solids (12.6% protein, N x 5.70).....	.133	.533	.621	.834	.411	.212	.245	.457	.610	.312	.745	.621	.301
Shredded wheat (10.1% protein, N x 5.83).....	.085	.405	.449	.684	.331	.139	.204	.343	.481	.236	.577	.523	.236
Whole wheat with added germ (12.8% protein, N x 5.83).....	.136				.466		.246		.755	.481		.742	.371

Table continued on the following page

Appendix Table 6.   AMINO ACID CONTENT OF FOODS PER 100 GM. EDIBLE PORTION (*Continued*)

ITEM, PROTEIN CONTENT, AND NITROGEN CONVERSION FACTOR	TRYPTO-PHAN	THREO-NINE	ISO-LEUCINE	LEUCINE	LYSINE	SULFUR CONTAINING			PLENYL-ALANINE	TYRO-SINE	VALINE	ARGININE	HISTIDINE
						Meth-ionine	Cystine	Total					
	Gm.	Gm.	Gm.	Gm.	Gm.	Gm.	Gm.	Gm.	Gm.	Gm.	Gm.	Gm.	Gm.
Fruits (Protein, N x 6.25):													
Abiu (1.7% protein)	0.028				0.085	0.013							
Avocados (1.3% protein)	.014				.074	.012							
Bananas, ripe:													
Common (1.2% protein)	.018				.055	.011				0.031			
Dwarf (1.2% protein)	.012				.049	.004							
Dates (2.2% protein)	.061	0.061	0.074	0.077	.065	.027			0.063				
Grapefruit (0.5% protein)	.001				.006	.000					.094	.049	0.049
Guavas, common (1.0% protein)	.010				.030	.010							
Limes (0.8% protein)	.003				.015	.002							
Mamey (0.5% protein)	.006				.040	.007							
Mangos (0.7% protein)	.014				.093	.008							
Muskmelons (0.6% protein)	.001				.015	.002							
Oranges, sweet (0.9% protein)	.003				.024	.003							
Orange juice (0.8% protein)	.003				.021	.002							
Oranges, mandarin including tangerines (0.8% protein)	.005				.028	.004							
Papayas (0.6% protein)	.012	.027	.056	.059	.038	.002							
Pineapple (0.4% protein)	.005				.009	.001							
Plantain or baking banana (1.1% protein)	.010				.050	.005							
Soursop (1.0% protein)	.011				.060	.007	.016	.021	.049		.065	.045	
Sugarapple (1.8% protein)	.009				.071	.008							
Vegetables:													
Immature Seeds (Protein, N x 6.25):													
Corn, sweet, white or yellow:													
Raw (3.7% protein)	.023	.151	.137	.407	.137	.072	.062	.134	.207	.124	.231	.174	.095
Canned, solids and liquid (2.0% protein)	.012	.082	.074	.220	.074	.039	.033	.072	.112	.067	.125	.094	.052
Cowpeas (9.4% protein)	.099	.353	.465	.653	.617	.131			.523		.513	.615	.310
Lima beans:													
Raw (7.5% protein)	.097	.338	.460	.605	.474	.080	.083	.163	.389	.259	.485	.454	.247
Canned, solids and liquid (3.8% protein)	.049	.171	.233	.306	.240	.041	.042	.083	.197	.131	.246	.230	.125
Peas:													
Raw (6.7% protein)	.056	.245	.308	.418	.316	.054	.073	.127	.257	.163	.274	.595	.109
Canned, solids and liquid (3.4% protein)	.028	.125	.156	.212	.160	.027	.037	.064	.131	.083	.139	.302	.055

	Gm.	Gm.	Gm.	Gm.	Gm.	Gm.	Gm.	Gm.	Gm.	Gm.	Gm.	Gm.	Gm.
Leafy Vegetables, Raw (Protein, N x 6.25):													
Amaranth (3.5% protein)	0.038	0.056	**0.164**	**0.206**	0.141	0.025	0.024	0.049	0.096	0.105	0.136	0.134	0.069
Beet greens (2.0% protein)	.024	.076	**.084**	**.129**	.108	.034	———	———	.116	———	.101	.083	.026
Brussels sprouts (4.4% protein)	.044	.153	**.186**	**.194**	.197	.046	———	.041	.148	.030	.193	.279	.106
Cabbage (1.4% protein)	.011	.039	**.040**	**.057**	.066	.013	.028	———	.030	———	.043	.105	.025
Chard (1.4% protein)	.014	.058	**.060**	**.076**	.055	.004	.006	.022	.046	.040	.055	.035	.018
Chicory (1.6% protein)	.024	.114	**.121**	**.218**	.052	.016	.059	.105	.124	.151	.195	.258	.024
Collards (3.9% protein)	.055	.139	**.133**	**.252**	.202	.046	.036	.071	.158	———	.184	.202	.087
Kale (3.9% protein)	.042	———	———	———	.121	.035	———	———	———	———	———	———	.062
Lettuce (1.2% protein)	.012	.060	**.075**	**.062**	.070	.004	.035	.059	.074	.121	.108	.167	.041
Mustard greens (2.3% protein)	.037	———	———	———	.111	.024	———	———	———	———	———	———	———
Parsley, curly garden (2.5% protein)	.050	———	———	———	.160	.012	———	———	———	———	———	———	———
Spinach (2.3% protein)	.037	.102	**.107**	**.176**	.142	.039	.046	.085	.099	.073	.126	.116	.049
Turnip greens (2.9% protein)	.045	.125	**.107**	**.207**	.129	.052	.045	.097	.146	.105	.149	.167	.051
Watercress (1.7% protein)	.028	.084	**.076**	**.131**	.091	.010	———	———	.062	.036	.084	.053	.034
Starchy Roots and Tubers (Protein, N x 6.25):													
Apio arracacia (1.2% protein)	.008	———	———	———	.042	.003	———	———	———	———	———	———	———
Cassava:													
Flour (1.6% protein)	.021	.044	**.045**	**.066**	.066	.010	.018	.028	.045	.030	.049	.159	.025
Root (1.1% protein)	.014	.030	**.031**	**.045**	.045	.007	.012	.019	.031	.021	.033	.110	.017
Potatoes:													
Raw (2.0% protein)	.021	.079	**.088**	**.100**	.107	.025	.019	.044	.088	.036	.107	.099	.029
Canned, solids and liquid (1.7% protein)	.018	.067	**.075**	**.085**	.091	.021	.016	.037	.075	.030	.091	.084	.024
Flour (7.1% protein)	.076	.279	**.311**	**.353**	.378	.089	.068	.157	.314	.127	.379	.350	.102
Sweetpotatoes (Ipomaea batatas):													
Raw (1.8% protein)	.031	.085	**.087**	**.103**	.085	.033	.029	.062	.100	.081	.135	.094	.036
Dehydrated (5.0% protein)	.087	.235	**.241**	**.286**	.236	.093	.080	.173	.278	.225	.374	.261	.099
Taro (1.9% protein)	.035	.089	**.099**	**.169**	.110	.021	———	———	.099	———	.114	.118	.032
Yam (Dioscorea spp.) (2.1% protein)	.035	———	———	———	.110	.034	———	———	———	———	———	———	———
Yautia malanga (1.7% protein)	.023	———	———	———	.067	.016	———	———	———	———	———	———	———
Other Vegetables (Protein, N x 6.25):													
Asparagus:													
Raw (2.2% protein)	.027	.066	**.080**	**.096**	.103	.032	———	———	.069	———	.106	.123	.036
Canned, solids and liquid (1.9% protein)	.023	.057	**.069**	**.083**	.089	.027	———	———	.060	———	.092	.106	.031

Table continued on the following page

Appendix Table 6. AMINO ACID CONTENT OF FOODS PER 100 GM. EDIBLE PORTION (Continued)

All values in Gm. Columns Methionine, Cystine, and Total are grouped under "SULFUR CONTAINING".

ITEM, PROTEIN CONTENT, AND NITROGEN CONVERSION FACTOR	TRYPTOPHAN	THREONINE	ISOLEUCINE	LEUCINE	LYSINE	Methionine	Cystine	Total	PHENYLALANINE	TYROSINE	VALINE	ARGININE	HISTIDINE
Vegetables—Continued													
Other Vegetables (Protein, N x 6.25)—Continued													
Beans, snap:													
Raw (2.4% protein)	0.033	0.091	0.109	0.139	0.126	0.035	0.024	0.059	0.057	0.050	0.115	0.101	0.045
Canned, solids and liquid (1.0% protein)	.014	.038	.045	.058	.052	.014	.010	.024	.024	.021	.048	.042	.019
Beets:													
Raw (1.6% protein)	.014	.034	.051	.055	.086	.006			.027		.049	.028	.022
Canned, solids and liquid (0.9% protein)	.008	.019	.029	.031	.048	.003			.015		.028	.016	.012
Broccoli (3.3% protein)	.037	.122	.126	.163	.147	.050			.119		.170	.192	.063
Carrots:													
Raw (1.2% protein)	.010	.043	.046	.065	.052	.010	.029	.039	.042	.020	.056	.041	.017
Canned, solids and liquid (0.5% protein)	.004	.018	.019	.027	.022	.004	.012	.016	.018	.008	.023	.017	.007
Cauliflower (2.4% protein)	.033	.102	.104	.162	.134	.047			.075	.034	.144	.110	.048
Celery (1.3% protein)	.012				.021	.015	.006	.021		.016			
Chayote (0.6% protein)	.008				.038	.001							
Cowpeas, yardlong, immature pod (3.4% protein)	.034				.203	.021							
Cucumbers (0.7% protein)	.005	.019	.022	.030	.031	.007			.016		.024	.053	.001
Cushaw (1.5% protein)	.014				.044	.008							
Eggplant (1.1% protein)	.010	.038	.056	.068	.030	.006			.048		.065	.037	.019
Mallow (3.7% protein)	.144	.155		.259	.155	.030			.166		.181	.189	.063
Mushrooms:													
(Agaricus campestris)[1]	.006	.156	.532	.281	.088	.167			.018		.378	.235	.027
(Lactarius spp.)[2]	.006		.201	.139	.076	.021			.065		.116	.021	.030
Okra (1.8% protein)	.018	.066	.069	.101	.064	.022	.017	.039	.039	.079	.091	.093	.014
Onions, mature (1.4% protein)	.021	.022	.021	.037		.013				.046	.031	.180	
Peppers (1.2% protein)	.009	.050	.046	.046	.051	.016			.055		.033	.024	.014
Pricklypears (1.1% protein)	.009	.053	.044	.057	.044	.008			.059		.041	.032	.016
Pumpkin (1.2% protein)	.016	.028	.044	.063	.058	.011			.032	.016	.045	.043	.019
Radishes (1.2% protein)	.005	.059			.034	.002					.030		
Seepweed (2.6% protein)	.027	.089	.113	.152	.089	.013			.116		.091	.062	
Soybean sprouts (6.2% protein)		.159	.225	.265	.211	.045			.186		.225	.225	.036
Squash, summer (0.6% protein)	.005	.014	.019	.027	.023	.008			.016				.133
Tomatoes and cherry tomatoes (1.0% protein)	.009		.029	.041	.042	.007			.028	.014	.022	.027	.009
Turnips (1.1% protein)		.033	.020		.057	.012			.020	.029	.028	.029	
Waxgourd, Chinese (0.4% protein)	.002				.009	.003							.015
Miscellaneous Food Items:													
Vegetable patty or steak (principally wheat protein) (15% protein, N x 5.70)	.142	.411	.884	1.079	.321	.253			.811		.705	.597	.321
Yeast:													
Baker's, compressed ([3], N x 6.25)	.122	.655	.655	1.151	.914	.248	.120	.368	.607	.580	.840	.536	.353
Brewer's, dried ([4], N x 6.25)	.710	2.353	2.398	3.226	3.300	.836	.548	1.384	1.902	1.902	2.723	2.250	1.251
Primary, dried:													
(Saccharomyces cerevisiae) ([4], N x 6.25)	.636	2.353	2.708	3.300	3.337	.851	.444	1.295	1.813	2.472	2.553	1.931	1.103
(Torulopsis utilis) ([4], N x 6.25)	.636	2.331	3.323	3.707	3.648	.710	.422	1.132	2.361	2.464	2.901	3.337	1.251

[1] Total nitrogen is 0.58%. This is equivalent to 2.4% protein on the basis that 2/3 of the nitrogen is protein nitrogen. If total nitrogen is used for the calculation, the protein content is 3.6%.

[2] Total nitrogen is 0.69%. This is equivalent to 2.9% protein on the basis that 2/3 of the nitrogen is protein nitrogen. If total nitrogen is used for the calculation, the protein content is 4.3%.

[3] Total nitrogen is 2.1%. This is equivalent to 10.6% protein on the basis that 4/5 of the nitrogen is protein nitrogen. If total nitrogen is used for the calculation, the protein content is 13.1%.

[4] Total nitrogen is 7.4%. This is equivalent to 36.9% protein on the basis that 4/5 of the nitrogen is protein nitrogen. If total nitrogen is used for the calculation, the protein content is 46.1%.

Appendix Table 7. FOLACIN CONTENT OF FOODS
Per 100 Gm. Edible Portions and in Specified Units[*][a][b]

ITEM NUMBER	FOOD AND DESCRIPTION	PER 100 GM. EDIBLE PORTION		PER SPECIFIED UNIT			
		Free Folacin (μg.)	Total Folacin[c] (μg.)	Approximate Measure	Weight (gm.)	Free Folacin (μg.)	Total Folacin[c] (μg.)
CEREAL GRAINS AND THEIR PRODUCTS							
1	barley, pot	9	20	1 c.	200	18	40
2	corn, whole-grain	15	19				
3	cornmeal, degermed	9	24	1 c.	122	11	29
4	macaroni, dry	4	12	8-oz. pkg.	227	9	27
	rice						
5	brown	12	16	1 c.	185	22	30
6	white	–[d]	10	1 c.	185	–	18
7	parboiled	9	11	1 c.	185	17	20
8	rice bran	–	39				
9	rice germ	–	64				
10	rice flour, sifted	31	78	1 c.	88	27	69
11	sorghum, grain	18	27				
12	spaghetti, dry	4	12	8-oz. pkg.	227	9	27
13	wheat, whole-grain	39	52				
	wheat flour						
14	whole	40	54	1 c.	120	48	65
15	clear	29	32				
	patent						
16	bread, sifted	19	25	1 c.	115	22	29
17	all-purpose, sifted	18	21	1 c.	115	21	24
18	wheat bran	134	258				
19	wheat germ	257	328				
	breakfast cereals, dry						
20	farina	–	24	1 c.	180	–	43
21	farina, wheat germ added	17	34	1 c.	180	31	61
22	oatmeal	16	52	1 c.	80	13	42
	breakfast cereals, ready-to-eat; not fortified with folacin						
23	cornflakes	9	12	1 oz.	28	3	3
24	oats, with added wheat gluten	8	22	1 oz.	28	2	6
25	rice, puffed	8	23	1 oz.	28	2	6
26	rice, with added protein concentrate and wheat gluten	14	31		28	4	9
27	wheat germ, toasted	125	420	1 oz.	28	35	118
28	wheat and malted barley granules	15	54	1 oz.	28	4	15
29	wheat, shredded	10	50	1 oz.	28	3	14
	bakery products						
	bread						
30	rye	6	23	1 slice	25	2	6
31	white	13	39	1 slice	25	3	10
32	whole-wheat	27	58	1 slice	28	8	16
	cakes						
33	chocolate with icing	4	6	1 slice (3″ high; 2⅜″ arc)	99	4	6
34	sponge	3	7	1 slice (3″ high; 2¼″ arc)	44	1	3
	cookies						
35	chocolate chip	4	9	1 cookie	10	<0.5	1
36	shortbread	4	9	1 cookie	8	<0.5	1

[*]From: Perloff, B. P., and Butrum, R. R.: Folacin in selected foods. J. Am. Diet. Assoc., 70:161, 1977.
[a]Measure and weight apply to edible part of food only.
[b]Assays using *L. casei* except when studies using *L. casei* could not be found. Reducing agent such as ascorbic acid used except for items 100, 107, 111, 140, 187 and 197.
[c]Recommend using total folacin for diet calculations.
[d]Dash denotes value not available.

Table continued on the following page

Appendix Table 7. FOLACIN CONTENT OF FOODS (Continued)

ITEM NUM-BER	FOOD AND DESCRIPTION	PER 100 GM. EDIBLE PORTION		PER SPECIFIED UNIT			
		Free Folacin (μg.)	Total Folacin (μg.)	Approximate Measure	Weight (gm.)	Free Folacin (μg.)	Total Folacin (μg.)
	CEREAL GRAINS AND THEIR PRODUCTS (*Continued*)						
	doughnuts						
37	cake type	5	8	1 doughnut	32	2	3
38	yeast-leavened	5	22	1 doughnut	35	2	8
39	pie, apple	2	4	1/6 of pie	158	3	6
	LEGUMINOUS SEEDS AND THEIR PRODUCTS						
	beans, common, mature seeds						
	white						
40	raw, dry	25	129	1 c.	205	51	264
41	canned, baked with tomato sauce	8	24	1 c.	255	20	61
	red						
42	raw, dry	24	133	1 c.	185	44	246
43	cooked	–	37	1 c.	185	–	68
	pinto, mature seeds, dry						
44	raw, dry	57	216	1 c.	190	108	410
45	cooked	–	59	1 c.	190	–	112
46	canned, drained	–	51	1 c.	190	–	97
	beans, Lima, mature seeds						
47	raw, dry	25	113	1 c.	190	48	215
48	cooked	–	43	1 c.	190	–	82
49	beans, mung, mature seeds, dry	26	133	1 c.	210	55	279
50	beans, mungo, mature seeds, dry	28	108				
	chickpeas or garbanzos, mature seeds						
51	raw, dry	32	199	1 c.	200	64	398
52	roasted	22	139				
53	canned, drained	–	102				
	cowpeas, mature seeds						
54	raw, dry	69	133	1 c.	170	117	226
55	canned, drained	–	80	1 c.	165	–	132
56	lentils, mature seeds, dry	19	36	1 c.	190	36	68
57	peanuts, roasted	24	106	1 c.	144	35	153
58	peanut butter	20	79	1 tbsp.	16	3	13
59	pigeon peas, mature seeds, dry	20	110				
60	soybeans, mature seeds, dry	75	171	1 c.	210	158	359
	soybean products, fermented						
61	natto	95	126				
62	tempeh	12	156				
63	soy sauce	8	28	1 tbsp.	18	1	5
	NUTS AND SEEDS (OTHER THAN LEGUMINOUS SEEDS)						
64	almonds	33	96	1 c.	142	47	136
65	Brazil nuts, shelled	1	4	1 c.	140	1	6
66	cashew nuts, roasted	8	68	1 c.	140	11	95
67	coconut, shredded	10	24	1 c.	130	13	31
68	filberts (hazelnuts), shelled	23	72	1 c.	135	31	97
69	pecans, shelled	13	24	1 c.	108	14	26
70	pistachio nuts	10	58				
71	sesame seeds	49	96	1 tbsp.	8	4	8
72	walnuts, English, shelled	52	66	1 c.	100	52	66
	VEGETABLES						
73	asparagus, raw	58	64	1 c.	135	78	86
74	bean sprouts, canned	7	10	1 c.	125	9	12
	beans, snap						
	green						
75	raw	33	44	1 c.	110	36	48
76	cooked, drained	–	40	1 c.	125	–	50
77	frozen	8	33	1 c.	125	10	41
	yellow or wax						
78	raw	32	40	1 c.	110	35	44
79	frozen	8	34	1 c.	125	10	42

Appendix Table 7.   FOLACIN CONTENT OF FOODS (*Continued*)

ITEM NUM-BER	FOOD AND DESCRIPTION	PER 100 GM. EDIBLE PORTION		PER SPECIFIED UNIT			
		Free Folacin (μg.)	*Total Folacin* (μg.)	*Approximate Measure*	*Weight* (gm.)	*Free Folacin* (μg.)	*Total Folacin* (μg.)
VEGETABLES (*Continued*)							
80	beans, Lima, frozen	9	31	1 c.	160	14	50
	beets, common, red						
81	raw	69	93	1 c.	135	93	126
82	cooked	38	78	1 c.	170	65	133
	broccoli						
	spears						
83	raw	51	69	3 med.	354	181	244
84	cooked	27	56	1 med.	180	49	101
85	flower, raw	102	105				
86	stem, raw	35	59				
	Brussels sprouts						
87	raw	55	78	6 med.	114	63	89
88	cooked	6	36	1 c. (7–8	155	9	56
	cabbage						
	common varieties						
89	raw	33	66	1 c.	90	30	59
90	cooked	2	18	1 c.	145	3	26
91	red, raw	23	34	1 c.	90	21	31
	cabbage, Chinese (also called celery cabbage or petsai)						
92	raw	42	83	1 c.	75	32	62
93	cooked	5	19				
	carrots						
94	raw	14	32	1 med.	59	8	19
95	cooked	2	24	1 c.	155	3	37
	cauliflower						
96	raw	31	55	1 c.	100	31	55
97	cooked	2	34	1 c.	125	2	42
98	celery, raw	6	12	1 c.	100	6	12
99	chicory greens, raw	33	52				
100	collards, raw	—	102	1 c.	55	—	56
	corn, sweet						
101	raw, whole-kernel	27	33	1 c.	165	45	54
102	frozen	2	21	1 c.	162	3	35
103	cucumber, raw, pared	12	15	1 small	128	15	19
	eggplant						
104	raw	9	31				
105	cooked	2	16	1 c.	200	4	32
106	endive, raw	—	49	1 c.	50	—	24
107	kale, raw	44	60	1 c.	110	48	66
	lettuce, raw						
108	leaf or head	34	37	1 c.	55	19	20
109	romaine	60	179	1 c.	55	33	98
110	mushrooms, raw	20	23	1 c.	68	14	16
111	okra, raw	10	24	1 c.	100	10	24
112	onion, mature, dry	10	25				
112a	onion, mature, chopped			1 c.	170	17	42
112b	onion, mature, chopped			1 tbsp.	10	1	2
	onion, young green, raw						
113	bulbs and white portion of top	40	36	1 tbsp.	6	2	2
114	tops only (green portion), chopped	52	80	1 tbsp.	6	3	5
	onion, Welsh, raw						
115	bulbs and white portion of top	16	66				
116	tops only (green portion)	49	105				
117	parsnips, raw	57	67	1 c.	130	74	87
118	parsley, raw	41	116	1 tbsp.	4	2	5
119	peas, green, frozen	17	53	1 c.	145	25	77
120	peppers, hot, mature, red, raw	23	52				
121	peppers, sweet, immature, green, raw	8	19	1 med.	164	13	31
	potatoes						
122	raw	11	19	1 med.	122	13	23
	cooked						

Table continued on the following page

Appendix Table 7. FOLACIN CONTENT OF FOODS (*Continued*)

ITEM NUM-BER	FOOD AND DESCRIPTION	PER 100 GM. EDIBLE PORTION		PER SPECIFIED UNIT			
		Free Folacin (μg.)	Total Folacin (μg.)	Approximate Measure	Weight (gm.)	Free Folacin (μg.)	Total Folacin (μg.)
	VEGETABLES (*Continued*)						
	potatoes, (*Continued*)						
123	French-fried	8	22	10 pieces	50	4	11
124	hashed brown	3	17	1 c.	155	5	26
125	mashed	5	10	1 c.	210	10	21
	pumpkin						
126	raw	5	36				
127	cooked	2	19	1 c.	245	5	47
128	radishes, common, raw	18	24	4 small	36	6	9
	rutabagas						
129	raw	23	27	1 c.	140	32	38
130	cooked	9	21				
130a	cooked, cubed			1 c.	170	15	36
130b	cooked, mashed			1 c.	240	22	50
	spinach						
131	raw	119	193	1 c.	55	65	106
132	cooked	60	91	1 c.	180	108	164
	squash, summer						
133	raw	23	31	1 c.	130	30	40
134	frozen, cooked	2	10	1 c.	210	4	21
	sweet potatoes						
135	raw	33	50	1 med.	146	48	73
136	cooked	7	18	1 med.	146	10	26
137	tomatoes, raw	21	39	1 med.	135	28	53
138	tomato juice, canned	10	26	1 c.	243	24	63
139	turnips, raw	17	20	1 c.	130	22	26
140	turnip greens, raw	–	95	1 c.	55	–	52
	FRUITS						
141	apples, raw	3	8	1 med.	166	5	13
142	applesauce, sweetened	1	1	1 c.	255	3	3
143	apricots, dried	10	14	1 c.	130	13	18
143a	apricots, dried			10 halves	35	4	5
144	avocados, raw	31	51	½ med.	115	36	59
145	bananas, raw	22	28	1 med.	119	26	33
146	blueberries, raw	2	6	1 c.	145	3	9
	cantaloupe, *see* muskmelon						
147	cherries, raw	6	8	1 c.	117	7	9
147a	cherries, raw			10 cherries	68	4	5
148	cranberries, raw	1	2	1 c.	91	1	2
149	currants, dried	4	11				
150	dates, dried	14	21	1 c.	178	25	37
150a	dates, dried			10 dates	80	11	17
151	figs, dried	3	9	1 large	21	1	2
152	grapefruit, raw	8	11	½ med.	98	8	11
153	grapefruit juice, fresh or frozen reconstituted	8	21	1 c.	247	20	52
154	grapes, red or white, raw	4	7	1 c.	152	6	11
155	grape juice, canned or frozen reconstituted	2	2	1 c.	253	5	5
156	lemon, raw	12	12	1 med.	74	9	9
157	lemonade	2	5	1 c.	248	5	12
158	limes, raw	6	4	1 lime	67	4	3
159	muskmelon or cantaloupe	30	30	½ med.	272	82	82
160	nectarines, raw	7	5	1 med.	138	10	7
161	oranges, raw	32	46	1 med.	141	45	65
162	orange juice, fresh or frozen reconstituted	34	55	1 c.	248	84	136
163	peaches, raw	2	8	1 med.	100	2	8
164	pears, raw	5	14	1 med.	164	8	23
165	pineapple, raw	9	11	1 c.	155	14	17
166	plantain (baking banana), raw	2	16	1 med.	263	5	42
167	plums, raw	4	6	1 med.	55	2	3
168	prunes, dried, softenized, raw	1	4	1 med.	26	<0.5	1
169	raisins, natural (unbleached), raw	3	4	1 c.	145	4	6

Appendix Table 7. FOLACIN CONTENT OF FOODS (*Continued*)

ITEM NUM-BER	FOOD AND DESCRIPTION	PER 100 GM. EDIBLE PORTION		PER SPECIFIED UNIT			
		Free Folacin (µg.)	*Total Folacin* (µg.)	*Approximate Measure*	*Weight* (gm.)	*Free Folacin* (µg.)	*Total Folacin* (µg.)
FRUITS (*Continued*)							
170	rhubarb, raw	9	7	1 c.	122	11	9
171	strawberries, raw	15	16	1 c.	149	22	24
172	tangerines, raw	19	21	1 med.	86	16	18
173	watermelon, raw	2	8	1 wedge, 4″ × 8″	426	9	34
MEAT							
	beef, separable lean						
174	raw	4	7				
175	cooked	–	4	3 oz.	85	–	3
	beef, ground						
176	raw	3	7				
177	cooked	–	4	3 oz.	85	–	3
	kidney						
178	beef, raw	63	80				
	lamb						
179	raw	24	42				
180	cooked	–	32	3 oz.	85	–	27
	lamb						
181	raw	1	4				
182	cooked	–	3	3 oz.	85	–	3
	liver						
	beef, lamb, or pork						
183	raw	80	219				
184	cooked	–	145	3 oz.	85	–	123
	pork						
	separable lean						
185	raw	3	8				
186	cooked	–	5	3 oz.	85	–	4
187	ham, smoked	–	11	3 oz.	85	–	9
	veal						
188	raw	4	5				
189	cooked	–	3	3 oz.	85	–	3
	sausages, cold cuts, and luncheon meats						
190	beerwurst	1	3	1 slice (1 oz.)	28	<0.5	1
191	bologna	2	5	1 slice (1 oz.)	28	1	1
192	frankfurters, unheated	2	4	1 (5″ long, ¾″ diam.)	45	1	2
193	head cheese	1	2	1 slice (1 oz.)	28	<0.5	1
194	liverwurst	20	30	1 slice (1 oz.)	28	6	8
	luncheon meats						
195	boiled ham	1	4	1 slice (1 oz.)	28	<0.5	1
196	pork, spiced	1	3	1 slice (1 oz.)	28	<0.5	1
197	sausage, pork, raw	–	14	3 oz.	85	–	12
POULTRY							
	chicken, without skin						
	dark meat						
198	raw	5	11				
199	cooked	–	7	3 oz.	85	–	6
	light meat						
200	raw	3	6				
201	cooked	–	4	3 oz.	85	–	3
	liver, chicken						
202	raw	–	364				
203	cooked	–	240	3 oz.	85	–	204
	turkey, without skin						
	dark meat						
204	raw	8	11				
205	cooked	–	7	3 oz.	85	–	6
	light meat						
206	raw	4	9				
207	cooked	–	5	3 oz.	85	–	4

Table continued on the following page

Appendix Table 7. FOLACIN CONTENT OF FOODS (*Continued*)

ITEM NUM-BER	FOOD AND DESCRIPTION	PER 100 GM. EDIBLE PORTION		PER SPECIFIED UNIT			
		Free Folacin (µg.)	Total Folacin (µg.)	Approximate Measure	Weight (gm.)	Free Folacin (µg.)	Total Folacin (µg.)
FISH AND SHELLFISH							
208	cod, frozen	6	18	3 oz.	85	5	15
209	crab, frozen	2	20	3 oz.	85	2	17
210	haddock, frozen	4	10	3 oz.	85	3	8
211	halibut, frozen	4	12	3 oz.	85	3	10
212	lobster, canned	8	17	3 oz.	85	7	14
213	ocean perch, frozen	5	9	3 oz.	85	4	8
	salmon						
214	canned	10	20	3 oz.	85	8	17
215	frozen	4	26	3 oz.	85	3	22
216	sardines, canned	13	16	1 fish	12	2	2
217	scallops, frozen	18	16	3 oz.	85	15	14
	shrimp						
218	canned	8	15	3 oz.	85	7	13
219	frozen	8	11	3 oz.	85	7	9
220	smelt, frozen	6	16	3 oz.	85	5	14
221	sole, frozen	5	11	3 oz.	85	4	9
222	tuna, canned	8	15	3 oz.	85	7	13
EGGS AND EGG PRODUCTS							
	eggs						
	whole						
223	raw	46	65	1 med.	44	20	29
224	hard-cooked	–	49	1 med.	44	–	22
225	white, raw	3	16	1 med.	29	1	5
226	yolk, raw	121	152	1 med.	15	18	23
227	eggnog	<0.5	1	½ c.	128	–	1
DAIRY PRODUCTS							
228	butter	1	3	1 tbsp.	14	<0.5	<0.5
	cheeses, natural						
229	Cheddar	1	18	1 c. shredded	113	1	20
229a	Cheddar			1 oz.	28	<0.5	5
230	cottage	–	12	1 c. packed	245	–	29
231	cream	–	13	3-oz. pkg.	85	–	11
231a	cream			1 cu. in.	16	–	2
232	cheese spread, pasteurized process	3	7	1 oz.	28	1	2
	cream, fluid						
233	half-and-half	2	2	1 c.	242	5	5
234	light coffee or table	1	2	1 c.	240	2	5
235	sour, cultured	–	11	1 c.	230	–	25
236	whipping, light	2	4	1 c.	239	5	10
237	ice cream, vanilla	2	2	1 c.	133	3	3
	milk, cow's, fluid						
238	whole, pasteurized	5	5	1 c.	244	12	12
239	skim, raw	3	–	1 c.	245	7	–
240	evaporated	4	8	1 c.	252	10	20
241	milk, goat's	1	1	1 c.	244	2	2
242	milk, human	3	5	1 fl. oz.	31	1	2
243	yogurt	<0.5	11	1 c.	245	–	27
MIXED DISHES, FROZEN							
244	beef with one vegetable	2	5	1 pkg.	254	5	13
245	beef with two vegetables, soup, dessert	5	12	1 pkg.	456	23	55
246	beef with three vegetables	8	24	1 pkg.	327	26	78
247	chicken, fried, with one vegetable	6	12	1 pkg.	205	12	25
248	chicken, fried, with two vegetables, dessert	6	18	1 pkg.	315	19	57
249	haddock with one vegetable	6	18	1 pkg.	273	16	49
250	ham with two vegetables, dessert	5	15	1 pkg.	314	16	47
251	lasagna	–	22	10-oz. portion	280	–	62

Appendix Table 7. FOLACIN CONTENT OF FOODS (*Continued*)

ITEM NUM-BER	FOOD AND DESCRIPTION	PER 100 GM. EDIBLE PORTION		PER SPECIFIED UNIT			
		Free Folacin (µg.)	Total Folacin (µg.)	Approximate Measure	Weight (gm.)	Free Folacin (µg.)	Total Folacin (µg.)
MIXED DISHES, FROZEN (*Continued*)							
	pizza						
252	cheese	–	37	⅛ pie, 13¾″ diam.	65	–	24
253	pepperoni	–	38	⅛ pie, 13¾″ diam.	67	–	25
254	sausage	–	35	⅛ pie, 13¾″ diam.	67	–	23
255	pork with one vegetable, one fruit, dessert	2	7	1 pkg.	303	6	21
256	poultry, Oriental style with rice, vegetables	2	4	1 pkg.	415	8	17
257	shrimp, Oriental style with rice, vegetables	4	13	1 pkg.	388	16	50
258	shrimp with one vegetable	8	14	1 pkg.	264	21	37
259	shrimp with two vegetables	9	22	1 pkg.	234	21	51
260	spaghetti with meatballs, one vegetable, dessert	6	18	1 pkg.	354	21	64
261	turkey with one vegetable	4	11	1 pkg.	264	11	29
262	turkey with two vegetables, dessert	6	14	1 pkg.	346	21	48
BABY FOODS—STRAINED, CANNED							
263	applesauce	<0.5	1				
263a	applesauce			1 jar	134	–	1
263b	applesauce			1 oz.	28	–	<0.5
264	apricots	<0.5	1				
264a	apricots			1 jar	134	–	1
264b	apricots			1 oz.	28	–	<0.5
265	bananas	1	2				
265a	bananas			1 jar	134	1	3
265b	bananas			1 oz.	28	<0.5	1
266	beans, green or wax	1	6				
266a	beans, green or wax			1 jar	128	1	8
266b	beans, green or wax			1 oz.	28	<0.5	2
267	beef with broth	1	6				
267a	beef with broth			1 jar	99	1	6
267b	beef with broth			1 oz.	28	<0.5	2
268	beets	2	10				
268a	beets			1 jar	128	3	13
268b	beets			1 oz.	28	1	3
269	carrots	1	2				
269a	carrots			1 jar	128	1	3
269b	carrots			1 oz.	28	<0.5	1
270	chicken with broth	1	2				
270a	chicken with broth			1 jar	99	1	2
270b	chicken with broth			1 oz.	28	<0.5	1
271	corn, creamed	1	3				
271a	corn, creamed			1 jar	128	1	4
271b	corn, creamed			1 oz.	28	<0.5	1
272	egg yolk	8	20				
272a	egg yolk			1 jar	94	8	19
272b	egg yolk			1 oz.	28	2	6
273	fruit, mixed	1	1				
273a	fruit, mixed			1 jar	134	1	1
273b	fruit, mixed			1 oz.	28	<0.5	<0.5
274	ham with broth	<0.5	6				
274a	ham with broth			1 jar	99	<0.5	6
274b	ham with broth			1 oz.	28	<0.5	2
275	lamb with vegetables	1	8				
275a	lamb with vegetables			1 jar	99	1	8
275b	lamb with vegetables			1 oz.	28	<0.5	2
276	oatmeal	–	4				

Table continued on the following page

Appendix Table 7. FOLACIN CONTENT OF FOODS (*Continued*)

ITEM NUM-BER	FOOD AND DESCRIPTION	PER 100 GM. EDIBLE PORTION		PER SPECIFIED UNIT			
		Free Folacin (μg.)	Total Folacin (μg.)	Approximate Measure	Weight (gm.)	Free Folacin (μg.)	Total Folacin (μg.)
BABY FOODS—STRAINED, CANNED (*Continued*)							
276a	oatmeal			1 jar	135	–	5
276b	oatmeal			1 oz.	28	–	1
277	peas	1	7				
277a	peas			1 jar	128	1	9
277b	peas			1 oz.	28	<0.5	2
278	spinach, creamed	2	4				
278a	spinach, creamed			1 jar	128	3	5
278b	spinach, creamed			1 oz.	28	1	1
279	squash	1	6				
279a	squash			1 jar	128	1	8
279b	squash			1 oz.	28	<0.5	2
280	sweet potatoes	1	3				
280a	sweet potatoes			1 jar	128	1	4
280b	sweet potatoes			1 oz.	28	<0.5	1
281	turkey with broth	2	4				
281a	turkey with broth			1 jar	99	2	4
281b	turkey with broth			1 oz.	28	1	1
282	veal with broth	2	7				
282a	veal with broth			1 jar	99	2	7
282b	veal with broth			1 oz.	28	1	2
283	vegetables, mixed	1	4				
283a	vegetables, mixed			1 jar	128	1	5
283b	vegetables, mixed			1 oz.	28	<0.5	1
MISCELLANEOUS							
284	barbecue sauce	3	4	1 c.	250	8	10
285	candy, milk chocolate, plain	4	7	1 oz.	28	1	2
286	margarine	2	2				
286a	margarine			1 c.	227	5	5
286b	margarine			1 tbsp.	14	<0.5	<0.5
287	mayonnaise	1	3	1 tbsp.	14	<0.5	<0.5
288	rice pudding	5	–	1 c.	255	13	–
	soups, commercial, canned						
289	asparagus, cream of	5	19	1 c.	245	12	47
290	beef broth	1	4	1 c.	240	2	10
291	clam chowder	3	7	1 c.	250	8	18
292	mushroom, cream of	1	3	1 c.	245	2	7
293	vegetable beef	2	6	1 c.	250	5	15
294	strawberry jam	7	8	1 tbsp.	20	1	2
295	tapioca, dry	2	8				
295a	tapioca, dry			1 c.	152	3	12
295b	tapioca, dry			1 tbsp.	8	<0.5	1
296	tapioca pudding	2	–	1 c.	255	5	–
297	tomato catsup	2	5				
297a	tomato catsup			1 c.	273	5	14
297b	tomato catsup			1 tbsp.	15	<0.5	1
	yeast						
298	baker's dry, active	140	4090	1 pkg.	7	10	286
299	brewer's, debittered	175	3909	1 tbsp.	8	14	313

Appendix Table 8. VITAMIN E CONTENT OF FOODS PER 100 GM. EDIBLE PORTION*

FOOD AND DESCRIPTION	NUMBER OF SAMPLES	TOTAL VITAMIN E	TOCOPHEROLS			
			Alpha	*Beta*	*Gamma*	*Delta*
			←————————— *mg./100 gm. food* —————————→			
ANIMAL PRODUCTS						
Meat (mammalian)						
beef						
muscle, skeletal, raw	9	0.43	0.41		0.02	
ground						
raw	1		0.79			
fried	1	0.63	0.37			
canned	3		0.60			
roast, cooked	3		0.14			
steak						
raw	1	0.63	0.47		<0.16	
broiled	1	0.55	0.13			
heart, raw	5		0.60			
liver						
raw	115	0.67	0.67	0	0	0
broiled	1	1.62	0.63			
veal						
muscle, skeletal						
raw	33	0.15				
very young, raw	12		0.08			
cutlet						
raw	2	0.08				
pan fried	1	0.24	0.05			
heart, raw	20	0.34	0.33	tr	tr	
liver, raw	16	0.35	0.33	tr	tr	
lamb						
chop						
raw	1	0.77	0.62		0.15	
broiled	1	0.32	0.16			
cutlet, broiled	1		0.22			
roast, leg, precooked, reheated	1		0.05			
liver, raw	10	0.79				
mutton						
muscle, skeletal, raw	4	0.46	0.43		0.03	
kidney, raw	4	0.41				
pork						
muscle, skeletal, raw	7	0.10	0.08		0.02	
chop						
raw	3	0.48				
pan fried	1	0.60	0.16			
loin						
raw	1		0.40			
canned	3		0.29			
ham, fried	1	0.52	0.28			
bacon						
raw	3	0.57	0.48			
fried	1	0.59	0.53			
heart, raw	200	0.63 (range: 0.3—1.34)				
liver, raw	263	0.47 (range: 0.06—1.76)				

From McLaughlin, P. J., and Weihrauch, J. L.: Vitamin E content of foods, J. Am. Diet. Assoc., 75: 647, 1979.

*Blanks indicate a lack of information. Zeros indicate an author tested for that form and stated that none was present. A dash means no detectable amount was reported. Trace (tr) means an amount too small to be measured was present. Brackets mean that numbers apply to columns they are centered between.

Table continued on the following page

Appendix Table 8.   VITAMIN E CONTENT OF FOODS PER 100 GM. EDIBLE
PORTION* (*Continued*)

FOOD AND DESCRIPTION	NUMBER OF SAMPLES	TOTAL VITAMIN E	TOCOPHEROLS			
			Alpha	*Beta*	*Gamma*	*Delta*
		←——————— mg./100 gm. food ———————→				

ANIMAL PRODUCTS (*Continued*)

Meat (mammalian), concluded

rabbit

muscle, skeletal

FOOD AND DESCRIPTION	NUMBER OF SAMPLES	TOTAL VITAMIN E	Alpha	Beta	Gamma	Delta
mature, raw	4		0.40			
young, raw	4	0.54				
liver						
mature, raw	6		1.69			
young, raw	9	1.46				
caribou, muscle, raw	2		0.02			
polar bear, meat, raw	1		0.04			
seal, meat, raw	3		0.15			
whale						
meat, frozen, raw	13		0.28			
liver, frozen, raw	10		0.81			
sausage and luncheon meats						
bologna	1	0.49	0.06			
knackwurst, knockwurst	10	0.57				
liver paste, canned	10	0.35				
liverwurst	1	0.69	0.35			
luncheon meat, canned	10	0.52				
salami	1	0.68	0.11			
sausage						
pork, fried	2	0.32	0.16			
beef, fried	1		0.15			
Poultry						
chicken						
meat						
raw	23	0.34	0.29			
cooked	3	0.55	0.35			
frozen fried, not heated	2	1.12	0.25			
frozen fried, oven heated	3	0.94	0.19			
frozen raw	1		0.42			
cooked, canned	3		0.28			
eviscerated carcass, raw	>2	0.98				
heart, raw	3		1.19			
liver, raw	75	1.44				
duck, white Peking, eviscerated						
carcass						
adult, raw	>2	2.80				
young, raw	>2	0.70				
goose, Toulouse, eviscerated carcass, raw	>2	1.74				
pigeon						
breast, raw	4		0.06			
liver, raw	4		1.54			
quail, Japanese domesticated,						
eviscerated carcass, raw	>2	0.70				
turkey, raw						
eviscerated carcass	>2	1.43				
breast	33		0.09			
thigh	1		0.64			
skin	1		0.40			
heart	1		0.16			
liver	5	2.90				
Eggs						
chicken						
yolk, raw	66	3.12	2.05		1.03	0.03
whole large, raw	66	1.06	0.70		0.35	0.01
whole, cooked	8		0.77			
powder	3	5.46				
pheasant, yolk, raw	2		4.86			
turkey, yolk, raw	290	2.90				

Appendix Table 8. VITAMIN E CONTENT OF FOODS PER 100 GM. EDIBLE PORTION* (*Continued*)

FOOD AND DESCRIPTION	NUMBER OF SAMPLES	TOTAL VITAMIN E	TOCOPHEROLS			
			Alpha	*Beta*	*Gamma*	*Delta*
		←————— *mg./100 gm. food* ————→				

ANIMAL PRODUCTS (*Continued*)

Dairy products
butter

United States (U.S.)	4	1.58	1.58			
foreign	644	2.40 (range: 0.5—5.0)	2.40			
cheese, various	3		0.64			
cream, sweet, fluid	7	0.63				
ice cream, chocolate	2	1.06	0.37			
ice cream, vanilla	2	0.35	0.06			
milk, cow—fluid, whole						
U.S. commercial	3	0.09	0.06		0.01	0
U.S. producer	1644	0.11				
U.S. producer calculated at milk fat content of 3.34%	1636	0.09				
foreign, commercial	206		0.16		⏜0.03	
chocolate	1		0.09			
buttermilk	2	0.07				
condensed, reconstituted	8	0.11				
evaporated	16	0.18				
skim	4	tr	tr			
dry						
whole	4	1.08				
buttermilk	3	0.40				
milk, human, fluid	448	0.99	0.88	0.02	0.07	0.02†
milk, sheep, fluid, whole	41	0.14				

Finfish
fillet

carp (*Cyprinus carpio*)						
raw	1		0.63			
with skin, raw	1	0.31				
cod, Atlantic (*Gadus morhua*)						
raw	10		0.23			
dark meat, raw	3		1.16			
white meat, frozen	1		0.24			
flounder, winter (*Pseudopleuronectes americanus*), frozen	20		0.36			
haddock (*Melanogrammus aeglefinus*)						
raw	2		0.39			
broiled	1	1.20	0.60			
halibut, Atlantic (*Hippoglossus hippoglossus*), raw	2		0.85			
halibut, bastard (*Paralichthys olivaceus*), raw	1		0.14			
herring (*Clupea harengus*)						
raw	3		1.07			
light meat, frozen 4-5 months	10	2.00	2.00			
dark meat, frozen 4-5 months	4	2.30	2.30			
ling (*Molva molva*), raw	1		0.30			
mackerel, Atlantic (*Scomber scombrus*)						
dark meat, raw	1		1.52			
canned	6	1.2				
mackerel, jack (*Trachurus japonicus*)						
raw	1		0.36			
ocean perch (*Sebastes marinus*), raw	1		1.25			
pollock (*Pollachius virens*), raw	2		0.31			
sablefish (*Anaplopoma fimbria*), frozen	1		4.35			

†Also present, trace of gamma-tocotrienol.

Table continued on the following page

Appendix Table 8. VITAMINE E CONTENT OF FOODS PER 100 GM. EDIBLE PORTION* *(Continued)*

FOOD AND DESCRIPTION	NUMBER OF SAMPLES	TOTAL VITAMIN E	TOCOPHEROLS			
			Alpha	*Beta*	*Gamma*	*Delta*
		←————— *mg./100 gm. food* —————→				

ANIMAL PRODUCTS *(Continued)*

Finfish, concluded
fillet, continued

salmon, unspecified, steak, broiled	1	1.81	1.35			
skipjack, unspecified, with skin, raw	1	1.47				
trout, rainbow (*Salmo gairdneri*), with skin, raw	1	0.20				
wolffish, Atlantic (*Anarhichas lupus*), raw	1		2.1			
wrasse, European (*Labrus bergylta*), raw	1		0.60			
yellowtail (*Seriola quinqueradiata*), raw	2		0.18			
frozen, 60 days	3		0.11			

liver

carp, raw	1		0.84			
cod, Atlantic						
raw	4		15.85			
canned	2		2.45			
haddock						
raw	2		6.25			
canned	4	17.5				
halibut, bastard, raw	1		0.34			
herring, raw	3		5.97			
mackerel, Atlantic, raw	1		3.10			
mackerel, jack, raw	1		1.21			
ocean perch, raw	1		16.5			
pollock, raw	4		8.40			
skipjack, raw	1	2.61				
trout, rainbow, raw	1	0.12				
tuna (*Thunnus thynnus*), raw	1		5.0			
turbot (*Rhombus lupus*), raw	1		3.0			
wolffish, Atlantic, raw	2		29.50			
wrasse, European, raw	2		14.40			
yellowtail						
raw	2		0.94			
frozen, 60 days	3		0.64			

Shellfish
molluscs

mussel, common (*Mytilus edulis*)						
fresh, raw	7		0.74			
frozen	1		2.5			
mussel, horse (*Volsella modiolus*), fresh, raw	1		0.58			
mussel, ribbed (*Volsella demissa*), fresh, raw	1		0.50			
oyster (*Crassostrea virginica*), fresh, raw	3		0.85			
oyster, Australian, raw	1		0.26			
limpet (*Patella vulgata*), raw	2		14.00			
periwinkle, common (*Littorina litorea*), fresh, raw	4		3.90			
squid (*Ommestrephes todarus*), raw	1		1.2			
whelk (*Bucinnum undatum*), raw	1		0.8			

crustaceans

crab, queen (*Chioncectes opilio*)						
frozen, raw	2	2.25				
frozen, cooked	1	1.22				
lobster (*Homarus americanus*), muscle, raw	3		1.47			
prawn (*Pandalus borealis*), raw	1		2.85			

Appendix Table 8. VITAMINE E CONTENT OF FOODS PER 100 GM. EDIBLE PORTION* *(Continued)*

FOOD AND DESCRIPTION	NUMBER OF SAMPLES	TOTAL VITAMIN E	TOCOPHEROLS			
			Alpha	*Beta*	*Gamma*	*Delta*
		←————— *mg./100 gm. food* —————→				

ANIMAL PRODUCTS *(Continued)*

Fats and oils
mammalian

beef tallow	1		2.65			
butter oil, cow						
U.S.	1643	2.83				
Butter oil, cow						
Japanese	28	2.61	2.48	0	0.13	0
foreign, summer	300	3.71				
foreign, winter	297	2.28				
caribou tallow	3		0.37			
ghee, cow or buffalo, fresh	34	3.00				
pork lard, commercial	12	1.34	1.20		0.07†	
seal oil	5		8.9			
whale, commercial oil	3		4.53			
poultry						
chicken fat, raw	83	2.73 (range: 0.1—30.0)				
turkey fat, raw	17	2.87				
finfish, commercial oil						
anchovy *(Engraulis ringens)*	3		29.08			
capelin *(Mallotus villosus)*	2		14.0			
cod, Atlantic, liver	7	21.96	21.96			
herring	5		9.22			
menhaden, Atlantic *(Brevoortia tyrannus)*	1		7.5			
dogfish, spiny, liver	2		25.0			
shark, Greenland *(Somniosus microcephalus)*, liver	2		50.0			
finfish, non-commercial oil						
anchovy	2		74.55			
haddock	1	0.7	0.6			
haddock, liver	1		18.0			
ocean perch	5	18.74				
salmon, chinook *(Oncorhynchus tshawytscha)*	2		19.15			
skipjack						
liver	1	90.0				
trout, rainbow						
meat and skin	1	12.5				
liver	1	5.2				
wolffish, Atlantic						
liver	1		185.5			
meat	2		35.5			
wrasse, European, liver	3	250.67	250.67			
shellfish oil						
limpet	1		150.0			
prawn	1		95.0			
squid, commercial oil	1		21.0			

FOOD AND DESCRIPTION	NUMBER OF SAMPLES	TOTAL VITAMIN E	TOCOPHEROLS				TOCOTRIENOLS		
			Alpha	*Beta*	*Gamma*	*Delta*	*Alpha*	*Beta*	*Gamma*
		←——————— *mg./100 gm. food* ———————→							

PLANT PRODUCTS

Beans and peas
beans

broad *(Vicia faba)*									
raw	1		0.05	0	0.40				
flour, dry	1		1.00		2.50	0		0	

†Also present, trace of gamma-tocotrienol.

Appendix Table 8. VITAMIN E CONTENT OF FOODS PER 100 GM. EDIBLE PORTION* (*Continued*)

FOOD AND DESCRIPTION	NUMBER OF SAMPLES	TOTAL VITAMIN E	TOCOPHEROLS				TOCOTRIENOLS		
			Alpha	Beta	Gamma	Delta	Alpha	Beta	Gamma
			←———————————— mg./100 gm. food ————————————→						

PLANT PRODUCTS (*Continued*)

Beans and peas, concluded
beans, continued
chickpea (*Cicer-arietinum*),

dry	5	3.11							
French (*Phaseolus vulgaris*),									
raw	3	<0.10							
great northern (*P. vulgaris*)									
dry	1	2.30							
sprouts only	1	0.06							
green (*P. vulgaris*)									
fresh	1	0.11	0.02	—	0.09	—	—	—	—
dry	2	0.51							
sprouts only	2	0.04							
canned	1	0.05	0.03						
freeze dried	1	6.25							
frozen, not cooked	1	0.24	0.09						
frozen, cooked	6	0.25	0.13						
kidney (*P. vulgaris*)									
dry	2	2.08	tr	—	2.08	tr	—	—	—
sprouts only	1	0.05							
Lima (*P. lunatus*) large									
dry	1	7.68	tr	—	7.15	0.53	—	—	—
mung (*P. aureus*)									
dry	1	1.97							
navy (*P. vulgaris*)									
dry	3	2.26	0.34		1.92				
sprouts only	1	0.06							
pinto (*P. vulgaris*)									
dry	1	1.40							
sprouts only	1	0.21							
snap (*P. vulgaris*)									
dry	3	1.55							
sprouts only	3	0.11							
wax (*P. vulgaris*), canned, boiled	1		0.29						
sprouts only	1	0.20							
scarlet runner (*P. coccineus*)									
raw	2	<0.1							
soy (*Glycine max*)									
dry	4	20.43	0.85	—	10.97	8.61	—	—	—
sprouts only	1	0.09							
sulphur									
dry	1	0.78							
sprouts only	1	0.07							
lentils, (*Lens culinaris*),									
dry	1	1.27							
peas (*Pisum sativum*)									
fresh	13	2.71	0.13		2.58				
dry	8	2.27	0.09	0	2.09	0.09			
canned	5	2.63							
frozen, not cooked	4	0.64	0.12		0.52	0			
cooked	1	0.65	0.12						
sprouts only	6	0.14							

Appendix Table 8. VITAMIN E CONTENT OF FOODS PER 100 GM. EDIBLE
PORTION* (*Continued*)

FOOD AND DESCRIPTION	NUMBER OF SAMPLES	TOTAL VITAMIN E	TOCOPHEROLS				TOCOTRIENOLS		
			Alpha	Beta	Gamma	Delta	Alpha	Beta	Gamma
			←————————————— mg./100 gm. food ————————————→						
PLANT PRODUCTS (*Continued*)									
Cocoa products									
butter, natural and Dutch	9	19.86	1.79	tr	17.39	0.43	0.25		—
powder, natural and Dutch	4	2.25	0.2						
chocolate									
dark, sweet	2	6.0	0.7						
milk									
12%, milk	2	5.6	0.7						
20%, milk	2	6.3	0.7						
bar	1	4.2	1.1						
Fruits									
apple (*Pyrus* sp.)									
whole, raw	9	0.66	0.59						
flesh only, raw	9		0.27						
stewed with sugar	1		0.05						
juice, canned	1		0.01						
apricot (*Prunus armeniaca*), canned, sweetened	1		0.89						
avocado (*Persea americana*)									
California Fuerte, raw	4		1.61						
California Hass, raw	2		1.07						
banana (*Musa sapientum*), raw	6	0.32	0.27						
blackberry (*Rubus* sp.)									
wild, raw	2		3.5		4.7	4.5			
cultivated, raw	3		0.6		1.1	1.0			
cherry (*Prunus avium*), raw	1		0.13						
currant									
black (*Ribes nigrum*), raw	1		1.0						
red (*R. rubrum*), raw	1		0.1						
damson (*Prunus instititia*), raw	1		0.7						
gooseberry (*Ribes grossularia, uva-crispa*), raw	7		0.37						
grapefruit (*Citrus paradisi*)									
raw	1	0.26	0.25		⌒<0.01				
juice, canned	1	0.18	0.04						
mango (*Mangifera indica*), raw	1		1.12						
muskmelon (*Cucumis melo*), raw	2	0.31	0.14						
orange (*Citrus sinensis*)									
raw	2	0.24	0.24		⌒—	—			
juice, fresh	1	0.2	0.04						

Table continued on the following page

Appendix Table 8. VITAMIN E CONTENT OF FOODS PER 100 GM. EDIBLE PORTION* (*Continued*)

FOOD AND DESCRIPTION	NUMBER OF SAMPLES	TOTAL VITAMIN E	TOCOPHEROLS				TOCOTRIENOLS		
			Alpha	*Beta*	*Gamma*	*Delta*	*Alpha*	*Beta*	*Gamma*
					mg./100 gm. food				
PLANT PRODUCTS (*Continued*)									
Fruits, concluded									
pear (*Pyrus communis*) flesh									
and skin, raw	3		0.5						
flesh, raw	3		<0.1						
pineapple (*Ananas comosus*), flesh	5	0.10	0.10						
raspberry (*Rubus idaeus*), raw	1		0.3		1.5	2.7			
strawberry (*Fragaria* sp.)									
raw	3	0.26	0.12	0.08		—			
frozen, sliced	1	0.40	0.21						
tomato (*Lycopersicum esculentum*)									
raw	10	0.49	0.34	0.13		0.02			
juice, canned	1	0.71	0.22						
Cereal grains and their products									
barley (*Hordeum vulgare*)									
whole grain	8	2.98	0.57	0.27		tr	1.23	0.90	
pearled	2	0.76	0.02	tr	tr	—	0.37	0.27	0.10
buckwheat (*Fagopyrum* sp.), flour	1	7.91	0.32	—	7.14	0.45	—	—	—
bulgur	1	1.40	0.06	0.12	—	—	0.14	1.08	—
corn (*Zea mays*)									
whole	127	5.81 (range: 0.9—11.16)	0.49	0	4.56	tr	0.21	0.09	0.46
flour	1	1.47	0.12		0.33		0.32		0.70
grits	1	1.38	0.12		0.36		0.34		0.56
meal	5	1.80	0.15		0.52		0.41		0.72
meal, cooked	1	0.42	0.08						
starch	1	0							
processed products									
flakes	4		0.10		0.29				
puffed	1		0.09		0.34				
shredded	1		0.08		0.26				
hominy grits, cooked	1	0.15	0.04						
millet, unspecified	1	1.75	0.05	tr	1.3	0.4	—	—	—
oats (*Avena sativa*)									
whole grain	9	2.05	1.09	0.20		0.01	0.67	0.08	—
dry cereal	1	1.53	0.60						
granular	2		0.09		0.23		0.11		
meal	6	2.31	1.51	0.11		—	0.63	0.05	
shredded	1		0.08		0.06		0		
rice (*Oryza sativa*)									
brown, dehulled	6	2.04	0.68	—	0.37	tr	—	—	0.98
white, milled	5	0.39	0.11	—	0.07	tr	0.05	—	0.15
bran	1	14.92							
germ	1	8.73							
grits	1		0.04		0.10				
meal	1		0.10		0.27				
processed cereal, dry	1	0.28	0.04						
puffed or expanded	5		0.06		0.35				
shredded	1		0.02		0.02	0.01			

Appendix Table 8. VITAMIN E CONTENT OF FOODS PER 100 GM. EDIBLE PORTION* (*Continued*)

FOOD AND DESCRIPTION	NUMBER OF SAMPLES	TOTAL VITAMIN E	TOCOPHEROLS				TOCOTRIENOLS		
			Alpha	*Beta*	*Gamma*	*Delta*	*Alpha*	*Beta*	*Gamma*
		←——————————————— *mg./100 gm. food* ———————————————→							

PLANT PRODUCTS (*Continued*)

Cereal grains and their products, concluded

FOOD AND DESCRIPTION	NUMBER OF SAMPLES	TOTAL VITAMIN E	*Alpha*	*Beta*	*Gamma*	*Delta*	*Alpha*	*Beta*	*Gamma*
rye (*Secale cereale*)									
whole grain	5	3.80	1.28	0.53	—	—	1.07	0.91	—
flour									
dark	1	6.68	1.41	0.60	—	—	2.89	1.78	—
light	3	0.93	0.43	0.16	—	—	0.17	0.16	—
medium	1	3.18	0.79	0.56	—	—	0.85	0.98	—
semolina, boiled	1		0.06						
triticale (*Triticum aestivum* x *Secale cereale*)									
whole grain	5		0.90						
flour	5		0.20						
wheat (*Triticum aestivum*)									
whole grain	106	4.57 (range: 0.58—5.2)	1.01	0.68	—	—	0.31	2.56	—
bran	65	9.12	1.49	1.11			0.91	5.60	
flour									
unbleached	71	2.31	0.25	0.17	0	0	0.12	1.77	
bleached	21	0.42	0.03	0.04	0	0	0	0.35	
cake	6	0.23	0.04	0.03	—	—	tr	0.17	
cracker	7	2.81	0.65	0.38	—	—	0.15	1.63	
whole wheat	1	3.95	0.82	0.66	—	—	0.27	2.20	—
low grade	61	4.24	1.08	0.82	—	—	0.20	2.14	—
germ	20	27.56 (range: 21.8—33.2)	14.07	8.14	0	0	0	1.06	
breakfast cereals									
farina	2	0.94							
flakes	13	2.11	0.42	0.24	0.23	tr	0.03	1.18	—
puffed	3	0.67							
shredded	10	2.15	0.36	0.28	0.26			1.25	
whole wheat	10	4.05	1.06	0.52	0.30			2.17	
wheat, durum (*T. durum*)									
whole grain	2	5.20	0.89	0.43	—	—	0.60	3.28	
flour	2	2.12	0.26	0.13	—	—	0.21	1.52	

Nuts, peanuts and seeds

FOOD AND DESCRIPTION	NUMBER OF SAMPLES	TOTAL VITAMIN E	*Alpha*	*Beta*	*Gamma*	*Delta*	*Alpha*	*Beta*	*Gamma*
almond (*Prunus amygdalus*)									
shelled, raw	5	24.48	23.96		0.51				
blanched	1	20.63							
roasted	1	5.65							
meal	1	33.4	31.7	0.3	0.9	—	0.5	—	—
Brazil nut (*Bertholletia excelsa*), raw	1		6.5		11.0				
cashew (*Anacardium occidentale*)									
shelled, raw	1	4.20	0.19	—	3.84	0.17	—	—	—
roasted, dry or oil	1	11							
chestnut (*Castanea sativa*), raw	1		0.5†		7.0				
coconut (*Cocos nucifera*), raw	1		0.7		0.25		tr		
filbert (*Corylus* sp.), raw	2		23.75		1.7†		tr		

†Approximately.

Table continued on the following page

Appendix Table 8.   VITAMIN E CONTENT OF FOODS PER 100 GM. EDIBLE PORTION* (*Continued*)

FOOD AND DESCRIPTION	NUMBER OF SAMPLES	TOTAL VITAMIN E	TOCOPHEROLS				TOCOTRIENOLS		
			Alpha	Beta	Gamma	Delta	Alpha	Beta	Gamma
			←——————————— mg./100 gm. food ———————————→						
PLANT PRODUCTS (*Continued*)									
Nut, peanuts, and seeds, concluded									
mixed									
dry roasted	1	12							
oil roasted	1	12							
peanut (*Arachis hypogaea*)‡									
shelled, raw	5	16.37	8.33	—	8.04	—	—	—	—
oil roasted	2	11.60	6.94						
dry roasted	2	11.85	7.80						
paprika seed (*Capsicum annum*), raw	1	9.60							
pecan (*Carya illincensis*)									
shelled, raw	3	19.86	1.24	—	18.62	—	—	—	—
pistachio (*Pistacia vera*), shelled									
raw	1		5.21						
poppy seed (*Papaver somniferum*), raw	1	11.0	1.8	—	9.2	—	—	—	—
sesame seed (*Sesamum indicum*), raw	1	22.7	—		22.7	—	—	—	—
sunflower seed (*Helianthus annuus*)									
hulled, raw	1	52.18	49.45	2.73⏜		—	—	—	—
walnut, English (*Juglans regia*)									
shelled, raw	3	19.62	0.84	—	17.84	0.94	—	—	—
Vegetables									
artichoke, Jerusalem (*Helianthus tuberosus*), tuber, raw	4		0.19						
asparagus (*Asparagus officinalis*)									
fresh, raw	5	2.10	1.98	0.05	0.07	—			
canned	2		0.38						
frozen	1	1.59	1.40	0.07	0.12	—	—	—	—
beet (*Beta vulgaris*)									
root, raw	1		<0.03						
root, canned	1		0.03						
leaf, raw	4		1.5						
broccoli (*Brassica oleracea*), fresh	1	0.64	0.46	—	0.18				
Brussels sprouts (*B. oleracea*)									
fresh, raw	11	0.88	0.88						
cooked	2	0.85	0.85						
cabbage, common (*B. oleracea*), raw	23	1.67	1.67	—	tr	tr	—	—	—
cabbage, Chinese (*B. chinersis*), raw	1	0.13	0.12	0.01⏜		—			
carrot (*Daucus carota*)									
raw	13	0.51	0.44	0.02	—	0.01	0.04	tr	
cooked	1	0.46	0.42						

‡A legume.

Appendix Table 8. VITAMIN E CONTENT OF FOODS PER 100 GM. EDIBLE
PORTION* (*Continued*)

FOOD AND DESCRIPTION	NUMBER OF SAMPLES	TOTAL VITAMIN E	TOCOPHEROLS				TOCOTRIENOLS		
			Alpha	*Beta*	*Gamma*	*Delta*	*Alpha*	*Beta*	*Gamma*
			←———————————mg./100 gm. food———————————→						

PLANT PRODUCTS (*Continued*)

Vegetables, continued

cauliflower (*B. olera-cea*), fresh	2	0.09	0.03	—	0.05	0.01	—	—	—
celery (*Apium graveolens*), stalk and pale leaf, raw	10	0.73	0.36	0.01		0.36			
corn, sweet (*Zea mays*)									
canned	1	0.62	0.04	—	0.16	tr	0.12	—	0.30
frozen	1	0.64	0.03	—	0.09	tr	0.14	—	0.38
cress (*Lepidium sativum*), raw	5		0.7						
cucumber (*Cucumis sativus*), whole, raw	4	0.31	0.15	0.11		0.05			
dandelion leaf (*Taraxacum officinale*), raw	4		2.5						
eggplant (*Solanum me-longena*), raw	1		0.03	tr		—			
garlic (*Allium sativum*), raw	1		0.01	tr		0.09			
leek (*A. porrum*), white, raw	10		0.92						
lettuce (*Lactuca sativa*), raw	17	0.75	0.40		0.35	—			
mint (*Mentha spicata*), leaf, raw	3		5.0						
mushroom (*Agaricus bisporus*), raw	6	0.29	0.08	0.09		—	0.12		
boletus, edible yellow (steinpilz), raw	1	0.60	0.04	0.11		0.06	0.39		
chanterelle (pfifferling), raw	1	0.08	0.03	0.02	0	0.03			
morel, raw	1	0.63	0.05	0.12	0	0.46			
lorchel, raw	1	0.14	0.03	0	0	0.11			
mustard greens (*Sinapis alba*), raw	10		2.01						
nasturtium (*Tropaeolum majus*), leaf, raw	6		2.5						
nettle (*Urtica dioica*), leaf, raw	21		14.5						
onion (*Allium cepa*)									
raw	8	0.31	0.12	0.01		0.18			
frozen French fried rings, not heated	2	5.4	0.56						
oven heated	2	6.3	0.69						
white pickled in vinegar	1		0.19						

Table continued on the following page

Appendix Table 8.   VITAMIN E CONTENT OF FOODS PER 100 GM. EDIBLE
PORTION* (*Continued*)

FOOD AND DESCRIPTION	NUMBER OF SAMPLES	TOTAL VITAMIN E	TOCOPHEROLS				TOCOTRIENOLS		
			Alpha	*Beta*	*Gamma*	*Delta*	*Alpha*	*Beta*	*Gamma*
			←		*mg./100 gm. food*				→

PLANT PRODUCTS (*Continued*)

Vegetables, concluded									
parsley (*Petroselinum hortense*), raw	15	2.53	1.74	0.18		0.61			
parsnip (*Pastinaca sativa*), raw	2		1.0						
pepper, sweet (*Caosicum* sp.), raw	2		0.68	0.01		—			
potato, white (*Solanum tuberosum*)									
raw	5	0.07	0.06	tr		—			
baked	1	0.06	0.03						
boiled	1	0.06	0.04						
chips	2	7.31	4.27						
French fried	2		0.19						
potato, sweet (*Ipomoea batatas*), raw	4	4.60	4.56	0.03		0.01			
pumpkin (*Cucurbita pepo*), raw	1		1.02	0.14		—			
radish (*Raphanus sativus*)									
root, raw	4		—	tr		tr			
leaf, raw	2	3.76	3.06	0.02		0.68			
raisin, Sultana (*Vitis vinifera*), raw	1		0.7						
rhubarb (*Rheum hybridum*), raw	3		0.2						
rutabaga (*Brassica napus*)									
raw	3		<0.03						
steamed	1		0.15						
shallots (*Allium ascalonicum*), green, raw	1		0.21						
spinach (*Spinacia oleracea*)									
fresh, raw	11	3.00	1.88	—	0.14	0.98	—	—	—
leaf, canned	1	0.06	0.02						
squash, marrow type (*Cucurbita pepo*), steamed	1		0.12						
tea leaf (*Camellia sinensis*)	1		25.90	0.07		1.02			
turnip (*Brassica rapa*)									
root, raw	2		<0.03						
greens, raw	1	2.30	2.24	0.06					
watercress (*Nasturtium officinale*), leaf and stalk, raw	6		1.0						
Vegetable oils									
almond	4	40.09	39.17	—	0.92	—			
apricot kernel	6	50.48	3.99		43.03	2.72			
avocado	15	17.23	12.55	—	4.23	tr	—		—
barley	11	150.29	25.77	5.59	5.05	tr	67.25	40.21	6.41

Appendix Table 8.   VITAMIN E CONTENT OF FOODS PER 100 GM. EDIBLE
PORTION* (*Continued*)

FOOD AND DESCRIPTION	NUMBER OF SAMPLES	TOTAL VITAMIN E	TOCOPHEROLS				TOCOTRIENOLS		
			Alpha	*Beta*	*Gamma*	*Delta*	*Alpha*	*Beta*	*Gamma*
		←————————— *mg./100 gm. food* —————————→							

PLANT PRODUCTS (*Continued*)

Vegetable oils, continued

FOOD AND DESCRIPTION	NUMBER OF SAMPLES	TOTAL VITAMIN E	*Alpha*	*Beta*	*Gamma*	*Delta*	*Alpha*	*Beta*	*Gamma*
Brazil nut	4	24.22	7.10	—	17.12	—			
castor bean (*Ricinus communis*) refined	6	67.40	1.91		26.04#	38.64**			
cherry seed (*Prunus* sp.)	2	35.14	6.5		21.1	7.5			
coconut, refined	13	3.58	0.35	0	0.17	0.35	1.29	0.10	1.32
corn refined commercial	46	83.17 (range: 40.0—150.88)	14.26	0.38	64.90	2.75	0.58	—	—
crude commercial	8	116.71	13.71	tr	98.04	4.95			
partially hydrogenated commercial	2	47.45	17.30						
cottonseed (*Gossypium* sp.) refined	22	65.24 (range: 25.9—94.0)	35.26	0	29.98	0	0	0	0
crude	42	105.52 (range: 34.4—147.5)	51.34	0	54.17	0			
filbert	14	47.24	47.24						
grapefruit	1	26.5							
grapeseed (*Vitis vinifera*)	17	61.82 (range: 19.4—115.6)	28.82		30.79	2.01			
oat (*Avena sativa*)	12	40.89	9.54		14.69	2.47	11.20	2.50	0.49
olive (*Olea europaea*)	31	12.64 (range: 0—24.0)	11.92	0	0.72	0	—	—	—
orange flavedo	1	390	390						
palm (*Elaeis guineensis*) refined	10	35.53	18.32	0	0	0	11.46	0	5.75
non-hydrogenated	9	38.40	19.12	0	0	0	13.10	0	6.18
hydrogenated	1	9.7	5.58	0	0	0	2.52	0	1.60
crude	15	58.74 (range: 9.42—80.45)	16.72	tr	0	0	11.18	2.46	22.74¶
palm kernel refined	3	6.20							
crude	3	21.06							
peach kernel (*Amygdalus persica*)	1	15.00	13.35		1.65	—			

**Approximately.
#Nearly all gamma-tocopherol.
¶In addition, 5.64 mg./100 gm. of delta-tocotrienol is present in crude palm oil. None was found in refined palm oil.

Table continued on the following page

Appendix Table 8. VITAMIN E CONTENT OF FOODS PER 100 GM. EDIBLE PORTION* (Continued)

FOOD AND DESCRIPTION	NUMBER OF SAMPLES	TOTAL VITAMIN E	TOCOPHEROLS				TOCOTRIENOLS		
			Alpha	Beta	Gamma	Delta	Alpha	Beta	Gamma
		←——————— mg./100 gm. food ———————→							
PLANT PRODUCTS (Continued)									
Vegetable oils, concluded									
peanut									
refined	24	25.00 (range: 9.4—54.0)	11.62	—	12.98	0.33	0	0	0
crude	23	37.88 (range: 14.8—93.4)	14.41	—	22.52	0.94			
hydrogenated	4	22.89	10.04	0	12.85	0	0		0
pecan	2	23.34	0.89	—	22.45	—	—	—	—
rapeseed (Brassica sp.)									
refined	45	44.81 (range: 14.6-85.3)	17.65		27.04	0.04	—	—	—
crude	38	62.75 (range: 36.6—100.0)	25.79	—	36.56	0.40			
hydrogenated	2	50.10	16.24		33.86	0			
rice									
bran	4	51.0	36.39	tr	present	tr	tr		
germ	2	171.87	103.12	—	34.89	18.41			
rye	3	192.11	71.42	16.74		0	53.24	50.55	—
safflower seed (Carthamus tinctorius)									
refined	22	38.10 (range: 24.8—69.77)	34.05		3.50	0.49	—	—	—
crude	4	51.63	38.25		7.45	5.93			
hydrogenated	2	23.2	18.8						
sesame									
refined	5	29.07	1.38	0.37	25.24	2.08	—	—	—
crude	5	74.60	28.82	0	45.66	tr	—	—	—
soybean (Glycine sp.)									
refined	84	93.74 (range: 25.0—163.9)	10.99		62.40	20.38	0	0	0
crude	34	110.56 (range: 52.9—166.6)	10.47	—	66.69	33.40	—	—	—
hydrogenated	3	103.0	9.58		66.27	27.15			
sunflower seed									
refined	33	63.62 (range: 26.8—90.0)	59.50		3.54	tr	—	—	—
crude	35	68.19 (range: 27.1-124.3)	62.26	—	5.85	tr			
tomato seed	2	59.3	3.8		20.5	35.0			
walnut (Juglans sp.)	4	32.07	0.44	—	27.83	3.80			
wheat germ	22	254.58 (range: 165.6—300.0)	149.44	81.19	—				
Margarine									
coconut, sunflower, palm oils—									
stick	1	11.1	8.8	0.6	0.8	0.4	0.5	tr	tr

Appendix Table 8. VITAMIN E CONTENT OF FOODS PER 100 GM. EDIBLE PORTION* (*Continued*)

FOOD AND DESCRIPTION	NUMBER OF SAMPLES	TOTAL VITAMIN E	TOCOPHEROLS				TOCOTRIENOLS		
			Alpha	*Beta*	*Gamma*	*Delta*	*Alpha*	*Beta*	*Gamma*
			←		*mg./100 gm. food*				→

PLANT PRODUCTS (*Continued*)

Margarine, concluded

corn oil—stick	6	57.65	12.89	42.46		2.30			
corn oil—tub	3	46.38	10.91	33.86		1.61			
corn oil—diet imitation, tub	2	30.0							
corn, soybean, cottonseed oils—stick	7	68.18	11.38	49.09		7.71			
safflower, soybean oils									
stick	1		17.75						
tub	1	48.8	11.7	29.0		8.1			
safflower, soybean, cottonseed oils, stick	1		16.43						
soybean oil									
stick	1		3.14						
tub	1	32.4	2.3	24.2		5.9			
diet imitation tub	1	9.71	0.8	7.11		1.8			
soybean, cottonseed oils									
stick	18	45.49	11.15	26.43		7.91			
tub	9	74.32	8.60	50.11		15.61			
liquid	2		2.53						
diet	2		5.62						

Other oil products

mayonnaise	4	58.0	20.74						
salad dressing, mayonnaise type	2	30.0							
salad dressing, other (Italian, French, Thousand Island)	4	47.5							
sandwich spread	2	34.5							
shortening, vegetable, soybean	4	98.28	13.97	—	76.07	7.67			
tartar sauce	2	51.5							

PROCESSED, MIXED AND MISCELLANEOUS FOODS

Baked products

bread									
white, U.S.	55	1.19	0.12	0.01	0.43	0.20	0.05	0.38	
whole wheat, U.S.	10	0.90	0.10	0.09	0.23	0.13		0.35	
biscuit mix, dry	10	2.48	0.27	tr	1.60	0.50		0.11	
cake—from soft wheat flour	6	7.27	0.85		4.86	1.56		tr	
various, unfrosted	3	8.49	2.69		5.80				
cookies, various	8	5.45	2.57						
crackers from soft wheat flour	7	1.82	0.37	0.24	0.09	0.03	0.09	1.00	
cupcakes, chocolate	1	2.0	0.14						
doughnuts	10	4.05	0.72	tr	2.23	0.74		0.36	
pies—apple, blueberry, and lemon cream	6	7.29	1.59						

Table continued on the following page

Appendix Table 8. VITAMIN E CONTENT OF FOODS PER 1OO GM. EDIBLE
PORTION* (*Continued*)

FOOD AND DESCRIPTION	NUMBER OF SAMPLES	TOTAL VITAMIN E	TOCOPHEROLS				TOCOTRIENOLS		
			Alpha	*Beta*	*Gamma*	*Delta*	*Alpha*	*Beta*	*Gamma*
		←————————————— mg./100 gm. food ——————————————→							
PROCESSED, MIXED, AND MISCELLANEOUS FOODS (*Continued*)									
Baked products, concluded									
pie shell	1	0.87	0.49		0.38				
pretzel sticks	1	0.77	0.15						
rolls									
hamburger	10	0.53	0.04	0.01	0.26	0.11	0.11		
from white patent flour	25	6.65	0.78	tr	3.57	1.23	0.21	0.86	
dough before baking from white patent flour	25	5.43	0.66	tr	2.70	1.05	0.18	0.84	
Infant and baby foods									
infant formulas, normal dilution									
milk-fat based, unfortified	14	0.04	0.03	0	tr				
vitamin E-fortified	1	0.70	0.70	0	0				
non-milk fat based; made with soybean oil, unfortified	11	1.94	0.46	0	1.32	0.06			
soybean oil, vitamin E-fortified	4	2.20	0.55	0	1.33	0.32			
corn oil, unfortified	1	1.87	0.28		1.55	0.02			
corn, coconut, and olive oils, unfortified	2	1.49	0.20		1.27	0			
soybean, corn, and coconut oils, vitamin E-fortified	1	1.14	0.51		0.57	0.06			
coconut, corn, and soybean oils, vitamin E-fortified	1	1.38	0.44		0.87	0.06			
assorted fat-based	53	0.87 (range: 0.003—1.94)	0.32	0	0.51	0.03	tr	tr	
infant cereals									
barley	2	0.64	0.10		0.57				
high protein	2	1.36	0.27		0.13	0.12	0.32	0.08	
mixed	2	1.01	0.16		0.38	0	0.40	0.32	
oat flakes	1	2.72	0.90				1.39	0.05	
oatmeal	2	0.85	0.19		0.35				
rice	2	0.83	0.26						
baby foods, strained, breakfast, cereal with fruit or egg	8	0.39	0.25		0.08	0.04			
desserts	8	0.23	0.23		0	0			
fruits	14	0.68	0.58		0.06	0.04			
meats	14	0.42	0.39		0.02	0.01			

Appendix Table 8. VITAMIN E CONTENT OF FOODS PER 100 GM. EDIBLE
PORTION* (*Continued*)

FOOD AND DESCRIPTION	NUMBER OF SAMPLES	TOTAL VITAMIN E	TOCOPHEROLS				TOCOTRIENOLS		
			Alpha	*Beta*	*Gamma*	*Delta*	*Alpha*	*Beta*	*Gamma*
		←			*mg./100 gm. food*				→

PROCESSED, MIXED, AND
MISCELLANEOUS FOODS (*Continued*)
Infant and baby foods, concluded

dinners									
meat and vegetable mixtures	29	0.31	0.22	0.05	0.02				
egg yolk	3	1.66	0.60	0.59	0.47				
vegetables	40	0.73	0.45	0.22	0.06				

Mixed dishes*

canned convenience foods									
beans									
Lima, with ham	2	0.47	0	0.47	0				
refried	2	0.50	0	tr	0.50				
beef									
corned, hash	4	0.04	0.03	0.01	0				
Mexican	4	0.14	0.06	0.08	0				
sloppy Joe	2	0.27	0.13	0.14	0				
stew	4	0.38	0.15	0.19	0.04				
chicken with dumplings	2	0.10	tr	0.10	tr				
ravioli	2	0.48	0.16	0.26	0.06				
chow mein and meat	3	0.05	tr	tr	0.05				
frozen convenience foods									
beef and vegetables	19		0.56						
chicken and vegetables	17		0.38						
pasta and cheese or beef	5		0.16						
pork or ham and vegetables	2		0.43						
scallops, deep fried	1	6.4	0.6						
shrimp, deep fried	1	6.6	0.4						
home prepared foods									
beans									
baked	2	1.08	0.22	0.86	0				
Lima with ham	1	1.55	0.20	1.13	0.22				
beef and vegetable stew	10	0.55	0.21	0.17	0.17				
chicken and dumplings	1	1.27	0.08	0.98	0.20				
sandwiches									
beef	2	0.50	0.07	0.35	0.08				
beef and cheese	2	0.18	0.05	0.10	0.03				
egg salad	1	1.14	0.09	0.94	0.11				
ham									
plain	1	1.86	0.88	0.82	0.17				
salad	1	0.59	tr	0.47	0.12				
with cheese	2	0.65	0.04	0.50	0.11				

** Listed by type and main ingredients.

Table continued on the following page

Appendix Table 8.　VITAMIN E CONTENT OF FOODS PER 100 GM. EDIBLE PORTION* (*Continued*)

FOOD AND DESCRIPTION	NUMBER OF SAMPLES	TOTAL VITAMIN E	TOCOPHEROLS				TOCOTRIENOLS		
			Alpha	*Beta*	*Gamma*	*Delta*	*Alpha*	*Beta*	*Gamma*
		←———————————————*mg./100 gm. food*———————————————→							

PROCESSED, MIXED, AND MISCELLANEOUS FOODS (*Continued*)

Mixed dishes, concluded

FOOD AND DESCRIPTION	NUMBER OF SAMPLES	TOTAL VITAMIN E	*Alpha*	*Beta*	*Gamma*	*Delta*	*Alpha*	*Beta*	*Gamma*
pork, hot									
dog	1	0.14	0.14	tr	tr				
tuna salad	1	1.49	tr	1.27	0.22				
turkey	1	1.05	0.04	0.84	0.17				
Miscellaneous									
candy, toffee	1		0.17						
coffee, instant	1	0.48	0						
jam and jelly	2		0.09						
molasses, cane	4		0.41						
mustard, pre-									
pared	1	4.15	1.75						
pasta									
macaroni	2	0.27	0.02	0.02			0.02	0.21	
spaghetti	1	1.20							
peanut butter	2	20.0	7.0		11.0	0.5			
seaweed (dry)									
kelp (*Lami-*									
naria sp.)	3	0.87	0.87						
dulse (*Rho-*									
dymenia									
palmata)	1	3.5	3.5						
laver (*Por-*									
phyra um-									
bilicalis)	1	<1.0	<1.0						
yeast, baker's									
(*Saccharo-*									
myces sp.)									
dried or com-									
pressed	5		0.08						

Appendix Table 9.   CALCIUM AND PHOSPHORUS CONTENT OF FOODS

Food	Amount	Calcium, mg	Phosphorus, mg
Meat, fish, poultry			
Beef	1 oz	3	56
Pork	1 oz	3	70
Chicken	1 oz	4	74
Liver	1 oz	4	137
Fish, average	1 oz	12	76
Tuna	1/4 cup	2	95
Sardines, canned, with bones	1 oz	86	101
Salmon, canned, with bones	1 oz	74	98
Luncheon meat	1 oz	3	53
Bacon, strip	1–5 g	1	11
Meat substitutes			
Eggs	1	28	90
Dried beans, average, cooked	1/2 cup	44	144
Lentils, cooked	1/2 cup	25	119
Peanuts and peanut butter	1 tbsp	11	60
Milk	1 cup		
Whole milk		290	227
2% milk		297	232
Skim milk		302	247
Buttermilk		285	219
Chocolate milk		280	251
Hot cocoa		298	270
Other dairy products			
Yogurt, plain, low-fat	8 oz	415	326
Cheddar cheese	1 oz	204	145
Swiss cheese	1 oz	272	171
Processed American cheese	1 oz	174	211
Cottage cheese, creamed	1/4 cup	31	69
Half-and-half	2 tbsp	32	28
Vanilla ice cream	1/2 cup	88	67
Sherbet	1/2 cup	51	37
Cereal and grain products			
Bread, white	1 slice	21	24
Bread, whole wheat	1 slice	23	52
Bread products made from white flour			
Biscuit	2-in. diameter	42	61
Doughnut, cake	1 average	13	61
Doughnut, raised	1 average	11	23
Pancake	4-in. diameter	45	63
Sweet roll	1 average	35	57
Waffle	5-in. diameter	85	130
Cereal, refined	1/2 cup cooked; 3/4 cup dry	35	57
Cereal, whole grain	1/2 cup cooked; 3/4 cup dry	14	109
Crackers, saltines	5 2-in. squares	2	15
Crackers, graham	2 2 1/2 in. squares	6	21

Table continued on the following page

Appendix Table 9. CALCIUM AND PHOSPHORUS CONTENT OF FOODS *(Continued)*

Food	Amount	Calcium, mg	Phosphorus, mg
Cereal and grain products *(Continued)*			
Macaroni; spaghetti; noodles	1/2 cup cooked	8	47
Rice	1/2 cup cooked	7	21
Vegetables	100 g; about 1/2 cup cooked		
Artichokes		51	69
Asparagus		21	50
Bean sprouts		17	48
Broccoli		88	62
Brussels sprouts		32	72
Cabbage		44	20
Corn		4	48
Cress		61	48
Greens			
Beet greens		99	25
Collards		152	39
Dandelion greens		140	42
Kale		134	46
Mustard greens		183	50
Spinach		98	30
Swiss chard		73	24
Turnip greens		184	37
Leeks		52	50
Lima beans		47	121
Mushrooms		6	116
Okra		92	41
Parsnips		45	62
Peas		20	66
Potatoes, white		9	65
Rutabagas		59	31
Winter squash		28	48
Other vegetables, average		25	26
Fruit			
Blackberries	5/8 cup	32	19
Orange	1 small	41	20
Raspberries	2/3 cup	30	22
Rhubarb	3/8 cup	78	15
Tangerine	1 large	40	18
Fresh fruit, average	1/2 cup or 1 medium	16	20
Canned fruit, average	1/2 cup	10	12
Fruit juice	1/2 cup	10	13
Fats and oils			
Butter or margarine	1 tsp	1	1
Nondairy cream substitute, nondairy powder	1 tsp	Tr	8
French dressing	1 tbsp	2	2
Gravy	1 tbsp	...	2
Mayonnaise	1 tsp	1	1
Sweets			
Candy, sugar	1/2 oz	...	...
Candy, milk chocolate	1/2 oz	26	28
Honey	1 tbsp	4	3

Appendix Table 9.   CALCIUM AND PHOSPHORUS CONTENT OF FOODS (*Continued*)

Food	Amount	Calcium, mg	Phosphorus, mg
Sweets (*Continued*)			
Jelly	1 tbsp	2	2
Sugar, white	1 tbsp	. . .	. . .
Sugar, brown	1 tbsp	9	6
Syrup, maple	1 tbsp	33	3
Desserts			
Assorted cookies	1 2-in.	7	32
Cake, white	2 in. by 3 in. by 2 in.	34	46
Pie, cream	1/8 of 9-in. pie	62	88
Pie, fruit	1/8 of 9-in. pie	23	30
Snack foods			
Popcorn	1 cup	2	39
Potato chips	5	3	15
Beverages			
Beer	8 oz	10	62
Carbonated beverages			
Colas, average	8 oz	7	42
Ginger ale, average	8 oz	3	. . .
Coffee	6 oz	5	5
Tea	6 oz	5	4

From Mayo Clinic Diet Manual. A Handbook of Dietary Practices. 5th ed. Philadelphia, W.B. Saunders Company, 1981.

SELECTED BIBLIOGRAPHY

Adams, C. F.: Nutritive Value of American Foods in Common Units. Agriculture Handbook No. 456. Washington, D. C., United States Department of Agriculture, 1975.

Church, C. F., and Church, H. N. (Editors): Bowes and Church's Food Values of Portions Commonly Used. Twelfth edition. Philadelphia, J. B. Lippincott Company, 1975.

United States Agriculture Research Service, Consumer Food Economics Institute: Composition of Foods: Dairy and Egg Products; Raw, Processed, Prepared. Agriculture Handbook No. 8-1. Washington, D. C., United States Department of Agriculture, 1976.

Appendix Table 10. SODIUM AND POTASSIUM CONTENT OF FOODS

Food	Approximate amount	Weight gm	Sodium mEq	Potassium mEq
Meat				
Meat (cooked)				
Beef	1 ounce	30	0.8	2.8
Ham	1 ounce	30	14.3	2.6
Lamb	1 ounce	30	0.9	2.2
Pork	1 ounce	30	0.9	3.0
Veal	1 ounce	30	1.0	3.8
Liver	1 ounce	30	2.4	3.2
Sausage, pork	2 links	40	16.5	2.8
Beef, dried	2 slices	20	37.0	1.0
Cold cuts	1 slice	45	25.0	2.7
Frankfurters	1	50	24.0	3.0
Fowl				
Chicken	1 ounce	30	1.0	3.0
Goose	1 ounce	30	1.6	4.6
Duck	1 ounce	30	1.0	2.2
Turkey	1 ounce	30	1.2	2.8
Egg	1	50	2.7	1.8
Fish	1 ounce	30	1.0	2.5
Salmon				
Fresh	1/4 cup	30	0.6	2.3
Canned	1/4 cup	30	4.6	2.6
Tuna				
Fresh	1/4 cup	30	0.5	2.2
Canned	1/4 cup	30	10.4	2.3
Sardines	3 medium	35	12.5	4.5
Shellfish				
Clams	5 small	50	2.6	2.3
Lobster	1 small tail	40	3.7	1.8
Oysters	5 small	70	2.1	1.5
Scallops	1 large	50	5.7	6.0
Shrimp	5 small	30	1.8	1.7
Cheese				
Cheese, American or Cheddar type	1 slice	30	9.1	0.6
Cheese foods	1 slice	30	15.0	0.8
Cheese spreads	2 tablespoons	30	15.0	0.8
Cottage cheese	1/4 cup	50	5.0	1.1
Peanut butter	2 tablespoons	30	7.8	5.0
Peanuts, unsalted	25	25	...	4.5
Fat				
Avocado	1/8	30	...	4.6
Bacon	1 slice	5	2.2	0.6
Butter or magarine	1 teaspoon	5	2.2	...
Cooking fat	1 teaspoon	5	...	...
Cream				
Half and half	2 tablespoons	30	0.6	1.0
Sour	2 tablespoons	30	0.4	...
Whipped	1 tablespoon	15	0.3	1.0
Cream cheese	1 tablespoon	15	1.7	...
Mayonnaise	1 teaspoon	5	1.3	...

From Mayo Clinic Diet Manual, 5th ed. Philadelphia, W.B. Saunders Co., 1981.

Appendix Table 10.   SODIUM AND POTASSIUM CONTENT OF FOODS (*Continued*)

Food	Approximate amount	Weight gm	Sodium mEq	Potassium mEq
Fat (*Continued*)				
Nuts				
Almonds, slivered	5 (2 teaspoons)	6	...	0.8
Pecans	4 halves	5	...	0.8
Walnuts	5 halves	10	...	1.0
Oil, salad	1 teaspoon	5	...	...
Olives, green	3 medium	30	31.3	0.4
Bread				
Bread	1 slice	25	5.5	0.7
Biscuit	1 (2″ diameter)	35	9.6	0.7
Muffin	1 (2″ diameter)	35	7.3	1.2
Cornbread	1 (1 1/2″ cube)	35	11.3	1.7
Roll	1 (2″ diameter)	25	5.5	0.6
Bun	1	30	6.6	0.7
Pancake	1 (4″ diameter)	45	8.8	1.1
Waffle	1/2 square	35	8.5	1.0
Cereals				
Cooked	2/3 cup	140	8.7	2.0
Dry, flake	2/3 cup	20	8.7	0.6
Dry, puffed	1 1/2 cups	20	...	1.5
Shredded wheat	1 biscuit	20	...	2.2
Crackers				
Graham	3	20	5.8	2.0
Melba toast	4	20	5.5	0.7
Oyster	20	20	9.6	0.6
Ritz	6	20	9.5	0.5
Rye-Krisp	3	30	11.5	3.0
Saltines	6	20	9.6	0.6
Soda	3	20	9.6	0.6
Dessert				
Commercial gelatin	1/2 cup	100	2.2	...
Ice cream	1/2 cup	75	2.0	3.0
Sherbet	1/3 cup	50	...	...
Angel food cake	1 1/2″ × 1 1/2″	25	3.0	0.6
Sponge cake	1 1/2″ × 1 1/2″	25	1.8	0.6
Vanilla wafers	5	15	1.7	...
Flour products*				
Cornstarch	2 tablespoons	15	...	...
Macaroni	1/4 cup	50	...	0.8
Noodles	1/4 cup	50	...	0.6
Rice	1/4 cup	50	...	0.9
Spaghetti	1/4 cup	50	...	0.8
Tapioca	2 tablespoons	15	...	...
Vegetable*				
Beans, dried (cooked)	1/2 cup	90	...	10.0
Beans, lima	1/2 cup	90	...	9.5
Corn				
Canned†	1/3 cup	80	8.0	2.0
Fresh	1/2 ear	100	...	2.0
Frozen	1/3 cup	80	...	3.7
Hominy (dry)	1/4 cup	36	4.1	...

Table continued on the following page

Appendix Table 10.   SODIUM AND POTASSIUM CONTENT OF FOODS (*Continued*)

Food	Approximate amount	Weight *gm*	Sodium *mEq*	Potassium *mEq*
Vegetable (*Continued*)				
Parsnips	2/3 cup	100	0.3	9.7
Peas				
Canned[†]	1/2 cup	100	10.0	1.2
Dried	1/2 cup	90	1.5	6.8
Fresh	1/2 cup	100	…	2.5
Frozen	1/2 cup	100	2.5	1.7
Popcorn	1 cup	15	…	…
Potato				
Potato chips	1 oz	30	13.0	3.7
White, baked	1/2 cup	100	…	13.0
White, boiled	1/2 cup	100	…	7.3
Sweet, baked	1/4 cup	50	0.4	4.0
Milk				
Whole milk	1 cup	240	5.2	8.8
Evaporated whole milk	1/2 cup	120	6.0	9.2
Powdered whole milk	1/4 cup	30	5.2	10.0
Buttermilk	1 cup	240	13.6	8.5
Skim milk	1 cup	240	5.2	8.8
Powdered skim milk	1/4 cup	30	6.9	13.5
Vegetable A[*]				
Asparagus				
Cooked	1/2 cup	100	…	4.7
Canned[†]	1/2 cup	100	10.0	3.6
Frozen	1/2 cup	100	…	5.5
Bean sprouts	1/2 cup	100	…	4.0
Beans, green or wax				
Fresh or frozen	1/2 cup	100	…	4.0
Canned[†]	1/2 cup	100	10.0	2.5
Beet greens	1/2 cup	100	3.0	8.5
Broccoli	1/2 cup	100	…	7.0
Cabbage, cooked	1/2 cup	100	0.6	4.2
Raw	1 cup	100	0.9	6.0
Cauliflower, cooked	1 cup	100	0.4	5.2
Celery, raw	1 cup	100	5.4	9.0
Chard, Swiss	3/5 cup	100	3.7	8.0
Collards	1/2 cup	100	0.8	6.0
Cress, garden (cooked)	1/2 cup	100	0.5	7.2
Cucumber	1 medium	100	0.3	4.0
Eggplant	1/2 cup	100	…	3.8
Lettuce	Varies	100	0.4	4.5
Mushrooms, raw	4 large	100	0.7	10.6
Mustard greens	1/2 cup	100	0.8	5.5
Pepper, green or red				
Cooked	1/2 cup	100	…	5.5
Raw	1	100	0.5	4.0
Radishes	10	100	0.8	8.0
Sauerkraut	2/3 cup	100	32.0	3.5
Spinach	1/2 cup	100	2.2	8.5
Squash	1/2 cup	100	…	3.5

Appendix Table 10. SODIUM AND POTASSIUM CONTENT OF FOODS (*Continued*)

Food	Approximate amount	Weight gm	Sodium mEq	Potassium mEq
Vegetable A (*Continued*)				
Tomatoes	1/2 cup	100	...	6.5
Tomato juice†	1/2 cup	100	9.0	5.8
Turnip greens	1/2 cup	100	0.7	3.8
Turnips	1/2 cup	100	1.5	4.8
Vegetable B*				
Artichokes	1 large bud	100	1.3	7.7
Beets	1/2 cup	100	1.8	5.0
Brussels sprouts	2/3 cup	100	...	7.6
Carrots, cooked	1/2 cup	100	1.4	5.7
Raw	1 large	100	2.0	8.8
Dandelion greens	1/2 cup	100	2.0	6.0
Kale, cooked	3/4 cup	100	2.0	5.6
Frozen	1/2 cup	100	1.0	5.0
Kohlrabi	2/3 cup	100	...	6.6
Leeks, raw	3–4	100	...	9.0
Okra	1/2 cup	100	...	4.4
Onions, cooked	1/2 cup	100	...	2.8
Pumpkin	1/2 cup	100	...	6.3
Rutabagas	1/2 cup	100	...	4.4
Squash, winter				
Baked	1/2 cup	100	...	12.0
Boiled	1/2 cup	100	...	6.5
Fruit				
Apple				
Fresh	1 small	80	...	2.3
Sauce	1/2 cup	120	...	2.5
Juice	1/2 cup	120	...	3.1
Apricots				
Canned	1/2 cup	120	...	6.0
Dried	4 halves	20	...	5.0
Fresh	3 small	120	...	8.0
Nectar	1/3 cup	80	...	3.0
Banana	1/2 small	60	...	4.8
Berries, fresh				
Blackberries	3/4 cup	100	...	3.0
Blueberries	1/2 cup	80	...	1.5
Boysenberries	1 cup	120	...	3.2
Gooseberries	3/4 cup	120	...	4.0
Loganberries	3/4 cup	100	...	4.4
Raspberries	3/4 cup	100	...	4.5
Strawberries	1 cup	150	...	6.3
Cherries				
Canned	1/2 cup	120	...	4.0
Fresh	15 small	80	...	2.7
Dates				
Pitted	2	15	...	2.5
Figs				
Canned	1/2 cup	120	...	4.6
Dried	1 small	15	...	2.5
Fresh	1 large	60	...	3.0

Table continued on the following page

Appendix Table 10.   SODIUM AND POTASSIUM CONTENT OF FOODS (*Continued*)

Food	Approximate amount	Weight gm	Sodium mEq	Potassium mEq
Fruit (*Continued*)				
Fruit cocktail	1/2 cup	120	...	5.0
Grapes				
Canned	1/3 cup	80	...	2.2
Fresh	15	80	...	3.2
Juice				
Bottled	1/4 cup	60	...	2.8
Frozen	1/3 cup	80	...	2.4
Grapefruit				
Fresh	1/2 medium	120	...	3.6
Juice	1/2 cup	120	...	4.1
Sections	3/4 cup	150	...	5.1
Mandarin orange	3/4 cup	200	...	6.5
Mango	1/2 small	70	...	3.4
Melon				
Cantaloupe	1/2 small	200	...	13.0
Honeydew	1/4 medium	200	...	13.0
Watermelon	1/2 slice	200	...	5.0
Nectarine	1 medium	80	...	6.0
Orange				
Fresh	1 medium	100	...	5.1
Juice	1/2 cup	120		5.7
Sections	1/2 cup	100	...	5.1
Papaya	1/2 cup	120	...	7.0
Peach				
Canned	1/2 cup	120	...	4.0
Dried	2 halves	20	...	5.0
Fresh	1 medium	120	...	6.2
Nectar	1/2 cup	120	...	2.4
Pear				
Canned	1/2 cup	120	...	2.5
Dried	2 halves	20	...	3.0
Fresh	1 small	80	...	2.6
Nectar	1/3 cup	80	...	0.9
Pineapple				
Canned	1/2 cup	120	...	3.0
Fresh	1/2 cup	80	...	3.0
Juice	1/3 cup	80		3.0
Plums				
Canned	1/2 cup	120	...	4.5
Fresh	2 medium	80	...	4.1
Prunes	2 medium	15	...	2.6
Juice	1/4 cup	60	...	3.6
Raisins	1 tablespoon	15	...	2.9
Rhubarb	1/2 cup	100	...	6.5
Tangerines				
Fresh	2 small	100	...	3.2
Juice	1/2 cup	120	...	5.5
Sections	1/2 cup	100	...	3.2

*Value for products without added salt.
†Estimated average based on addition of salt, approximately 0.6% of the finished product.

Appendix Table 11.   FOODS HIGH IN IRON*

FOOD	AVERAGE SERVING		IRON, MG.	
	Weight Gm.	Approximate Measure	Per Serving	Per 100 Gm.
Almonds	15	12–15	0.7	4.4
Apricots, dried	30	5 halves	1.5	4.9
Bacon, cooked	25	4–5 slices	0.8	3.3
Beans, dried	30 (dry)	½ cup (cooked)	2.1	6.9
Lima, dried	30 (dry)	½ cup (cooked)	2.3	7.5
Beef, rib roast, cooked	60	2 ounces	1.8	3.0
Corned, medium fat	60	2 ounces	2.6	4.3
Dried	30	1 ounce	1.5	5.1
Beet greens, cooked	75	½ cup	2.4	3.2
Bologna	30	1 slice	0.7	2.2
Bran flakes, 40 per cent	15	½ cup	0.8	5.1
Brazil nuts	15	2 medium	0.5	3.4
Breaded, whole wheat	25	1 slice	0.6	2.2
Cashews	15	6–8	0.8	5.0
Chard	75	½ cup	1.9	2.5
Chocolate, bitter	30	1 square	1.3	4.4
Sweetened, plain	30	1 square	0.8	2.8
Clams	60	2 ounces	4.2	7.0
Cocoa	7	1 tablespoon	0.8	11.6
Coconut, fresh	15	½ ounce	0.3	2.0
Dried	15	2 tablespoons	0.5	3.6
Cornmeal, degermed, enriched	15 (dry)	½ cup (cooked)	0.4	2.9
Cress, garden	10	5–8 sprigs	0.3	2.9
Currants, dried	30	2 tablespoons	0.8	2.7
Dandelion greens	75	½ cup	2.3	3.1
Dates	30	3–4	0.6	2.1
Egg, whole	50	1	1.4	2.7
Yolk	20	1	1.4	7.2
Figs, dried	30	2 small	0.9	3.0
Flour, all-purpose, enriched	15	2 tablespoons	0.4	2.9
Flour, whole wheat	15	2 tablespoons	0.5	3.3
Ham, smoked	60	2 ounces	1.7	2.9
Hazelnuts	15	10–12	0.6	4.1
Heart, beef	60	2 ounces	2.8	4.6
Kale	75	¾ cup	1.7	2.2
Kidney, beef	60	2 ounces	4.7	7.9
Lamb, leg	60	2 ounces	1.9	3.1
Lentils, dry	30 (dry)	½ cup (cooked)	2.2	7.4
Liver, beef	60	2 ounces	4.7	7.8
Liver sausage	30	1 slice	1.6	5.4
Molasses, light	20	1 tablespoon	0.9	4.3
Oatmeal	15 (dry)	½ cup (cooked)	0.7	4.5
Oysters, raw	60	2 ounces	3.4	5.6
Parsley	10	10 small sprigs	0.4	4.3
Peaches, dried	30	3 halves	1.9	6.9
Peas, dry	30 (dry)	½ cup (cooked)	1.4	4.7
Pecans	15	12 halves	0.4	2.4
Popcorn	15	1 cup, popped	0.4	2.7
Pork loin, cooked	60	2 ounces	1.8	3.0
Pork sausage	60	2 ounces	1.4	2.3
Prunes, dried	30	4 prunes	1.2	3.9
Raisins, dried	50	5 tablespoons	1.7	3.3
Rice, brown	15 (dry)	½ cup (cooked)	0.3	2.0
Rye, whole meal	15	1 tablespoon	0.6	3.7
Sardines	60	2 ounces	1.6	2.7
Shrimp, canned	60	2 ounces	1.9	3.1

*From Mayo Clinic Diet Manual. 3rd Ed. Philadelphia, W. B. Saunders Company, 1961, pp. 188–189.

Table continued on the following page

Appendix Table 11. FOODS HIGH IN IRON (*Continued*)

FOOD	AVERAGE SERVING		IRON, MG.	
	Weight Gm.	*Approximate Measure*	*Per Serving*	*Per 100 Gm.*
Syrup, table blends	20	1 tablespoon	0.8	4.1
Soybeans, dried	25	2 tablespoons	2.0	8.0
Flour, medium fat	15	3 tablespoons	2.0	13.0
Spinach, cooked	75	½ cup	1.5	2.0
Sugar, brown	15	1 tablespoon	0.4	2.6
Tongue, beef	60	2 ounces	1.7	2.8
Turkey	60	2 ounces	2.3	3.8
Turnip greens	75	½ cup	1.8	2.4
Veal roast, cooked	60	2 ounces	2.2	3.6
Walnuts	15	8 to 15 halves	0.3	2.1
Wheat flakes	15	½ cup	0.5	3.0
Shredded, plain	30	1 biscuit	1.1	3.5
Whole meal	15	½ cup (cooked)	0.5	3.4
Yeast, compressed	30	1 ounce	1.5	4.9
Dried brewer's	15	2 tablespoons	2.7	18.2

Appendix Table 12. ZINC CONTENT OF FOODS PER 100 GM. EDIBLE PORTION

FOOD AND DESCRIPTION	ZINC	FOOD AND DESCRIPTION	ZINC
	mg.		*mg.*
apples, raw	0.05*	chicken, broiler-fryer, continued	
applesauce, unsweetened	0.1	cooked, dry heat	1.2
bananas, raw	0.2	chickpeas or garbanzos, mature	
beans, common, mature, dry		seeds, dry	
raw	2.8	raw	2.7
boiled, drained	1.0	boiled, drained	1.4
beans, Lima, mature, dry		chocolate sirup	0.9
raw	2.8	clams	
boiled, drained	0.9	soft shell	
beans, snap, green		raw	1.5
raw	0.4	cooked	1.7
boiled, drained	0.3	hard shell	
canned, solids and liquid	0.2	raw	1.5
canned, drained solids	0.3	cooked	1.7
beef, separable lean		surf, canned, solids and liquid	1.2
raw	4.2	cocoa, dry powder	5.6
cooked, dry heat	5.8	coffee	
cooked, moist heat	6.2	dry, instant	0.6
beef, separable fat, raw	0.5	fluid beverage	0.03
beef, ground (77% lean)		cookies, vanilla wafers	0.3
raw	3.4	cooking oil, see oils	
cooked	4.4	corn, field, whole-grain, yellow,	
beverages, carbonated,		or white	2.1
nonalcoholic		corn, sweet, yellow	
bottled	<0.01	raw	0.5
canned	0.08	boiled, drained	0.4
bran, see wheat		corn, canned, whole kernel, yellow	
breads		brine pack, solids and liquid	0.3
rye	1.6	brine pack, drained solids	0.4
white	0.6	vacuum pack, solids and liquid	0.4
whole wheat	1.8	corn chips	1.5
butter	0.1	corn grits, white, degermed,	
cabbage, common		dry form	0.4
raw	0.4	corn flakes	0.3
boiled, drained	0.4	cornmeal, white or yellow	
cake, white, without icing	0.2	bolted (nearly whole grain)	1.8
carrots		degermed	
raw	0.4	dry form	0.8
cooked or canned, drained solids	0.3	cooked	0.1
cheese, Cheddar type	4.0	cornstarch	0.03
chicken, broiler-fryer		cowpeas (blackeye), mature, dry	
breast, meat only		raw	2.9
raw	0.7	boiled, drained	1.2
cooked, dry heat	0.9	crabs, blue and Dungeness	
breast		raw	4.0
raw (81% meat, 12% skin,		steamed	4.3
7% fat)	0.7	crackers	
cooked, dry heat (89% meat,		Graham	1.1
11% skin)	0.9	saltines	0.5
drumstick, thigh, back, meat only		doughnuts, cake-type	0.5
raw	1.8	eggs, fresh	
cooked, dry heat	2.8	whites	0.02
drumstick		yolks	3.0
raw (85% meat, 13% skin,		whole	1.0
2% fat)	1.7	farina, regular	
cooked, dry heat (84% meat,		dry form	0.5
16% skin)	2.5	cooked	0.06
wing, meat only		fish, white varieties, flesh only	
raw	1.6	raw	0.7
cooked, dry heat	2.4	cooked, fillet	1.0
neck, meat only		cooked, steak	0.8
raw	2.7	gizzard	
cooked, moist heat	3.0	chicken	
skin		raw	2.9
raw	1.0	cooked, drained	4.3

*Data given to two decimal places if food contained less than 0.1 mg. zinc.

From Murphy, E.W., Willis, B.W., and Watt, B.K.: Provisional tables on the zinc content of foods. J. Am. Diet. Assoc., 66:345, 1975.

Table continued on the following page

Appendix Table 12. ZINC CONTENT OF FOODS PER 100 GM. EDIBLE PORTION (*Continued*)

FOOD AND DESCRIPTION	ZINC	FOOD AND DESCRIPTION	ZINC
	mg.		*mg.*
gizzard, continued		peas, green, immature	
turkey		raw	0.9
raw	2.8	boiled, drained	0.7
cooked, drained	4.1	canned, drained solids	0.8
granola	2.1	peas, green mature seeds, dry	
heart		raw	3.2
chicken		boiled, drained	1.1
raw	2.9	popcorn	
cooked, drained	4.8	unpopped	3.9
turkey		popped	
raw	2.8	plain	4.1
cooked, drained	4.8	oil and salt added	3.0
ice cream	0.5	pork	
lamb, separable lean		trimmed lean cuts, separable lean	
raw	3.0	raw	2.7
cooked, dry heat	4.3	cooked	3.8
cooked, moist heat	5.0	Boston butt, separable lean	
separable fat, raw	0.5	raw	3.2
lard	0.2	cooked	4.5
lentils, mature, dry		ham or picnic, separable lean	
raw	3.1	raw	2.8
boiled, drained	1.0	cooked	4.0
lettuce, head or leaf	0.4	loin, separable lean	
liver		raw	2.2
beef		cooked	3.1
raw	3.8	separable fat, raw	0.5
cooked	5.1	potatoes	
calf		raw	0.3
raw	3.8	boiled, drained	0.3
cooked	6.1	rice	
chicken		brown	
raw	2.4	dry form	1.8
cooked	3.4	cooked	0.6
turkey		white, regular	
raw	2.7	dry form	1.3
cooked	3.4	cooked	0.4
lobster, crayfish		white, parboiled	
raw	1.8	dry form	1.1
cooked or canned	2.2	cooked	0.3
macaroni		white, precooked quick	
dry form	1.5	dry form	0.7
cooked, tender stage	0.5	cooked	0.2
margarine	0.2	cereal, ready-to-eat, Puffed,	
milk		or flakes	1.4
fluid, whole or skim	0.4	rolls, hamburger	0.6
canned, evaporated	0.8	salad dressing	0.2
dry, nonfat	4.5	salmon, canned, (77% solids, 23%	
oatmeal or rolled oats		liquid)	0.9
dry form	3.4	sausages and cold cuts	
cooked	0.5	bologna, beef	1.8
oat cereal, puffed, ready-to-eat	3.0	Braunschweiger	2.8
oil, salad or cooking	0.2	frankfurters	
onions, mature or green, raw	0.3	made with beef	2.0
oranges, raw	0.2	made with beef and pork	1.6
orange juice		shrimp	
canned, unsweetened	0.07	raw	1.5
fresh or frozen	0.02	boiled, peeled, deveined	2.1
oysters, raw or frozen		canned, drained solids	2.1
Atlantic	74.7	spinach	
Pacific	9.0	raw	0.8
peaches		boiled, drained	0.7
raw	0.2	canned	
canned, drained slices	0.1	solids and liquid	0.6
peanuts		drained solids	0.8
raw	2.9	sugar, white, granulated	0.06
roasted	3.0	tea	
peanut butter	2.9	dry leaves	3.3

Appendix Table 12.   ZINC CONTENT OF FOODS PER 100 GM. EDIBLE PORTION (*Continued*)

FOOD AND DESCRIPTION	ZINC	FOOD AND DESCRIPTION	ZINC
	mg.		*mg.*
tea, continued		veal (continued)	
fluid beverage	0.02	cooked, moist heat	4.2
tomatoes, ripe		separable fat, raw	0.5
raw	0.2	wheat, whole grain	
boiled, solids and liquid	0.2	hard	3.4
canned, solids and liquid	0.2	soft	2.7
tuna fish, canned in oil		white	2.2
85% solids, 15% oil	1.0	durum	2.7
drained solids	1.1	wheat flours	
turkey		whole	2.4
light meat		80% extraction	1.5
raw	1.6	all-purpose	0.7
cooked, dry heat	2.1	bread flour	0.8
dark meat		cake or pastry flour	0.3
raw	3.1	wheat bran, crude	9.8
cooked, dry heat	4.4	wheat germ, crude	14.3
neck meat		wheat cereal, whole-meal (see	
raw	5.0	also farina)	
cooked	6.4	dry form	3.6
skin		cooked	0.5
raw	1.3	wheat cereals, ready-to-eat	
cooked	2.1	bran flakes, 40%	3.6
veal		flakes	2.3
separable lean		germ, toasted	15.4
raw	2.8	Puffed	2.6
cooked, dry heat	4.1	Shredded	2.8

Appendix Table 13.   OXALATE CONTENT OF FOODS PER 100 GM. EDIBLE PORTION

FOOD	OXALATE mg.	FOOD	OXALATE mg.
Cereal and Cereal Products		*Vegetables, continued*	
Bread, white	4.9	Pokeweed	476.0
Cake, fruit	11.8	Potatoes, white boiled	0.0
Cake, sponge	7.4	Potatoes, sweet	56.0
Cornflakes	2.0	Radishes	0.3
Crackers, soybean	207.0	Rice, boiled	0.0
Egg noodle (chow mein)	1.0	Rutabagas	19.0
Grits (white corn)	41.0	Spinach, boiled	750.0
Macaroni, boiled	1.0	Spinach, frozen	600.0
Oatmeal, porridge	1.0	Squash, summer	22.0
Spaghetti, boiled	1.5	Tomatoes, raw	2.0
Spaghetti in tomato sauce	4.0	Turnips, boiled	1.0
Wheat germ	269.0	Watercress, early fine curled	10.0
Milk and Milk Products		*Fruits*	
Butter	0.0	Apples, raw	3.0
Cheese, cheddar	0.0	Apricots	2.8
Margarine	0.0	Avocado	0.0
Milk	0.15	Banana, raw	trace
Meats and Eggs		Berries:	
Bacon, streaky fried	3.3	Black	18.0
Beef, canned corned	0.0	Blue	15.0
Beef, topside roast	0.0	Dew	14.0
Chicken, roast	0.0	Green goose	88.0
Eggs, boiled	0.0	Raspberries, black	53.0
Fish:		Raspberries, red	15.0
Haddock	0.2	Strawberries, canned	15.0
Plaice	0.3	Strawberries, raw	10.0
Sardines	4.8	Cherries:	
Ham	1.6	Bing	0.0
Hamburger, grilled	0.0	Sour	1.1
Lamb, roast	trace	Currants:	
Liver	7.1	Black	4.3
Pork, roast	1.7	Red	19.0
Vegetables		Fruit salad, canned	12.0
Asparagus	5.2	Grapes:	
Beans, green boiled	15.0	Concord	25.0
Beans in tomato sauce	19.0	Thompson seedless	0.0
Beetroot, boiled	675.0	Lemon peel	83.0
Beetroot, pickled	500.0	Lime peel	110.0
Broccoli, boiled	trace	Mangoes	0.0
Brussels sprouts, boiled	0.0	Melons:	
Cabbage, boiled	0.0	Cantaloupe	0.0
Carrots, canned	4.0	Casaba	0.0
Cauliflower, boiled	1.0	Honeydew	0.0
Celery	20.0	Watermelon	0.0
Chard, Swiss	645.00	Nectarines	0.0
Chive	1.1	Orange, raw	4.0
Collards	74.0	Peaches:	
Corn, yellow	5.2	Alberta	5.0
Cucumber, raw	1.0	canned	1.2
Dandelion greens	24.6	Hiley	0.0
Eggplant	18.0	Stokes	1.2
Escarole	31.0	Pears:	3.0
Kale	13.0	Bartlett, canned	1.7
Leek	89.0	Pineapple, canned	1.0
Lettuce	3.0	Plums:	
Lima beans	4.3	Damson	10.0
Mushrooms	2.0	Golden gage	1.1
Mustard greens	7.7	Green gage	0.0
Okra	146.0	Preserves:	
Onion, boiled	3.0	Red plum jam	0.5
Parsley, raw	100.0	Strawberry jam	9.4
Parsnips	10.0	Prunes, Italian	5.8
Peas, canned	1.0	Rhubarb:	
Pepper, green	16.0	canned	600.0
		stewed, no sugar	860.0

Appendix Table 13. OXALATE CONTENT OF FOODS PER 100 GM. EDIBLE PORTION (*Continued*)

FOOD	OXALATE mg.	FOOD	OXALATE mg.
Nuts		*Juices continued*	
Peanuts, roasted	187.0	Grapefruit juice	0.0
Pecans	202.0	Orange juice	0.5
		Pineapple juice	0.0
Confectionery		Tomato juice	5.0
Chocolate, plain	117.0		
Jelly, with allowed fruit	0.0	*Beverages, alcoholic*	
Marmalade	10.8	Beer:	
Sweets, boiled (plain candies)	0.0	bottled	0.0
		draft	1.0
Beverages, Non-alcoholic		Lager draft, Tuborg Pilsner	4.0
Barley water, bottled	0.0	Stout, Guiness Draft	2.0
Coca-Cola	trace	Cider	0.0
Coffee (0.5 g Nescafe/100 ml)	3.2	Sherry, dry	trace
Lemon Squash drink (lemonade)	1.0	Wine:	
Lucozade, bottled (soda)	0.0	Port	trace
Orange squash drink (orangeade)	2.5	Rose	1.5
Ovaltine drink, 2 gm in 100 ml	10.0	White	0.0
Pepsi-Cola	trace		
Ribena, concentrate	2.0	*Miscellaneous*	
(black currant drink)		Cocoa, dry powder	623.0
Tea, Indian:		Coffee powder (Nescafe)	33.0
2 min. infusion	55.0	Chicken noodle soup	1.0
4 min. infusion	72.0	Lemon juice	1.0
6 min. infusion	78.0	Lime juice	0.0
Tea, rosehip	4.0	Ovaltine, powder canned	35.0
		Oxtail soup	1.0
Juices		Pepper	419.0
Apple juice	trace	Tomato soup	3.0
Cranberry juice	6.6	Vegetable soup	5.0
Grape juice	5.8		

Adapted from: Ney, D. M., et al.: The low oxalate diet book for the prevention of oxalate kidney stones, San Diego, University of California, 1981, pp. 19–23.

Appendix Table 14. EXCESS OF ACIDITY OR ALKALINITY IN FOODS*

NEUTRAL FOODS

Butter	Lard	Sugar, white
Candy, plain	Oil, olive and salad	Tapioca
Coffee	Postum	Tea
Cornstarch		

FOODS WITH ACID ASH

| POOD | SIZE OF SERVING | | NORMAL ACID, CC. | |
	Weight Gm.	Approximate Measure	Per Serving	Per 100 Gm.
Bread				
White	25	1 slice	1.2	4.8
Whole Wheat	25	1 slice	1.5	6.1
Rye	25	1 slice	1.3	5.2
Cake, plain	75	1 piece	1.7	2.3
Cereal				
Cornflakes	15	½ cup	0.3	2.1
Farina	15 (dry)	½ cup (cooked)	1.4	9.6
Macaroni	15 (dry)	½ cup (cooked)	1.8	12.0
Oatmeal	15 (dry)	½ cup (cooked)	2.0	13.1
Puffed wheat	15	1 cup	1.6	10.8
Puffed rice	15	1 cup	1.4	9.0
Rice	15 (dry)	½ cup (cooked)	1.2	7.8
Shredded wheat	15	½ biscuit	1.8	12.2
Fat, mayonnaise	15	1 tablespoon	0.3	2.3
Fruit				
Cranberries	100	½ cup	+	+
Plums	100	½ cup	+	+
Prunes	100	½ cup	+	+
Meat				
Bacon	30	5 strips	5.9	19.6
Beef, roast	60	2 ounces	10.6	17.7
Cheese, Cheddar	30	1 ounce	1.7	5.5
Cheese, cottage	70	2 heaping tablespoons	3.2	4.5
Chicken	60	2 ounces	10.7	17.8
Eggs	50	1	7.7	15.4
Fish, halibut	60	2 ounces	12.4	20.7
Ham	60	2 ounces	9.1	15.2
Lamb	60	2 ounces	11.1	18.5
Pork	60	2 ounces	9.8	16.3
Veal	60	2 ounces	11.3	18.8
Nuts				
Brazil nuts	15	2 medium	1.7	11.0
Peanut butter	15	1 tablespoon	0.7	4.7
Peanuts	15	16–17 nuts	0.9	6.0
Walnuts, English	15	4–8 nuts	1.3	8.4
Vegetables				
Corn	100	½ cup	3.6	3.6
Lentils, dried	30	½ cup (cooked)	1.8	6.0
Cream	75	⅓ cup	0.8	1.0
Fruit				
Apple	100	1 small	3.8	3.8
Apricots, raw	100	2–3	6.8	6.8
Apricots, dried	30	4–6 halves	10.9	36.3
Banana	100	1 small	7.9	7.9
Blackberries, raw	100	⅝ cup	5.0	5.0
Blueberries, raw	100	⅝ cup	2.7	2.7
Cantaloupe	150	½ melon	9.0	6.0
Cherries, fresh	100	15 large	7.0	7.0
Currants, fresh	100	¾ cup	7.5	7.5
Dates, dried	30	3–4	2.9	9.7
Figs, dried	30	2 small	10.8	36.0
Gooseberries	100	⅔ cup	4.1	4.1
Grapefruit	100	½ medium	6.0	6.0
Grapes	100	1 bunch	6.0	6.0
Lemon	30	1 ounce	1.2	4.0
Lime	30	1 ounce	1.2	4.0

*From Mayo Clinic Diet Manual. 3rd ed. Philadelphia, W. B. Saunders Company, 1961, pp. 182–184.

Appendix Table 14. EXCESS OF ACIDITY OR ALKALINITY IN FOODS (*Continued*)

FOODS WITH ALKALINE ASH

Fruit (continued)				
Loganberries	100	⅔ cup	5.0	5.0
Mango	100	1 small	5.0	5.0
Nectarines	100	2 small	6.2	6.2
Olives, green. and ripe	30	3 medium	6.5	21.5
Orange	100	1 small	5.0	5.0
Peach, raw	100	1 medium	7.0	7.0
Pear, raw	100	1 medium	3.3	3.3
Persimmon	100	1 medium	7.5	7.5
Pineapple, raw	100	½ cup	6.5	6.5
Pineapple juice	200	1 cup, scant	6.0	3.0
Raisins	30	3 tablespoons	4.5	15.0
Raspberries, black and red	100	¾ cup	6.0	6.0
Strawberries	100	10 large	3.5	3.5
Tangerine	100	1 large	5.5	5.5
Watermelon	600	1 slice	22 8	3.8
Ice cream	70	⅓ cup	0.5	0.7
Jam	20	1 rounded teaspoon	0.7	3.3
Milk	240	½ pint	4.8	2.0
Nuts				
Almonds	15	12–15 nuts	1.8	12.0
Chestnuts	15	2 large	1.5	10.0
Coconut, fresh	15	1 piece	0.6	4.0
Sweets				
Molasses, medium	20	1 tablespoon	7.0	35.0
Vegetables				
Asparagus	75	6–8 tips	2.3	3.0
Beans, baked	100	½ cup	2.8	2.8
Beans, lima	75	⅓ cup	9.8	13.1
Beans, navy, pea	30	½ cup (cooked)	5.4	18.0
Beans, snap	75	⅓ cup	2.5	3.3
Beets	75	⅓ cup	7.9	10.5
Beet greens	75	⅓ cup	20.3	27.0
Broccoli	75	½ cup	3.0	4.0
Cabbage, cooked	75	⅓ cup	3.3	4.4
Carrots	75	½ cup	5.2	6.9
Cauliflower	75	½ cup	1.5	2.0
Celery	30	3 strips	2.5	8.4
Chard, Swiss	75	½ cup	12.0	16.0
Cucumber	50	½ medium	4.0	8.0
Dandelion greens	75	⅓ cup	14.7	19.6
Eggplant	75	⅓ cup	3.0	4.0
Endive, curly	50	10 leaves	4.5	9.0
Kale	75	⅓ cup	7.4	9.8
Kohlrabi	75	⅓ cup	8.3	11.1
Lettuce	50	5 leaves	3.0	6.0
Mushrooms	75	⅓ cup	2.3	3.1
Okra	75	⅓ cup	2.0	2.6
Onions	75	⅓ cup	0.1	0.1
Parsnips	75	⅓ cup	6.0	8.0
Peas	75	⅓ cup	0.7	0.9
Peppers	30	3 strips	0.6	2.0
Potato, white	100	1 small	9.0	9.0
Potato, baked	100	1 small	10.6	10.6
Potato, mashed	100	½ cup	9.6	9.6
Pumpkin	75	⅓ cup	5.9	7.8
Radish	50	5	1.5	3.0
Rutabagas	75	⅓ cup	6.4	8.5
Salsify	75	½ cup	2.2	2.9
Sauerkraut	75	½ cup	4.3	5.7
Squash, summer	75	⅓ cup	0.8	1.0
Squash, winter	75	⅓ cup	2.3	3.0
Sweet potato	100	1 small	6.0	6.0
Tomatoes or juice	75	½ large or ⅓ cup	3.8	5.0
Turnip greens	75	⅓ cup	1.7	2.3
Turnip	75	⅓ cup	1.7	2.3
Water cress	50	10 leaves	4.0	8.0

Appendix 15

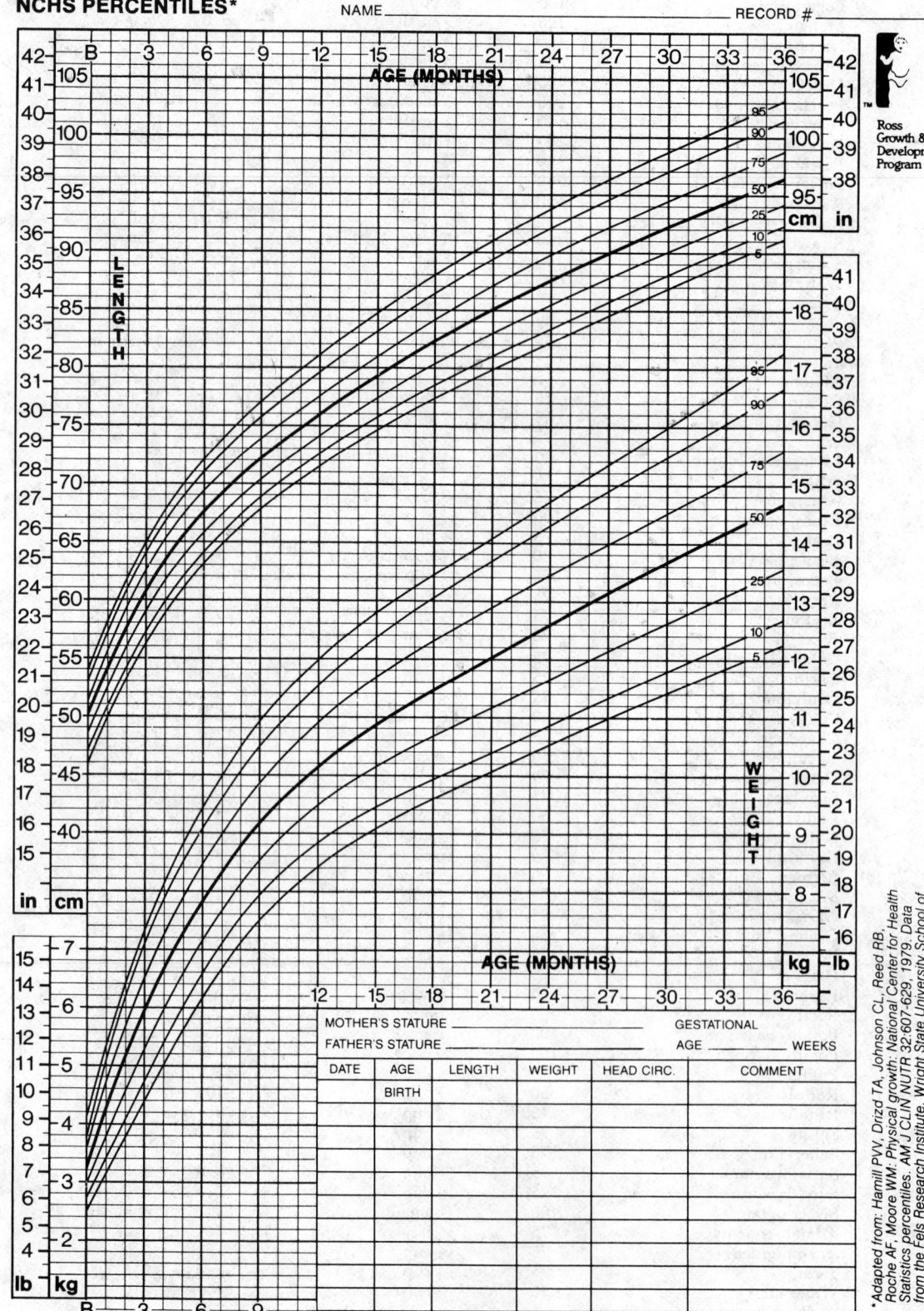

BOYS: BIRTH TO 36 MONTHS
PHYSICAL GROWTH
NCHS PERCENTILES*

NAME _____ RECORD # _____

Ross
Growth &
Development
Program

MOTHER'S STATURE _____ GESTATIONAL
FATHER'S STATURE _____ AGE _____ WEEKS

DATE	AGE	LENGTH	WEIGHT	HEAD CIRC.	COMMENT
	BIRTH				

* Adapted from: Hamill PVV, Drizd TA, Johnson CL, Reed RB,
Roche AF, Moore WM: Physical growth: National Center for Health
Statistics percentiles. AM J CLIN NUTR 32:607-629, 1979. Data
from the Fels Research Institute, Wright State University School of
Medicine, Yellow Springs, Ohio.

© 1982 ROSS LABORATORIES

Appendix 16

BOYS: BIRTH TO 36 MONTHS
PHYSICAL GROWTH
NCHS PERCENTILES*

NAME _____   RECORD # _____

*Adapted from: Hamill PVV, Drizd TA, Johnson CL, Reed RB, Roche AF, Moore WM. Physical growth: National Center for Health Statistics percentiles. AM J CLIN NUTR 32:607-629, 1979. Data from the Fels Research Institute, Wright State University School of Medicine, Yellow Springs, Ohio.
© 1982 ROSS LABORATORIES

DATE	AGE	LENGTH	WEIGHT	HEAD CIRC.	COMMENT

ROSS LABORATORIES
COLUMBUS, OHIO 43216
DIVISION OF ABBOTT LABORATORIES, USA

G105/DECEMBER 1982

Appendix 17

GIRLS: BIRTH TO 36 MONTHS
PHYSICAL GROWTH
NCHS PERCENTILES*

NAME _____ RECORD # _____

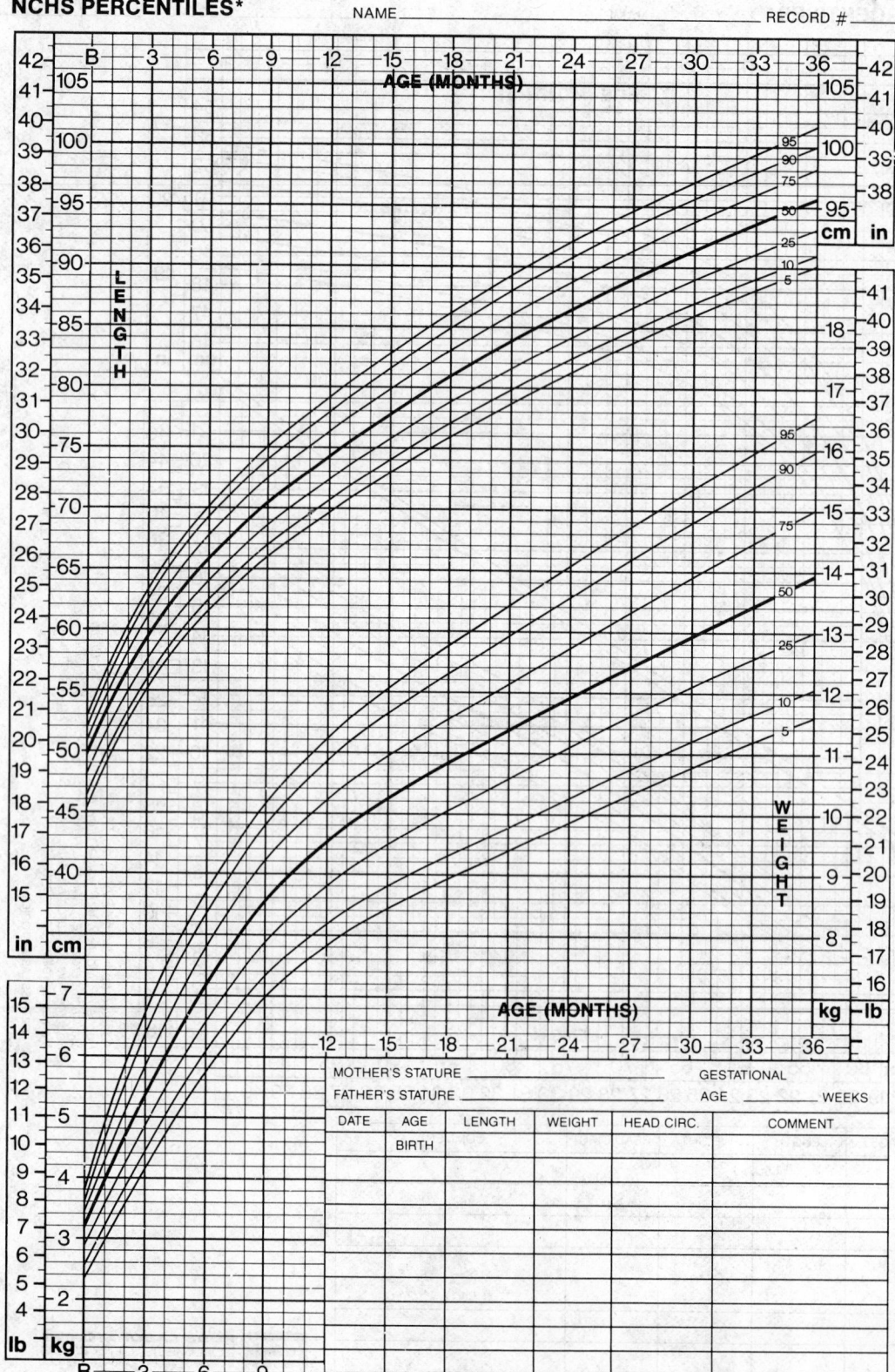

Ross
Growth &
Development
Program

*Adapted from: Hamill PVV, Drizd TA, Johnson CL, Reed RB,
Roche AF, Moore WM: Physical growth: National Center for Health
Statistics percentiles. AM J CLIN NUTR 32:607-629, 1979. Data
from the Fels Research Institute, Wright State University School of
Medicine, Yellow Springs, Ohio.
© 1982 ROSS LABORATORIES

MOTHER'S STATURE _____ GESTATIONAL
FATHER'S STATURE _____ AGE _____ WEEKS

DATE	AGE	LENGTH	WEIGHT	HEAD CIRC.	COMMENT
	BIRTH				

Appendix 18

GIRLS: BIRTH TO 36 MONTHS
PHYSICAL GROWTH
NCHS PERCENTILES*

NAME _____   RECORD # _____

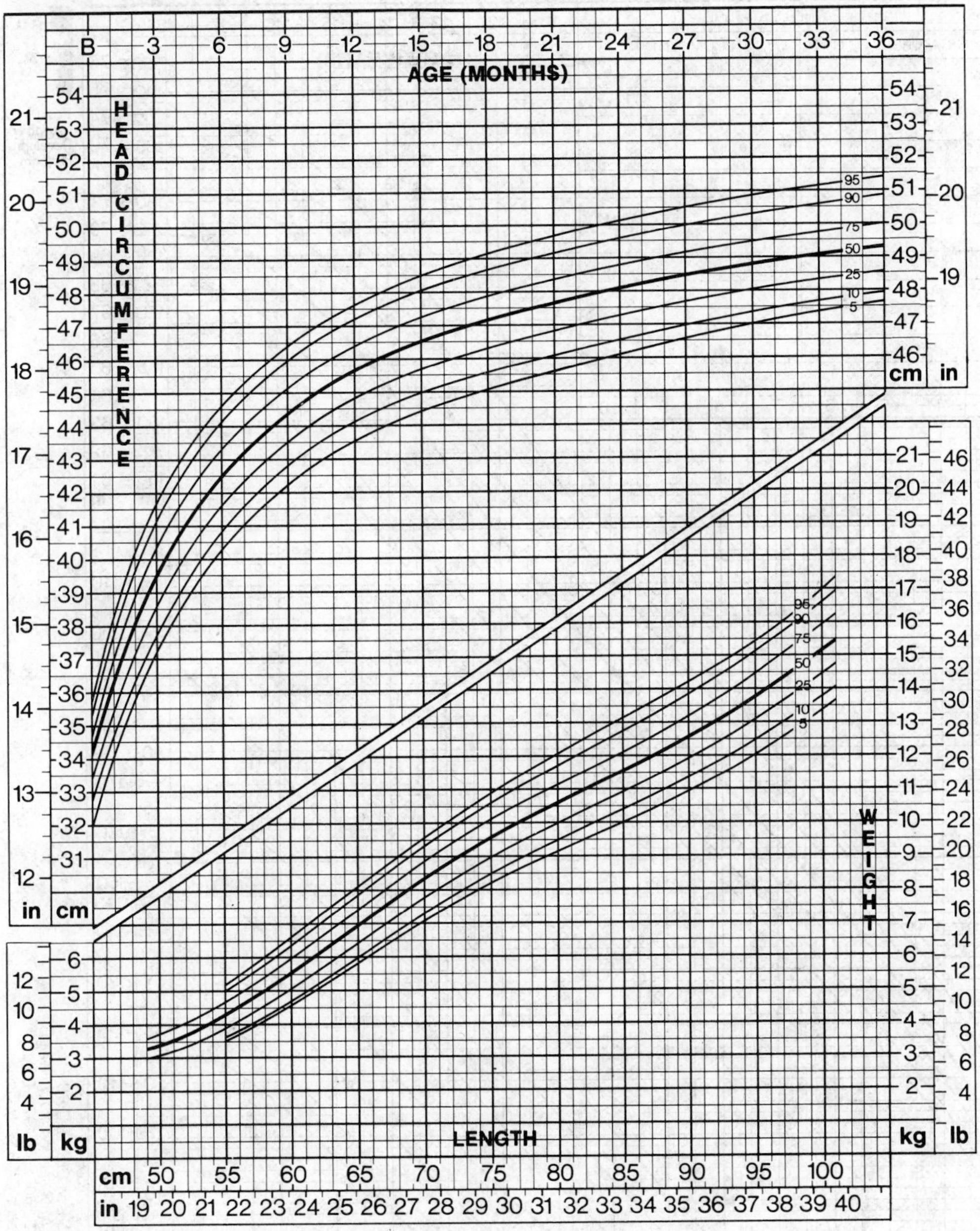

AGE (MONTHS)

HEAD CIRCUMFERENCE

95
90
75
50
25
10
5

cm   in

WEIGHT

LENGTH

cm   50   55   60   65   70   75   80   85   90   95   100
in   19 20 21 22 23 24 25 26 27 28 29 30 31 32 33 34 35 36 37 38 39 40

*Adapted from: Hamill PVV, Drizd TA, Johnson CL, Reed RB, Roche AF, Moore WM. Physical growth: National Center for Health Statistics percentiles. AM J CLIN NUTR 32:607-629, 1979. Data from the Fels Research Institute, Wright State University School of Medicine, Yellow Springs, Ohio.
© 1982 ROSS LABORATORIES

DATE	AGE	LENGTH	WEIGHT	HEAD CIRC.	COMMENT

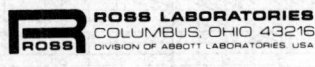

ROSS LABORATORIES
COLUMBUS, OHIO 43216
DIVISION OF ABBOTT LABORATORIES, USA

G106/DECEMBER 1982

Appendix 19

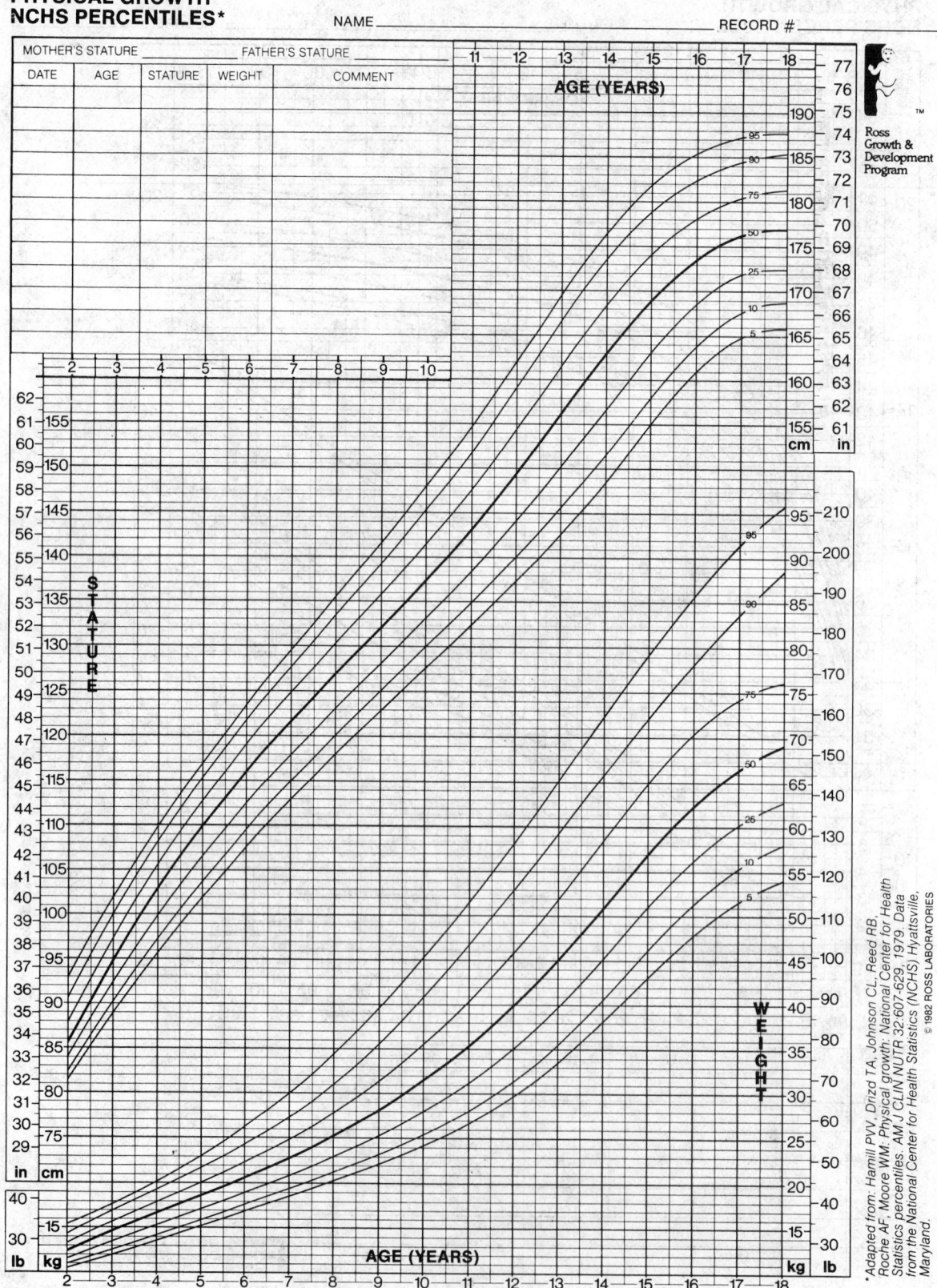

BOYS: 2 TO 18 YEARS
PHYSICAL GROWTH
NCHS PERCENTILES*

NAME _____ RECORD # _____

Ross
Growth &
Development
Program

* Adapted from: Hamill PVV, Drizd TA, Johnson CL, Reed RB, Roche AF, Moore WM: Physical growth: National Center for Health Statistics percentiles. AM J CLIN NUTR 32:607-629, 1979. Data from the National Center for Health Statistics (NCHS) Hyattsville, Maryland.

© 1982 ROSS LABORATORIES

Appendix 20

**BOYS: PREPUBESCENT
PHYSICAL GROWTH
NCHS PERCENTILES***

NAME_____   RECORD #_____

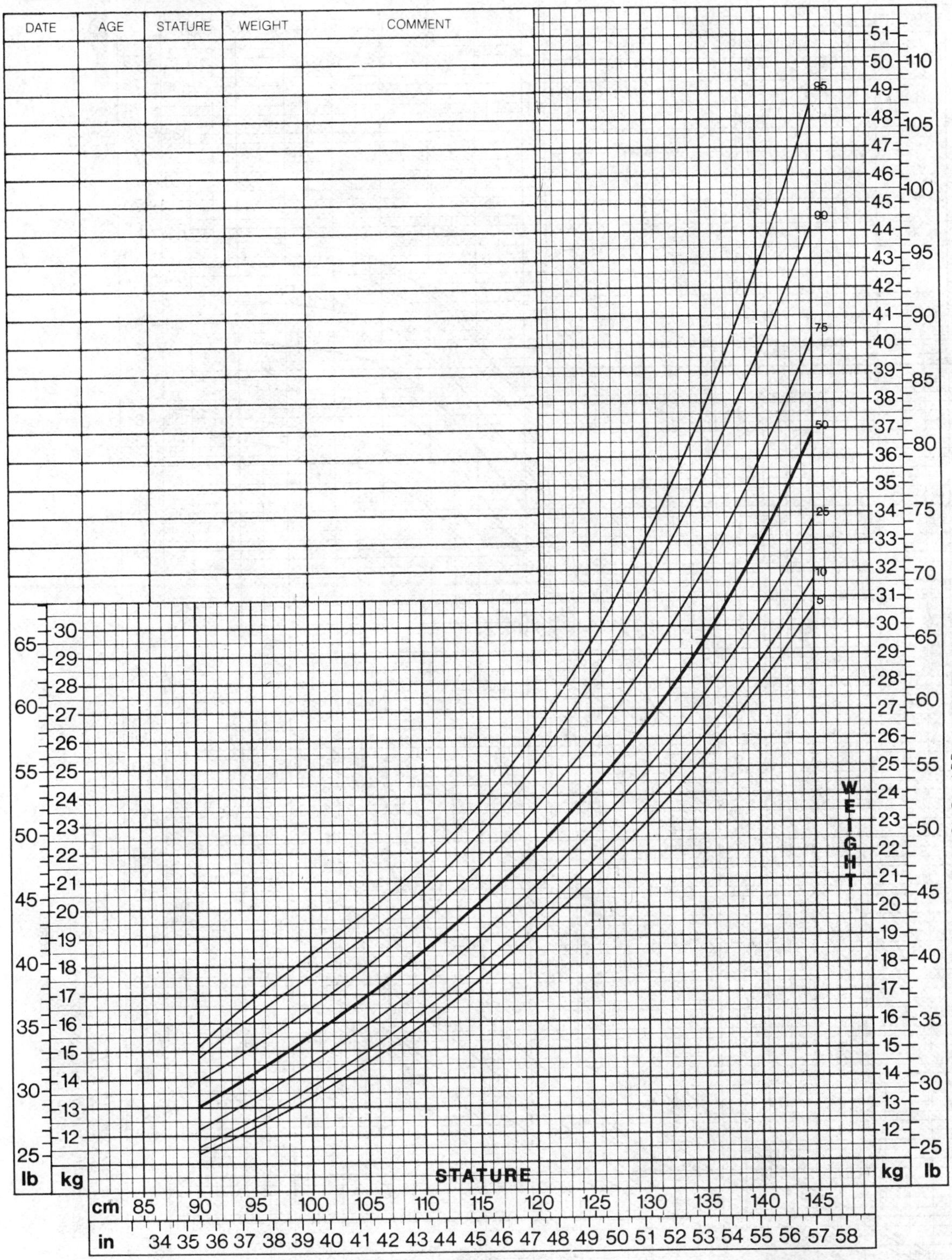

DATE	AGE	STATURE	WEIGHT	COMMENT

STATURE

cm 85 90 95 100 105 110 115 120 125 130 135 140 145

in 34 35 36 37 38 39 40 41 42 43 44 45 46 47 48 49 50 51 52 53 54 55 56 57 58

WEIGHT

*Adapted from: Hamill PVV, Drizd TA, Johnson CL, Reed RB, Roche AF, Moore WM: Physical growth: National Center for Health Statistics percentiles. AM J CLIN NUTR 32:607-629, 1979. Data from the National Center for Health Statistics (NCHS), Hyattsville, Maryland.

© 1982 ROSS LABORATORIES

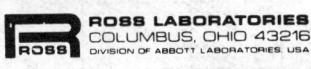

ROSS LABORATORIES
COLUMBUS, OHIO 43216
DIVISION OF ABBOTT LABORATORIES, USA

G107/DECEMBER 1982

Appendix 21

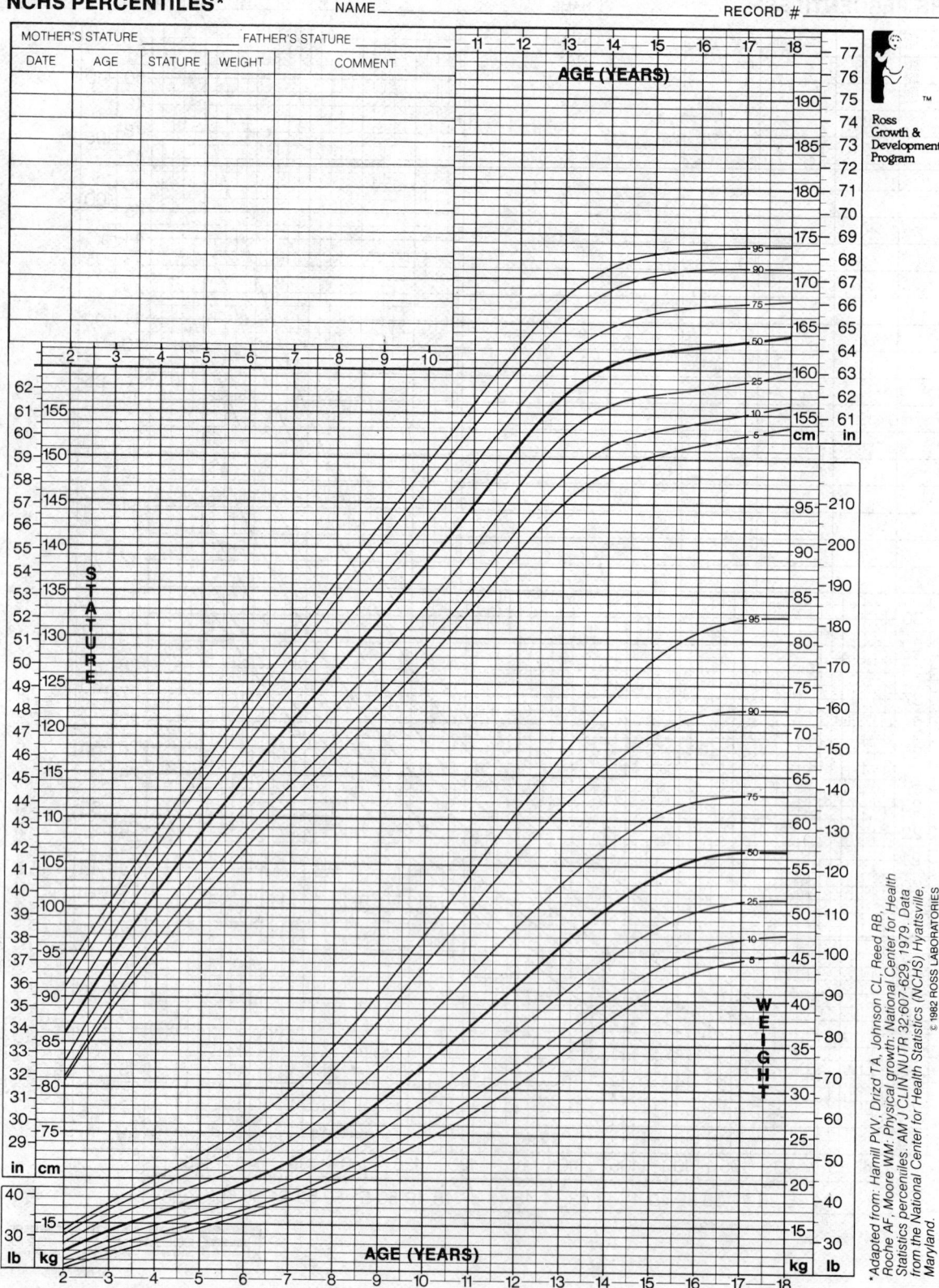

GIRLS: 2 TO 18 YEARS
PHYSICAL GROWTH
NCHS PERCENTILES*

NAME _____ RECORD # _____

*Adapted from: Hamill PVV, Drizd TA, Johnson CL, Reed RB, Roche AF, Moore WM: Physical growth: National Center for Health Statistics percentiles. AM J CLIN NUTR 32:607-629, 1979. Data from the National Center for Health Statistics (NCHS), Hyattsville, Maryland.

© 1982 ROSS LABORATORIES

Ross Growth & Development Program

Appendix 22

GIRLS: PREPUBESCENT
PHYSICAL GROWTH
NCHS PERCENTILES*

NAME_____ RECORD #_____

DATE	AGE	STATURE	WEIGHT	COMMENT

STATURE

cm 85 90 95 100 105 110 115 120 125 130 135 140 145

in 34 35 36 37 38 39 40 41 42 43 44 45 46 47 48 49 50 51 52 53 54 55 56 57 58

WEIGHT

*Adapted from: Hamill PVV, Drizd TA, Johnson CL, Reed RB, Roche AF, Moore WM: Physical growth: National Center for Health Statistics percentiles. AM J CLIN NUTR 32:607-629, 1979. Data from the National Center for Health Statistics (NCHS) Hyattsville, Maryland.

© 1982 ROSS LABORATORIES

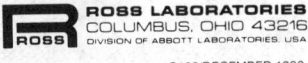

ROSS LABORATORIES
COLUMBUS, OHIO 43216
DIVISION OF ABBOTT LABORATORIES, USA

G108/DECEMBER 1982

Appendix Table 23. HEIGHT IN CM. OF YOUTHS AGED 12 TO 18 YEARS

Sex and age	Average age	n	N	$\overline{X}$	s	$s_{\overline{x}}$	Percentile						
							5th	10th	25th	50th	75th	90th	95th
Male									In centimeters				
12 years	12.10	43	144	151.1	8.18	1.44	138.6	141.2	146.1	150.5	153.9	159.9	163.8
12 1/4 years	12.24	150	465	150.2	7.87	0.65	138.3	140.1	144.1	149.5	155.9	161.0	162.7
12 1/2 years	12.50	187	577	151.5	8.33	0.87	138.0	140.4	145.9	152.6	156.8	161.2	165.1
12 3/4 years	12.76	184	589	154.3	7.48	0.62	142.3	146.1	149.6	153.7	158.0	164.4	167.6
13 years	12.99	165	520	154.7	9.37	0.67	136.9	143.0	148.1	155.4	161.4	166.6	170.3
13 1/4 years	13.25	154	511	158.9	8.55	0.82	146.2	148.5	153.0	157.8	164.9	171.1	174.4
13 1/2 years	13.49	162	524	159.7	9.11	1.06	144.7	148.2	153.3	158.8	165.3	173.2	176.1
13 3/4 years	13.75	158	478	161.4	8.44	0.68	148.1	149.9	155.8	161.8	167.5	173.1	174.6
14 years	14.00	135	465	164.0	7.90	0.69	151.4	153.2	157.8	164.2	169.8	173.6	177.0
14 1/4 years	14.26	159	503	165.4	10.01	1.15	148.5	152.5	157.9	165.1	172.7	178.5	182.1
14 1/2 years	14.50	155	487	167.5	7.96	0.79	153.5	156.6	161.5	169.4	173.0	176.5	178.7
14 3/4 years	14.76	151	467	167.1	8.46	0.99	152.7	155.2	162.3	167.7	173.5	176.5	180.8
15 years	15.00	155	489	169.4	7.59	0.59	156.3	158.7	163.7	169.4	174.8	178.1	181.4
15 1/4 years	15.25	169	511	171.4	7.57	0.62	159.2	160.8	166.5	171.7	176.5	180.5	183.1
15 1/2 years	15.50	159	493	171.2	6.89	0.43	159.8	162.8	166.8	171.2	174.7	179.5	185.0
15 3/4 years	15.75	150	461	171.9	7.04	0.70	159.1	163.9	167.6	172.6	176.1	181.0	183.0
16 years	16.01	134	456	172.9	6.13	0.53	161.5	164.5	170.1	173.7	177.0	179.6	181.3
16 1/4 years	16.24	157	541	174.5	7.33	0.82	162.4	163.9	170.4	175.1	178.8	184.0	186.5
16 1/2 years	16.50	135	413	174.3	6.56	0.44	165.1	166.8	170.5	173.9	178.4	182.4	184.5
16 3/4 years	16.75	122	401	174.7	6.78	0.66	164.6	166.1	169.8	174.4	179.6	183.1	185.4
17 years	17.00	136	479	175.1	6.94	0.61	163.2	166.4	170.5	175.6	179.7	183.7	186.3
17 1/4 years	17.26	125	435	176.4	6.97	0.71	162.6	167.5	172.1	176.7	181.3	184.3	188.0
17 1/2 years	17.50	111	396	175.4	7.15	0.89	162.9	165.8	170.3	175.2	180.1	185.4	187.8
17 3/4 years	17.75	113	409	175.1	7.32	0.77	162.7	167.2	170.3	175.3	179.7	184.7	189.3
18 years	17.97	76	275	176.0	6.46	0.63	165.7	167.3	171.3	175.8	180.4	185.3	186.4
Female													
12 years	12.10	42	153	154.5	7.05	1.38	142.2	145.9	150.8	153.8	157.3	167.0	167.9
12 1/4 years	12.27	142	520	153.8	7.20	0.64	141.0	143.6	149.5	153.9	158.5	162.5	165.6
12 1/2 years	12.50	140	511	155.6	7.69	0.60	141.8	145.4	151.7	155.5	160.4	164.6	168.3
12 3/4 years	12.75	147	517	156.0	6.82	0.57	143.6	147.5	151.8	156.3	160.5	164.5	166.6
13 years	13.01	166	578	157.1	7.30	0.43	143.8	148.3	152.5	157.3	162.7	166.7	169.2
13 1/4 years	13.25	144	461	158.3	7.54	0.73	145.3	146.8	152.6	158.6	163.4	166.7	169.5
13 1/2 years	13.50	146	500	159.2	6.08	0.42	149.6	152.1	155.2	158.8	163.3	167.7	170.2
13 3/4 years	13.76	148	499	159.3	6.67	0.56	147.5	149.5	155.2	159.9	164.2	167.5	169.4
14 years	14.01	138	452	159.8	6.59	0.53	149.1	151.5	155.9	160.3	164.1	167.2	170.5
14 1/4 years	14.25	159	510	161.3	6.00	0.62	150.8	153.4	157.6	161.2	164.7	168.4	170.8
14 1/2 years	14.51	137	415	161.2	6.66	0.63	150.3	152.6	157.1	161.2	165.4	170.3	172.2
14 3/4 years	14.76	130	457	162.5	6.43	0.69	153.6	154.7	157.7	162.9	167.2	170.0	174.1
15 years	14.99	133	449	161.3	5.73	0.53	151.7	154.6	157.5	160.7	164.8	169.4	171.4
15 1/4 years	15.25	135	479	162.2	6.68	0.58	151.3	153.2	157.3	163.2	166.7	170.3	171.8
15 1/2 years	15.51	114	433	161.8	7.27	0.92	151.8	153.2	156.4	161.3	167.4	171.1	173.5
15 3/4 years	15.75	136	526	162.9	7.19	0.84	150.8	152.8	158.1	163.3	167.8	170.7	175.1
16 years	16.01	141	474	161.9	6.38	0.71	152.4	153.6	157.5	161.6	166.6	169.8	172.2
16 1/4 years	16.24	138	491	163.6	6.17	0.51	152.7	155.8	160.2	164.8	166.8	170.7	173.6
16 1/2 years	16.50	112	341	161.5	6.51	0.70	151.3	153.0	157.2	161.8	166.1	170.2	172.2
16 3/4 years	16.76	135	450	162.9	6.52	0.52	151.5	154.0	158.6	162.8	167.3	171.7	173.0
17 years	17.00	135	477	163.0	6.48	0.71	151.5	154.5	158.9	163.4	167.0	171.1	173.3
17 1/4 years	17.24	125	461	162.7	6.62	0.52	151.5	153.8	157.8	164.2	166.9	171.3	173.6
17 1/2 years	17.51	111	415	162.9	6.02	0.59	152.7	155.7	158.4	162.6	168.1	171.4	172.8
17 3/4 years	17.75	90	325	162.9	5.90	0.87	152.4	154.4	158.3	163.1	167.4	169.9	171.7
18 years	17.97	79	306	163.0	6.77	0.74	152.5	154.6	158.2	162.5	167.6	171.4	175.3

From National Center for Health Statistics: Height and Weight of Youths 12–17 Years, United States. In Vital and Health Statistics, Series 11, no. 124. Health Services and Mental Health Administration. Washington, D.C., U.S. Government Printing Office, 1973.

NOTE: n = sample size; N = estimated number of youths in population in thousands; $\overline{X}$ = mean; s = standard deviation; $s_{\overline{x}}$ = standard error of the mean.

Appendix Table 24. PERCENTILES FOR WEIGHT FOR HEIGHT OF YOUTHS AGED 12 TO 18 YEARS

Weight in Kg. of Youths Aged 12 Years at Last Birthday

Sex and height	n	N	$\bar{X}$	s	$s_{\bar{x}}$	Percentile						
						5th	10th	25th	50th	75th	90th	95th
Male						In kilograms						
Under 130 cm	5	15	*	*	*	*	*	*	*	*	*	*
130.0-134.9 cm	4	8	*	*	*	*	*	*	*	*	*	*
135.0-139.9 cm	34	111	32.50	3.741	0.727	26.6	27.6	30.2	31.6	34.7	37.7	39.4
140.0-144.9 cm	80	241	34.28	3.635	0.601	28.1	30.0	31.8	34.1	36.5	38.6	40.7
145.0-149.9 cm	123	386	39.27	6.243	0.615	32.1	33.2	35.7	38.2	40.9	46.1	52.5
150.0-154.9 cm	156	513	42.90	6.314	0.480	34.9	36.1	38.2	42.1	46.0	51.6	56.3
155.0-159.9 cm	135	432	47.35	7.551	0.769	38.3	39.4	41.9	46.2	50.5	57.4	61.9
160.0-164.9 cm	65	201	50.82	8.735	1.388	42.1	42.7	44.9	48.4	56.0	61.1	67.1
165.0-169.9 cm	29	88	55.75	8.811	2.031	43.3	46.4	49.0	54.4	59.9	68.3	76.6
170.0-174.9 cm	8	21	62.37	4.503	1.993	54.0	58.1	60.1	61.0	66.0	69.1	69.5
175.0-189.9 cm	3	10	*	*	*	*	*	*	*	*	*	*
180.0-184.9 cm	1	2	*	*	*	*	*	*	*	*	*	*
185.0-189.9 cm	-	-	-	-	-	-	-	-	-	-	-	-
190.0-194.9 cm	-	-	-	-	-	-	-	-	-	-	-	-
195.0 cm. and over	-	-	-	-	-	-	-	-	-	-	-	-
Female												
Under 130 cm	-	-	-	-	-	-	-	*	*	*	*	*
130.0-134.9 cm	3	10	*	*	*	*	*	*	*	*	*	*
135.0-139.9 cm	12	44	29.41	3.372	0.914	25.0	25.0	26.4	28.9	32.1	34.1	34.2
140.0-144.9 cm	32	116	38.30	7.314	1.194	28.8	30.6	33.3	36.8	41.4	49.2	55.1
145.0-149.9 cm	72	258	39.78	6.205	0.975	31.8	32.8	35.5	38.5	42.8	48.3	50.6
150.0-154.9 cm	147	517	44.00	7.421	0.677	34.4	35.8	38.9	42.8	47.4	52.9	57.4
155.0-159.9 cm	144	525	48.74	8.369	0.714	37.9	39.2	43.0	46.8	53.8	60.7	63.5
160.0-164.9 cm	95	336	53.06	8.010	0.658	42.5	43.9	47.2	51.1	57.2	65.6	69.6
165.0-169.9 cm	31	117	54.89	7.022	1.384	43.9	47.1	50.4	53.1	59.7	64.5	71.3
170.0-174.9 cm	11	42	63.66	14.501	6.214	48.7	50.1	50.8	56.7	82.2	86.0	86.1
175.0-179.9 cm	-	-	-	-	-	-	-	-	-	-	-	-
180.0-184.9 cm	-	-	-	-	-	-	-	-	-	-	-	-
185.0-189.9 cm	-	-	-	-	-	-	-	-	-	-	-	-
190.0-194.9 cm	-	-	-	-	-	-	-	-	-	-	-	-
195.0 cm. and over	-	-	-	-	-	-	-	-	-	-	-	-

From National Center for Health Statistics: Height and Weight of Youths 12–17 Years, United States. In Vital and Health Statistics, Series 11, no. 124. Health Services and Mental Health Administration. Washington, D.C., U.S. Government Printing Office, 1973.

NOTE: n = sample size; N = estimated number of youths in population in thousands; X = mean; s = standard deviation; $s_{\bar{x}}$ = standard error of the mean.

Table continued on the following page

Appendix Table 24. PERCENTILES FOR WEIGHT FOR HEIGHT OF YOUTHS AGED 12 TO 18 YEARS (*Continued*)

Weight in Kg. of Youths aged 13 Years at Last Birthday

Sex and height	n	N	$\overline{X}$	s	$s_{\overline{x}}$	Percentile						
						5th	10th	25th	50th	75th	90th	95th
Male						In kilograms						
Under 130 cm----------	-	-	-	-	-	-	-	-	-	-	-	-
130.0-134.9 cm--------	2	5	*	*	*	*	*	*	*	*	*	*
135.0-139.9 cm--------	6	25	32.62	5.624	7.716	27.2	27.6	28.9	31.0	34.9	43.1	43.2
140.0-144.9 cm--------	18	56	36.54	5.852	1.607	30.0	30.5	32.1	36.1	39.2	41.7	53.2
145.0-149.9 cm--------	65	204	39.03	5.270	0.662	32.4	33.9	36.1	37.9	41.2	44.5	46.4
150.0-154.9 cm--------	99	312	42.58	6.724	0.865	34.8	36.2	37.9	41.0	45.5	49.4	61.0
155.0-159.9 cm--------	131	421	47.27	7.482	0.717	37.8	39.2	41.7	45.8	51.1	58.7	61.7
160.0-164.9 cm--------	125	393	53.01	9.324	0.916	41.5	43.7	46.9	50.4	58.2	64.4	72.5
165.0-169.9 cm--------	91	285	55.92	8.560	0.833	46.3	47.5	49.3	53.6	59.4	69.0	75.0
170.0-174.9 cm--------	63	215	62.01	10.362	1.033	51.2	51.6	53.7	60.1	67.0	76.0	85.0
175.0-179.9 cm--------	19	68	67.92	12.085	3.428	56.3	57.9	60.1	63.3	70.3	88.3	89.0
180.0-184.9 cm--------	5	15	*	*	*	*	*	*	*	*	*	*
185.0-189.9 cm--------	-	-	-	-	-	-	-	-	-	-	-	-
190.0-194.9 cm--------	-	-	-	-	-	-	-	-	-	-	-	-
195.0 cm. and over----	-	-	-	-	-	-	-	-	-	-	-	-
Female												
Under 130 cm----------	-	-	-	-	-	-	-	-	-	-	-	-
130.0-134.9 cm--------	1	3	*	*	*	*	*	*	*	*	*	*
135.0-139.9 cm--------	-	-	-	-	-	-	-	-	-	-	-	-
140.0-144.9 cm--------	15	51	37.13	7.317	2.259	26.6	27.5	30.5	36.7	40.1	44.5	56.1
145.0-149.9 cm--------	47	165	42.23	6.880	0.888	34.7	35.6	38.2	40.5	44.2	53.6	57.6
150.0-154.9 cm--------	98	329	44.32	7.029	0.787	35.6	36.5	39.2	42.9	47.3	53.7	57.9
155.0-159.9 cm--------	152	499	49.75	8.757	0.699	39.1	39.9	43.8	48.4	53.8	61.0	65.9
160.0-164.9 cm--------	156	515	53.16	8.399	0.522	41.2	43.9	47.7	52.2	57.0	63.8	68.5
165.0-169.9 cm--------	86	284	58.17	9.125	0.921	46.2	47.4	52.2	58.1	61.5	69.3	76.2
170.0-174.9 cm--------	24	87	58.11	13.209	2.343	46.2	47.1	48.4	52.9	65.3	68.6	96.8
175.0-179.9 cm--------	3	10	*	*	*	*	*	*	*	*	*	*
180.0-184.9 cm--------	-	-	-	-	-	-	-	-	-	-	-	-
185.0-189.9 cm--------	-	-	-	-	-	-	-	-	-	-	-	-
190.0-194.9 cm--------	-	-	-	-	-	-	-	-	-	-	-	-
195.0 cm. and over----	-	-	-	-	-	-	-	-	-	-	-	-

NOTE: n = sample size; N = estimated number of youths in population in thousands; $\overline{X}$ = mean; s = standard deviation; $s_{\overline{x}}$ standard error of the mean.

Appendix Table 24. PERCENTILES FOR WEIGHT FOR HEIGHT OF YOUTHS AGED 12 TO 18 YEARS (*Continued*)

Weight in Kg. of Youths Aged 14 Years at Last Birthday

Sex and height	n	N	$\overline{X}$	s	$s_{\overline{x}}$	Percentile						
						5th	10th	25th	50th	75th	90th	95th
Male						In kilograms						
Under 130 cm	-	-	-	-	-	-	-	-	-	-	-	-
130.0-134.9 cm	-	-	-	-	-	-	-	-	-	-	-	-
135.0-139.9 cm	2	7	*	*	*	*	*	*	*	*	*	*
140.0-144.9 cm	3	13	*	*	*	*	*	*	*	*	*	*
145.0-149.9 cm	11	42	40.51	1.829	0.644	36.9	38.6	39.6	40.6	42.0	42.5	42.7
150.0-154.9 cm	45	135	43.63	6.277	1.182	36.2	37.0	39.0	41.4	48.0	51.7	55.3
155.0-159.9 cm	83	261	47.42	7.822	0.872	37.7	38.7	41.8	46.1	51.2	58.0	62.7
160.0-164.9 cm	96	299	52.28	6.785	0.584	42.5	44.0	47.5	52.1	56.3	61.5	65.1
165.0-169.9 cm	134	432	58.07	9.416	1.054	47.7	49.3	51.6	55.4	62.3	70.6	75.7
170.0-174.9 cm	144	435	62.37	11.516	1.095	49.7	51.0	55.0	59.4	65.6	79.2	86.3
175.0-179.9 cm	71	228	65.54	9.704	1.306	50.9	55.1	58.5	64.7	69.9	74.5	84.0
180.0-184.9 cm	25	81	72.44	13.014	2.298	59.6	60.0	65.1	69.4	77.0	83.0	94.3
185.0-189.9 cm	3	9	*	*	*	*	*	*	*	*	*	*
190.0-194.9 cm	1	3	*	*	*	*	*	*	*	*	*	*
195.0 cm. and over	-	-	-	-	-	-	-	-	-	-	-	-
Female												
Under 130 cm	-	-	-	-	-	-	-	-	-	-	-	-
130.0-134.9 cm	-	-	-	-	-	-	-	-	-	-	-	-
135.0-139.9 cm	1	2	*	*	*	*	*	*	*	*	*	*
140.0-144.9 cm	2	6	*	*	*	*	*	*	*	*	*	*
145.0-149.9 cm	17	52	42.00	5.879	1.683	32.0	35.3	36.3	42.3	47.5	49.5	51.1
150.0-154.9 cm	64	196	48.26	6.797	0.926	37.7	39.2	42.5	47.9	53.3	55.9	58.8
155.0-159.9 cm	157	508	51.35	7.705	0.520	41.2	43.4	46.3	49.6	55.6	62.2	64.3
160.0-164.9 cm	186	603	54.59	8.810	0.707	43.0	45.0	48.4	53.0	59.7	66.7	70.7
165.0-169.9 cm	114	372	58.46	10.185	0.955	45.9	47.5	52.1	56.8	61.8	70.5	76.4
170.0-174.9 cm	36	121	64.37	15.821	2.814	49.2	52.1	56.2	59.8	70.5	72.9	99.4
175.0-179.9 cm	7	28	61.33	5.496	2.620	51.7	52.0	57.7	59.8	64.6	70.2	70.6
180.0-184.9 cm	2	7	*	*	*	*	*	*	*	*	*	*
185.0-189.9 cm	-	-	-	-	-	-	-	-	-	-	-	-
190.0-194.9 cm	-	-	-	-	-	-	-	-	-	-	-	-
195.0 cm. and over	-	-	-	-	-	-	-	-	-	-	-	-

NOTE: n = sample size; N = estimated number of youths in population in thousands; $\overline{X}$ = mean; s = standard deviation; $s_{\overline{x}}$ = standard error of the mean.

Table continued on the following page

Appendix Table 24. PERCENTILES FOR WEIGHT FOR HEIGHT OF YOUTHS
AGED 12 TO 18 YEARS (*Continued*)

Weight in Kg. of Youths Aged 15 Years at Last Birthday

Sex and height	n	N	$\overline{X}$	s	$s_{\overline{x}}$	Percentile						
						5th	10th	25th	50th	75th	90th	95th
Male						In kilograms						
Under 130 cm----------	-	-	-	-	-	-	-	-	-	-	-	-
130.0-134.9 cm--------	-	-	-	-	-	-	-	-	-	-	-	-
135.0-139.9 cm--------	-	-	-	-	-	-	-	-	-	-	-	-
140.0-144.9 cm--------	-	-	-	-	-	-	-	-	-	-	-	-
145.0-149.9 cm--------	1	2	*	*	*	*	*	*	*	*	*	*
150.0-154.9 cm--------	10	30	45.72	8.582	3.550	35.7	39.2	42.6	44.7	46.0	48.7	76.1
155.0-159.9 cm--------	34	99	52.81	10.552	1.695	40.3	43.1	46.7	49.2	56.7	69.6	76.3
160.0-164.9 cm--------	71	206	53.01	8.417	0.986	42.7	44.1	46.9	51.5	56.3	65.3	68.8
165.0-169.9 cm--------	132	404	57.72	8.503	0.819	48.0	48.8	53.1	56.4	61.3	67.1	73.3
170.0-174.9 cm--------	176	574	62.88	8.464	0.633	51.6	53.4	56.7	61.9	67.2	72.9	78.1
175.0-179.9 cm--------	118	374	65.80	9.457	1.045	53.1	55.6	59.7	64.3	69.5	80.2	89.2
180.0-184.9 cm--------	51	144	72.00	11.928	1.724	54.6	60.3	64.4	70.2	78.4	84.4	96.6
185.0-189.9 cm--------	14	48	74.21	15.035	5.200	58.3	58.5	62.9	70.7	84.6	92.4	110.8
190.0-194.9 cm--------	6	15	83.39	16.431	10.332	66.4	66.7	69.6	73.8	103.0	105.7	106.2
195.0 cm. and over----	-	-	-	-	-	-	-	-	-	-	-	-
Female												
Under 130 cm----------	-	-	-	-	-	-	-	-	-	-	-	-
130.0-134.9 cm--------	-	-	-	-	-	-	-	-	-	-	-	-
135.0-139.9 cm--------	-	-	-	-	-	-	-	-	-	-	-	-
140.0-144.9 cm--------	2	5	*	*	*	*	*	*	*	*	*	*
145.0-149.9 cm--------	15	51	47.91	7.875	3.623	36.0	39.4	42.1	45.4	52.7	55.7	66.3
150.0-154.9 cm--------	69	242	49.69	8.895	1.190	39.1	40.6	44.3	48.1	52.8	60.5	68.3
155.0-159.9 cm--------	111	400	51.52	8.473	0.934	41.4	43.5	46.3	50.8	55.1	59.8	65.2
160.0-164.9 cm--------	137	509	57.03	10.828	0.875	45.1	47.3	50.2	55.0	60.2	71.7	77.7
165.0-169.9 cm--------	109	398	60.71	10.357	1.053	47.5	49.3	55.1	58.4	65.7	74.1	81.0
170.0-174.9 cm--------	49	188	65.27	10.730	1.880	49.7	53.6	57.2	61.2	71.6	85.3	86.4
175.0-179.9 cm--------	7	23	63.30	8.872	4.807	49.7	49.9	53.8	62.4	71.1	71.9	79.2
180.0-184.9 cm--------	3	26	*	*	*	*	*	*	*	*	*	*
185.0-189.9 cm--------	1	3	*	*	*	*	*	*	*	*	*	*
190.0-194.9 cm--------	-	-	-	-	-	-	-	-	-	-	-	-
195.0 cm. and over----	-	-	-	-	-	-	-	-	-	-	-	-

NOTE: n = sample size: N = estimated number of youths in population in thousands; $\overline{X}$ = mean; s = standard deviation: $s_{\overline{x}}$ = standard error of the mean.

Appendix Table 24. PERCENTILES FOR WEIGHT FOR HEIGHT OF YOUTHS
AGED 12 TO 18 YEARS (*Continued*)

Weight in Kg. of Youths Aged 16 Years at Last Birthday

Sex and height	n	N	$\bar{X}$	s	$s_{\bar{x}}$	5th	10th	25th	50th	75th	90th	95th
						Percentile						
						In kilograms						
Male												
Under 130 cm----------	-	-	-	-	+	-	-	-	-	-	-	-
130.0-134.9 cm--------	-	-	-	-	+	-	-	-	-	-	-	-
135.0-139.9 cm--------	-	-	-	-	-	-	-	-	-	-	-	-
140.0-144.9 cm--------	-	-	-	-	-	-	-	-	-	-	-	-
145.0-149.9 cm--------	1	1	*	*	*	*	*	*	*	*	*	*
150.0-154.9 cm--------	4	12	*	*	*	*	*	*	*	*	*	*
155.0-159.9 cm--------	11	33	49.89	7.323	3.572	42.0	42.2	44.7	46.8	54.4	59.8	67.2
160.0-164.9 cm--------	32	108	53.09	6.459	1.273	44.2	44.9	48.2	51.4	58.0	60.9	66.1
165.0-169.9 cm--------	87	275	59.39	9.178	0.981	48.5	49.8	52.7	58.0	63.9	69.3	75.9
170.0-174.9 cm--------	166	552	62.66	7.556	0.629	51.6	53.8	57.5	61.6	67.1	73.1	78.0
175.0-179.9 cm--------	149	511	67.33	9.018	0.856	56.3	58.2	61.0	65.4	72.5	80.1	83.8
180.0-184.9 cm--------	72	227	72.38	12.485	1.993	58.3	59.3	64.4	68.9	76.5	90.2	96.9
185.0-189.9 cm--------	29	95	81.06	14.268	3.265	63.7	66.6	69.7	78.4	90.3	97.0	111.4
190.0-194.9 cm--------	3	10	*	*	*	*	*	*	*	*	*	*
195.0 cm. and over----	2	7	*	*	*	*	*	*	*	*	*	*
Female												
Under 130 cm----------	-	-	-	-	-	-	-	-	-	-	-	-
130.0-134.9 cm--------	--	-	-	-	-	-	-	-	-	-	-	-
135.0-139.9 cm--------	-	-	-	-	-	-	-	-	-	-	-	-
140.0-144.9 cm--------	2	5	*	*	*	*	*	*	*	*	*	*
145.0-149.9 cm--------	10	33	52.58	8.198	3.191	43.9	44.1	44.9	51.0	54.5	72.0	72.1
150.0-154.9 cm--------	57	178	51.79	10.457	1.053	41.4	42.0	45.8	48.9	54.1	61.5	83.3
155.0-159.9 cm--------	117	354	53.20	7.766	0.734	44.0	45.6	48.4	51.6	56.4	61.9	69.0
160.0-164.9 cm--------	160	547	57.71	11.129	1.246	46.1	47.3	51.5	55.5	61.2	69.5	75.1
165.0-169.9 cm--------	122	450	61.72	11.998	0.802	47.1	48.8	53.3	59.1	67.3	78.7	86.7
170.0-174.9 cm--------	53	170	63.61	8.734	1.126	52.9	53.8	58.1	62.1	66.8	73.8	84.2
175.0-179.9 cm--------	14	45	72.55	15.012	5.224	58.6	58.8	61.7	65.9	80.6	99.1	105.5
180.0-184.9 cm--------	1	2	*	*	*	*	*	*	*	*	*	*
185.0-189.9 cm--------	-	-	-	-	-	-	-	-	-	-	-	-
190.0-194.9 cm--------	-	-	-	-	-	-	-	-	-	-	-	-
195.0 cm. and over----	-	-	-	-	-	-	-	-	-	-	-	-

NOTE: n = sample size; N = estimated number of youths in population in thousands; $\bar{X}$ = mean; s = standard deviation; $s_{\bar{x}}$ = standard error of the mean.

Table continued on the following page

Appendix Table 24. PERCENTILES FOR WEIGHT FOR HEIGHT OF YOUTHS
AGED 12 TO 18 YEARS (*Continued*)

Weight in Kg. of Youths Aged 17 Years at Last Birthday

Sex and height	n	N	$\bar{X}$	s	$s_{\bar{x}}$	Percentile						
						5th	10th	25th	50th	75th	90th	95th
Male						In kilograms						
Under 130 cm ---------	-	-	-	-	-	-	-	-	-	-	-	-
130.0-134.9 cm--------	-	-	-	-	-	-	-	-	-	-	-	-
135.0-139.9 cm--------	-	-	-	-	-	-	-	-	-	-	-	-
140.0-144.9 cm--------	-	-	-	-	-	-	-	-	-	-	-	-
145.0-149.9 cm--------	-	-	-	-	-	-	-	-	-	-	-	-
150.0-154.9 cm--------	1	3	*	*	*	*	*	*	*	*	*	*
155.0-159.9 cm--------	11	39	54.63	9.397	3.414	43.8	46.4	48.2	49.7	57.8	69.9	73.2
160.0-164.9 cm--------	25	81	57.75	6.503	1.355	49.7	51.1	52.5	56.9	61.6	70.1	70.8
165.0-169.9 cm--------	63	248	62.57	8.344	1.224	50.2	53.2	56.4	61.5	66.9	72.7	77.3
170.0-174.9 cm--------	115	396	67.06	11.163	0.704	53.3	55.5	59.5	64.6	71.9	80.9	91.6
175.0-179.9 cm--------	151	537	68.37	9.907	0.831	56.9	58.9	61.5	66.5	73.6	79.4	88.4
180.0-184.9 cm--------	80	297	73.31	12.454	1.335	59.6	61.0	65.1	71.2	78.4	91.8	102.7
185.0-189.9 cm--------	36	133	76.03	9.171	1.301	62.4	66.3	70.5	75.3	80.8	90.3	92.9
190.0-194.9 cm--------	7	25	81.40	10.985	7.588	62.9	62.9	67.8	87.3	90.3	90.6	90.6
195.0 cm. and over----	-	-	-	-	-	-	-	-	-	-	-	-
Female												
Under 130 cm----------	-	-	-	-	-	-	-	-	-	-	-	-
130.0-134.9 cm--------	-	-	-	-	-	-	-	-	-	-	-	-
135.0-139.9 cm--------	-	-	-	-	-	-	-	-	-	-	-	-
140.0-144.9 cm--------	2	5	*	*	*	*	*	*	*	*	*	*
145.0-149.9 cm--------	8	26	43.49	3.939	1.604	38.6	38.8	40.1	45.1	45.7	51.1	51.2
150.0-154.9 cm--------	43	151	49.96	6.508	0.827	41.6	42.3	44.6	48.9	53.5	59.2	64.1
155.0-159.9 cm--------	103	385	54.71	9.903	0.775	44.4	45.5	48.7	53.2	57.7	61.6	76.2
160.0-164.9 cm--------	133	506	57.79	10.620	1.028	46.8	48.0	50.2	55.4	61.5	72.3	82.3
165.0-169.9 cm--------	116	433	60.63	10.117	1.182	47.9	50.3	55.1	59.3	65.1	69.4	71.6
170.0-174.9 cm--------	51	186	62.18	9.132	1.407	50.6	52.9	55.5	60.2	65.7	76.1	82.7
175.0-179.9 cm--------	12	47	65.76	8.405	2.229	54.9	56.7	60.1	61.7	75.2	75.9	83.0
180.0-184.9 cm--------	1	2	*	*	*	*	*	*	*	*	*	*
185.0-189.9 cm--------	-	-	-	-	-	-	-	-	-	-	-	-
190.0-194.9 cm--------	-	-	-	-	-	-	-	-	-	-	-	-
195.0 cm. and over----	-	-	-	-	-	-	-	-	-	-	-	-

NOTE: n = sample size; N = estimated number of youths in population in thousands; $\bar{X}$ = mean; s = standard deviation; $s_{\bar{x}}$ = standard error of the mean.

Appendix Table 25. 1983 METROPOLITAN HEIGHT AND WEIGHT TABLES

	MEN					WOMEN			
Height		Small	Medium	Large		Height		Small	Medium	Large
Feet	Inches	Frame	Frame	Frame	Feet	Inches	Frame	Frame	Frame
5	2	128–134	131–141	138–150	4	10	102–111	109–121	118–131
5	3	130–136	133–143	140–153	4	11	103–113	111–123	120–134
5	4	132–138	135–145	142–156	5	0	104–115	113–126	122–137
5	5	134–140	137–148	144–160	5	1	106–118	115–129	125–140
5	6	136–142	139–151	146–164	5	2	108–121	118–132	128–143
5	7	138–145	142–154	149–168	5	3	111–124	121–135	131–147
5	8	140–148	145–157	152–172	5	4	114–127	124–138	134–151
5	9	142–151	148–160	155–176	5	5	117–130	127–141	137–155
5	10	144–154	151–163	158–180	5	6	120–133	130–144	140–159
5	11	146–157	154–166	161–184	5	7	123–136	133–147	143–163
6	0	149–160	157–170	164–188	5	8	126–139	136–150	146–167
6	1	152–164	160–174	168–192	5	9	129–142	139–153	149–170
6	2	155–168	164–178	172–197	5	10	132–145	142–156	152–173
6	3	158–172	167–182	176–202	5	11	135–148	145–159	155–176
6	4	162–176	171–187	181–207	6	0	138–151	148–162	158–179

Weights for adults age 25 to 59 years based on lowest mortality. For determination of frame size see Appendix 26. Weight in pounds according to frame size in indoor clothing (5 pounds for men and 3 pounds for women) wearing shoes with 1-inch heels.

Source of basic data *1979 Build Study*, Society of Actuaries and Association of Life Insurance Medical Directors of America. Courtesy of the Metropolitan Life Insurance Company, 1983.

Appendix 26. DETERMINATION OF FRAME SIZE

METHOD 1

Height is recorded without shoes on.

Wrist circumference is measured just distal to the styloid process at the wrist crease on the right arm using a tape measure.

The following formula is used:

$$r = \frac{\text{Height (cm.)}}{\text{Wrist circumference (cm.)}}$$

Frame size can be determined as follows:

Males	Females
$r > 10.4$ small	$r > 11.0$ small
$r = 9.6\text{–}10.4$ medium	$r = 10.1\text{–}11.0$ medium
$r < 9.6$ large	$r < 10.1$ large

Source: Grant, J. P.: Handbook of Total Parenteral Nutrition. Philadelphia, W. B. Saunders Company, 1980, p. 15.

METHOD 2

The patient's right arm is extended forward perpendicular to the body, with the arm bent so the angle at the elbow forms 90° with the fingers pointing up and the palm turned away from the body. The greatest breadth across the elbow joint is measured with a sliding caliper along the axis of the upper arm, on the two prominent bones on either side of the elbow. This is recorded as the elbow breadth. The following tables give the elbow breadth measurements for medium-framed men and women of various heights. Measurements lower than those listed indicate a small frame size; higher measurements indicate a large frame size.

MEN		WOMEN	
Height in 1" Heels	Elbow Breadth	Height in 1" Heels	Elbow Breadth
5'2"–5'3"	2½"–2⅞"	4'10"–4'11"	2¼"–2½"
5'4"–5'7"	2⅝"–2⅞"	5'0"–5'3"	2¼"–2½"
5'8"–5'11"	2¾"–3"	5'4"–5'7"	2⅜"–2⅝"
6'0"–6'3"	2¾"–3⅛"	5'8"–5'11"	2⅜"–2⅝"
6'4"	2⅞"–3¼"	6'0"	2½"–2¾"

Source: Metropolitan Life Insurance Co., 1983.

Appendix Table 27. SUGGESTED DESIRABLE WEIGHTS FOR HEIGHTS AND RANGES OF ADULT MALES AND FEMALES

	METRIC				NONMETRIC				
	MEN Weight (kg.)*		WOMEN Weight (kg.)*			MEN Weight (lb.)*		WOMEN Weight (lb.)*	
HEIGHT (m.)	Average	Acceptable Weight	Average	Acceptable Weight	HEIGHT (ft., in.)	Average	Acceptable Weight	Average	Acceptable Weight
1.45			46.0	42–53	4 10				
1.48			46.5	42–54	4 11			102	92–119
1.50			47.0	43–55	5 0			104	94–122
1.52			48.5	44–57	5 1			107	96–125
1.54			49.5	44–58	5 2	123	112–141	110	99–128
1.56			50.4	45–58	5 3	127	115–144	113	102–131
1.58	55.8	51–64	51.3	46–59	5 4	130	118–148	116	105–134
1.60	57.6	52–65	52.6	48–61	5 5	133	121–152	120	108–138
1.62	58.6	53–66	54.0	49–62	5 6	136	124–156	123	111–142
1.64	59.6	54–67	55.4	50–64	5 7	140	128–161	128	114–146
1.66	60.6	55–69	56.8	51–65	5 8	145	132–166	132	118–150
1.68	61.7	56–71	58.1	52–66	5 9	149	136–170	136	122–154
1.70	63.5	58–73	60.0	53–67	5 10	154	140–174	140	126–158
1.72	65.0	59–74	61.3	55–69	5 11	158	144–179	144	130–163
1.74	66.5	60–75	62.6	56–70	6 0	162	148–184	148	134–168
1.76	68.0	62–77	64.0	58–72	6 1	166	152–189	152	138–173
1.78	69.4	64–79	65.3	59–74	6 2	171	156–194		
1.80	71.0	65–80			6 3	176	160–199		
1.82	72.6	66–82			6 4	181	164–204		
1.84	74.2	67–84							
1.86	75.8	69–86							
1.88	77.6	71–88							
1.90	79.3	73–90							
1.92	81.0	75–93							

*Height without shoes, weight without clothes.

From Bray, G. A. (ed.): Obesity in America. NIH Publication No. 79–359, U.S. Dept. of Health, Education and Welfare, Public Health Service, National Institutes of Health. Washington, D.C., U.S. Government Printing Office, 1979. Adapted from the recommendations of the Fogarty Center Conference on Obesity, 1973.

Appendix 28.   ARM ANTHROPOMETRY FOR CHILDREN

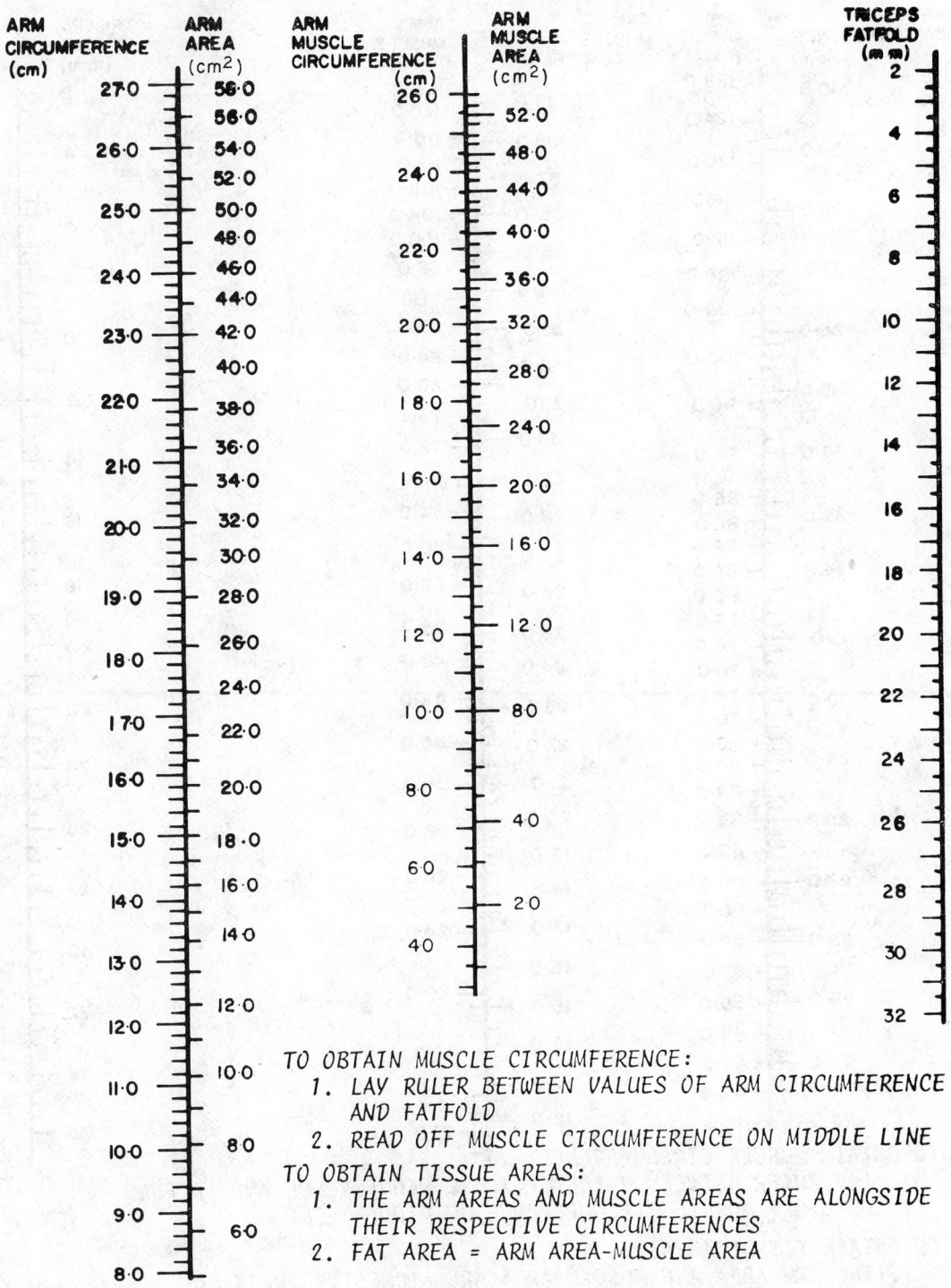

TO OBTAIN MUSCLE CIRCUMFERENCE:
1. LAY RULER BETWEEN VALUES OF ARM CIRCUMFERENCE AND FATFOLD
2. READ OFF MUSCLE CIRCUMFERENCE ON MIDDLE LINE

TO OBTAIN TISSUE AREAS:
1. THE ARM AREAS AND MUSCLE AREAS ARE ALONGSIDE THEIR RESPECTIVE CIRCUMFERENCES
2. FAT AREA = ARM AREA-MUSCLE AREA

(From: Gurney, J. M., and Jelliffe, D. B.: Arm anthropometry in nutritional assessment: nomogram for rapid calculation of muscle circumference and cross-sectional muscle fat areas. Am. J. Clin. Nutr., 26:913, 1973.)

Appendix 29.   ARM ANTHROPOMETRY FOR ADULTS

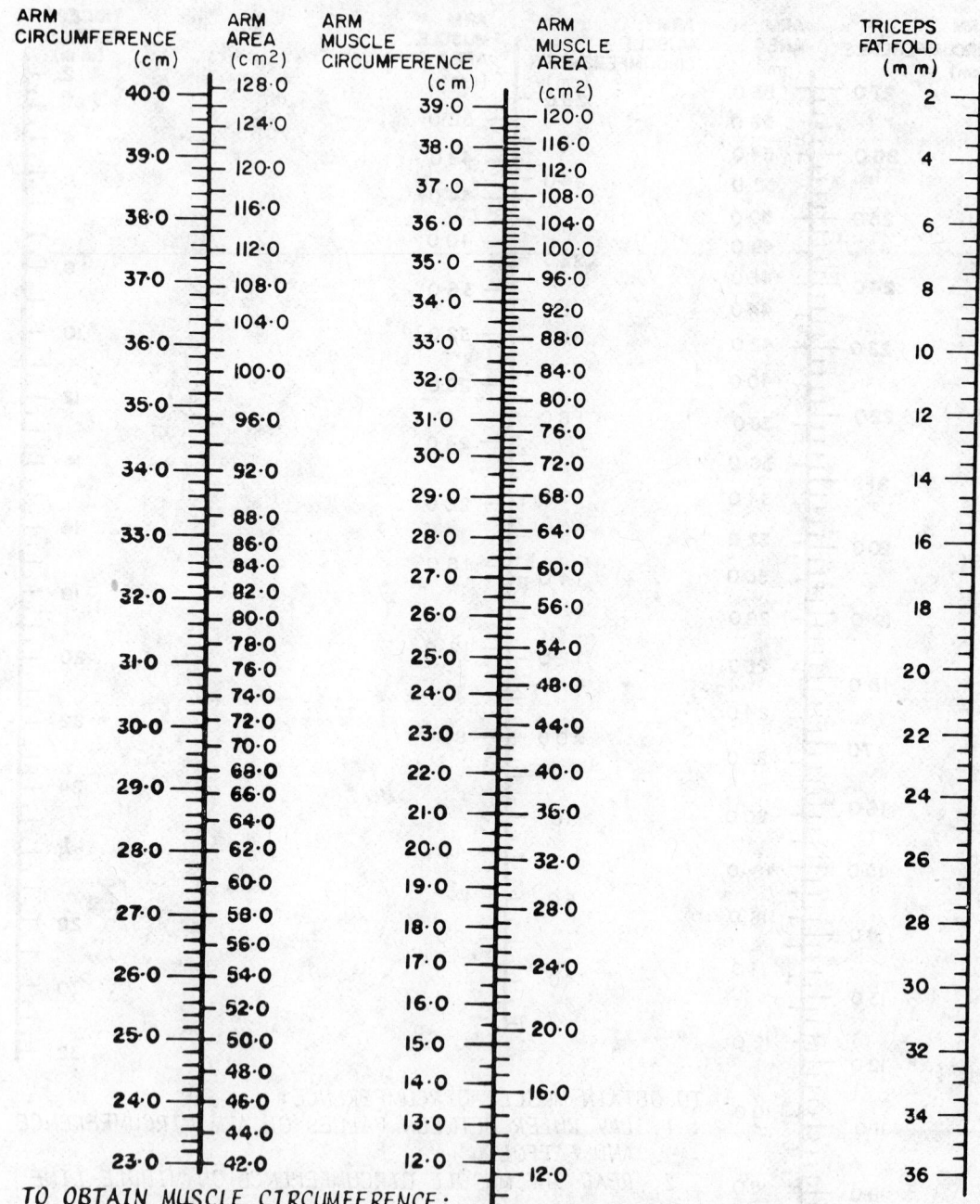

TO OBTAIN MUSCLE CIRCUMFERENCE:
   1. LAY RULER BETWEEN VALUE OF ARM CIRCUMFERENCE AND FATFOLD
   2. READ OFF MUSCLE CIRCUMFERENCE ON MIDDLE LINE

TO OBTAIN TISSUE AREAS:
   1. THE ARM AREA AND MUSCLE AREA ARE ALONGSIDE THEIR
      RESPECTIVE CIRCUMFERENCES
   2. FAT AREA = ARM AREA-MUSCLE AREA

(From: Gurney, J. M., and Jelliffe, D. B.: Arm anthropometry in nutritional assessment: nomogram for rapid calculation of muscle circumference and cross-sectional muscle fat areas. Am. J. Clin. Nutr., *26*:912, 1973.)

Appendix Table 30.   TRICEPS SKINFOLD THICKNESS: YOUTH, 1–17 YEARS, UNITED STATES: 1971–1974

Race and Age in Years	Number in Sample	Estimated Population in Thousands	Mean	Standard Deviation	Percentile								
					5th	10th	15th	25th	50th	75th	85th	90th	95th

Triceps Skinfold in Millimeters

MALES

Race and Age in Years	Number in Sample	Estimated Population in Thousands	Mean	Standard Deviation	5th	10th	15th	25th	50th	75th	85th	90th	95th
WHITE													
1	211	1,402	10.7	3.0	7.0	7.0	7.5	8.0	10.0	12.0	14.0	15.0	16.5
2	217	1,461	9.9	2.6	6.0	6.5	7.0	8.0	10.0	12.0	12.5	13.0	14.7
3	226	1,536	9.9	2.6	6.5	7.0	7.0	8.0	10.0	11.0	12.5	13.5	14.5
4	229	1,547	9.6	2.4	6.0	7.0	7.0	8.0	10.0	11.0	12.0	12.5	14.0
5	207	1,319	9.8	3.2	6.0	6.5	7.0	7.5	9.0	11.0	12.5	13.5	15.0
6	126	1,343	8.9	3.1	5.5	5.6	6.0	7.0	9.0	10.0	12.0	12.5	14.0
7	125	1,718	9.1	3.5	5.0	6.0	6.0	7.0	8.0	10.5	12.0	13.5	17.0
8	116	1,644	9.1	3.3	5.0	5.5	6.0	7.0	8.5	10.5	12.0	13.0	16.0
9	117	1,636	11.1	4.8	5.5	6.5	6.5	7.5	10.0	14.0	17.0	17.0	19.0
10	148	1,909	11.1	4.2	5.5	6.0	7.0	8.0	10.0	14.0	15.5	17.0	19.5
11	132	1,823	12.5	6.5	6.0	6.0	7.0	8.0	10.0	15.0	19.0	20.5	24.5
12	152	1,970	12.4	6.1	6.0	6.0	7.0	8.5	11.0	14.0	18.0	21.0	27.0
13	129	1,697	11.7	6.7	5.0	5.0	6.0	7.0	10.0	14.0	19.0	22.0	25.5
14	134	1,730	10.9	6.4	4.0	5.0	6.0	7.0	9.0	13.0	18.0	20.0	24.0
15	124	1,728	10.2	6.1	4.0	5.0	6.0	6.0	8.0	12.0	15.0	19.0	24.0
16	128	1,752	10.1	5.2	4.0	5.0	5.0	6.5	9.0	12.5	15.0	17.0	22.0
17	139	1,831	9.3	5.4	4.5	5.0	5.5	6.0	7.5	11.0	13.0	15.0	19.0
BLACK													
1	72	280	9.4	3.4	4.5	6.0	7.0	8.0	8.0	11.0	12.0	13.0	15.0
2	77	267	10.1	3.2	4.5	6.0	6.5	8.0	10.0	12.0	14.0	15.0	15.0
3	72	212	9.1	2.6	6.0	6.5	6.5	7.0	9.0	10.5	12.0	12.0	13.0
4	74	260	8.0	2.6	5.0	5.0	5.0	6.5	7.0	9.0	10.0	10.5	15.0
5	64	226	7.7	3.4	4.5	5.0	5.0	5.0	7.0	9.0	10.0	12.0	15.5
6	52	321	7.1	1.8	4.0	4.0	5.0	6.0	7.0	8.0	9.0	9.0	9.0
7	38	253	7.5	3.2	4.0	4.0	4.0	5.0	6.5	9.0	11.5	13.0	15.0
8	33	203	7.8	3.4	4.0	5.0	5.0	6.0	6.5	10.0	11.0	11.0	12.5
9	52	383	8.2	3.9	3.5	4.0	4.5	6.0	7.0	8.0	12.0	13.0	18.0
10	33	251	9.1	5.3	5.0	5.0	6.0	6.0	7.5	10.0	13.0	15.0	20.0
11	43	313	8.0	5.0	4.0	4.0	5.0	5.0	6.0	8.5	11.0	12.0	15.0
12	47	316	9.4	7.0	4.0	4.0	4.5	6.0	7.5	10.7	11.0	15.0	24.0
13	45	281	8.2	4.4	4.0	5.0	5.0	5.0	7.0	8.5	11.0	19.0	19.0
14	39	282	6.6	2.6	3.5	3.5	3.5	5.0	6.5	7.0	8.0	9.0	12.0
15	43	310	8.9	6.1	4.0	4.5	5.0	5.0	6.5	9.0	10.0	21.0	21.0
16	41	267	7.2	4.8	4.0	4.0	4.0	5.0	6.0	7.5	8.0	11.0	15.0
17	35	235	8.7	5.8	3.5	3.5	5.0	5.0	7.0	10.5	12.0	12.0	23.2

FEMALES

Race and Age in Years	Number in Sample	Estimated Population in Thousands	Mean	Standard Deviation	5th	10th	15th	25th	50th	75th	85th	90th	95th
WHITE													
1	189	1,328	10.2	2.8	6.0	7.0	7.0	8.0	10.0	12.0	13.0	13.5	15.5
2	203	1,434	10.6	2.6	7.0	7.5	8.0	9.0	10.0	12.0	13.5	14.0	15.0
3	211	1,438	11.1	2.6	7.0	8.0	8.5	9.0	11.0	13.0	13.5	14.0	15.0
4	204	1,339	10.8	2.6	7.5	8.0	8.0	9.0	10.5	12.0	13.0	14.5	16.0
5	224	1,416	10.7	3.7	6.0	7.0	8.0	8.5	10.0	12.0	13.0	15.0	17.5
6	125	1,445	10.6	3.3	6.5	7.0	7.5	8.0	10.5	12.0	13.0	14.0	16.0
7	122	1,507	10.9	4.2	4.0	6.0	7.0	8.0	11.0	12.0	15.0	15.5	17.5
8	117	1,507	12.4	4.7	7.0	8.0	8.0	9.0	11.5	15.0	16.5	18.0	22.0
9	129	1,751	13.6	4.6	7.5	8.0	9.0	10.0	13.0	16.0	18.0	20.0	22.0
10	148	1,855	13.4	4.8	7.5	8.0	8.5	10.0	12.5	15.5	19.0	20.0	23.0
11	122	1,569	14.9	6.1	8.0	8.5	9.0	10.0	13.0	17.5	20.5	24.5	28.5
12	128	1,506	15.2	5.6	8.0	9.0	10.0	11.0	14.0	18.5	20.0	23.0	26.0
13	153	1,886	16.2	6.8	7.0	8.0	10.0	11.5	15.0	20.0	24.0	25.0	28.5
14	132	1,731	17.8	7.3	9.0	9.5	10.5	13.0	16.7	21.0	24.0	28.5	33.0
15	125	1,752	17.7	6.7	9.0	10.5	11.0	13.0	17.0	21.0	24.0	25.0	28.5
16	141	1,933	18.2	6.6	10.0	10.5	12.5	14.0	17.0	21.0	24.0	26.0	32.1
17	117	1,549	19.8	8.0	10.0	12.0	12.5	13.5	19.0	24.0	26.5	29.5	35.0

From the National Center for Health Statistics, Department of Health and Human Services. Health and Nutrition Examination Survey I, 1971–1974.

Table continued on the following page

Appendix Table 30. TRICEPS SKINFOLD THICKNESS: YOUTH, 1–17 YEARS, UNITED STATES: 1971–1974 (*Continued*)

Race and Age in Years	Number in Sample	Estimated Population in Thousands	Mean	Standard Deviation	Percentile								
					5th	10th	15th	25th	50th	75th	85th	90th	95th

Triceps Skinfold in Millimeters

FEMALES

BLACK

1	73	257	10.0	3.0	5.5	5.5	7.0	8.0	10.0	12.0	13.0	14.0	15.0
2	66	261	10.0	2.3	7.0	8.0	8.0	8.0	10.0	11.0	12.0	14.0	15.5
3	78	245	9.7	2.9	6.0	7.0	7.0	8.0	10.0	11.0	12.0	13.0	14.0
4	73	246	8.8	2.7	5.0	6.0	7.0	7.0	8.0	10.5	12.0	13.0	14.0
5	88	265	9.4	3.9	5.0	5.0	6.5	7.0	8.0	10.0	12.0	13.5	17.0
6	50	336	9.0	3.1	5.5	6.0	6.0	8.0	8.0	10.0	11.5	12.0	13.0
7	46	241	10.1	4.0	5.0	6.0	7.0	7.5	9.0	11.0	17.5	18.0	18.0
8	35	293	11.5	5.1	5.0	6.5	7.0	8.0	10.0	13.5	18.0	18.0	23.0
9	41	247	10.2	5.1	5.5	6.0	6.0	6.5	8.0	12.0	18.0	18.0	20.0
10	48	303	11.7	5.6	6.5	6.5	7.0	7.5	10.0	16.0	18.0	19.0	24.0
11	42	315	12.7	6.4	4.0	5.0	6.5	7.5	10.0	18.0	22.0	23.0	23.0
12	47	284	13.6	7.6	5.5	6.0	6.0	7.5	12.0	17.0	22.0	25.0	30.0
13	44	287	16.1	7.0	7.0	8.5	10.0	11.0	14.0	18.0	24.0	24.0	33.5
14	50	265	15.9	6.7	8.0	8.0	9.0	10.5	14.0	20.5	24.0	24.5	24.5
15	46	411	14.0	7.6	6.5	6.5	8.0	10.0	12.5	16.0	16.5	20.0	32.8
16	33	203	18.9	8.0	8.0	8.0	10.0	12.0	19.0	24.0	24.5	33.0	33.1
17	39	239	16.9	6.6	7.5	9.0	11.0	12.0	14.5	20.0	24.0	28.0	31.0

Appendix Table 31. TRICEPS SKINFOLD THICKNESS: ADULTS, UNITED STATES: 1971–1974

Race and Age in Years	Number in Sample	Estimated Population in Thousands	Mean	Standard Deviation	Percentile								
					5th	10th	15th	25th	50th	75th	85th	90th	95th

Triceps Skinfold in Millimeters

MALES

Race and Age in Years	Number in Sample	Estimated Population in Thousands	Mean	Standard Deviation	5th	10th	15th	25th	50th	75th	85th	90th	95th
WHITE	4,344	54,694	12.2	5.8	5.0	6.0	6.5	8.0	11.0	15.0	18.0	20.0	23.0
18–19	203	3,206	11.3	5.9	5.0	5.5	6.0	7.0	9.0	15.0	18.0	20.0	23.0
20–24	423	7,094	11.5	6.0	4.0	5.0	6.0	7.0	10.0	15.0	18.0	21.0	23.0
25–34	672	11,594	12.7	6.2	5.0	6.0	6.5	8.0	12.0	16.0	18.5	21.0	24.0
35–44	569	9,516	12.6	5.4	5.0	6.0	7.0	9.0	12.0	15.5	17.5	20.0	23.0
45–54	628	10,039	12.6	5.9	5.5	6.5	7.0	8.5	11.0	15.0	18.0	20.0	26.0
55–64	505	8,275	11.7	5.0	5.0	6.0	7.0	8.0	11.0	14.0	16.5	18.0	21.0
65–74	1,344	4,970	12.0	5.4	5.0	6.0	7.0	8.0	11.0	15.0	17.0	19.0	22.0
BLACK	847	5,753	10.6	7.0	3.5	4.0	4.5	6.0	8.5	13.0	16.0	20.0	23.0
18–19	52	404	8.9	6.7	2.0	4.0	5.0	5.1	7.0	8.0	12.0	21.0	24.0
20–24	80	866	10.0	7.9	3.0	4.0	4.0	6.0	8.0	11.0	13.0	18.0	24.0
25–34	119	1,232	11.8	8.4	4.0	4.0	4.0	5.0	10.0	15.0	20.0	22.0	23.0
35–44	87	1,005	11.3	6.5	4.0	4.5	5.0	7.0	10.0	14.0	17.0	18.4	22.0
45–54	130	1,057	10.0	5.1	4.0	4.0	5.0	6.0	10.0	12.5	14.0	16.0	20.0
55–64	85	703	10.7	7.2	3.0	4.0	4.5	5.0	8.0	14.0	20.0	22.0	26.0
65–74	294	486	9.7	5.4	4.0	4.5	5.0	6.0	9.0	12.0	14.0	15.0	19.5

FEMALES

Race and Age in Years	Number in Sample	Estimated Population in Thousands	Mean	Standard Deviation	5th	10th	15th	25th	50th	75th	85th	90th	95th
WHITE	6,757	59,923	22.9	8.1	11.0	13.0	14.5	17.0	22.0	28.0	31.0	34.0	37.0
18–19	208	3,159	18.9	6.6	9.5	12.0	13.0	14.5	18.0	22.5	24.0	26.5	33.5
20–24	956	7,972	19.8	7.7	10.0	11.0	12.0	14.0	19.0	24.0	27.9	30.5	34.0
25–34	1,539	12,161	21.8	8.0	11.0	12.5	14.0	16.0	20.5	26.0	30.0	33.0	36.5
35–44	1,302	10,111	23.7	8.3	12.0	14.0	15.9	18.0	22.5	29.0	32.0	35.1	38.5
45–54	705	10,879	25.3	8.1	13.0	15.0	17.0	20.0	25.0	30.0	33.5	35.5	39.5
55–64	551	9,037	24.6	7.9	11.5	14.5	16.0	19.0	24.0	30.0	33.0	34.1	38.0
65–74	1,496	6,603	23.3	7.3	12.0	14.0	16.0	18.0	23.0	28.0	31.0	33.0	35.5
BLACK	1,557	7,302	23.7	10.3	9.0	11.0	12.0	15.5	23.0	30.5	34.0	36.6	41.0
18–19	70	504	16.2	7.3	8.0	9.0	9.0	11.5	14.0	20.0	25.0	29.0	32.0
20–24	259	1,073	19.3	8.7	9.0	10.0	11.5	12.5	17.0	24.5	28.6	32.0	36.0
25–34	335	1,646	22.5	9.6	8.5	10.0	12.0	14.0	22.0	30.0	32.6	34.1	40.0
35–44	334	1,318	25.8	9.2	11.5	13.0	16.0	20.0	25.5	32.0	35.0	36.5	41.0
45–54	126	1,237	26.8	9.8	12.0	14.0	17.0	20.0	26.0	34.0	37.1	40.0	42.2
55–64	115	871	28.2	12.9	10.0	11.0	13.0	19.0	28.0	34.0	40.0	45.0	51.5
65–74	318	652	23.8	9.0	7.5	11.5	15.0	17.5	24.0	30.0	32.2	35.5	40.0

From the National Center for Health Statistics, Department of Health and Human Services, Health and Nutrition Examination Survey I, 1971–1974.

Appendix Table 32. PERCENTILES FOR UPPER ARM CIRCUMFERENCE AND ESTIMATED UPPER ARM MUSCLE CIRCUMFERENCE OF WHITES IN THE UNITED STATES HEALTH AND NUTRITION EXAMINATION SURVEY I, 1971–1974 *

Age group	Arm circumference (mm)							Arm muscle circumference (mm)						
	5	10	25	50	75	90	95	5	10	25	50	75	90	95
Males														
1–1.9	142	146	150	159	170	176	183	110	113	119	127	135	144	147
2–2.9	141	145	153	162	170	178	185	111	114	122	130	140	146	150
3–3.9	150	153	160	167	175	184	190	117	123	131	137	143	148	153
4–4.9	149	154	162	171	180	186	192	123	126	133	141	148	156	159
5–5.9	153	160	167	175	185	195	204	128	133	140	147	154	162	169
6–6.9	155	159	167	179	188	209	228	131	135	142	151	161	170	177
7–7.9	162	167	177	187	201	223	230	137	139	151	160	168	177	190
8–8.9	162	170	177	190	202	220	245	140	145	154	162	170	182	187
9–9.9	175	178	187	200	217	249	257	151	154	161	170	183	196	202
10–10.9	181	184	196	210	231	262	274	156	160	166	180	191	209	221
11–11.9	186	190	202	223	244	261	280	159	165	173	183	195	205	230
12–12.9	193	200	214	232	254	282	303	167	171	182	195	210	223	241
13–13.9	194	211	228	247	263	286	301	172	179	196	211	226	238	245
14–14.9	220	226	237	253	283	303	322	189	199	212	223	240	260	264
15–15.9	222	229	244	264	284	311	320	199	204	218	237	254	266	272
16–16.9	244	248	262	278	303	324	343	213	225	234	249	269	287	296
17–17.9	246	253	267	285	308	336	347	224	231	245	258	273	294	312
18–18.9	245	260	276	297	321	353	379	226	237	252	264	283	298	324
19–24.9	262	272	288	308	331	355	372	238	245	257	273	289	309	321
25–34.9	271	282	300	319	342	362	375	243	250	264	279	298	314	326
35–44.9	278	287	305	326	345	363	374	247	255	269	286	302	318	327
45–54.9	267	281	301	322	342	362	376	239	249	265	281	300	315	326
55–64.9	258	273	296	317	336	355	369	236	245	260	278	295	310	320
65–74.9	248	263	285	307	325	344	355	223	235	251	268	284	298	306
Females														
1–1.9	138	142	148	156	164	172	177	105	111	117	124	132	139	143
2–2.9	142	145	152	160	167	176	184	111	114	119	126	133	142	147
3–3.9	143	150	158	167	175	183	189	113	119	124	132	140	146	152
4–4.9	149	154	160	169	177	184	191	115	121	128	136	144	152	157
5–5.9	153	157	165	175	185	203	211	125	128	134	142	151	159	165
6–6.9	156	162	170	176	187	204	211	130	133	138	145	154	166	171
7–7.9	164	167	174	183	199	216	231	129	135	142	151	160	171	176
8–8.9	168	172	183	195	214	247	261	138	140	151	160	171	183	194
9–9.9	178	182	194	211	224	251	260	147	150	158	167	180	194	198
10–10.9	174	182	193	210	228	251	265	148	150	159	170	180	190	197
11–11.9	185	194	208	224	248	276	303	150	158	171	181	196	217	223
12–12.9	194	203	216	237	256	282	294	162	166	180	191	201	214	220
13–13.9	202	211	223	243	271	301	338	169	175	183	198	211	226	240
14–14.9	214	223	237	252	272	304	322	174	179	190	201	216	232	247
15–15.9	208	221	239	254	279	300	322	175	178	189	202	215	228	244
16–16.9	218	224	241	258	283	318	334	170	180	190	202	216	234	249
17–17.9	220	227	241	264	295	324	350	175	183	194	205	221	239	257
18–18.9	222	227	241	258	281	312	325	174	179	191	202	215	237	245
19–24.9	221	230	247	265	290	319	345	179	185	195	207	221	236	249
25–34.9	233	240	256	277	304	342	368	183	188	199	212	228	246	264
35–44.9	241	251	267	290	317	356	378	186	192	205	218	236	257	272
45–54.9	242	256	274	299	328	362	384	187	193	206	220	238	260	274
55–64.9	243	257	280	303	335	367	385	187	196	209	225	244	266	280
65–74.9	240	252	274	299	326	356	373	185	195	208	225	244	264	279

*Percentiles are not yet available for the black population for upper arm circumference or arm muscle circumference.

From Frisancho, A.R.: New norms of upper limb fat and muscle areas for assessment of nutritional status. Am. J. Clin. Nutri., *34*:2540, 1981.

Appendix Table 33. PERCENTILES FOR ESTIMATES OF UPPER ARM FAT AREA AND UPPER ARM MUSCLE AREA OF WHITES IN THE UNITED STATES HEALTH AND NUTRITION EXAMINATION SURVEY I, 1971 TO 1974 *

Age group	Arm muscle area percentiles (mm²)							Arm fat area percentiles (mm²)						
	5	10	25	50	75	90	95	5	10	25	50	75	90	95
Males														
1–1.9	956	1014	1133	1278	1447	1644	1720	452	486	590	741	895	1036	1176
2–2.9	973	1040	1190	1345	1557	1690	1787	434	504	578	737	871	1044	1148
3–3.9	1095	1201	1357	1484	1618	1750	1853	464	519	590	736	868	1071	1151
4–4.9	1207	1264	1408	1579	1747	1926	2008	428	494	598	722	859	989	1085
5–5.9	1298	1411	1550	1720	1884	2089	2285	446	488	582	713	914	1176	1299
6–6.9	1360	1447	1605	1815	2056	2297	2493	371	446	539	678	896	1115	1519
7–7.9	1497	1548	1808	2027	2246	2494	2886	423	473	574	758	1011	1393	1511
8–8.9	1550	1664	1895	2089	2296	2628	2788	410	460	588	725	1003	1248	1558
9–9.9	1811	1884	2067	2288	2657	3053	3257	485	527	635	859	1252	1864	2081
10–10.9	1930	2027	2182	2575	2903	3486	3882	523	543	738	982	1376	1906	2609
11–11.9	2016	2156	2382	2670	3022	3359	4226	536	595	754	1148	1710	2348	2574
12–12.9	2216	2339	2649	3022	3496	3968	4640	554	650	874	1172	1558	2536	3580
13–13.9	2363	2546	3044	3553	4081	4502	4794	475	570	812	1096	1702	2744	3322
14–14.9	2830	3147	3586	3963	4575	5368	5530	453	563	786	1082	1608	2746	3508
15–15.9	3138	3317	3788	4481	5134	5631	5900	521	595	690	931	1423	2434	3100
16–16.9	3625	4044	4352	4951	5753	6576	6980	542	593	844	1078	1746	2280	3041
17–17.9	3998	4252	4777	5286	5950	6886	7726	598	698	827	1096	1636	2407	2888
18–18.9	4070	4481	5066	5552	6374	7067	8355	560	665	860	1264	1947	3302	3928
19–24.9	4508	4777	5274	5913	6660	7606	8200	594	743	963	1406	2231	3098	3652
25–34.9	4694	4963	5541	6214	7067	7847	8436	675	831	1174	1752	2459	3246	3786
35–44.9	4844	5181	5740	6490	7265	8034	8488	703	851	1310	1792	2463	3098	3624
45–54.9	4546	4946	5589	6297	7142	7918	8458	749	922	1254	1741	2359	3245	3928
55–64.9	4422	4783	5381	6144	6919	7670	8149	658	839	1166	1645	2236	2976	3466
65–74.9	3973	4411	5031	5716	6432	7074	7453	573	753	1122	1621	2199	2876	3327
Females														
1–1.9	885	973	1084	1221	1378	1535	1621	401	466	578	706	847	1022	1140
2–2.9	973	1029	1119	1269	1405	1595	1727	469	526	642	747	894	1061	1173
3–3.9	1014	1133	1227	1396	1563	1690	1846	473	529	656	822	967	1106	1158
4–4.9	1058	1171	1313	1475	1644	1832	1958	490	541	654	766	907	1109	1236
5–5.9	1238	1301	1423	1598	1825	2012	2159	470	529	647	812	991	1330	1536
6–6.9	1354	1414	1513	1683	1877	2182	2323	464	508	638	827	1009	1263	1436
7–7.9	1330	1441	1602	1815	2045	2332	2469	491	560	706	920	1135	1407	1644
8–8.9	1513	1566	1808	2034	2327	2657	2996	527	634	769	1042	1383	1872	2482
9–9.9	1723	1788	1976	2227	2571	2987	3112	642	690	933	1219	1584	2171	2524
10–10.9	1740	1784	2019	2296	2583	2873	3093	616	702	842	1141	1608	2500	3005
11–11.9	1784	1987	2316	2612	3071	3739	3953	707	802	1015	1301	1942	2730	3690
12–12.9	2092	2182	2579	2904	3225	3655	3847	782	854	1090	1511	2056	2666	3369
13–13.9	2269	2426	2657	3130	3529	4081	4568	726	838	1219	1625	2374	3272	4150
14–14.9	2418	2562	2874	3220	3704	4294	4850	981	1043	1423	1818	2403	3250	3765
15–15.9	2426	2518	2847	3248	3689	4123	4756	839	1126	1396	1886	2544	3093	4195
16–16.9	2308	2567	2865	3248	3718	4353	4946	1126	1351	1663	2006	2598	3374	4236
17–17.9	2442	2674	2996	3336	3883	4552	5251	1042	1267	1463	2104	2977	3864	5159
18–18.9	2398	2538	2917	3243	3694	4461	4767	1003	1230	1616	2104	2617	3508	3733
19–24.9	2538	2728	3026	3406	3877	4439	4940	1046	1198	1596	2166	2959	4050	4896
25–34.9	2661	2826	3148	3573	4138	4806	5541	1173	1399	1841	2548	3512	4690	5560
35–44.9	2750	2948	3359	3783	4428	5240	5877	1336	1619	2158	2898	3932	5093	5847
45–54.9	2784	2956	3378	3858	4520	5375	5964	1459	1803	2447	3244	4229	5416	6140
55–64.9	2784	3063	3477	4045	4750	5632	6247	1345	1879	2520	3369	4360	5276	6152
65–74.9	2737	3018	3444	4019	4739	5566	6214	1363	1681	2266	3063	3943	4914	5530

*Percentiles are not yet available for the black population for arm fat areas

From Frisancho, A.R.: New norms of upper limb fat and muscle areas for assessment of nutritional status. Am. J. Clin. Nutri., *34*:2540, 1981.

Appendix Table 34.   PERCENTAGE OF BODY FAT BASED ON FOUR SKINFOLD MEASUREMENTS *

Skinfolds (mm)	Males (age in years)				Females (age in years)			
	17–29	30–39	40–49	50+	16–29	30–39	40–49	50+
15	4·8	—	—	—	10·5	—	—	—
20	8·1	12·2	12·2	12·6	14·1	17·0	19·8	21·4
25	10·5	14·2	15·0	15·6	16·8	19·4	22·2	24·0
30	12·9	16·2	17·7	18·6	19·5	21·8	24·5	26·6
35	14·7	17·7	19·6	20·8	21·5	23·7	26·4	28·5
40	16·4	19·2	21·4	22·9	23·4	25·5	28·2	30·3
45	17·7	20·4	23·0	24·7	25·0	26·9	29·6	31·9
50	19·0	21·5	24·6	26·5	26·5	28·2	31·0	33·4
55	20·1	22·5	25·9	27·9	27·8	29·4	32·1	34·6
60	21·2	23·5	27·1	29·2	29·1	30·6	33·2	35·7
65	22·2	24·3	28·2	30·4	30·2	31·6	34·1	36·7
70	23·1	25·1	29·3	31·6	31·2	32·5	35·0	37·7
75	24·0	25·9	30·3	32·7	32·2	33·4	35·9	38·7
80	24·8	26·6	31·2	33·8	33·1	34·3	36·7	39·6
85	25·5	27·2	32·1	34·8	34·0	35·1	37·5	40·4
90	26·2	27·8	33·0	35·8	34·8	35·8	38·3	41·2
95	26·9	28·4	33·7	36·6	35·6	36·5	39·0	41·9
100	27·6	29·0	34·4	37·4	36·4	37·2	39·7	42·6
105	28·2	29·6	35·1	38·2	37·1	37·9	40·4	43·3
110	28·8	30·1	35·8	39·0	37·8	38·6	41·0	43·9
115	29·4	30·6	36·4	39·7	38·4	39·1	41·5	44·5
120	30·0	31·1	37·0	40·4	39·0	39·6	42·0	45·1
125	30·5	31·5	37·6	41·1	39·6	40·1	42·5	45·7
130	31·0	31·9	38·2	41·8	40·2	40·6	43·0	46·2
135	31·5	32·3	38·7	42·4	40·8	41·1	43·5	46·7
140	32·0	32·7	39·2	43·0	41·3	41·6	44·0	47·2
145	32·5	33·1	39·7	43·6	41·8	42·1	44·5	47·7
150	32·9	33·5	40·2	44·1	42·3	42·6	45·0	48·2
155	33·3	33·9	40·7	44·6	42·8	43·1	45·4	48·7
160	33·7	34·3	41·2	45·1	43·3	43·6	45·8	49·2
165	34·1	34·6	41·6	45·6	43·7	44·0	46·2	49·6
170	34·5	34·8	42·0	46·1	44·1	44·4	46·6	50·0
175	34·9	—	—	—	—	44·8	47·0	50·4
180	35·3	—	—	—	—	45·2	47·4	50·8
185	35·6	—	—	—	—	45·6	47·8	51·2
190	35·9	—	—	—	—	45·9	48·2	51·6
195	—	—	—	—	—	46·2	48·5	52·0
200	—	—	—	—	—	46·5	48·8	52·4
205	—	—	—	—	—	—	49·1	52·7
210	—	—	—	—	—	—	49·4	53·0

*Measurements made on the right side of the body, using biceps, triceps, subscapular and suprailiac skinfolds.
From Durnin, J. V. G. A., and Wormersley, J.: Body fat assessed from total body density and its estimation from skinfold thickness: measurements on 481 men and women aged from 16–72 years. Br. J. Nutr., *32*:77, 1974.

Appendix Table 35. EXPECTED 24-HR. URINE CREATININE EXCRETION OF NORMAL ADULT MEN AND WOMEN OF DIFFERENT HEIGHTS *

MEN[†]					WOMEN				
Height		Ideal Weight	Creatinine Coefficient	24-hr. Urine Creatinine	Height		Ideal Weight	Creatinine Coefficient	24-hr. Urine Creatinine
in.	cm.	kg.	mg./kg.	gm.	in.	cm.	kg.	mg./kg.	gm.
62	157.5	56.0	23	1.29	58	147.3	46.0	17	0.782
63	160.0	57.6		1.32	59	149.9	47.2		0.802
64	162.5	59.0		1.36	60	152.4	48.6		0.826
65	165.1	60.3		1.39	61	154.9	49.9		0.848
66	167.6	62.0		1.43	62	157.5	51.3		0.872
67	170.2	63.8		1.47	63	160.0	52.6		0.894
68	172.7	65.8		1.51	64	162.6	54.3		0.923
69	175.3	67.6		1.55	65	165.1	55.9		0.950
70	177.8	69.4		1.60	66	167.6	57.8		0.983
71	180.3	71.4		1.64	67	170.2	59.6		1.01
72	182.9	73.5		1.69	68	172.7	61.5		1.04
73	185.4	75.6		1.74	69	175.3	63.3		1.08
74	188.0	77.6		1.78	70	177.8	65.1		1.11
75	190.5	79.6		1.83	71	180.3	66.9		1.14
76	193.0	82.2		1.89	72	182.9	68.7		1.17

*Creatinine:height index is defined as the 24-hr. creatinine excretion of the patient divided by the expected 24-hr. creatinine excretion of a normal adult of the same height.

[†]From Bistrian, B. R., et al.: Therapeutic index of nutritional depletion in hospitalized patients. Surg. Gynecol. Obstet., *141*:512, 1973.

From Bistrian, B.R.: Nutritional assessment and therapy of protein-calorie malnutrition in the hospital. J. Am. Diet. Assoc., *71*:393, 1977.

Appendix Table 36. GUIDELINES FOR EVALUATION OF BIOCHEMICAL MEASUREMENTS OF NUTRITIONAL STATUS

NUTRIENT	DETERMINATION	CLASSIFICATION CATEGORY		
		LESS THAN ACCEPTABLE		
		Deficient	Low	ACCEPTABLE[a]
Energy/protein	Total lymphocyte count (number per cubic mm.) for person 21+ years of age	< 2000 per mm.³ [b]		1500–4000 per mm.³ average[c] 20–53% of white blood cells (WBC)
	Serum total protein (gm./100 ml.)[d]			
	0–11 mo.		< 5.0	≥ 5.0
	1–5 yr.		< 5.5	≥ 5.5
	6–17 yr.		< 6.0	≥ 6.0
	Adult	< 6.0	6.0–6.4	≥ 6.5
	Pregnant, 2nd and 3rd trimester	< 5.5	5.5–5.9	≥ 6.0
	Serum albumin (gm./100 ml.)[d]			
	0–11 mo.		< 2.5	≥ 2.5
	1–5 yr.		< 3.0	≥ 3.0
	6–17 yr.		< 3.5	≥ 3.5
	Adult	< 3.0	3.0–3.4	≥ 3.5
	Pregnant, 1st trimester	< 3.0	3.0–3.9	≥ 4.0
	Pregnant, 2nd and 3rd trimester	< 3.0	3.0–3.4	≥ 3.5
	Serum thyroxine–binding prealbumin (mg./100 ml.)			20–50[e]
	Serum transferrin (mg./100 ml.) can be estimated from total iron binding capacity (TIBC) by following formula: transferrin (mg./100 ml.) = $\dfrac{\text{TIBC } (\mu g./100 \text{ ml.})}{1.45}$			180–260[f]
	Serum retinol-binding protein (μg./ml.)			37.2 ± 7.3[g]
Lipids	Serum triglycerides (mg./100 ml.)			
	1–19 yr.			≤ 150
	20 yr.+			≤ 150
	Serum cholesterol (mg./100 ml.)			
	1–19 yr.			≤ 180
	20 yr.+			≤ 240
Magnesium	Serum magnesium (mg./100 ml.)			1.8–3.0[h]
	Urinary magnesium (mg./100 ml.)			7.2–24
Zinc	Serum zinc (μg./100 ml.)			101–139 μg./ml.[h]
Phosphorus	Serum phosphorus (mg./100 ml.)			
	Infant			5.0–6.5[h]
	Child			4.0–7.0
	Adult			2.0–4.5
Iodine	Urinary iodine (μg./gm. creatinine[d])	> 25	25–49	≥ 50
	Protein-bound iodine (PBI) (μg./100 ml.)			4.0–8.0[e]
Iron	Hemoglobin (gm./100 ml.)[d]			
	6–23 mo.	< 9.0	9.0–9.9	≥ 10.0
	2–5 mo.	< 10	10.0–10.9	≥ 11.0
	6–12 yr.	< 10	10.0–11.4	≥ 11.5
	13–16 yr., male	< 12	12.0–12.9	≥ 13.0
	13–16 yr., female	< 10	10.0–11.4	≥ 11.5
	> 16 yr., male	< 12	12.0–13.9	≥ 14.0
	> 16 yr., female	< 10	10.0–11.9	≥ 12.0
	Pregnant, 2nd trimester	< 9.5	9.5–10.9	≥ 11.0
	Pregnant, 3rd trimester	< 9.0	9.0–10.4	≥ 10.5
	Hematocrit (%)[d]			
	6–23 mo.	< 28	28–30	≥ 31
	2–5 yr.	< 30	30–33	≥ 34
	6–12 yr.	< 30	30–35	≥ 36
	13–16 yr., male	< 37	37–39	≥ 40

Appendix Table 36. GUIDELINES FOR EVALUATION OF BIOCHEMICAL MEASUREMENTS OF NUTRITIONAL STATUS (*Continued*)

NUTRIENT	DETERMINATION	CLASSIFICATION CATEGORY LESS THAN ACCEPTABLE — Deficient	Low	ACCEPTABLE[a]
Iron (Continued)	Hematocrit (%)[d]			
	13–16 yr., female	< 31	31–35	≥ 36
	> 16 yr., male	< 37	37–43	≥ 44
	> 16 yr., female	< 31	31–37	≥ 38
	Pregnant, 2nd trimester	< 30	30–34	≥ 35
	Pregnant, 3rd trimester	< 30	30–32	≥ 33
	Serum iron (μg./100 ml.)[d]			
	0–5 mo.		—	—
	6–23 mo.		< 30	≥ 30
	2–5 yr.		< 40	≥ 40
	6–12 yr.		< 50	≥ 50
	> 12 yr., male		< 60	≥ 60
	> 12 yr., female		< 40	≥ 40
	Transferrin saturation (%)[d]			
	0–5 mo.		—	—
	6–23 mo.		< 15	≥ 15
	2–12 yr.		< 20	≥ 20
	> 12 yr., male		< 20	≥ 20
	> 12 yr., female		< 15	≥ 15
	Mean corpuscular volume (MCV) (femtoliters)			80–94[h]
	Mean corpuscular hemoglobin concentration (MCHC) (%)			32–36[h]
Vitamin A	Plasma carotene (μg./100 ml.)[d]		< 10	≥ 10
	0–5 mo.		< 10	≥ 10
	6–11 mo.		< 30	≥ 30
	1–17 yr.		< 40	≥ 40
	Adult	< 20[i]	20–39	≥ 40
	Pregnant, 2nd trimester		30–79	≥ 80
	Pregnant, 3rd trimester		40–79	≥ 80
	Plasma vitamin A (retinol) (μg./100 ml.)			
	0–5 mo.	< 10		≥ 20[c]
	6 mo.–17 yr.	< 20		≥ 30[c]
	Adult	< 10		≥ 20[c]
Vitamin D	Alkaline phosphatase (units/100 ml.)			
	Infant			5–15 Bodansky units
				14–42 King Armstrong units[c]
	Adult			3–5 Bodansky units
				8–14 King Armstrong units[c]
		Elevated in rickets, osteomalacia, and calcium deficiency		
		Decreased with excessive vitamin D and calcium		
Vitamin E	Serum tocopherol (mg./100 ml.)[j,k]			
	All ages	< 0.5	0.5–0.7	> 0.7
	Red cell hemolysis in H₂O₂(%)[j]			
	All ages	> 20	10–20	< 10
	Prothrombin time (seconds or %)			
	Adult			11–18 seconds or 70–100% of control[l]
	Child			70–100% of control but normally not done on children

Table continued on the following page

Appendix Table 36. GUIDELINES FOR EVALUATION OF BIOCHEMICAL MEASUREMENTS OF NUTRITIONAL STATUS (*Continued*)

| NUTRIENT | DETERMINATION | CLASSIFICATION CATEGORY | | ACCEPTABLE[a] |
| | | LESS THAN ACCEPTABLE | | |
		Deficient	*Low*	
Thiamin	Urinary thiamin (μg./gm. creatinine)[d]			
	1–3 yr.	< 120	120–175	≥ 176
	4–6 yr.	< 85	85–120	≥ 121
	7–9 yr.	< 70	70–180	≥ 181
	10–12 yr.	< 60	60–180	≥ 181
	13–15 yr.	< 50	50–150	≥ 151
	Adult	< 27	27–65	≥ 66
	Pregnant, 2nd trimester	< 23	23–54	≥ 55
	Pregnant, 3rd trimester	< 21	21–49	≥ 50
	RBC transketolase-TPP-effect (ratio of % increase)[j,k]			
	All ages	≥ 25	15–25	< 15
Riboflavin	Urinary riboflavin (μg./gm. creatinine)[d]			
	1–3 yr.	< 150	150–499	≥ 500
	4–6 yr.	< 100	100–299	≥ 300
	7–9 yr.	< 85	85–269	≥ 270
	10–15 yr.	< 70	70–199	≥ 200
	Adult	< 27	27–79	≥ 80
	Pregnant, 2nd trimester	< 39	39–119	≥ 120
	Pregnant, 3rd trimester	< 30	30–89	≥ 90
	RBC glutathione reductase-FAD-effect (ratio)[j]			
	All ages	> 1.4	1.2–1.4	< 1.2
Niacin	Urinary N-methylnicotinamide (mg./gm. creatinine)[m]			
	Adult	< 0.5	0.5–1.59	≥ 1.6
	Pregnant, 2nd trimester	< 0.6	0.6–1.99	≥ 2.0
	Pregnant, 3rd trimester	< 0.8	0.8–2.49	≥ 2.5
	Urinary 2-pyridone: N-methyl-nicotinamide ratio			
	All ages	< 1.0		1.0–4.0[c]
Folacin	Red cell folacin (ng./ml.)[d]			
	All ages	< 140	140–159	≥ 160–650
	Serum folacin (ng./ml.)[d]	< 3.0	3.0–5.9	≥ 6.0
	FIGLU excretion (mg.)	Deficient subjects will excrete 5–10 times as much as acceptable		5.20[c]
Pyridoxine	Tryptophan load (mg. xanthurenic acid excreted)[j,k]			
	Adult	> 50	—	< 25
	Urinary pyridoxine (μg./gm. creatinine)[j,k]			
	1–3 yr.	< 90	—	≥ 90
	4–6 yr.	< 75	—	≥ 75
	7–9 yr.	< 50	—	≥ 50
	10–12 yr.	< 40	—	≥ 40
	13–15 yr.	< 30	—	≥ 30
	16+	< 20	—	≥ 20
	Plasma pyridoxal (ng./ml.)			
	Adult[n]	< 5.0	5–8	≥ 8.0
	Transaminase index (ratio)[j,k] EGOT[o]			
	Adult	> 1.5	—	≤ 1.5
	EGPT[p]			
	Adult	> 1.25	—	≤ 1.25
Vitamin B_{12}	Serum vitamin B_{12} (pg./ml.)[j,k]			
	All ages	< 100	100–149	≥ 150
	Urinary methylmalonic acid (mg./24 hr.)	In deficiency can be 500 mg./24 hour		12 mg.[c]

Appendix Table 36. GUIDELINES FOR EVALUATION OF BIOCHEMICAL
MEASUREMENTS OF NUTRITIONAL STATUS (*Continued*)

| | | CLASSIFICATION CATEGORY | | |
| | | LESS THAN ACCEPTABLE | | |
NUTRIENT	DETERMINATION	Deficient	Low	ACCEPTABLE[a]
Vitamin B$_{12}$ (*Continued*)				
	Serum Biotin (μg./100 ml.)			
	Infants			140–155
	Adult			120–240
	Pantothenic acid (mg./gm. creatinine)	<2.0		$\geq$2.0[n]
Vitamin C	Serum vitamin C (mg./100 ml.)[j]			
	$\geq$1 yr.	<0.20	0.2–0.29	$\geq$0.3

[a]Excessively high levels may indicate abnormal clinical status or toxicity.

[b]Bistrian, B. R., et al.: Cellular immunity in semi-starved states in hospitalized adults. Am. J. Clin. Nutr., *28*:1148, 1975.

[c]Wallach, J.: Interpretation of Diagnostic Tests. Boston, Little, Brown and Company, 1974.

[d]From the Ten-State Nutrition Survey, 1968–70.

[e]Ingenbleek, Y., et al.: Measurement of pre-albumin as an index of protein-calorie malnutrition. Lancet, *2*:106, 1972.

[f]Jacobs, A., and Worwood, M.: Iron Biochemistry and Medicine. New York, Academic Press, 1974.

[g]Smith, F., et al.: Depressed plasma retinol-binding protein levels in cystic fibrosis. J. Lab. Clin. Med., *80*:423, 1972.

[h]Harper, H. A.: Review of Physiological Chemistry. 16th ed. Los Altos, Lange Medical Publications, 1975.

[i]May indicate unusual diet or malabsorption.

[j]From: Sauberlich, H. E., Dowdy, R. P., and Skala, J. H.: Laboratory Tests for Assessment of Nutritional Status. Cleveland, Ohio, CRC Press, 1973.

[k]Criteria may vary with different methodology.

[l]Garb, S.: Laboratory Tests in Common Use. 6th ed. New York, Springer Publishing Co., Inc., 1976.

[m]From: ICNND Manual for Nutrition Surveys. 2nd ed. Washington, D.C., U.S. Government Printing Office, 1963.

[n]From Sauberlich, H. E.: Laboratory procedures used in vitamin nutritional assessment. Nutritional assessment— present status, future directions and prospects. Report of 2nd Ross Conference on Medical Research. Columbus, Ohio, Ross Laboratories, 1981.

[o]Erythrocyte glutamic oxalacetic transaminase.

[p]Erythrocyte glutamic pyruvic transaminase.

Appendix 37. PHYSICAL SIGNS AND NUTRITIONAL TERMS ASSOCIATED WITH MALNUTRITION*

GENERAL APPEARANCE

Apathy. Unreactive, unresponsive, disinterested and inattentive to surroundings.

Clinical Marasmus. Evidence of pronounced wasting of subcutaneous fat without edema. Significant apathy may be present. Frequently the face and eyes of the child may appear unusually bright due to the combination of wasting and prominence of the eyes. The child is usually considerably underdeveloped in relation to age, and there may or may not be associated hair changes such as dyspigmentation, thinness, ease in plucking or signs of avitaminosis.

Irritability. Hyperresponsive; excessive or overreaction to minor stimuli, particularly manifest through crying or unusual indication of fear as a result of minor or relatively insignificant happenings.

Kwashiorkor. Pitting edema at least on the pretibial region; underweight, undersize, underdeveloped for age. Muscular wasting may be present but masked by edema. Apathy of some degree is present. Changes in the hair are usually noted, such as thinning, easily pluckable with dyspigmentation or flag sign, and change in texture to silken, sparse hair. Dermatosis with desquamation of the so-called flaky-paint type, with or without hyperpigmentation. In severe cases the dermatosis may resemble a relatively severe burn but lacks erythema.

Pallor. Paleness and loss of color of skin, nail beds, mucosa and lips.

Pre-kwashiorkor. An underweight, undersized, underdeveloped child, without the evident pronounced wasting present in marasmus. Child is thin and undersized but has relatively normal body proportions and rather poor muscle tone, and hair changes may be present. Not apathetic, though would not be described as alert.

HAIR

Dry Staring. Dry, wirelike, unkempt, stiff hair, often brittle, sometimes may exhibit some bleaching of the normal color.

Dyspigmentation. Definite change from normal pigment of the hair, most usually evident distally and best seen by carefully combing hair strands upward and viewing the orderly array of hair in good light. Dyspigmentation includes both change of pigment (usually lightening of color) and depigmentation. Not to be confused with dyed or tinted hair. Dyspigmentation is often bandlike in character and usually is associated with some change in texture of hair in the depigmented band. In some ethnic groups, particularly among Negroid groups, the pigment may be slightly reddish in color. In others, especially among straight black-haired peoples, the bandlike depigmentation ("flag sign") is common.

Easily Pluckable. Easily pluckable hair is that in which the shafts are readily removed with minimum tug when a few strands are grasped between the finger and thumb and gently pulled. In such cases there is a lack of reaction of the child, indicating a lack of pain associated with removing of the hair.

SKIN

Crackled Skin. Definite scales larger in size than those seen in xerosis. It is often congenital and is most prominent in cool weather. It is non-nutritional in origin.

Dependent Edema. The presence of abnormally large amounts of fluid in the intercellular tissue spaces of the body; usually applied to demonstrable accumulation of excessive fluid in the subcutaneous tissues that are dependent upon position and gravity.

Dermatitis with Desquamation, or Crazy-pavement Type. Under this heading should be recorded those desquamating changes of the skin, usually with increased pigmentation, that occur on the extremities, especially legs, thighs and buttocks, but may occur over the trunk in association with kwashiorkor. (These have been termed "flaky-paint" dermatoses.) Small, circumscribed bleblike lesions are sometimes seen in association with kwashiorkor and on occasion may precede the desquamation. In addition, any "crazy-pavement" type of lesions observed should be noted. These are characterized by a thin-appearing epithelium marked by striations usually resembling in outline the microscopic picture of epithelial cells. Not to be confused, however, with ichthyosis (scaly skin).

Follicular Hyperkeratosis. This lesion has been likened to the "gooseflesh" that is seen on chilling, but it is not generalized and does not disappear with brisk rubbing of the skin. Readily felt, as it presents a "nutmeg grater" feel. Follicular hyperkeratosis is more readily detected by the sense of touch than by the eye. The skin is rough, with papillae formed by keratotic plugs that project from the hair follicles. The surrounding skin is dry and lacks the usual amount of moisture or oiliness. Differentiation from adolescent folliculosis can usually be made through recognition of the normal skin between the follicles in the adolescent disorder. It is distinguished from perifolliculosis by the ring of capillary congestion that occurs about each follicle in scorbutic perifolliculosis.

Pellagrous Dermatitis. Symmetrical lesions typical of acute or chronic, mild or severe pellagra are observed; lesions are usually red, often swollen or blistered like sunburn, pigmented, scaly over exposed areas, clearly demarcated from normal skin.

Purpura or Petechia. Small localized extravasations of blood, red or purplish in color, depending on time elapsed since formation. Usually distributed at sites of pressure, and may be perifollicular.

Xerosis. Xerosis is a clinical term used to describe a dry and crinkled skin that is accentuated by pushing the skin parallel to its surface. In more pronounced cases it is often mottled and pigmented and may appear as scaly or alligator-like pseudo-

---

*From: Christakis, G. (ed.): Nutritional Assessment in Health Programs. Washington, D.C., American Public Health Association, Inc., 1973, pp. 26–27.

Appendix 37. PHYSICAL SIGNS AND NUTRITIONAL TERMS ASSOCIATED
WITH MALNUTRITION (*Continued*)

plaques, usually not greater than 0.5 cm. in diameter. Nutritional significance is not established. Differential diagnosis must be made from changes due to dirt and exposure and ichthyosis.

SKELETAL

Bowleg. An outward curve of one or both legs at or below the knee (genu varum).

Costochondral Beading. Palpable and visible enlargement of the costochondral junctions.

Cranial Bossing. Abnormal prominence or protrusion of frontal or parietal areas.

Enlarged Joints. When the more obvious ends of long bones are enlarged; i.e., the wrist, ankles, knees.

Winged Scapula. A scapula having a prominent vertebral border.

MUSCLE

Muscle Wasting. Appearance indicates abnormal loss of muscle substance, as exhibited by unusual prominence of bony skeleton, undue degree of folding of the skin of the buttocks, or the abnormal flabby feel (sometimes described as jelly-like) of the child with poor muscle tone.

EYES

Bitot's Spots. Bitot's spots are small, circumscribed grayish or yellowish gray, dull, dry, foamy superficial lesions of the conjunctiva. They most often occur on the lateral aspect of the bulbar conjunctiva in the interpalpebral area. Do not confuse with pterygium.

Blepharitis. Inflammation of eyelids.

Keratomalacia. Softening of the cornea.

Thickened Opaque Bulbar Conjunctivae. All degrees of thickening may occur. The blueness of the sclera may disappear and the bulbar conjunctivae develop a wrinkled appearance with increase in vascularity. The thickened conjunctivae may result in a glazed, porcelain-like appearance, obscuring the vascularity.

Xerosis Conjunctivae. The conjunctivae, upon exposure by holding the lids open and having the subject rotate the eyes, appear dull and lusterless and exhibit a striated or roughened surface.

FACE

Angular Lesions. Present bilaterally when mouth is held half open. May appear as pink or moist whitish macerated angular lesions that blur the mucocutaneous junction. Angular fissures are recorded when there is definite break in continuity of epithelium at the angles of the mouth.

Angular Scars. Scars at the angles that, if recent, may be pink; if old, may appear blanched.

Cheilosis. Cheilosis is present when the lips are swollen, tense or puffy and, where it appears, the buccal mucosa extends out onto the lips. These lesions are also denuded. This category may be used to record vertical fissuring of the lips but not for lesions of the angles of the mouth only.

Nasolabial Seborrhea. Definite greasy yellowish scaling or filiform excrescences in the nasolabial area that become more pronounced on slight scratching with the fingernail or a tongue blade.

MOUTH

Filiform Papillary Atrophy. Filiform papillae exceedingly low or absent, giving the tongue a smooth appearance that remains after scraping slightly with an applicator stick. "Mild" involves less than one fourth of the tongue (tip and lateral margins only); "moderate" involves one fourth to three fourths of the tongue; "severe" involves over three fourths of the tongue.

Glossitis. Glossitis is any increase in redness, fissuring or swelling with color change (break in lingual mucosa) or diffuse involvement of mucosa. Geographic tongue has the typical irregularly shaped and distributed areas of atrophy with irregular white patches resembling leukoplakia. Glossitis is usually associated with some sensation of pain or burning, particularly upon eating.

Magenta Color. The color of alkaline phenolphthalein.

Swollen Gums. Swollen, red interdental papillae, with more than one papilla involved.

TEETH

Carious Teeth. Molecular decay of a bone, in which it becomes friable, thinned and dark and gradually breaks down, with the formation of pus.

Fluorosis. Opaque paper-white areas in the enamel of the tooth, ranging in size from a few flecks to entire enamel surface. In the latter case brown stain is a frequent accompaniment, as is attrition of opposing surfaces. The most severe forms of fluorosis include discrete or confluent pitting, with widespread brown staining and a general corroded appearance.

GLANDS

Parotid Enlargement. Because of various types of facial configuration, parotid enlargement may be easily missed in certain populations. Check by palpation, moving the gland with fingers upward and backward toward the ear. Check if bilateral.

Thyroid Enlargement. Thyroid enlargement is when a visually perceptible enlargement that is definitely palpable with or without swallowing is noted. It is preferable to examine the subject with his head slightly extended in order to detect thyroid enlargements.

ORGANS

Hepatomegaly. Liver edges more than 2 cm. below the costal margin. (In children, the liver edge may normally be palpable.)

Splenomegaly. Spleen is palpable.

Appendix Table 38. CANADA'S FOOD GUIDE

VARIETY	ENERGY BALANCE	MODERATION
Choose different kinds of foods from within each group in appropriate numbers of servings and portion sizes.	Needs vary with age, sex and activity. Balance energy intake from foods with energy output from physical activity to control weight. Foods selected according to the Guide can supply 4000–6000 kJ (kilojoules) (1000–1400 kilocalories). For additional energy, increase the number and size of servings from the various food groups and/or add other foods.	Select and prepare foods with limited amounts of fat, sugar and salt. If alcohol is consumed, use limited amounts.

MILK AND MILK PRODUCTS	MEAT, FISH, POULTRY AND ALTERNATIVES: 2 SERVINGS	BREADS AND CEREALS: 3–5 SERVINGS	FRUITS AND VEGETABLES: 4–5 SERVINGS
Children up to 11 years — 2–3 servings Adolescents — 3–4 servings Pregnant and nursing women — 3–4 servings Adults — 2 servings Skim, 2%, whole, buttermilk, reconstituted dry or evaporated milk may be used as a beverage or as the main ingredient in other foods. Cheese may also be chosen. *Some Examples of One Serving* 250 mL (1 cup) milk 175 mL (¾ cup) yoghurt 45 g (1½ ounces) cheddar or process cheese In addition, a supplement of vitamin D is recommended when milk is consumed which does not contain added vitamin D.	*Some Examples of One Serving* 60 to 90 g (2–3 ounces) cooked lean meat, fish, poultry or liver 60 mL (4 tablespoons) peanut butter 250 mL (1 cup) cooked dried peas, beans or lentils 125 mL (½ cup) nuts or seeds 60 g (2 ounces) cheddar cheese 125 mL (½ cup) cottage cheese 2 eggs	whole grain or enriched. Whole grain products are recommended. *Some Examples of One Serving* 1 slice bread 125 mL (½ cup) cooked cereal 175 mL (¾ cup) ready-to-eat cereal 1 roll or muffin 125 to 175 mL (½–¾ cup) cooked rice, macaroni, spaghetti or noodles ½ hamburger or weiner bun	Include at least two vegetables. Choose a variety of both vegetables and fruits—cooked, raw or their juices. Include yellow, green or green leafy vegetables. *Some Examples of One Serving* 125 mL (½ cup) vegetables or fruits—fresh, frozen or canned 125 mL (½ cup) juice—fresh, frozen or canned 1 medium-sized potato, carrot, tomato, peach, apple, orange or banana

Appendix Table 39. CALCULATION OF THE CALORIC DISTRIBUTION OF A DIET

To calculate the number of grams of carbohydrate, protein and fat needed to make up a diet that has a particular distribution of calories:

total kcal. in the diet × % of kcal. desired from a particular nutrient = number of kcal. to come from that nutrient

$$\frac{\text{number of kcal. from a nutrient}}{\text{number of kcal. per gm. of that nutrient}} = \text{grams of nutrient required}$$

For example, to calculate the required number of grams of protein, carbohydrate and fat for this diet:
total kcal. = 2400
20% of kcal. = protein
50% of kcal. = carbohydrate
30% of kcal. = fat
2400 kcal. × 20% = 480 kcal. from protein

$$\frac{480 \text{ kcal. from protein}}{4 \text{ kcal./gm. of protein}} = 120 \text{ gm. of protein}$$

2400 kcal. × 50% = 1200 kcal. from carbohydrate

$$\frac{1200 \text{ kcal. from carbohydrate}}{4 \text{ kcal./gm. of carbohydrate}} = 300 \text{ gm. carbohydrate}$$

2400 kcal. × 30% = 720 kcal. from fat

$$\frac{720 \text{ kcal. from fat}}{9 \text{ kcal./gm. of fat}} = 80 \text{ gm. of fat}$$

The final diet contains 120 gm. protein, 300 gm. carbohydrate and 80 gm. fat.

To calculate the caloric distribution of a diet of known composition:
gm. protein in diet × 4 kcal./gm. protein = number of kcal. from protein
gm. carbohydrate in diet × 4 kcal./gm. carbohydrate = number of kcal. from carbohydrate
gm. fat in diet × 9 kcal./gm. fat = number of kcal. from fat
kcal. from protein + kcal. from carbohydrate + kcal. from fat = total kcal. in the diet

$$\frac{\text{kcal. from nutrient}}{\text{total kcal. in the diet}} \times 100 = \% \text{ of total kcal. from nutrient}$$

For example, to calculate the caloric distribution of a diet that contains 100 gm. fat, 100 gm. protein and 300 gm. carbohydrate:
100 gm. protein × 4 kcal./gm. protein = 400 kcal. from protein
300 gm. carbohydrate × 4 kcal./gm. carbohydrate = 1200 kcal. from carbohydrate
100 gm. fat × 9 kcal./gm. fat = 900 kcal. from fat
400 kcal. + 1200 kcal. + 900 kcal. = 2500 kcal. = total kcal. in diet

$$\frac{400 \text{ kcal. from protein}}{2500 \text{ total kcal. in diet}} \times 100 = 16\% \text{ of kcal. from protein}$$

$$\frac{1200 \text{ kcal. from carbohydrate}}{2500 \text{ total kcal. in diet}} \times 100 = 48\% \text{ of kcal. from carbohydrate}$$

$$\frac{900 \text{ kcal. from fat}}{2500 \text{ total kcal. in diet}} \times 100 = 36\% \text{ of kcal. from fat}$$

Appendix 40. MILLIEQUIVALENTS AND MILLIGRAMS OF SODIUM, SODIUM CHLORIDE AND POTASSIUM

TO CONVERT MILLIGRAMS TO MILLIEQUIVALENTS

1. Divide milligrams by atomic weight

Example: 1,000 mg sodium $= \dfrac{1,000}{23} = 43.5$ mEq sodium

Mineral	Atomic weight
Sodium	23
Potassium	39

TO CONVERT SPECIFIC WEIGHT OF SODIUM TO SODIUM CHLORIDE

1. Multiply by 2.54

Example: 1,000 mg sodium $= 1,000 \times 2.54 = 2,540$ mg sodium chloride (2.5 gm)

TO CONVERT SPECIFIC WEIGHT OF SODIUM CHLORIDE TO SODIUM

1. Multiply by 0.393

Example: 2.5 gm sodium chloride $= 2.5 \times 0.393 = 1,000$ mg sodium

Milligrams	Sodium Values Milliequivalents	Grams of Sodium Chloride
500	21.8	1.3
1,000	43.5	2.5
1,500	75.3	3.8
2,000	87.0	5.0

From Mayo Clinic Diet Manual. 4th ed. Philadelphia, W. B. Saunders Company, 1971

Appendix 41. THE METRIC SYSTEM AND EQUIVALENTS

The metric system is a standardized system of measurement that is used internationally. However, the United States also employs another system of measurement based on the old English system. In the field of dietetics, both systems are used. The following charts give equivalents for common household measures. With this information it is possible to calculate measure and weigh in either system.

EQUIVALENT LEVEL MEASURES AND WEIGHTS

60 drops	=	1 tsp.
		5 cc.
		5 gm.
1 tsp.	=	5 gm.
3 tsp.	=	1 tbsp.
		15 cc.
		15 gm.
1 dessert spoon	=	10 cc.
2 tbsp.	=	30 cc.
		30 gm.
		1 oz. (fluid)
4 tbsp.	=	¼ cup
		60 cc.
		60 gm.
8 tbsp.	=	½ cup
		120 cc.
		120 gm.
16 tbsp.	=	1 cup
		240 gm.
		250 ml.
		8 oz. (fluid)
		½ lb.
2 cups	=	1 pt.
		480 gm.
		500 ml.
		16 oz. (fluid)
		1 lb.
4 cups	=	2 pt.
		1 qt.
		1000 or 960 cc.
		1000 ml.
		1 kg.
		2.2 lb.
4 qt.	=	1 gal.
8 qt.	=	1 peck
2 gal.	=	1 peck
4 pecks	=	1 bushel
8 gal.	=	1 bushel

EQUIVALENTS IN GRAMS

For easy computing purposes, the cubic centimeter (cc.) is considered equivalent to 1 gram:

$$1 \text{ cc.} = 1 \text{ gm.}$$

Also for easy computing purposes, one ounce equals 30 gm. or 30 cc.

1 qt.	=	960 gm.
1 pt.	=	480 gm.
1 cup	=	240 gm.
½ cup	=	120 gm.
1 soup cup	=	120 gm.
1 glass (8 oz.)	=	240 gm.
½ glass (4 oz.)	=	120 gm.
1 orange juice glass	=	100 to 120 gm.
1 tbsp.	=	15 gm.
1 tsp.	=	5 gm.

Appendix 42. ABBREVIATIONS

Along with the specialized vocabulary that is employed in the medical, dietetic and nursing fields, there are acceptable forms of abbreviations. Here is a list of abbreviations commonly used.

aa: Gr. *ana;* of each
a.c.: L. *ante cibum;* before meals
ad., add: L. *adde, addatur,* or *addantur;* add or added
ad. lib.: L. *ad libitum;* at pleasure, as desired
aq.: L. *aqua;* water
aq. dest.: L. *aqua destillata;* distilled water
b.i.d., bis in d.: L. *bis in die;* twice a day
c.: L. *cum;* with
c.: cup
cc.: cubic centimeter
Cent.; cent.; C.: centigrade, Celsius
cm.: centimeter
dilut.: L. *dilutus;* dilute
div.: L. *divide;* divide
fac.: make
gm.: gram
gr.: L. *granum;* grain
gtt.: L. *guttae;* drops
h.s.: L. *hora somni;* at hour of sleep, 8 P.M.
I.U.: international unit
kcal.: kilocalorie
kg.: kilogram

kJ.: kilojoule
lb.: pound
μg.: microgram
mcg.: microgram
μU.: microunit
mEq.: milliequivalent
mg.: milligram
mil. or ml.: milliliter
mM.: millimole
mOsm.: milliosmole
oz.: ounce
p.r.n.: L. *pro re nata;* may be repeated according to instructions
pt.: pint
pulv.: L. *pulvis;* powder
q.d.: L. *quaque die;* every day
Q.I.D., q.i.d.: L. *quater in die;* four times daily
q. 3h.: every three hours
q.s.: L. *quantum satis;* a sufficient quantity
qt.: quart
R.E.: retinol equivalent
s.: L. *sine;* without
sol.: solution
ss.: L. *semis;* half
stat.: L. *statim;* immediately
t., tsp.: teaspoon
T., tbsp.: tablespoon
t.i.d.: L. *ter in die;* three times a day

Appendix 43. GENERAL NUTRITION REFERENCES

JOURNALS

American Journal of Nursing
American Journal of Public Health
Borden's Review of Nutrition Research
Dairy Council Digest
Journal of the American Dietetic Association
Journal of the American Medical Association
Journal of Nutrition
Journal of Nutrition Education

Journal of Parenteral and Enteral Nutrition
Nursing Outlook
Nutrition Action
Nutrition Reviews
Nutrition Today
The American Journal of Clinical Nutrition
World Health

RELIABLE RESOURCES FOR NUTRITION INFORMATION AND VISUAL AIDS

American Diabetes Association, 18 E. 48th Street, New York 10017.

American Dietetic Association, 430 N. Michigan Avenue, Chicago, Illinois 60611.

American Heart Association, 44 E. 23rd Street, New York 10010.

American Home Economics Association, 1600 20th Street N.W., Washington, D.C. 20009.

American Institute of Baking, Consumer Service Department, 400 E. Ontario Street, Chicago, Illinois 60611.

Borden Company, 350 Madison Avenue, New York 10017.

Campbell Soup Company, Home Economics Department, 385 Memorial Avenue, Camden, New Jersey 08103.

Center for Science in the Public Interest, 1755 S St., NW, Washington, D.C. 20009.

Cereal Institute, Inc., 135 South LaSalle Street, Chicago, Illinois 60603.

Department of Food and Nutrition, American Medical Association, 535 N. Dearborn Street, Chicago, Illinois 60610.

Extension Service, Department of Home Economics, State Colleges and Universities.

Food and Nutrition Board, National Research Council, National Academy of Sciences, 2101 Constitution Avenue, NW, Washington, D.C. 20418.

Food and Nutrition News, National Live Stock and Meat Board, Chicago, Illinois 60603.

Food and Nutrition Section, American Public Health Association, 1790 Broadway, New York 10019.

General Foods Corporation, 250 North Street, White Plains, New York 10602.

General Mills, Inc., 9200 Wayzata Blvd., Minneapolis, Minnesota 55426.

Gerber Products, Department of Nutrition, Fremont, Michigan 49412.

John Hancock Life Insurance Company, 200 Berkley Street, Boston, Massachusetts 02117.

Mead Johnson & Company, 2404 W. Pennsylvania Street, Evansville, Indiana 47721.

Metropolitan Life Insurance Company, Health and Welfare Division, 1 Madison Avenue, New York 10010.

National Dairy Council, 111 North Canal Street, Chicago, Illinois 60606.

Nutrition Foundation, Inc., 99 Park Avenue, New York 10016.

Nutrition News, National Dairy Council, Chicago, Illinois 60606.

Poultry and Egg National Board, 250 West 57th Street, New York 10010.

Ross Laboratories, Columbus, Ohio 43216.

State Department of Health, Nutrition Division.

Superintendent of Documents, U.S. Government Printing Office, Washington, D.C. 20402.

United Fresh Fruit and Vegetable Association, Washington, D.C.

U.S. Department of Agriculture, Washington, D.C. 20250.

U.S. Department of Health, Education and Welfare: Food and Drug Administration, Public Health Service, Office of Public Affairs, Washington, D.C. 20204.

INDEX

Note: Page numbers in *italic* refer to illustrations; references to tables are indicated by *t*.

Food (*Continued*)
    nutrient composition of, values of, 850–876*t*
    pesticide residues on, 366–368
    pharmacological agents in, reactions to, 635*t*
    postoperative introduction of, 691
    preoperative restriction of, 690
    preparation of, cancer correlation with, 742
    production of, energy in, 22, *22*
    "residue" of, 447
    restored, 365
    safety of, laws and rules regulating, 359,
        363–370
        history of, 364*t*
    specific dynamic action of, 19
    supply data for, 344, 345*t*
    toxins in, natural, 366, 367*t*
        reactions to, 635*t*
Food advertising, influence of, on children's food
        habits, 299
    regulating of, 370
Food assistance and nutrition programs,
        352–354, 353*t*
Food-borne microorganisms, toxigenic and
        pathogenic, 365, 365*t*
Food Consumption Surveys (FCS), 344–349, 346*t*
Food diary, 197
Food frequency questionnaire, 194, 196*t*
Food guide, daily, 223, 227*t*, 230*t*
    modification of, 231–232*t*
Food patterns, 334–336
    development of, 335
    of nationality groups in North America,
        336–340, 336–340*t*
    religious restriction of, 340, 342
Food plans, USDA, 355
Food record, 197
    in food allergy, 639, *641*
Food Stamp Program, 353*t*, 354
    for elderly, 329
Formula, 274
    composition of, 275–277*t*
        vs. human milk and premature formulas,
            771*t*
    concentrated, for infant with congenital heart
        disease, 795, 796*t*
    cow's milk–based, 278
        alternatives to, 649, 650*t*
    defined, 719–720*t*, 725
    for enteral feeding, 715
        composition of, 716, 717–720*t*
        selection of, factors in, 725*t*
    for inborn errors of metabolism, 809*t*
    for parenteral nutrition, nutrient requirements
        and composition of, 728, 729*t*
    nutrient levels of, 279*t*
    phenylalanine-restricted, 803, 809*t*
    premature infant, composition of, 769, 771*t*
        vs. standard formula, 770*t*
    preparation of, 278
    rehydration, for diarrhea, 783*t*
    soy-based, 278
    vitamin and mineral adequacy of, 284, 285,
        797*t*
    whole protein, lactose-free, 717–718*t*
        high-calorie, 719*t*
        milk-based, 718*t*
Formula diets, 531
Fortified foods, 365
Fractures, nutritional care for, 699–701
Frame size, determination of, 963*t*
Free radical, aging process and, 320
Fructose, 24, 25, 27*t*, *28*
    absorption of, 81, *83*

Fructose (*Continued*)
    as sweetener for diabetic food, 499
    intolerance to, 808*t*, 825
    metabolism of, cellular, 93, *95*
Fructose-free diet, foods eliminated in, 825*t*
Fruit, 843–844
Fruitarian diet, 343

Galactokinase deficiency, 807*t*, 823
Galactose, 25, 27*t*
    absorption of, 81, *83*
    metabolism of, cellular, 93, *95*
Galactose-free diet, food list for, 824*t*
Galactosemia, 807*t*, 820, *823*
Galactose-1-phosphate uridyl transferase defi-
        ciency, 823
Gallbladder, diseases of, nutritional care in,
        474–475
    physiology and function of, 473–474, *474*
    resection of, 695
Gangliosides, 44
Gastric acidity, factors affecting, 428*t*
    foods stimulating, 432
Gastric gavage, of low-birth-weight infant, 766
Gastric inhibitory polypeptide (GIP), 76, 77*t*
Gastric juice, digestive enzymes in, 82*t*
Gastric partitioning surgery, 538, *538*
Gastric resection, partial, *693*
Gastric surgery, 692–695, *693*
    nutritional care in, 694, 695*t*
Gastric ulcer, 428–436, *429*. See also *Peptic ulcer.*
Gastrin, function of, 76, 76*t*
Gastritis, acute, 427
    chronic, 427
Gastroenteritis, eosinophilic, 451
Gastroesophageal reflux esophagitis, 425
Gastrointestinal activity, regulation of, 75–78
    hormonal mechanisms of, 76, 76–77*t*
    neural mechanisms of, 75
Gastrointestinal allergy, 451
Gastrointestinal biopsy, in food allergy, 640
Gastrointestinal disorders, food intolerance due
        to, 635*t*
    nutritional assessment in, 423–424, 424*t*
Gastrointestinal mucosa, drug effects on, 412
    factors damaging, 432
Gastrointestinal system
    absorption in, 78–87, *86*
    aging changes in, 321
    involvement of, in cystic fibrosis, 786
    medication reactions in, 412
Gastropathy, of diabetic on dialysis, 625
Gastroplasty, 538
Gavage, gastric, of low-birth-weight infant, 766
Gestational age, 755
Gliadin-containing derivatives, 456*t*
Glomerulonephritis, acute, 602
    chronic, 602
Glucagon, blood glucose regulation by, 33
    function of, 77*t*
    in therapy of diabetes, 486
Glucocorticoids
    blood glucose regulation by, 33
    deficiency of, in Addison's disease, 508
    metabolism effect of, 509
        on fat, 49
        on protein, 61
Gluconeogenesis, 31
    metabolism of muscle and liver during, 91, *91*
Glucose, 24, 25, 27*t*, *28*
    absorption of, 81, *83*